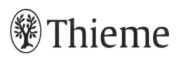

Atlas of Pediatric Head and Neck and Skull Base Surgery

Dan M. Fliss, MD
Professor and Chairman
Department of Otolaryngology Head and Neck Surgery and Maxillofacial Surgery
Director
Interdisciplinary Center for Head and Neck Surgical Oncology
Tel Aviv Sourasky Medical Center
Tel Aviv, Israel

Ari DeRowe, MD
Director
Pediatric Otolaryngology Unit
Dana-Dwek Children's Hospital
Tel Aviv Sourasky Medical Center
Tel Aviv, Israel

1080 illustrations

Thieme
Stuttgart • New York • Delhi • Rio de Janeiro

Library of Congress Cataloging-in-Publication Data is available from the publisher

© 2021. Thieme. All rights reserved.

Georg Thieme Verlag KG
Rüdigerstraße 14, 70469 Stuttgart
Germany
www.thieme.de
+49 [0]711 8931 421
customerservice@thieme.de

Cover design: Thieme Publishing Group
Typesetting by DiTech Process Solutions, India

Printed in Germany by CPI Books   5 4 3 2 1

ISBN 978-3-13-241427-3

Also available as an e-book:
eISBN 978-3-13-241434-1

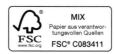

This book is dedicated to my beloved parents, Dr. Adolf and Thea Fliss. I would also like to dedicate this to my devoted wife, Maayana, for her patience and support during its completion.

To my children Naomi, Ehud, Ruth, and Yael and my beautiful grandchildren Ariel, Lavi, Abigail, Tammuz, and Ari.

None of this would have been possible without their dedication and support.

Dan M. Fliss

Contents

Section I   Introduction

Section II   Head and Neck

Contents

Contents

Section III   Skull Base and Craniofacial

27 Endoscopic Treatment of Juvenile Angiofibroma: Surgical Technique 274

Ahmad Safadi, Alberto Schreiber, Dan M. Fliss, Piero Nicolai

28 Juvenile Angiofibroma with Intracranial Extension............................. 282

Philippe Lavigne, Carl H. Snyderman, Paul A. Gardner

29 Expanded Endonasal Approaches for Treatment of Malignancy in Children ... 289

Meghan Wilson, Carl H. Snyderman, Paul A. Gardner, Elizabeth C. Tyler-Kabara

Section IV Airway, Voice, and Swallowing

45 Surgery of Laryngomalacia 435

Yoram Stern, Moshe Hain

46 Unilateral and Bilateral Vocal Fold Paralysis 442

Carol Nhan, Jean-Paul Marie, Karen B. Zur

47 Endoscopic Airway Surgery 450

K. A. Stephenson, M. E. Wyatt

Contents

48 Surgical Approach to Juvenile Onset Recurrent Respiratory Papillomatosis 463

Seth M. Pransky, Jeffrey D. Bernstein

49 Laryngotracheal Reconstruction 475

Diego Preciado, George Zalzal

50 Partial Cricotracheal Resection 486

Ian N. Jacobs

Section VI   Reconstruction

Videos

Preface

The need for specialized care of the airway in dedicated children's hospitals led to the foundation of pediatric otolaryngology as a subspecialty. Since then, it has become a burgeoning subspecialty that coincided with the realization that children are not small adults. Their pathology, physiology, and developmental concerns are unique and require additional training to provide quality of care. The surgery is also distinct, sometimes completely different from adult surgery. There can be subtle differences in surgical techniques that impact the surgical results.

As we follow the growth of pediatric otolaryngology as a subspecialty, we can see it is further branching out. Presently we are seeing pediatric otolaryngology group practices with subspecialties such as airway surgeons, head and neck surgeons, otologists, etc. Thus, there is a need for more detailed descriptions of surgical techniques. This is how the concept of an atlas on pediatric head and neck and skull base surgery was born.

Working together with the publisher, we approached the leading pediatric otolaryngologists worldwide to share their experiences in pediatric head and neck surgery. The result is an up-to-date atlas with a plethora of pearls and insights. Common surgical cases have been presented in a new light, and uncommon cases have been presented in a step-by-step manner with high-quality photos and illustrations that can be very helpful for fellows as well as seasoned surgeons.

Our appreciation extends to all the authors who have generously contributed chapters to this book. Our warmest acknowledgments are accorded to Mrs. Irit Sturm for her invaluable aid in the compilation of the notes and her assistance throughout the production process of this book.

Atlas of Pediatric Head and Neck and Skull Base Surgery incorporates basic surgical techniques along with state-of-the-art advances. This book will be a valuable resource for otolaryngology head and neck and skull base surgery residents, attending pediatric otolaryngology fellows, as well as seasoned surgeons. As the field of pediatric otolaryngology continues to blossom, we hope that this atlas will contribute to the excellence of care that is expected from us by our patients and their parents.

Dan M. Fliss, MD
Ari DeRowe, MD

Contributors

Avraham Abergel, MD
Deputy Director
Department of Otolaryngology–Head and Neck Surgery
Tel Aviv Sourasky Medical Center
Affiliated to the Sackler School of Medicine
Tel Aviv University
Tel Aviv, Israel

Uri Amit, MD, B. Pharm
Resident
Occupational Medicine
Maccabi Health Services
Tel Aviv, Israel

Max M. April, MD, FAAP, FACS
Professor of Otolaryngology and Pediatrics
Director
Millstone Family Fellowship in Pediatric Otolaryngology
NYU Langone Health
New York, USA

Darrin V. Bann, MD, PhD
Clinical Resident
Department of Otolaryngology–Head and Neck Surgery
Penn State Health
Milton S. Hershey Medical Center
Hershey, Pennsylvania, USA

Christine Barron, MD
Resident
The Ohio State University School of Medicine
Columbus, Ohio, USA

Oded Ben-Ari, MD, MHA
Surgeon
Department of Otolaryngology Head and Neck and
    Maxillofacial Surgery
Tel Aviv Sourasky Medical Center
Affiliated to Sackler School of Medicine
Tel Aviv University
Tel Aviv, Israel

David Ben-Nun, MD
Resident Physician
Department of Internal Medicine
University of Texas at Austin Dell Medical School
Austin, Texas, USA

Jeffrey D. Bernstein, MD
Resident Physician
Division of Otolaryngology–Head and Neck Surgery
UC San Diego Health
La Jolla, California, USA

Narin N. Carmel Neiderman, MD
Physician
Department of Otolaryngology
Tel Aviv Sourasky Medical Center
Affiliated to the Sackler School of Medicine
Tel Aviv University
Tel Aviv, Israel

Paolo Castelnuovo, MD, FRCSEd, FACS
Full Professor and Chairman
Divison of Otorhinolaryngology
Department of Biotechnology and Life Sciences
HNS and FDRC
University of Insubria
Ospedale di Circolo e Fondazione Macchi
Varese, Italy

Oren Cavel, MD
Head
Department of ENT
Hôpital Universitaire Des Enfants Reine Fabiola
Université Libre de Bruxelles
Brussels, Belgium

Baishakhi Choudhury, MD
Assistant Professor
Otology, Neurotology, and Lateral Skull Base Surgery
Department of Otolaryngology–Head and Neck Surgery
Loma Linda University Health
Loma Linda, California, USA

Sam J. Daniel, MDCM, FRCSC
Professor
Pediatric Surgery and Otolaryngology
McGill University
Montreal, Quebec, Canada

Ari DeRowe, MD
Director
Pediatric Otolaryngology Unit
Dana-Dwek Children's Hospital
Tel Aviv Sourasky Medical Center
Tel Aviv, Israel

Vaninder K. Dhillon, MD
Assistant Professor
Department of Otolaryngology–Head and Neck Surgery
Division of Endocrine Head and Neck Surgery
Division of Laryngology
Suburban Hospital
Johns Hopkins University
Bethesda, Maryland, USA

Gillian R. Diercks, MD, MPH
Instructor
Department of Otolaryngology–Head and Neck Surgery
Harvard Medical School
Boston, Massachusetts, USA

Irit Duek, MD
Department of Otolaryngology Head and Neck Surgery
    and Maxillofacial Surgery
Tel Aviv Sourasky Medical Center
Sackler School of Medicine
Tel Aviv University
Tel Aviv, Israel

Marisa Earley, MD
Assistant Professor and Residency Program Director
Department of Otolaryngology Head and Neck Surgery
University of Texas Health San Antonio
San Antonio, Texas, USA

Yaniv Ebner, MD
Director
Cleft Lip and Palate Center
Meir Medical Center
Kfar Saba, Israel

Najjar Esmat, MD
Senior ENT Head and Neck Surgeon
Department of ENT Head and Neck Surgery
Rabin Medical Center-Beilinson
Petah Tikva, Israel

Gadi Fishman, MD
Director
Pediatric Otolaryngology Clinics
Acting Director
Pediatric Otolaryngology Unit
Tel Aviv Sourasky Medical Center
Affiliated to Sackler Medical Faculty
Tel Aviv University
Tel Aviv, Israel

Ron Flaishon, MD
Head of Ambulatory Anesthesia
Department of Anesthesia, Intensive Care and Pain
Tel Aviv Sourasky Medical Center
Tel Aviv, Israel

Dan M. Fliss. MD
Professor and Chairman
Department of Otolaryngology Head and Neck Surgery
    and Maxillofacial Surgery
Director
Interdisciplinary Center for Head and Neck Surgical
    Oncology
Tel Aviv Sourasky Medical Center
Tel Aviv, Israel

Christine Fordham, MD
Pediatric Otolaryngologist
Presbyterian Medical Group
Albuquerque, New Mexico, USA

Itzhak Fried, MD, PhD
Professor
Department of Neurosurgery
Tel Aviv Sourasky Medical Center
Affiliated to Sackler School of Medicine
Tel Aviv University
Tel Aviv, Israel

David R. Friedmann, MD, MSc
Assistant Professor
Department of Otolaryngology–Head and Neck Surgery
NYU Grossman School of Medicine
Director of Resident Research
Department of Otolaryngology
NYU Langone Health
New York, New York, USA

Stefania Gallo, MD
Medical Doctor
Divison of Otorhinolaryngology
Department of Biotechnology and Life Sciences
University of Insubria
Ospedale di Circolo e Fondazione Macchi
Varese, Italy

Paul A. Gardner, MD
Professor
Departments of Neurological Surgery and Otolaryngology
Co-Director
Center for Cranial Base Surgery
University of Pittsburgh Medical Center
Pittsburgh, Pennsylvania, USA

Mohammad Abraham Kazemizadeh Gol, MD
Otolaryngology Specialist
Maryland ENT Center
Baltimore, Maryland, USA

Gabriel Gomez, MD
Assistant Professor of Clinical Otolaryngology
Department of Otolaryngology–Head and Neck Surgery
Keck School of Medicine of USC
Los Angeles, California, USA

Golda Grinblat, MD
Otologist and Skull Base Surgeon
Gruppo Otologico
Piacenza and Rome, Italy;
Otology and Neurotology Consultant
Hillel Yaffe Medical Center
Affiliated to the Technion University
Haifa, Israel

Eyal Gur, MD
Chief of Plastic Reconstructive and Aesthetic Surgery
Tel Aviv Sourasky Medical Center
Affiliated to the Sackler School of Medicine
Tel Aviv University
Tel Aviv, Israel

Moshe Hain, MD
Pediatric Otolaryngologist
Department of Otolaryngology
Schneider Children's Hospital
Petach Tikva, Israel

Ophir Handzel, MD
Director
Cochlear Implant Center
Department of Otolaryngology–Head and Neck Surgery
Tel Aviv Sourasky Medical Center
Affiliated to the Sackler School of Medicine
Tel Aviv University
Tel Aviv, Israel

Ben Hartley, MBBS, BSc, FRCS
Consultant Paediatric Otolaryngologist
Great Ormond Street Hospital for Children
Senior Lecturer
University College London
London, United Kingdom

Contributors

Christopher Hartnick, MD
Professor
Department of Otology and Laryngology
Harvard Medical School
Division Director
Pediatric Otolaryngology
Chief Quality Officer for Otolaryngology
Massachusetts Eye and Ear Infirmary
Boston, Massachusetts, USA

Roy Hod, MD
Senior Physician
Department of Pediatric Otolaryngology
Schneider Children's Medical Center
Petach Tiqwa, Israel

Gilad Horowitz, MD
Staff Physician
Head and Neck Unit
Department of Otolaryngology Head and Neck
    and Maxillofacial Surgery
Tel Aviv Sourasky Medical Center
Affiliated to Sackler School of Medicine
Tel Aviv University
Tel Aviv, Israel

Ian N. Jacobs, MD
Endowed Chair in Pediatric Otolaryngology and Pediatric
Airway Disorders
Medical Director of the Center for Pediatric Airway
    Disorders
Division of Otolaryngology (ENT)
Children's Hospital of Philadelphia
Philadelphia, Pennsylvania, USA

Daniel J. Kedar, MD
Surgeon
Plastic Reconstructive and Aesthetic Surgery
Laboratory of Nerve Regeneration
Tel Aviv Sourasky Medical Center
Affiliated to the Sackler School of Medicine
Tel Aviv University
Tel Aviv, Israel

Shay Keren, MD
Consultant Ophthalmologist
Department of Ophthalmology
Tel Aviv Sourasky Medical Center
Affiliated to Sackler School of Medicine
Tel Aviv University
Tel Aviv, Israel

Paul Krakovitz, MD, FACS
Vice President and Chief Medical Officer
Specialty Based Care
Adjunct Associate Professor of Surgery
Intermountain Healthcare
Salt Lake City, Utah, USA

Sonia Kumar, FRCS (ORL-HNS), MA Hons (Oxon),
    M Med Sci
Consultant Pediatric and Adult ENT Surgeon
John Radcliffe Hospital
Oxford, United Kingdom

Gil Lahav, MD
Division of Otology
Department of Otolaryngology–Head and Neck Surgery
Kaplan Medical Center
The Hebrew University of Jerusalem
Jerusalem , Israel

Philippe Lavigne, MD
Cranial Base Surgery Fellow
Department of Otolaryngology
University of Pittsburgh Medical Center
Pittsburgh, Pennsylvania, USA

Amir Laviv, DMD
Specialist in Oral and Maxillofacial Surgery
Senior Lecturer
Department of Oral and Maxillofacial Surgery
The Maurice and Gabriela Goldschleger School
    of Dental Medicine
Tel Aviv University
Tel Aviv, Israel

Igal Leibovitch, MD
Professor of Ophthalmology
Director of Oculoplastic and Orbital Surgery Institute
Tel Aviv Medical Center
Tel Aviv University
Tel Aviv, Israel

David Leshem, MD
Head of Pediatric Plastic and Craniofacial Surgery Unit
Department of Plastic and Reconstructive Surgery
Tel Aviv Sourasky Medical Center
Affiliated to Sackler Medical Faculty
Tel Aviv University
Tel Aviv, Israel

Jessyka G. Lighthall, MD
Director
Facial Plastic and Reconstructive Surgery
Co-Director
Facial Nerve Disorders
Clinic Assistant Professor of Surgery
Division of Otolaryngology-Head and Neck Surgery
Milton S. Hershey Medical Center
Pennsylvania State University
Hershey, Pennsylvania, USA

Davide Locatelli, MD
Full Professor and Chairman
Divison of Neurosurgery
Department of Biotechnology and Life Sciences
University of Insubria
Ospedale di Circolo e Fondazione Macchi
Varese, Italy

Justin Loloi, BS
MD Candidate
Milton S. Hershey Medical Center
Pennsylvania State University
Hershey, Pennsylvania, USA

Jean-Paul Marie, MD, PhD
Head
Departments of Otolaryngology Head and Neck Surgery
    and Audiophonology
Rouen University Hospital
Head
Experimental Surgical Research Laboratory,
    EA 3830 GRHV
Rouen Normandy University
Rouen, France

Anna H. Messner MD, FACS, FAAP
Bobby Alford Endowed Chair in Pediatric Otolaryngology
Professor
Baylor College of Medicine
Chief of Pediatric Otolaryngology
Texas Children's Hospital
Houston, Texas, USA

Craig Miller, MD
Otolaryngologist
Department of Otolaryngology–Head and Neck Surgery
University of Washington
Seattle, Washington, USA

Lindsey Moses, MD
Resident
Department of Otolaryngology
NYU Langone Medical Center
New York, USA

Nidal Muhanna, MD
Director
Department of Otolaryngology
Tel Aviv Sourasky Medical Center
Affiliated to Sackler Medical Faculty
Tel Aviv University
Tel Aviv, Israel

Oded Nahlieli, DMD
Professor and Chairman
Department of Oral and Maxillofacial Surgery
Barzilai University Medical Center
Ashkelon, Israel;
Faculty of Medicine
Ben Gurion University of the Negev
Beer Sheva, Israel;
Adjunct Professor
Eastman Institute for Oral Health University of Rochester
Rochester, New York, USA

Piero Nicolai, MD
Professor and Chairman
Section of Otorhinolaryngology–Head and Neck Surgery
Department of Neurosciences
University of Padova Azienda Ospedale Università Padova
Padova, Italy

Carol Nhan, MD, FRCSC
Assistant Professor
Division of Pediatric Otolaryngology
Ste-Justine Hospital
University of Montreal;
Assistant Professor
Division of Pediatric Otolaryngology
Montreal Children's Hospital
McGill University Health Center
McGill University Health Center
Montreal, Quebec, Canada

Yahav Oron, MD
Otolaryngologist, Head and Neck Surgeon
Department of Otolaryngology Head and Neck
    and Maxillofacial Surgery
Tel Aviv Sourasky Medical Center
Affiliated to Sackler School of Medicine
Tel Aviv University
Tel Aviv, Israel

Reema Padia, MD
Assistant Professor
Department of Otolaryngology
University of Pittsburgh School of Medicine
Co-Surgical Director
Vascular Anomalies Center
UPMC Children's Hospital of Pittsburgh
Pittsburgh, Pennsylvania, USA

Sanjay R. Parikh, MD, FACS
Professor
Department of Otolaryngology–Head and Neck Surgery
University of Washington
Associate Surgeon-in-Chief
Seattle Children's Hospital
Seattle, Washington, USA

Aviyah Peri, MD
Doctoral Student
Department of Otolaryngology Head and Neck Surgery
    and Maxillofacial Surgery
Tel Aviv Sourasky Medical Center
Tel Aviv University
Tel Aviv, Israel

Diego Preciado, MD, PhD
Vice Chief of Pediatric Otolaryngology
Director of Pediatric Otolaryngology Fellowship
Professor of Surgery and Pediatrics (with tenure)
Children's National Hospital
Washington, D.C., USA

Gianluca Piras, MD
Otologist and Skull Base Surgeon
Gruppo Otologico
Piacenza and Rome, Italy

Contributors

Seth M. Pransky, MD
Pediatric Otolaryngologist
Pediatric Otolaryngology Head and Neck Surgery
Pediatric Specialty Partners
San Diego, California, USA

Reza Rahbar, DMD, MD
Associate Otolaryngologist-in-Chief
Airway Disorder Chair in Pediatric Otolaryngology
Boston Children's Hospital
Professor of Otolaryngology
Harvard Medical School
Boston, Massachusetts, USA

Eyal Raveh, MD
Senior Physician
Chief of Department of Pediatric Otolaryngology
Schneider Children's Medical Center
Petach Tiqwa, Israel

Vadim Reiser, DMD
Director Oral and Maxillofacial Surgery Unit
Department of Otolaryngology Head and Neck Surgery
    and Maxillofacial Surgery
Tel Aviv Sourasky Medical Center
Affiliated to Sackler School of Medicine
Tel Aviv University
Tel Aviv, Israel

Barak Ringel, MD
Resident
Department of Otolaryngology Head and Neck and
    Maxillofacial Surery
Tel Aviv Sourasky Medical Center
Affiliated to the Sackler School of Medicine
Tel Aviv University
Tel Aviv, Israel

J. Thomas Roland, Jr., MD
Mendik Foundation Chairman
Department of Otolaryngology–Head and Neck Surgery
Professor of Otolaryngology and Neurosurgery
Co-Director
NYU Cochlear Implant Program and NYU NF2 Center
NYU Grossman School of Medicine
New York, USA

Jessica Ruggiero, MD
Medical Doctor
Divison of Otorhinolaryngology
Department of Biotechnology and Life Sciences
University of Insubria
Ospedale di Circolo e Fondazione Macchi
Varese, Italy

Jonathon O. Russell, MD, FACS
Assistant Professor
Director of Endoscopic and Robotic Thyroid and
    Parathyroid Surgery
Head and Neck Endocrine Surgery
Department of Otolaryngology–Head and Neck Surgery
Johns Hopkins
Chair
Endocrine Technology Committee, Endocrine Section
American Head and Neck Society
Baltimore, Maryland, USA

Alessandra Russo, MD
Otologist and Skull Base Surgeon
Gruppo Otologico
Piacenza and Rome, Italy

Michael Rutter, MD
Professor
Department of Pediatric Otolaryngology–Head
    and Neck Surgery
Cincinnati Children's Hospital Medical Center
Cincinnati, Ohio, USA

Ahmad Safadi, MD
Senior Staff
Department of Otolaryngology Head and Neck
    and Maxillofacial Surgery
Tel Aviv Sourasky Medical Center
Affiliated to Sackler School of Medicine
Tel Aviv University
Tel Aviv, Israel

Mario Sanna, MD
Professor of Otolaryngology
Department of Head and Neck Surgery
University of Chieti
Chieti, Italy;
Director
Gruppo Otologico
Piacenza and Rome, Italy

Alberto Schreiber, MD, PhD
Assistant Professor
Unit of Otorhinolaryngology–Head and Neck Surgery
Spedali Civili of Brescia
University of Brescia
Brescia, Italy

Claudia Schweiger, MD, PhD
Professor
Department of Otolaryngology–Head and Neck Surgery
Hospital de Clínicas de Porto Alegre
Porto Alegre, Brazil

Craig Senders, MD
Director of Pediatric Otolaryngology
Director of the Cleft and Craniofacial Program
UC Davis Children's Hospital
Sacramento, California, USA

Shahaf Shilo, MD
Medical Doctor
Department of Otolaryngology Head and Neck
    and Maxillofacial Surgery
Tel Aviv Sourasky Medical Center
Affiliated to Sackler School of Medicine
Tel Aviv University
Tel Aviv, Israel

Amir Shuster, DMD
Specialist in Oral and Maxillofacial Surgery
Department of Otolaryngology Head and
    Neck Surgery and Maxillofacial Surgery
Tel Aviv Sourasky Medical Center
Department of Oral and Maxillofacial Surgery
The Maurice and Gabriela Goldschleger School of
    Dental Medicine
Tel Aviv University
Tel Aviv, Israel

Shelly I. Shiran, MD
Acting Director Pediatric MRI
Radiology Department
Tel Aviv Sourasky Medical Center
Affiliated to Sackler Medical Faculty
Tel Aviv University
Tel Aviv, Israel

Carl H. Snyderman, MD, MBA
Professor
Departments of Otolaryngology and Neurological Surgery
Co-Director
Center for Cranial Base Surgery
University of Pittsburgh Medical Center
Pittsburgh, Pennsylvania, USA

Blake Smith, MD
Attending Surgeon
Otolaryngology–Head and Neck Surgery
The Southeast Permanente Medical Group
Atlanta, Georgia, USA

**K. A. Stephenson, FRCS ORL-HNS (Eng.), FC ORL
    (SA), MMed**
Young Otolaryngologists of IFOS (YO-IFOS) Networking
    Committee Chairperson
ENT UK Global Health Committee member
Consultant Paediatric ENT Surgeon
Birmingham Children's Hospital
Birmingham, United Kingdom

Yoram Stern, MD
Director
Upper Airway Unit
Department of Otolaryngology
Schneider Children's Hospital
Petach Tikva, Israel

Abdelkader Taibah, MD
Neurosurgeon, Skull Base Surgeon, and Otologist
Gruppo Otologico
Piacenza and Rome, Italy

Mary Roz Timbang, MD
Resident
Otolaryngology, Head and Neck Surgery
UC Davis Medical Center
Sacramento, California, USA

Ralph P. Tufano, MD, MBA, FACS
Charles W. Cummings MD Professor
American Thyroid Association Board of Directors
Director of the Division of Head and Neck
    Endocrine Surgery
Director of AHNS Fellowship in Advanced Head and
    Neck Endocrine Surgery
Department of Otolaryngology–Head and Neck Surgery
The Johns Hopkins Medical Institutions
Baltimore, Maryland, USA

Elizabeth C. Tyler-Kabara, MD, PhD
Associate Professor
Departments of Neurological Surgery
The University of Texas at Austin Dell Medical School
Austin, Texas, USA

Omer J. Ungar, MD
Otolaryngologist, Head and Neck Surgeon
Department of Otolaryngology Head and Neck
    and Maxillofacial Surgery
Tel Aviv Sourasky Medical Center
Affiliated to Sackler School of Medicine
Tel Aviv University
Tel Aviv, Israel

Tulio A. Valdez, MD, MSc
Associate Professor of Otolaryngology
Otolaryngology–Head and Neck Surgery Divisions
Stanford University
Stanford, California, USA

Robert F. Ward, MD
Pediatric Otolaryngology Division Chief
Professor of Otolaryngology–Head and Neck Surgery
Department of Otolaryngology–Head and Neck Surgery
NYU Langone Medical Center
New York, USA

Anton Warshavsky, MD
Staff Head and Neck Surgeon
Department of Otolaryngology Head and Neck
    and Maxillofacial Surgery
Tel Aviv Sourasky Medical Center
Affiliated to Sackler School of Medicine
Tel Aviv University
Tel Aviv, Israel

Oshri Wasserzug, MD
Senior Surgeon
Pediatric ENT Unit
Department of Otolaryngology–Head and Neck Surgery
Sourasky Medical Center
Tel Aviv, Israel

Avi A. Weinbroum, MD
Professor of Anesthesiology and Perioperative Medicine
Pain Consultant
The Sackler Faculty of Medicine
Tel Aviv University
Tel Aviv, Israel

Contributors

Anat Wengier, MD
Resident
Department of Otolaryngology Head and Neck Surgery
    and Maxillofacial Surgery
Tel Aviv Sourasky Medical Center
Sackler School of Medicine
Tel Aviv University
Tel Aviv, Israel

Meghan Wilson, MD
Assistant Professor
Department of Otolaryngology–Head and Neck Surgery
Departments of Pediatrics and Neurosurgery
Penn State Health
Milton S. Hershey Medical Center
Hershey, Pennsylvania, USA

Nikolaus E. Wolter, MD, MSc, FRCSC
Staff Otolaryngologist
Department of Otolaryngology–Head and Neck Surgery
The Hospital for Sick Children
Assistant Professor of Otolaryngology–Head and
    Neck Surgery
University of Toronto
Toronto, Ontario, Canada

**M.E. Wyatt, MA (Cantab), FRCS, FRCS (Oto), FRCS
    (ORL - HNS)**
Consultant Paediatric ENT Surgeon
Great Ormond Street Hospital
Honorary Senior Lecturer
University College London
London, United Kingdom

Annabelle Tay Sok Yan, MBBS, MMED, MRCS
Pediatric Otolaryngologist
Department of Otolaryngology
National University Hospital
National University of Singapore
Singapore

Ravit Yanko, MD
Senior Surgeon
Department of Plastic and Reconstructive Surgery
Tel Aviv Sourasky Medical Center
Tel Aviv, Israel

Arik Zaretski, MD
Head and Neck Reconstruction Service
Department of Plastic Surgery
Tel Aviv Sourasky Medical Center
Affiliated to Sackler Medical Faculty
Tel Aviv University
Tel Aviv, Israel

Carlton J. Zdanski, MD, FACS
The Herbert H. Thorp and Julian T. Mann Distinguished
    Professor of Otolaryngology/Head and Neck Surgery
Chief of Pediatric Otolaryngology–Head and Neck Surgery
Associate Pediatric Surgeon-in-Chief
Surgical Director of The North Carolina Children's
    Airway Center
University of North Carolina at Chapel Hill
Chapel Hill, North Carolina, USA

Sivan Zissman, MD
Surgeon
Pediatric Plastic and Craniofacial Surgery Unit
Department of Plastic and Reconstructive Surgery
Tel Aviv Sourasky Medical Center
Affiliated to Sackler Medical Faculty
Tel Aviv University
Tel Aviv, Israel

George Zalzal, MD, FACS,FAAP
Chief
Division of Otolaryngology
Children's National Medical Center
Professor of Otolaryngology and Pediatrics (with tenure)
George Washington University
Washington, D.C., USA

Jacopo Zocchi, MD
Medical Doctor
Divison of Otorhinolaryngology
Department of Biotechnology and Life Sciences
University of Insubria
Ospedale di Circolo e Fondazione Macchi
Varese, Italy

Karen B. Zur, MD
Interim Chief
Division of Pediatric Otolaryngology
Director of Pediatric Voice Program
Associate Director
Center for Pediatric Airway Disorders
Children's Hospital of Philadelphia
Philadelphia, Pennsylvania, USA

Section I

Introduction

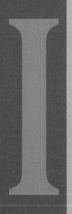

1 Pediatric Anatomy

Roy Hod, Najjar Esmat

Summary

In general, the anatomy of the head and neck and specifically pediatric anatomy has always been challenging for dissectors and surgeons. In this chapter, we have tried to emphasize and simplify the complexities of head and neck anatomy.

Keywords: Neck muscles, fascia, ear, laryngeal muscles

1.1 Introduction

What makes pediatric otolaryngology distinct from its adult discipline—Otolaryngology/Head and Neck Surgery—are the special problems that present in children with an often unique approach to their management. The specific problems that a pediatric otolaryngologist may encounter include airway disorders that present congenitally or iatrogenically, swallowing disorders that may change with growth and development, head and neck tumors in children and infants, hearing loss that may be congenital or acquired, and other congenital anomalies that may present in the head and neck. The differential diagnosis, the approach to the child and parent, and the overall surgical management may diverge significantly from adults.

1.2 Fasciae of the Neck

In the neck, the superficial layer of cervical fascia is a single layer of fascia that underlies the skin and contains the platysma muscle and cutaneous nerves and vessels. It is usually thin. Its primary surgical significance is that it provides a fascial pad that protects underlying structures when a skin incision is made. In exceptionally lean people, however, the paucity of this layer may not protect underlying structures, such as the accessory nerve, so the surgeon should be wary when operating on such patients. The deep layer is formed from 3 sheets: these are the superficial (investing), middle (pretracheal or visceral), and deep (prevertebral) layers of the deep cervical fascia. The *superficial layer* of deep fascia underlies the platysma muscle and completely invests or encircles all of the superficial neck structures. For these reasons, the superficial layer is also known as the *investing layer* of deep fascia. In the region of the sternocleidomastoid and trapezius muscles, it splits and envelops the individual muscles. The superficial layer of the deep cervical fascia also invests the strap muscles and parotid and submandibular glands. The *middle layer* of the deep cervical fascia encloses the visceral structures of the neck: the trachea, esophagus, and thyroid gland. Hence, the synonym for the

middle layer is the *pretracheal* or *visceral fascia*. The *deep layer* of the deep cervical fascia surrounds the deep muscles of the neck and cervical vertebrae. This layer is also known by its descriptive term, the *prevertebral fascia*. The muscles enclosed by the prevertebral fascia include the deep muscles of the neck: the levator scapulae; scalenus anterior, middle, and posterior; and longus colli and capitis, which lie on the anterior aspect of the cervical vertebrae. In addition, within the prevertebral fascia are the phrenic nerve and brachial plexus, located near the anterior and middle scalene muscles and the sympathetic chain lying anterior to the longus colli muscle. The superficial layer of deep fascia, along with the middle and deep layers, envelops the carotid and jugular vessels and vagus nerve to form the carotid sheath (▶ Fig. 1.1).

1.3 Muscles of the Neck

The muscles of the neck are grouped as follows:
- Superficial muscles (platysma, sternocleidomastoid).
- Medial muscles, or muscles of the hyoid bone:
  (1) muscles located above the hyoid bone (mylohyoid, digastric, stylohyoid, geniohyoid); (2) muscles located below the hyoid bone (sternohyoid, sternothyroid, thyrohyoid, omohyoid).
- Deep muscles: (1) lateral, attached to the ribs (scalenus anterior, medius, and posterior); (2) prevertebral muscles (longus cervicis, longus capitis, rectus capitis anterior and lateralis).

1.3.1 Superficial Muscles

- Platysma is a subcutaneous muscle of the neck lying directly under the fascia as a thin sheet. It arises on the level of the second rib from the pectoral and deltoid fascia, runs upward over the clavicle, and then attaches to the edge of the mandible and the parotid and masseteric fascia. It runs partly continuous with the muscles of the mouth. A triangular space not covered with the muscle remains on the midline.
  Innervation: n. facialis.
  Action: Pulling the skin of the neck, the muscle protects the subcutaneous veins from compression; it can also depress the angle of the mouth, which is important for facial expression (▶ Fig. 1.2).
- The sternocleidomastoid muscle lies immediately under the platysma and is separated from it by the cervical fascia. It originates from the sternal manubrium and the sternal end of the clavicle. Both heads fuse proximally and the muscle is attached to the mastoid process and linea nuchae superior of the occipital

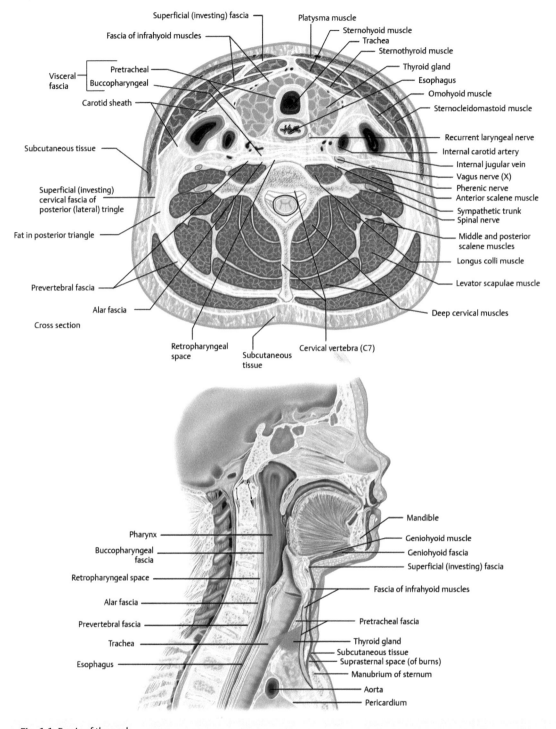

Fig. 1.1 Fascia of the neck.

bone. This muscle originated as part of the trapezius muscle, and it, therefore, has innervation in common with the trapezius (n. accessory and C2).

Action: In unilateral contraction, the muscle flexes the cervical segment of the spine to the same side; the head is raised at the same time, and the face turned to the opposite side. In bilateral contraction, the muscles hold the head in a vertical position (head-holder); that is why the muscle itself and the place of its attachment (the mastoid process) are most developed in man,

Fig. 1.2 Superficial muscles.

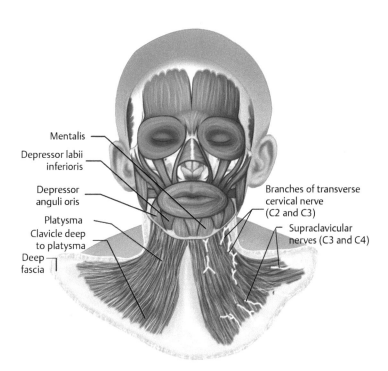

Mentalis

Depressor labii inferioris

Depressor anguli oris

Platysma

Clavicle deep to platysma

Deep fascia

Branches of transverse cervical nerve (C2 and C3)

Supraclavicular nerves (C3 and C4)

Sternocleidomastoid muscle (SCM)

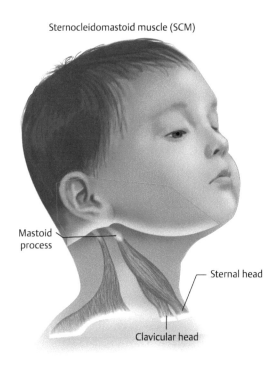

Mastoid process

Sternal head

Clavicular head

Fig. 1.3 Sternocleidomastoid muscle.

who walks erect. Bilateral contraction may also bend the cervical spine forward and simultaneously raise the face. When the head is fixed, the muscle can raise the chest in respiration (an accessory muscle of inspiration) (▶ Fig. 1.3).

1.3.2 Middle Muscles or Muscles of the Hyoid Bone

Muscles located above the hyoid bone—these muscles lie between the mandible and the hyoid bone.

- The mylohyoid muscle is a flat muscle with parallel fibers that arise from the mandibular mylohyoid line, run medially, and terminate on the tendinous line, raphe, stretching from the inner surface of the chin to the body of the hyoid bone on the midline along the border between both mylohyoid muscles. The posterior part of the muscle is attached to the body of the hyoid bone. Both mylohyoid muscles meet and form the floor of the mouth, which closes the bottom of the oral cavity.
- The digastric muscle consists of two bellies connected by a round intermediate tendon. The whole muscle is shaped like an arch concave upwards. The anterior belly, venter anterior, located on the inferior surface of the oral diaphragm, arises in the digastric fossa of the mandible and runs back and laterally to the hyoid bone.

The posterior belly, venter posterior, arises in the mastoid notch of the temporal bone and descends obliquely forward and medially, gradually narrowing, to the tendon by means of which it is joined to the anterior belly.

The intermediate tendon is attached to the body and greater horn of the hyoid bone by a fascial loop.

- The stylohyoid muscle descends obliquely from the styloid process of the temporal bone to the body of the hyoid bone and embraces the intermediate tendon of the digastric muscle with two slips.
- The geniohyoid muscle lies above the mylohyoid muscle laterally of the raphe. It stretches from the spina mentalis of the mandible to the body of the hyoid bone. It is a derivative of the anterior longitudinal muscle of the trunk.

  Action: All the four muscles described above raise the hyoid bone. When the bone is steadied, three muscles (mylohyoid, geniohyoid, and digastric) lower the mandible and thus are antagonists of the muscles of mastication. The hyoid bone is steadied by muscles lying below it (sternohyoid, omohyoid, etc.). The same three muscles, the mylohyoid in particular, on contraction during swallowing raise the tongue and press it to the palate, as a result of which food is pushed into the pharynx (▸Fig. 1.4).

Muscles located below the hyoid bone—these muscles are related to the system of the straight muscles of the neck and are situated on both sides of the midline directly under the skin, in front of the larynx, trachea, and thyroid gland. They stretch between the hyoid bone and the sternum. An exception is the omohyoid muscle that extends to the scapula and in origin is a muscle displaced from the trunk to the shoulder girdle (truncofugal) (▸Fig. 1.5).

- The sternohyoid muscle originates from the posterior surface of the sternal manubrium, sternoclavicular joint, and the sternal end on the clavicle, runs upward as a flat band, and joins its contralateral fellow and attaches to the inferior edge of the hyoid bone. Between the medial borders of both sternohyoid

muscles is a narrow vertical space closed by fascia; this is the linea alba cervicalis.

Action: Pulls the hyoid bone downward (▸Fig. 1.6).

Innervation: C1–3.

- The sternothyroid muscle lies under the sternohyoid muscle and is broader. It arises from the posterior surface of the manubrium sterni and the cartilage of the first rib; its medial border touches that of its fellow. It then ascends and attaches to the lateral surface of the thyroid cartilage (to its linea obliqua) (▸Fig. 1.7).

Action: Lowers the larynx.

Innervation: C1–3.

- The thyrohyoid muscle seems to be a continuation of the sternothyroid muscle from which it is separated by a tendinous intersection. It stretches from the oblique

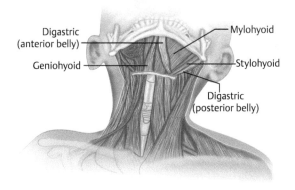

Fig. 1.4 Suprahyoid muscles and ligament.

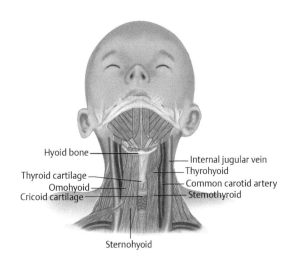

Fig. 1.5 Strap muscles.

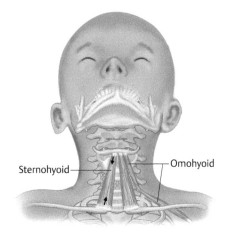

Fig. 1.6 Sternohyoid muscle.

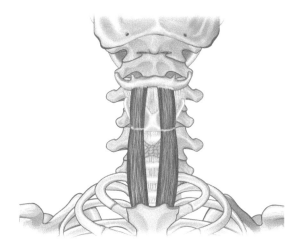

Fig. 1.7 Sternohyoid muscle with insertion to thyroid cartilage.

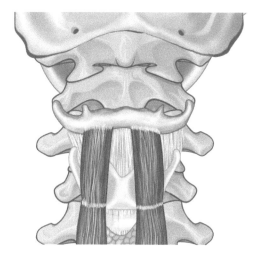

Fig. 1.8 Thyrohoid muscle.

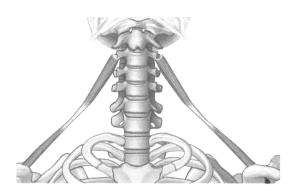

Fig. 1.9 Omohyoid muscle.

line of the thyroid cartilage to the body and greater horn of the hyoid bone (▶ Fig. 1.8).
Action: Pulls the larynx upwards when the hyoid bone is steadied.
Innervation: C1–3.

• The omohyoid muscle is a long narrow muscle consisting of two bellies joined almost at a right angle by an intermediate tendon. The inferior belly arises medially of the scapular notch, overlaps the spatium antescalenum under the cover of sternocleidomastoid muscle where it joins the superior belly by means of the intermediate tendon; the superior belly rises almost perpendicular and is attached to the body of the hyoid bone (▶ Fig. 1.9).

Action: The omohyoid muscle lies in the thickness of the cervical fascia, which it tightens on contraction and thus aids in dilation of the large veins situated under the fascia. It also pulls the hyoid bone downwards.
Innervation: C1–3.

1.3.3 Deep Muscles

I. Lateral muscles attached to the ribs, the scalene muscles. The three scalene muscles are altered intercostal muscles, which explains their attachment to the ribs:

1. The scalenus anterior muscle arises from the anterior tubercles of the transverse processes of the third to sixth cervical vertebrae and is attached to the scalene tubercle of the first rib and the sulcus of the subclavian artery.
Innervation: C5–7.
2. The scalenus medius muscle is the largest scalene muscle. It originates from the anterior tubercles of the transverse processes of all the cervical vertebrae and is attached to the first rib behind the sulcus of the subclavian artery.
Innervation: C2–8.
3. The scalenus posterior muscle arises from the posterior tubercles of the three lower cervical vertebrae and is attached to the outer surface of the second rib.
Innervation: C5–8.
Action: The scalene muscles raise the upper ribs and act as muscles of inspiration. When the ribs are steadied, bilateral contraction of the muscles accomplish forward flexion of the cervical spine; in unilateral contraction, they flex and rotate this segment of the spine to their side (▶ Fig. 1.10).

II. Prevertebral muscles:

1. The longus cervicis muscle is triangular and lies on the anterior surface of the spine, on both sides of it. Three portions are distinguished in it: (1) vertical portion corresponding to the base of the triangle stretching from the anterior surface of the bodies of the upper three thoracic and the lower three cervical

vertebrae to the anterior surface of the bodies of the second, third, and fourth cervical vertebrae; (2)

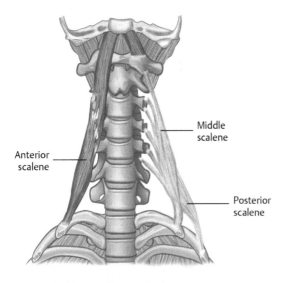

Fig. 1.10 Scalene muscles.

superior oblique portion stretching from the anterior tubercles of the transverse processes of the third, fourth, and fifth cervical vertebrae to the anterior tubercle of the atlas and the body of the axis; (3) inferior oblique portion arising from the bodies of the upper thoracic vertebrae and attached to the anterior tubercles of the transverse processes of the fifth and sixth cervical vertebrae.
Innervation: C3–8.

2. The longus capitis muscle overlaps the upper part of longus colli. It originates from the anterior tubercles of the transverse processes of the third, fourth, fifth, and sixth cervical vertebrae and is attached to the basilar part of the occipital bone.
Innervation: C1–3.

3. The rectus capitis anterior and the rectus lateralis muscles stretch from the lateral mass of the atlas (anterior muscle) and its transverse process (lateral muscle) to the occipital bone (▶ Fig. 1.11).
Innervation: C1.
Action: Rectus capitis anterior and longus capitis flex the head forward. Longus colli flexes the cervical spine on bilateral contraction of all its fibers; in unilateral

Fig. 1.11 Prevertebral muscles.

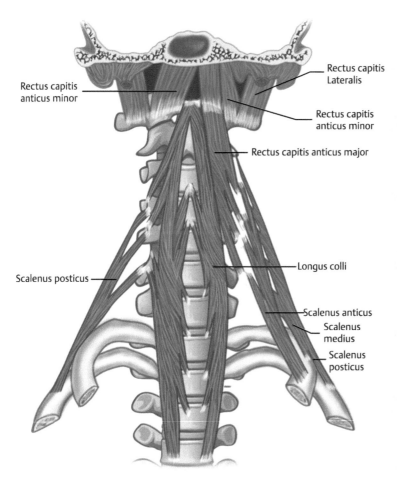

contraction the spine is flexed laterally; the oblique portions take part in rotation and flexion of the head to the side; rectus capitis lateralis helps this muscle.

1.4 Topography of the Neck

The neck (collum) is divided into four regions: posterior, lateral, the region of the sternocleidomastoid muscle, and the anterior region.

The posterior region is behind the lateral border of the trapezius muscle and is the nape, or nucha.

The lateral region is behind the sternocleidomastoid muscle and is bounded in front by this muscle, below by the clavicle, and behind by the trapezius muscle.

The sternocleidomastoid region corresponds to the projection of this muscle.

The anterior region is in front of the sternocleidomastoid muscle and is bounded posteriorly by this muscle, in front by the midline of the neck, and above by the border of the mandible. A small area behind the mandibular angle and in front of the mastoid process is called the fossa retromandibularis. It lodges the posterior part of the parotid gland, nerves, and vessels.

The anterior and lateral regions are divided into a number of triangles by the omohyoid muscle descending obliquely from front to back and crossing the sternocleidomastoid muscle.

The omoclavicular triangle or subclavian triangle is distinguished in the lateral region of the neck; it is bounded by the sternocleidomastoid muscle in front, the inferior belly of the omohyoid muscle above, and the clavicle below.

Two triangles are distinguished in the anterior region of the neck: (1) the fossa carotica or carotis trigone (transmitting the carotid artery), formed by the sternocleidomastoid muscle posteriorly, the posterior belly of the digastric muscle in front and above, and the superior belly of the omohyoid muscle in front and below; and (2) the submandibular trigone (lodging the submaxillary gland), formed by the inferior border of the mandible above and the two bellies of the digastric muscle.

Triangular slits or spaces form between the scalene muscles; they transmit nerves and vessels of the upper limb.

- Between the anterior and middle scalene muscles is spatium interscalenum; bounded by the first rib below (it transmits the subclavian artery and the brachial plexus).
- In front of the anterior scalene muscle is spatium antescalenum covered in front by the sternothyroid and sternohyoid muscles (it transmits the subclavian vein, the suprascapular artery, and the omohyoid muscle).

1.4.1 Muscles of the Head

- Muscles of mastication: derivatives of the first visceral (mandibular) arch.
  Innervation: trigeminal nerve.
- Muscles of facial expression: derivatives of the second visceral (hyoid) arch.
  Innervation: facial nerve.

1.4.2 Muscles of Mastication

The four muscles of mastication on each side are related genetically (they originate from a single visceral arch, the mandibular arch), morphologically (they are all attached to the mandible that they move when they contract), and functionally (they accomplish the chewing movements of the mandible, which determines their location).

- The masseter muscle is thick and quadrangular. It arises from the inferior border of the zygoma and the zygomatic arch and is attached to the masseteric tuberosity and the external surface of the mandibular ramus.
- The temporal muscle is wide at its origin and occupies the whole temporal fossa of the skull up to the temporal line. The muscle fibers converge like a fan and form a strong tendon that passes under the zygomatic arch and is attached to the coronoid process of the mandible.
- The lateral pterygoid muscle arises from the inferior surface of the greater wing of the sphenoid bone and the pterygoid process. It is directed almost horizontally backward and laterally and is attached to the neck of the mandibular condylar process and to the capsule and articular disk of the temporomandibular joint.
- The medial pterygoid muscle arises in the pterygoid fossa of the pterygoid process, passes downward and laterally, and attaches to the medial surface of the mandibular angle, symmetrically with the masseter muscle, at the pterygoid tuberosity (▶Fig. 1.12).

Action: The temporal, masseter, and medial pterygoid muscles pull the mandible to the maxilla when the mouth is open and thus close the mouth. On simultaneous contraction of both lateral pterygoid muscles, the mandible protrudes forward. Movement in the opposite direction is accomplished by the posterior fibers of the temporal muscle, which pass almost horizontally forward. Unilateral contraction of the lateral pterygoid muscle displaces the mandible to the contralateral side of the mouth.

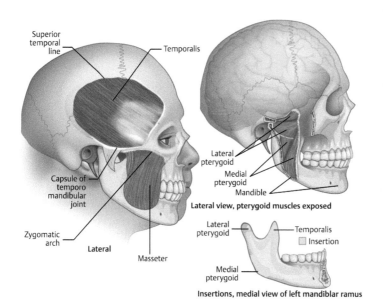

Fig. 1.12 Mastication muscles.

Superior temporal line — Temporalis

Capsule of temporo mandibular joint

Zygomatic arch

Lateral

Masseter

Lateral pterygoid
Medial pterygoid
Mandible

Lateral view, pterygoid muscles exposed

Lateral pterygoid — Temporalis
☐ Insertion

Medial pterygoid

Insertions, medial view of left mandiblar ramus

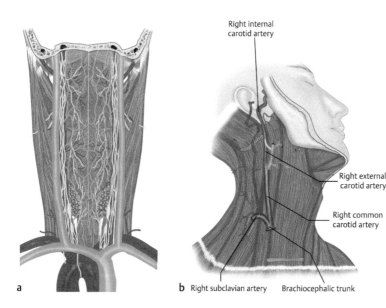

Fig. 1.13 **(a)** Blood supply to prevertebral. **(b)** Common and internal carotid artery.

Right internal carotid artery

Right external carotid artery

Right common carotid artery

a

b Right subclavian artery   Brachiocephalic trunk

1.4.3 Blood Supply of the Head and Neck

Carotid Artery

The common carotid arteries are major blood vessels that supply blood to the *head and neck region*. There is one common carotid artery on either side of the body and these arteries differ in their origin. The left common carotid artery arises from the aortic arch within the superior mediastinum, while the right common carotid artery arises from the brachiocephalic artery posterior to the right sternoclavicular joint.

The common carotid artery ascends lateral to the trachea and esophagus within a deep cervical fascia, the carotid sheath, medial to the internal jugular vein, and anterior to the vagus nerve.

Branches

At the level of the superior border of the laryngeal thyroid cartilage, the artery divides into two terminal branches (▶Fig. 1.13a, b):
- External carotid artery: This artery arises at the level of the intervertebral disc, between C3 and C4, and ascends slightly anteriorly before inclining posterolaterally. In the carotid triangle, it is anteromedial to the internal carotid artery. The external carotid gives off eight main branches, which supply regions of the head and neck.

- Internal carotid artery: This runs from its origin at the carotid bifurcation to the anterior perforated substance, where it bifurcates into the anterior and middle cerebral arteries at the Circle of Willis. It supplies the forehead, nose, eyes, and the ipsilateral cerebral hemisphere.

External Carotid Artery

The external carotid artery supplies the areas of the head and neck external to the cranium. After arising from the common carotid artery, it travels up the neck, posterior to the mandibular neck, and anterior to the lobule of the ear. The artery ends within the parotid gland, by dividing into the **superficial temporal artery** and the **maxillary artery**. Before terminating, the external carotid artery gives off six branches:

1. Superior thyroid artery.
2. Lingual artery.
3. Facial artery.
4. Ascending pharyngeal artery.
5. Occipital artery.
6. Posterior auricular artery.

The facial, maxillary, and superficial temporal arteries are the major branches of note. The maxillary artery supplies the deep structures of the face, while the facial and superficial temporal arteries generally supply superficial areas of the face (▶ Fig. 1.14).

1. Superior thyroid artery: The superior thyroid artery is the origin of the superior laryngeal artery that supplies the larynx. The main artery also supplies the thyroid gland, infrahyoid muscles, and the sternocleidomastoid muscle (▶ Fig. 1.15).
2. Ascending pharyngeal artery: The ascending pharyngeal artery ascends superiorly along the pharynx while branching off to the pharynx, prevertebral muscles, the middle ear, and the cranial meninges (▶ Fig. 1.16).

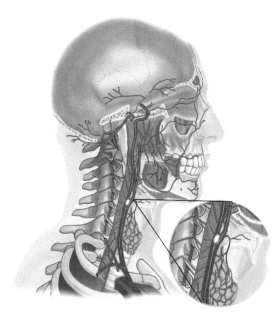

Fig. 1.15 Super thyroid artery.

Fig. 1.14 External carotid artery and branches.

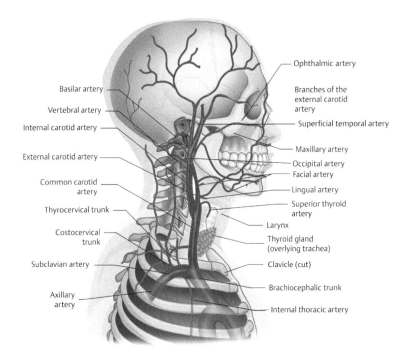

Basilar artery

Vertebral artery

Internal carotid artery

External carotid artery

Common carotid artery

Thyrocervical trunk

Costocervical trunk

Subclavian artery

Axillary artery

Ophthalmic artery

Branches of the external carotid artery

Superficial temporal artery

Maxillary artery

Occipital artery

Facial artery

Lingual artery

Superior thyroid artery

Larynx

Thyroid gland (overlying trachea)

Clavicle (cut)

Brachiocephalic trunk

Internal thoracic artery

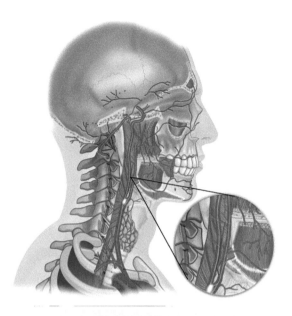

Fig. 1.16 Ascending pharyngeal artery.

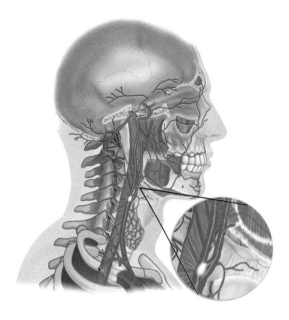

Fig. 1.17 Lingual artery.

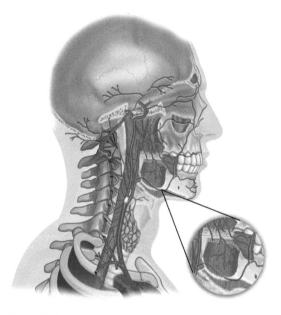

Fig. 1.18 Facial artery.

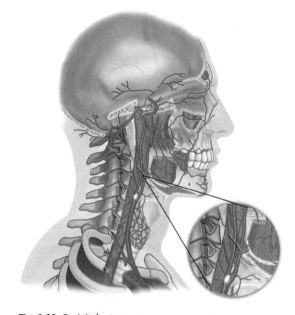

Fig. 1.19 Occipital artery.

3. Lingual artery: The lingual artery is covered by the hypoglossal nerve (CN XII), the stylohyoid muscle, and the posterior belly of the digastric muscle. It runs beneath the hyoglossus muscles and branches into the deep lingual and sublingual arteries that supply the intrinsic muscles of the tongue and the floor of the mouth (▶ Fig. 1.17).

4. Facial artery: The facial artery runs around the middle of the mandible before it enters the face, where it branches into the tonsils, palate, and the submandibular glands (▶ Fig. 1.18).

5. Occipital artery: The occipital artery supplies the posterior region of the scalp and grooves the base of the skull as it travels. Initially, it passes deep into the posterior belly of the digastric muscle (▶ Fig. 1.19).

6. Posterior auricular artery: The posterior auricular artery runs behind the external acoustic meatus and the mastoid process, separating the two structures.

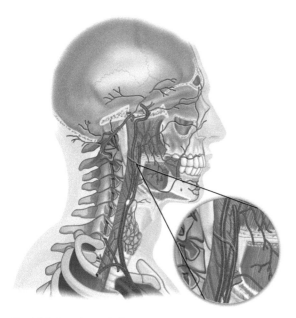

Fig. 1.20 Posterior auricular artery.

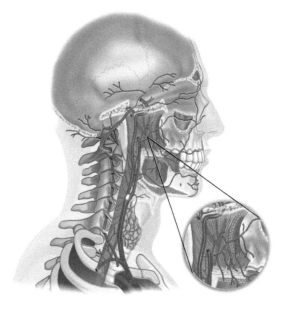

Fig. 1.21 Maxillary artery.

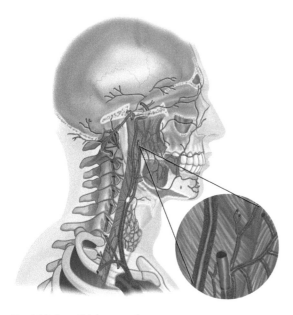

Fig. 1.22 Superficial temporal artery.

It supplies the adjacent musculature, the parotid gland, the facial nerve (CN VII), the ear, and the scalp (▶ Fig. 1.20).

7. Maxillary artery: The maxillary artery (▶ Fig. 1.21) is the larger of the two terminal branches that can precede one another depending on which anatomist you ask. Its branches supply:
   - External acoustic meatus.
   - Tympanic membrane.
   - Dura mater.
   - Calvaria.
   - Mandible.
   - Gingivae.
   - Teeth.
   - Temporal muscle.
   - Pterygoid muscle.
   - Masseter muscle.
   - Buccinator muscle.

8. Superficial temporal artery: The superficial temporal artery supplies only the temporal region of the scalp, as it is the smaller terminal branch and does not have additional named branches or divisions (▶ Fig. 1.22).

1.5 Major Salivary Glands

- The parotid: This gland is bilateral, paired, and sits on either side of the face in the preauricular area, behind and upon the mandibular ramus. There it is encapsulated by the masseteric fascia deriving from the deep cervical fascia. The parotid plexus, branches of the facial nerve, passes through the parotid gland and divides it into a superficial and a deep part but does not innervate it. The parotid duct (Stensen's duct) drains the saliva into the oral cavity opposite the upper second molar tooth. In its course it crosses the masseter and pierces through the buccinator.

  The parotid is bordered anteriorly by the masseter muscle and the mandibular ramus and superiorly by the external acoustic meatus and the condyle of the mandible in the glenoid fossa. Posterior to the gland is the mastoid process of the temporal bone and the sternocleidomastoid muscle. On the medial side, which is not covered by the capsule, the styloid process is visible (▶ Fig. 1.23).

Blood supply: The maxillary arteries and superficial temporal arteries.

Innervation: Sensory—auriculotemporal nerve. Parasympathetic—glossopharyngeal nerve. Sympathetic—direct fibers of the external carotid plexus.

- The submandibular gland: It is situated both superiorly and inferiorly to the posterior aspect of the mandible in the submandibular triangle of the neck and makes up part of the floor of the oral cavity.

  The mylohyoid muscle runs through the lobules of the gland and sections it off into superficial and deep parts. The superficial portion of the submandibular gland can be seen in the submandibular triangle of the neck and is covered by the investing layer of deep cervical fascia. The deep portion of the submandibular gland is that which limits the inferior aspect of the oral cavity. It lies between the hyoglossus muscle and the mandible. It ends at the posterior border of the sublingual gland.

  Its duct (Wharton's duct) opens at the lingual papilla, which can be found on either side of the lingual frenulum. It runs along the gland and is approximately 4 centimeters in length (▶ Fig. 1.24).

Blood supply: The facial and lingual arteries.

Innervation: Parasympathetic (stimulated)—facial nerve fibers to submandibular.

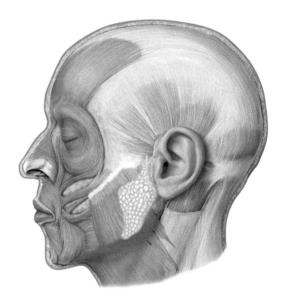

Fig. 1.23 Parotid salivary gland.

Fig. 1.24 Submandibular salivary gland.

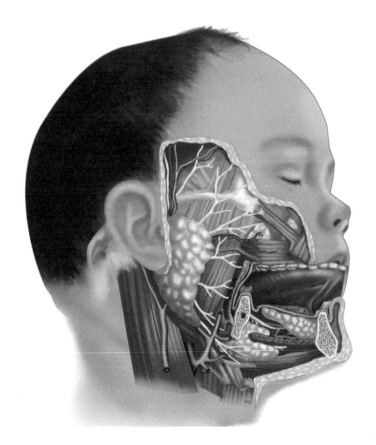

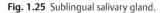

Fig. 1.25 Sublingual salivary gland.

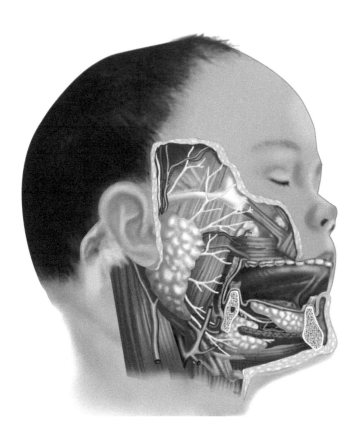

Sympathetic (inhibited)—superior cervical ganglion fibers.[3] The sublingual gland lies bilaterally in the floor of the mouth (over mylohyoid muscle), is covered only by the mucous membrane, and forms a sublingual fold between the tongue and the inner surface of the mandible.

The gland is bordered by the mandible anteroinferiorly, the genioglossus muscle posteroinferiorly and covered superiorly by the tongue (▶ Fig. 1.25).

Blood supply: Lingual artery, which branches into the sublingual artery.

Facial artery, which gives rise to the submental artery.

Innervation: Via the chorda tympani, which carries fibers that originate from the facial nerve.

1.6 The Larynx

The larynx is situated on the level of the fourth, fifth, and sixth cervical vertebrae immediately below the hyoid bone, on the anterior surface of the neck, and forms here a clearly visible eminence. To the back of it is the pharynx with which it communicates directly through an opening called

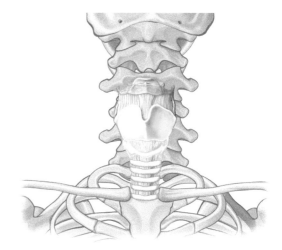

Fig. 1.26 The larynx (ant border).

the inlet of the larynx. On both sides of the larynx pass large vessels of the neck, while in front it is covered with muscles of the infrahyoid group, the cervical fascia, and the superior parts of the lateral lobes of the thyroid (▶ Fig. 1.26).

1.6.1 Cartilages of the Larynx

The larynx is composed of six individual cartilages of which three are paired and three are unpaired. The hyaline cartilages consist of:

- Thyroid cartilage (unpaired).
- Cricoid cartilage (unpaired).
- Arytenoid cartilage (paired).

The elastic cartilages are the following:
- Epiglottis (unpaired).
- Corniculate cartilage (paired).
- Cuneiform cartilage (paired).

1. The cricoid cartilage is hyaline and shaped like a signet ring with a wide plate (lamina) at the back and an arch in front and on the sides. It is a complete circle of cartilage and is attached superiorly via the median cricothyroid ligament to the inferior aspect of the thyroid cartilage. The cricotracheal ligament also attaches it to the trachea inferiorly.
2. The thyroid cartilage is the largest of the laryngeal cartilages; it is hyaline in structure and consists of two laminae of which the two lower thirds fuse in the midline, while the most superior third remains unfused and creates the laryngeal notch. The site of union of the laminae (the thyroid angle) in children and females is rounded, and there is, therefore, no conspicuous prominence in them as in adult males (Adam's apple). In the superior border on the midline is the thyroid notch.
   The cartilaginous superior and inferior horns are created by the projections of the posterior superior and inferior borders of the cartilage, respectively. The thyrohyoid membrane connects the entire superior aspect of the cartilage to the hyoid bone.
3. The arytenoid cartilages are directly related to the vocal cords and muscles. They are pyramidal in shape and have three faces. The cricoid lamina articulates with these cartilages on its lateral superior aspect. The three processes of a single arytenoid cartilage include the apex, which is most superior, balances the corniculate cartilage, and attaches to the aryepiglottic fold; the vocal process, which sits anteriorly and is the posterior attachment of a vocal cord; and the muscular process, which sits laterally and holds the posterior and lateral insertions of the cricoarytenoid muscles.
4. The corniculate cartilages are seated on the apices of the arytenoid cartilages in the thickness of the aryepiglottic folds.
5. The cuneiform cartilages are directly in front of the corniculate cartilages, and in the aryepiglottic folds, they do not attach themselves to any other cartilages, just muscles and ligaments.

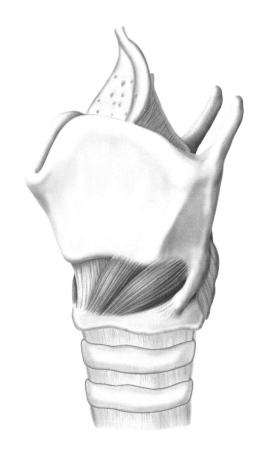

Fig. 1.27 Thyroid cartilage.

6. The epiglottis cartilage, also known as the epiglottis, is a leaf-shaped lamina of elastic cartilaginous tissue situated between the hyoid bone and the dorsal part of the tongue anteriorly and the laryngeal inlet posteriorly, while the superior tip is left standing free (▶ Fig. 1.27).

1.6.2 Ligaments and Membranes of the Larynx

The ligaments and membranes of the larynx (▶ Fig. 1.28a, b) are as follows:
   Major extrinsic ligaments:
- Two lateral thyrohyoid ligaments.
- Single median thyrohyoid ligament.
- Median cricothyroid ligament.
- Cricotracheal ligament.
- Thyrohyoid membrane.

Major intrinsic ligaments:
- Vocal ligament.
- Conus elasticus.

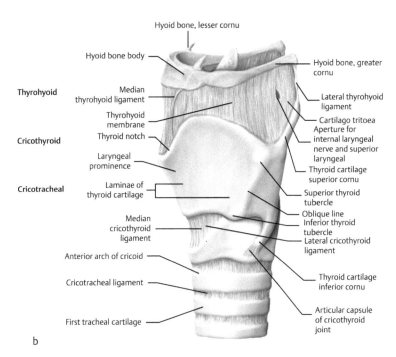

Fig. 1.28 (a) Intrinsic membranes of larynx. **(b)** Extrinsic membranes of larynx.

Greater cornu of hyoid

Thyrohyoid membrane

Opening for neurovascular bundle

Quadrangular membrane

Corniculate cartilage

Muscular process of arytenoid cartilage

Vocal process of arytenoid cartilage

Cut surface of hyoid bone

Epiglottis

Thyroepiglottic ligament

Cut surface of thyroid cartilage

Vestibular ligament

Vocal ligament

Cricovocal membrane

Cricoid cartilage

a

Hyoid bone, lesser cornu

Hyoid bone body

Thyrohyoid

Median thyrohyoid ligament

Thyrohyoid membrane

Cricothyroid

Thyroid notch

Laryngeal prominence

Cricotracheal

Laminae of thyroid cartilage

Median cricothyroid ligament

Anterior arch of cricoid

Cricotracheal ligament

First tracheal cartilage

Hyoid bone, greater cornu

Lateral thyrohyoid ligament

Cartilago tritoea

Aperture for internal laryngeal nerve and superior laryngeal

Thyroid cartilage superior cornu

Superior thyroid tubercle

Oblique line

Inferior thyroid tubercle

Lateral cricothyroid ligament

Thyroid cartilage inferior cornu

Articular capsule of cricothyroid joint

b

- Quadrangular membrane.
- Vestibular ligament.

The ligament is formed of yellowish elastic fibers passing parallel to one another. Children and young boys have, in addition, intersecting elastic fibers, which disappear in adults.

1.6.3 Muscles of the Larynx

The muscles of the larynx move its cartilages and thus change the width of its cavity and the width of the rima glottidis bounded by the vocal ligaments. According to function, they may, therefore, be grouped as follows: (1) constrictors; (2) dilators; (3) muscles altering the tension of the vocal ligaments.

Some of the muscles can be related to more than one group because of their mixed character.

Constrictors

- The lateral cricoarytenoid muscle—ailing from the arch of the cricoid cartilage, this muscle distally attaches itself to the muscular process of the arytenoid cartilage. It acts as an adductor of the vocal folds (▶Fig. 1.29).

- The thyroarytenoid muscle originates upon the posterior aspect of the thyroid cartilage. It inserts into the muscular process of the arytenoid cartilage, just as the posterior and lateral cricoarytenoid muscles do. It shortens and relaxes the vocal cords (▶Fig. 1.30).[3] The transverse arytenoid muscle is an unpaired muscle. Originates from the muscular process of the arytenoid cartilage and fastens itself to the muscular process of the opposing arytenoid cartilage. On contraction, it narrows the posterior part of the rima glottides (▶Fig. 1.31).
- The oblique arytenoid muscle has no origin as it stretches itself between the two arytenoid cartilages and inserts into both of their apices. On simultaneous contraction, it narrows the laryngeal inlet and vestibule (▶Fig. 1.32).

Dilators

- The posterior cricoarytenoid muscle is triangular in shape. It originates in the lamina of the cricoid cartilage and inserts into the muscular process of the arytenoid cartilage. On contraction, it opens the rima glottides (▶Fig. 1.33).
- The thyroepiglottic muscle originates from the inner surface of the lamina of the thyroid cartilage and is

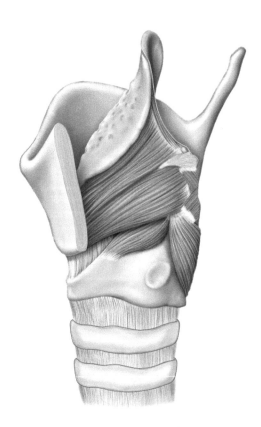

Fig. 1.29 Lateral cricoarytenoid muscle.

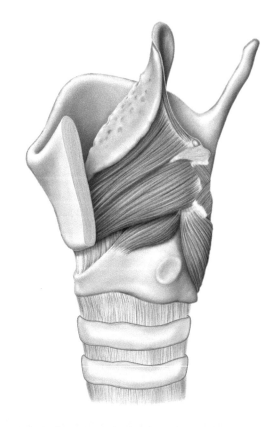

Fig. 1.30 Thyroarytenoid muscle.

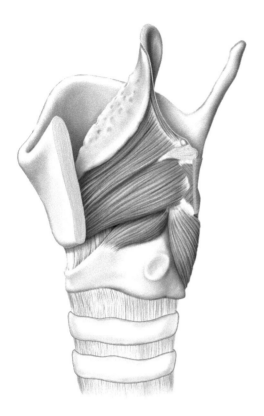

Fig. 1.31 Transverse arytenoid muscle.

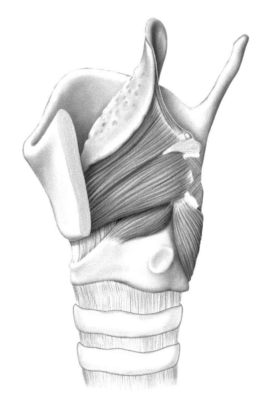

Fig. 1.32 Oblique arytenoid muscles.

inserted on the margin of the epiglottis and is partly continuous with the aryepiglottic fold. It acts as the dilator of the laryngeal inlet and vestibule (▶ Fig. 1.34).

Muscles Altering the Tension of the Vocal Ligaments

- The cricothyroid muscle originates on the anterior cricoid cartilage and inserts into the inferior border of the thyroid cartilage and its inferior horn. Upon contraction, it lengthens and tenses the vocal ligaments (▶ Fig. 1.35).
- The vocalis muscle—the proximal attachment of the vocalis muscle is upon the vocal process of the arytenoid cartilage. It inserts distally upon the vocal ligament and acts by tensing the anterior vocal ligament and relaxing the posterior vocal ligament.

Innervation

The motor and sensory innervation of the larynx in its entirety comes from the vagus nerve (CN X). The three branches that are contributed include the internal laryngeal nerve, the recurrent laryngeal nerve, and the external laryngeal nerve.

Blood Supply

The arterial supply of the larynx is provided by the superior laryngeal artery and the inferior laryngeal artery. The

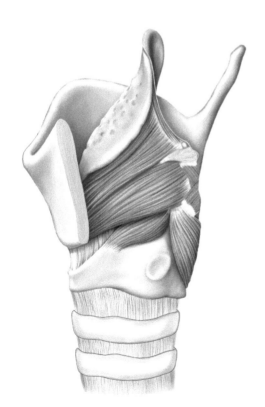

Fig. 1.33 Posterior cricoarytenoid muscle.

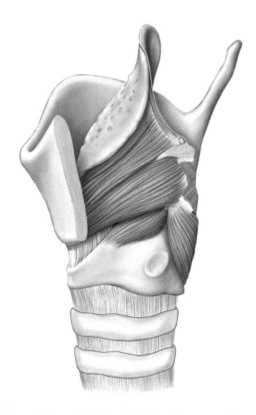

Fig. 1.34 Thyroepiglottic muscle.

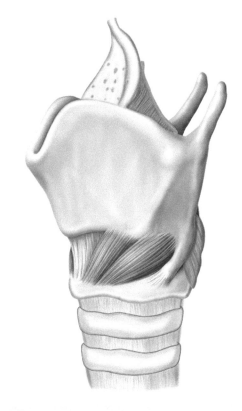

Fig. 1.35 Cricothyroid muscle.

venous drainage is managed by the superior laryngeal vein and the inferior laryngeal vein.

1.6.4 Anatomical Differences Between Pediatric and Adult Larynx

The anatomical differences between pediatric and adult larynx is shown in ▶ Fig. 1.36a, b.

Infant Larynx

- Position: Infant larynx is situated higher in the neck. Vocal cords lie at C3/C4 level and during swallowing go up to C1/C2 level. In adults, vocal cords lie at C5 level.
- Cartilages: Laryngeal cartilages in infants are soft and collapse easily.
  - Epiglottis: It is omega shaped.
  - Arytenoids: They are relatively large and cover a significant part of glottis.
  - Thyroid: It is flat.
  - Cricoid: The diameter of cricoid is smaller than glottis.
- Cricothyroid and thyrohyoid spaces: They are very narrow. Hyoid bone overlaps thyroid and thyroid overlaps cricoid.

- Size: The larynx of an infant is smaller and has a narrow lumen.
- Shape: It is conical and funnel-shaped.
- Submucosal tissue: It is thick and loose and becomes easily edematous in response to trauma or inflammation.

1.7 Facial Nerve

1.7.1 Components and Branches

The facial nerve contains many different types of fibers, including general sensory (afferent) fibers, special sensory fibers, visceral/autonomic motor (efferent) fibers, and somatic motor fibers. General sensory fibers in the facial nerve are responsible for transmitting signals to the brain from the external acoustic meatus, as well as the skin over the mastoid and lateral pinna. Special sensory fibers in the facial nerve are responsible for receiving and transmitting taste information from the anterior two-thirds of the tongue.

Visceral/autonomic motor fibers in the facial nerve are responsible for innervating the lacrimal gland, submandibular gland, sublingual gland, and the mucous

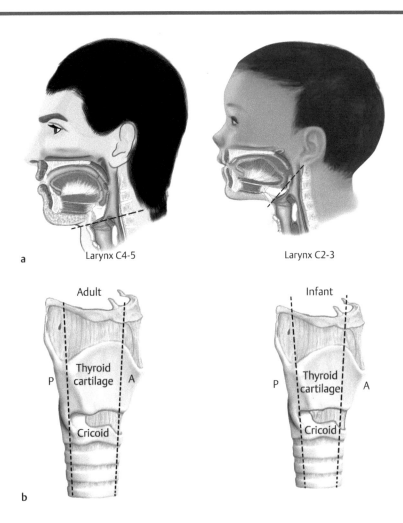

Fig. 1.36 (a) Larynx position—adult/infant. **(b)** Larynx shape—adult/infant.

a   Larynx C4-5   Larynx C2-3

Adult   Infant

P   Thyroid cartilage   A   P   Thyroid cartilage   A

Cricoid   Cricoid

b

membranes of the nasal cavity and hard and soft palates, allowing for the production of tears, saliva, etc., from these locations. Somatic motor fibers in the facial nerve are responsible for innervating the muscles of facial expression and muscles in the scalp, as well as the stapedius muscle in the ear, the posterior belly of the digastric muscle, and the stylohyoid muscle.

The facial nerve roots enter the facial canal in petrous part of temporal bone, where the small sensory and large motor roots fuse, forming the facial nerve. This united nerve enlarges at the geniculate ganglion, which contains cell bodies for sensory neurons.

As the facial nerve continues to travel along the bony canal, two branches emerge: nerve to stapedius that innervates the stapedius muscle and chorda tympani that is responsible for transmitting taste sensation and innervating the submandibular gland.

The facial nerve exits skull via stylomastoid foramen. In a child, the facial nerve is more superficial than in an adult (and therefore more prone to disruption from trauma or surgery); it gives off the posterior auricular nerve that is

Table 1.1 Branches of facial nerve

With facial canal	• Nerve to the stapedius muscle • Chroda tympani
At its exit from the stylomastoid foramen	• Posterior auricular • Digastric • Stylohyoid
On the face	• Temporal • Zygomatic • Buccal • Mandibular • Cervical

meant to supply the occipital belly of the occipitofrontalis muscle and some of the auricular muscles, and nerves to the posterior belly of the digastric and the stylohyoid. The nerve then enters the parotid gland, from whence it gives off five terminal branches—the temporal, zygomatic, buccal, marginal mandibular, and cervical branches—which emerge from around the parotid gland and innervate structures across the entire face (▸Table 1.1 and ▸Fig. 1.37).

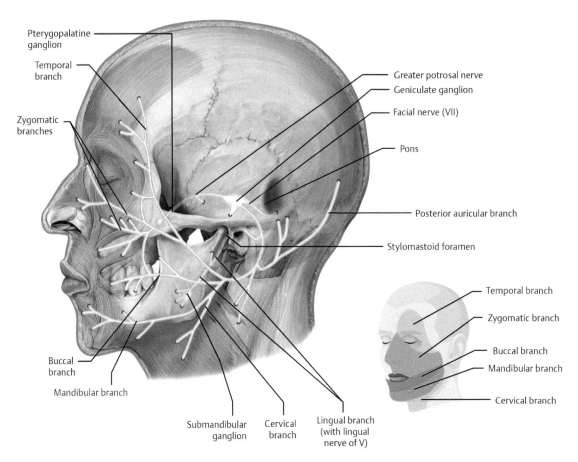

Fig. 1.37 Facial nerve.

1.8 The Organ of Hearing

See ▶ Fig. 1.38 for reference.

1.8.1 The External Ear

The external ear consists of the auricle and the external auditory meatus (▶ Fig. 1.39a, b). The auricle is formed of elastic cartilage covered with skin. This cartilage determines the external shape of the auricle and its projections: the free curved margin called the helix, the antihelix, located parallel to it, the anterior prominence, the tragus, and the antitragus situated behind it. Downward the ear it terminates as the lobule that has no cartilage. In the depression on the lateral surface of the auricle (the concha auriculae), behind the tragus, is the external auditory meatus.

The external auditory meatus consists of two parts: cartilaginous and bony.

The cartilaginous auditory meatus is a continuation of the auricular cartilage in the form of a groove open upward and to the back. Its internal end is joined by means of connective tissue with the edge of the tympanic part of the temporal bone. The cartilaginous auditory meatus constitutes two-thirds of the whole external auditory meatus.

The bony auditory meatus that constitutes two-thirds of the entire length of the auditory meatus opens to the exterior by means of the porus acusticus externus on the periphery of which runs a circular bony tympanic groove.

The direction of the whole auditory meatus is frontal in general but it does not advance in a straight line; it winds in the form of letter "S" both horizontally and vertically. Because of the curves of the auditory meatus, the deeply situated tympanic membrane can only be seen by pulling the auricle backward, outward, and upward. The skin that covers the auricle continues into the external auditory meatus. In the cartilaginous part of the meatus, the skin is very rich both in sebaceous glands and in a particular kind of glands, the ceruminous glands, which produce cerumen (ear wax).

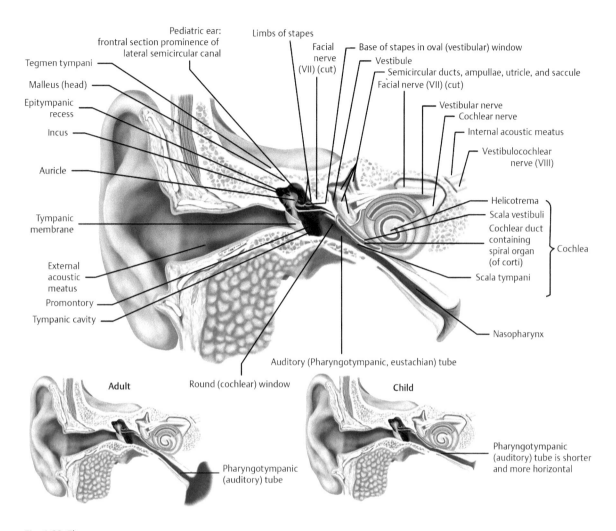

Fig. 1.38 The ear.

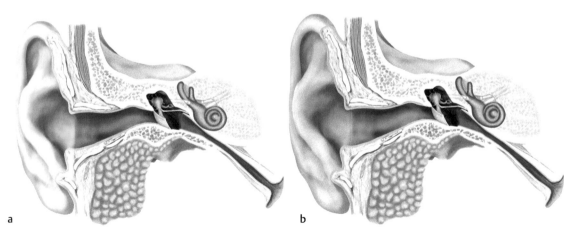

a   b

Fig. 1.39 **(a)** The auricle. **(b)** External auditory canal.

1.8.2 The Tympanic Membrane

The tympanic membrane is located at the junctions of the external and middle ears. It is a thin fibrous structure, and has an external surface that is exposed to the external environment and lined by stratified squamous epithelium, and an inner surface (facing the tympanum) that is lined by low columnar epithelium. The tympanic membrane is an oval structure that is situated at an angle relative to the external acoustic meatus, but in newborns it is almost horizontal.

At the center of the tympanic membrane, there is a depression known as the umbo. This concavity is created by the attachment of the malleus to the center of the tympanum.

The superior part of the tympanic membrane, between the mallear folds, is known as pars flaccida and is relatively loose. The remainder of the membrane is held tight by the tensor tympani muscle, and is therefore known as the pars tensa (▶ Fig. 1.40).

1.8.3 The Middle Ear

The middle ear consists of the tympanic cavity and the auditory tube through which it communicates with the nasopharynx.

The tympanic cavity is a pneumatized (air-filled) region, situated in the base of the pyramid of the temporal bone between the external auditory meatus and the labyrinth (internal ear). It contains a chain of three small ossicles transmitting sound vibrations from the tympanic membrane to the labyrinth (▶ Fig. 1.41).

The three tiny auditory ossicles in the tympanic cavity are called the malleus, incus, and stapes.

- The malleus has a rounded head (caput mallei) which by means of a neck (collum mallei) is joined to the handle (manubrium mallei) (▶ Fig. 1.42).
- The incus has a body (corpus inoudis) and two diverging processes: a short (crus breve) and a long process (crus longum). The short process projects backward and abuts upon the fossa. The long process

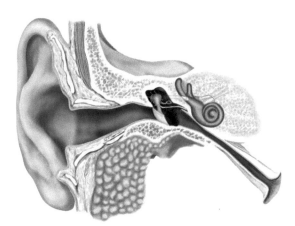

Fig. 1.40 Tympanic membrane.

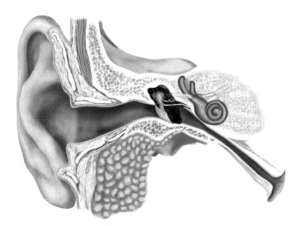

Fig. 1.41 Middle ear cavity.

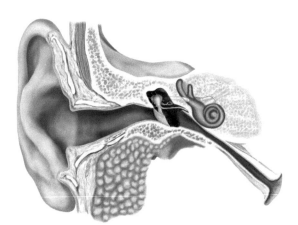

Fig. 1.42 Malleus.

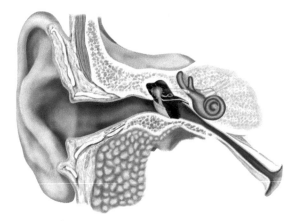

Fig. 1.43 Incus.

runs parallel to the handle of the malleus, medially and posteriorly of it and has a small oval thickening on its end, the lenticular process (processus lenticularis), which articulates with the stapes (▶Fig. 1.43). The stapes justifies its name in shape and consists of a small head (caput stapedis), carrying an articulating surface for the lenticular process of the incus and two limbs: an anterior, less curved limb (crus anterius), and a posterior more curved limb (crus posterius). The limbs are attached to an oval base (basis stapedis) fitted into the fenestra vestibule (▶Fig. 1.44).

In places where the auditory ossicles articulate with one another, two true joints of limited mobility are formed: the incudomalleolar joint (articulation incudomallearis) and the incudostapedial joint (articulatio incudostapedia).

The base of the stapes is joined with the edges of fenestra vestibuli by means of connective tissue to form the tymanostapedial syndesmosis. The auditory ossicles are attached, moreover, by several separate ligaments. The mobility of the ossicles becomes gradually reduced from malleus to stapes, as the result of which the organ of Corti located in the internal ear is protected from excessive concussions and harsh sounds.

The chain of ossicles performs two functions: (1) the conduction of sound through the bones and (2) the mechanical transmission of sound vibrations to the fenestra cochlea. The latter function is accomplished by two small muscles connected with the auditory ossicles and located in the tympanic cavity; they regulate the movement of the chain of ossicles. One of them, the tensor tympani muscle, lies in the canal for the tensor tympany constituting the upper part of the musculotubal canal of the temporal bone; its tendon is fastened to the handle of the malleus near the neck. This muscle pulls the handle of the malleus medially, thus tensing the tympanic membrane. At the same time

all the system of ossicles moves medially and the stapes presses into the fenestra cochlea. The muscle is innervated from the third division of the trigeminal nerve by a small branch of the nerve supplied to the tensor tympani muscle. The other muscle, the stapedius muscle, is lodged in the pyramid of the tympanum and fastened to the posterior limb of the stapes at the head. In function, this muscle is an antagonist of the preceding one and accomplishes a reverse movement of the ossicle in the middle ear in the direction of the fenestra cochlea. The stapedius muscle is innervated from the facial nerve, which, passing nearby, sends small branch to the muscle.

The auditory or Eustachian tube lets the air pass from the pharynx into the tympanic cavity, thus equalizing the pressure in this cavity with the atmospheric pressure, which is essential for the proper conduction of the vibrations to the labyrinth. The auditory tube consists of osseous and cartilaginous parts that are joined with each other. At the site of their junction, called the isthmus of the tube, the canal of the tube is narrowest. The bony part of the tube, beginning with its tympanic, occupies the large inferior portion of the muscular-tube canal of the temporal bone. The cartilaginous part, which is a continuation of the bony part, is formed of elastic cartilage.

The tube widens downward and terminates on the lateral wall of the nasopharynx as the pharyngeal opening (ostium pharyngeum tubae auditivae); the edge of the cartilage pressing into the pharynx forms the torus tubarius.

1.8.4 The Inner Ear

The inner ear (which consists of a series of interlinked cavities termed *labyrinths*) is located in the depth of the pyramid of the temporal bone between the tympanic cavity and the internal auditory meatus.

It can be divided into three general parts:
1. Cochlear component that is concerned with hearing.
2. Vestibular component (comprised of the utricle and saccule) that deals with balance while stationary.
3. Semicircular component that regulates balance while in motion.
    - The vestibule, which forms the middle part of the labyrinth, is a hollow cavity located between the cochlea and the semicircular canals. It is located medial to the tympanic cavity, posterior to the cochlea, and anterior to the semicircular canals. It contains three recesses:
        - Elliptical recess, which is closer to the ampullae of the anterior and lateral semicircular canals.
        - Cochlear recess, which is adjacent to the cochlea.
        - Spherical recess, which is adjacent to the opening of the scala vestibuli.

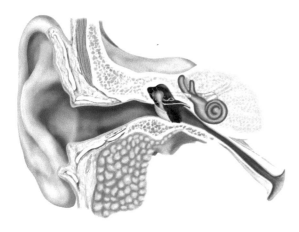

Fig. 1.44 Stapes.

Six orifices open into the vestibule: five belonging to the semicircular canals and one resulting from the scala vestibuli of the cochlea. There are smaller openings on the side adjacent to the internal acoustic meatus that serve as conduits for the vestibular part of CN VIII (vestibulocochlear). The vestibule communicates with the middle ear via the fenestra vestibuli (oval window) (▶Fig. 1.45).

• The semicircular canals are three arch-like bony passages situated in three mutually perpendicular planes. The anterior semicircular canal is directed vertically at right angles to the axis of the pyramid of the temporal bone; the posterior semicircular canal, which is also

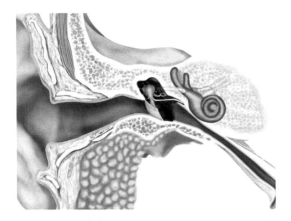

Fig. 1.45 The vestibule.

vertical, is situated nearly parallel to the posterior surface of the pyramid, while the lateral canal lies horizontally, protruding toward the tympanic cavity.

At one end of each canal is an enlargement called the bony ampulla. The ampullae of all three canals open into the vestibule independently. However, the non-ampullated ends of the anterior and posterior canals fuse to form the common bony crus. The non-ampullated end of the lateral semicircular canal is known as the simple bony crus (▶Fig. 1.46).

The bony labyrinth may easily be separated as a whole from the spongy substance of the pyramid surrounding it in the skulls of children.

• The cochlea is like a spiral bony canal that, beginning from the vestibule, winds up like the shell of a snail into two-and-a-half coils. The bony pillar around which the coils wind lies horizontally and is called the modiolus. An osseous spiral lamina projects from the modiolus into the cavity of the canal along the entire length of its coils. This lamina together with the cochlear duct divides the cavity of the cochlea into two sections: the scala vestibuli that communicates with the vestibule and the scala tympani that opens on the skeletonized bone into the tympanic cavity through the fenestra cochlea. Near this fenestra in the scala tympani is a very small inner orifice of the aqueduct of the cochlea, whose external opening lies on the inferior surface of the pyramid of the temporal bone (▶Fig. 1.47).

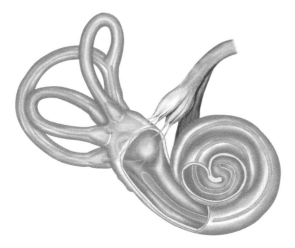

Fig. 1.46 The semicircular canals.

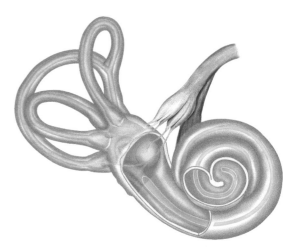

Fig. 1.47 The cochlea.

1.9 Thyroid Gland

The thyroid develops as a small mass in the tongue, which invaginates around the fifth week of embryonic development (▶ Fig. 1.48). This point of origin and invagination is called the foramen cecum. The thyroid gland migrates inferiorly through the developing neck and is intimately associated with the hyoid bone. By the seventh week, the thyroid gland reaches its final destination in the neck just inferior to the cricoid cartilage anterior to the trachea. The thyroid gland is functional by the tenth to twelfth week of development. Abnormal migration of the thyroid gland may result in ectopic thyroid tissue. The tract of the migration of the thyroid gland, termed the *thyroglossal duct,* normally collapses and atrophies. If the duct fails to undergo atrophy, it may result in a thyroglossal duct cyst. The thyroglossal duct cyst derives from persistence of the embryonic thyroglossal duct anywhere between the foramen cecum and the thyroid gland. Most commonly, the thyroglossal duct cyst is found just above the thyroid lamina and below the hyoid bone. Because of the attachments to the base of the tongue, thyroglossal duct remnants will move superiorly in the neck when the tongue is protruded; the thyroglossal duct remnant may contain ectopic thyroid tissue, and occasionally, the cyst contains all of the functioning thyroid tissue. Because of the potential for permanent hypothyroidism after surgical excision, many authors advocate routine preoperative assessment of the thyroid. Ultrasound of the neck provides information regarding the consistency of the cystic lesion and can also be used to assess for the presence of thyroid tissue in its normal position lower in the neck. It is important to note that the possibility of malignancy, usually arising from thyroid tissue, is present within these lesions, although very rare. Thyroglossal duct cysts often present as a midline neck mass that can become infected with upper respiratory tract infections that can cause rapid enlargement, erythema, and drainage. Surgical excision is the treatment of choice. Because the thyroglossal duct remnants are intimately associated with the central part of the hyoid, removal of the midportion of the hyoid, along with the thyroglossal duct (within the base of the tongue to the foramen cecum) and the cyst—a procedure first described by Sistrunk—is recommended to minimize the risk of recurrence.

Fig. 1.48 Thyroid gland.

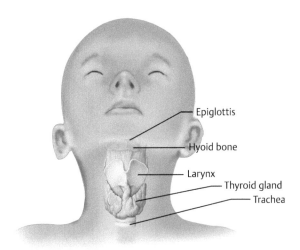

Epiglottis

Hyoid bone

Larynx

Thyroid gland

Trachea

2 The Distinctive Anatomical Features of the Pediatric Skull Base

Oren Cavel, Dan M. Fliss, Irit Duek

Summary

Pediatric skull base and craniofacial surgery presents a unique challenge since the potential benefits of therapy must be balanced against the cumulative impact of treatment on craniofacial growth and the potential for serious psychosocial issues.

The unique demands and physiologic consequences of skull base surgery in pediatrics merit special attention and the distinctive anatomical features of the pediatric skull base must be well understood and anticipated for the prevention of distinct surgical complications.

Keywords: Developmental anatomy, pediatric skull base, surgery

2.1 Introduction

Compared to adults, the size of the cranial base and maxillofacial complex in children is smaller, the cranial bone is thinner, and the floor of the frontal and middle cranial fossa may be flatter.[1] Anatomic landmarks that are found in the fully developed cranium of adults can be absent or different in babies. Examples of those are a more anteriorly located pterion, an absent superior orbital fissure, and undeveloped mastoid process. In addition, neurovascular elements in children are thinner and more fragile than in adults,[2] whereas the brain itself is denser and less amendable to physical manipulation.

2.2 Cranial Fossae

The human skull grows rapidly during the first four years of life (▶Fig. 2.1). The maximal growth rate at birth slopes down to a minimum in pre-puberty, and returns to a smaller second spike at puberty. The growth of the skull base is slower than that of the calvaria, with the anterior, middle, and posterior fossae each developing at different rates. The anterior fossa undergoes ossification starting at birth, when it is still cartilaginous, until the third year of life when it nearly attains adult structure. During the second year of life the mastoid starts to project inferiorly from the squamous and petrous parts of the temporal bone and undergoes pneumatization up until adolescence, with the middle fossa reaching its final size approximately at the age of 10. The posterior fossa is the last to attain mature form. It is comprised mainly of the occipital

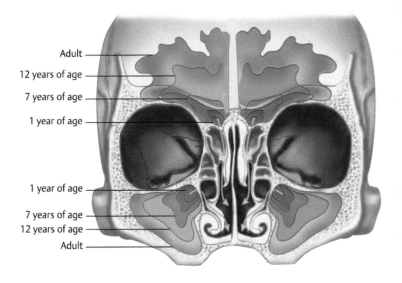

Fig. 2.1 Maxillary and frontal sinuses development.

Adult
12 years of age
7 years of age
1 year of age

1 year of age
7 years of age
12 years of age
Adult

bone with a lesser contribution of the sphenoid anteriorly and the temporal bone laterally. There are four synchondroses which begin to fuse during the second year of life but do not fuse completely until the age of 4 at the posterior junction (exo-occipital and squamous segment) and age of 8 at the anterior junction (basi-occipital and exo-occipital). At the age of 10 the posterior fossa nearly achieves adult proportions. The spheno-occipital synchondrosis, which is the main axis of skull base growth, fuses at the ages 12 to 15 and ossifies only at early adulthood.

2.3 Anterior Skull Base

All the adult structures are present at the small nasal cavity of the newborn, resulting in a relatively narrow and delicate airway passage. The nasal turbinates are voluminous such that the middle meatus is hardly functional. Some of the children are born with a supreme turbinate that usually involutes with growth. The cavum in the newborn lies low and the choana is round with a 6 mm diameter. Its size grows and its shape changes until the age of 12 years, when the sphenoid sinus is usually well developed. The opening of the Eustachian tube is first located behind the inferior turbinate at the level of the hard palate. At the age of 4 years it reaches its final location behind the posterior end of the middle turbinate.[3]

2.4 Paranasal Sinus Development

The paranasal sinus development is a complex and extremely variable process (Table 2.1). It begins with evaginations from the lateral nasal wall (except from the sphenoid sinus). During the seventh week of gestation several projections develop into the nasal capsule; the maxilloturbinals form the inferior turbinate; the ethmoturbinals form the middle, superior, and supreme (26%) turbinates. The furrows between those projections form the nasal meatus and the infundibulum. The nasoturbinal develops into the agger nasi; and the uncinate process develops on the superior–posterior border of the agger nasi. The attachments of these structures to the lateral nasal wall form the lamellae. During the first pneumatization, the furrows continue to grow and contribute to the pneumatization of the ethmoid bone, maxillary bone, frontal bone, and agger nasi. The second pneumatization occurs postnatally, mostly completed by the age of 12 to 14 years.[4]

2.5 Maxillary Sinus Development

The maxillary sinus is the first to develop, during the tenth week of gestation. It begins as an outpouching of the lateral wall within the infundibulum, posterior to the developing uncinate process. After the nasal capsule is resorbed, the maxillary sinus enters the developing maxillary process. At birth, the maxillary sinus has a spherical size, with a length of 10 mm and a height of 3 to 4 mm and its floor is higher than the floor of the nasal cavity (▶ Fig. 2.2). Further growth follows the development of the maxilla and the descent of the teeth, until the sinus floor reaches a position that is 5 to 10 mm lower than the nasal floor. Permanent teeth eruption starts with the first molar at the age of 6 and usually ends with the third molar at 15 to 20 years of age.

Table 2.1 Development of the paranasal sinuses

Sinus	Gestational month when development starts	Status at birth	Growth	Clinically significant size at	First radiologic evidence	Fully developed
Maxillary	2	At birth; Vol: 6–8 ml	Rapid growth from birth to 3 years; from 7 to 12 years	Birth	4–6 months after birth	15 years
Ethmoid	3	At birth; Anterior: 5 × 2 x 2 mm Posterior: 5 × 4 x 2 mm	Reaches adult size by 12 years	Birth	1 year	12 years
Frontal	4	Single cell in ethmoid bone	Invades frontal bone at 4 years. Variable growth	3 years	6 years	18–20 years
Sphenoid	3	Not present	Reaches sella turcica at 7 years; dorsum sellae late teens; basisphenoid adult	8 years	4 years	12–15 years

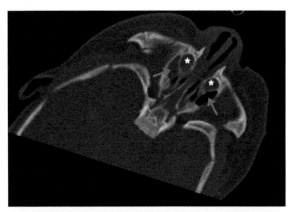

Fig. 2.2 A newborn axial computed tomography (CT) scan demonstrating elongated maxillary sinuses (*blue arrows*). In this case nasolacrimal ducts were obstructed and enlarged (*yellow asterisks*).

2.6 Ethmoid Sinus Development

The ethmoid sinus development begins during the fourth fetal month with multicentric origin: the anterior ethmoid cells (majority) evaginate from the lateral nasal wall at the middle meatus. The posterior ethmoid cells evaginate from the nasal mucosa of the superior and supreme meatus. The ethmoid sinus is well developed at birth but continues to develop until the ethmoid has reached almost adult size and the septae gradually ossify by the age of 12 years. The ethmoid cells are classified according to the skeletal structures they pneumatize: Within the ethmoid bone (intramural cells): conchal, bullar, infundibular, and frontal recess cells. Beyond the ethmoid bone (extramural cells): agger nasi cells, frontal sinus cells, orbital cells, maxillary cells (Haller cells), palatine bone, and sphenoid bone cells.

2.7 Frontal Sinus Development

The frontal sinus begins to develop during the fourth month of gestation, after the development of the frontal recess which is found between the uncinate process and the anterior attachment of the middle turbinate. The frontal sinus develops in several ways, which explains the great variation in its drainage systems: By direct extension of the whole frontal recess; from the laterally placed anterior ethmoid cells within the frontal recess; from the ethmoid infundibular cells; from one or more of the anterior group of ethmoid cells arising in the frontal furrows. At birth the small frontal cell has not yet penetrated and pneumatized the frontal bone,[5] a process that

occurs between 6 months and 2 years. Until the age of 6 years the frontal sinus is small and its opening wide. It reaches its final size at adolescence and as the left and the right sinuses develop independently, asymmetry is the rule (▶ Fig. 2.1).

2.8 Sphenoid Sinus Development

It is the only sinus that does not arise as an outpouching from the lateral nasal wall. During the third fetal month the nasal mucosa invaginates into the posterior portion of the cartilaginous nasal capsule forming a small presphenoid recess and in the fifth fetal month the sinus ostium develops. At birth the sphenoid sinus is absent and the bone is full of marrow. During the second and third years the pre-sphenoid recess becomes the sphenoethmoid recess and usually only at the age of 8 to 10 years a real sinus cavity may be observed. The definitive form of the sinus is attained at puberty.

2.9 Lateral Skull Base

The otic capsule and its content as well as the ossicular chain acquire their definitive size and shape during the fetal life and are completely formed and developed in the newborn.[3] On the other hand, the mastoid cavity and the external auditory canal evolve in size, shape, and directions during the first years of life. Knowledge of the distinctive features of the newborn ear is crucial for the otologic surgeon.

2.10 The External Auditory Canal

In the newborn, the external auditory canal (EAC) is short, straight, and its walls are mostly collapsible. It is oriented medially and inferiorly. Its bony part is mostly composed of a U-shaped tympanic ring in the concavity of which is a groove, the tympanic sulcus, for the attachment of the circumference of the tympanic membrane. During the first year of life, two bony prominences on the inner part of the tympanic ring grow toward each other from the anterior and posterior walls. Those bony growths fuse and delimit inferiorly and medially the tympanic foramen (foramen of Huschke). Gradually, until the age of 5 years, the foramen closes in 95% of children.[6] The bony spurs that first fused progressively spread as the bony EAC continues to elongate inward and inferiorly and acquires its curvature until the age of 6 to 9.[7] The original tympanic ring, as seen at term, will remain, in the adult, at the deep end of the external auditory meatus[8] (▶Fig. 2.3, ▶Fig. 2.4 and ▶Fig. 2.5).

2.11 The Tympanic Membrane

At birth, the tympanic membrane (TM) is already at its adult size but it is oriented inferior-medially and is almost horizontal. It creates a wide open angle with the EAC, which makes otoscopy difficult. In the first 3 years of life it gradually reaches its more vertical position.

2.12 The Middle Ear Cleft

The middle ear cavity, including the ossicles, reaches its adult size at birth. Mesenchymal remnants are abundant in the attic and dissipate in the first few months of life. The Eustachian tube of the neonate is shorter, narrower, and has a more horizontal course. The antrum is present at birth as a small cell located 1 mm deep to the cribrose area of the supra meatal triangle and starts to pneumatize.[3] The mastoid portion is at first quite flat, and the mastoid process appears around the age of 1 year and elongates with the gradual pneumatization of the mastoid cells along childhood. Mastoid growth and pneumatization are also

Fig. 2.3 The facial nerve course and the relations between the facial nerve, the antrum, and the tympanic bone in the newborn.

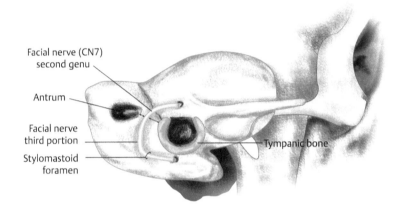

Facial nerve (CN7) second genu
Antrum
Facial nerve third portion
Stylomastoid foramen
Tympanic bone

Fig. 2.4 The foramen tympanicum. TMJ, temporomandibular joint.

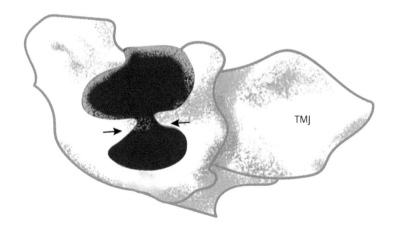

TMJ

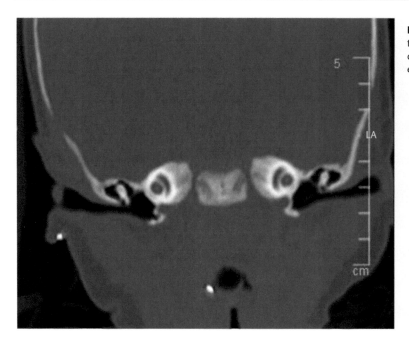

Fig. 2.5 Coronal computed tomography (CT) scan of a neonate demonstrating the undeveloped bony external auditory canal.

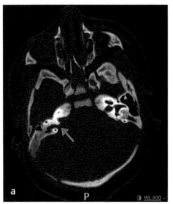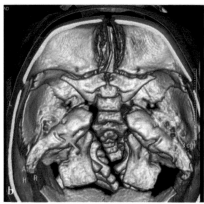

Fig. 2.6 Axial computed tomography **(a)** and 3D reconstruction images **(b)** demonstrating the wide neonate petromastoid canal (*blue arrows*).

evident medially. While at birth the superior semicircular canal seems prominent into the middle fossa and the petromastoid canal (PMC) passing between its two limbs is wide[9] (►Fig. 2.6), with time the mastoid grows and usually fills the space so that only a narrow PMC remains and the subarcuate eminence seems flatter. The spine of Henle does not exist at birth. The curvature of the second genu of the facial nerve is less pronounced in the newborn as the nerve passes 2 mm away from the floor of the antrum and 4 mm from the superior posterior angle of the tympanic ring at a depth of 5 to 6 mm (►Fig. 2.7). The course of the facial nerve becomes shallower and reaches 2 mm depth before the stylomastoid foramen. The foramen is located at the outer surface of the bone at a horizontal line tangential to the lower rim of the tympanic EAC about 4 mm from its posterior border (►Fig. 2.8). At that level, the facial nerve, which is hidden by the anterior part of the posterior belly of the digastric muscle, sharply turns forward.[3,10]

2.13 Highlights

- Several differences exist between adults and children with regard to skull base morphology, which may influence treatment decision-making, presurgical planning, and the choice of surgical approach.
- Unique anatomic considerations in children include smaller craniofacial complex, cranial fossa and paranasal sinuses, stage of tooth eruption, absence of anatomic landmarks such as the superior orbital fissure and mastoid pneumatization, and the fragility of neurovascular elements.
- Another important anatomic consideration is the developmental stage of the paranasal sinuses, which develop in a complex and extremely variable process.

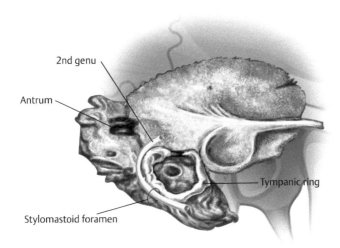

Fig. 2.7 The temporal bone of the neonate.

2nd genu

Antrum

Tympanic ring

Stylomastoid foramen

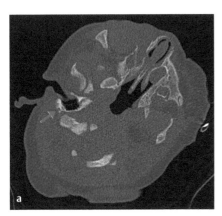

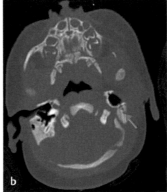

Fig. 2.8 (a, b) Axial computed tomography (CT) scans demonstrating a superficial stylomastoid foramen (*blue arrows*) located 4 mm posterior to the EAC meatus.

References

[1] Brockmeyer D, Gruber DP, Haller J, Shelton C, Walker ML. Pediatric skull base surgery. 2. Experience and outcomes in 55 patients. Pediatr Neurosurg 2003;38(1):9–15

[2] Gil Z, Constantini S, Spektor S, et al. Skull base approaches in the pediatric population. Head Neck 2005;27(8):682–689

[3] Bobin S. Particularités anatomiques et physiologiques de l'enfant. In: Garabédian EN, Bobin S, Monteil JP, Triglia JM, eds. ORL L'enfant. 2nd ed. Paris: Flammarion Médecine-Sciences 2006: 3–5

[4] Gruber DP, Brockmeyer D. Pediatric skull base surgery. 1. Embryology and developmental anatomy. Pediatr Neurosurg 2003;38(1):2–8

[5] Marianowski R, Triglia J-M. Particularités anatomiques et physiologiques des fosses nasales de l'enfant. In: Garabédian EN, Bobin S, Monteil JP, Triglia JM, eds. ORL L'enfant. 3rd ed. Paris: Flammarion Médecine-Sciences. 2006: 99–101

[6] Lacout A, Marsot-Dupuch K, Smoker WRK, Lasjaunias P. Foramen tympanicum, or foramen of Huschke: pathologic cases and anatomic CT study. AJNR Am J Neuroradiol 2005;26(6):1317–1323

[7] Wright CG. Development of the human external ear. J Am Acad Audiol 1997;8(6):379–382

[8] Anson BJ, Bast TH, Richany SF. The fetal and early postnatal development of the tympanic ring and related structures in man. Ann Otol Rhinol Laryngol 1955;64(3):802–823

[9] Koral K, Vachha B, Gimi B, et al. MRI of the petromastoid canal in children. J Magn Reson Imaging 2014;39(4):966–971

[10] Beauvillain C, Simon C, Wesoluch M, Legent F. Facial nerve anatomy in neonates. Second and third parts: surgical applications Ann Otolaryngol Chir Cervicofac 1982;99(6):223–230 http://www.ncbi.nlm.nih.gov/pubmed/7125478

3 Special Considerations in Pediatric Anesthesia and Pain Control

Uri Amit, Ron Flaishon, Avi A. Weinbroum

Summary

The provision of anesthesia to children requires unique considerations. The limited airway anatomy, their exceptional reaction to pathology or instruments and therefore possible functional incompetence may be even dangerous during ear, nose and throat interventions. While the anesthetist is physically close to the child at all times during surgery, this "protective proximity" no longer exists after the intervention is complete, although threats to the child's breathing capabilities continue during the postoperative period. These factors influence modes of anesthesia and the drugs to be used.

Postoperative pain therapy is an essential part of the perioperative care in patients of all ages, and more so in a sick or traumatized child. Appropriate pain control ultimately determines whether or not the outcome will be favorable (complete recovery vs. morbidity and vs. mortality), as well as length of hospital stay, and costs. Otolaryngologic surgery inevitably poses special challenges to the young patient's ability to cope with upper airway restrictions if inadequate types or doses of analgesics, especially opioids, are used. This also holds true preoperatively, in cases of trauma or selected endocrinologic conditions. Pain assessment in children is thus as essential as it is in adults. However, while verbal and written self-assessments are applicable for grown-ups, pictograms provide a feasible protocol for children starting at 3 years of age. Additional recommended scores have been found reliable pain assessment in younger children, with the aim of replacing or refining the judgment of others regarding the child's pain status.

This chapter will discuss various aspects of anesthesia and perioperative care in the pediatric population. It will discuss pain expression at various ages, and appropriate drugs and their protocols, adverse events that must be identified and prevented, and modes of age-specified pain assessments.

Keywords: Pediatric, ENT, ORL, anesthesia, pain, assessment, airways, control, opioids

3.1 Introduction

Children at any age are subject to otolaryngological (ORL) interventions, which are the most common surgeries in this cohort. ENT (ear, nose, and throat) interventions involving the airways may pose life-threatening episodes. These are especially critical because pediatric airways compared to adult airways are smaller and much less robust to resist sudden obstruction. Furthermore, airways of smaller children will react more intensely, and abrupt vagal response may ensue. At the time of the scheduled operation, children frequently suffer from accompanying illnesses such as upper respiratory tract infection (URTI), obstructive sleep apnea (OSA), rhinitis, and various viral infections. These illnesses lead to increased anesthesia risks because of the intensity of their response to anesthetics or surgical stimuli. Pain irritates the respiratory system as well, via its neuro-hormonal and immunological components; the choice of pain management following specific procedures, e.g., tonsillectomy, may be limited. Thus, whenever discussing pediatric ENT anesthesia and perioperative pain control, airway protection is a concern to the anesthetist who needs to walk the child through a safe perioperative process with as little discomfort and pain as possible.

3.2 Perioperative Considerations

3.2.1 Airway Risks versus Safety

ENT interventions are of different types and complexities; even if not emergent ones, they are seldom done in a healthy child. The most frequent operations between the age of 2 and 5 years are auricular paracentesis and adeno- and/or tonsillectomy.1 Other interventions may include insertion of ventilation tubes, conchotomy, otopexy, tympanoplasty, myringoplasty, and functional endoscopic sinus surgery (FESS). As a rule, surgery that comprises large areas of the face or oral cavity may pose significant risk to the patient's airways. Oral or facial SOL removal, or trauma, is considered a major surgery in adults as well. These interventions require special attention, including pre-incisional team case-debate, especially in pediatric patients.

The different types of interventions are out of the scope of this chapter; the cardinal anesthesia aspects that are relevant to pediatric ENT procedures are:
- Emergency vs. scheduled intervention.
- Extensive vs. limited area of intervention.
- Surgery that involves or not the child's airways.
- Previous airways status, e.g., chronic URTI, asthma, whizzing, or external treatment (irradiation).

These outlooks will be briefly highlighted as the discussion proceeds.

Airway control is a top priority in the child. From the anesthesia point of view, the following circumstances are valid as *absolute contraindications* for *ambulatory* otorhinolaryngology (ORL) operations:[2–5]
- Chronic comorbidity with unstable course.
- Disease with need of prolonged monitoring.
- Increased risk of postoperative bleeding.

3.2.2 Detriments in the ENT Pediatric Population

Common causes are the URTI that are viral infections (e.g., rhino-, corona-, influenza, etc.). The invasion of the virus into the epithelium and the mucous membrane of the respiratory system leads to an inflammatory response, followed by edema, excessive secretions, containing tachykinins and neuropeptides, and bronchial (smooth muscle) constriction ("bronchial hyper-reactivity"). There is characteristic hyper-reactive response of the respiratory tract to endotracheal tube (ETT) insertion and to volatile anesthetics, e.g., desflurane.[6] At the same time, a major advantage of desflurane over other inhalational agents is that its blood-gas partition coefficient (0.42) is lower than the others', predicting rapid induction and recovery from desflurane-based general anesthesia (GA). However, due to the above-mentioned airway irritation, possibly leading to breath holding, coughing, excessive secretions, and laryngospasm,[7] its use in such subpopulation is not recommended.

The "airway susceptibility" is characterized by productive cough, purulent secretion from the nose, shortness of breath, and fever, all causing perioperative respiratory adverse events (AEs),[8] lasting >6 weeks. Neither blood count nor acute phase parameters, such as C-reactive protein (CrP) or procalcitonin (PCT), are of value in predicting the outcome of an infection or perioperative complication risk.[2,9]

There are potential characteristic risks for respiratory AEs:
- Patient influences:
  - Age: Younger kids are more susceptible than older ones; history of premature birth is an additional factor.
  - Associated respiratory illnesses: URTI ≤2 weeks, recurrent wheezing, current/past asthma, nocturnal dry cough, wheezing during exercise, hay fever, current/past eczema, family history of asthma, and passive/active smoker are all deteriorating issues.
  - Other Bronchopulmonary diseases: Bronchopulmonary dysplasia (BPD), cystic fibrosis.
  - Diverse pathologies: Previous history of apnea, OSA, obesity, syndromes associated with airway obstruction (e.g., Down syndrome), anemia (hematocrit <30%), unfasted patient.
- Surgical factors: Shared airway procedures (e.g., ENT + dental + upper airways); blood or secretions present or expected in upper airways; sudden surgical stimulation; emergency procedure.
- *Anesthesia-related factors*: Premedication with benzodiazepines (BZD) (e.g., midazolam); topical airway use of lidocaine; inhalational induction of anesthesia; invasive airway management (ETT > laryngeal mask airway [LMA] > facemask); less experienced anesthetist with airway management; insufficient supervision ratio for trainees (e.g., supervisor absence during critical periods of anesthesia); desflurane administration; high-dose opioid administration; administration of neuromuscular blocking agents; low nurse-to-patient ratio in the recovery area (<1:1); mixed anesthetic clinical practice (adult/pediatric > solely pediatric). All these are to be considered perioperatively by the anesthetist.[10]

3.3 Perioperative Anesthesia Considerations in the ENT Child

The following few safety key points in the ENT pediatric population are worth memorizing:
- In the spontaneously breathing child, if respiration is not disabling/dangerous, it is best to secure ventilation and oxygenation until the anesthetist takes over.
- Avoid excessive BZDs and opioids pre- and postoperatively so that respiration and cooperation are reduced.
- Always titter analgesia; always monitor drugs' effects.

ENT perioperative anesthetic and pain considerations in the pediatric cohort will be discussed for the following three specific periods:
1. Preoperative evaluation and preparation for anesthesia.
2. Intraoperative anesthesia/analgesia regimens.
3. Postoperative patient-tailored adequate pain treatment and prevention of AEs.

The reader is referred to a detailed review regarding perioperative anesthesia considerations.[11] In their Clinical Practice Guidelines for Pediatric Tonsillectomy of the French Society of ENT and Head and Neck Surgery (SFORL 2009), the authors highlight aspects that reflect outcome, starting with the appropriate indications for tonsillectomy, and the eventuality of OSA, all during the preoperative assessment. The surgical techniques to be used are important, as well as the intervention being performed in an in- or out-patient facility, modes of postoperative follow-up, and how to manage complications.

3.3.1 Preoperative Evaluation and Preparation for Anesthesia

Any patient requiring anesthesia is subject to physician-patient interview, physical examination, auxiliary testing if necessary, and explanatory discussion, all taking place before obtaining the patient's consent. All preoperative phases of preparation of the child involve parents' or guardian's participation. Indeed, the intimate relationship between the two affects the overall acceptance of the unfamiliar and frightening environment and refusal expressible by the child. Thus, psychological (= non-pharmacological) and pharmacological approaches are essential for the smooth transition of the child from his known, secure, and loving surrounding into an unfamiliar environment that may upset the child.

Standardized Provision of Detailed History

This is the most important screening instrument used to prepare patients for anesthesia.[12] Earlier reports have offered various standardized questionnaires; they are helpful, sometimes even essential. Besides providing information regarding organ dysfunction, allergies, passive smoking, previous exposure to anesthetics, and their eventual consequences, parents need to also provide relevant behavioral and medical information about the child.[12]

Important issues relevant to the operated child are *obesity* and *metabolic syndrome*, which represent problematic current public health issues worldwide. In a recent National Health and Nutrition survey, it was suggested that 17% of the children and adolescents in the United States are obese and overweight,[13–15] compared to ~20% of the European obese and overweight children.[16,17] The WHO defines pediatric overweight and obesity according to standard deviations (BMI Z-scores) from the mean adult BMI values, whereas the United States defines BMI ≥85th percentile as overweight and BMI ≥95th percentile as obesity.[18] Pediatric obesity is a special challenge to the anesthetist mainly due to respiratory, pharmacological, and metabolic changes.[19,20]

Physical Examination

This should focus on signs and symptoms that may be relevant to anesthesia, above all the *respiratory* and *cardiac systems,* with emphasis on auscultation. Since ENT surgery may involve the upper respiratory system, particular attention should be paid to its examination. The anatomy of the face and the skull should also be considered. It is important to allow the child to have a break when possible, in-between examinations, which would minimize confounding information and excessive agitation. It is highly advisable to conduct the exam while the primary caregiver stays next to the child. Early team sessions, and meetings with the guardian who delivers informative and behavioral experiences, are essential.[21–23]

History of Bronchial Asthma and URTI

Asthma is the most common condition in childhood that warrants particular attention, and therefore meticulous questioning and auscultation. Preoperative X-ray of the lung is not diagnostic in children with asthma.[24] Existing algorithms help in individual decision when an intervention should be postponed in a child with URTI/asthma, and for how long.[6,8,25] Briefly, in the presence of watery or purulent congestion, and where airways are not involved during surgery conducted by an expert or ETT is not part of the surgical plan, one may proceed. If fever or malaise or purulent congestion is detected, that is where risks overweigh benefits, surgery should be postponed for

10 to 14 days and the child then re-examined. Recent (<30 days) asthmatic breakthrough and pulse therapy need to be analyzed individually; airway functioning and breathing conditions must be thoughtfully evaluated before a decision is made. This is because non-emergency pediatric interventions, especially ENT ones, are dangerous, possibly lethal, if performed during periods of airway irritation. Systemic steroid pretreatment for asthmatic patients, especially those treated with systemic steroid within previous 6 months, was suggested upon intervening for nasal polyp, otolaryngological and oral surgery.[26] These children should not be operated under ambulatory conditions.

Obstructive Sleep Apnea (OSA)

The obese child is another concern for the anesthetist.[27] Adenotonsillectomy (ATE) is one of the most frequent surgical interventions in children with OSA.[28] This combination of illnesses still lacks guidelines and recommendations of care.[29] The risk for postoperative hypoxia[30] and the known increased sensitivity to μ-receptor-agonist opioids[31] are to be judiciously considered in all children, especially in those suffering from URTI, OSA, or obesity. In a pilot study aiming at identifying perioperative risk factors for respiratory complications in children with ATE with heavy OSA, the presence of only 1 out of 4 risk factors led to an increase in ~35% of complication rates vs. children without any risk. They require strict follow-up and preoperative preparations if factors are known by history.[32] The above-mentioned 4 risk factors are:

- Age < 2 years.
- Intraoperative laryngospasm or other airway reactions.
- Postoperative occurrences of SpO_2 <90%.
- Apnea-hypopnea index (AHI) >24.

Interval between Vaccination and Intervention

There are currently no evidence-based recommendations regarding such intervals.[33] Common clinical attitude recommends 5- to 7-day interval.

Blood Sampling

Blood sampling induces considerable stress in the child; it should be carried out only when necessary.[34] Indeed, a systematic review found that routine laboratory examinations deliver no additional information after a conscientiously carried out history or clinical examination that showed no pathologies which would influence the anesthetist's decision-making.[34] Nevertheless, preoperative evaluation of the hemostatic and coagulation system is crucial in ORL patients, in order to minimize the risk of postoperative bleeding. The most common coagulation pathology in childhood is the autosomal dominant inherited von Willebrand syndrome;[35,36] specific consultation is warranted. Finally, for those with known or newly onset cardiac disease, the anesthetist should consult a pediatric cardiologist before final decisions regarding surgery and anesthesia are taken.[12]

3.3.2 Trauma Patients

Trauma to facial soft tissue or bones, infection, or SOL involving facial muscles or oral cavity frequently limits the opening of the mouth, and may obstruct air passage through the glottis, mainly due to inflammation, edema, and hemorrhage, and may induce trismus of the masseter muscles (tonic contraction of the muscles of mastication, "lock-jaw"). Myofascial pain syndrome (previously known as myofascial pain and dysfunction syndrome [MFPDS]) may follow spasm of the masticatory muscles (medial, internal and lateral, or external pterygoids, temporalis, and masseter). Such pain may also intensify trismus. The limitation in opening the mouth is a "warning sign" to any sort of deep uncontrolled sedation—not analgesia, which, if adequately administered, rather moderates these pain-potentiated phenomena. The current practice to rely on the Mallampati score is better played down in such cases because unexpected airway obstruction may hide beyond an incomplete oropharyngeal opening.

Upon attending those admitted to the emergency department (ED), a quick, safe, multi-task, and integrating approach would enable appropriate analgesia and diagnostic procedures before further decision is made. Under these circumstances, maintenance of spontaneous breathing is the rule of thumb during any analgesic treatment. The best mode of sedating and reducing pain is the use of a safe pharmacological approach that would comfort the child, and minimize refusal, like during the placement of an IV line (if not placed by pre-hospital staff). In case the child does not allow it because of fear or anxiety, or is uncooperative for any reason, it should be corrected immediately, except when those are signs of hypoxia. LA paste (e.g., Emla cream, a lidocaine and prilocaine topical compound) is worth applying to the back of the hand/foot, so that a few minutes later a vein can be painlessly accessed. This would allow not only injecting measured doses of medications, but also administering fluids if necessary. It is recommended not to use large doses of BZDs or opioids IV in face/oral traumatized or burnt children, especially those who require ED observation or transfer to the imaging department. As mentioned below, rectal (PR), sublingual, or intranasal (IN) administration of drugs (e.g., ketamine) is worth using in the absence of an IV line.[37] Drug titration that aims at reaching a low grade of sedation—where the child is calm, painless, and arousable—is best, provided oxygen is supplemented, SpO_2 is monitored, and an anesthetist/pediatrician monitors the patient all the way from the time the sedative is administered to the induction of anesthesia or panned awakening. An airway device and a laryngoscope must be placed next to any sedated ENT patient.

Oncological Interventions: Anesthesia Considerations

Tumor of the superior chest, the thymus, or surrounding lymph nodes can easily compress the superior vena cava, causing venous stasis. Signs of superior vena cava syndrome (SVCS), including swelling and cyanosis of the upper body, and symptoms of the superior mediastinal syndrome (SMS), associated with cardiopulmonary stress or dyspnea and cough, dysphagia, orthopnea, and hoarseness, although none are of acute severity, may worsen respiration following sedation or analgesics administration. Tracheostomy may be necessary—and therefore tools should be ready for use—if optimal ventilation or oxygenation require assisted ventilation obtainable via ETT or LMA.

The presence of a tumor in the oral cavity or near the airways, or a history of past or recent radiation therapy to the head, face, or neck, is risky to the patient's life.[38] Effects of past head or neck irradiation include fibrosis and stiffness of soft tissues, which can lead to limited mouth opening, neck extension, or oropharyngeal manipulation. Such chronic (or recent) changes also may include airway mucosal fibrosis, chronic subglottic edema, supra- and subglottic narrowing, or stenosis, growth retardation of cartilaginous structures of the larynx or hypoplasia of the jaw in children of any age, xerostomia, and chondronecrosis of the epiglottis, the arytenoids, and the trachea.[39–41] These medical records require full attention of the teams; imaging of the areas is an essential source of information and provision of safety data, so that the anesthetist may not be surprised and the child endangered upon inducing GA.

Since radiation habitually alters neck anatomy, thus affecting airway management, Delbridge et al[41] reported that smaller ETTs than those predicted (by age and weight) were required in adults whose neck had been irradiated in infancy, due to significant tracheal stenosis. Giraud et al[42] reported of the use of LMAs in adults who had earlier received oral or cervical radiotherapy. The authors found a high rate of restricted mouth opening as well, difficulty with LMA insertion, and laryngeal collapse, making ventilation with an LMA difficult or even impossible. Specific complications in children, however, have not been reported, probably because such outcomes after irradiation require time to develop. Nevertheless, when caring for a child who has undergone radiotherapy to the neck, similar potential airway difficulties must be kept in mind during preoperative examination and upon inducing anesthesia to the patient. Psychological preparation of the child and the guardian (see below) enables focusing on the consequences and their correlates in this subpopulation.

High-dose chemotherapy and total body irradiation (TBI), as for hematopoietic stem cell transplantation (HSCT), may cause mucositis of sufficient severity to jeopardize airways' patency, because of pseudomembrane formation, supraglottic edema, bleeding, and aspiration of blood and secretions, all contributing to malfunctioning airway reflexes.[43,44] When discussing how to manage the airways,[44] besides the need to have their clear picture, one needs to avoid airway trauma and maintain the oral mucosa constantly wet.[38] Even when mucositis is not severe, radiation therapy, glucocorticoids, chemotherapy, and chronic graft versus host disease (CGVHD) that are often combined can provoke airway mucosa damage because of its friability. All these need to be reported and evidenced preoperatively, much before instrumenting the airways. The oral cavity and dental areas should be handled in a precautious and highly attentive manner.[45] The original lesions and those following instrumentation generate soaring pain that needs attention preoperatively. Patients should be kept in hospital for a judicious postoperative surveillance.

Endocrine and Neuroendocrine Tumors

These tumors include thyroid tumors (30%, adenomas and carcinomas) and pituitary tumors (20%, craniopharyngiomas and pituitary adenomas). Carcinoma of the thyroid usually presents with a single thyroid nodule.[46] Craniopharyngiomas, which are the most common pituitary tumor, frequently cause headaches, visual disturbances, and pan-hypopituitarism, including diabetes insipidus.[47] The former may affect free approach to the airways; they need to be evidenced by X-ray of CT, whereby description of airways format and exact width of the trachea need to be obtained preoperatively.

The use of corticosteroids is discussed next.

Preoperative Decision-Making

As occurring in adults, surgery may accompany decisional conflicts among the medical staff, parenteral uncertainty, and the fear from negative consequences, so that emotional distress and delays in decision-making at any step of the course may come up.[48] Interestingly, a decisional regret may reflect earlier postoperative complications.[49,50] Shared decision-making is thus recommended to improve quality of care and satisfaction, as well as patient's or parent's anxiety, decreasing the health care system costs as well.[48–52]

It is therefore relevant that while patients and caregivers should provide medical history and health details minutely, they should also be provided with all information and instructions regarding the nature of the procedure, benefits, risks, and expected postoperative course of the intervention. Discussion of anesthesia details, including tracheostomy, when applicable, involves perioperative emotional support that should be provided to patients and families; a preoperative meeting with a communication and/or feeding specialist for post-interventional rehabilitation may then be necessary as well.[53,54]

Fasting Regulations

Guidelines for preoperative fasting times before elective interventions are currently well defined:[12,55–57] 6 h for food, 4 h for milk/breast milk/formula diet, and 2 h or less for clear liquids (water, tea, clear juices, lemonade). The latter option (≤2 h) positively affects the child both physically and psychologically.

Non-Pharmacological Preoperative Preparation

Periprocedural psychological evaluation is essential in the pediatric population. When supporting their children perioperatively,[58] parents sense helplessness and are anxious; these are transmitted to their children (of any age).[59] Parents' coaching and application of emotional pre-interventional preparation are therefore of positive potential benefits.[60]

Specific methodologies, inducing psychological embracement, that aim at reducing mothers' and children's built-up fear are beyond the scope of this discussion. It is, however, essential to point out that these are to be addressed before surgery, thus avoiding untrue promises to the child or parents.[53,54]

Pre-interventional preparation of the mature, and even the less mature, child, by visual description of the interventional steps decreases the stress and anxiety associated with the procedure. This should be performed in a quiet environment, with the availability of cognitive-behavioral interventions among participants. If the child is hospitalized, the meeting should be held away from the child's room.[61] Explanations and illustrations of postoperative pain and the ways to control it are an essential component in this gathering.

Based on the case, every anesthesia team must decide for itself regarding whether anesthesia should be induced in the presence of the parents or not. While no clear clinical advantage has been evidenced using this approach,[62,63] the Modified Yale Preoperative Anxiety Scale has shown that children who were allowed to be accompanied also by a clown showed significantly lower anxiety scores.[64] These opportunities should be discussed with the child preoperatively.

Preoperative Pharmacological Preparation

Preoperative pharmacological approaches aim at coadjuvating the mother-child tranquility, thus strengthening the child's confidence and acceptance of the sites of intervention (emergency medicine, operating room [OR], day-care area, or out of the OR suite). It has been proven that a calm child is accompanied by a calm parent, the latter reflecting on the former's behavior and vice versa. While explanations, discussions, and assurances can generate calm and cooperation, and a grown-up child can also benefit from them, pharmacological aid will optimize the child's serenity. The pharmacological approach consists of various sedatives administered ahead of the time of the intervention, titrated to the desired stage of tranquility while communication is preserved and vital functions remain unaffected. Importantly, if preoperative pain is present and is scored high by the child, its control is an integral part of reduction in tension and hindrance. Noteworthy is the fact that combining drugs of various neuropharmacological activities may potentiate each other; this may be undesired, and the child's surveillance is necessary while cautiously augmenting the doses.[65]

It has been stated that more than 3 weeks of exogenous corticosteroid therapy (>20 mg/d prednisone or equivalent) can produce measurable suppression and inability to self-generate stress response for up to 1 year.[66] Although the need for, and benefit of, intraoperative "stress dose" corticosteroid therapy has been questioned,[66–70] preoperatively obtaining the history of dosage, duration, and last use of exogenous corticosteroids is warranted. With this information, the anesthetist can better decide whether a stress dose of steroids will be necessary.[66]

Variable lengths of glucocorticoid-induced adrenal suppression have been reported in the pediatric oncology literature as well,[71–77] ranging from 2 to 8 months. Such a variance may reflect varying glucocorticoid protocols, doses, and tapering protocols. In a study of 24 children who were treated with prednisolone, persistent adrenal suppression was measured in 46% of the cohort at 2 weeks, and 13% of children 20 weeks after cessation of prednisolone.[75] The stress response being unpredictable, steroid coverage need to be provided during stressful conditions 1 to 2 months after cessation of glucocorticoids.[71] The usual replacement regimen is 1 to 2 mg/kg of hydrocortisone (Solu-Cortef) or of dexamethasone (0.05–0.1 mg/kg) IV.[78] Preoperative multidisciplinary consultation should therefore be held to decide perioperative use of corticosteroids.[61]

Premedication

Various drugs were found efficacious in lessening children's anxiety in the pre-procedural period. Best sedative status is attained after IV/PR/IN/intraoral bolus administration of certain drugs: the effect is achieved almost immediately, where the degree of needs vs. effects and the duration of action are timely pre-determined. Unlike past use of oral drugs (e.g., chloral hydrate, diazepam), whose clinical sedative effects were long and unpredictable, current protocols provide pharmacological certainty as well as patient's safety. Following are few examples.

Midazolam

This is a short-acting anxiolytic, which can be administered either IV/IM, orally, rectally, or intranasally.[79,80]

Nevertheless, midazolam has recently been challenged due to both the amnesic and undesirable cognitive postoperative effects it may induce,[81] and increased risk of post-sevoflurane agitation (when combined).[82,83] The use of the drug remains at the anesthetist's discretion.

Alfa$_2$ Agonists

Clonidine is rather a viable alternative:[84] it produces better early postoperative pain relief (especially when combined with other analgesics), and reduces shivering and postoperative confusion and agitation compared to midazolam.[85] Furthermore, similarly to its handling in adults, IV BZDs (mostly midazolam) are currently rarely used preoperatively, rather intraoperatively.

When pre-ENT procedure MRI is required, although the procedure is not painful but lasts relatively long, and there is need for a calm and immobile patient within a tunnel-like apparatus, and where noise may annoy or frighten the child, some sedation is warranted. Parents are rarely permitted to stay aside the bed during the entire examination. The efficacious use (infusion) of dexmedetomidine, an alfa$_2$ agonist, has been reported to cause no delay in discharging the child home. Besides within-the-normal-range slight changes in blood pressure (BP) and heart rate (HR) induced by the drug, no other untoward effects were noted, particularly those related to respiration and maintenance of patent airways.[86–89] It also provides an opioid-sparing effect and lowers emergence delirium compared to other drug combinations.[90] Comparatively, CT imaging is currently an ultra-short procedure so that children can be left alone for a very brief period and may need no sedation, unless uncooperative. Finally, the unwanted effects of dexmedetomidine may include initial hypertension, hypotension, and rare nausea, bradycardia, atrial fibrillation, and hypoxia, all occurring mostly during or shortly after the drug's loading dose and depending on its rate of infusion.[91] Such overdose may also cause first- or second-degree atrioventricular block (AVB). Nevertheless, it was reported at a dose 60-time higher than the prescribed dose that was infused to a small child (<6 month) for 1 h during imaging. No hypotension, hypertension, and changes in HR or in respiration/oxygenation were noted. Safe discharge was delayed by 2 h after discontinuation of the infusion.[92] Dexmedetomidine exhibits linear kinetics when infused in dose ranges of 0.2 to 0.7 µg/kg/h for <24 h (as approved by the FDA). For pharmacokinetics and dynamics of the drug see;[93] doses are specified in ▶ Table 3.1.

Ketamine

Either alone or not, this drug has been proven to produce efficacious sedation and analgesia, to a better grade than fentanyl, when given IN in the ED, or when added to LA or deposited intraorally.[94,95] This is besides the common pharmacological routes (IV, IM, PR). From the safety standpoint, ketamine is superior to any opioid for ENT children reaching for help in the ED or in pre-hospital area, mainly because it is devoid of respiratory depression or hemodynamic instability. Intraoral ketamine was indeed found to induce prolonged sedo-analgesic effect when given as a mouthwash liquid.[94] When mixed with LA, it provided better analgesic results than when each drug was used alone.[96,97] The dose ranges of ketamine are specified in ▶Table 3.1.[37]

Table 3.1 Recommended drugs and doses for children at ages from 6 months to 13 years

Drugs Numbers indicate different protocols	Dosage PO ALL are of IR form	Dosage IV * = Regimens used in OR, NICU, PICU	Remarks	Special considerations or precautions
Morphine 1) 2) 3)	0.3 mg/kg Q3–4h[231] 0.2–0.5mg/kg/dose Q4h PRN[232]	0.1 mg/kg Q3–4h[231] *Initial dose: 10–20 µg/kg/h[232] Max: 150 µg/kg/h 0.05–0.1 mg/kg/dose Q2–4h PRN	• PO potency = ⅓ of the IVs • Various regimens not covered here (ED, IT, PCA)	• CNS and respiratory depression is dose-limiting factor • Dose adjustment required in renal impairment
Hydromorphone 1) 2)	0.06 mg/kg Q3–4h[231] 0.03–0.08 mg/kg/dose Q4h PRN[232]	0.015 mg/kg Q3–4h[231] 0.015 mg/kg/dose Q4h PRN[232]	Drug 4–6 times more potent than MO	• WHO guidelines suggest PO dosage 0.06–0.2 mg/kg[21]
Fentanyl 1) 2)	NA	*Initial dose: 1–2 µg/kg/h[232] Max: 10 µg/kg/h 0.5–1 µg/kg/dose Q1–2h PRN Continuous infusion: 1–5 µg/kg/h: titrate slowly to effect[233] Bolus: 1–2 µg/kg/dose Q2–4h PRN	100 times more potent than MO	• Potential addiction • Withdrawal may cause agitation and hyperalgesia • Slow IV administration to avoid chest wall rigidity
Oxycodone 1) 2)	0.2 mg/kg Q34h[231] 0.05–0.15 mg/kg/dose Q4h PRN or as scheduled[232] Max: 10 mg/dose	NA	• 1.5 times more potent than MO • Slow release form available for BID use	High addictive potential
Methadone 1) 2)	0.1 mg/kg Q8–12h 0.2 mg/kg Q12h[231]	0.05–0.1 mg/kg Q8–12h *0.1 mg/kg Q6–8h[231]	Rarely induces euphoria; long-lasting effect[21]	Variable pharmacokinetics; half-life long; needs to be titrated Note possible use: 0.1 mg/kg/dose IV/PO Q6h[232]
Levorphanol	0.04 mg/kg Q6–8h[231]	0.02 mg/kg Q6–8h[231]	Eight times more potent than MO and longer half-life	
Naloxone	NA	For *respiratory depression*[232]: Start by titration (1–2 µg/kg) 0.001–0.01 mg/kg/dose (1–10 µg/kg/dose), repeatable Q2–3min Max: 0.4 mg/dose Rapid, full reversal of *Narcotic OD*: 0.1 mg/kg/dose IV, repeatable Q2–3min PRN Max: 2 mg/dose	• For opioid AEs reversal • Reversal of PCA-induced pruritus: 0.25–2 µg/kg/h IV infusion[233]	May cause severe pain, distress, agitation, which limits dosage

(continued)

Table 2.1 (*continued*) Recommended drugs and doses for children at ages from 6 months to 13 years

Drugs Numbers indicate different protocols	Dosage PO ALL are of IR form	Dosage IV * = Regimens used in OR, NICU, PICU	Remarks	Special considerations or precautions
Flumazenil		0.01 mg/kg/dose[233] Max: 0.2 mg/dose; repeatable Q1min Max total dose: 1 mg	Lasting effect: <1 h[233]	• BZD OD reversal • Contraindicated in patients with history of seizures
Paracetamol 1) 2)	10–15 mg/kg/dose Q4–6h PRN[232]	10–15 mg/kg 10 mg/kg/dose Q6h PRN[233]	PR: 15–20 mg/kg Q6h PR: 10–15 mg/kg/dose Q6–12h PRN[233]	• Hepatotoxicity dose-dependent • <50 mg/kg/d is safe
Ibuprofen 1) 2)	10 mg/kg Q8h[234] 10 mg/kg/dose Q6h as scheduled or PRN[232] Max: 800 mg/dose; 3200 mg/d	NA	• Taken on full stomach to prevent gastritis and bleeding • Hydration avoids AKI	
Metimazol (dipyrone)	Up to 20 mg/kg Q8h[234] Single dose of 500 mg	Up to 20 mg/kg Q8h in small infusion[234]	Not FDA approved (but used worldwide) d/t rare occurrences of agranulocytosis and bone marrow suppression	Intraoperative administration optimally affects handling of postoperative pain
Clonidine 1) 2) 3)	0.02 µg/kg up to TID[234] 1.5–5 µg/kg/dose Q8h[232] Titration mode[22]: Days 1–3: 0.002 mg/kg (max: 0.1 mg) qhs Days 4–6: 0.002 mg/kg, BID; Days 7–9: 0.002 mg/kg, TID Increase dose every 2–4 days by 0.002 mg/kg	*1–2 µg/kg by bolus *0.18–3.16 µg/kg/h 1 µg/kg/h with midazolam 50 µg/kg/h alone[235]	• Very slow bolus injection; better by slow infusion • Also used IN, IT, PR, ED, caudal or spinal block[235] • Intraoperative administration optimally aids handling of postoperative pain	• Lowers emergence delirium • May affect BP and HR • Increase dose Q2–4d by 0.002 mg/kg until the following[22]: 1. AEs noted (rarely) 2. Titratable rapidly if dose tolerated 3. Average dose in 1 study (for spasticity): 0.02 mg/kg/d 4. 0.002–0.004 mg/kg Q4h PRN for breakthrough pain if autonomic storm occurs (diagnosed by facial flushing, muscle stiffening, tremor, and hyperthermia)
Dexmedetomidine 1) 2) 3) 4)		*Bolus 0.7–1 µg/kg infused over 10 min *<1.5 µg/kg/h for >24 h is safe w/o hemodynamic changes upon discontinuation[236] Initial dose: 0.2–0.5 µg/kg/h if starting w/o bolus[232] If using loading dose: 1–2 µg/kg over 10 min, then 2 µg/kg/h Max: 2 µg/kg/h Infusion: 0.1 µg/kg/h[233] Max: 2 µg/kg/h Bolus: 1 µg/kg over 10 min Maintenance 0.6 µg/kg/h, titrate to effect (usually 0.2–1 µg/kg/h)[237]	0.2–0.7 µg/kg/h/<24 h is the FDA-approved dose (d/t linear kinetics) Change dose once >Q 30 min to prevent hypotension	• Possible changes in blood pressure and heart rate • Minimizes emergence delirium • Off-label usability for any sedation/interventional procedures; this use's safety and efficacy have not been verified

(*continued*)

Table 2.1 (*continued*) Recommended drugs and doses for children at ages from 6 months to 13 years

Drugs Numbers indicate different protocols	Dosage PO ALL are of IR form	Dosage IV * = Regimens used in OR, NICU, PICU	Remarks	Special considerations or precautions

Gabapentin
1)
 	
2)
	Days 1–3: 2 mg/kg;
	Max dose: 100 mg;
	TID[22]
	Days 4–6: 4 mg/kg, TID
	Increase Q2–4d by 5–6 mg/kg/d
	Max total dose: 50–72 mg/kg/d (2400–3600 mg/d)
	Day 1–3: 5 mg/kg/dose qhs
	Day 4–6: 2.5 mg/kg/dose AM and midday, and 5 mg/kg qhs
	Day 7–9: 2.5 mg/kg/dose AM and midday, and 10 mg/kg qhs;
	Day 10–12: 5 mg/kg/dose AM and midday, and 10 mg/kg qhs[230,238–241]
		NA	Slow titration minimizes AEs	Titration until the following:[22]
				1. Effective analgesia is reached (as low a dose as 30–45 mg/kg/d)
				2. Side effects ensue (nystagmus, sedation, tremor, ataxia, swelling)
				3. Max total dose is reached
				4. Children <5 years of age may require 30% higher mg/kg/d dosage (e.g., 45–60 mg/kg/d) than adults
				5. If pain symptoms appear (mostly in evening/night) administer half total daily dose qhs
				6. Titrate more rapidly for severe pain as long as tolerated; titrate gradually if sedation occurs
				7. Another protocol suggests dose increase Q4 days by 5 mg/kg/d until:[230,238–241]
				  a. effective analgesia has been reached;
				  b. side effects are tolerated;
				  c. a total dose of 75 mg/kg/d is reached (maximum of 3600 mg/d);
				  d. give half of the total daily dose as the evening dose;
				  e. titrate more rapidly for severe pain[242]

Pregabalin	Dose titration is essential[243] Days 1–3: 1 mg/kg (50 mg max)/night Days 4–6: 1 mg/kg BID[22] Increase dose/2–4 days up to 3 mg/kg/dose, BID or TID Max dose: 6 mg/kg	NA	Slow titration minimizes AEs	Possible AEs: sedation, dizziness, nausea, abdominal cramps, sweating
Dimenhydrinate	NA	0.5 mg/kg[163]		Antihistamine with an anticholinergic effect used for PONV
Ondansetron 1) 2)	0.1 mg/kg Max dose: 4 mg[162] 0.15 mg/kg/dose Q8h PRN[233] Max dose: 8 mg	0.1 mg/kg; Max dose: 4 mg[162] 0.15 mg/kg/dose Q8h PRN[233] Max dose: 8 mg	PO and IV equal dosing d/t optimal GI absorption although pharmacokinetics may vary	

(continued)

Table 2.1 (*continued*) Recommended drugs and doses for children at ages from 6 months to 13 years

Drugs Numbers indicate different protocols	Dosage PO ALL are of IR form	Dosage IV * = Regimens used in OR, NICU, PICU	Remarks	Special considerations or precautions
Dexamethasone	*Asthma*: 0.6 mg/kg/dose IV/PO twice 24–36 h apart[232] Max: 16 mg/dose *Croup*: single dose of 0.6 mg/kg/dose IV/PO	*PONV*: 0.15 mg/kg Max dose: 4 mg[162] *Extubation or Airway Edema*: 0.25–0.5 mg/kg/dose Q6h[232] Max dose: 8 mg/dose *Croup*: single dose of 0.6 mg/kg/dose IV/PO	Wide variety of dose regimens according to etiology	• Other steroids (hydrocortisone TID) can be used • For dose conversion see[232]
Ketamine 1) 2)	3–6 mg/kg/dose[244] 0.2–0.5 mg/kg/dose BID, TID Max:<50 mg/dose TID[245] *Intranasal* 5 mg/kg[246] *Topical* (skin, oral) alone/drug combination 1–10%[247,248]	*Initial dose: bolus 0.25 mg/kg, then 0.3–0.5 mg/kg/h[232] Max dose: 2 mg/kg/h Starting with infusion: 1–2 mg/kg/h, then 1–2 mg/kg/dose Q2h PRN[233] 2–4 mg/kg[232]*IM* for procedural sedation	Also available for intraoral, buccal, intranasal, rectal, topical and inhalational regimens[37]	• Rarely induces psychomimetic AEs • BZD and atropine rarely required • Intraoperative administration optimally affects handling of postoperative pain
Propofol 1) 2)	NA	*Bolus: 2–4 mg/kg, repeatable *Infusion: 50–200 µg/kg/min[232]	No analgesic effect	• Fast onset, short duration (<5 min) • High dose or fast infusion leads to Propofol Infusion Syndrome (PRIS)
Midazolam	0.25–0.5 mg/kg/dose[233] Max dose: 20 mg/dose	0.1 mg/kg/dose Q1h PRN[233] Max dose: 5 mg/dose	*Intranasal* 0.2–0.3 mg/kg/dose[233] Max: 10 mg/dose	Sedative, amnesic
Lignocaine 1) 2)	–	0.2 mg/kg *Resuscitation*: 1 mg/kg bolus IV/IO[232]	*LA dose*: <4 mg/kg; combined with adrenaline <7 mg/kg	Duration of action <2–4 h; don't repeat dose above max dosage
Marcaine	NA	NA	For *LA/RA* only Max dose: 2 mg/kg	Longer than lidocaine onset time and duration of action (>6 h)
Lactulose (66.7g%)[175,249] 1) Infants <1 years 2) Children (1–6 years) 3) Children/ toddlers (7–14 years)	Initial dose: Up to 5 mL Maintenance: Up to 5 mL Initial dose: 5–10 mL Maintenance: 5–10 mL Initial dose: 15 mL Maintenance: 10–15 mL	NA	• Used diluted or undiluted • Large amounts of fluid intake are necessary (1.5–2 L/d/70 kg)	Contraindications: • Hypersensitivity to the active substance/excipients • Galactosaemia • Bowel obstruction • Intolerants to lactose

Abbreviations: AEs, adverse events; AKI, acute kidney injury; BID, twice daily; BZD, benzodiazepines; d, day(s); ED, epidural/ly; qhs, at night sleep; h, hour/s/ly; ICU, intensive care unit; IN, intranasally; IO, intra osseous; IR, immediate release; IT, intrathecal/ly; IV, intravenous; kg, kilogram; LA, local anesthesia/anesthetic; mg, milligram; ml, milliliter; min, minute(s); NA, not applicable; NICU, neonatal ICU; OD, overdose; OR, operating room; PICU, pediatric ICU; PO, oral/ly; PR, rectal/ly; PRN, as needed; Q, every; RA = regional anesthesia/anesthetic.

3.3.3 Intraoperative Anesthesia and Analgesia Regimens

Emergency Interventions

Among the ENT emergency cases, several would present to the anesthetist already intubated or tracheotomized, and well sedated. The old but only accepted emergency mode of controlling the airways safely when oral cavity, glottis, or facial muscles are suspiciously involved in the trauma is the Rapid Sequence Induction (RSI). This procedure requires an open IV line in order to quickly induce deep hypnosis and muscle relaxation conjoint with the RSI. The patient should be awake—or slightly sedated—and breathing spontaneously up to the instant when the anesthetist and his aid take over the control of the airways, inserting an ETT. The choice of ETT or LMA for securing the airways depends on the case, the magnitude of the intervention, and the facial area involved. Recent data have shown the usability of LMAs in ENT cases:[98]

however, the choice about which device is safer for a specific case is left to the mutual decision of the anesthetist and the surgeon. Medium to high dose of ketamine may also induce deep anesthesia, still preserving airway patency and their reflexes, and allowing safe takeover of airway control. The opinion of the present authors is, however, that in either case, an early slow titration of fentanyl or morphine at low doses is favorable for reducing pain and anxiety, while maintaining the child calm but awake, breathing spontaneously, and cooperating with its surroundings. From the safety point of view, the use of an LMA can offer advantages over ETT in children with difficult airway susceptibility, avoiding the need for muscle relaxation, and allowing rapid and smooth removal of the device at the end of surgery.[99] The LMA thus provides some advantages over the ETT concerning comfort, complication prevention, and avoidance of postoperative airway problems.[100] Some authors argue that when operating "round the LMA,"[101] as in children with acute infection, the use of LMA can still be judiciously considered in selected cases.[6,8]

Induction of Anesthesia

Difficult airway cart is an essential tool in the OR where ENT intervention is to take place. The suggested content includes:[20]

- Rigid laryngoscope blades of different sizes and designs.
- Glide scope.
- Fiberoptic or video laryngoscope.
- Flexible fiberoptic kit.
- Tracheal tubes of various sizes/forms.
- Guides (light wands) and forceps.
- LMAs or ILMAs of various sizes for non-invasive and assist ventilation.
- Emergency surgical airway tools.
- EtCO$_2$ detector.

Intraoperative Drugs

General Anesthesia (GA) and IV Drugs

ENT interventions are rarely carried out under regional anesthesia (RA), especially in children. The main choice for maintenance of anesthesia is GA. The agents to be used during GA are at the discretion of the attending physician. The IV-based GA technique includes the classic opioids, muscle relaxants, or remifentanil and propofol infusions, using appropriate formulae of TCI (Target Controlled Infusion).[102] These protocols frequently require supplementations of multimodal drugs, or readjustments of the TCI dose formula. Ketamine is currently administered intraoperatively, starting with a pre-incisional bolus, and followed by an infusion until skin closure, or for up to 72 h postoperatively.[103] Remifentanil is optimal

for dose adjustment regimen, since it is used at as low a dose as the site concentration. Nevertheless, remifentanil may induce POH (Postoperative Hyperalgesia) and OIH (Opioid-Induced Hyperalgesia), which are highly upsetting, especially for a child waking-up into severe pain, which would influence the parent's emotional state as well. It is highly advisable to prevent such occurrence by adjuvating the drug and coadjuvating it with ketamine or pregabalin.[104] Intraoperative TCI-programmed infusion of propofol + remifentanil may be highly recommended in toddlers; this technique further enables inserting the reinforced or conventional LMA, favoring the spontaneous respiration technique,[105] or assist/control ventilation.

Ketamine

Perioperative systemic ketamine is optimal for many reasons. It has been proven effective in decreasing intraoperative opioid usage, postanesthesia care unit (PACU) pain intensity, and analgesic requirements, the latter throughout early (6–24 h) and late (1–3 months) periods after surgery.[106] Peritonsillar infiltration of ketamine at the end of tonsillectomy proved to decrease PACU and early (6–24 h) pain intensity, as well as analgesic requirements.[107] Ketamine IV, either alone (0.5 mg/kg) or with fentanyl (1 µg/kg), when administered in children undergoing tonsillectomy, improved postoperative pain control without delaying home discharge.[108] Systemic pre-incisional bolus of ketamine followed by an infusion until closure of the wound is of common practice.[106,109]

Dexmedetomidine

This drug is of value for both pre- and intraoperative use.[110] The latter was reported to be of equivalent effects to total postoperative rescue opioid (MO) requirements in pediatric patients undergoing tonsillectomy and adenoidectomy (at single intraoperative doses of dexmedetomidine 0.75 or 1 µg/kg vs. MO 50 or 100 µg/kg infused over 10 min after endotracheal intubation). Furthermore, the combination of dexmedetomidine 1 µg/kg and MO 100 µg/kg was further shown to increase the time to first postoperative analgesic need, and reduce the need for further analgesia doses, without increasing discharge times.[111]

Lidocaine

Data regarding the benefits of lidocaine and its regimens are reported all over this chapter.

ETT is frequently associated with elevation in blood pressure and pulse, cough reflexes, occasional dysrhythmias, increased intracranial pressure, and increased intraocular pressure. Preintubation IV lidocaine blunts most of these. There is no documentation of harmful effects of such prophylactic use if pharmacological dose is not exceeded.[112]

GA and Inhalational Agents

There is little evidence regarding which technique, inhalational or IV GA, is superior for the child.[113] Desflurane can act as an airway irritant and may stimulate airway smooth muscles via a tachykinin pathway (see above).[114,115] It was also found to enhance postoperative hyperalgesia.[116,117] Nevertheless, desflurane induces quicker GA because of its low blood-gas partition coefficient compared to other inhalation agents.[7] For these and other reasons TIVA is advantageous, particularly in the preschool children.[118] Other pros of TIVA use vs. inhalation agents are:

- Avoidance of volatile anesthetics = reduction in the risk for PONV and postoperative agitation.
- Application of propofol = antiemetic properties, preventive effect in children with airway susceptibility, no air contamination by airway leakage.
- Usability of opioids at very low doses, with or without ketamine.
- Availability of an IV access = security advantage during the critical periods of induction and emergence.

Recovery from Anesthesia

It is essential to discuss, though briefly, the end-surgery safety criteria in the pediatric population. ENT interventions would cause discomfort to the patient, especially if tubes are left, either to drain fluids from the site of surgery, to secure the airways, or allowing passage to the stomach. Children may fight these parts insistently. In addition, in cases of fractured face bones or lacerations that underwent adaptation, or were sutured, extubation should be handled judiciously: the patient must be fully awake, responding to commands, be free of secretion or bleeding, and breath to satisfaction. Only then the artificial airway can be removed, but the patient should remain attended by the anesthetist while still in the OR. When all parameters are stable, especially respiration and oxygenation, the child can be transferred to the PACU. A metal scissor should be next to the head of the patient in case the maxilla and mandible are closely attached to maintain optimal approximation. These highlight the importance of full and adequate preoperative explanation to the child and parent when emerging from surgery.

Overall, anesthesia recovery milestones in children must be adjusted for the child's age, developmental stage, medical status, surgical procedure, and social circumstances.[53] The more the staff gets to know the child and guardian preoperatively, the better the postoperative handling is.

Finally, the patient may recover from anesthesia, breath spontaneously, but still appear deeply sedated or unresponsive to voice or touch stimuli. While close medical surveillance is essential and airways secured, one may use appropriate antagonists: naloxone or flumazenil. These must be administered IV at small increasing doses, leaving enough time after each portion to detect the pharmacological effect. For doses see ▶ Table 3.1.[119-122]

Anesthesia and Emergence and Respiratory AEs

Serious anesthesia-related complications of tonsil and adenoid surgery occur rarely, but can be life threatening. The most common of these potentially serious complications are airway problems, e.g., laryngospasm, bronchospasm. In addition, oral endotracheal intubation and mouth gag placement may be detected postoperatively as injuries to oropharyngeal tissues, teeth, or to the temporomandibular joints.[38,123] These may be detrimental if not identified immediately upon awakening the child. LMA placement in patients who had been treated by radiation or chemotherapy may injure the oropharyngeal mucosa as well (see above). In a meta-analysis of 17 studies, the estimated incidence of respiratory complications following ATE was 9%; however, there was a wide variation in the types and severity of complications reported in the individual studies, so that direct relationship is unworkable.[124] The risk of respiratory compromise is however accepted to be the greatest among children with OSA.[125]

The post-tonsil and adenoid surgery respiratory mishaps are worth mentioning.[124,126-129] These may include:
- Common events:
  - Upper airway obstruction.
  - Laryngospasm.
  - Airway edema.
  - Central apnea/hypoventilation (including breath holding, as inhalational agents' effects, and narcotic-associated hypoventilation).
- Less common events:
  - Bronchospasm (more common in children with underlying history of asthma).
  - Negative pressure pulmonary edema (also termed "post-obstructive pulmonary edema").

Patient-related conditions that can easily lead to postoperative respiratory complications include the following:[124,126,130-135]
- OSA.
- Obesity.
- Age <3 years.
- Craniofacial abnormalities affecting the pharyngeal airway.
- Neurologic disorders (e.g., cerebral palsy).
- History of asthma.
- Recent upper respiratory infection.

Most respiratory complications occur in the immediate postoperative period and usually can be managed with simple interventions. These include:
- Immediate provision of supplemental oxygen.
- Suctioning.
- Repositioning of the patient.
- Positive pressure ventilation or intubation (rare).

Hill et al indicated the importance of intra- and postoperative factors that seem predictive of postoperative airway problems. The most frequent one is desaturation or the need for positive pressure ventilation.[32] Other events would be:

- Intraoperative laryngospasm, requiring treatment (increase in FiO_2, positive pressure ventilation [PPV]).
- Intra- and postoperative oxygen desaturation (<90% on room air) in the PACU.
- PACU stay >100 min.

In another study, encompassing ambulatory children with severe OSA undergoing ATE, a preoperative AHI of ≥15, and O_2 saturation nadir <80% was also individualized as predictors for postoperative desaturation, oxygen requirement, and prolonged length of stay (>24 h).[136]

3.3.4 Postoperative Patient-Tailored Management

Postoperative Care

Care includes various aspects to which both the surgeon and the anesthetist must stick:
- Provision of maximal safety both immediately and after discharge.
- Pain relief.
- Management of nausea and vomiting.
- Assisting the return to normal diet and activity.

Postoperative Patient's Safety

The modalities by which safety is accomplished would vary according to the following:
- Patient characteristics:
  - Age.
  - Comorbidities.
  - Need for airway protection.
  - Level of communication, etc.
- Extension of the intervention.
- Type and mode of administration of the anesthetics and analgesic.
- Grade of the ward (PACU, ICU, pediatric ward) where the patient is transferred to postoperatively.
- The knowhow and experience of the staff, who need to be familiar with the patient's pathologies and drugs' AEs in the pediatric population.

The decision of where the patient is to be discharged to postoperatively should be based on several grounds:
- The child's medical history.
- Size and extend of the intervention.
- Intraoperative respiratory or cardiac mishaps.
- Risk of appearance or life-threatening AEs.
- Bed availability (PICU throughput, overcrowding).

Interestingly, intravenous induction with propofol (2–4 mg/kg) with added lignocaine (0.2 mg/kg) is effective for the clearheaded recovery and for antiemetic effects in children.[137]

3.3.5 Postoperative Complications

This review does not discuss pure surgically related acute or chronic complications. The complications covered herein are anesthesia-related during the immediate postoperative period.

Among other surgeries, tonsillectomy, an extremely common pediatric surgical procedure, is associated with significant morbidity and mortality. The postoperative challenges include: respiratory complications, post-tonsillectomy bleeding, nausea, vomiting, and significant pain. Most of these interventions are managed in ambulatory settings; meticulous triage is therefore needed. Comparatively, large numbers of pediatric patients do undergo adeno- and tonsillectomies in ambulatory settings despite the increase in rates of complications in younger patients and in patients suffering from various comorbidities. This double sword data is the probable result of an appropriate triage made regarding patients' underling conditions, although it is not yet concluded who truly warrants postoperative hospitalization.[138]

Bleeding

This occurrence, as after adeno- or tonsillectomy, can evolve in a life-threatening emergency, because of the danger of hemorrhagic shock and acute airway obstruction, accompanied by aspiration. As mentioned above, the child would better be extubated in the OR, and released from PACU after oroglottic cavities have been inspected and secured dry, and breathing is satisfactory.

The re-admission of a bleeding child is an emergency case, which needs to follow well-defined algorithms, following the guidelines emitted by the European Resuscitation Council (ERC) and the German Resuscitation Council (GRC).[139] The decision about how to manage the case—in the OR, or bedside under close observation—depends on the state of the surgical site and on the child's conditions.[140] It is worth noting that older children tend to bleed more post-tonsillectomy, if tonsillitis is present, and after co-ablation techniques.[141] Breathing room air needs to be enriched with oxygen throughout the time. However, mask-and-bag ventilation should be avoided, in order to prevent the oral blood from being pushed and aspirated into the bronchial tree. Note that the child and the parent are probably alarmed; the patient breathes quickly and shallowly. Positioning the patient in half-sitting position may aid mechanically spontaneous breathing. Oxygen source is put in front of the patient's face, but distantly, so that he does not panic. The only recommended way to improve oxygenation while protecting the airways is the RSI with a cuffed tube, which minimizes blood dripping into the bronchial system.[142] Suction equipment must be set ready to remove blood from the oropharynx upon the insertion of the laryngoscope (see above). A primary clinical evaluation of blood loss or the circulatory performance is the peripheral capillary refill time (standard value: <2 s), as well as examining the pulse oximetry reading, which also depicts distal perfusion, heart frequency, and blood pressure range (primarily noninvasive). Use of the recently introduced non-invasive hemoglobin detector is advisable in these emergency cases, although acute bleed is underestimated by any hemoglobin count.[143,144]

Electro-cautery and suturing are the common management techniques in treating post-tonsillectomy bleed. Other alternatives are out of the scope of this chapter; blood products may be needed and therefore be prepared in advance.[140,141]

Respiratory Adverse Events

Several risk factors and perioperative respiratory problems are illustrated above. In essence, the teams need to identify pre-existing oral and airway abnormalities on the one hand (e.g., obesity), and potential risk factors during (e.g., surgery near the airway) and immediately after ENT interventions (e.g., intermittent apnea episodes) that may invigorate respiratory mishaps, on the other hand. Experienced pediatric anesthetist and availability of PACU, PICU, and on-ward qualified medical staff are essential to prevent life-threatening conditions from terminating in death.[145]

Respiratory AEs were estimated to cause one-third of all perioperative cardiac arrests.[146] The clinical appearances that represent the advent of postoperative respiratory complications are:
- Laryngospasm (primary cause for cardiac arrest).
- Bronchospasm.
- Airway obstruction.
- Apnea (e.g., d/t reflex or excessive inhalation drug).
- Desaturation.

While respiratory risk factors are closely associated with the type of ENT intervention, they may also be specific to the patient's characteristics.[147] Those associated with the patient itself include:
- URTI in the last 2 preoperative weeks.
- Pulmonary disease (e.g., bronchial asthma).
- OSA.
- Upper airway obstruction (e.g., hypertrophy of the tonsils).
- Age <3 years.
- Passive smoking.
- Obesity/morbid obesity.
- Rare craniofacial abnormality.
- Orphan diseases and syndromes.
- Neuromuscular diseases.

Some anesthesia-related risk factors that affect postoperative outcome also need to be mentioned. Among the most relevant ones are:
- Interventional invasiveness of the airway (endotracheal intubation, surgery around the LMA).
- Relatively low FiO_2.

- Choice of anesthetics (see above).
- Experience/inexperience of the anesthetist.

Noteworthy: the occurrence of short apnea incidences may quickly lead to hypoxia and myocardial depression in young children, because they tolerate hypoxemia much less than adults. This is mainly due to the smaller lung reserve volume and the functional residual capacity (FRC) and the higher central sensitivity to hypoxemia, which leads to immediate cardiac depression.[148,149]

The principal management of respiratory insufficiency is definitive and secured airway, such as ETT, including re-anesthesia, muscle relaxation, and PPV. Some desaturation cases can be managed with oxygen enrichment,[148,150] or verbal encouragement on the attainment of increasing oxygen input. Even in these cases, and as mentioned above, a preoperative chest X-ray and electrocardiogram were found to be of little predictive values, and are not cost-effective screening tests for postoperative respiratory complications.

Agitation (Emergence Delirium, ED)

This is defined as a dissociative state of consciousness in which the child is motorically hyperactive without a recognizable reason, is touchy, uncooperative, cries disconsolately, shouts, and/or hits around himself.[151] In some reports, this incidence reaches 80% of the operated children who have behaved normally preoperatively. These children can also suffer from later long-term and persistent postoperative behavioral disorders.[152] Agitation typically appears 30 to 60 min after the end of anesthesia, lasting between 5 and 60 min; the event is thus self-limiting. Emergency delirium is stressful to the child, the guardian, and to the medical team; it can also endanger the surgical result and child's life.[153]

Among preventive strategies, if susceptible, perioperative pain therapy is the first to opt. Use of propofol instead of volatile anesthetics, IV analgesics like fentanyl, ketamine, as well as alpha$_2$ receptor agonists (clonidine or dexmedetomidine), has also proven to exert preventive effects.[153,154] Consoling the child and comforting the parent are of importance in these cases.

Postoperative Nausea and Vomiting (PONV)

Postoperative feeling of sickness and/or vomiting is one of the most frequent post-surgical complications in children in general, particularly when surgery takes place in the orofacial surrounding. In the absence of antiemetics intake, the incidence reaches >50%.[155] PONV is an age-dependent complication: children <3 years are involved only seldom. The peak incidence lies between 6 and 10 years; the incidence among adolescents approaches adults' values.[156] Importantly, children <4-year-old are unable to describe sickness without vomiting as a disturbance, and would vomit when crying a lot.[157] Furthermore, frequent PONV can lead to additional complications: electrolyte loss, dehydration and acidosis, bleeding complications, airway aspiration and their obstruction, and to esophageal rupture.[158]

Overall, PONV may affect up to 30% to 80% of high-risk populations. Post-discharge nausea and vomiting (PDNV), especially in the ambulatory setting, may be under-recognized by the anesthetist. The common risk factors for PONV in infancy are as follows:[159]

- Operation duration >30 min.
- Age ≥3 years.
- ORL combined with eye surgery.
- Positive PONV history of motion sickness of the child.

With the existence of one of the four indicative factors, the PONV risk would rise by 10% over the initial 30%, reaching a 70% risk by the presence of all 4 factors.[160] The suggested preventive remedies are:

- Use of TIVA rather than inhalational GA.
- Avoidance of opioids, rather use of multimodal protocols.
- Preventing conditions and avoidance of drugs generating PONV.
- Perioperative use of antiemetics in a sequential manner:
    - Dexamethasone, ondansetron, or dimenhydrinate;[161–166] for specific doses see ▶ Table 3.1.
    - bA single-dose administration of *steroids* (1 mg/kg, max 50 mg dexamethasone) before performing tonsillectomy was advised in children. It was proven to reduce emesis and pain on POD1, to improve oral intake, and minimize pain following cold surgical technique. Steroids reduce tissue damage and postoperative pain by suppressing fibrin deposition, capillary dilation, edema formation, and leukocyte migration.[167,168] Nevertheless, a study regarding prophylaxis of PONV following ATE found an increase in postoperative bleeding rate of 24% in patients given "high-dose dexamethasone," i.e., 0.5 mg/kg IV. Prophylactic dose of 0.15 mg/kg dexamethasone reliably prevented PONV, while avoiding the risk for postoperative bleeding.[169,170]

For further therapeutic regimens see ▶ Table 3.1; for PONV-detailed risk factor findings in adults and children refer to reference number 171.[171]

Most postoperative gastrointestinal dismotility events appertain indeed to PONV. Nevertheless, the abundant use of analgesics, especially opioids, induces constipation, bloating, intestinal cramps, and inability to eat/drink, and even provokes complete ileus. These phenomena need to be correctly identified and appropriately treated; young children may not be able to describe such discomfort. Factors impeding normal restoration of motility include:

- Longer operation period.
- Prolonged opioid analgesics usage.

- Long nasogastric catheter maintenance.
- Presence of systemic inflammation.[172]

Treatment may include dopamine receptor antagonists (see above and in ▶ Table 3.1), and macrolides as potent stimulants currently in use in adults.[173] Lactulose may be used cautiously; it is contraindicated in cases of galactosemia or bowel obstruction. Its dosages are reported in ▶ Table 3.1.[166,174,175]

3.4 Pain Management in ENT-Operated Children

Pain is always a concern to the surgical patient; it further imposes bustle to the child and the accompanying person, generating fear even when groundless. Pain is also a public health concern of major implications, not just because of the physical and emotional impacts on the child and family, but also due to the potential morbidity and mortality thereby involved. As detailed below, proper assessment of pain is a challenge in the pediatric population, due to lack of verbalization, communication, or possible improper specification/characterization of pain, leading to its mis- or under-estimation. This makes satisfactory treatment arduous, sometimes even erroneously over-treating it, when using opioids. Pain plan is therefore best discussed in details starting preoperatively. The severity of postoperative pain, and the eventuality of a long-lasting pain should also be discussed.

Throat pain, particularly experienced during swallowing, is common following *tonsillectomy*.[176–179] Throat pain may lead the patient to restrict intake of liquids, resulting in dehydration and, potentially, re-admission to the hospital.[180] This pain typically persists for 7 and even 14 days postoperatively, and is scored moderate to severe.[181] Otalgia is also a frequent complaint following *tonsillectomy* and *adenoidectomy*.[177] Ear pain is referred from the pharynx as well, and can be even more disturbing than throat pain.

3.4.1 Pain Handling Highlights

- Most guidelines for the management of postoperative pain are based on ongoing experience and evolving evidence that, however, are still of limited satisfaction. Optimal postoperative pain management begins in the preoperative period where patient assessment and caregiver's information are integrated with the medical staff's experience and understanding of the case as a whole.
- Multimodal regimens are the most recommended approaches, although the exact modes, doses, and components vary depending on three factors: (1) patient, (2) settings, and (3) surgical procedure.
- Despite the ongoing clamor for opioids restriction, pediatric analgesia is still based on perioperative

opioids, for which the effectiveness of opioid-sparing multimodal adjuvants, as shown by the present authors in adults, is highly desirable.

- Maximal pain scores were found to independently associate with (1) usage of high opioid dose in the PACU; (2) use of non-opioids or opioids on ward; (3) gender (female displaying lower scores).

Preoperative clear verbal instructions about pain control, wound care, mobilization, and resumption of activities are essential. Several institutions have built special areas where teams meet the child with the parent, and explain, both verbally and by illustrations, all that concerns surgery, anesthesia, and pain control. All these need to be feasible for those who need emergency interventions as well.

Overall, the type of the intervention and its postoperative consequences affect both the duration and the intensity of pain that correspondingly influence the amounts of analgesic and the modes of their administration. Multimodal analgesia, the preferred regimen of analgesia, combines opioids and NSAIDs to various degrees. Adjuvants are essential to both potentiate and reduce opioid amounts, and minimize consequential AEs. This chapter will also briefly discuss alternative approaches to pain reduction.

3.4.2 Pain Assessment

This paragraph is of high importance because research has demonstrated that children are at particular risk for oligoanalgesia.

Pain assessment may encounter difficulties in children who are unable to self-report pain and specify its severity, type, and location. There are no physical signs that are specific indicators of pain, and its diagnosis must rely on physiological, behavioral, and self-report methods.[182]

Various models have been established in order to enable pain scoring in children; their utility depends on the age of the child and psychological/intellectual progress. Pain scores are to be explained to the parent preoperatively (see above), the latter being a mediator, buffer, and interpreter of the child's verbal or mimic pain expression/behavior when incapable of articulating themselves (due to age or intellectuality/maturity deficits). The parent/guardian is, thus, an essential component in the chain of medical cooperation with the child during the entire perioperative period.

To best outline modes of pain assessment, one has to remember:

- Pain assessment is optimal when knowing the child and parent well, being familiar with the population and heritage or culture they come from.
- Well-organized pain services, dedicated for children, which provide prompt pain assessment and management 24/7.

- Pain assessment needs to be done bed-side; although frequently considered an objective process (mainly in adults), pain evaluation frequently becomes intersubjective with nurse or physician's engagement along with verbal and visual communication of the child, family, or ward nurse. These enable better understanding of the origin and type of the pain experienced by the grown-up child, or body expression or parent report for those who are non-communicable or of small age.

For advanced knowledge, please refer to Chou R, et al.[183]

Pain Assessment vs. Patient's Age
Newborn and Toddlers (<3 Years)[184]

Most ways of identifying the presence of pain and its intensity in these children are based on mimics vs. tranquility of the child, and behavioral changes, as reported by the caregiver. See below specific tools, all of which are based on changes in behavior. It is recommended to familiarize with one/two techniques and apply each adequately based on the child's characteristics.

- For the neonate, the *CRIES* scale is a qualitative scale, indicating degrees of Crying, oxygen Requirement, Increased vital signs, Expression (e.g., grimace), or Sleeplessness.
- The behavior rating scale for assessing pain in children also applies to premature children (Premature Infant Pain Profile, *PIPP*), or to those with severe physical and learning impairments. They are characterized by brow bulge, eye squeeze, and nasal-labial furrow.[185,186,187]
- The Neonatal Infant Pain Scale (*NIPS*) uses another group of changes in neonates: facial expression, respiration pattern, extremity muscle tone, and state of arousal.
- The Neonatal Pain, Agitation, and Sedation Scale (*N-PASS*) is a crying/irritability componential scale, added to behavioral state (e.g., movements), facial expression, muscle tone of the extremities, and vital signs.

Young Children (3–6 Years)

While most children at these ages translate pain to a visual representation, some may also be capable of quantifying their pain. Pain is less quantifiable by VAS or NRS, but is based on a series of faces showing an increase in distress or pain (such as r-FLACC).[188,189]

Older Children (8–11 Years)

The reliability of pain assessment increases with age and the cognitive ability of the child; these enable quantification, where 0–100 VAS, horizontal, or the 0–10 NRS is usable.

Adolescents and Toddlers

Adolescents can rate pain using an NRS without the use of other accessory tools. In this age group, a description of intensity and characteristics of pain are also obtainable, based on history on the one hand and new experiences on the other, involving:

- Description: Is the pain sharp, stabbing, dull, burning, or tingling?
- Location and radiation: Where does the pain start and spread to?
- Intensity: Pain scale of 1 to 10?
- Duration and constancy: Steady or comes and goes pain?
- Frequency: How often does the pain occur?
- Factors that worsen or relieve pain: What makes the pain better or worse?

3.4.3 Specific Pain Assessment Tools

The following are pain models, used in young children (excluded are the most well-known pain VAS or NRS that are used by adolescents and adults), who are *unable* to quantify, qualify, or locate pain:

- *Pain-location tools*: Several graphic-based pain-location tools have been used to determine the location of pain in children and adolescents. They have been originally created for chronic and neuropathic pain. They are pre- and postoperative implements, and include:
  - The Adolescent and Pediatric Pain Tool.[190]
  - The Pediatric Pain Questionnaire.[191]
  - The simple *PainDETECT* questionnaire (PD-Q),[192] which is not a time-consuming clinical examination like the grading system.[193]

These tools typically use a graphic outline of the body, and the small patient is asked to "color" in the areas where he/she is experiencing pain. It may be concluded that although the quality of the included studies is debatable, they evidenced reliable located pain scoring both in small and older children.[194]

- *Observational tools*: The observational tools help assessing pain in infants and children who are unable to self-report. These pain scales are of similar characters and are based on scoring facial expressions, ability to be consoled, level of interaction with the surroundings, limb and trunk motor responses, and verbal responses[195,196,197] (see below).

Pain Assessment in the Non-Communicating Children

Nonverbal and/or Neurologically Impaired (NI) Children

These children present unique challenges when evaluating the presence and severity of pain; they cannot self-report them properly. Since not appraised by the medical staff, they frequently remain undertreated. Nevertheless, these children present consistent corpse expressions enabling assessment of pain, although each child will display a unique set of behavioral responses that need acquaintance before the intervention. These expressions necessitate input from their care provider/parent who is knowledgeable of the child's standard behavioral patterns in response to painful and non-painful (such as hunger) events.[22]

The specific behaviors that are associated with pain in nonverbal children/NI include:

- Vocalization (crying, moaning).
- Facial expression (e.g., grimacing).
- Un-consoled.
- Increased movement, tone and posture (arching, stiffening), and physiological responses (sweating).
- Atypical behavior, such as laughing, withdrawing, or lack of facial expression.

The Non-Communicating Children's Pain Checklist—Postoperative Version (*NCCPC-PV*)

This is another tool usable for nonverbal children.[198] Its items include postoperative vocalization of the child (moaning, crying), non-happy socialization (like withdrawal from contact), facial (grimaces or strange mimics), activity (moving or not), abnormal tone of body and limbs, and physiological signs (e.g., shivering, abnormal breath). These items are similar to other tools that are used in small or incapacitated children, where nurses or parents help de-codify the child's behavior.

Individualized Numeric Rating Scale (INRS)

Based on the parent's/caregiver's description of the child's daily responses to its surroundings, nurses can supplement this tool to other information, and assess pot-interventional level of pain. The INRS[188,199] principally relies on parent's consideration of whether the child appears in pain, and how severe it is, and what grade (0–10) is to be applied to each of the 6 items (facial expression, interpersonal reaction, cry or vocalization, consolability, and appearance of tears, seating, or gasping). Overall, the ability to recover specific behaviors is an important feature for children with atypical pain behaviors; these are referable by the caregiver and are absent in other tools. This further highlights the importance of becoming acquainted with the child's preoperative mode of behavior.

Psychometric Properties of the Modified Preverbal or Early Verbal Pediatric Pain Scale (M-PEPPS)

This is a set of tools applicable to the *emergency department* pediatric population.[200] Its analysis on 118 children proved the M-PEPPS instrument to be a reliable tool for emergency nurses measuring pediatric pain. The M-PEPPS captures the range of expressions of pediatric pain and it measures the single construct of pain, rather than multiple constructs, such as pain and anxiety.

Follow several *observational pain tools* in children.[95–197]

Revised FLACC (r-FLACC)

This is a Face, Legs, Activity, Cry, Consolability reaction tool.[188] It is useful in pre-verbal (small) children, as well as for children with cognitive disability. The nurse can assess scores together with the parent, also inquiring if behaviors are uncommon, which indicates pain in the child. Each of the five categories, (F) Face; (L) Legs; (A) Activity; (C) Cry; (C) Consolability, is scored from 0 to 2, resulting in a total score between 0 and 10. When the patient is awake, observe the legs and body uncovered for 1 to 2 min. Activity, tenseness, and body tone after consolation should remain normal. If the child is asleep, similarly reposition him, then touch the body and assess for tenseness and tone changes in response to touch.

Specifications of the scores:

- *Face*: No particular expression or smile = 0.
  Occasional grimace or frown, withdrawn, disinterested, appears sad or worried = 1.
  Frequent to constant frown, clenched jaw, quivering chin; distressed-looking face: expression of fright or panic = 2.
- *Legs*: Normal position or relaxed = 0.
  Uneasy, restless, tense, occasional tremors = 1.
  Kicking, or legs drawn up, marked increase in spasticity, constant tremors or jerking = 2.
- *Activity*: Lying quietly, normal position,
  moves easily = 0.
  Squirming, shifting back and forth, tense, mildly agitated (e.g., head back and forth, aggression), shallow and splinting respirations, intermittent sighs = 1.
  Arched, rigid, or jerking; severe agitation, head banging; shivering (not rigors), breath-holding, gasping or sharp intake of breath; severe splinting = 2.
- *Cry*: No cry (awake or asleep) = 0.
  Moans or whimpers, occasional complaint, occasional verbal outburst or grunt = 1.

Crying steadily, screams or sobs, frequent complaints; repeated outbursts, constant grunting = 2.
- Consolability: Content, relaxed = 0.
  Reassured by occasional touching, hugging, or being talked to, distractible = 1.
  Difficult to console or comfort, pushing away caregiver, resisting care or comfort measures = 2.

Wong Baker Pain Rating Scale[201]

This is a scale (for children between 3 and 8 years of age (and less if able to use this format) (▶Fig. 3.1). The scale needs being explained to the child and parent preoperatively, when discussing pain and its control. The scale uses facial expressions, thus delivering information even without saying anything.

Specifically, the face appears happy because the child has no pain (no hurt) or is sad because he has some or a lot of pain; these are the "0" or "1" face, respectively. Face "2" means it hurts a little more. Face "3" hurts even more; face "4" hurts a whole lot, while face "5" means it hurts as much as you can imagine, although you do not have to be crying because you feel this bad. When asked, the child will choose a face that best describes how he is feeling.

CHEOPS Scale (Children's Hospital of Eastern Ontario Pain Scale for Postoperative Pediatric Pain)

This quantifies postoperative pain in pediatric patients at 1 to 5 years of age, alternatively to the less used Behavioral Observational Pain Scale (*BOPS*) that enables pain scoring using the previously mentioned scales, although grading is numerically different. Scores ≥5 in the CHEOPS scale require re-administration of analgesia.[202]

Following are the specifics of the tool:

- *Cry*: ranging from no crying (+1), through moaning or quietly vocalizing silent cry or crying gently, or whimpering (+2), to full-lunged cry, sobbing, or screaming (+3).
- *Facial expression*: Smiling (0), expression of neutral facial (+1), or grimacing (+2).

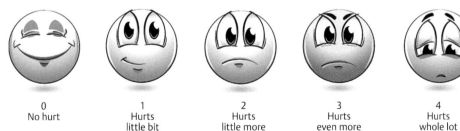

| 0 | 1 | 2 | 3 | 4 | 5 |
| No hurt | Hurts little bit | Hurts little more | Hurts even more | Hurts whole lot | Hurts worst |

Fig. 3.1 The Wong Baker pain rating scale.

- Child emitting *verbal responses*: Positive statements, or talks about things without complaint (0); the child not talking, or complains, but not about pain (+1); or complains about pain and/or other subjects (+2).
- *Torso*: Neutral/resting position (+1); body in motion or shifting or in serpentine fashion (+1), or body shuddering/shaking involuntarily/in a vertical or upright position, or is restrained (+2).
- *Wound evaluation*: Child not touching/reaching for the wound (+1); reaching/touching/grabbing the wound gently; arms are restrained (+2).
- *Legs*: Relaxed in any position (1); demonstrating uneasiness or restlessness and/or striking out with foot or feet (+2). The child may depict tensed legs and/or pull up legs tightly to body and keep them there, stand, crouching/kneeling, or legs are restrained (+2).

Nursing Assessment of Pain Intensity (NAPI)

This measure is useful in newborns and toddlers. The NAPI is a scale adapted by Stevens[203] from the CHEOPS pain rating scale (see above). The scale specifically looks at pain *intensity,* using a 0–3 scale of behavioral categories of (1) verbal/vocal behavior, (2) body movement, (3) facial expression, and (4) touching of the surgical site. In the mentioned study, NAPI evaluated the use of an assessment flow sheet to better manage children's pain; however, reliability and validity of the tool were not addressed by the author. High inter-rater reliability (90–99%) and some support for validity were reported for the original CHEOPS when used following surgery in young children (1–7 years). It provides fine discrimination between pain and no-pain observations in the presence of low caregiver burden. Neither of the two tools are useable in infants <1 month.[204]

Noteworthy: the r-FLACC (see above) has received the highest clinical utility score followed by the NAPI.[205] Both scales are based on the above-mentioned physio-behavioral alterations detectable in a painful child.

3.4.4 Analgesia Modus Operandi

Basically, non-pharmacological cognitive/behavioral therapies have become acceptable vis-à-vis pharmacological therapies tailored to the severity of pain and the child's age. The former are particularly fruitful if management has been initiated preoperatively, especially when involving toddlers and mature children. The latter are based on evidence-based recommendations for pain treatment, including non-opioid analgesics, opioid analgesics and adjuvant medicines to improve the management of pain in children in otolaryngology services upon request. Since the former are operable in few medical centers only, the interested readers may refer to the cited references.[206,207]

3.4.4.1 Non-Pharmacologic Therapy

This approach to pain includes:
- Physical measures: massage, heat and cold stimulation, and acupuncture.
- Behavioral measures: exercise, operant conditioning, relaxation, biofeedback, desensitization, and art and play therapy.
- Cognitive measures: distraction, imagery, hypnosis, and psychotherapy.

Biofeedback and Hypnosis

Biofeedback is an integrative technique that may help patients cope with pain.[208] Both biofeedback[209] and *hypnosis*[210] have increasingly become popular as modalities for the treatment of chronic, non-cancer pain as well. Although biofeedback rarely cures such pain, it can help patients self-regulate and influence pain perception.[211] Noteworthy, only few have investigated acute, perioperative biofeedback in the pediatric population, probably none did so following ENT-related interventions. These non-pharmacological behavioral adjuncts have been suggested as efficient safe means in reducing discomfort and adverse effects in patients undergoing percutaneous vascular and renal procedures in a prospective, randomized, single-center study. The authors found that structured attention and self-hypnotic relaxation proved beneficial during the invasive medical procedures. Hypnosis had more pronounced effects on pain and anxiety reduction, and it also improved hemodynamic stability.[210] Bayat et al found that adjuvants (e.g., ketamine) combined with non-pharmacological techniques can limit the use of drugs (and hence AEs), as well as improve children's participation and satisfaction.[212] A survey of the use of complementary and alternative medical therapies by pediatric pain management services affiliated with major universities[213] was conducted among 43 pediatric anesthesia fellowship programs, where 38 institutions (86%) offered one or more complementary and alternative medical therapies for their patients. Those therapies included biofeedback (65%), guided imagery (49%), relaxation therapy (33%), massage (35%), hypnosis (44%), acupuncture (33%), art therapy (21%), and meditation (21%). The results indicated a high prevalence in the integration of complementary and alternative medical therapies in pediatric pain management programs.

In another study[214] it was demonstrated that during invasive medical procedures, hypnotizability did not vary with age. Patients receiving attention and hypnosis had greater pain reduction during the procedure.

Cognitive-Procedural Analgesia

Non-pharmacologic measures are useful in reducing stress and anxiety in children undergoing invasive procedures. A meta-analysis reported strong evidence that cognitive-behavioral therapy (i.e., distraction, hypnosis, and combined cognitive-behavioral interventions) reduced pain and distress associated with needle-related procedures in children.[215]

Pharmacological Therapy

As mentioned above, pain management in children must consider (1) baseline illness, (2) type and extension of operation, (3) outcome or surgery, (4) site and availability of monitoring, (5) availability of pharmacological and non-pharmacological means.

Despite the common practice, it was recently reported that oral MO plus ibuprofen or each drug alone were inadequate for relieving musculoskeletal pain in pediatric patients in the emergency department. MO-treated children experienced more side effects than those given ibuprofen, but no serious AEs were reported.[216] The best practice of preventing and treating pain in children involves using multimodal (opioid-sparing) analgesia, which may include analgesics and adjuvants, procedural interventions, rehabilitation, psychological and integrative therapies that act synergistically for more effective pediatric pain control with fewer side effects than a single analgesic or modality.[217]

Opioids

In cases where the glottis and oral areas are the sites of operation, ICU surveillance is recommended, mainly for airway protection, since edema and potential obstruction to spontaneous breathing may ensue, and upper airway reflexes may become ineffective. IV analgesics are commonly used in PICU, e.g., continuous infusion (fentanyl or remifentanil, with or without ketamine), PCA-MO alone or PCA-MO + ketamine, the latter pending the patient's age and level of comprehension and cooperation, with or without the addition of alpha$_2$ agonists. In less severe cases, which however still require surveillance, IV paracetamol, or dipyrone, is the basic analgesia protocol, and can coadjuvate opioid therapy. Non-opioids are also of rescue value to counteract breakthrough pain, if used as IV boluses, rectal deposition, or oral instillation. All these regimens and modes of administration are applicable for ketamine as well. These compounds are strong and fast enough for breakthrough pain control; however, distinction among types and intensities of pain must be made by the attending nurse or the physician. Lists and doses of drugs usable postoperatively are provided in ▶ Table 3.1.

Indeed, in a randomized study,[218] 98 children undergoing tonsillectomy were treated with either IV paracetamol infusion (15 mg/kg, starting 15 min before the end of surgery) or added to IV bolus of ketamine (0.25 mg/kg). The CHEOPS pain scales were significantly lower in the ketamine compared to the control group up to 6 postoperative hours, but not at 12 h. Adjuvant rescue analgesic and incidence of PONV were similar between the two groups.

Opioid administration by any route, especially IV (by bolus or infusion), may induce unwanted consequences. This is of importance mainly after perioral surgery or in an obese child. Special attention is required during the first hours of opioid administration, to detect sedation allergy or other types of reactions, and until a stable and acceptable analgesic status has been established. Additional amounts of drugs added to reach the desired analgesia stage, may induce untoward effects, e.g., PONV, depressed respiration, or hypotension, which are especially undesired following many of the ENT interventions.

A recent FDA contraindication has cautioned the use of codeine after tonsillectomy and other pediatric ORL surgeries; it is directed to lay primary caregiver's attitude. Thus, based on currently available evidence, a preventative multimodal strategies to manage pain, and PONV, without increasing the risk of post-tonsillectomy bleeding, is therefore essential.[219]

Local and Systemic Adjuvant Drugs

Several regimens are mentioned briefly; some may be used in the emergency department (peri-interventionally), and others are intended to be applied postoperatively.

- The 5% EMLA Cream is superior to all other topical anesthetic agents used before an IV line is placed.[220]
- The electronic dental anesthesia (EDA) is an application of electric current that loads the nerve stimulation pathway to the extent that pain stimulus is blocked. This suits grown-ups and cooperative adolescents.
- TENS was also shown to reduce pain in dental procedures, with limited use as mentioned above.[221,222]
- Transtracheal block with lidocaine is a good alternative to IV propofol in toddlers or those consenting to such a maneuver, when no muscle blockage is neccesary.[223]
- Lidocaine sprayed over the laryngoscope blade and/or the trachea lowers hemodynamic response to intubation.[224] A study found that the effects of lidocaine gel compared to mouthwash and saline were of similar analgesic efficacy;[225] ketamine provided better results (see above).
- The use of intraoral lidocaine also lowers the severity of post-intubation sore throat.[226]

3.4.5 The WHO's Two-Step Pain Strategy

The WHO suggests that the choice of analgesics in children (non-specifically indicated for ATE) can be based on two-step factors:[21]

1. Pain intensity.
2. The child's response to previously administered agents (the reader is referred to the 2012 World Health Organization guidelines[21]).

Following the above WHO principle, pain intensity may be categorized as:

- Mild pain: It is generally adequately treated with acetaminophen and NSAIDs. Oral paracetamol can be given several hours before the operation or rectally at the completion of surgery.
- Severe pain: It will respond to opioids.
- Moderate-to-severe pain: It is generally treated with opioids (e.g., MO, oxycodone, hydromorphone, fentanyl, and methadone in grown-ups for oncological patients).[227]

The First Step: Mild Pain

Paracetamol and ibuprofen are the medicines of choice as first-step cases. This bears strong recommendations, but low-quality evidence.

For children with *mild* pain, of ≥3 months of age, and who can take oral medication, paracetamol and ibuprofen are the medicines of choice. For those below that age, the only option is paracetamol. No other NSAIDs are safe. Ibuprofen is less convincingly safe than paracetamol in acute pain, especially for continuous and persisting pain. Noteworthy, both drugs are potentially toxic: renal and gastrointestinal toxicity, and bleeding with ibuprofen as with other NSAIDs, and hepatotoxicity and acute overdose associated with paracetamol. Nevertheless, both medicines are the first-line treatment in the pediatric pain management strategy for mild pain. They are available in child-appropriate dosage forms, such as oral liquids, and are relatively inexpensive. However, the oral solid dosage forms have precedence because they are better accepted by the child, require only a small quantity of water for administration, and ensure a more accurate dosage than traditional tablets.

The Second Step: Moderate-to-Severe Pain

If pain is moderate or severe, MO is the medicine of choice for the second step, although other strong opioids can be considered when necessary (e.g., AEs). The first-step drugs should be bypassed based on the clinical judgment of the severity of a child's pain, the disability caused by pain, the cause of pain, expected prognosis, and other aspects. Guidance on the use of related drugs is provided under sections 3.6–3.13 (pp. 41–50) and Annex 1 (p, 66) of the WHO Guidelines.[21]

3.4.6 Late Pain Control

Except for pain following ATE, other common head and neck operations also are painful for a varying period.[228] Among 251 patients (50 adenoidectomy, 51 ATE, 19 myringoplasty, 52 myringotomy, 43 strabismus, and 36 tongue tie divisions), myringoplasty, strabismus surgery, and ATE children of various ages depicted moderate pain, whereas adenoidectomy, tongue tie, and myringotomy ones had mild pain on POD0. ATE patients continued to suffer from moderate pain for an average of 9 days, with this intervention being the biggest challenge in postoperative pain management among the ENT surgeries; the other surgical groups suffered from mild pain for 1–3 days. Behavioral manifestations were dependent on pain scores. Home oral analgesics varied widely (see above and ►Table 2.1). Post-discharge PONV were low in all groups, with unplanned medical re-attendance rate of 16%.

Pain Regimens Highlights

- Regular, standardized age-dependent pain scoring and its timely assessments are the most important pilaster in pain treatment.
- Minimize opioid and sedative use.
- Use local anesthesia, including compounded topical creams, if feasible, with or without adjuvants (e.g., ketamine).[229]
- Multimodal pain therapy should be age-tailored and weight-oriented. All coadjuvant are best administered starting preoperatively (clonidine, dexamethasone, dexmedetomidine, gabapentinoids, ketamine).
- NSAIDs: Minimize their use, especially after tonsillectomy.

PONV prophylaxis (e.g., dexamethasone, ondansetron) helps the child feel better overall, even tolerating pain.

Gabapentinoids inhibit neural excitation by binding to the $\alpha\text{-}_2\text{-}\delta$ subunit of voltage-dependent Ca^{2+} ion channels in the CNS. They are currently applied in children as well as for adults.[106] They can be initiated preoperatively to calm the suffering and anxious child[104,106,230] and provide good night sleep.[104]

3.5 Conclusion

ENT surgery in the pediatric population is not much different from that in adults, with respect to preoperative preparation, anesthesia precautions, postoperative pain control and drug usage, and the need for nursing and close observation soon after surgery. Nevertheless, while the grown-ups are more capable of adjusting and assisting themselves when sensing difficulty or changes in respiration or cognition, the children are mostly dependent on parents' or nurses' support. Optimization of the bonding between these two parties is fruitful for perioperative trust, confidence, and improved medical provision. Age, intellect, and emotion-based preoperative preparations, techniques and analgesia reassurances, and preoperative calming down of the child, together with similar attention and assurance of the parent, all confer safe and smooth induction of anesthesia and calm emergence from it. Safe induction is of utmost importance; intraoperative managements, both the technique and the drugs thereby used, are to be carefully chosen by the anesthetist and judiciously administered. Proper management of pediatric postoperative pain is largely nurse- and parent-assured; it relies on continuous and/or PRN modes of IV treatment, and various enteral regimens. The capability of coadjuvating opioids with ketamine, dextromethorphan, or gabapentinoids (orally used only), when applicable (age, patient's and parents' cooperation), helps to diminish opioid usage, and their AEs, such as PONV, respiratory depression, or deep sedation. This improves the child's overall feeling and hastens recovery. This latter significantly ameliorate pain tolerance and strengthens patient- and parent-staff mutual aid, thereby accelerating recovery and discharge home.

References

[1] Statistisches Bundesamt. Gesundheit—Fallpauschalenbezogene Krankenhausstatistik (DRG-Statistik) Operationen und Prozeduren der vollstationären Patientinnen und Patienten in Krankenhäusern 2011. Wiesbaden: Statistisches Bundesamt; 2012. Artikelnummer: 5231401117014. Available at https://www.destatis.de/DE/Publikationen/Thematisch/Gesundheit/Krankenhaeuser/OperationenProzeduren5231401117014.pdf; accessed December 30, 2017. [German]

[2] Strauß JM, Gäbler R, Schmidt J, Mehler J, Giest J. Empfehlungen zur ambulanten Anästhesie bei Neugeborenen, Säuglingen und Kleinkindern. Anästh Intensivmed 2007;48:S67–S70

[3] Brennan LJ. Modern day-case anaesthesia for children. Br J Anaesth 1999;83(1):91–103

[4] Windfuhr JP, Hübner R, Sesterhenn K. Kriterien zur stationären Krankenhausbehandlung der Adenotomie. HNO 2003;51(8):622–628

[5] Spencer DJ, Jones JE. Complications of adenotonsillectomy in patients younger than 3 years. Arch Otolaryngol Head Neck Surg 2012;138(4):335–339

[6] Becke K. Anesthesia in children with a cold. Curr Opin Anaesthesiol 2012;25(3):333–339

[7] Smiley RM. An overview of induction and emergence characteristics of desflurane in pediatric, adult, and geriatric patients. Anesth Analg 1992;75(4, Suppl):S38–S44, discussion S44–S46

[8] von Ungern-Sternberg BS, Boda K, Chambers NA, et al. Risk assessment for respiratory complications in paediatric anaesthesia: a prospective cohort study. Lancet 2010;376(9743):773–783

[9] Jaye DL, Waites KB. Clinical applications of C-reactive protein in pediatrics. Pediatr Infect Dis J 1997;16(8):735–746, quiz 746–747

[10] von Ungern-Sternberg BS. Respiratory complications in the pediatric postanesthesia care unit. Anesthesiol Clin 2014;32(1):45–61

[11] Lescanne E, Chiron B, Constant I, et al; French Society of ENT (SFORL). French Association for Ambulatory Surgery (AFCA). French Society for Anaesthesia, Intensive Care (SFAR). Pediatric tonsillectomy: clinical practice guidelines. Eur Ann Otorhinolaryngol Head Neck Dis 2012;129(5):264–271

[12] Becke K, Giest J, Strauß JM. Handlungsempfehlungen zur präoperativen Diagnostik, Impfabstand und Nüchternheit im Kindesalter. Anästh Intensivmed 2007;48:62–66

[13] NCD Risk Factor Collaboration (NCD-RisC). Worldwide trends in body-mass index, underweight, overweight, and obesity from 1975 to 2016: a pooled analysis of 2416 population-based measurement studies in 128·9 million children, adolescents, and adults. Lancet 2017;390(10113):2627–2642

[14] Ogden CL, Carroll MD, Lawman HG, et al. Trends in obesity prevalence among children and adolescents in the United States, 1988–1994 through 2013–2014. JAMA 2016;315(21):2292–2299

[15] Mazur A, Caroli M, Radziewicz-Winnicki I, et al. Reviewing and addressing the link between mass media and the increase in obesity among European children: The European Academy of Paediatrics (EAP) and The European Childhood Obesity Group (ECOG) consensus statement. Acta Paediatr 2018;107(4):568–576

[16] World Health Organization. The WHO child Growth standards. Available at: http://www.who.int/childgrowth/standards/en/; accessed December 30, 2017

[17] World Health Organization. Growth reference data for 5–19 years. Available at: http://www.who.int/growthref/en/; accessed December 30, 2017

[18] Kuczmarski RJ, Ogden CL, Guo SS, et al. 2000 CDC Growth Charts for the United States: methods and development. Vital Health Stat 11 2002;246(246):1–190

[19] Veyckemans F. Child obesity and anaesthetic morbidity. Curr Opin Anaesthesiol 2008;21(3):308–312

[20] Apfelbaum JL, Hagberg CA, Caplan RA, et al; American Society of Anesthesiologists Task Force on Management of the Difficult Airway. Practice guidelines for management of the difficult airway: an updated report by the American Society of Anesthesiologists Task Force on Management of the Difficult Airway. Anesthesiology 2013;118(2):251–270

[21] http://apps.who.int/iris/bitstream/10665/44540/1/9789241548120_Guidelines.pdf; accessed December 30, 2017

[22] Hauer J, Houtrow AJ; Section on hospice and palliative medicine, council on children with disabilities. Pain Assessment and treatment in children with significant impairment of the central nervous system. Pediatrics 2017;139(6):e20171002: Review

[23] Becke K. Anesthesia for ORL surgery in children. GMS Curr Top Otorhinolaryngol Head Neck Surg 2014;13:Doc04

[24] Tantisira KG, Fuhlbrigge AL, Tonascia J, et al; Childhood Asthma Management Program Research Group. Bronchodilation and bronchoconstriction: predictors of future lung function in childhood asthma. J Allergy Clin Immunol 2006;117(6):1264–1271

[25] Tait AR, Malviya S. Anesthesia for the child with an upper respiratory tract infection: still a dilemma? Anesth Analg 2005;100(1):59–65

[26] Ie K, Yoshizawa A, Hirano S, et al. [A survey of perioperative asthmatic attack among patients with bronchial asthma underwent general anesthesia] Arerugi 2010;59(7):831–838

[27] Gislason T, Benediktsdóttir B. Snoring, apneic episodes, and nocturnal hypoxemia among children 6 months to 6 years old. An epidemiologic study of lower limit of prevalence. Chest 1995;107(4):963–966

[28] Ishman SL. Evidence-based practice: pediatric obstructive sleep apnea. Otolaryngol Clin North Am 2012;45(5):1055–1069

[29] Schwengel DA, Sterni LM, Tunkel DE, Heitmiller ES. Perioperative management of children with obstructive sleep apnea. Anesth Analg 2009;109(1):60–75

[30] Nixon GM, Kermack AS, McGregor CD, et al. Sleep and breathing on the first night after adenotonsillectomy for obstructive sleep apnea. Pediatr Pulmonol 2005;39(4):332–338

[31] Brown KA, Laferrière A, Lakheeram I, Moss IR. Recurrent hypoxemia in children is associated with increased analgesic sensitivity to opiates. Anesthesiology 2006;105(4):665–669

[32] Hill CA, Litvak A, Canapari C, et al. A pilot study to identify pre- and peri-operative risk factors for airway complications following adenotonsillectomy for treatment of severe pediatric OSA. Int J Pediatr Otorhinolaryngol 2011;75(11):1385–1390

[33] Short JA, van der Walt JH, Zoanetti DC. Immunization and anesthesia: an international survey. Paediatr Anaesth 2006;16 (5):514–522

[34] Munro J, Booth A, Nicholl J. Routine preoperative testing: a systematic review of the evidence. Health Technol Assess 1997;1(12): i–iv, 1–62

[35] Eisert S, Hovermann M, Bier H, Göbel U. Preoperative screening for coagulation disorders in children undergoing adenoidectomy (AT) and tonsillectomy (TE): does it prevent bleeding complications? Klin Padiatr 2006;218(6):334–339

[36] Close HL, Kryzer TC, Nowlin JH, Alving BM. Hemostatic assessment of patients before tonsillectomy: a prospective study. Otolaryngol Head Neck Surg 1994;111(6):733–738

[37] Kronenberg RH. Ketamine as an analgesic: parenteral, oral, rectal, subcutaneous, transdermal and intranasal administration. J Pain Palliat Care Pharmacother 2002;16(3):27–35

[38] Raber-Durlacher JE, Barasch A, Peterson DE, Lalla RV, Schubert MM, Fibbe WE. Oral complications and management considerations in patients treated with high-dose chemotherapy. Support Cancer Ther 2004;1(4):219–229

[39] Lefor AT. Perioperative management of the patient with cancer. Chest 1999;115(5, Suppl):165S–171S

[40] Tartaglino LM, Rao VM, Markiewicz DA. Imaging of radiation changes in the head and neck. Semin Roentgenol 1994;29(1):81–91

[41] Delbridge L, Sutherland J, Somerville H, Steinbeck K, Stevens G. Thyroid surgery and anaesthesia following head and neck irradiation for childhood malignancy. Aust N Z J Surg 2000;70(7): 490–492

[42] Giraud O, Bourgain JL, Marandas P, Billard V. Limits of laryngeal mask airway in patients after cervical or oral radiotherapy. Can J Anaesth 1997;44(12):1237–1241

[43] Chaimberg KH, Cravero JP. Mucositis and airway obstruction in a pediatric patient. Anesth Analg 2004;99(1):59–61

[44] Drew B, Peters C, Rimell F. Upper airway complications in children after bone marrow transplantation. Laryngoscope 2000;110(9):1446–1451

[45] Majorana A, Schubert MM, Porta F, Ugazio AG, Sapelli PL. Oral complications of pediatric hematopoietic cell transplantation: diagnosis and management. Support Care Cancer 2000;8(5):353–365

[46] Dinauer CA, Breuer C, Rivkees SA. Differentiated thyroid cancer in children: diagnosis and management. Curr Opin Oncol 2008; 20(1):59–65

[47] Ohmori K, Collins J, Fukushima T. Craniopharyngiomas in children. Pediatr Neurosurg 2007;43(4):265–278

[48] Légaré F, O'Connor AM, Graham ID, Wells GA, Tremblay S. Impact of the Ottawa Decision Support Framework on the agreement and the difference between patients' and physicians' decisional conflict. Med Decis Making 2006;26(4):373–390

[49] Clark JA, Wray NP, Ashton CM. Living with treatment decisions: regrets and quality of life among men treated for metastatic prostate cancer. J Clin Oncol 2001;19(1):72–80

[50] Lorenzo AJ, Pippi Salle JL, Zlateska B, Koyle MA, Bägli DJ, Braga LH. Decisional regret after distal hypospadias repair: single institution prospective analysis of factors associated with subsequent parental remorse or distress. J Urol 2014;191(5, Suppl):1558–1563

[51] Hess EP, Knoedler MA, Shah ND, et al. The chest pain choice decision aid: a randomized trial. Circ Cardiovasc Qual Outcomes 2012;5(3):251–259

[52] Arterburn D, Wellman R, Westbrook E, et al. Introducing decision aids at Group Health was linked to sharply lower hip and knee surgery rates and costs. Health Aff (Millwood) 2012;31(9):2094–2104

[53] Strychowsky JE, Albert D, Chan K, et al. International Pediatric Otolaryngology Group (IPOG) consensus recommendations: routine peri-operative pediatric tracheotomy care. Int J Pediatr Otorhinolaryngol 2016;86:250–255

[54] Curley MA, Harris SK, Fraser KA, Johnson RA, Arnold JH. State behavioral scale: a sedation assessment instrument for infants and young children supported on mechanical ventilation. Pediatr Crit Care Med 2006;7(2):107–114

[55] Andersson H, Hellström PM, Frykholm P. Introducing the 6-4-0 fasting regimen and the incidence of prolonged preoperative fasting in children. Paediatr Anaesth 2018;28(1):46–52

[56] Scheuber K, Becke K. Ambulante Anästhesie–Kinder in der ambulanten Anästhesie. Anasthesiol Intensivmed Notfallmed Schmerzther 2013;48(3):192–198, quiz 199

[57] Falconer R, Skouras C, Carter T, Greenway L, Paisley AM. Preoperative fasting: current practice and areas for improvement. Updates Surg 2014;66(1):31–39

[58] Kleiber C, Craft-Rosenberg M, Harper DC. Parents as distraction coaches during i.v. insertion: a randomized study. J Pain Symptom Manage 2001;22(4):851–861

[59] Power N, Liossi C, Franck L. Helping parents to help their child with procedural and everyday pain: practical, evidence-based advice. J Spec Pediatr Nurs 2007;12(3):203–209

[60] Chartrand J, Tourigny J, MacCormick J. The effect of an educational pre-operative DVD on parents' and children's outcomes after a same-day surgery: a randomized controlled trial. J Adv Nurs 2017;73(3):599–611

[61] Latham GJ, Greenberg RS. Anesthetic considerations for the pediatric oncology patient—part 2: systems-based approach to anesthesia. Paediatr Anaesth 2010;20(5):396–420

[62] Yip P, Middleton P, Cyna AM, Carlyle AV. Non-pharmacological interventions for assisting the induction of anaesthesia in children. Cochrane Database Syst Rev 2009(3):CD006447

[63] Vagnoli L, Caprilli S, Messeri A. Parental presence, clowns or sedative premedication to treat preoperative anxiety in children: what could be the most promising option? Paediatr Anaesth 2010;20(10):937–943

[64] Vagnoli L, Caprilli S, Robiglio A, Messeri A. Clown doctors as a treatment for preoperative anxiety in children: a randomized, prospective study. Pediatrics 2005;116(4):e563–e567

[65] Hong P, Maguire E, Purcell M, Ritchie KC, Chorney J. Decision-making quality in parents considering adenotonsillectomy or tympanostomy tube insertion for their children. JAMA Otolaryngol Head Neck Surg 2017;143(3):260–266

[66] Jabbour SA. Steroids and the surgical patient. Med Clin North Am 2001;85(5):1311–1317

[67] Brown CJ, Buie WD. Perioperative stress dose steroids: do they make a difference? J Am Coll Surg 2001;193(6):678–686

[68] Stam H, Grootenhuis MA, Last BF. Social and emotional adjustment in young survivors of childhood cancer. Support Care Cancer 2001;9(7):489–513– Review

[69] Tasch MD. Corticosteroids and anesthesia. Curr Opin Anaesthesiol 2002;15(3):377–381

[70] Marik PE, Varon J. Requirement of perioperative stress doses of corticosteroids: a systematic review of the literature. Arch Surg 2008;143(12):1222–1226

[71] Einaudi S, Bertorello N, Masera N, et al. Adrenal axis function after high-dose steroid therapy for childhood acute lymphoblastic leukemia. Pediatr Blood Cancer 2008;50(3):537–541

[72] Kuperman H, Damiani D, Chrousos GP, et al. Evaluation of the hypothalamic-pituitary-adrenal axis in children with leukemia before and after 6 weeks of high-dose glucocorticoid therapy. J Clin Endocrinol Metab 2001;86(7):2993–2996

[73] Felner EI, Thompson MT, Ratliff AF, White PC, Dickson BA. Time course of recovery of adrenal function in children treated for leukemia. J Pediatr 2000;137(1):21–24

[74] Rix M, Birkebaek NH, Rosthøj S, Clausen N. Clinical impact of corticosteroid-induced adrenal suppression during treatment for acute lymphoblastic leukemia in children: a prospective observational study using the low-dose adrenocorticotropin test. J Pediatr 2005;147(5):645–650

[75] Mahachoklertwattana P, Vilaiyuk S, Hongeng S, Okascharoen C. Suppression of adrenal function in children with acute lymphoblastic leukemia following induction therapy with corticosteroid and other cytotoxic agents. J Pediatr 2004;144(6):736–740

[76] Petersen KB, Müller J, Rasmussen M, Schmiegelow K. Impaired adrenal function after glucocorticoid therapy in children

with acute lymphoblastic leukemia. Med Pediatr Oncol 2003; 41(2):110–114

[77] Cunha CdeF, Silva IN, Finch FL. Early adrenocortical recovery after glucocorticoid therapy in children with leukemia. J Clin Endocrinol Metab 2004;89(6):2797–2802

[78] Ghazal EA, Mason LJ, Cote CJ. Preoperative evaluation, premedication, and induction of anesthesia. In: Cote CJ, Lerman J, Todres ID, eds. A Practice of Anesthesia for Infants and Children, 4th ed. Philadelphia, PA: Saunders Elsevier; 2009: 37

[79] Kain ZN, Mayes LC, Wang SM, Caramico LA, Hofstadter MB. Parental presence during induction of anesthesia versus sedative premedication: which intervention is more effective? Anesthesiology 1998;89(5):1147–1156, discussion 9A–10A

[80] Bahetwar SK, Pandey RK, Saksena AK, Chandra G. A comparative evaluation of intranasal midazolam, ketamine and their combination for sedation of young uncooperative pediatric dental patients: a triple blind randomized crossover trial. J Clin Pediatr Dent 2011;35(4):415–420

[81] Lönnqvist PA, Habre W. Midazolam as premedication: is the emperor naked or just half-dressed? Paediatr Anaesth 2005;15(4):263–265

[82] Tesoro S, Mezzetti D, Marchesini L, Peduto VA. Clonidine treatment for agitation in children after sevoflurane anesthesia. Anesth Analg 2005;101(6):1619–1622

[83] Cole JW, Murray DJ, McAllister JD, Hirshberg GE. Emergence behaviour in children: defining the incidence of excitement and agitation following anaesthesia. Paediatr Anaesth 2002;12(5): 442–447

[84] Bergendahl H, Lönnqvist PA, Eksborg S. Clonidine in paediatric anaesthesia: review of the literature and comparison with benzodiazepines for premedication. Acta Anaesthesiol Scand 2006;50(2):135–143

[85] Bergendahl HT, Lönnqvist PA, Eksborg S, et al. Clonidine vs. midazolam as premedication in children undergoing adenotonsillectomy: a prospective, randomized, controlled clinical trial. Acta Anaesthesiol Scand 2004;48(10):1292–1300

[86] Mahmoud M, Mason KP. Dexmedetomidine: review, update, and future considerations of paediatric perioperative and periprocedural applications and limitations. Br J Anaesth 2015; 115(2):171–182

[87] Zhang W, Fan Y, Zhao T, Chen J, Zhang G, Song X. Median effective dose of intranasal dexmedetomidine for rescue sedation in pediatric patients undergoing magnetic resonance imaging. Anesthesiology 2016;125(6):1130–1135

[88] Ahmed SS, Unland T, Slaven JE, Nitu ME, Rigby MR. Successful use of intravenous dexmedetomidine for magnetic resonance imaging sedation in autistic children. South Med J 2014;107(9):559–564

[89] Plambech MZ, Afshari A. Dexmedetomidine in the pediatric population: a review. Minerva Anestesiol 2015;81(3):320–332 Review

[90] Song J, Ji Q, Sun Q, Gao T, Liu K, Li L. The opioid-sparing effect of intraoperative dexmedetomidine infusion after craniotomy. J Neurosurg Anesthesiol 2016;28(1):14–20

[91] Ebert TJ, Hall JE, Barney JA, Uhrich TD, Colinco MD. The effects of increasing plasma concentrations of dexmedetomidine in humans. Anesthesiology 2000;93(2):382–394

[92] Max BA, Mason KP. Extended infusion of dexmedetomidine to an infant at sixty times the intended rate. Int J Pediatr 2010;2010:825079

[93] Yazbek-Karam VG, Aouad MM. Perioperative uses of dexmedetomidine. Middle East J Anesthesiol 2006;18(6):1043–1058

[94] Canbay O, Celebi N, Uzun S, Sahin A, Celiker V, Aypar U. Topical ketamine and morphine for post-tonsillectomy pain. Eur J Anaesthesiol 2008;25(4):287–292

[95] Smith DJ, Westfall DP, Adams JD. Assessment of the potential agonistic and antagonistic properties of ketamine at opiate receptors in the guinea-pig ileum. Neuropharmacology 1982;21(7):605–611

[96] Hosseini Jahromi SA, Hosseini Valami SM, Hatamian S. Comparison between effect of lidocaine, morphine and ketamine spray on post-tonsillectomy pain in children. Anesth Pain Med 2012;2(1):17–21

[97] Kaviani N, Khademi A, Ebtehaj I, Mohammadi Z. The effect of orally administered ketamine on requirement for anesthetics and postoperative pain in mandibular molar teeth with irreversible pulpitis. J Oral Sci 2011;53(4):461–465

[98] Mandel JE. Laryngeal mask airways in ear, nose, and throat procedures. Anesthesiol Clin 2010;28(3):469–483

[99] Gravningsbråten R, Nicklasson B, Raeder J. Safety of laryngeal mask airway and short-stay practice in office-based adenotonsillectomy. Acta Anaesthesiol Scand 2009;53(2):218–222

[100] Sierpina DI, Chaudhary H, Walner DL, et al. Laryngeal mask airway versus endotracheal tube in pediatric adenotonsillectomy. Laryngoscope 2012;122(2):429–435

[101] Lalwani K, Richins S, Aliason I, Milczuk H, Fu R. The laryngeal mask airway for pediatric adenotonsillectomy: predictors of failure and complications. Int J Pediatr Otorhinolaryngol 2013;77(1):25–28

[102] Lerman J. TIVA, TCI, and pediatrics: where are we and where are we going? Paediatr Anaesth 2010;20(3):273–278

[103] Loftus RW, Yeager MP, Clark JA, et al. Intraoperative ketamine reduces perioperative opiate consumption in opiate-dependent patients with chronic back pain undergoing back surgery. Anesthesiology 2010;113(3):639–646

[104] Weinbroum AA. Postoperative hyperalgesia: A clinically applicable narrative review. Pharmacol Res 2017;120:188–205

[105] Kain ZN, Caldwell-Andrews AA, Weinberg ME, et al. Sevoflurane versus halothane: postoperative maladaptive behavioral changes: a randomized, controlled trial. Anesthesiology 2005;102(4):720–726

[106] Weinbroum AA. Non-opioid IV adjuvants in the perioperative period: pharmacological and clinical aspects of ketamine and gabapentinoids. Pharmacol Res 2012;65(4):411–429

[107] Yenigun A, Et T, Aytac S, Olcay B. Comparison of different administration of ketamine and intravenous tramadol hydrochloride for postoperative pain relief and sedation after pediatric tonsillectomy. J Craniofac Surg 2015;26(1):e21–e24

[108] Elshammaa N, Chidambaran V, Housny W, Thomas J, Zhang X, Michael R. Ketamine as an adjunct to fentanyl improves postoperative analgesia and hastens discharge in children following tonsillectomy: a prospective, double-blinded, randomized study. Paediatr Anaesth 2011;21(10):1009–1014

[109] Dahmani S, Michelet D, Abback PS, et al. Ketamine for perioperative pain management in children: a meta-analysis of published studies. Paediatr Anaesth 2011;21(6):636–652

[110] Cho HK, Yoon HY, Jin HJ, Hwang SH. Efficacy of dexmedetomidine for perioperative morbidities in pediatric tonsillectomy: A meta-analysis. Laryngoscope 2018;128(5):E184–E193

[111] Olutoye OA, Glover CD, Diefenderfer JW, et al. The effect of intraoperative dexmedetomidine on postoperative analgesia and sedation in pediatric patients undergoing tonsillectomy and adenoidectomy. Anesth Analg 2010;111(2):490–495

[112] Lev R, Rosen P. Prophylactic lidocaine use preintubation: a review. J Emerg Med 1994;12(4):499–506

[113] Lerman J, Jöhr M. Inhalational anesthesia vs total intravenous anesthesia (TIVA) for pediatric anesthesia. Paediatr Anaesth 2009;19(5):521–534

[114] Satoh JI, Yamakage M, Kobayashi T, Tohse N, Watanabe H, Namiki A. Desflurane but not sevoflurane can increase lung resistance via tachykinin pathways. Br J Anaesth 2009;102(5):704–713

[115] TerRiet MF, DeSouza GJA, Jacobs JS, et al. Which is most pungent: isoflurane, sevoflurane or desflurane? Br J Anaesth 2000;85(2):305–307

[116] Joly V, Richebe P, Guignard B, et al. Remifentanil-induced postoperative hyperalgesia and its prevention with small-dose ketamine. Anesthesiology 2005;103(1):147–155

[117] Guignard B, Coste C, Costes H, et al. Supplementing desflurane-remifentanil anesthesia with small-dose ketamine reduces perioperative opioid analgesic requirements. Anesth Analg 2002; 95(1):103–108

[118] Becke K. Narkoseeinleitung bei Kindern. Anästh Intensivmed 2010;6:347–360

57

[119] Weinbroum AA, Weisenberg M, Rudick V, Geller E, Niv D. Flumazenil potentiation of postoperative morphine analgesia. Clin J Pain 2000;16(3):193–199

[120] Weinbroum AA, Flaishon R, Sorkine P, Szold O, Rudick V. A risk-benefit assessment of flumazenil in the management of benzodiazepine overdose. Drug Saf 1997;17(3):181–196 Review

[121] Weinbroum A, Halpern P, Geller E. The use of flumazenil in the management of acute drug poisoning--a review. Intensive Care Med 1991;17(Suppl 1):S32–S38

[122] Pergolizzi J, Aloisi AM, Dahan A, et al. Current knowledge of buprenorphine and its unique pharmacological profile. Pain Pract 2010;10(5):428–450

[123] Mathew R, Asimacopoulos E, Walker D, Gutierrez T, Valentine P, Pitkin L. Analysis of clinical negligence claims following tonsillectomy in England 1995 to 2010. Ann Otol Rhinol Laryngol 2012;121(5):337–340

[124] De Luca Canto G, Pachêco-Pereira C, Aydinoz S, et al. Adenotonsillectomy Complications: A Meta-analysis. Pediatrics 2015;136(4):702–718

[125] Weatherly RA, Mai EF, Ruzicka DL, Chervin RD. Identification and evaluation of obstructive sleep apnea prior to adenotonsillectomy in children: a survey of practice patterns. Sleep Med 2003;4(4):297–307

[126] Tom LW, DeDio RM, Cohen DE, Wetmore RF, Handler SD, Potsic WP. Is outpatient tonsillectomy appropriate for young children? Laryngoscope 1992;102(3):277–280

[127] Cohen D, Dor M. Morbidity and mortality of post-tonsillectomy bleeding: analysis of cases. J Laryngol Otol 2008;122(1):88–92

[128] Orestes MI, Lander L, Verghese S, Shah RK. Incidence of laryngospasm and bronchospasm in pediatric adenotonsillectomy. Laryngoscope 2012;122(2):425–428

[129] Peng A, Dodson KM, Thacker LR, Kierce J, Shapiro J, Baldassari CM. Use of laryngeal mask airway in pediatric adenotonsillectomy. Arch Otolaryngol Head Neck Surg 2011;137(1):42–46

[130] Roland PS, Rosenfeld RM, Brooks LJ, et al; American Academy of Otolaryngology–Head and Neck Surgery Foundation. Clinical practice guideline: Polysomnography for sleep-disordered breathing prior to tonsillectomy in children. Otolaryngol Head Neck Surg 2011;145(1, Suppl):S1–S15

[131] Rosen GM, Muckle RP, Mahowald MW, Goding GS, Ullevig C. Postoperative respiratory compromise in children with obstructive sleep apnea syndrome: can it be anticipated? Pediatrics 1994;93(5):784–788

[132] Liang C, Ruiz AG, Jensen EL, Friedman NR. Indications, clinical course, and postoperative outcomes of urgent adenotonsillectomy in children. JAMA Otolaryngol Head Neck Surg 2015;141(3):236–244

[133] Nafiu OO, Green GE, Walton S, Morris M, Reddy S, Tremper KK. Obesity and risk of peri-operative complications in children presenting for adenotonsillectomy. Int J Pediatr Otorhinolaryngol 2009;73(1):89–95

[134] Leong AC, Davis JP. Morbidity after adenotonsillectomy for paediatric obstructive sleep apnoea syndrome: waking up to a pragmatic approach. J Laryngol Otol 2007;121(9):809–817

[135] Lavin JM, Shah RK. Postoperative complications in obese children undergoing adenotonsillectomy. Int J Pediatr Otorhinolaryngol 2015;79(10):1732–1735

[136] Keamy DG, Chhabra KR, Hartnick CJ. Predictors of complications following adenotonsillectomy in children with severe obstructive sleep apnea. Int J Pediatr Otorhinolaryngol 2015; 79(11):1838–1841

[137] Fujii Y. Clinical management of postoperative vomiting after strabismus surgery in children. Curr Drug Saf 2010;5(2):132–148

[138] Amoils M, Chang KW, Saynina O, Wise PH, Honkanen A. Postoperative Complications in Pediatric Tonsillectomy and Adenoidectomy in Ambulatory vs Inpatient Settings. JAMA Otolaryngol Head Neck Surg 2016;142(4):344–350

[139] Biarent D, Bingham R, Richmond S, et al; European Resuscitation Council. European Resuscitation Council guidelines for resuscitation 2005. Section 6. Paediatric life support. Resuscitation 2005;67(Suppl 1):S97–S133

[140] El Rassi E, de Alarcon A, Lam D. Practice patterns in the management of post-tonsillectomy hemorrhage: An American Society of Pediatric Otolaryngology survey. Int J Pediatr Otorhinolaryngol 2017;102:108–113

[141] Lane JC, Dworkin-Valenti J, Chiodo L, Haupert M. Postoperative tonsillectomy bleeding complications in children: A comparison of three surgical techniques. Int J Pediatr Otorhinolaryngol 2016;88:184–188

[142] Schmidt J, Strauß JM, Becke K, Giest J, Schmitz B. Handlungsempfehlung zur Rapid-Sequence-Induction im Kindesalter. Anästh Intensivmed 2007;48:S88–S93

[143] Liu XY, Yang XQ, Xiao HJ, Ding J. [Comparison between continuous noninvasive hemoglobin monitoring and venous blood hemoglobin monitoring in children with kidney disease] Beijing Da Xue Xue Bao 2017;49(5):778–782

[144] Gamal M, Abdelhamid B, Zakaria D, et al. Evaluation of noninvasive hemoglobin monitoring in trauma patients with low hemoglobin levels. Shock 2018;49(2):150–153

[145] Deutsche Gesellschaft für Anästhesiologie und Intensivmedizin eV; Berufsverbandes Deutscher Anästhesisten eV. Mindestanforderungen an den anästhesiologischen Arbeitsplatz. Anästh Intensivmed. 2013;54:39–42

[146] Bhananker SM, Ramamoorthy C, Geiduschek JM, et al. Anesthesia-related cardiac arrest in children: update from the Pediatric Perioperative Cardiac Arrest Registry. Anesth Analg 2007;105(2):344–350

[147] Mamie C, Habre W, Delhumeau C, Argiroffo CB, Morabia A. Incidence and risk factors of perioperative respiratory adverse events in children undergoing elective surgery. Paediatr Anaesth 2004;14(3):218–224

[148] Christensen RE, Haydar B, Voepel-Lewis TD. Pediatric cardiopulmonary arrest in the postanesthesia care unit, rare but preventable: Analysis of data from Wake Up Safe, the Pediatric Anesthesia Quality Improvement Initiative. Anesth Analg 2017;124(4):1231–1236

[149] Serebrovskaya TV, Xi L. Intermittent hypoxia in childhood: the harmful consequences versus potential benefits of therapeutic uses. Front Pediatr 2015;3:44

[150] Biavati MJ, Manning SC, Phillips DL. Predictive factors for respiratory complications after tonsillectomy and adenoidectomy in children. Arch Otolaryngol Head Neck Surg 1997;123(5): 517–521

[151] Vlajkovic GP, Sindjelic RP. Emergence delirium in children: many questions, few answers. Anesth Analg 2007;104(1):84–91

[152] Kain ZN, Caldwell-Andrews AA, Maranets I, et al. Preoperative anxiety and emergence delirium and postoperative maladaptive behaviors. Anesth Analg 2004;99(6):1648–1654

[153] Dahmani S, Stany I, Brasher C, et al. Pharmacological prevention of sevoflurane- and desflurane-related emergence agitation in children: a meta-analysis of published studies. Br J Anaesth 2010;104(2):216–223

[154] Pieters BJ, Penn E, Nicklaus P, Bruegger D, Mehta B, Weatherly R. Emergence delirium and postoperative pain in children undergoing adenotonsillectomy: a comparison of propofol vs sevoflurane anesthesia. Paediatr Anaesth 2010;20(10):944–950

[155] Tramèr M, Moore A, McQuay H. Prevention of vomiting after paediatric strabismus surgery: a systematic review using the numbers-needed-to-treat method. Br J Anaesth 1995;75(5):556–561

[156] Sossai R, Jöhr M, Kistler W, Gerber H, Schärli AF. Postoperative vomiting in children. A persisting unsolved problem. Eur J Pediatr Surg 1993;3(4):206–208

[157] Büttner W, Finke W, Hilleke M, Reckert S, Vsianska L, Brambrink A. Entwicklung eines Fremdbeobach-tungsbogens zur Beurteilung des postoperativen Schmerzes bei Säuglingen. [Development of an observational scale for assessment of postoperative pain in infants] Anasthesiol Intensivmed Notfallmed Schmerzther 1998;33(6):353–361 [German]

[158] Antonis JH, Poeze M, Van Heurn LW. Boerhaave's syndrome in children: a case report and review of the literature. J Pediatr Surg 2006;41(9):1620–1623

[159] Eberhart LH, Geldner G, Kranke P, et al. The development and validation of a risk score to predict the probability of

postoperative vomiting in pediatric patients. Anesth Analg 2004;99(6):1630–1637

[160] Rüsch D, Eberhart LH, Wallenborn J, Kranke P. Nausea and vomiting after surgery under general anesthesia: an evidence-based review concerning risk assessment, prevention, and treatment. Dtsch Arztebl Int 2010;107(42):733–741

[161] Becke K, Kranke P, Weiss M, Kretz FJ. Risikoeinschätzung, Prophylaxe und Therapie von postoperativem Erbrechen im Kindesalter. Anästh Intensivmed 2007;9:S95–S98– [German]

[162] Kizilcik N, Bilgen S, Menda F, et al. Comparison of Dexamethasone-dimenhydrinate and dexamethasone-ondansetron in prevention of nausea and vomiting in postoperative patients. Aesthetic Plast Surg 2017;41(1):204–210

[163] Gheini S, Ameli S, Hoseini J. Effect of oral dimenhydrinate in children with acute gastroenteritis: A clinical trial. Oman Med J 2016;31(1):18–21

[164] Wimmer S, Neubert A, Rascher W. The safety of drug therapy in children. Dtsch Arztebl Int 2015;112(46):781–787– Review

[165] Sawicka KM, Goez H, Huntsman RJ. Successful treatment of paroxysmal movement disorders of Infancy with dimenhydrinate and diphenhydramine. Pediatr Neurol 2016;56:72–75

[166] Höhne C. Postoperative nausea and vomiting in pediatric anesthesia. Curr Opin Anaesthesiol 2014;27(3):303–308– Review

[167] Schimmer B, Parker K. ACTH. Adrenocortical steroids and their synthetic analogs. In: Hardman J, Limbird L, eds. Goodman and Gilman's The Pharmacological Basis of Therapeutics. New York, NY: McGraw-Hill; 1996: 1459–85

[168] Melby JC. Drug spotlight program: systemic corticosteroid therapy: pharmacology and endocrinologic considerations. Ann Intern Med 1974;81(4):505–512

[169] Czarnetzki C, Elia N, Lysakowski C, et al. Dexamethasone and risk of nausea and vomiting and postoperative bleeding after tonsillectomy in children: a randomized trial. JAMA 2008;300(22):2621–2630

[170] Becke K, Kranke P, Weiss M, Kretz FJ, Strauß J. Prophylaxe von postoperativer Übelkeit und Erbrechen im Kindesalter bei Adeno-Tonsillektomien mit Dexamethason. Stellungnahme des Wissenschaftlichen Arbeitskreises Kinderanästhesie der Deutschen Gesellschaft für Anästhesiologie und Intensivmedizin (DGAI). Anästh Intensivmed 2009;7:496–497

[171] Geralemou S, Gan TJ. Assessing the value of risk indices of postoperative nausea and vomiting in ambulatory surgical patients. Curr Opin Anaesthesiol 2016;29(6):668–673

[172] Ay AA, Kutun S, Ulucanlar H, Tarcan O, Demir A, Cetin A. Risk factors for postoperative ileus. J Korean Surg Soc 2011;81(4):242–249

[173] Asrani VM, Yoon HD, Megill RD, Windsor JA, Petrov MS. Interventions that affect gastrointestinal motility in hospitalized adult patients: a systematic review and meta-analysis of double-blind placebo-controlled randomized trials. Medicine (Baltimore) 2016;95(5):e2463

[174] Becke K. [Pediatric anesthesia in ear nose throat (ENT) surgery] Laryngorhinootologie 2014;93(Suppl 1):S150–S166– [German]

[175] Stoicea N, Gan TJ, Joseph N, et al. Alternative therapies for the prevention of postoperative nausea and vomiting. Front Med (Lausanne) 2015;2:87: Review

[176] Isaacson G. Tonsillectomy care for the pediatrician. Pediatrics 2012;130(2):324–334

[177] Le T, Drolet J, Parayno E, Rosmus C, Castiglione S. Follow-up phone calls after pediatric ambulatory surgery for tonsillectomy: what can we learn from families? J Perianesth Nurs 2007;22(4):256–264

[178] Fortier MA, MacLaren JE, Martin SR, Perret-Karimi D, Kain ZN. Pediatric pain after ambulatory surgery: where's the medication? Pediatrics 2009;124(4):e588–e595

[179] Huth MM, Broome ME. A snapshot of children's postoperative tonsillectomy outcomes at home. J Spec Pediatr Nurs 2007;12(3):186–195

[180] Schmidt R, Herzog A, Cook S, O'Reilly R, Deutsch E, Reilly J. Complications of tonsillectomy: a comparison of techniques. Arch Otolaryngol Head Neck Surg 2007;133(9):925–928

[181] Stewart DW, Ragg PG, Sheppard S, Chalkiadis GA. The severity and duration of postoperative pain and analgesia requirements in children after tonsillectomy, orchidopexy, or inguinal hernia repair. Paediatr Anaesth 2012;22(2):136–143

[182] Rodríguez MC, Villamor P, Castillo T. Assessment and management of pain in pediatric otolaryngology. Int J Pediatr Otorhinolaryngol 2016;90:138–149

[183] Chou R, Gordon DB, de Leon-Casasola OA, et al. Management of Postoperative Pain: A Clinical Practice Guideline From the American Pain Society, the American Society of Regional Anesthesia and Pain Medicine, and the American Society of Anesthesiologists' Committee on Regional Anesthesia, Executive Committee, and Administrative Council. J Pain 2016;17(2):131–157

[184] Papadatou D. Symptom care, pain assessment. In: Oxford Textbook of Palliative Care for Children, 1st ed. Goldman A, Hain R, Liben S, eds. Oxford University Press, 2006:Section 3, Chapter 34

[185] Johnston C, Campbell-Yeo M, Rich B, et al. Therapeutic touch is not therapeutic for procedural pain in very preterm neonates: a randomized trial. Clin J Pain 2013;29(9):824–829

[186] Ohlsson A, Shah PS. Paracetamol (acetaminophen) for prevention or treatment of pain in newborns. Cochrane Database Syst Rev 2016;10:CD011219

[187] Anand KJS, Hall RW, Desai N, et al; NEOPAIN Trial Investigators Group. Effects of morphine analgesia in ventilated preterm neonates: primary outcomes from the NEOPAIN randomised trial. Lancet 2004;363(9422):1673–1682

[188] Malviya S, Voepel-Lewis T, Burke C, Merkel S, Tait AR. The revised FLACC observational pain tool: improved reliability and validity for pain assessment in children with cognitive impairment. Paediatr Anaesth 2006;16(3):258–265

[189] Field MJ, Behrman RE, Eds. Institute of Medicine (U.S.). In: Committee on Palliative and End-of-Life Care for Children and Their Families. When Children Die: Improving Palliative and End-of-Life Care for Children and Their Families. Washington (DC), National Academies Press (US), 2003

[190] Fernandes AM, De Campos C, Batalha L, Perdigão A, Jacob E. Pain assessment using the adolescent pediatric pain tool: a systematic review. Pain Res Manag 2014;19(4):212–218– Review

[191] Daher A, Versloot J, Costa LR. The cross-cultural process of adapting observational tools for pediatric pain assessment: the case of the Dental Discomfort Questionnaire. BMC Res Notes 2014;7:897

[192] Freynhagen R, Baron R, Gockel U, Tölle TR. painDETECT: a new screening questionnaire to identify neuropathic components in patients with back pain. Curr Med Res Opin 2006;22(10):1911–1920

[193] Treede RD, Jensen TS, Campbell JN, et al. Neuropathic pain: redefinition and a grading system for clinical and research purposes. Neurology 2008;70(18):1630–1635

[194] Chidambaran V, Sadhasivam S. Pediatric acute and surgical pain management: recent advances and future perspectives. Int Anesthesiol Clin 2012;50(4):66–82

[195] Berde CB, Sethna NF. Analgesics for the treatment of pain in children. N Engl J Med 2002;347(14):1094–1103

[196] Breau LM, Camfield C, McGrath PJ, Rosmus C, Finley GA. Measuring pain accurately in children with cognitive impairments: refinement of a caregiver scale. J Pediatr 2001;138(5):721–727

[197] Breau LM, McGrath PJ, Camfield CS, Finley GA. Psychometric properties of the non-communicating children's pain checklist-revised. Pain 2002;99(1–2):349–357

[198] Breau LM, Finley GA, McGrath PJ, Camfield CS. Validation of the non-communicating children's pain checklist-postoperative version. Anesthesiology 2002;96(3):528–535

[199] Solodiuk J, Curley MA. Pain assessment in nonverbal children with severe cognitive impairments: the Individualized Numeric Rating Scale (INRS). J Pediatr Nurs 2003;18(4):295–299

[200] Strout TD, Baumann MR. Reliability and validity of the modified preverbal, early verbal pediatric pain scale in emergency department pediatric patients. Int Emerg Nurs 2011;19(4): 178–185

[201] Wong DL, Hockenberry-Eaton M, Wilson D, Winkelstein ML, Schwartz P. Wong's Essentials of Pediatric Nursing, 6th ed. St. Louis, MO: Mosby; 2001: 301

[202] McGrath PJ, Johnson G, Goodman JT, Dunn J, Chapman J. CHEOPS: A behavioral scale for rating postoperative pain in children. In: Fields HL, Dubner R, Cervero F, eds. Advances in Pain Research and Therapy. New York, NY: Raven Press; 1985: 395–402

[203] Stevens B. Development and testing of a pediatric pain management sheet. Pediatr Nurs 1990;16(6):543–548

[204] Schade JG, Joyce BA, Gerkensmeyer J, Keck JF. Comparison of three preverbal scales for postoperative pain assessment in a diverse pediatric sample. J Pain Symptom Manage 1996;12(6):348–359

[205] Voepel-Lewis T, Malviya S, Tait AR, et al. A comparison of the clinical utility of pain assessment tools for children with cognitive impairment. Anesth Analg 2008;106(1):72–78

[206] Casanova-García C, Lerma Lara S, Pérez Ruiz M, Ruano Domínguez D, Santana Sosa E. Non-pharmacological treatment for neuropathic pain in children with cancer. Med Hypotheses 2015;85(6):791–797

[207] Cunin-Roy C, Bienvenu M, Wood C. [Non-pharmacological methods for the treatment of pain in children and adolescents] Arch Pediatr 2007;14(12):1477–1480

[208] Cosio D, Lin EH. https://www.practicalpainmanagement.com/treatments/psychological/biofeedback/biofeedback-information-pain-management; accessed December 30, 2017

[209] Schwartz M, Andrasik F, eds. Biofeedback: A practitioner's guide. 3rd ed. New York, NY: Guilford Press; 2005

[210] Lang EV, Benotsch EG, Fick LJ, et al. Adjunctive non-pharmacological analgesia for invasive medical procedures: a randomised trial. Lancet 2000;355(9214):1486–1490

[211] Willmarth E, Willmarth K. Biofeedback and hypnosis in pain management. 2005. http://www.resourcenter.net/images/AAPB/Files/Biofeedback/2005/BIOF3301_20–24.pdf accessed December 30 2017

[212] Bayat A, Ramaiah R, Bhananker SM. Analgesia and sedation for children undergoing burn wound care. Expert Rev Neurother 2010;10(11):1747–1759

[213] Lin YC, Lee AC, Kemper KJ, Berde CB. Use of complementary and alternative medicine in pediatric pain management service: a survey. Pain Med 2005;6(6):452–458

[214] Lutgendorf SK, Lang EV, Berbaum KS, et al. Effects of age on responsiveness to adjunct hypnotic analgesia during invasive medical procedures. Psychosom Med 2007;69(2):191–199

[215] Kussman BD, Devavaram P, Hansen DD, et al. Anesthetic implications of primary cardiac tumors in infants and children. J Cardiothorac Vasc Anesth 2002;16(5):582–586

[216] Le May S, Ali S, Plint AC, et al; Pediatric Emergency Research Canada (PERC). Oral analgesics utilization for children with musculoskeletal injury (OUCH Trial): An RCT. Pediatrics 2017;140(5):e20170186

[217] Tan GX, Tunkel DE. Tunkel. Control of pain after tonsillectomy in children: A review. JAMA Otolaryngol Head Neck Surg 2017;143(9):937–942

[218] Kimiaei Asadi H, Nikooseresht M, Noori L, Behnoud F. The Effect of administration of ketamine and paracetamol versus paracetamol singly on postoperative pain, nausea and vomiting after pediatric adenotonsillectomy. Anesth Pain Med 2016;6(1):e31210

[219] Lauder G, Emmott A. Confronting the challenges of effective pain management in children following tonsillectomy. Int J Pediatr Otorhinolaryngol 2014;78(11):1813–1827

[220] Kravitz ND. The use of compound topical anesthetics: a review. J Am Dent Assoc 2007;138(10):1333–1339, quiz 1382

[221] Blanton PL, Jeske AH. Dental local anesthetics: alternative delivery methods. J Am Dent Assoc 2003;134(2):228–234

[222] Harvey M, Elliott M. Transcutaneous electrical nerve stimulation (TENS) for pain management during cavity preparations in pediatric patients. ASDC J Dent Child 1995;62(1):49–51

[223] Rajan S, Puthenveettil N, Paul J. Transtracheal lidocaine: An alternative to intraoperative propofol infusion when muscle relaxants are not used. J Anaesthesiol Clin Pharmacol 2014;30(2):199–202

[224] Lee SY, Min JJ, Kim HJ, Hong DM, Kim HJ, Park HP. Hemodynamic effects of topical lidocaine on the laryngoscope blade and trachea during endotracheal intubation: a prospective, double-blind, randomized study. J Anesth 2014;28(5):668–675

[225] Taghavi Gilani M, Miri Soleimani I, Razavi M, Salehi M. Reducing sore throat following laryngeal mask airway insertion: comparing lidocaine gel, saline, and washing mouth with the control group. Braz J Anesthesiol 2015;65(6):450–454

[226] Fuller PB. The relationship between preintubation lidocaine and postanesthesia sore throat. AANA J 1992;60(4):374–378

[227] World Health Organization. Common Surgical Problems—Pain Control, the Pocket Book of Hospital Care for Children: Guidelines for the Management of Common Childhood Illnesses. 2nd ed. Geneva; 2013: 262

[228] Wilson CA, Sommerfield D, Drake-Brockman TF, von Bieberstein L, Ramgolam A, von Ungern-Sternberg BS. Pain after discharge following head and neck surgery in children. Paediatr Anaesth 2016;26(10):992–1001

[229] Weinbroum AA, Zur E. Patient-tailored combinations of systemic and topical preparations for localized peripheral neuropathic pain: a two-case report. J Pain Palliat Care Pharmacother 2015;29(1):27–33

[230] Hauer J. Identifying and managing sources of pain and distress in children with neurological impairment. Pediatr Ann 2010;39(4):198–205, quiz 232–234

[231] Gutstein HB, Akil H. Opioids, analgesia and pain management. In: Goodman and Gilman's Pharmacological basis of therapeutics, 12th ed, New York, NY: McGraw-Hill; 2011:498

[232] Klick JC, Hauer J. Pediatric palliative care. Curr Probl Pediatr Adolesc Health Care 2010;40(6):120–151

[233] 2016 Pediatric Medication Handbook. The Children's Hospital of the King's Daughters, Norfolk, VA, US. http://www.chkd.org/uploadedFiles/Documents/Medical_Professionals/PedMedHandbook.pdf; accessed December 30, 2017

[234] Hearn L, Derry S, Moore RA. Single dose dipyrone (metamizole) for acute postoperative pain in adults. Cochrane Database Syst Rev 2016;4:CD011421

[235] Basker S, Singh G, Jacob R. Clonidine in paediatrics: a review. Indian J Anaesth 2009;53(3):270–280

[236] Gerlach AT, Murphy CV, Dasta JF. An updated focused review of dexmedetomidine in adults. Ann Pharmacother 2009;43(12):2064–2074

[237] https://reference.medscape.com/drug/precedex-dexmedetomidine-342932: Dexmedetomidine dosing information; accessed December 30, 2017

[238] Hauer JM, Solodiuk JC. Gabapentin for management of recurrent pain in 22 nonverbal children with severe neurological impairment: a retrospective analysis. J Palliat Med 2015;18(5): 453–456

[239] Amin SM. Evaluation of gabapentin and dexamethasone alone or in combination for pain control after adenotonsillectomy in children. Saudi J Anaesth 2014;8(3):317–322

[240] Tsai KC, Yang YL, Fan PC. Gabapentin for postoperative vomiting in children requiring posterior fossa tumor resection. Pediatr Neonatol 2015;56(5):351–354

[241] Amin SM, Amr YM. Comparison between preemptive gabapentin and paracetamol for pain control after adenotonsillectomy in children. Anesth Essays Res 2011;5(2):167–170

[242] Schechter NL, Berde CB, Yaster M. Pain in infants, children, and adolescents. 2nd ed. Lexi-Comp's Pediatric Dosage Handbook.

15th ed. Philadelphia, PA: Lippincott Williams and Wilkins; 2003: 471–86

[243] Gray P, Kirby J, Smith MT, et al. Pregabalin in severe burn injury pain: a double-blind, randomised placebo-controlled trial. Pain 2011;152(6):1279–1288

[244] Gutstein HB, Johnson KL, Heard MB, Gregory GA. Oral ketamine preanesthetic medication in children. Anesthesiology 1992;76(1):28–33

[245] Bredlau AL, Thakur R, Korones DN, Dworkin RH. Ketamine for pain in adults and children with cancer: a systematic review and synthesis of the literature. Pain Med 2013;14(10):1505–1517

[246] Gyanesh P, Haldar R, Srivastava D, Agrawal PM, Tiwari AK, Singh PK. Comparison between intranasal dexmedetomidine and intranasal ketamine as premedication for procedural sedation in children undergoing MRI: a double-blind, randomized, placebo-controlled trial. J Anesth 2014;28(1):12–18

[247] Sawynok J. Topical and peripheral ketamine as an analgesic. Anesth Analg 2014;119(1):170–178

[248] McNulty JP, Hahn K. Compounded oral ketamine. Int J Pharm Compd 2012;16(5):364–368

[249] Pashankar DS. Childhood constipation: evaluation and management. Clin Colon Rectal Surg 2005;18(2):120–127

4 Imaging of the Pediatric Head and Neck

Shelly I. Shiran

Summary

When evaluating head and neck pathology in children judicious use of imaging modalities can aid the physician with diagnosis, treatment planning, and follow-up. As in any aspect of caring for children, referring a child to imaging requires risk versus benefit assessment and avoiding unnecessary examinations.

Important Safety considerations include level of radiation exposure, need for sedation, and intravenous (IV) contrast related complications. The absence of ionizing radiation or need of sedation makes ultrasound (US) the initial imaging of choice for most cases of pediatric neck pathology.

A cross-sectional imaging study is indicated for either further assessment of an US diagnosed lesion or as initial evaluation for suspected skull base or facial pathology. When this is indicated a child may be referred to computed tomography (CT) study or magnetic resonance imaging (MRI) study depending on the diagnostic question. CT will be the initial study of choice in the setting of head trauma or cases of complicated sinusitis and mastoiditis where contrast injection is indicated. In the setting of suspected skull base or facial mass, referring a child to an MRI study for initial evaluation can be justified. It is important to note that in pathologies involving skull and facial bones MRI and CT studies have a complementary role.

Keywords: Imaging modalities, imaging safety, CT, MRI, US

4.1 Introduction

When evaluating head and neck pathology in children, the use of imaging modalities can aid the physician with diagnosis, treatment planning, and follow-up. Specifically, for the pediatric ENT surgeon, the use of imaging is crucial for surgery planning and for image-guided navigation systems. The modalities available for imaging the pediatric head and neck can be divided into two groups on the basis of related exposure of the patient to ionizing radiation. Radiography, fluoroscopy, CT and nuclear medicine (NM) studies all expose the imaged patient to different degrees of ionizing radiation; US and MRI do not.

When imaging children there are unique safety issues regarding radiation exposure and sedation, which differ from the adult population and need to be addressed when referring a child for a diagnostic study. In the following chapter, safety issues will be discussed, the different imaging modalities will be described, and the proper diagnostic workup will be recommended.[1–3]

4.2 Pediatric Imaging Safety

4.2.1 Radiation Safety

In the last 20 years, following the increased usage of CT studies in medicine, there has been increased awareness of radiation burden from imaging studies especially in the pediatric population.[4,5] Children are more sensitive to radiation effect due to higher effective dose per delivered dose in a smaller patient compared to a larger patient (infant vs. adult), and due to a longer expected life span for carcinogenic changes to take place. This highlighted the importance of reducing the radiation exposure to children by adjusting the technique.[6] Since the society of pediatric radiology launched the "Image gently" campaign,[7] pediatric imaging centers adopted dedicated protocols adjusted to child's size and age to reduce the delivered effective dose, in compliance with two major concepts:

1. The linear, no-threshold model, which states that no level of radiation exposure is without risk.
2. The ALARA (As Low As Reasonably Achievable) concept, where studies are performed with lowest radiation dose possible to still produce a diagnostic study. This has become an important guideline in pediatric radiology practice.[2]

In recent years two large cohort studies were published that demonstrated relative increased risk for developing certain malignancies following diagnostic CT exposure in childhood.[8,9] These studies gained media attention and caused concern to parents. The main teaching points from these studies are that the relative increased risk per mGy of exposure is small but present, this relative increased risk is more substantial the younger the patient is at the time of exposure, especially below 5 years of age and that there is an accumulative effect from multiple studies. For sake of discussion, mGy is the measuring unit for radiation exposure and mSv is the measuring unit for effective dose (1 mSv = 1 mGy). Pearce et al[9] demonstrated excessive relative risk (ERR) of 0.023 per mGy (range 0.010–0.049) for brain tumors. However, for patients who received a cumulative dose of 50–74 mGy (mean dose 60.42 mGy) the ERR for developing brain cancer was 2.82 (1.33–6.03). In their study patients received 5 to 10 mGy per brain CT, which puts a child in relative increased risk to develop brain tumor after having 5 to 10 CT studies of the head. One should remember that these studies evaluated exposure to CT imaging prior to low-dose pediatric protocols adjustments. In an attempt to assess the impact of head and neck CT in children, Chen et al[10] reviewed the literature and found limited data regarding the effect of otolaryngological imaging (i.e., temporal bone, sinus, neck). In modern pediatric imaging facilities, the expected effective dose from a single brain CT is around 2 mSv and the expected dose from a facial or temporal bone CT is around 1 mSv. ▶ Table 4.1 lists the expected effective dose from additional common imaging studies. With these lower dose imaging protocols and by avoiding multiple repeat studies, the actual increased relative risk for the individual patient should be very small. In addition, advances in technology and post processing algorithms bring to the medical world new faster CT machines that will further decrease radiation exposure as these will become more prevalent in imaging facilities.

4.2.2 Sedation

In recent years there have been experimental animal studies followed by retrospective population studies that raised concern regarding increased risk for neurodevelopmental pathology in children who were exposed to anesthetic substances in early infancy. To date, no scientific evidence is available to support a change in pediatric anesthesia practice, and the scientific community is awaiting results of large population prospective studies that are being performed. However, as young children need sedation for several imaging studies, this concern should be addressed.[11] Out of all imaging studies performed, the largest number of children requiring sedation is at the MRI suit. MRI is sensitive to motion artifact and a good quality MRI study requires cooperation of the patient with holding still for a substantial length of time, 20 to 60 min, depending on the type of study. For young children, this means that sedation is required; a child can be sedated with moderate sedation or general anesthesia depending on the child's clinical condition and the anesthesiologist preference. Efforts to decrease the number of children requiring sedation for their MRI study include the development of motion-insensitive fast imaging sequences, as well as developing age-appropriate protocols.

It is possible to image neonates without sedation with proper feeding prior to the study, careful attention to noise and light reduction, using ear muffles, wrapping and swaddling the patients and keeping them warm. Infants and children up to 6-year-old usually require sedation. For children 6- to 10-year-old the ability to hold still may vary. In some pediatric imaging centers, a "test" study or a mock exam can be performed for each child prior to the scheduled study to decide whether sedation is needed. Using an MRI video and audio system, which creates a movie theater experience by wearing specialized goggles, can further decrease the need for sedation. Sedation is also needed for non-cooperative children undergoing a CT study, though these are much shorter studies in the range of a few minutes. Future newer faster CT scanners may obliviate the need for sedation completely. Additional studies that may require sedation are PET-CT and interventional radiology procedures.

4.3 The Imaging Modalities

4.3.1 Ultrasound

The absence of ionizing radiation or need of sedation makes US the initial imaging of choice for most cases of pediatric neck pathology that require additional evaluation to supplement the physical exam. US is an imaging modality based on detection and display of acoustic energy reflected from interfaces within the body. On US, fluid is hypoechoic (dark) with through-transmission, fat is hyperechoic (bright), air and bone will create acoustic shadowing, eliminating evaluation of deeper structures (▶ Fig. 4.1a). An US study may be sufficient for diagnosis, especially in evaluation of a focal mass, parotid space lesions (▶ Fig. 4.2a), or thyroid pathology.[12] In addition to US a Doppler study can be obtained that will add information regarding vascularity of a focal lesion (▶ Fig. 4.1a and ▶ Fig. 4.2b) and patency of the carotid sheath vessels. US is an excellent method for

Table 4.1 Mean effective dose for patients from common pediatric radiology studies with correlation to effective dose from natural background radiation

Examination	Dose (mSv)	Time period for equivalent effective dose from natural background radiation
Chest PA radiograph	0.02	2.4 days
Skull lateral radiograph	0.02	2.4 days
Panoramic dental radiograph	0.015	1.8 days
Barium swallow	0.6	72 days
Head CT	2.0	240 days
Facial bones CT	1.0	120 days
Temporal bones CT	1.0	120 days
FDG-PET-CT	15	1800 days

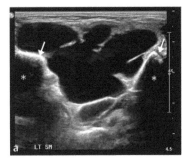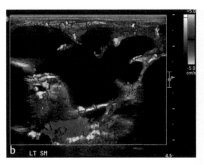

Fig. 4.1 A 2-year-old girl presented with left submandibular swelling. A US study **(a)** demonstrates a multilobulated space-occupying lesion of low echogenicity consistent with fluid. Increased echogenicity in soft tissue deep into the lesion compared to soft tissue anterior to the lesion is related to enhanced through-transmission typical to fluid. The dark regions (*) on both sides of the image are related to acoustic shadowing from mandible (*arrows*). A US-Doppler study **(b)** demonstrates no flow within the lesion. The findings are consistent with a lymphatic malformation.

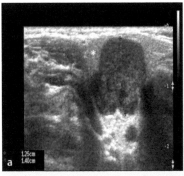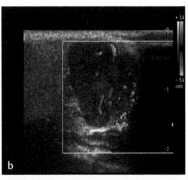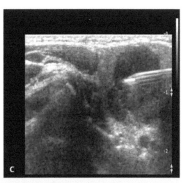

Fig. 4.2 A 10-year-old girl presented with a right-sided parotid focal mass. A US study **(a)** demonstrates a focal, round, space-occupying lesion which is hypoechoic compared to normal parotid tissue (*). A US-Doppler study **(b)** demonstrated increased vascularity within the lesion. A US-guided fine needle biopsy was performed, with the needle appearing as a linear hyperechoic structure with acoustic shadowing, positioned within the lesion **(c)**. Pleomorphic adenoma was diagnosed.

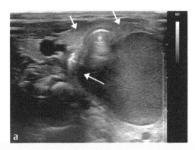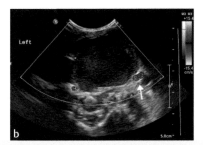

Fig. 4.3 A 4-week-old infant had feeding difficulties and left neck swelling. A US study **(a)** demonstrated a large cystic mass in the left neck with internal low-level echoes which reflect complicated fluid. The mass extended to the retropharyngeal space (*arrow*) displacing the trachea (*), which can be recognized by the echogenic artifact of air within it. There was also mass effect and displacement of the thyroid gland (*short arrows*). A US-Doppler study **(b)** demonstrated no internal vascularity. The left carotid sheath vessels were effaced and displaced laterally and posteriorly (*arrow*). To evaluate the full extent of this space-occupying lesion and to better characterize it, an MRI study was performed ▶Fig. 4.15).

guiding procedures such as fine needle aspiration (FNA) (▶Fig. 4.2c) or abscess drainage.

It is also a preferred method for following progression or regression of a lesion. When a diffuse pathologic process is evaluated, US may not be able to assess the full extent and additional cross-sectional imaging, such as CT or MRI, will be needed. This is especially important for processes extending towards skull base, as US cannot penetrate the skull base bone, and for lesions involving retropharyngeal space or extending into the mediastinum (▶Fig. 4.3).

In recent years US has gained popularity as a bedside tool in the hand of the emergency room or ICU physician for point-of-care US; this may serve for assessing intubation tube placement.[13] Studies published in recent years are suggesting expanding US interrogation of the neck to include assessment of laryngeal structures, as the vocal cords can be assessed in children through the uncalcified cartilage (▶Fig. 4.4), and assessment of tonsillar and peritonsillar infections (▶Fig. 4.5).

In the adult literature, the use of contrast-enhanced US of the neck is being evaluated for differentiating benign from malignant thyroid nodules or lymph nodes; this may expand to the pediatric population in the future.

The main limitation of US is that the quality of the study and related interpretation depends on the skills of the examiner; it is advisable to have children examined by specifically trained personnel.

4.3.2 Cross-sectional Imaging

A cross-sectional imaging study is indicated for either further assessment of a US diagnosed lesion (▶Fig. 4.5) or as initial evaluation for suspected skull base pathology. When this is indicated a child may be referred to CT study or MRI study depending on the diagnostic question.

Computed Tomography

With the development of multi-detector CT (MDCT) the scan time has decreased significantly to the point where

children can be scanned with very short sedation time or no sedation at all. CT with IV contrast injection will allow good evaluation of the soft tissue of the neck, although, differentiating between soft tissue structures is more challenging in infants and young children than in

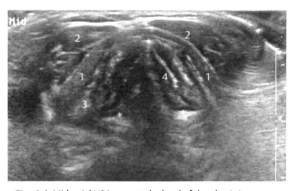

Fig. 4.4 Mid-axial US image at the level of the glottis in an 8-year-old boy. The thyroid cartilage has an inverse V shape and hyperechoic margins (1). Anterior to the thyroid cartilage the anterior superficial muscles of the neck are visible (2). Deep to the thyroid cartilage the paraglottic fat is hyperechoic (3), the muscles and process of the true vocal cords are relative hypoechoic (4). The arytenoids are seen as two triangular structures deep into the vocal folds (*).

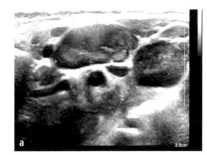
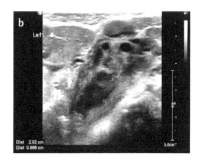
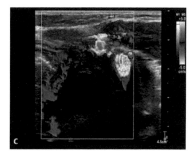
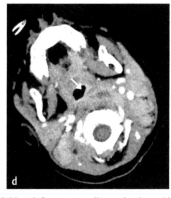
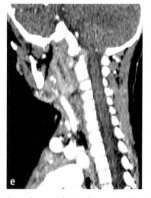

Fig. 4.5 An 18-month-old child with fever, torticollis, and enlarged lymph nodes on physical examination. A US study was performed to assess for lymphadenitis. The US study demonstrated enlarged reactive lymph nodes in the left neck without areas of necrosis **(a)**. Deep to the carotid space a hypoechoic oval lesion was demonstrated with increased echogenicity of the adjacent fat **(b)** and no internal vascularity on Doppler study **(c)** suspected for a retropharyngeal abscess. A contrast-enhanced CT study was performed; an axial image at the level of the oropharynx **(d)** and a sagittal reformat image **(e)** demonstrate a retropharyngeal phlegmon involving nasopharyngeal and oropharyngeal spaces on the left with central hypodensity consistent with abscess formation. There is mild airway effacement (*arrow* on d) and extensive enlargement of lymph nodes in the left neck **(d)**.

adults due to lower amount of visceral fat. The exam is performed with very thin, sub-millimeter, section thickness creating isotropic voxels, which enable multi-plane reformats to be created based on the axial data with similar spatial resolution. In addition, three-dimensional (3D) image reconstruction, including volume-rendered imaging and virtual bronchoscopy, can be obtained. Due to high contrast between air and soft tissue, CT is well suited for airway evaluation (▶ Fig. 4.6). CT is excellent for assessing the bone structure and calcifications in the soft tissue. The superior bone detail in a CT study makes it indispensable when evaluating pathologies of skull base and facial bones (▶ Fig. 4.7).

Availability of CT and the speed of the exam make it particularly useful in the emergency room setting, as in the setting of trauma or pre-surgical evaluation of acute retropharyngeal abscess (▶ Fig. 4.5). Facial trauma is one of the few indications for CT as the initial study of choice (▶ Fig. 4.8).

When there is a specific diagnostic question related to the blood vessels of the neck, a CT angiogram (CTA) can be performed with excellent diagnostic information, saving an invasive angiogram for when treatment procedures are needed (▶ Fig. 4.9 and ▶ Fig. 4.10). The study requires at least a 24-gauge angiocatheter, preferably in the hand. Low osmolar, nonionic iodine contrast media is injected with the timing of the scan aimed at optimizing enhancement of the investigated vessels.

In addition to radiation concern there are contrast-related safety issues. The main adverse effects from a contrast-enhanced CT or CTA study are either allergic reactions ranging from mild urticaria to anaphylactic shock, or contrast-induced nephropathy which is especially important in children with underlying renal disease.

Magnetic Resonance Imaging

Magnetic resonance imaging (MRI) is based on magnetic spin properties of protons. Different sequences highlight different tissue properties and thereby allow superb soft

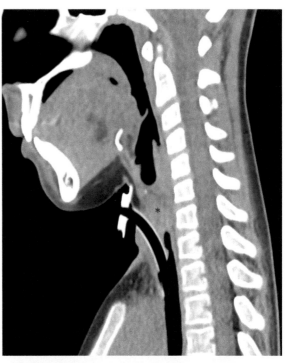

Fig. 4.6 A 6-year-old child with chronic tracheostomy was evaluated for possible tracheoplasty surgery. A sagittal reformat image from a non-enhanced neck CT demonstrates thick granulation tissue (*) obstructing the sub-glottic trachea above the tracheostomy tube.

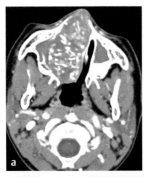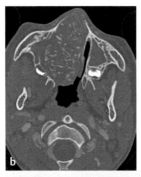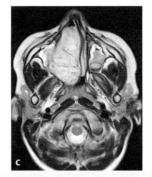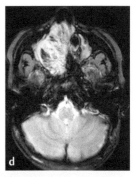

Fig. 4.7 A 14-year-old boy with nasal obstruction was diagnosed with nasal chondrosarcoma. A contrast-enhanced CT was performed [soft tissue window **(a)**; bone window **(b)**] demonstrating a mass in the right sinonasal region with multiple calcifications of "ring and arc" pattern typical for chondral lesions. The typical pattern of calcification is harder to discern on the MRI study of the face. They appear as some linear areas of hypointense signal on axial T2W image **(c)** correlated to increased susceptibility artifact on susceptibility weighted image (SWI) **(d)** consistent with either calcifications or hemosiderin deposits.

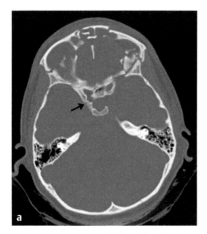 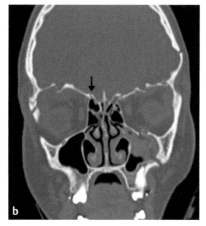 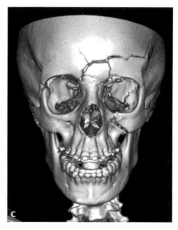

Fig. 4.8 A 12-year-old child after high-impact head trauma. A non-contrast CT study of the head was done and bone window images [axial **(a)**; coronal reformat **(b)**] demonstrate comminuted fractures of bilateral orbital roof and lateral wall, left orbital floor, left lateral maxillary wall, bilateral frontal sinuses with involvement of anterior and posterior walls. Fracture lines extend to involve sphenoid and ethmoid roof (*arrows*). A non-displaced fracture is seen in the occipital bone. Based on the axial images a 3D volume rendering image can be created **(c)**.

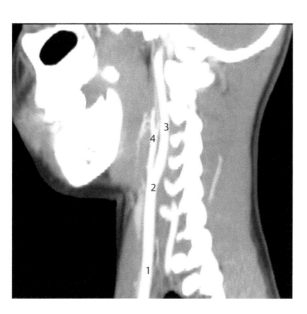

Fig. 4.9 CTA of the neck with MIP reformat of a normal carotid bifurcation. Common carotid artery (CCA, 1), carotid bifurcation (2), internal carotid artery (ICA, 3), external carotid artery (ECA, 4). CTA, Computed tomography angiography; MIP, maximum intensity projection.

tissue contrast and more specific characterization of pathologic tissue.

The basic MRI sequences are T1-weighted (T1W), T2-weighted (T2W), and proton density–weighted (PD) with possible addition of fat suppression or fluid suppression. On T1-weighted images fluid will be hypointense (dark); fat, high concentration of protein, acute blood products, and melanin will appear hyperintense (bright). On T2-weighted images fluid will be hyper-intense; fibrotic changes, calcifications, and hemosiderin will be hypo-intense (▶Fig. 4.11).

In recent years diffusion-weighted imaging (DWI), which is based on hydrogen proton diffusivity in tissue, is a sensitive adjunct for diagnosis of lesions and is now an important part of head and neck imaging protocol. Based on the diffusion-weighted signal an apparent diffusion coefficient (ADC) can be calculated. ADC values tend to be high in areas of increased tissue permeability or excess free water, such as in areas of necrosis, and tend to be low in areas of high cellularity, such as in tumors (▶Fig. 4.12), or areas of high viscosity, such as pus or in dermoid cyst (▶Fig. 4.13).

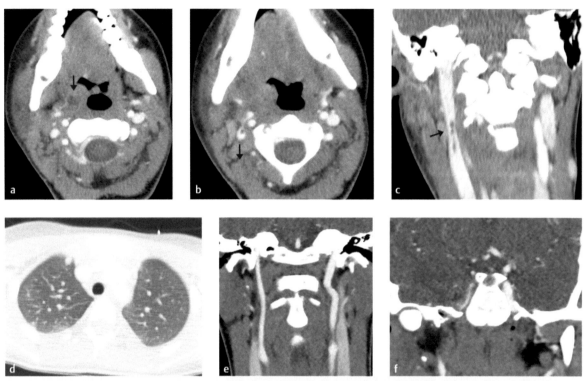

Fig. 4.10 A 13-year-old girl was hospitalized with sepsis and neck swelling. A contrast-enhanced CT study of the neck demonstrated fat stranding and soft tissue swelling involving all spaces of the right neck. Swelling with central hypodensity is seen in the right tonsillar region (*arrow*, **a**), a filling defect is noted in the right internal jugular vein (IJV) (*arrow*, **b** and **c**) consistent with thrombus. In addition, lung windows through the lung apex **(d)** revealed nodular opacities consistent with septic emboli. The findings were consistent with Lemierre's syndrome. The patient developed sixth cranial nerve palsy, and a follow-up CTA **(e, f)** demonstrated mild narrowing of the right neck internal carotid artery (ICA) and significant narrowing of the intracranial cavernous ICA, related to skull base extension of the infectious process.

Diffusion imaging has an important role in assessing tumor characteristics and is being investigated as a tool for treatment response evaluation in adult head and neck cancer[14] on its own and in conjugation with perfusion study; the role of these advanced techniques in pediatric head and neck cancer will likely expand. Another important role for diffusion imaging is in the diagnosis of cholesteatoma (▶Fig. 4.14).

MR angiography (MRA) can be added for evaluation of the neck vasculature; this can be performed without injection of contrast using time of flight (TOF) or phase-contrast techniques or post-contrast dynamic MRA (▶Fig. 4.15).

Intravenous gadolinium–based contrast injection will further highlight pathologic processes and is indispensable for diagnosis and follow-up of oncologic pathologies; however, a few safety issues regarding gadolinium should be addressed. Due to the association between chronic renal insufficiency, gadolinium administration, and the development of nephrogenic systemic sclerosis (NSF), patients with renal insufficiency should have their GFR calculated and if below 30, IV gadolinium administration should be avoided, unless crucial for patient care.[15] In recent years data has been accumulated regarding gadolinium retention in basal ganglia and dentate nuclei of the brain following multiple administrations, but no correlation to specific morbidity has been found to date. Based on safety profile of different gadolinium agents, they have been divided into three groups (ACR NSF safety group), where group 2 agents are recommended for use in pediatric patients when gadolinium injection cannot be avoided. MRI safety requires also screening for any device or object that may interact with the magnetic field, for example, odontogenic braces or cardiac pacemaker. Odontogenic braces may cause significant artifact that can obscure facial and skull base structures. Referring a child with braces to an MRI study requires removal of the braces prior to the study.

Additional limitations of MRI are high cost and relative decreased availability worldwide.

4.3.3 Radiography and Fluoroscopy

Radiography and fluoroscopy are two imaging modalities whose use has decreased significantly in head and neck imaging since the introduction of direct endoscopic inspection as part of the routine ENT physical exam.

Plain films are still useful for assessing the upper airway due to excellent contrast between the air column and the adjacent soft tissue. A good-technique lateral film of the neck with optimal positioning (neutral position, closed

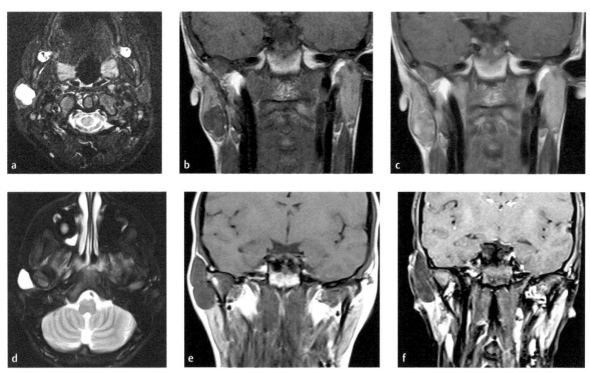

Fig. 4.11 Two patients with focal right parotid space lesion. ▶Fig. 4.10**a–c** are from a staging MRI prior to surgery for resection of pleomorphic adenoma of the right parotid space (same patient as ▶Fig. 4.2). Axial T2W image with fat suppression **(a)** demonstrates very high T2 signal in the lesion, which is well circumscribed. Coronal T1W image **(b)** shows the lesion with low T1 signal compared to the parotid gland. Coronal T1W image post gadolinium injection **(c)** demonstrates marked enhancement. The imaging features are typical for pleomorphic adenoma and in this case no extra parotid extension is demonstrated. ▶Fig. 4.10**d–f** are from an MRI study of a 3-year-old boy with facial swelling. On axial T2W image with fat suppression **(d)** the signal is hyperintense and isointense to CSF. On Coronal T1W image **(e)** the signal is hypointense, slightly higher than CSF. These features are consistent with fluid with minimal increased protein concentration compared to simple fluid. T1W image after gadolinium injection **(f)** demonstrates no enhancement. The anatomic position and the signal characteristics are consistent with first branchial cleft cyst. These two cases demonstrate the importance of analyzing the signal characteristics in all the study sequences in order to arrive at a proper diagnosis or differential diagnosis.

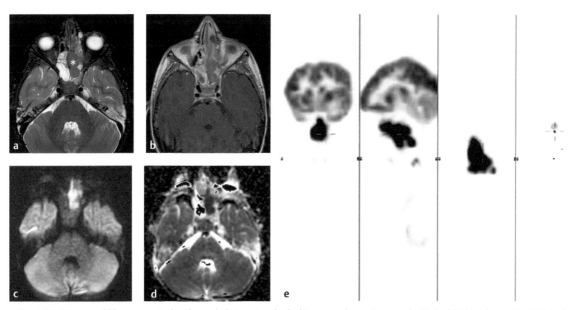

Fig. 4.12 A 5-year-old boy presented with nasal obstruction, had a biopsy, and was diagnosed with Burkitt lymphoma. An MRI study was performed prior to the biopsy. Axial T2W image with fat suppression **(a)** helps to differentiate between the hypointense tumor mass in the left sinonasal space (*, **a**) to the hyperintense mucosal thickening and fluid in the right sinonasal space. The mass is homogenous and mildly enhancing on the T1W image after gadolinium injection **(b)**. Axial diffusion-weighted imaging (DWI) **(c)** and apparent diffusion coefficient (ADC) **(d)** images demonstrate high signal on DWI and low signal on ADC consistent with restricted diffusion, which is typical in tumors where there is high nucleus-to-cytoplasm ratio. The FDG-PET study **(e)** demonstrates high uptake of FDG in the sinonasal region without additional tumor sites.

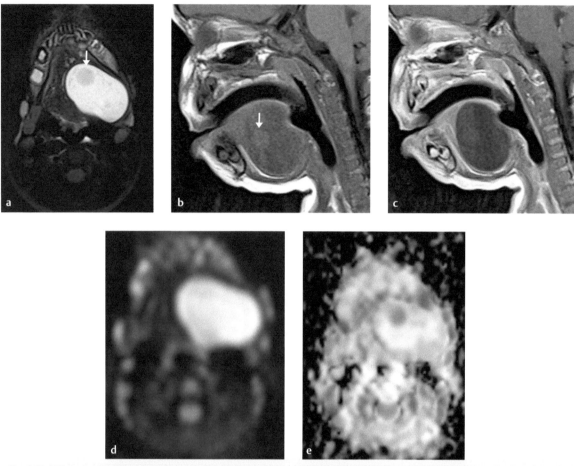

Fig. 4.13 MRI study of a child with floor-of-mouth dermoid cyst. Axial T2W image **(a)** demonstrates a well-circumscribed large cystic mass with areas of internal nodular T2 hypointensity (*arrow*). Sagittal T1W image **(b)** and sagittal T1W post-contrast image **(c)** demonstrate slight increased T1 signal in the internal nodule (*arrow*, **b**) and no enhancement. Diffusion-weighted imaging (DWI) image **(d)** and apparent diffusion coefficient (ADC) map **(e)** demonstrate that the mass is mostly cystic with focal-restricted diffusion in the internal nodule. These complex imaging features suggested that this cystic mass is a dermoid cyst, as was proven post-surgical excision, and not a ranula as was presumed by the referring physician.

mouth, inspiratory phase) will allow evaluation of the size of the adenoids and tonsils and related airway narrowing, pathologic thickening of the retropharyngeal soft tissue (as can be seen in retropharyngeal abscess), and evaluation of the epiglottis, aryepiglottic folds, and sub-glottic airway (▶ Fig. 4.16). The sub-glottic trachea is well seen on chest X-rays, which allows evaluation for sub-glottic stenosis (▶ Fig. 4.17).

Fluoroscopy is still a valuable technique for assessing the swallow mechanism using videofluoroscopy technique, and for evaluation of the esophagus. Airway fluoroscopy in children with stridor will demonstrate physiologic respiratory cycle change in airway caliber in case of laryngomalacia or tracheomalacia, although this is usually evaluated on laryngoscopy and bronchoscopy. Referral to interventional radiology fluoroscopy guided procedures in children is reserved mainly for treating vascular malformations, or for embolization prior to tumor resection, as in juvenile nasopharyngeal angiofibroma (JNA) (▶ Fig. 4.18). In modern fluoroscopy machines, a pulse technique is used to reduce the delivered radiation dose, and a time limit for the exam is kept, to avoid direct radiation effects such as erythema.

4.3.4 Nuclear Medicine

Nuclear medicine studies for evaluation of head and neck pathology include mainly thyroid scintigraphy and

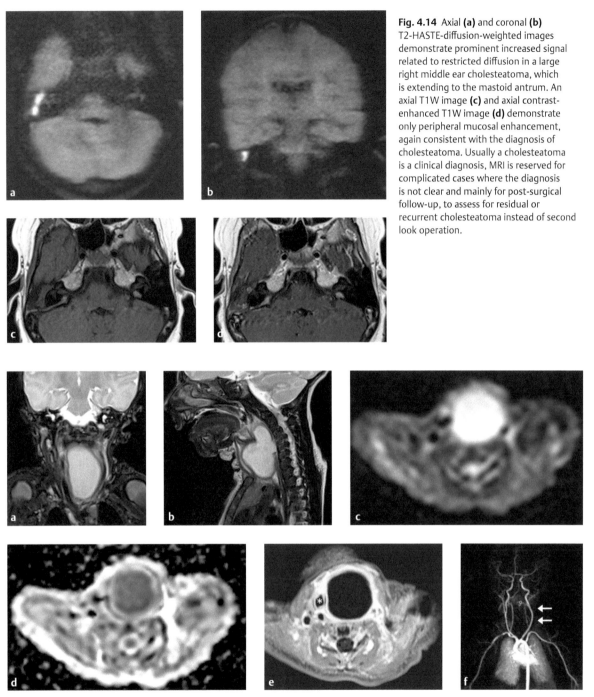

Fig. 4.14 Axial **(a)** and coronal **(b)** T2-HASTE-diffusion-weighted images demonstrate prominent increased signal related to restricted diffusion in a large right middle ear cholesteatoma, which is extending to the mastoid antrum. An axial T1W image **(c)** and axial contrast-enhanced T1W image **(d)** demonstrate only peripheral mucosal enhancement, again consistent with the diagnosis of cholesteatoma. Usually a cholesteatoma is a clinical diagnosis, MRI is reserved for complicated cases where the diagnosis is not clear and mainly for post-surgical follow-up, to assess for residual or recurrent cholesteatoma instead of second look operation.

Fig. 4.15 A 4-week-old infant had feeding difficulties and left neck swelling. A US study demonstrated a large cystic mass in the left neck (same patient as ▶ Fig. 4.3). Coronal T2W image with fat suppression **(a)** and sagittal T2W image **(b)** demonstrate the full extent of the lesion, from the level of the oropharynx-hypopharynx junction to the level of the chest inlet. DWI **(c)** and ADC **(d)** images demonstrate that the fluid within the mass is restricted, consistent with high viscosity. Fat-suppressed T1W image post-contrast injection **(e)** demonstrates enhancement of the cyst wall with no internal enhancement, and displacement of the trachea (*). Contrast-enhanced time-resolved MRA study **(f)** shows the left CCA and carotid bifurcation mildly displaced to the left (*arrows*) but of normal caliber. On pathology a thyroglossal duct cyst was diagnosed. This is an unusual large size and posterior position for a thyroglossal duct cyst.

positron emission tomography (PET) using 18F-fluorode-oxyglucose (FDG).

Thyroid scintigraphy provides anatomic and physiologic data in patients with thyroid-related pathology. In neonates with hypothyroidism, imaging with technetium-99m pertechnetate (99mTc) is preferred for relatively lower radiation dose and better anatomic evaluation (►Fig. 4.19). Imaging with Iodine-123 (123-I) is performed when measurement of uptake is needed.

PET-CT is an important tool for evaluating malignancy. In the pediatric neck PET-CT has an important role in staging and treatment response in lymphoma and sarcoma patients (►Fig. 4.12e). For patients who need to be evaluated with a diagnostic CT in addition to a PET-CT study, the PET-CT study should be performed with a diagnostic CT protocol including IV contrast injection, thereby eliminating the need for a repeat exam and decreasing the overall radiation exposure for the patient.[16] In recent years PET-MRI machines are being evaluated in research centers with possible advantages related to decreased radiation dose and

better soft tissue evaluation in comparison to PET-CT.[17] The complexity of the exam, longer sedation times, and additional costs may postpone widespread use of this fusion modality.

4.4 The Imaging Diagnostic Workup

As in any aspect of caring for children, referring a child to imaging requires risk versus benefit assessment. The first rule is to avoid unnecessary examinations. For example, CT of the sinonasal structures is not indicated for routine evaluation of acute sinusitis, which is a clinical diagnosis, and should be reserved for cases of treatment failure or complications. The second rule is to choose the proper imaging study for the specific clinical question. For children US would be the initial imaging study of choice in most of suspected pathologies of the neck, and in many cases, will suffice for diagnosis and treatment decisions. For example, in a child presenting with a focal palpated mass US will demonstrate it to be cystic or solid and Doppler investigation will demonstrate lack or presence of vascularity (►Fig. 4.1). CT will be the initial study of choice in the setting of head trauma for assessment of facial and skull fractures as well as intracranial injury; in this setting, usually a non-contrast study is performed (►Fig. 4.8). Cases of complicated sinusitis and mastoiditis should be assessed with contrast-enhanced CT study, preferably with a CTV protocol (►Fig. 4.20 and ►Fig. 4.21).[18-20]

A neonate with dyspnea and suspected nasal obstruction is one of the rare justified indications for facial CT study in the neonatal period (►Fig. 4.22).

After initial diagnostic imaging is performed either by US or CT, in some cases additional imaging is needed. When evaluating inflammatory or neoplastic pathology, due to superb soft tissue delineation, an MRI study would be the next step, allowing further characterization of the pathologic process as well as assessment of intracranial extension. In the setting of suspected skull base or facial mass, referring a child to an MRI study for initial evaluation can be justified. It is important to note that in pathologies involving skull and facial bones MRI and CT studies have a complementary role (►Fig. 4.23).

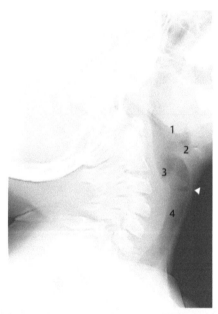

Fig. 4.16 Lateral neck X-ray with moderate tonsillar enlargement (1). The vallecula (2), pyriform sinus (3), trachea (4), and laryngeal ventricle (*arrowhead*) are well delineated.

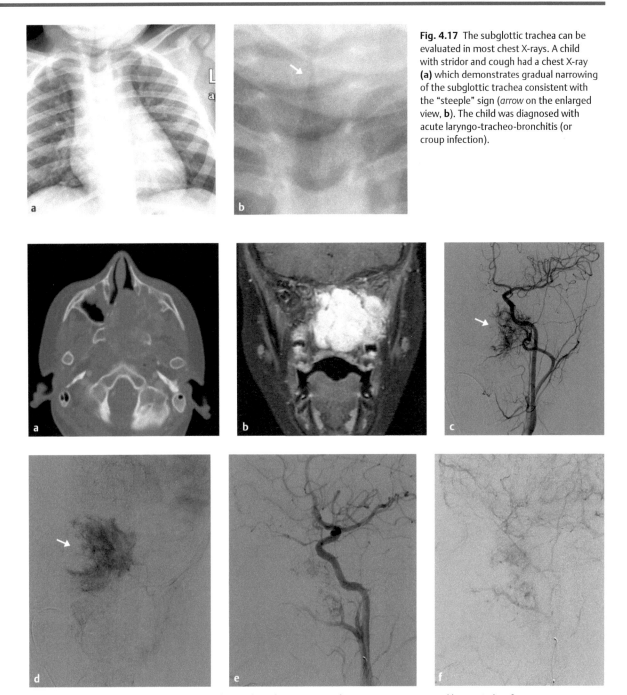

Fig. 4.17 The subglottic trachea can be evaluated in most chest X-rays. A child with stridor and cough had a chest X-ray **(a)** which demonstrates gradual narrowing of the subglottic trachea consistent with the "steeple" sign (*arrow* on the enlarged view, **b**). The child was diagnosed with acute laryngo-tracheo-bronchitis (or croup infection).

Fig. 4.18 A 13-year-old boy with nose bleeding and an obstructing nasal mass on inspection. Axial bone window from contrast-enhanced CT **(a)** shows a large soft tissue mass centered on the pterygo-palatine fossa (PPF) with invasion and destruction of adjacent bone. Coronal post-contrast fat-suppressed T1W MRI image demonstrates avid enhancement **(b)**. These are typical features of Juvenile nasopharyngeal angiofibroma (JNA). Presurgery conventional angiography for embolization purpose was performed. Left CCA injection of iodine based contrast demonstrates extensive tumor enhancement (*arrow*, **c**) with late persistent tumor blush (*arrow*, **d**). Post embolization images **(e, f)** show significant reduction in tumor blush.

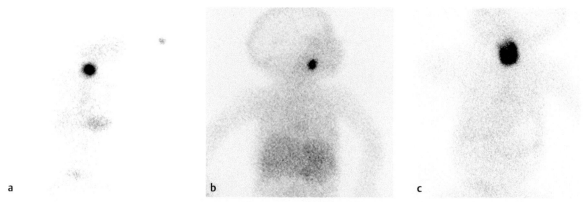

Fig. 4.19 Thyroid scintigraphy with technetium-99m pertechnetate (99mTc) in three neonates with hypothyroidism. Normal anatomic position and uptake **(a)**, ectopic thyroid positioned at the lingual region **(b)**, normal anatomic position with enlargement and increased uptake **(c)** suggesting dyshormonogenesis.

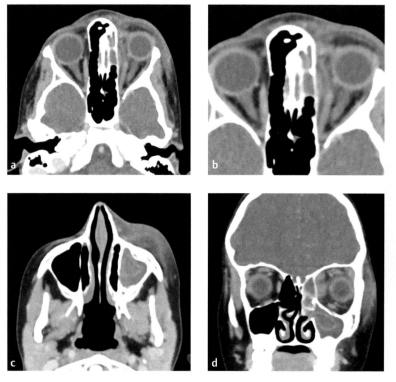

Fig. 4.20 A 9-year-old boy with periorbital cellulitis and eye movement limitation on ophthalmologic examination was referred for contrast-enhanced CT study. Axial image of the orbits **(a)**, an enlarged view **(b)**, axial image of the maxillary sinus **(c)**, and coronal reformat image **(d)** demonstrate extensive pre-malar and periorbital soft tissue stranding with intraorbital involvement along the lamina papyracea of the left orbit. There is related thickening and lateral displacement of the left medial rectus muscle. There is mucosal thickening, increased secretions and no aeration of the left maxillary sinus, anterior ethmoid air cells and frontal cells (not shown), consistent with sinusitis. This pattern of paranasal sinus involvement with normal aeration in all other air cells suggests left anterior pathway obstruction. The child was diagnosed with intraorbital cellulitis related to complicated sinusitis.

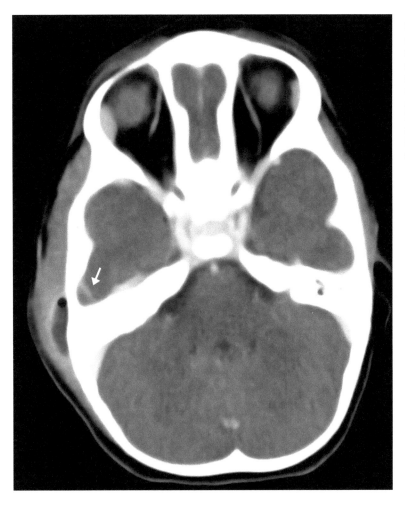

Fig. 4.21 A 4-year-old girl was referred to a CT study due to suspected complicated mastoiditis. Contrast-enhanced CT demonstrates extensive stranding and thickening of the retro auricular soft tissue of the right scalp with a prominent sub-periosteal abscess. There is intracranial extension with an associated epidural abscess (*arrow*). There are no filling defects in the right sigmoid sinus, excluding sinus vein thrombosis.

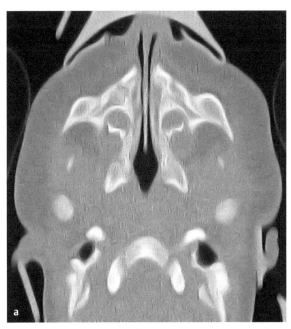

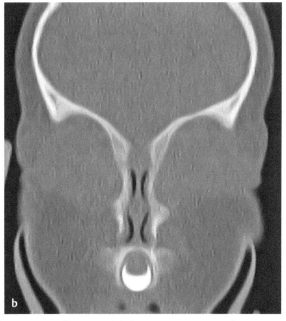

Fig. 4.22 A newborn with difficulty breathing and suspected nasal obstruction. Axial CT image **(a)** demonstrates severe pyriform aperture stenosis. The coronal reformate image **(b)** demonstrates associated single mega incisor. The significant noise in the images is related to low dose protocol.

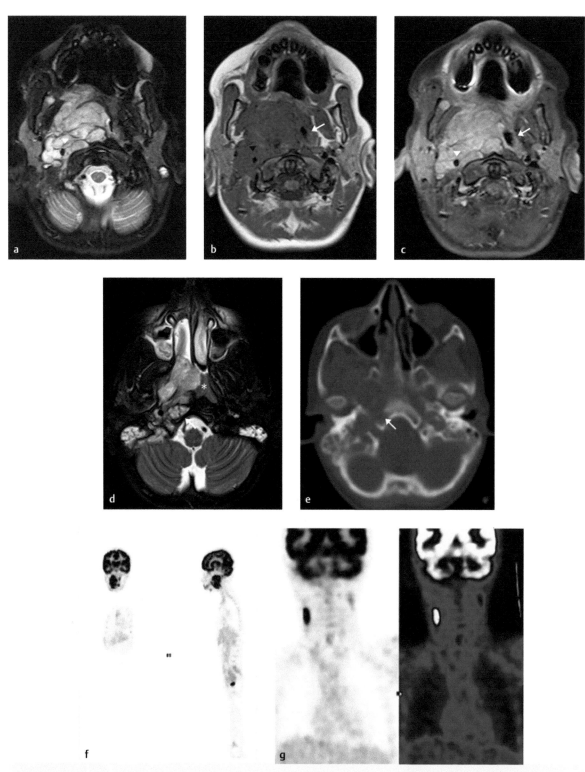

Fig. 4.23 A 4-year-old boy with right parameningeal rhabdomyosarcoma. Axial T2W image with fat suppression **(a)**, axial T1W image **(b)**, and Axial T1W image with fat suppression after gadolinium injection **(c)**, demonstrate a large multispatial multilobulated mass involving the retropharyngeal, parapharyngeal, oropharyngeal, and carotid spaces on the right with displacement and severe narrowing of the airway column (*arrow*). The Internal jugular vein (IJV) is completely effaced and the internal carotid artery (ICA) is encased and slightly narrowed (*short arrow*). At the level of the nasopharynx an axial T2W image with fat suppression **(d)** shows extension of the mass to the nasopharyngeal space with a distinct border differentiating it from adenoidal tissue (*). There is thinning of the clivus on the right (*arrow*), and skull base invasion through the jugular fossa (*short arrow*). A bone window CT at the same level **(e)** demonstrates the aggressive invasion of the tumor to the bone as opposed to effacement. A PET-CT study **(f, g)** shows high FDG uptake in the tumor and in an ipsilateral lymph node.

References

[1] Som PM, Hugh DC, eds. Head and Neck Imaging. 5th ed. Elsevier Mosby; 2011

[2] Coley BD, ed. Caffey's Pediatric Diagnostic Imaging. 12th ed. Elsevier Saunders; 2013

[3] King SJ, Boothroyd AE, eds. Pediatric ENT Radiology. In: Leuven ALB, Heidelberg AS, eds. Medical Radiology/Diagnostic Imaging. Springer; 2002

[4] Brenner DJ, Hall EJ. Computed tomography: an increasing source of radiation exposure. N Engl J Med 2007;357(22):2277–2284

[5] Brenner DJ. Estimating cancer risks from pediatric CT: going from the qualitative to the quantitative. Pediatr Radiol 2002;32(4): 228–1, discussion 242–244

[6] Frush DP, Donnelly LF, Rosen NS. Computed tomography and radiation risks: what pediatric health care providers should know. Pediatrics 2003;112(4):951–957

[7] Goske MJ, Applegate KE, Bulas D, et al; Alliance for Radiation Safety in Pediatric Imaging. Image Gently: progress and challenges in CT education and advocacy. Pediatr Radiol 2011;41(Suppl 2):461–466

[8] Mathews JD, Forsythe AV, Brady Z, et al. Cancer risk in 680,000 people exposed to computed tomography scans in childhood or adolescence: data linkage study of 11 million Australians. BMJ 2013;346:f2360

[9] Pearce MS, Salotti JA, Little MP, et al. Radiation exposure from CT scans in childhood and subsequent risk of leukaemia and brain tumours: a retrospective cohort study. Lancet 2012;380(9840):499–505

[10] Chen JX, Kachniarz B, Gilani S, Shin JJ. Risk of malignancy associated with head and neck CT in children: a systematic review. Otolaryngol Head Neck Surg 2014;151(4):554–566

[11] Callahan MJ, MacDougall RD, Bixby SD, Voss SD, Robertson RL, Cravero JP. Ionizing radiation from computed tomography versus anesthesia for magnetic resonance imaging in infants and children: patient safety considerations. Pediatr Radiol 2018;48(1):21–30

[12] Wunsch R, von Rohden L, Cleaveland R, Aumann V. Small part ultrasound in childhood and adolescence. Eur J Radiol 2014;83(9):1549–1559

[13] Green JS, Tsui BCH. Applications of ultrasonography in ENT: airway assessment and nerve blockade. Anesthesiol Clin 2010;28(3):541–553

[14] Srinivasan A, Dvorak R, Perni K, Rohrer S, Mukherji SK. Differentiation of benign and malignant pathology in the head and neck using 3T apparent diffusion coefficient values: early experience. AJNR Am J Neuroradiol 2008;29(1):40–44

[15] Penfield JG. Nephrogenic systemic fibrosis and the use of gadolinium-based contrast agents. Pediatr Nephrol 2008; 23(12):2121–2129

[16] Wong TZ, Paulson EK, Nelson RC, Patz EF Jr, Coleman RE. Practical approach to diagnostic CT combined with PET. AJR Am J Roentgenol 2007;188(3):622–629

[17] Kim S, Salamon N, Jackson HA, Blüml S, Panigrahy A. PET imaging in pediatric neuroradiology: current and future applications. Pediatr Radiol 2010;40(1):82–96

[18] Ludwig BJ, Foster BR, Saito N, Nadgir RN, Castro-Aragon I, Sakai O. Diagnostic imaging in nontraumatic pediatric head and neck emergencies. Radiographics 2010;30(3):781–799

[19] Meuwly JY, Lepori D, Theumann N, et al. Multimodality imaging evaluation of the pediatric neck: techniques and spectrum of findings. Radiographics 2005;25(4):931–948

[20] Capps EF, Kinsella JJ, Gupta M, Bhatki AM, Opatowsky MJ. Emergency imaging assessment of acute, nontraumatic conditions of the head and neck. Radiographics 2010;30(5):1335–1352

Section II

Head and Neck

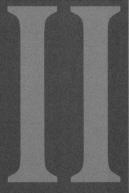

II

5 Surgery of Head and Neck Infection

Roy Hod, Eyal Raveh

Summary

Neck infections are commonly seen in the pediatric population. Characteristic findings of neck infection include fever, sore throat, and a warm, tender neck mass. A computed tomography (CT) scan is the gold standard for diagnosis and surgical planning, but the specificity is low. Ultrasonography (US) is a less-invasive alternative that may be equally effective in certain cases. Infections are typically polymicrobial. A neck abscess is usually treated with surgical drainage and intravenous antibiotics. Intravenous antibiotics without surgical drainage in a clinically stable neck may be effective in selected cases. Diagnosis may be more challenging in younger children and in retropharyngeal infections. Complications of deep neck infections are uncommon but carry severe sequelae.

Keywords: Deep space neck infection, abscess, computed tomography, retropharyngeal infection, peritonsillar abscess, parapharyngeal abscess, atypical mycobacterium

5.1 Introduction

Deep neck infections (DNIs) are commonly encountered in both children and adults. However, the presentation, progression, and management differ greatly in these two groups. The morbidity and mortality rates of DNIs have improved dramatically since the initiation of antibiotic therapy and the understanding of deep neck anatomy. Infectious and inflammatory conditions of the upper aerodigestive tract are the primary cause of DNIs. Dental infections are the most common cause of DNIs in adults, whereas oropharyngeal infections are the most common cause in children.[1-4] Diagnosis and treatment are dependent on the age of the child, the location of the infection, and the etiological agent involved. In the pediatric population, acute rhinosinusitis is a common cause of retropharyngeal lymphadenitis. Oral surgical procedures and endoscopic instrumentation may iatrogenically traumatize the pharyngo-esophageal lumen and incite an upper airway infection. Sialadenitis, with or without ductal obstruction, can precipitate infectious spread. Foreign bodies trapped within the upper aerodigestive tract may initiate infections that spread to the deep neck. Superficial infections, such as skin cellulitis, may spread along fascial planes into deeper neck compartments. Penetrating trauma may introduce pathogens into the fascial planes. Congenital or acquired lesions such as branchial cleft cysts, thyroglossal duct cysts, or laryngoceles may become infected and result in spread of infection. Congenital cysts account for 10 to 15% of DNIs in the pediatric population, and these should be suspected, especially in the setting of recurrent DNIs.

5.2 Anatomy

An understanding of deep infections of the neck requires knowledge of the anatomy of the superficial and deep cervical neck fascia and spaces. It is their relationship to each other that forms the potential neck spaces that can harbor or limit infection and abscess formation.[5-7] DNIs may be broadly classified as involving the suprahyoid spaces, infrahyoid space, or spaces involving the entire neck:

- *Suprahyoid spaces*: Submandibular space, pharyngo-maxillary (lateral pharyngeal) space, masticator space, parotid space, and peritonsillar space.
- *Infrahyoid space*: Visceral space.
- *Spaces involving the entire neck*: Retropharyngeal space, prevertebral space, vascular (carotid) space, and "danger" space.

Infections in these spaces exert fatal effect either by local airway occlusion or extension to vital areas such as the mediastinum or carotid sheath. Fascial planes divide the neck into true and potential spaces. The deep cervical fascia of the neck can be divided into a superficial, middle (pretracheal), and deep layer (prevertebral), which envelop various structures in the neck and dictate potential routes for spread of infections. Of primary importance for deep neck space infections are the submandibular, peritonsillar, parapharyngeal, and retropharyngeal spaces (▶ Fig. 5.1).

5.3 Clinical Presentation and Preoperative Evaluation

Children with deep space neck infections more commonly present with fever, neck mass, odynophagia, dysphagia, sore throat, and decreased oral intake. These symptoms are usually present for approximately 2 to 5 days. Less common symptoms include agitation, cough, dehydration, drooling, snoring, stridor, dyspnea,

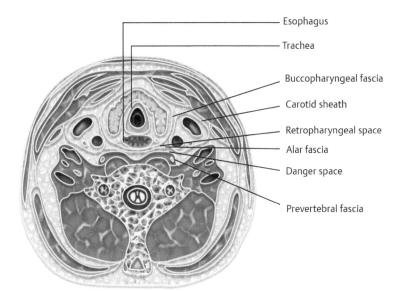

Fig. 5.1 Cross-section of the neck illustrating visceral structures and fascial planes.

Esophagus
Trachea
Buccopharyngeal fascia
Carotid sheath
Retropharyngeal space
Alar fascia
Danger space
Prevertebral fascia

and torticollis.[8,9] Important points in the history include the duration and progression of the symptoms, a recent upper respiratory tract infection, procedures performed to the neck (i.e., dental surgery, intubation), prior antibiotic therapy, recent travel, and a possible immunocompromised state. The average age at presentation is 4 to 5 years, with peritonsillar abscesses typically presenting in older children and retropharyngeal abscesses seen in younger children.[9–13]

Physical examination should assess for the presence of erythema, tenderness, and fluctuance of the neck mass, as well as lymphadenopathy, tracheal deviation, and neck stiffness. The examination of the oral cavity and pharynx should be performed with attention to the tonsillar size and symmetry, dentition, palatal edema, and uvular deviation. Though potentially life-threatening, airway compromise secondary to a DNI is very rare. An important sign of airway compromise is "tripoding," which refers to a child in the seated position with their elbows or hands on their knees, leaning forward with the neck extended and head tilted slightly backward.

Though not mandatory, laboratory tests may be helpful in the work-up of a child with a potential DNI. Leukocytosis, with or without a left shift, is typically seen on a complete blood count. Other helpful laboratory tests include a C-reactive protein (which can aid in determining progression of infection over time), a monospot test, and Epstein-Barr virus (EBV) titers. In cases of more chronic infection, a PPD (TB and atypical TB) skin test should be considered. It is also important to consider other causes of inflammation such as congenital, neoplastic, or inflammatory conditions.[14]

Contrast-enhanced CT scans is the gold standard in the evaluation of DNIs (▶ Fig. 5.2 and ▶ Fig. 5.3). CT scan

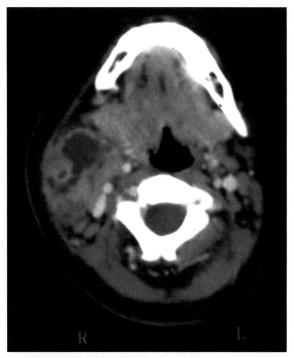

Fig. 5.2 Contrast-enhanced axial CT showing a right parapharyngeal abscess.

provides important valuable information of the site and extent of infection. It has a sensitivity of 100% in determining the precise location of an infectious process (abscess) and a sensitivity of 88 to 95% in the ability to differentiate between cellulitis and an abscess.[15] It is also valuable in locating the relative position of the major vessels. CT scan of the chest may be helpful

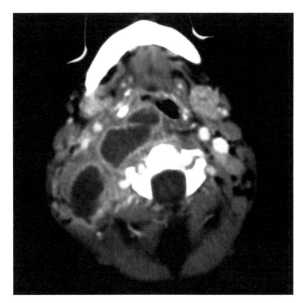

Fig. 5.3 Contrast-enhanced axial CT showing a right parapharyngeal abscess.

if extension of abscess into the mediastinum is suspected. The role for magnetic resonance imaging (MRI) is under debate. MRI was shown to be superior to CT in demonstrating disease extension, the spaces involved, and source of infection, as it is less degraded by artifacts. Ultrasound scans may also aid in the diagnosis of an abscess. However, the quality of the scan is highly operator-dependent, and there is poorer visualization of structures in the upper oropharynx.[11,12] Imaging techniques are performed according to the location of the DNI, the child's medical condition, and whether or not clinical improvement has been seen following initiation of antibiotic treatment.

5.4 Pathogens

The types of bacteria found in neck infections vary regionally and continue to evolve over time. The microbiology of DNI often yields a mixture of aerobic and anaerobic organisms that are representative of oropharyngeal flora. Group A betahemolytic streptococcus (GABHS), *Staphylococcus aureus*, and anaerobes are the most commonly isolated bacteria in neck abscess cultures.[5,7,10,14,18] The location of the abscess has been correlated with specific bacteria. Peritonsillar, retropharyngeal, and parapharyngeal abscesses tend to be caused by GABHS, while submandibular and superficial neck abscesses are more commonly associated with *S. aureus*.

Other less common causes of neck infections and lymphadenopathy include atypical mycobacterium, actinomycosis, fusobacterium necrophorum (Lemierre's syndrome), histoplasmosis, toxoplasmosis, and aspergillosis.[10]

Empiric therapy for DNIs varies greatly, but should include adequate coverage of Gram-positive, Gram-negative, and anaerobic organisms. Typical choices for empiric therapy include ampicillin-sulbactam, clindamycin with a third-generation cephalosporin, trimethoprim-sulfamethoxazole, vancomycin with a third-generation cephalosporin, and linezolid. Clindamycin with a third-generation cephalosporin is a commonly used antibiotic choice, as it provides good Gram-positive and anaerobic coverage, and usually covers MRSA.[9,13,15,18,19]

5.5 Treatment

Treatment for deep neck abscesses depends on whether lymphadenitis or a suppurative abscess is suspected. In general, lymphadenitis and cellulitis are treated with antibiotics, whereas a neck abscess in a clinically unstable child is treated with immediate surgical drainage.[7,8,11,13] Controversy exists over the best management of a clinically stable child with a neck abscess. Clinical stability typically implies the child is without signs of systemic toxicity, airway compromise, or evidence of spread to adjacent tissue spaces.[11,13,20] Many studies have shown good treatment outcomes with medical management of a CT-defined neck abscess. McClay et al found that 10 of 11 children (91%) with a CT-defined neck abscess improved with intravenous antibiotics alone.[17] Complications of a neck abscess are uncommon but can carry severe morbidity and mortality. They are typically associated with a delay in diagnosis or treatment. Airway obstruction and death can occur. Rupture of a retropharyngeal or parapharyngeal abscess may result in severe pneumonitis. Septic venous thrombosis can occur, leading to septic emboli, septic shock, or neurovascular compromise. Carotid artery rupture may also result from an unresolved abscess. Spread of an infection along the danger space can rapidly lead to mediastinitis.

Most DNIs are located medial to the great vessels, while lymphadenitis is more commonly seen lateral to them. Children with clinical evidence of an abscess lateral to the great vessels typically undergo a transcervical incision and drainage under general anesthesia. The primary benefits of incision and drainage include obtaining cultures for culture-directed antibiotic therapy, removing free pus from the neck, and creating an external tract to prevent the re-accumulation of pus. External incision and drainage has been reported to be 99% successful.[12] The risks of the surgery depend on the location of the abscess, but primarily include injury to the marginal mandibular nerve, accessory nerve, vagus nerve, or great vessels.[10]

5.6 Site-Specific Surgical Technique

5.6.1 Retropharyngeal Infection

This space refers to the lymph node containing space that lies anterior to the alar fascia and posterior to the pharynx and esophagus. Posterior to it is the potential space. These infections are unique in their presentation, diagnosis, and treatment. Retropharyngeal infections tend to occur in a younger age group (26–42 months), possibly due to the regression of these nodes by the age of 5. These nodes receive drainage from the sinuses, nose, adenoids, and nasopharynx, which may explain why these infections often follow an upper respiratory infection, and are more commonly caused by *Streptococcus*. Trauma to the pharynx and esophagus, either from foreign body ingestion or from an iatrogenic cause, such as intubation, may also result in the development of a retropharyngeal infection.[8–10] A diagnosis may be difficult to make, given the children are typically younger and a neck mass is not always present on examination. Fever and malaise, the most common presenting symptoms, are nonspecific. However, symptoms such as torticollis, decreased range of movement of the neck, unilateral bulging of posterior pharyngeal wall, dysphagia, voice changes, or drooling should raise the clinical suspicion of a retropharyngeal infection. Though symptoms of airway obstruction while awake are rare, many children demonstrate an acute onset of snoring and obstructive apnea during sleep.[9,10] Lateral neck films and CT scans are both useful tests in the diagnosis of a retropharyngeal infection/abscess. Lateral neck films (▶Fig. 5.4) are a good screening tool, with thickness of the posterior pharyngeal wall greater than 7 mm at C2 and 14 mm at C6 considered a positive finding in a child with a retropharyngeal infection/abscess.[12] These films must be taken with the child in neck extension and at the end of inspiration, or a falsely positive thickening of the posterior pharyngeal wall may be diagnosed.[16] This may be difficult to achieve in an uncooperative child.[9,10] CT scanning is the imaging method of choice in the management of a retropharyngeal abscess.[16] However, the same concerns with the specificity of predicting purulence in other regions of the neck apply to the retropharynx. Many studies demonstrate satisfactory outcomes with nonoperative management of retropharyngeal infections. However, prompt surgical drainage is necessary when no response to medical therapy is demonstrated, neurologic findings are compatible with progressive spinal cord compression, there is evidence of airway compromise, free pus is seen in the retropharyngeal space on imaging, or if the child appears toxic.[8,12,13,21]

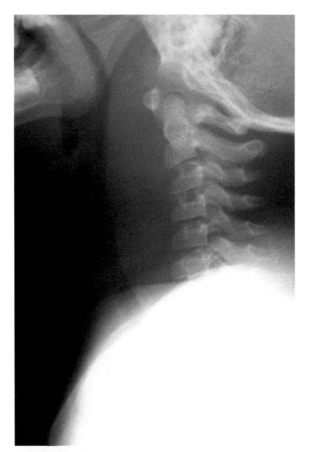

Fig. 5.4 Lateral neck X-ray demonstrating thickening of the retropharyngeal space.

Anesthesia and Preparation

- This procedure must be performed under general anesthesia with protection of the airway by an endotracheal tube (cuffed in older children or teenagers, and hypopharyngeal packing in uncuffed tubes). If an intraoral drainage is planned, the throat is packed with a gauze pack.
- If an external incision is planned, the skin is prepared with an antiseptic scrub of the surgeon's choice.
- The patient is placed in the supine position with extension of the head and neck to prevent aspiration of the abscess contents.

If there is a question concerning the presence of purulence, aspiration with an 18-gauge needle into the upper retropharyngeal space is indicated (▶Fig. 5.5).

- *Intraoral* aspiration and drainage are recommended if the abscess is limited to the upper retropharyngeal space and medial to the great vessels:
  - The incision is carried through the postero-lateral pharyngeal wall mucosa vertically through the edematous mucosa.

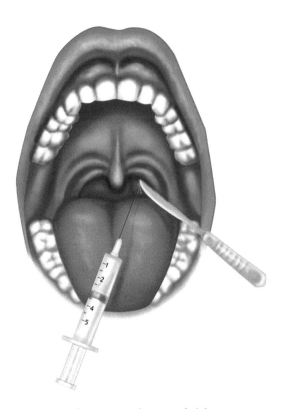

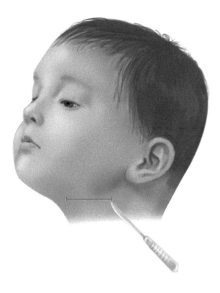

Fig. 5.6 Horizontal incision for external parapharyngeal abscess drainage.

Fig. 5.5 Intraoral aspiration and incision of a left retropharyngeal abscess.

– Dissection is then carried bluntly into the cavity. The cavity is cultured and drained completely.
• *External* drainage is used when the abscess extends inferiorly to the hyoid bone:
  – The incision is made horizontally with a modified apron-like fashion (▶ Fig. 5.6) with a horizontal limb at the midportion of the abscess cavity, and the vertical portion is carried along the anterior border of the sternocleidomastoid muscle superiorly.
  – The dissection is carried down to the sternocleidomastoid muscle, which is retracted laterally. The carotid sheath is identified, and most commonly its contents are reflected laterally, with the dissection into the abscess cavity continued anterior to the sheath.

However, if the approach is anterior to the carotid sheath, the sheath contents are retracted laterally, and the larynx, trachea, and thyroid gland are retracted medially.
• The dissection is then carried down to the prevertebral muscles behind the inferior constrictors. The cavity is opened with blunt dissection superiorly to inferiorly, and the contralateral extent is identified.

• The abscess cavity is irrigated with saline and antibiotic solution, and Jackson–Pratt drains are inserted, both superiorly and inferiorly.

5.6.2 Parapharyngeal Space (Lateral Pharyngeal Space)

This is a cone-shaped space with its base at the base of the skull, petrous portion of the temporal bone, and its apex at the hyoid bone. Infection of this space may originate from the teeth, tonsils, peritonsillar space, nose and sinuses, and penetrating wounds to the lateral pharyngeal wall. Signs and symptoms may include fever, trismus, swelling of the lateral pharyngeal wall in the region posterior to the tonsils, with occasional displacement of the tonsil medially or anteriorly. Surgical drainage is indicated when there is unsatisfactory response to antibiotic therapy, impending respiratory obstruction, or if there is extension of the abscess along the carotid sheath with impending rupture of the internal carotid artery.

Anesthesia and Preparation

• General anesthesia is used, preferably nasotracheal intubation. Oral endotracheal anesthesia is acceptable if the trismus is not too great.
• The skin is prepared with an antiseptic scrub.
• The surgeon should have a nerve stimulator available.

Procedure

- A horizontal incision or apron incision is made in the neck in the region of the infection, taking care to avoid the marginal mandibular nerve (▶ Fig. 5.6 and ▶ Fig. 5.7).
- The dissection is carried through the skin and platysma to identify the anterior border of the sternocleidomastoid muscle and the posterior and inferior aspects of the submandibular gland (▶ Fig. 5.7).
- The anterior border of the sternocleidomastoid muscle is retracted posteriorly and the carotid sheath structures are identified.
- The abscess is drained by blunt finger dissection along the anterior carotid sheath, retracting the sheath laterally and posteriorly. An elevator beneath the angle of the mandible facilitates exposure. Dissection extends superiorly to the cranial base.
- The area of purulence is drained; cultures are taken for aerobic, anaerobic bacteria and PCR analysis, and the wound is copiously irrigated with sterile saline with or without antibiotic solution.
- A Penrose or a drain is placed.
- There is also an option for an internal drainage, especially in children where a parapharyngeal abscess might coexist with a retropharyngeal abscess.

5.6.3 Peritonsillar Abscess

This space contains loose connective tissue lying between the capsule of the lingual tonsil medially and the superior constrictor muscle laterally. A peritonsillar abscess is the most common complication of tonsillitis. It typically occurs in older children (10–13 years), although cases have been reported in children as young as 14 months.[8] *Streptococcus* is the most commonly isolated pathogen.[8] The classic history is that of a unilateral sore throat, odynophagia, dysphagia, fever, drooling, referred otalgia, and a "hot potato" voice. Trismus and poor oral intake are common symptoms. A peritonsillar abscess is primarily diagnosed by physical examination. Findings include unilateral edema and erythema of the soft palate on the affected side, uvular deviation to the opposite side, and displacement of the tonsil medially and inferiorly. Rarely, a bilateral peritonsillar abscess may confound the diagnosis, as no uvular deviation is seen.[23] A CT scan may be helpful if the diagnosis is unclear or the child is too young for an adequate examination, though it is not routinely necessary. In older children and in adolescents, a peritonsillar abscess can often be drained under local anesthesia in an outpatient setting. Young children often require intraoperative drainage and hospital admission.

Fig. 5.7 (a–c) Apron incision for external parapharyngeal space abscess drainage.

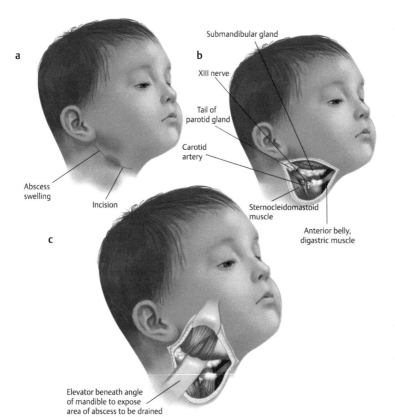

Needle drainage or incision and drainage under conscious sedation have been safely performed with minimal complications.[22-24] Indications for intervention are peritonsillar abscess with unsatisfactory response to antibiotic therapy or airway compromise.

Anesthesia and Preparation

- In younger children, a general anesthetic is necessary. In older children and teenagers, topical and local anesthesia is usually adequate for needle aspiration.
- If a hot tonsillectomy is to be performed, general anesthesia is usually necessary.
- If the patient requires a general anesthetic, the throat should be packed with a gauze pack.

Procedure

- The initial method of diagnosing and treating a peritonsillar abscess is with aspiration (▶ Fig. 5.8). A syringe with a 16- or 18-gauge needle is inserted at the junction of the soft palate and superior tonsillar pillar (the area most likely to have purulence and also the area that is least dangerous for aspiration). If there is bulging in another area, or if the initial aspiration in this area fails, then drainage is attempted inferiorly and more medially.
- Incision of the tonsillar pillar (▶ Fig. 5.8) is done over the most fluctuant area or at the site of a purulent needle aspirate.

Postoperative Care

- If only aspiration has been used, the patient may be given intravenous antibiotics until oral intake is satisfactory to ensure compliance with oral antibiotics.
- If a tonsillectomy or incision and drainage were performed, intravenous antibiotics are given until oral intake is satisfactory.

5.6.4 Atypical Mycobacterium

Also known as scrofula, this is the most common cause of persistent cervicofacial masses in children and commonly affects children under the age of 5. These infections present as a slowly enlarging neck mass with a violaceous color that persists for weeks after antibiotic therapy (▶ Fig. 5.9a, b). Infected nodes often erupt and form draining fistulae. Chest X-ray and PPD are usually normal.[25-27] Scrofula is spread locally and is not life-threatening. Diagnosis is best made clinically, or by tissue biopsy and culture, which may take 3 to 6 weeks to obtain.

Incision and drainage of these lesions result in a high rate of recurrence.

The treatment options for this condition might be watchful waiting, antibiotic therapy with clarithromycin for 3 to 6 months, or complete surgical excision which is mainly reserved for achieving good cosmetic results.

5.7 Conclusion

To conclude, DNIs represent a commonly encountered problem in children. Though there is debate about various treatment methods, prompt diagnosis and intervention is the key to managing these infections. If treated

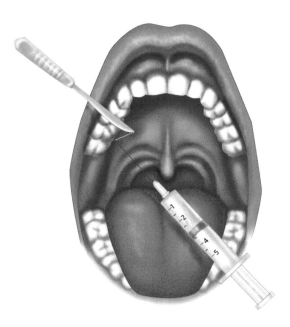

Fig. 5.8 Site of aspiration and incision of a right peritonsillar abscess.

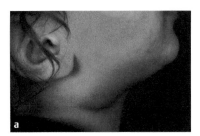
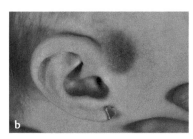

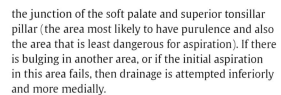

Fig. 5.9 (a, b) Atypical TB.

appropriately, they tend to resolve with minimal sequelae. However, if diagnosis and intervention is delayed, life-threatening complications may occur. Changes in technology and antibiotic resistance may alter the principles of management in the future.

5.8 Highlights

a. Pathology
- Deep neck infections are common in the pediatric population.
b. Complications
- Systemic toxicity.
- Airway compromise.
- Spread to adjacent tissue space.
- Mediastinitis.
- Septic venous thrombosis.
- Carotid artery blowout.
- Death.
c. Treatment
- Most deep neck infections (lymphadenitis/cellulitis) respond to antibiotic therapy.
- Deep neck abscesses usually requires surgical drainage.
d. Special preoperative considerations
- Imaging recommended (US, CT).
- General endotracheal anesthesia.
- If infection is intraoral: perform packing.
e. Special intraoperative considerations
- When working close to marginal mandibular branch of facial nerve or to recurrent laryngeal nerve, consider nerve monitoring.
f. Special postoperative considerations
- Hospitalization for antibiotic treatment and monitoring.
- Discharge home when child is stable and conditions permit.

References

[1] Boscolo-Rizzo P, Marchiori C, Montolli F, Vaglia A, Da Mosto MC. Deep neck infections: a constant challenge. ORL J Otorhinolaryngol Relat Spec 2006;68(5):259–265

[2] Brook I. Microbiology and management of peritonsillar, retropharyngeal, and parapharyngeal abscesses. J Oral Maxillofac Surg 2004;62(12):1545–1550

[3] Huang TT, Liu TC, Chen PR, Tseng FY, Yeh TH, Chen YS. Deep neck infection: analysis of 185 cases. Head Neck 2004;26(10):854–860

[4] Larawin V, Naipao J, Dubey SP. Head and neck space infections. Otolaryngol Head Neck Surg 2006;135(6):889–893

[5] Byrne M, Lee KJ. Neck spaces and fascial planes. In: Lee KJ, ed. Essential Otolaryngology. New York: McGraw-Hill; 2003:422–439

[6] Moore K, Dalley A. Fascia of the neck. In: Moore K, Dalley, A, eds. Clinically Oriented Anatomy, Philadelphia: Lippincott Williams & Wilkins; 1999:998–999

[7] Standring S, Berkovitz B. Neck. In: Standring S, ed. Gray's Anatomy: The Anatomical Basis of Clinical Practice, Edinburgh: Elsevier; 2005:531–566

[8] Cmejrek RC, Coticchia JM, Arnold JE. Presentation, diagnosis, and management of deep-neck abscesses in infants. Arch Otolaryngol Head Neck Surg 2002;128(12):1361–1364

[9] Coticchia JM, Getnick GS, Yun RD, Arnold JE. Age-, site-, and time-specific differences in pediatric deep neck abscesses. Arch Otolaryngol Head Neck Surg 2004;130(2):201–207

[10] Craig FW, Schunk JE. Retropharyngeal abscess in children: clinical presentation, utility of imaging, and current management. Pediatrics 2003;111(6 Pt 1):1394–1398

[11] Dodds B, Maniglia AJ. Peritonsillar and neck abscesses in the pediatric age group. Laryngoscope 1988;98(9):956–959

[12] Kirse DJ, Roberson DW. Surgical management of retropharyngeal space infections in children. Laryngoscope 2001;111(8):1413–1422

[13] Lalakea ML, Messner AH. Retropharyngeal abscess management in children: current practices. Otolaryngol Head Neck Surg 1999;121(4):398–405

[14] Roberson D, Kirse D. Infectious and inflammatory disorders of the neck. In: Wetmore RF, McGill TJ, Muntz HR, eds. Pediatric Otolaryngology. New York, NY: Thieme; 2000:969–991

[15] Nagy M, Pizzuto M, Backstrom J, Brodsky L. Deep neck infections in children: a new approach to diagnosis and treatment. Laryngoscope 1997;107(12 Pt 1):1627–1634

[16] Lazor JB, Cunningham MJ, Eavey RD, Weber AL. Comparison of computed tomography and surgical findings in deep neck infections. Otolaryngol Head Neck Surg 1994;111(6):746–750

[17] McClay JE, Murray AD, Booth T. Intravenous antibiotic therapy for deep neck abscesses defined by computed tomography. Arch Otolaryngol Head Neck Surg 2003;129(11):1207–1212

[18] Cabrera CE, Deutsch ES, Eppes S, et al. Increased incidence of head and neck abscesses in children. Otolaryngol Head Neck Surg 2007;136(2):176–181

[19] Ossowski K, Chun RH, Suskind D, Baroody FM. Increased isolation of methicillin-resistant Staphylococcus aureus in pediatric head and neck abscesses. Arch Otolaryngol Head Neck Surg 2006;132(11):1176–1181

[20] Sichel J-YMD, Dano I, Hocwald E, Biron A, Eliashar R. Nonsurgical management of parapharyngeal space infections: a prospective study. Laryngoscope 2002;112(5):906–910

[21] Gidley P, Stiernberg C. Deep space neck infections. In: Gwaltney J, Grandis JR, Sugar A, eds. Infectious Diseases and Antimicrobial Therapy of the Ears, Nose and Throat. Philadelphia, PA: WB Saunders; 1997:500–519

[22] Simons JP, Branstetter BF IV, Mandell DL. Bilateral peritonsillar abscesses: case report and literature review. Am J Otolaryngol 2006;27(6):443–445

[23] Suskind DL, Park J, Piccirillo JF, Lusk RP, Muntz HR. Conscious sedation: a new approach for peritonsillar abscess drainage in the pediatric population. Arch Otolaryngol Head Neck Surg 1999;125(11):1197–1200

[24] Bauer PW, Lieu JE, Suskind DL, Lusk RP. The safety of conscious sedation in peritonsillar abscess drainage. Arch Otolaryngol Head Neck Surg 2001;127(12):1477–1480

[25] Rahal A, Abela A, Arcand PH, Quintal MC, Lebel MH, Tapiero BF. Nontuberculous mycobacterial adenitis of the head and neck in children: experience from a tertiary care pediatric center. Laryngoscope 2001;111(10):1791–1796

[26] Lindeboom JA, Kuijper EJ, Bruijnesteijn van Coppenraet ES, Lindeboom R, Prins JM. Surgical excision versus antibiotic treatment for nontuberculous mycobacterial cervicofacial lymphadenitis in children: a multicenter, randomized, controlled trial. Clin Infect Dis 2007;44(8):1057–1064

[27] Tunkel DE. Surgery for cervicofacial nontuberculous mycobacterial adenitis in children: an update. Arch Otolaryngol Head Neck Surg 1999;125(10):1109–1113

6 Thyroidectomy

Vaninder K. Dhillon, Jonathon O. Russell, Ralph P. Tufano

Summary

This chapter summarizes the indications, techniques, and surgical considerations for pediatric patients undergoing thyroidectomy. Based upon the pathophysiology of thyroid disease in children, namely thyroid cancers, and the current 2015 American Thyroid Association (ATA) guidelines, we discuss the nuances of performing thyroid surgery in the pediatric population. Thyroidectomy technique and principles in the pediatric population are similar to an adult. We emphasize the importance of experienced surgeons expert in thyroid and neck anatomy in order to perform a safe, complete resection of the thyroid as well as a robust multidisciplinary team inclusive of pediatric endocrinologists who are familiar with caring for and managing a pediatric-centric patient population.

Keywords: Thyroidectomy, pediatric thyroid disease, pediatric patient, multidisciplinary team, endocrine surgeon, surgical technique, surgical considerations

6.1 Introduction

Thyroidectomy in the pediatric population is approached similarly to the adult population, and is not necessarily significantly more complex or difficult when done by experienced surgeons who are familiar with pediatric thyroid disease. The indications for thyroidectomy are the same as in adults for many associated thyroid diseases, both benign and neoplastic. Some of the benign diseases are Graves' disease, congenital hypothyroidism, and benign nodules that cause compressive symptoms. Among thyroid neoplasms are the well-differentiated ones like papillary thyroid carcinoma, and medullary and follicular thyroid carcinomas. For each of these thyroid cancers, there is a recommendation for total thyroidectomy for locoregional control.[1] For the pediatric population, the behavior of these neoplastic processes may be slightly different from that for adults, but the surgical technique for resection is the same.

The incidence of thyroid malignancy in the pediatric population is different than the adult population. Differentiated thyroid carcinoma (DTC) is 1% of all cancers in prepubertal children, and up to 7% in adolescents.[2] Thyroid cancer is the most common malignancy in childhood.[3] Compared to adults, children and adolescents with thyroid cancer may be more likely to present with disseminated disease.[4,5] Complete preoperative imaging of the thyroid and neck is important in a pediatric patient that may present with what appears as a solitary thyroid nodule with a biopsy diagnosis of carcinoma. Preoperative imaging may include ultrasound (US) but to be more inclusive, computed tomography (CT) is the standard of care in order to identify distant disease.[6,7] Prepubertal children with DTC have more extrathyroid extension, lymph node and lung metastasis than adolescents. Medullary thyroid cancer is more common in prepubertal patients, with the familial type more common.[4,8,9]

The risk factors for thyroid malignancy differ slightly compared to adults. Childhood exposure to ionizing radiation (especially in patients <5 years old), iodine deficiency, history of prior thyroid conditions, and genetic syndromes increase the risk for thyroid malignancy early on in life.[4]

The 2015 American Thyroid Association (ATA) guidelines created a separate guideline on pediatric thyroid nodules and DTC. Thyroid nodules diagnosed in children are uncommon compared to adult counterparts, but when they are discovered, there is a greater risk of up to 22–26% for malignancy, and a higher risk for regional lymph node involvement, extrathyroidal extension, and pulmonary metastasis.[4] The risk of recurrence in pediatric DTC not treated by total thyroidectomy and radioactive iodine (RAI) is up to 30%.[2]

In regard to gene rearrangements, the prevalence may be low in children, but when positive it is indicative of more aggressive disease. For example, the BRAF mutation is rare in children, but when positive, it indicates a more aggressive form of papillary thyroid carcinoma.[2,10] The RET oncogene mutation is also seen more commonly in pediatric papillary thyroid cancer.[2,10,11]

Overall, pediatric patients who present with a thyroid nodule should undergo imaging and a biopsy. If a fine needle aspiration (FNA) is positive for thyroid carcinoma, it is important to consider a CT scan of the neck and chest in order to thoroughly identify the extent of regional and distant disease. Once the extent of disease is determined, a complete plan including the surgical treatment can be shared with the patient's multidisciplinary team and discussed with the patient and family.

6.2 Preoperative Evaluation

According to the 2015 ATA guidelines, the preoperative evaluation of thyroid nodules should include clinical examination and US.[1,4] US characteristics and clinical context, despite the size of nodule(s), should warrant need for FNA. The risk profile suggestive of family history of thyroid disease or cancer and/or history of ionizing radiation exposure is considered a significant component for consideration of FNA in a child with a thyroid nodule.[4] Given that the prevalence of thyroid cancers is higher for the pediatric patient when a nodule exists, there is an overall lower threshold for FNA. US findings such as microcalcifications and any evidence of cervical lymphadenopathy are important. It is highly recommended that all FNA be done under US guidance. Diffuse thyroid enlargement should prompt US, as well as the presence of cervical lymph nodes. Indeterminate FNA has a higher risk for malignancy in children than in adults, and warrants a diagnostic lobectomy as compared to a total thyroidectomy, instead of a repeat FNA.[4]

The preoperative counseling for thyroid malignancies in children must take into account the goals of management. The goals of management for thyroid cancer are outlined nicely in Randolph et al's chapter on pediatric thyroid in his textbook, Surgery of the Thyroid and Parathyroid Glands.[12] According to the chapter, the principles of initial surgery are: (1) removal of primary lesion, (2) removal of any local invasive disease, (3) removal of involved cervical LN, (4) low morbidity, (5) permit accurate staging, (6) facilitate postoperative RAI when appropriate, (7) permit accurate long-term surveillance for recurrence, and (8) minimize risk for recurrence.[12] These goals of surgery are irrespective of age, but what's important is that experienced surgeons are involved in the initial surgical intervention for pediatric patients, given the fact that disease pathology often requires attention to the thyroid and quite possibly lymph nodes, with the least morbidity possible to clear all gross disease.

For pediatric patients with thyroid malignancy limited to the thyroid only, the general consensus is total thyroidectomy or near total thyroidectomy for papillary thyroid carcinoma, and lobectomy for micropapillary or follicular carcinoma <2 cm with no vascular invasion or other risk factors for aggressive behavior.[1] Papillary thyroid carcinoma has an increased incidence of bilateral (30%) and multifocal disease (65%) in children with an increased risk for recurrence.[11] A total thyroidectomy also allows optimization of RAI and thyroglobulin as a marker for surveillance. In children with follicular carcinoma, a lobectomy as mentioned above is regarded as appropriate surgical management, but if RAI is being considered, then a total thyroidectomy would be the recommendation. Some papers even show that a total thyroidectomy shows less risk of recurrence in children,[13] and even more importantly, increased survival.[14] Furthermore, pediatric patients who test positive for RET germline mutation should have a total thyroidectomy.[11] Lobectomy is indicated when FNA is benign, there is an increase in size of a nodule over time, compressive symptoms, cosmetic reasons patient/parent choice, and concern for unifocal malignancy.[4] According to the ATA, in children with no evidence of lymph node disease, there is no role for prophylactic lymph node dissection unless there is extrathyroidal extension of the primary, or MTC has been diagnosed.

It is important to complete a comprehensive history and physical during the preoperative evaluation with a pediatric patient. Part of that evaluation is establishing a one-on-one relationship with the patient at hand, as well as a sense of trust. A conversation about the patient's condition and frank discussion about the plan for surgical treatment should take place with the patient. Part of the comprehensive physical examination includes a full head and neck examination, including the thyroid and any cervical lymph nodes. An assessment of voice, swallow and breathing should also be made, and again if the child is old enough laryngeal examination should be considered. Laryngeal examination in the form of transnasal fiberoptic examination can be completed if the child is cooperative, but an alternative is transcutaneous laryngeal US. Transcutaneous laryngeal US is an accessible, and less invasive evaluation of the larynx using an in-office US probe over the skin and laryngeal skeleton that has been shown to be comparable to direct visualization.[15] A baseline voice assessment of the pediatric patient is just as important in order to establish expectations of voice use and vocal demands/ability after surgery. The involvement of a speech language pathology (SLP) early on is an important component of the preoperative evaluation. The prevalence of a multidisciplinary team dedicated to pediatric voice assessment is rare, but important.[16] Just as in adult patients, a preoperative voice assessment of a pediatric patient by both a specialist and an SLP team can elicit postoperative expectations and goals from the thyroid surgical standpoint.

6.3 Outcomes

The outcome postoperatively for children after total thyroidectomy is dependent on the completeness of the surgical resection and the experience of the surgeon. In accordance with Randolph et al's goals of management, it is imperative that a total thyroidectomy be complete, with low risk of morbidity to the patient.[12] It has been shown that if thyroidectomy is performed by high-volume surgeons, the complication rate is significantly less.[17] In a literature review examining over 20 case series reports on a total of 1800 pediatric patients, rates of permanent recurrent laryngeal nerve injury and permanent hypoparathyroidism were lowest in operations by high-volume thyroid surgeons.[18] There is a strong correlation of better outcome with high volume, high experience of the endocrine surgeon.

Overall, for patients with thyroid malignancy, prognosis for the pediatric population is very good with a 100% 10-year DSS.[4] The 2015 ATA guidelines stratify pediatric patients into ATA risk levels: low, intermediate, and high. Low-risk patients may have RAI omitted postoperatively, to avoid long-term morbidity of RAI without significantly altering disease-specific mortality and morbidity. Pediatric patients over adults are much more likely to present with advanced disease, including metastatic disease, but they still have better outcomes than adults.[4] Even those pediatric patients with pulmonary metastasis remain stable despite the number of RAI treatments, as compared to their adult counterparts.[4]

6.4 Multidisciplinary Team

The 2015 ATA guidelines highlight the importance of a multidisciplinary team involved in workup of pediatric thyroid patient, the need for a high-volume surgeon (30 or more endocrine procedure annually) to avoid complications, and the centralization of care for pediatric thyroid disease within a center.[2] This collaborative approach toward pediatric endocrine surgery has been endorsed by the American Thyroid Association in their management of pediatric thyroid cancer, with a recommendation rating of "B" (recommends, based on fair evidence).[4] The risks of surgery are known to occur less in the hands of experienced, high-volume surgeons. Those who are well versed in pediatric thyroidectomy should be performing these surgeries consistently. Experienced surgeons are more apt in removing all thyroid tissue safely without leaving remnant thyroid tissue behind. This is especially important when performing a thyroidectomy for familial MTC (prophylactic or therapeutic) and if one wishes to avoid RAI in PTC. Also important is that the surgeon be competent with performing comprehensive compartment-based nodal dissection when necessary.

The importance of surgeon volume and outcomes in pediatric thyroid patients is critical for best outcomes. Tuggle et al analyzed 607 pediatric patients undergoing thyroidectomy and parathyroidectomy using HCUP-NIS.[19] In this study, surgeons performing >30 cervical endocrine procedures per year in adults and children were defined as high volume irrespective of whether they were pediatric surgeons or not. High-volume surgeon was associated with better patient outcomes, with endocrine-specific complication rates of 5.6%, compared with 11.0% for pediatric surgeons and 9.5% for all other surgeons.[19] There was a significantly shorter hospital length of stay, and lower inpatient cost. Surgeon volume was an independent predictor of length of stay and cost, and surgeon specialty was not associated with outcomes in multivariate analysis.[19] These results suggest that the most important predictor of pediatric outcomes after cervical endocrine surgery is surgeon volume, not surgeon specialty, and that the best outcomes are achieved by surgeon experience in both adult and pediatric thyroid disease.

Preoperative counseling regarding the risks, benefits, and alternatives for a diagnostic lobectomy versus total thyroidectomy, and the need for central and lateral neck dissections if indicated, must be done in detail with the patient and their family. Risks include and are not limited to bleeding, infection, hypoparathyroidism, voice changes and possible airway difficulty, need for tracheostomy for airway management, thyroid hormone supplementation, and possibility of calcium supplementation postoperatively. The risks of central and lateral neck dissection are similar to the adult patient population. The risks should be outlined with the goals for complete resection of bulky disease for locoregional control.

Preoperative labs including calcium, vitamin D, PTH, albumin and TSH, FT4 are also drawn as baseline values.

6.5 Pediatric Anesthesia for Thyroidectomy

For all pediatric patients, preoperative evaluation is imperative with a dedicated pediatric anesthesiologist. Appropriate dosing of pediatric medications as well as induction using an age-appropriate endotracheal tube is important. If using a NIMS® endotracheal tube for intraoperative neural monitoring of the recurrent laryngeal nerve, it is important to discuss about the size of the tube with the anesthesiology team.

6.6 Surgical Technique/ Operative Planning

6.6.1 Goals

The surgical technique for thyroidectomy in pediatric patients is the same as adult patients at our institution. The goals of thyroidectomy in the pediatric population are to remove all disease to provide adequate staging, with the least morbidity to the parathyroid glands and the recurrent laryngeal nerves. Precision and meticulous attention to anatomy during any thyroidectomy is the key to optimal surgical outcome. Surgical precision requires attention to detail.

6.6.2 Anesthesia

It is important that for all pediatric patients, a pediatric anesthesiology team evaluates the patient prior to surgery and is available for the day of surgery to administer the age-appropriate anesthesia. The patient and family should be comfortable with the anesthesiology staff, and this is also important for a non-traumatic intubation. If using a NIMS monitoring endotracheal tube it must be positioned appropriately for neural monitoring during the procedure. After anesthesia induction, proper confirmation of the endotracheal tube placement is done prior to taping. The size of the endotracheal tube is dependent on the diameter of the tube in relation to the patient. We check for appropriate EMG connection with the neural monitor. A perioperative dose of dexamethasone may be delivered intravenously prior to incision, based upon weight. Antibiotics are given if a central or lateral neck dissection is part of the procedure but are typically not given before thyroid surgery alone.

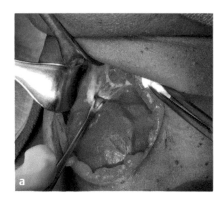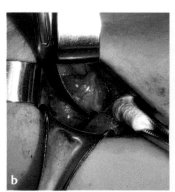

Fig. 6.1 **(a)** First example of the external branch of the superior laryngeal nerve trajectory upon taking down superior pole. **(b)** Second example of the external branch of the superior laryngeal nerve trajectory upon taking down superior pole.

6.6.3 Preparation/Planning the Incision

The patient is prepped and draped. We use a 2 to 3 cm transverse incision in the most natural skin crease that is not as easy to find in a pediatric patient compared to an adult. It is typically higher in the neck and often at the level of the cricoid. Despite this high location we feel it gives excellent access if just performing a thyroidectomy alone.

6.6.4 Incision and Flap Elevation

We incise skin and elevate subplatysmal flaps, superiorly to the thyroid notch and inferiorly to the clavicle. In an effort to lateralize the strap muscles we incise along the median raphe, and then elevate the sternohyoid muscle off the sternothyroid, and then the sternothyroid muscle off the thyroid capsule. The lateral extent of our dissection is the carotid artery on both sides. It is important to always begin on the side of the lesion in question, and in regard to cancer diagnosis in the thyroid, on the side that has the largest nodule with a cancer diagnosis.

6.6.5 Mobilization of Thyroid Gland

Once that side is decided, we begin by elevating off the fascia from the thyroid capsule laterally, and skeletonize the thyroid gland from superior lobe to inferiorly along the trachea.

6.6.6 Key Maneuvers

We perform key maneuvers in mobilization of the thyroid gland inferiorly by elevating it off midline trachea at the thyrothymic ligament as well as excising the Delphian node and pyramidal lobe protecting the cricothyroid musculature so we can identify hypovascular plane between the cricothyroid, inferior constrictor and superior pole. This plane is also referred to as Joll's space.[20] Once this space is developed and defined using blunt dissection, the external branch of the superior laryngeal nerve coursing over the inferior constrictor to the cricothyroid musculature can be identified in about 85%

of cases and stimulated. The trajectory of the external branch of the superior laryngeal nerve can take multiple routes and it is important to stimulate the nerve during dissection ▶Fig. 6.1a, b). The superior pole can then be taken down and along the plane of the thyroid capsule, and the thyroid can be rotated medially along the trachea.

6.6.7 Identifying the Recurrent Laryngeal Nerve and Parathyroid Glands

We identify the recurrent laryngeal nerve at the mid-thyroid lobe region, and then proceed to dissect superiorly toward the insertion point. We can also identify the inferior thyroid artery that courses perpendicular to the nerve, and rather than take this down, we can dissect bluntly deep into this and identify the recurrent laryngeal nerve. Identification of our parathyroid glands also allows mapping of the recurrent laryngeal nerve, as the superior parathyroid lies deep and caudal to the nerve, and the inferior parathyroid superficial to it. In taking down the thyroid capsule we identify and preserve the inferior thyroid artery-based pedicle of the superior and inferior parathyroid glands. Intracapsular parathyroids that can't be preserved in situ are removed and reimplanted at the end of surgery if necessary.

Once the recurrent laryngeal nerve is identified, it is important to trace the nerve beginning inferiorly and working superiorly, taking down the thyroid capsule meticulously. The goal is to protect the recurrent laryngeal nerve, stimulate and preserve it, while at the same time mobilizing the thyroid off Berry's ligament medially and rotating the gland over the trachea (▶Fig. 6.2).

6.6.8 Medialization of Thyroid Gland over Trachea

The RLN can be protected with a moist Kitner and gently pushed posteriorly to allow for complete removal of all tissue at Berry's ligament. Perforators at the cricothyroid, isthmus boundary as well as the cricothyroid joint are micro bipolared for hemostasis. We take down the isthmus, pyramidal lobe and Delphian nodes with the

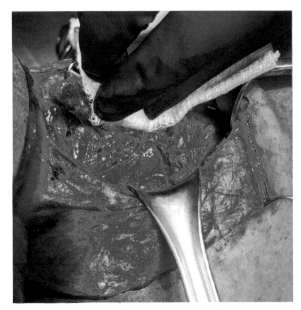

Fig. 6.2 Medialization of the thyroid lobe over the trachea. Identification of the recurrent laryngeal nerve.

total thyroidectomy specimen. Depending on the size of the total gland we can choose to take the specimen off the trachea in entirety or remove each lobe in sequence. Our goal is to achieve meticulous hemostasis along the entirety of the case, in order to preserve clear identification of tissue planes.

6.6.9 Removal of the Specimen, Reimplantation, and Re-evaluation of Nerves

Once the specimen is removed, we evaluate it grossly for number and size of thyroid nodules. We are also careful to identify any intracapsular parathyroid glands that may have been adherent to the thyroid capsule during dissection and/or whose vascular supply was from the thyroid gland itself, requiring intracapsular dissection of the parathyroid gland off the thyroid capsule and placement of the parathyroid gland in normal saline on ice for later auto reimplantation. We stimulate our vagus nerves and our recurrent laryngeal nerves bilaterally one last time, and place Surgicel within each side of the neck along with fibrin glue.

6.6.10 Closure of Wound

We reapproximate the strap muscles with a running 3–0 Vicryl stitch, making sure to reappose the fascia over the musculature appropriately. We then verify the absence of any further bleeding within the subplatysmal space before closing the skin with 3–0 vicryl subdermal sutures. We are sure to remove the patient from

extension before skin closure. We place tissue adhesive glue over the skin after everting the edges meticulously for final wound closure.

6.7 Postoperative Management

The most immediate consideration in postoperative management includes the integrity of the vocal fold function upon extubation. The concern for a lost signal with the intraoperative neural monitoring is rare but if present, flexible laryngoscopy immediately upon extubation is a good tool to confirm intact mobility of bilateral true vocal cords, as well as an assessment of postoperative laryngeal edema. Safe transfer of the patient to a pediatric unit or the recovery unit is the next step. During the hospital stay, the patient is monitored for pain, oral intake, as well as calcium surveillance with calcium blood draws every 6 to 8 hours. Immediately postoperatively in the PACU a PTH level is also drawn to be compared to the preoperative PTH.[21] This helps us determine a gradient for which concern for hypocalcemia, along with the calcium trend, may occur.[21,22] If patients undergo a neck dissection, a suction drain is placed in the compartments of the neck that underwent dissection. For lateral neck dissections we consult occupational therapy and physical therapy to assist in immediate postoperative range of motion exercises at the bedside prior to discharge.

The patient is usually inpatient for a day postoperatively, and discharged home with the possibility of JP drains if output >30 cc/24 hours. The need for calcium and calcitriol supplementation for home is dependent upon the serial calcium checks as an inpatient. Follow-up for drain removal is within 3 to 5 days postoperatively, and formal postoperative follow-up is within 2 to 3 weeks. Discharge instructions must be made available and detailed for pediatric patients and family members upon discharge, including a schedule and compliance of all home medications upon discharge, including age-appropriate dosages. Activity restrictions, diet, and showering should also be discussed. Communication about postoperative home care is important in both the preoperative consultation and prior to discharge. A contact number should be made available in case there are any immediate questions or concerns.

6.8 Conclusion

Pediatric thyroidectomy requires a multidisciplinary approach and a high-volume endocrine surgeon to complete a comprehensive and thorough surgical outcome. Pediatric thyroidectomy in our institution is technically similar to our adult population, but the importance of low morbidity with completeness of resection must be balanced among the long-term goals for a pediatric patient and the family. Having a multidisciplinary team is crucial in facilitating sound communication, patient satisfaction, and patient outcome. This chapter approaches pediatric thyroidectomy with these goals in mind.

6.9 Highlights

a. Indications
   - Graves' disease.
   - Benign nodules causing compressive symptoms.
   - Papillary thyroid carcinoma, medullary and follicular thyroid carcinomas.
   - MEN syndromes (prophylactic thyroidectomy).
b. Contraindications
   - Medical comorbidities.
   - Age <18 months.
   - Increased perioperative risk.
c. Complications
   - Hypocalcemia.
   - Vocal cord palsy/paralysis.
   - Hematoma/Seroma.
d. Special preoperative considerations
   - Pediatric anesthesiology team.
   - Pediatric nursing care/OR staff.
   - Multidisciplinary team/tumor board with surgeon, endocrinologist, oncologist, pediatrician.
   - Parent/child consultation/informed consent prior to surgery.
e. Special intraoperative considerations
   - Positioning of child.
   - Size of endotracheal tube (size of NIMS endotracheal tube for IONM).
   - IONM.
   - Incision/Scar placement.
   - Position of parathyroid glands (inferior parathyroid gland within potentially thymic tissue).
   - Size and integrity of the superior laryngeal nerves.
   - Size and integrity of the recurrent laryngeal nerves.
f. Special postoperative considerations
   - Postoperative pediatric floor/nursing care.
   - Pain control.
   - Rehabilitation.
   - Postoperative calcium management.
   - Compliance with thyroid hormone and calcium supplementation.
   - Discharge instructions for home (including activity, diet, shower, pain control, medications).

References

[1] Haugen BR, Alexander EK, Bible KC, et al. 2015 American Thyroid Association Management Guidelines for Adult Patients with Thyroid Nodules and Differentiated Thyroid Cancer: The American Thyroid Association Guidelines Task Force on Thyroid Nodules and Differentiated Thyroid Cancer. Thyroid 2016;26(1):1–133

[2] Hogan AR, Zhuge Y, Perez EA, Koniaris LG, Lew JI, Sola JE. Pediatric thyroid carcinoma: incidence and outcomes in 1753 patients. J Surg Res 2009;156(1):167–172

[3] Wang TS, Sosa J. Who should do Thyroid Surgery? In: Hanks JB, and Inabet W, eds. Controversies in Thyroid Surgery. Switzerland: Springer International Publishing; 2016: 57–64

[4] Francis GL, Waguespack SG, Bauer AJ, et al. Management Guidelines for Children with Thyroid Nodules and Differentiated Thyroid Cancer: The American Thyroid Association Guidelines Task Force on Pediatric Thyroid Cancer. Thyroid 2015;26(1):2016

[5] Feinmesser R, Lubin E, Segal K, Noyek A. Carcinoma of the thyroid in children: a review. J Pediatr Endocrinol Metab 1997;10(6):561–568

[6] Halac I, Zimmerman D. Thyroid nodules and cancers in children. Endocrinol Metab Clin North Am 2005;34(3):725–744, x

[7] Josefson J, Zimmerman D. Thyroid nodules and cancers in children. Pediatr Endocrinol Rev 2008;6(1):14–23

[8] Kloos RT, Eng C, Evans DB, et al; American Thyroid Association Guidelines Task Force. Medullary thyroid cancer: management guidelines of the American Thyroid Association. Thyroid 2009;19(6):565–612

[9] Wu LS, Roman SA, Sosa JA. Medullary thyroid cancer: an update of new guidelines and recent developments. Curr Opin Oncol 2011;23(1):22–27

[10] Prasad ML, Vyas M, Horne MJ, et al. NTRK fusion oncogenes in pediatric papillary thyroid carcinoma in northeast United States. Cancer 2016;122(7):1097–1107

[11] Nikiforov YE, Rowland JM, Bove KE, Monforte-Munoz H, Fagin JA. Distinct pattern of ret oncogene rearrangements in morphological variants of radiation-induced and sporadic thyroid papillary carcinomas in children. Cancer Res 1997;57(9):1690–1694

[12] Randolph G. Surgery of the Thyroid and Parathyroid Glands. Saunders; 2012

[13] Handkiewicz-Junak D, Wloch J, Roskosz J, et al. Total thyroidectomy and adjuvant radioiodine treatment independently decrease locoregional recurrence risk in childhood and adolescent differentiated thyroid cancer. J Nucl Med 2007;48(6):879–888

[14] Bilimoria KY, Bentrem DJ, Ko CY, et al. Extent of surgery affects survival for papillary thyroid cancer. Ann Surg 2007;246(3):375–381, discussion 381–384

[15] Wong KP, Au KP, Lam S, Lang BH. Lessons Learned After 1000 Cases of Transcutaneous Laryngeal Ultrasound (TLUSG) with Laryngoscopic Validation: Is There a Role of TLUSG in Patients Indicated for Laryngoscopic Examination Before Thyroidectomy? Thyroid 2017;27(1):88–94

[16] Kelchner LN, Brehm SB, de Alarcon A, Weinrich B. Update on pediatric voice and airway disorders: assessment and care. Curr Opin Otolaryngol Head Neck Surg 2012;20(3):160–164

[17] Gourin CG, Tufano RP, Forastiere AA, Koch WM, Pawlik TM, Bristow RE. Volume-based trends in thyroid surgery. Arch Otolaryngol Head Neck Surg 2010;136(12):1191–1198

[18] Thompson GB, Hay ID. Current strategies for surgical management and adjuvant treatment of childhood papillary thyroid carcinoma. World J Surg 2004;28(12):1187–1198

[19] Tuggle CT, Roman SA, Wang TS, et al. Pediatric endocrine surgery: who is operating on our children? Surgery 2008;144(6):869–877, discussion 877

[20] Clark OH, et al. Textbook of Endocrine Surgery. 3rd ed. Jaypee Brothers Medical Publishing; 2016

[21] Noureldine SI, Genther DJ, Lopez M, Agrawal N, Tufano RP. Early predictors of hypocalcemia after total thyroidectomy: an analysis of 304 patients using a short-stay monitoring protocol. JAMA Otolaryngol Head Neck Surg 2014;140(11):1006–1013

[22] Al Khadem MG, Rettig EM, Dhillon VK, Russell JO, Tufano RP. Postoperative IPTH compared with IPTH gradient as predictors of post-thyroidectomy hypocalcemia. Laryngoscope 2018; 128(3):769–774

7 Neck Dissection for Thyroid Cancer in Children

Vaninder K. Dhillon, Jonathon O. Russell, Ralph P. Tufano

Summary

This chapter summarizes the guidelines, techniques, and surgical considerations for pediatric patients undergoing neck dissection for thyroid cancer. Based upon the pathophysiology of lymph node disease in pediatric thyroid cancer, alongside the current 2015 American Thyroid Association (ATA) guidelines, we discuss the nuances of performing central and lateral neck dissection in the pediatric population. Neck dissection techniques and principles in the pediatric population are similar to an adult. We emphasize the importance of expertise from high-volume endocrine surgeons in performing neck dissections for the pediatric thyroid cancer patient, in order to complete a safe comprehensive resection of the neck. A robust multidisciplinary team like in our thyroidectomy patients, that are familiar with caring for and managing a pediatric-centric patient population, is crucial to the overall care as well.

Keywords: Neck dissection , pediatric thyroid cancer, pediatric patient, multidisciplinary team, endocrine surgeon, surgical technique, surgical consideration, lymph node disease

7.1 Introduction

Neck dissection in the pediatric population is primarily limited to malignancies of the thyroid gland.[1] Well-differentiated thyroid malignancies with evidence of lymph node disease must be addressed with a total thyroidectomy and respective neck dissection of the compartments involved. Total thyroidectomy by a high-volume surgeon is traditionally favored as the optimal treatment, with a neck dissection to remove regional lymph nodes as required.[1] The goal of a neck dissection for malignant thyroid disease is to ensure complete surgical resection of all gross tumor disease, as well as the frequent microscopic foci of cancer.[2,3] Removal of all tissue with well-differentiated thyroid carcinoma allows for improved adjuvant radioiodine ablation and monitoring of serum thyroglobulin levels to monitor for tumor recurrence.[4,5] A recent review of the medical management of differentiated thyroid carcinoma (DTC) in children supports this approach.[2]

This chapter discusses the importance of a neck dissection for malignant thyroid disease, both in the central neck and lateral neck. It will outline the indications for neck dissection, and the considerations for neck disease in a pediatric patient. There will be a discussion of surgical technique and the main steps involved at our institution. Highlights of the complications associated with neck dissection will also be discussed.

7.2 Guidelines for Pediatric Neck Dissection in Thyroid Malignancy

The indications for neck dissection in pediatric thyroid malignancies are similar to those in adults, although there should be higher index for suspicion for lymphadenopathy present in children. According to the American Thyroid Association (ATA), pediatric thyroid cancer demonstrates a higher prevalence of metastatic disease in the surrounding lymph nodes as compared to adults.[6] Pediatric patients presenting with a diagnosis of thyroid carcinoma should undergo a comprehensive evaluation for metastatic disease, including a screening ultrasound of the cervical lymph nodes as well as CT neck and chest to evaluate for disease in the retropharynx and distant sites.[6] While the latter may not be amenable to surgical intervention, the former should usually be managed by a thoughtful surgeon at the time of the index surgery. Patients with metastatic thyroid carcinoma to the cervical lymph nodes should undergo a comprehensive compartmental neck dissection.[7,8] Pediatric patients with medullary thyroid carcinoma should undergo bilateral central neck dissection prophylactically, similar to adults, as the risk for lymph node disease in the central neck is as high as 80 to 85%.[9,10] The recommendation for pediatric patients with a family history of MEN syndrome is a prophylactic thyroidectomy, but there are no current guidelines suggesting prophylactic neck dissection in this subgroup.[6,9] In consultation with a multidisciplinary team, factors such as age, calcitonin levels, exam findings, and RET mutation should be considered before determining the role of prophylactic central neck dissection in such cases.[6]

7.3 Anatomy of a Neck Dissection

The cervical anatomy of a pediatric patient is equivalent to that of an adult with some exceptions. While the trachea may be shorter and the neck more stout, the landmarks and compartmental borders in neck anatomy are equal when considering neck dissection in children. Neck dissections are divided into the lymphatic compartments being resected. Compartmentalization of lymph node dissection is important for adequate resection of all disease. The neck can be broadly divided into the central and lateral neck compartments. According to the ATA, the central neck is defined as the region bounded laterally by the carotid arteries, superiorly by the hyoid bone and inferiorly by the sternal notch.[11] The central neck can be divided into the right and left sides with the tracheal skeleton as the center. The technique of central neck dissection varies slightly as well, because the more oblique course of the recurrent laryngeal nerve on the right is not at the level of the esophageal muscularis. Instead, a complete dissection of the right central neck requires a full mobilization of the recurrent laryngeal nerve, removing nodes and fibrofatty tissue both caudad and cephalad to the nerve. On the left, however, the fibrofatty tissue of the central neck is all cephalad to the recurrent laryngeal nerve, and full mobilization of the nerve is therefore not required.[12] It is important to consider the implications of a composite resection and its morbidity. This may influence dissection technique to prevent morbidity to the nerve and possibilities of vocal cord weakness. Central neck dissection is further complicated by the near translucent quality of immature parathyroid glands, which can be very difficult to identify in young patients.

The lateral neck, on the other hand, is outlined as the compartment that includes anatomic neck levels 1 through 5. In accordance with the ATA task force on lateral neck dissection, if there is evidence of lateral neck disease in levels 2 to 4, then it is important to compartmentally resect levels 2A through 5B.[13,14] Level 2 is divided into A/B bounded by the accessory nerve (CN XI). Level 5 can likewise be divided by the accessory nerve, but is more frequently divided into these levels at the level of the cricoid. Dissection of levels 2B and 5A is not routinely done unless there is disease in adjacent nodal basins (i.e., 2a).[14] For children with evidence of bulky lymphadenopathy in the lateral neck and no evidence of central neck disease, a central neck dissection is most often performed unilateral to the side of lateral neck disease. There is a 20 to 40% risk for central neck disease in clinically N0 central neck if lateral neck is involved,[14] although "skip" metastases are also common. Again, the decision to perform a prophylactic central neck dissection should be considered cautiously, although many surgeons feel that the risks are justified given the high rate of occult disease.

Adequate exposure for compartmental clean out is crucial in any neck dissection, regardless of the compartment. For a central neck dissection, exposure up to the hyoid and down to the sternal notch with good visualization of the innominate artery is important. For the lateral neck, visualization of the accessory nerve (CN XI) is important in defining the boundary for level 2A and, importantly, 2B. If level 5 disease is involved then it may be necessary to transpose the accessory nerve in order to resect disease completely behind the sternocleidomastoid muscle up to the trapezius.

7.4 Considerations for Neck Dissection in the Pediatric Population

It is important to consider each pediatric patient with an individualized approach. Age and the appropriate level of maturity for each pediatric patient are important when approaching children in regards to evaluation and discussion. It is important to have a multidisciplinary team with pediatric inclined endocrinologists, oncologists, endocrine surgeons as well as all ancillary staff like speech therapists, psychologists, and nursing discussing patient care, expectations, and recommendations, and having a cohesive plan to present to each patient and their parents. A directed approach to imaging proven neck disease may occur if the child's health and limitations may limit a comprehensive dissection, but such decisions should be made among a multidisciplinary team. The imperative of such shared decision making is a strong recommendation by the ATA.[6] This is important in the preoperative as much as it is in the postoperative periods. As previously mentioned, similar considerations should be made for all pediatric patients undergoing a neck dissection.

In the preoperative evaluation, the following should be evaluated in a pediatric patient:

- Voice use, demand, and any preoperative voice concerns.
- Airway (concerns).
- Craniofacial abnormalities.
- Level of physical activity and baseline nutrition.
- Healing potential.
- Expectation (of patient and family).
- Medications and medical comorbidities.
- Genetic factors (RET oncogene mutation, bleeding diatheses, etc.).

7.5 Intraoperative Considerations

- Type and size of endotracheal tube used for intraoperative nerve monitoring (IONM).
- Degree of fibrosis and infiltration of thyroid tissue during resection.
- Consideration of recurrent laryngeal nerve status during dissection (with use of IONM).
- Parathyroid gland status and vasculature.
- Cranial nerves.
- Thoracic duct.
- Vascular structures, including great vessels.

7.6 Postoperative Considerations

- Pain control.
- Vocal fold weakness, voice quality.
- Hypoparathyroidism and need for calcium repletion.
- Hypothyroidism.
- Level of activity, rehabilitation with physical therapy/ occupational therapy.
- Nutritional status.
- Psychosocial component.
- Swallowing problems.
- The need for further therapy such as radioactive iodine (RAI).

7.7 Surgical Technique

Our surgical approach to the pediatric neck is similar to the adult. We adhere to the guidelines by the ATA Surgical Affairs Committee on their guidelines for central and lateral neck dissection.[11,13] A representative computed tomography (CT) neck and chest done preoperatively at our institution for every patient undergoing neck dissection allows for full evaluation of the neck anatomy in guiding the approach for dissection. This is especially important for identifying nodes that may not be fully visualized on preoperative ultrasonography, which is also critical. Specific areas of focus for CT review should therefore include the retropharyngeal nodes as well as nodes in level 7 (substernal) that may be accessible via a cervical incision with appropriate planning. Positioning of a pediatric patient is important with neck extension and mobility balanced with the size, body habitus, and flexibility of the child. The surgical approach to the neck is outlined below, divided into compartments.

7.7.1 Central Neck Dissection

The central neck compartment can be accessed through the thyroidectomy incision (▶Fig. 7.1). With our thyroidectomy approach we have already lateralized the carotid sheath contents and for the central neck dissection we begin by dissection over the carotid artery. We dissect inferiorly to the level of the innominate artery and superiorly to the level of the cricoid on the respective side. We identify our recurrent laryngeal nerve and dissection continues on the nerve, taking down fibrofatty tissue between the course of the nerve and the trachea. On the right-hand side, lymph node tissue lies both caudad and cephalad to the nerve and therefore the right recurrent laryngeal nerve should be transposed for the fibrofatty tissue to be resected medially to the trachea. Sensory branches will therefore be sacrificed, but fortunately do

not add morbidity to the resection. The posterior boundary of the compartment is the esophageal muscularis, and it is important to clean all fibrofatty tissue off this structure. In the rare case of invasive disease, the muscularis itself can be removed with caution. Esophageal defects created in this fashion should be closed primarily while inverting the mucosa. The superior extent of the dissection is to the inferior thyroid artery, the trunk that gives off blood supply to the superior parathyroid gland. It is important to preserve this trunk in order to retain vascular integrity to the superior parathyroid tissue. An example of a completed right central neck dissection can be seen in ▶Fig. 7.2. It is common to resect the inferior parathyroid glands during a central compartment resection, given the unpredictable location of these glands as compared to the superior parathyroid glands.[11] This is especially true with a pediatric dissection. When identified, they can be clipped and removed from the final specimen, then reimplanted at the end of the case. They are routinely stored on sterile ice until the time of reimplantation. Because these glands can be so difficult to identify once the dissection has begun, we may choose to harvest these inferior glands prophylactically if they are identified early in the dissection (e.g., during thyroidectomy). We utilize IONM through our neck dissections to assess the integrity of the recurrent laryngeal nerve. It is important to maintain a stable vagal and recurrent laryngeal nerve stimulus throughout the case in order to assure vocal fold function. The decision to stage the procedure if signal is lost so as to prevent the need for tracheostomy is one that should be discussed between

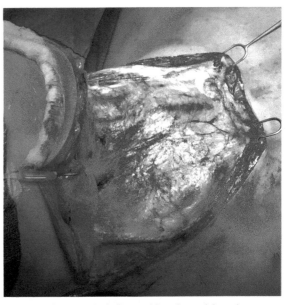

Fig. 7.1 Elevation of subplatysmal flaps for total thyroidectomy with bilateral central neck and lateral neck dissections.

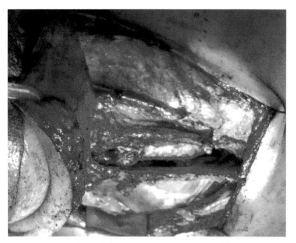

Fig. 7.2 Right central neck dissection.

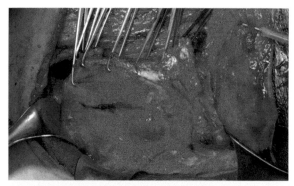

Fig. 7.3 Elevation of fibrofatty tissue medially from the floor of the neck over the carotid sheath.

the patient and the surgeon. Tracheostomy in this patient population is not without some risk, and, in cases where gross nerve integrity has been confirmed but physiologic activity is not noted, staging the contralateral thyroidectomy or central neck dissection may be appropriate.

7.7.2 Lateral Neck Dissection

The lateral neck dissection incorporates levels 2A through 5B in patients with evidence of lateral neck disease on preoperative evaluation. The incision for our lateral neck dissections is an extension of the thyroidectomy incision, approximately to the level of the mid-sternocleidomastoid muscle. This is done within a normal skin crease for cosmesis rather than curving the incision in the standard apron fashion. If level 2B is involved, however, the incision may be extended higher with a more vertical direction in order to gain adequate exposure to the compartment. We begin by elevating subplatysmal planes superiorly to one to two fingerbreadths below the angle of the mandible and inferiorly to the level of the clavicle. The subplatysmal fascia is incised at the inferior border of the submandibular gland (again, 1–2 fingerbreadths below the mandible so as to protect the marginal mandibular nerve) and we identify the digastric tunnel in order to follow it laterally to the internal jugular vein. We can then also identify our hypoglossal nerve just posterior to the digastric tendon. The sternocleidomastoid muscle is then incised medially so that fibrofatty tissue is elevated medially. We identify level 2A by tracing out the accessory nerve in a lateral-to-medial trajectory toward the internal jugular vein. This defines the boundaries of levels 2A and 2B and we can then proceed to dissect down to the floor of the neck using a Hemostatic scalpel blade or other dissecting instrumentation. We transpose the accessory nerve over level 2B during dissection and then proceed to elevated levels 2–5B from the medial

edge of the sternocleidomastoid muscle in an inferior direction. We can remove the fibrofatty tissue swiftly and identify our cervical rootlets. Following the rootlets inferiorly we are able to protect the contents of the floor of the neck including the phrenic nerve and the brachial plexus in level 4 which can be identified using the intraoperative nerve monitor. We identify and skeletonize the omohyoid, transversing in a diagonal direction at level 3–4 junction and are able to transpose this and retract during the rest of the inferior dissection, preserving it to the best of our ability. At the inferior aspect of level 4 we dissect out and preserve the transverse cervical vessels and, as we move medially toward the internal jugular vein, identify our thoracic duct. We use the Ligasure device, ties, or clips to take down all lymphatic channels that may be associated with the thoracic duct close to the internal jugular vein in order to seal these structures and protect from potential leak. Clips may make subsequent imaging and follow-up more difficult, however, and some authors discourage their use. Once the internal jugular vein is identified inferiorly we elevate the fibrofatty tissue medially over the carotid artery, vagus, and vein (▶Fig. 7.3). Once medialized we are able to stay over the anterior edge of the internal jugular and take down levels 2A/B and excise the tissue over the strap musculature to finally resect our specimen. It is important to evaluate the retrocarotid location for any occult lymphadenopathy. It is also important that all fibrofatty tissue is resected in levels 5B behind the sternocleidomastoid muscle. If 5A is involved we will plan for the dissection of the accessory nerve through the sternocleidomastoid muscle to the trapezius, with its transposition to allow for that compartment to be resected. This may leave more traction on the accessory nerve but our goal is to keep it intact. ▶Fig. 7.4 represents the completion of a lateral neck dissection. We perform a Valsalva at the end of the procedure in order to identify any chyle leak or bleeding from a major vessel. We stimulate all nerves for final confirmation of physiologic function including the vagus, accessory nerve, hypoglossal nerve, and the phrenic, and then proceed to close

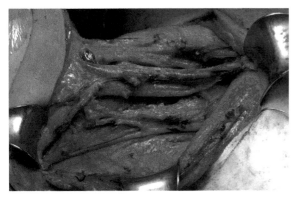

Fig. 7.4 Right lateral neck dissection (levels 2A/B through 5B) after resection with identification of landmarks.

the neck. We place a single size-10-blake drain into the lateral neck for every dissection, sutured to the skin. Subdermal closure is achieved using 3–0 vicryl interrupted sutures and the skin can be closed with a monocryl in a subcuticular fashion. Dermal glue can be placed over the incision.

7.7.3 Postoperative Surveillance

Postoperatively we monitor for the most common complications of a lateral neck dissection including hematoma, cranial nerve palsy (most commonly shoulder weakness), and chyle leak. It is important that pain is controlled with an appropriate pediatric staff and team in charge of pain management for children. It is important to get rehabilitation services including physical therapy involved early to help with ambulating and range of motion exercises. If level 5A is resected, there should be a lower threshold to get physical therapy involved in the rehabilitation early on, but we will routinely order physical therapy and occupational therapy for all patients with a lateral neck dissection. Children can be placed on a regular diet and chyle can be monitored with oral intake. The Blake drain remains in place as long as the output >30 cc/day and if necessary a child can go home with it as long as the parents and caregivers have adequate instructions on nursing care. Based upon the overall condition of the patient, an establishment of expectations during the convalescent period, and the comfort level of the parents in care at home, a pediatric patient can go home the next day after surgery.

7.7.4 Parathyroid Autoimplantation

If there are parathyroid glands clipped during a central neck dissection as previously discussed, it is common to reimplant the parathyroid glands. The inferior parathyroid glands are the most commonly resected and reimplanted. It is routine for us to review the final specimen before it is sent to pathology for any evidence of parathyroid tissue as well. A piece of suspected parathyroid tissue can be sent for frozen for confirmation, and reimplanted at the end of the case. Parathyroid autoimplantation is done by incising the ipsilateral sternocleidomastoid muscle (or the sternocleidomastoid muscle which is intact if resection is necessary) and created a pocket within the muscle to place the parathyroid tissue. We mince up the parathyroid tissue and place within the pocket, using a mattress 3–0 vicryl to suture the muscle and overlying fascia closed, and then clip on either side for identification purposes.

7.8 Conclusion

Neck dissection in the pediatric population is an important component of any child with thyroid malignancy. The approach to the pediatric neck is similar to that of an adult, but the ability to balance a comprehensive approach with low morbidity is dependent upon the experience and technique of a high-volume surgeon who is facile with the anatomy of the lateral neck and the nuances of a detailed dissection. Nodal yield is important as a low nodal yield has been associated with increased recurrence in some series.[15] As in pediatric thyroidectomy it is important to emphasize goals and expectations with patients and their families in a multidisciplinary fashion, and enable the child to participate as much as possible in their care. This chapter is meant to outline those expectations and surgical technique in order to achieve the best outcome for a child.

7.9 Highlights

a. Indications
   - All pediatric patients should undergo comprehensive evaluation for metastatic disease with US and CT of the neck.
   - All patients with evidence of neck disease should undergo compartmental neck dissection of the levels involved.
b. Contraindications
   - Surgically inoperable disease.
   - Medical comorbidities precluding surgery.
   - Surgical risks are higher than prognostic benefits.
c. Complications
   - Pain.
   - Scar.
   - Infection.
   - Hoarseness or change of voice.
   - Swallowing problems.

- Vocal cord paralysis.
- Airway compromise.
- Hypoparathyroidism.
- Hypothyroidism.
- Thoracic duct injury.
- Psychosocial difficulty (in coping).
- Nutritional status.
- Poor mobility postoperatively/poor rehabilitation potential.
- Poor wound healing.
- Recurrence.

d. Special preoperative considerations
- Voice use, demand, and any preoperative voice concerns.
- Airway (concerns).
- Craniofacial abnormalities.
- Level of physical activity and baseline nutrition.
- Healing potential.
- Expectation (of patient and family).
- Medications and medical comorbidities.
- Genetic factors (RET oncogene mutation, bleeding diatheses, etc.).

e. Special intraoperative considerations
- Type and size of endotracheal tube used for intra-operative nerve monitoring (IONM).
- Degree of fibrosis and infiltration of thyroid tissue during resection.
- Consideration of recurrent laryngeal nerve status during dissection (with use of IONM).
- Parathyroid gland status and vasculature.
- Cranial nerves.
- Thoracic duct.
- Vascular structures, including great vessels.

f. Special postoperative considerations
- Pain control.
- Vocal fold weakness, voice quality.
- Hypoparathyroidism and need for calcium repletion.
- Hypothyroidism.
- Level of activity, rehabilitation with physical therapy/occupational therapy.
- Nutritional status.
- Psychosocial component.
- Swallowing problems.
- The need for further therapy such as radioactive iodine (RAI).

References

[1] Jin X, Masterson L, Patel A, et al. Conservative or radical surgery for pediatric papillary thyroid carcinoma: a systematic review of the literature. Int J Pediatr Otorhinolaryngol 2015;79(10):1620–1624

[2] Rivkees SA, Mazzaferri EL, Verburg FA, et al. The treatment of differentiated thyroid cancer in children: emphasis on surgical approach and radioactive iodine therapy. Endocr Rev 2011;32(6):798–826

[3] Vermeer-Mens JC, Goemaere NN, Kuenen-Boumeester V, et al. Childhood papillary thyroid carcinoma with miliary pulmonary metastases. J Clin Oncol 2006;24(36):5788–5789

[4] Diesen DL, Skinner MA. Pediatric thyroid cancer. Semin Pediatr Surg 2012;21(1):44–50

[5] Scholz S, Smith JR, Chaignaud B, Shamberger RC, Huang SA. Thyroid surgery at Children's Hospital Boston: a 35-year single-institution experience. J Pediatr Surg 2011;46(3):437–442

[6] Francis GL, Waguespack SG, Bauer AJ, et al; American Thyroid Association Guidelines Task Force. Management guidelines for children with thyroid nodules and differentiated thyroid cancer. Thyroid 2015;25(7):716–759

[7] Welch Dinauer CA, Tuttle RM, Robie DK, McClellan DR, Francis GL. Extensive surgery improves recurrence-free survival for children and young patients with class I papillary thyroid carcinoma. J Pediatr Surg 1999;34(12):1799–1804

[8] Kloos RT, Eng C, Evans DB, et al; American Thyroid Association Guidelines Task Force. Medullary thyroid cancer: management guidelines of the American Thyroid Association. Thyroid 2009; 19(6):565–612

[9] Carty SE, Cooper DS, Doherty GM, et al; American Thyroid Association Surgery Working Group. American Association of Endocrine Surgeons. American Academy of Otolaryngology-Head and Neck Surgery. American Head and Neck Society. Consensus statement on the terminology and classification of central neck dissection for thyroid cancer. Thyroid 2009;19(11):1153–1158

[10] Scollo C, Baudin E, Travagli JP, et al. Rationale for central and bilateral lymph node dissection in sporadic and hereditary medullary thyroid cancer. J Clin Endocrinol Metab 2003;88(5):2070–2075

[11] Pai SI, Tufano RP. Central compartment neck dissection for thyroid cancer: technical considerations. ORL J Otorhinolaryngol Relat Spec 2008;70(5):292–297

[12] Stack BC Jr, Ferris RL, Goldenberg D, et al; American Thyroid Association Surgical Affairs Committee. American Thyroid Association consensus review and statement regarding the anatomy, terminology, and rationale for lateral neck dissection in differentiated thyroid cancer. Thyroid 2012;22(5):501–508

[13] Farrag T, Lin F, Brownlee N, Kim M, Sheth S, Tufano RP. Is routine dissection of level II-B and V-A necessary in patients with papillary thyroid cancer undergoing lateral neck dissection for FNA-confirmed metastases in other levels. World J Surg 2009;33(8):1680–1683

[14] Park JH, Lee YS, Kim BW, Chang HS, Park CS. Skip lateral neck node metastases in papillary thyroid carcinoma. World J Surg 2012;36(4):743–747

[15] Schneider DF, Mazeh H, Chen H, Sippel RS. Lymph node ratio predicts recurrence in papillary thyroid cancer. Oncologist 2013;18(2):157–162

8 Pediatric Parotidectomy

Darrin V. Bann, Meghan Wilson

Summary

In comparison to adults, parotid lesions in children are more likely to result from infectious or inflammatory conditions than neoplastic processes. The etiology of the condition may often be determined through a combination of imaging and fine needle aspiration biopsy. Pediatric parotid surgery may be performed safely and effectively, provided that the surgeon is cognizant of important anatomical differences in the position of the facial nerve in children compared to adults.

Keywords: Parotidectomy in children, pediatric parotidectomy, parotid mass, facial nerve anatomy

8.1 Introduction

In comparison to adults, lesions of the parotid gland are significantly less common in pediatric patients. Nonetheless, there are a multitude of conditions that may involve the parotid gland in children, many of which ultimately require surgical intervention. Pediatric parotid surgery is safe and effective, provided that important anatomical differences between children and adults are recognized. The purpose of this chapter is to review the anatomy and development of the parotid gland in children; provide an overview of common pathology affecting the parotid gland in the pediatric population; and to provide a guide for performing safe and effective parotid surgery in children.

8.2 Anatomy and Embryology

A thorough understanding of the embryology and anatomy of the parotid gland, facial nerve, and mastoid bone is essential to performing safe and effective parotid surgery in the pediatric population. Importantly, there are several anatomic differences between children and adults that must be considered as part of the surgical planning and approach.

Like all salivary glands, the parotid gland is derived from rests of oral ectoderm, which first appear between the fourth and sixth weeks of gestation. These ectodermal rests pierce the surrounding mesoderm, arborize, and subsequently form the acini of the gland. The developing facial nerve reaches the parotid gland around the seventh week of gestation, and by the eleventh to twelfth week of gestation, the nerve has been completely enveloped by the gland parenchyma. Because expanding parotid parenchyma envelops the facial nerve, there is no true "plane" dividing the superficial from the deep lobe of the gland. Head and neck lymphatic development occurs between the twelfth and fourteenth weeks of gestation, which is prior to encapsulation of the parotid gland by the surrounding mesenchyme and the deep cervical fascia.[1] Although the parotid gland is the first major salivary gland to develop embryologically, it is the last major salivary gland to be encapsulated by fascia. Therefore, the parotid gland is the only salivary gland to contain lymph nodes within the gland parenchyma. Typically, 2–20 nodes are found within the superficial portion of the gland and 1–4 nodes are located in the deep portion of the gland.[1]

Drainage of saliva from the parotid gland is accomplished by Stensen's duct, which arises from the anterolateral surface of the gland. The duct courses anteriorly superficial to the masseter muscle, before turning medially at the anterior border of the masseter to pierce the buccinator and enter the oral cavity. The Stensen's duct os is typically located across from the second maxillary molar. Detached accessory parotid glands may be identified along Stensen's duct in up to 21% of individuals.[2]

The saliva produced by the parotid gland is predominately serous in nature and is responsible for nearly 50% of stimulated saliva production. By contrast, only 30 to 40% of resting saliva production originates from the parotid. Salivary flow from the parotid gland is regulated by parasympathetic and sympathetic innervation. Parasympathetic innervation of the parotid gland originates in the inferior salivatory nucleus in the medulla. These fibers travel with cranial nerve IX to exit the skull at the jugular foramen. The fibers leave the glossopharyngeal nerve as Jacobsen nerve before re-entering the skull through the inferior tympanic canniliculus and passing through the middle ear space as the tympanic plexus. These nerves coalesce into the lesser petrosal nerve, which exits the skull base through the foramen ovale. The presynaptic fibers synapse in the otic ganglion, with the postsynaptic fibers traveling with the auriculotemporal nerve to innervate the parotid parenchyma. Postganglionic sympathetic innervation of the parotid gland occurs through the superior cervical plexus. Parasympathetic stimulation produces large quantities of low-protein, serous saliva while sympathetic stimulation produces a small and variable quantity of thick saliva.

As noted above, the facial nerve is intimately associated with the parotid gland. In adults, well-defined anatomic landmarks are used to identify the main trunk of the facial nerve during parotid surgery (▶ Table 8.1). However, in pediatric patients the facial nerve is far more superficial, often lying just deep to the subcutaneous tissue. In addition, in young children for whom the mastoid is poorly pneumatized, the facial nerve takes a more abrupt and horizontal course from the stylomastoid foramen to the parotid gland. Based on cadaveric dissections of three stillborn infants, Farroir and Santini[3] recommend searching for the facial nerve as it exits the stylomastoid foramen in a triangle bordered by the cartilaginous ear canal, the anterior border of the sternocleidomastoid muscle, and

Table 8.1 Landmarks and approaches to identifying the main trunk of the facial nerve

Younger children	Older children and adults
• Triangle bordered by: – Cartilaginous ear canal (superior) – Anterior border of SCM (posterior) – Posterior belly of digastric (inferior) • Identify peripheral branch and trace posteriorly	• 1 cm anterior, inferior, and deep to the tragal pointer • 6–8 mm deep to the tympanomastoid suture line • Identify peripheral branch and trace posteriorly

the digastric muscle (▶ Table 8.1). Although the length of the facial nerve trunk distal to the stylomastoid foramen in healthy newborns remains poorly defined, studies on human fetuses have indicated that the main trunk ranges in length between 9 and 26 mm.[4] Branching patterns of the facial nerve were initially described by Davis et al in 1956 based on cadaveric dissections in 350 craniofacial halves.[5] Most commonly, the facial nerve bifurcates (~80%) into superior and inferior divisions with a variable degree of anastomosis,[6] but trifurcation may also be identified (~20%) (▶ Fig. 8.1).[4] It is important to note that the marginal mandibular branch of the facial nerve also takes a more superior course over the mandible in children compared to adults.

Differences in the extracranial course of the facial nerve between children and adults result largely from the relative absence of the mastoid process in young children.

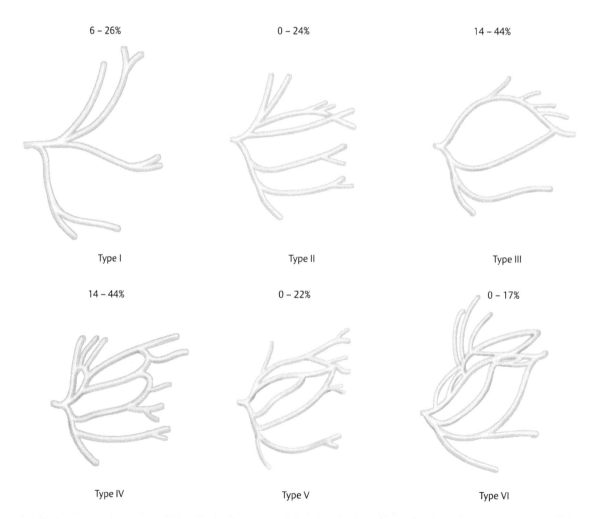

Fig. 8.1 Branching patterns of the facial nerve as described by Davis et al.[5] The percentage of individuals with each branching pattern is indicated above each illustration.[6] Type I: no anastomosis between the upper and lower division; Type II: anastomosis only between the branches of the upper division; Type III: single anastomosis between the upper and lower divisions; Type IV: combination of Type II and Type III; Type V: double anastomosis between the upper and lower divisions; Type VI: complex and numerous anastomoses between the two divisions.

The mastoid antrum is the first air cell to develop, and can be first recognized at 21 to 22 weeks of gestation with full development by 34 weeks. At birth, the antrum is typically the only fully developed air cell, representing an area of 2.9 cm^2.[7] Mastoid growth occurs at a rate of ~1 cm^2 per year up to age 6, at which point there is a more gradual increase in area until the mastoid reaches the adult size of approximately 12 cm^2.[8] As the mastoid air cell system increases in size and volume, the facial nerve subsequently takes a more medial and protected course behind the mastoid tip and tragal cartilage. Therefore, it is critical to consider patient age and the extent of mastoid development when dissecting towards the expected course of the facial nerve in pediatric patients.

8.3 Patient Evaluation

8.3.1 History and Physical Examination

Assessment of pediatric parotid gland disorders requires a detailed history regarding the course, onset, duration, severity, and frequency of symptoms. Parotid enlargement presenting in the perinatal period typically represents congenital lesions, while slowly enlarging, painless masses, especially those presenting in older children, may be more concerning for malignancy. By contrast, acute-onset painful swelling, particularly if associated with fever, suggests an infectious or inflammatory etiology. The quality and quantity of secretions should also be sought. Parents may attribute sialorrhea to the overproduction of saliva; however, this typically results from an inability to clear oral secretions and may be associated with underlying neuromuscular disorders. On the other hand, complaints of decreased salivary production, particularly in association with dry eye or dental caries, may suggest autoimmune conditions. Unilateral symptoms are generally suggestive of congenital, infectious, neoplastic, or traumatic disease processes, while bilateral or multiglandular involvement suggests systemic autoimmune or inflammatory disease. A history of trauma may be indicative of ductal disruption.

Physical examination for parotid lesions should always begin with a complete head-and-neck exam, including bimanual palpation of the parotid glands. The examiner should note the size, symmetry, consistency, and mobility of the parotid glands along with any nodularity, tenderness, and any overlying skin changes. The buccal mucosa should be carefully examined to identify the Stensen's duct orifice and scars, lesions, or bite marks that could potentially contribute to ductal obstruction. Saliva should be expressed by massaging the gland in a superior–anterior direction beginning at the angle of the mandible, noting the quantity, clarity, and viscosity of saliva. An absence of salivary flow may indicate ductal obstruction, while purulent fluid typically indicates bacterial parotitis. Erythema of the Stensen's duct orifice with clear saliva production is suggestive of viral sialadenitis. Although systematic evaluation of facial nerve function is sometimes challenging in pediatric patients, particularly young children who are unable or unwilling to follow commands, analysis and documentation of facial nerve function is essential to the evaluation of parotid lesions. Solid parotid gland lesions are more likely to be malignant in pediatric patients, and a history of a slowly growing mass combined with facial nerve weakness should immediately raise the concern for a malignant process.

8.3.2 Laboratory Evaluation

A thorough history and physical examination will guide the need for laboratory studies. Concern for an infectious etiology may indicate the need to evaluate white blood cell count, erythrocyte sedimentation rate, and/or C-reactive protein levels. By contrast, concern for an autoimmune etiology may necessitate serologic tests to evaluate for Sjögren's syndrome or sarcoidosis. Cystic multiglandular enlargement is suggestive of human immunodeficiency virus (HIV)–associated salivary gland disease and should prompt HIV testing. Serologic testing for Mumps may also be useful, particularly in unvaccinated children with parotid swelling.

8.3.3 Imaging Studies

Ultrasound remains the workhorse imaging modality for parotid lesions in children because it is inexpensive, widely available, and avoids radiation exposure.[9] In addition, ultrasound examinations can be performed rapidly on awake patients, potentially avoiding the need for sedation. It should be noted that ultrasound evaluation is highly user-dependent and therefore studies may vary significantly in quality. In experienced hands ultrasound can frequently identify sialoliths >2 mm and may help distinguish between benign and malignant lesions.[10] An important caveat regarding the use of ultrasound is that this modality has low specificity and accuracy regarding the diagnosis of solid parotid tumors,[11] although semi-quantitative ultrasound algorithms have been developed to more readily distinguish between benign and malignant solid masses.[12]

One particular advantage of ultrasound is that image-guided fine needle aspiration biopsy (FNAB) may be performed at the time of imaging, although sedation may be required, particularly for young children. A recent meta-analysis indicated that FNAB has a sensitivity and specificity of 88% and 99.5% with 19% probability of non-diagnostic or indeterminate cytology.[13] When applied specifically to pediatrics, a small study by Lee et al indicated that FNAB has a sensitivity of 100%, positive predictive value of 85%, and accuracy of 85.7% for the diagnosis of benign parotid lesions.[14] For superficial lesions that can be completely visualized on ultrasound and are confirmed to be benign on FNAB, additional imaging is often not required prior to surgical extirpation.[15] It is important to note that FNAB is contraindicated for vascular lesions due to the risk of bleeding.

Despite the advantages of ultrasound and its utility as an initial diagnostic modality, additional imaging studies are often required to evaluate for deep lobe lesions, involvement of the parapharyngeal space, cervical lymphadenopathy, and skull base extension. Computed tomography (CT) scanning with and without contrast is often the preferred modality of the evaluation of suspected inflammatory or obstructive conditions including sialolithiasis, sialadenitis, ranulas, and abscesses. Advantages of CT include the high degree of anatomic detail provided and operator-independent image acquisition permitting an unbiased analysis of the lesion and surrounding structures. Additionally, modern CT scanners have extremely rapid image acquisition times and therefore sedation is often not required. An important concern regarding the use of CT scanning, particularly among pediatric patients, is the development of secondary malignancies as a result of exposure to ionizing radiation. Several large studies have examined the risk of malignancy associated with CT scanning in pediatric patients and have indicated that CT scanning results in approximately one excess malignancy per 10,000 patients under 10 years of age exposed to CT scanning with a 10-year follow-up.[16–18] Despite the low risk of secondary malignancy, the risks and benefits of performing a CT scan should be carefully considered and dose-reduction protocols should be utilized to reduce the associated risk.[19]

In the case of solid parotid masses, where malignancy is a concern, magnetic resonance imaging (MRI) is the imaging modality of choice. MRI provides excellent soft tissue resolution, which can be used to identify tumor margins, depth of invasion, facial nerve involvement, and/or perineural spread. The use of gadolinium contrast combined with additional imaging protocols such as fat suppression, diffusion-weighted imaging, and dynamic contrast may be used to help distinguish between benign and malignant lesions. Importantly, many solid parotid masses have characteristic imaging characteristics on MRI, which may suggest diagnosis (▶Table 8.2). Generally, malignant lesions display reduced signal intensity on T2-weighted imaging associated with central necrosis, soft tissue invasion, perineural invasion, and variable contrast enhancement.[20,21] In pediatric populations a particular advantage of MRI is the lack of ionizing radiation. However, despite improvements in image acquisition time MRI remains a lengthy study that typically requires sedation or general anesthesia to minimize motion artifact. In addition, MRI is significantly more expensive than other imaging modalities and is frequently less readily available.

Imaging of the salivary ductal system has traditionally required sialography, which involves cannulation of Stensen's duct and injection of radio-opaque contrast material. However, the invasive nature of this study generally limits its applicability in pediatric patients. MR sialography can provide accurate mapping of first-, second-, and occasionally third-order branches using heavily T2-weighted imaging. Moreover, this modality may provide information regarding strictures, sialolithiasis, and acute or chronic sialadenitis.[22,23] Performing MR sialography adds minimal additional time to a traditional

Table 8.2 Imaging characteristics of parotid lesions[20,21]

Lesion	T1 intensity	T2 intensity	Contrast enhancement	Additional characteristics
Branchial cleft cyst	Hypointense	Hyperintense	No	Thickened wall may suggest infection
Lipoma	Hyperintense	Hypointense	No	Suppresses with fat suppression
Pleomorphic adenoma	Isointense	Hyperintense	Yes	No invasion of surrounding structures
Warthin tumor	Isointense	Hyperintense	No	
Lymphatic malformation	Isointense	Hyperintense	–	Multiple loculations
Capillary hemangioma	Heterogeneous hyperintensity	Hyperintense	Variable	Fluid–fluid levels indicate prior hemorrhage
Venous malformations	Isointense to slightly hyperintense	Hyperintense	Significant	"Salt and pepper" appearance on T2
Mucoepidermoid carcinoma	Heterogeneous	Hypointense	Variable	Invasion, lymphadenopathy
Adenoid cystic carcinoma	Hypointense to isointense	Hypointense to isointense	Yes	Perineural invasion

MRI studies, and therefore may be considered if the child is already undergoing general anesthesia. Advantages over traditional sialography include the lack of ionizing radiation and the non-invasive nature of the procedure.

Nuclear imaging can also play an important role in quantifying parotid gland function and in detecting aspiration in at-risk children. Tecnetium-99m pertechnetate (99mTc) concentrated in all major salivary glands after intravenous injection and is secreted in saliva. Therefore, 99mTc studies can be used to measure saliva secretion in response to sialogogues or to measure residual gland function following ductal ligation or in the cases of autoimmune glad destruction. As a sensitive test for aspiration, particularly in children who are unable to cooperate with videofluoroscopic swallow studies, 99mTc-labeled sulfur colloid is placed sublingually and the radiotracer is followed by dynamic imaging and chest images at the conclusion of the study. Aspiration is confirmed by the presence of the radiotracer in the bronchi or lungs.

8.3.4 Sialendoscopy

Sialendoscopy was first introduced in the early 1990s as a method to directly examine salivary ductal anatomy and remove or repair obstructive stones or strictures.[24,25] In general, sialendoscopes are either diagnostic, which contain only fiberoptic, light, and irrigation channels, or interventional, which include an additional working channel through which various instruments may be passed. Recent studies have indicated that sialendoscopy is safe and effective for the treatment of sialolithiasis and juvenile recurrent parotitis (JRP) in pediatric populations, although it should be noted that endoscopic treatment of JRP may not be more efficacious than conservative measures.[26,27] Some pediatric patients >8 years of age may also tolerate sialendoscopy under local anesthesia,[28] thereby obviating the need for sedation and general anesthesia. Accordingly, sialendoscopy is a potentially valuable and/or therapeutic tool for pediatric parotid disorders. The details of performing sialendoscopy are beyond the scope of this chapter, and the reader is referred to several excellent resources on the topic.[29,30]

8.3.5 Pediatric Parotid Gland Disorders

In pediatric populations, the parotid gland may be affected by a variety of congenital or acquired disorders (▶Table 8.3). Generally speaking, infectious or inflammatory etiologies are more common in children compared to adults; however, solid parotid lesions in children are more commonly malignant and therefore full evaluation of these lesions should not be delayed.

Table 8.3 Differential diagnosis of parotid lesions in pediatric patients

- Congenital
- Branchial cleft cyst
- Dermoid cysts
- Ductal cysts
- Benign neoplasms
- Vascular and lymphatic malformations
- Pleomorphic adenoma
- Warthin tumor
- Neurofibroma
- Angiolipoma
- Oncocytoma
- Hamartoma
- Lipoma
- Malignant neoplasms
- Mucoepidermoid carcinoma
- Rhabdomyosarcoma
- Adenoid cystic carcinoma
- Squamous cell carcinoma
- Adenocarcinoma
- Acinous carcinoma
- Lymphoma
- Metastatic neoplasms
- Infectious and inflammatory
- Acute parotitis
- Atypical mycobacterium (Mycobacterium avium)
- HIV
- Mumps
- Epstein-Barr virus
- Juvenile recurrent parotitis
- Sjögren's syndrome
- Sarcoidosis
- Sialolithiasis

8.3.6 Congenital Lesions

Congenital lesions of the parotid gland include first branchial cleft cysts, dermoid cysts, ductal cysts, and congenital venolymphatic malformations (▶Table 8.3). First branchial cleft cysts are divided into two types based on embryology, histology, and location. Type I cysts represent an ectodermal duplication of the membranous external auditory canal, pass lateral to the facial nerve, and end in a bony cul-de-sac near the mesotympanum. By contrast, type II cysts are composed of both ectoderm and mesoderm, and represent duplications of the external auditory canal and pinna. These cysts track medial to the facial nerve and end near the angle of the mandible. Because of their embryologic origin, Type II cysts may contain cartilage. First branchial cleft cysts may present with swelling near the angle of the mandible, parotid mass, or even otorrhea due to the presence of a fistula between the cyst and the external auditory canal. Treatment consists of surgical excision with facial nerve dissection and preservation.

Dermoid cysts of the parotid are rare, with only 18 cases reported in the literature.[31] Imaging by US, CT, or MRI typically reveals a "sack of marbles" appearance, due to fat globules within the cyst, which is considered nearly pathognomonic. Treatment consists of a superficial parotidectomy to avoid recurrence. Ductal cysts result from congenital ductal dilations manifesting as swelling of the parotid gland in infancy. These dilations can be visualized on sialography or US, and in the absence of repeated infections management consists of observation.

8.3.7 Acquired Lesions

Vascular and Lymphatic Anomalies

Vascular anomalies of the head and neck are classified as vascular tumors or vascular malformations. Vascular malformations are formed by arteries, veins, capillaries, lymphatics, or a combination of vessel types and grow proportionally with the child through expansion and vascular recruitment. Infantile hemangiomas are the most common pediatric parotid tumor and[32] overall, hemangiomas are found in 4 to 10% of children and 23% of premature infants.[33] Thirty percent of infantile hemangiomas are present at birth, with the remainder arising within the first 6 weeks of life. Characteristically, these lesions grow rapidly during the first 1 to 2 months of life and again at 4 to 6 months of age, followed by a growth plateau and then slowly progressive involution. Approximately 50% of lesions are expected to resolve by age 5, 70% by age 7, and 90% by age 9. For lesions that fail to resolve, oral propranolol at a dose of 1 to 2 mg/kg/day for at least 12 weeks has been shown to be a safe and effective treatment.[33,34] Biopsy is not necessary and should be avoided when classic imaging characteristics are seen. Surgical excision should be avoided whenever possible, except in the case of life-threatening hemangiomas unresponsive to medical management.[35] All children with segmental hemangiomas involving the parotid gland should undergo screening for PHACES (Posterior fossa abnormalities, Hemangiomas, Arterial abnormalities, Cardiac abnormalities, Eye abnormalities, Sternal defects) including MRI, ECG, and ophthalmology referral.

Lymphatic malformations present as a soft, compressible mass that arises within the perinatal period; 50% present within the first year, and 90% within the second year. These lesions are divided histologically into three categories based on the size of the lymphatic channels: microcystic lesions consisting of small cysts <2 cm, macrocystic lesions containing cysts >2 cm, and mixed lesions. Macrocystic lesions may often be eradicated through surgical excision. Sclerotherapy such as OK-432, doxycycline, or ethanol is also effective for the treatment of deep macrocystic lesions;[36] however, sclerotherapy should be avoided for superficial lesions due to the risk of ulceration. Microcystic lesions are typically more difficult to eradicate, as these lesions often do not respond to sclerotherapy and frequently require staged excision.

Benign Solid Tumors

Classically, solid parotid lesions in children were thought to have a higher likelihood of being malignant compared to similar lesions in adults, although more recent studies refuted this idea.[37,38] Pleomorphic adenomas are the most common benign solid tumor of the parotid gland, representing approximately 20% of all pediatric parotid masses.[37] These lesions present as painless, gradually enlarging masses in late childhood or adolescence with a slight female predominance.[39,40] These lesions occur most commonly in the superficial lobe; however, deep lobe pleomorphic adenomas have been reported.[39,40] MRI shows a T2 hyperintense lesion that enhances with gadolinium contrast (▶ Table 8.2). Histologically, pleomorphic adenomas are composed of varying quantities of epithelial and mesenchymal elements. Treatment consists of superficial parotidectomy with facial nerve preservation or complete excision of the tumor with a cuff of normal tissue. Although pleomorphic adenomas often appear to be well-encapsulated, simple enucleation is inappropriate due to the presence of microscopic pseudopodal extensions through the capsule, resulting in a high recurrence rate. In adult populations pleomorphic adenomas may undergo malignant transformation (carcinoma ex-pleomorphic adenoma); however, there are no reports of carcinoma ex-pleomorphic adenoma occurring in pediatric patients. None-the-less, carcinoma ex-pleomorphic adenoma may arise many decades after excision of the original lesion,[41] necessitating long-term follow-up.

Warthin tumors (papillary cystadenoma) are rare, accounting for 0 to 10% of benign pediatric parotid masses.[42,43] They present as slow-growing, painless masses that may occasionally be bilateral. On MRI, Warthin tumors are typically T2 hyperintense but in contrast to pleomorphic adenomas they do not exhibit significant contrast enhancement (▶ Table 8.2). Treatment consists of superficial parotidectomy with facial nerve dissection. Other rare benign tumors include neurofibroma, embryoma (sialoblastoma, congenital basal adenoma), monomorphic adenoma, lipoma, and teratoma. Sialoblastoma is notable for its aggressive local invasion and potential for distant metastasis if left untreated. These tumors are typically diagnosed at birth or shortly thereafter,[44,45] and prompt surgical excision is recommended to reduce the risk of local invasion or distant metastasis.

Malignant Neoplasms

Mucoepidermoid carcinoma (MEC) is the most common salivary gland malignancy in children, accounting for approximately 49 to 54% of all pediatric salivary gland malignancies.[46–48] MEC typically presents in late childhood to early adolescence as an enlarging, painless mass; presentation with facial palsy should immediately raise the concern for malignancy.[47,49] Importantly, MEC may arise as a second primary malignancy in children previously treated with chemotherapy and/or radiation therapy.[49–51] The majority of pediatric tumors are low- or intermediate-grade, with portends an excellent prognosis with a 5-year survival approaching 100%.[47,49] Treatment for low-grade tumors consists of wide local extirpation, while high-grade lesions typically require total parotidectomy with selective neck dissection and/or adjuvant radiation therapy. The facial nerve should be preserved except when directly invaded by tumor.

The second-most common pediatric salivary malignancy is acinic cell carcinoma, which comprises approximately 40% of all pediatric parotid malignancies.[48] Similar to MEC, acinic cell carcinoma typically presents as a slow-growing painless mass in late childhood or adolescence. Most tumors are low-grade at diagnosis, which has a favorable prognosis. Low-grade lesions rarely metastasize, and treatment consists of partial parotidectomy with facial nerve preservation. Adjuvant radiation therapy does not appear to improve survival and remains controversial.[48]

The remaining ~10% of pediatric parotid malignancies consist of adenoid cystic carcinoma, adenocarcinoma, and undifferentiated carcinoma.[46,48] Adenoid cystic carcinoma has a predilection for perineural invasion, and is commonly treated with excision followed by radiation therapy.[48] Adenocarcinoma and undifferentiated carcinoma most frequently present in childhood or early adolescence. These tumors tend to be highly aggressive and are associated with poor outcomes. Treatment consists of excision of local disease along with any associated nodal metastasis, followed by radiation therapy.

8.3.8 Infectious Conditions

Acute Suppurative Parotitis

Acute suppurative parotitis can occur at any age, even in the neonatal period although this predominantly occurs among premature infants.[52] Suppurative parotitis typically presents with acute onset swelling and induration of the parotid area extending to the angle of the mandible, erythema of the overlying skin, tenderness, and trismus. Infections are typically unilateral, but may be bilateral. In severe cases, parotitis may also be associated with fever and chills. Expression of purulent saliva from Stensen's duct is pathognomonic for acute bacterial parotitis. Purulent saliva should be cultured to confirm the diagnosis and to guide treatment.

Staphylococcus aureus is the most common causative agent; however, other bacteria have been isolated.[52,53] Predisposing factors include ductal obstruction by a sialolith, stricture, or parotid neoplasm; dehydration with resultant salivary stasis; and congenital ductal abnormalities. Medical management includes hydration, parotid massage, sialogogues, and antibiotics. Uncomplicated infections may be treated with oral amoxicillin/clavulonic acid or clindamycin, while more severe infections may require intravenous therapy with amoxicillin/sulbactam, clindamycin, vancomycin, and/or metronidazole. In cases of recurrent infection, sialendoscopy may be required to remove obstructing sialoliths, dilate areas of stricture, or deliver medical therapy (most often corticosteroids). Parotidectomy should only be undertaken for recurrent parotitis that cannot be managed through conventional means.

Parotid abscess is a rare complication of acute suppurative parotitis that typically presents with swelling, tenderness, trismus, and fever. Abscesses may occur in all age groups and are non-responsive to antibiotics. Although fluctuance may be present on physical examination, in many cases fluctuance is not clinically apparent due to the thick fascia overlying the parotid gland. Therefore, ultrasound is a valuable tool in the diagnosis of parotid abscess. Needle aspiration of the abscess may be performed under ultrasound guidance; however, definitive treatment of parotid abscess often requires incision and drainage, taking care not to injure the facial nerve.

Atypical Bacterial Infections

Atypical mycobacteria, also called non-tuberculous mycobacteria (NTM), are a collection of ubiquitous acid-fast bacteria that are an increasingly common cause of infection in developed countries.[54,55] Tap water is thought to serve as the major bacterial reservoir in human populations and prior studies have isolated NTM in 78 to 83% of chlorinated water samples from across the United States.[56,57] NTM infections in the head and neck typically occurs in immunocompetent children aged 1 to 5 years, with *Mycobacterium avium* complex being the most commonly isolated organisms.[58–60]

Treatment of atypical mycobacterial infections involves superficial parotidectomy with facial nerve preservation to completely remove the abscess, which is effective in 96% of cases.[61] Simple incision and drainage is contraindicated due to a high risk of skin fistula formation. Several groups have proposed medical management protocols as an alternative or adjunct to surgery, which may be beneficial in up to two-third of cases.[62,63] However, antibiotic courses of up to 12 weeks are often required to clear the infection and a majority (78%) of patients report adverse effects associated with antibiotic therapy.[63]

Actinomycosis of the parotid gland is a rare condition caused by Gram-positive anaerobic bacilli, usually from an odontogenic source. Patients may present with slow, painless enlargement of the parotid, mimicking neoplastic growth, or as a rapidly developing infection with overlying erythema and fever.[64,65] In either case, draining sinus tracts to the skin are common. Histologic examination of purulent material shows pathognomonic "sulfur granules." Cultures are often negative due to the strict anaerobic growth requirements; however, molecular testing may be used. Actinomycosis is rare in immunocompetent individuals so all affected children should be tested for underlying immune dysfunction. Treatment consists of IV penicillin G for 2 to 6 weeks followed by oral penicillin for 3 to 12 months. Surgery may be required to drain abscess cavities, debride fibrotic tissue in recalcitrant lesions, or to resect fistula tracts.

Cat scratch disease (CSD) presents as regional lymphadenopathy resulting from infection with *Bartonella helensae*. Due to the presence of intraparotid lymph nodes, CSD may present as tender swelling of the parotid gland, which may be mistaken for suppurative parotitis.[66,67] Diagnosis requires a high index of suspicion and meticulous history taking, which is often significant for a recent cat scratch or bite. Treatment consists of a 5-day course of azithromycin (10 mg/kg on day 1, 5 mg/kg days 2–4). Surgical therapy is rarely required.

Viral Infections

A number of viruses may cause parotitis including mumps, Epstein-Barr virus, parainfluenza virus, influenza virus, adenovirus, cytomegalovirus, human immunodeficiency virus (HIV), and coxsackievirus. Viral parotitis is usually self-limited and is managed conservatively with warm compresses, sialogogues, analgesia, and hydration. HIV produces cystic parotid gland enlargement, which is seen in up to 30% of HIV-infected children.[68] Cystic enlargement of the parotid gland is rare in the general population, and is therefore an indication for HIV testing.[69] Management of HIV-associated salivary gland disease consists of managing the underlying HIV infection with highly active antiretroviral therapy (HAART); however, repeated aspiration or even surgical extirpation may be required for large cysts that cause cosmetic deformity.

8.3.9 Inflammatory and Autoimmune Conditions

Juvenile Recurrent Parotitis

Juvenile recurrent parotitis (JRP) is an inflammatory condition of the parotid gland of unknown etiology and is the second-most common childhood salivary gland disease after mumps.[70,71] The disease is defined as non-obstructive, non-suppurative unilateral or bilateral inflammation of the parotid gland recurring at least twice before puberty.[72] The disease has a bimodal age of presentation, with the first peak in children 3 to 6 years of age and the second peak around age 10; however, there

may be considerable variation in the age of presentation.[71] A variety of factors have been implicated including dental malocclusion, congenital anatomic abnormalities, genetic factors, and immunologic abnormalities.[70,71] Exacerbations usually last from 4 to 7 days and patients have an average of 1 to 2 episodes per year, although some patients may have considerably more exacerbations.[70] Each exacerbation leads to destruction of the gland parenchyma with a corresponding drop in salivary production.[73] The disease typically resolves spontaneously after puberty, although rare cases persist through adulthood.

Diagnosis of JRP focuses on history and physical exam with the exclusion of other identifiable causes such as Sjögren's syndrome, viral infection, and immunodeficiency. Sialography remains the gold-standard imaging technique and shows sialectasia, as evidenced by punctate shadows, strictures, and kinks.[74] However, ultrasound is equally sensitive at detecting JRP and avoids exposure to ionizing radiation.[75] Medical treatment of JRP includes oral hydration, warm compresses, sialogogues, and gland massage.[73,75] Historically, treatments including ligation of Stensen's duct or total parotidectomy with facial nerve preservation have been abandoned due to unacceptable morbidity.[73] More recently, sialendoscopy has been proposed as a diagnostic and therapeutic modality for JRP, although it remains to be determined whether sialendoscopy per se confers any clinical benefit.[76] Ductal irrigation with corticosteroids, which is often performed as part of sialendoscopy procedures, effectively manages disease symptoms when performed alone, suggesting that sialendoscopy should be reserved to rule out additional pathology.[77] Other treatments, such as ductal irrigation with 48% iodinated oil have been tried with promising results.[73]

Sarcoidosis

Sarcoidosis is a rare, granulomatous condition that affects people of all racial and ethnic groups with a bimodal peak incidence at 25 to 29 years and 65 to 69 years of age.[78] The disease typically presents with hilar lymphadenopathy, pulmonary opacities, lesions of the skin, joints, and/or eyes. Occasionally, sarcoidosis may present as Heerfordt syndrome (uveo-parotid fever), which is characterized by anterior uveitis, parotid gland enlargement, facial palsy, and fever. Diagnostic testing includes a chest X-ray to evaluate for hilar adenopathy and serum angiotensin-converting enzyme levels, which are elevated in up to 60% of sarcoidosis patients.[78] In cases of parotid enlargement, biopsy showing non-caseating granulomas is diagnostic.

Sjögren's Syndrome

Primary Sjögren's syndrome is rare in children; however, the parotid gland is involved in 70% of pediatric patients. The disease is characterized by systemic autoimmune infiltration of glandular tissue. The most common presentation in children is recurrent bilateral parotitis, which may be associated with fever, arthralgia/arthritis, fatigue, and submandibular swelling.[79,80] Symptoms common in adults, such as keratoconjunctavitis and xerostomia are less common in children.[79] Serologic tests including SS-A (anti-Ro), SS-B (anti-La), antinuclear antibody (ANA), rheumatoid factor (RF), and erythrocyte sedimentation rate (ESR) are elevated in a majority of patients. Minor salivary gland biopsy, a mainstay of Sjögren's diagnosis in adults, is not indicated in children for whom the diagnosis is otherwise clear.[79] A diagnosis of Sjögren's syndrome should prompt referral to rheumatology, ophthalmology, and dentistry for management of complications relating to the disease. In adult patients, Sjögren's syndrome is associated with increased overall risk of malignancy, non-Hodgkin lymphoma, and thyroid cancer[81]; however, malignancies in association with Sjögren's syndrome appear to be rare in pediatrics.[80] Treatment focuses on symptom alleviation (sialogogues, parotid massage, hydration) and management of systemic effects of the disease.

Sialolithiasis

Sialolithiasis is rare in the pediatric population and only ~20% of stones occur in the parotid.[82] Approximately 83% of parotid stones are found within Stensen's duct.[82] The most common presenting symptoms are postprandial swelling and pain.[83] Stone removal may be conducted through sialendoscopic or open approaches, including transoral techniques for stones lodged within Stensen's duct or transfacial approaches for stones lodged within the gland parenchyma. Combined open and sialendoscopic approaches have also been reported, which may be beneficial for large stones.[84]

Sialorrhea

Sialorrhea is defined by anterior or posterior spillage of saliva secondary to excessive saliva production (primary sialorrhea) or dysfunctional swallowing of saliva (secondary sialorrhea). Anterior sialorrhea refers to spillage of saliva onto the lips or chin, while posterior sialorrhea refers to the spillage of saliva onto the larynx and glottis. Importantly, anterior sialorrhea may produce skin breakdown, infection, and social isolation, while posterior sialorrhea increases the risk of aspiration pneumonia. In the United States, cerebral palsy is the most common cause of sialorrhea, which is present in 10 to 40% of affected individuals.[85]

Medical management of sialorrhea includes glycopyrrolate or scopolamine patches to reduce saliva production. In cases that are refractory to medical management, a variety of surgical techniques have been utilized including rerouting of Wharton ducts, extirpation of the submandibular glands with ligation of Stensen's duct, or ligation of Wharton's and Stensen's ducts (four-duct ligation). The four-duct ligation procedure is minimally invasive and reduces drooling in a majority of patients at both the 1-month and 1-year timepoints.[86,87,88] Overall, many caregivers report an improvement in drooling symptoms following four-duct ligation, although only about 50% of caregivers would recommend the procedure after one year and long-term caregiver satisfaction is low.[88,89]

More recently, ultrasound-guided botulinum toxin type-A (Botox®) into salivary glands has been used as a non-surgical approach for sialorrhea management. Injections typically target the bilateral submandibular glands as well as the superficial lobe of both parotid glands with a total dose of 1 to 5.5 U/kg.[90] Typically, the parotid gland is injected in 2 to 3 locations;[90] however, some authors have utilized as many as 9 separate injection sites.[91] The submandibular gland is injected in 1 to 3 locations.[90] These procedures are often performed under general anesthesia; however, in our experience the procedure is well-tolerated by awake children with the use of topical lidocaine cream prior to injection. Success rates range from 30 to 75%, with a reported duration of 8 to 16 months.[92] The most common complication of Botox injection is treatment failure, which occurs in approximately 10% of cases. Other complications are rare and include dysphagia resulting from toxin diffusion into the surrounding neck muscles, increased saliva thickness, xerostomia, and pneumonia.[93]

8.4 Parotidectomy

8.4.1 Procedure

Parotid surgery in children is performed under general anesthesia with the use of intraoperative neuromonitoring. Long-acting paralytic agents such as rocuronium must be avoided to allow for facial monitoring during the procedure. It is important to note that while neuromonitoring may assist in the identification of the facial nerve and therefore shorten operative time, neuromonitoring does not reduce the rate of inadvertent facial nerve injury or predict facial nerve outcomes following surgery.[94-96] The patient is placed on the operating table in the supine position with the head rotated to the contralateral side. A shoulder roll should be placed to provide adequate extension of the neck. The surgical site should be draped so that the entire ipsilateral face can be visualized. For younger children with undeveloped mastoids, in whom the facial nerve is more superficial, an incision should be designed in a neck crease approximately 1.5 to 2 cm below the mandible, curving posteriorly over the sternocleidomastoid before turning superiorly and ending on the mastoid prominence (▶Fig. 8.2a). Because the mastoid air cells generally reach adult size by early adolescence,[8] the traditional modified Blair incision may be used for older children (▶Fig. 8.2b).

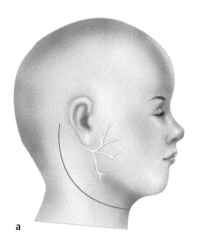
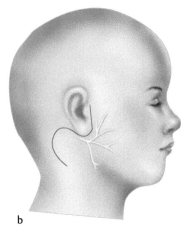

a   b

Fig. 8.2 Pediatric parotidectomy incisions. (**a**) In younger children, a cervical incision should be used. The incision starts on the mastoid prominence, descends inferiorly over the sternocleidomastoid, and ends in a neck crease 2–2.5 cm below the mandible. (**b**) A traditional modified Blair incision may be used for adolescents.

In younger children, the superior flap is raised in a sub-platysmal plane until the ramus of the mandible is reached. Because the facial nerve runs in a more superficial plane in young children, further flap elevation onto the face is delayed until the main trunk of the facial nerve has been identified. To accomplish this, the anterior border of the sternocleidomastoid is followed superiorly to its insertion on the mastoid process. The greater auricular nerve is encountered well below the mastoid and should be spared. Just deep into the insertion of the sternocleidomastoid, the posterior belly may be seen coursing in an anterior and slightly inferior vector. The facial nerve in young children is located within a triangle of fibrofatty tissue bordered by the sternocleidomastoid posteriorly, the posterior belly of the digastric inferiorly, and the cartilaginous ear canal anteriorly (▶ Fig. 8.3).[3] The nerve at this level measures approximately 1 mm in diameter and is followed anteriorly in a plane parallel to the superior border of the digastric, keeping in mind that there may be minimal parotid tissue overlying the nerve. The pes anserinus is typically located posterior to the mandibular ramus, often obviating the need for additional flap elevation.[3]

In older children skin flaps are raised superficial to the parotid fascia to reduce the incidence of gustatory sweating (Frye syndrome) postoperatively. The parotid gland is then separated from the cartilaginous ear canal and subsequently from the anterior border of the sternocleidomastoid. Attention is then turned to the identification of the facial nerve, which is found 1 cm anterior, inferior, and deep to the tragal pointer at the depth of the posterior belly of the digastric muscle. Alternatively, the nerve may be found approximately 6 to 8 mm deep into the tympanomastoid suture line.

Once the nerve is identified, soft tissue dissection should proceed by spreading tissue parallel to the nerve, only cutting through glandular tissue when the precise location of the nerve and its branches is known. Dissection is continued anteriorly until the anterior border of the neoplasm or lesion is reached, at which point the lesion is extirpated. All efforts should be made to

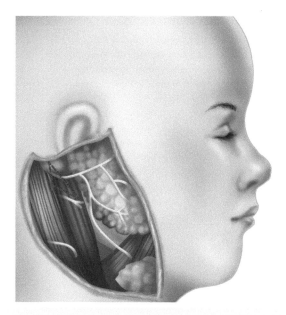

Fig. 8.3 Identification of the facial nerve in young children. The main trunk of the facial nerve may be found in a fibrofatty triangle bordered by the sternocleidomastoid posteriorly, the cartilaginous external auditory canal superiorly, and the posterior belly of the digastric muscle inferiorly.

identify and preserve the facial nerve, even in the case of malignant lesions. Sacrifice of the facial nerve is only indicated in patients with preoperative facial nerve paresis or paralysis, for whom postoperative recovery is unlikely.

In rare cases of a deep lobe parotid tumor, a superficial parotidectomy must be performed first to identify and release the facial nerve. Once the nerve has been dissected, it is gently retracted superiorly to permit access to the deep lobe of the gland. If the parotid tissue lateral to the nerve is not involved, it may be pedicled anteriorly and returned to its original position during closure to restore the normal contour of the face. After the nerve is retracted, the deep parotid tissue is swept inferiorly and delivered into the field. For very large lesions involving the deep lobe, a mandibulotomy may be required to improve surgical access. If this is the case, fixation plates should be fitted and screw holes drilled prior to performing the mandibulotomy to preserve occlusion.

After extirpation of the lesion, hemostasis should be ensured and the wound should be irrigated, taking care not to injure the facial nerve. The integrity of the facial nerve should be confirmed both by visual inspection and by electrical stimulation. The wound should be closed over a negative pressure suction drain, which is brought out through a separate stab incision. The incision itself is closed in layers and the skin is closed with absorbable suture. A bulky dressing is placed over the parotid and secured with an elastic compression bandage.

8.4.2 Postoperative Management

In our practice, children are observed at least overnight. A facial nerve exam is performed as soon as the child has recovered from anesthesia and is able to participate in the examination. Postoperative weakness may occur, particularly in the lower division;[97,98] however, even partial function generally indicates good functional outcomes. Weakness generally resolves within 1 to 2 months.[97,98] The drain is placed next to bulb suction and removed once drainage is <15 mL per 24-hour period. The compression dressing is ideally left in place for 24 hours if tolerated by the child and the wound should be kept clean and dry for at least 24 hours after drain removal. The incision should be cleaned twice daily with ½ strength hydrogen peroxide and then covered with a thin layer of petroleum jelly.

8.4.3 Complications

Significant complications are rare following parotidectomy in pediatric patients. In a study of 90 pediatric parotidectomy patients, seroma was the most common postoperative complication (7%) and resolved with observation.[98] Hematoma was the next-most common complication and was observed in only 2 patients (2%); salivary fistula, wound infection, and wound dehiscence each occurred in 1 patient.[98] Long-term complications such as gustatory sweating (Frey syndrome) also appear to be uncommon; however, small sample sizes preclude accurate estimation of the true incidence.[97] Fortunately, Frey syndrome is frequently manageable through the application of non-scented antiperspirant or via botulinum toxin injections.

8.5 Conclusion

In pediatric populations, parotidectomy is most commonly performed for infectious or inflammatory conditions. However, benign and malignant neoplastic processes do occur in children and should be considered in the evaluation of children presenting with a parotid mass. Imaging studies, particularly MRI, may be useful in determining the likely etiology of a lesion, and fine needle aspiration biopsy frequently provides sufficient sample for a more definitive diagnosis. When performing a parotidectomy in children, care must be taken to avoid injury to the facial nerve, which travels in a more superficial plane compared to adults. Nonetheless, parotidectomy can be performed safely in pediatric populations with a low incidence of postoperative complications.

8.6 Highlights

a. Indications
   - Congenital masses, cysts, and lymphovascular malformations.
   - Benign or malignant tumors.
   - Recurrent infectious parotitis or parotid abscess.
   - Sialolithiasis.
b. Contraindications
   - No absolute contraindications.
c. Complications
   - Surgical site infection.
   - Wound dehiscence.
   - Skin flap necrosis.
   - Hematoma.
   - Sialocele.
   - Salivary fistula.
   - Gustatory sweating (Frey syndrome).
   - Facial nerve injury/paralysis.
d. Special preoperative considerations
   - General endotracheal anesthesia.
   - Neuromonitoring for evaluation of facial nerve integrity.
   - Avoid use of long-acting paralytics.
e. Special interoperative considerations
   - Superficial course of facial nerve in children.
   - Only cut parotid tissue when the location of the facial nerve is known.
   - Facial nerve sacrifice only for malignant lesions with preoperative facial nerve paralysis.
f. Special postoperative considerations
   - Overnight hospitalization.
   - Postoperative facial nerve exam.
   - Compression dressing for 24 hours.
   - Suction drain removal when ouput is <15 mL/ 24 hours.

References

[1] Som P, Miletich I. The embryology of the salivary glands: An update. Neurographics. 2015;5(4):167–177
[2] Frommer J. The human accessory parotid gland: its incidence, nature, and significance. Oral Surg Oral Med Oral Pathol 1977;43(5):671–676
[3] Farrior JB, Santini H. Facial nerve identification in children. Otolaryngol Head Neck Surg 1985;93(2):173–176

[4] Kalaycioğlu A, Yeginoğlui G, Ertemoğlu Öksüz C, Uzun Ö, Kalkişim SN. An anatomical study on the facial nerve trunk in fetus cadavers. Turk J Med Sci 2014;44(3):484–489

[5] Davis RA, Anson BJ, Budinger JM, Kurth LR. Surgical anatomy of the facial nerve and parotid gland based upon a study of 350 cervicofacial halves. Surg Gynecol Obstet 1956;102(4):385–412

[6] Gataa IS, Faris BJ. Patterns and surgical significance of facial nerve branching within the parotid gland in 43 cases. Oral Maxillofac Surg 2016;20(2):161–165

[7] Qvarnberg Y. Acute otitis media: a prospective clinical study of myringotomy and antimicrobial treatment. Acta Otolaryngol Suppl 1981;375:1–157

[8] Cinamon U. The growth rate and size of the mastoid air cell system and mastoid bone: a review and reference. Eur Arch Otorhinolaryngol 2009;266(6):781–786

[9] Sodhi KS, Bartlett M, Prabhu NK. Role of high resolution ultrasound in parotid lesions in children. Int J Pediatr Otorhinolaryngol 2011;75(11):1353–1358

[10] Gritzmann N, Rettenbacher T, Hollerweger A, Macheiner P, Hübner E. Sonography of the salivary glands. Eur Radiol 2003;13(5):964–975

[11] Wu S, Liu G, Chen R, Guan Y. Role of ultrasound in the assessment of benignity and malignancy of parotid masses. Dentomaxillofac Radiol 2012;41(2):131–135

[12] Yonetsu K, Ohki M, Kumazawa S, Eida S, Sumi M, Nakamura T. Parotid tumors: differentiation of benign and malignant tumors with quantitative sonographic analyses. Ultrasound Med Biol 2004;30(5):567–574

[13] Liu CC, Jethwa AR, Khariwala SS, Johnson J, Shin JJ. Sensitivity, specificity, and posttest probability of parotid fine-needle aspiration: a systematic review and meta-analysis. Otolaryngol Head Neck Surg 2016;154(1):9–23

[14] Lee DH, Yoon TM, Lee JK, Lim SC. Clinical utility of fine needle aspiration cytology in pediatric parotid tumors. Int J Pediatr Otorhinolaryngol 2013;77(8):1272–1275

[15] Brennan PA, Herd MK, Howlett DC, Gibson D, Oeppen RS. Is ultrasound alone sufficient for imaging superficial lobe benign parotid tumours before surgery? Br J Oral Maxillofac Surg 2012;50(4):333–337

[16] Pearce MS, Salotti JA, Little MP, et al. Radiation exposure from CT scans in childhood and subsequent risk of leukaemia and brain tumours: a retrospective cohort study. Lancet 2012;380(9840):499–505

[17] Mathews JD, Forsythe AV, Brady Z, et al. Cancer risk in 680,000 people exposed to computed tomography scans in childhood or adolescence: data linkage study of 11 million Australians. BMJ 2013;346:f2360

[18] Chen JX, Kachniarz B, Gilani S, Shin JJ. Risk of malignancy associated with head and neck CT in children: a systematic review. Otolaryngol Head Neck Surg 2014;151(4):554–566

[19] Greenwood TJ, Lopez-Costa RI, Rhoades PD, et al. CT Dose Optimization in Pediatric Radiology: A Multiyear Effort to Preserve the Benefits of Imaging While Reducing the Risks. Radiographics 2015;35(5):1539–1554

[20] Mamlouk MD, Rosbe KW, Glastonbury CM. Paediatric parotid neoplasms: a 10 year retrospective imaging and pathology review of these rare tumours. Clin Radiol 2015;70(3):270–277

[21] Christe A, Waldherr C, Hallett R, Zbaeren P, Thoeny H. MR imaging of parotid tumors: typical lesion characteristics in MR imaging improve discrimination between benign and malignant disease. AJNR Am J Neuroradiol 2011;32(7):1202–1207

[22] Kalinowski M, Heverhagen JT, Rehberg E, Klose KJ, Wagner HJ. Comparative study of MR sialography and digital subtraction sialography for benign salivary gland disorders. AJNR Am J Neuroradiol 2002;23(9):1485–1492

[23] Gadodia A, Seith A, Sharma R, Thakar A. MRI and MR sialography of juvenile recurrent parotitis. Pediatr Radiol 2010;40(8):1405–1410

[24] Katz P. [Endoscopy of the salivary glands] Ann Radiol (Paris) 1991;34(1–2):110–113

[25] Katz P. [New method of examination of the salivary glands: the fiberscope] Inf Dent 1990;72(10):785–786

[26] Rosbe KW, Milev D, Chang JL. Effectiveness and costs of sialendoscopy in pediatric patients with salivary gland disorders. Laryngoscope 2015;125(12):2805–2809

[27] Ramakrishna J, Strychowsky J, Gupta M, Sommer DD. Sialendoscopy for the management of juvenile recurrent parotitis: a systematic review and meta-analysis. Laryngoscope 2015;125(6):1472–1479

[28] Konstantinidis I, Chatziavramidis A, Tsakiropoulou E, Malliari H, Constantinidis J. Pediatric sialendoscopy under local anesthesia: limitations and potentials. Int J Pediatr Otorhinolaryngol 2011;75(2):245–249

[29] Faure F, Froehlich P, Marchal F. Paediatric sialendoscopy. Curr Opin Otolaryngol Head Neck Surg 2008;16(1):60–63

[30] Thottam PJ, Schaitkin B, Mehta DK. Pediatric sialendoscopy. Oper Tech Otolaryngol--Head Neck Surg 2015;26(3):150–155

[31] Yigit N, Karslioglu Y, Yildizoglu U, Karakoc O. Dermoid cyst of the parotid gland: report of a rare entity with literature review. Head Neck Pathol 2015;9(2):286–292

[32] Weiss I, O TM, Lipari BA, Meyer L, Berenstein A, Waner M. Current treatment of parotid hemangiomas. Laryngoscope 2011;121(8):1642–1650

[33] Li G, Xu DP, Sun HL, et al. Oral propranolol for parotid infantile hemangiomas. J Craniofac Surg 2015;26(2):438–440

[34] Sadykov RR, Podmelle F, Sadykov RA, Kasimova KR, Metellmann HR. Use of propranolol for the treatment infantile hemangiomas in the maxillofacial region. Int J Oral Maxillofac Surg 2013;42(7):863–867

[35] Sinno H, Thibaudeau S, Coughlin R, Chitte S, Williams B. Management of infantile parotid gland hemangiomas: a 40-year experience. Plast Reconstr Surg 2010;125(1):265–273

[36] Wiegand S, Eivazi B, Zimmermann AP, Sesterhenn AM, Werner JA. Sclerotherapy of lymphangiomas of the head and neck. Head Neck 2011;33(11):1649–1655

[37] Orvidas LJ, Kasperbauer JL, Lewis JE, Olsen KD, Lesnick TG. Pediatric parotid masses. Arch Otolaryngol Head Neck Surg 2000;126(2):177–184

[38] Stevens E, Andreasen S, Bjørndal K, Homøe P. Tumors in the parotid are not relatively more often malignant in children than in adults. Int J Pediatr Otorhinolaryngol 2015;79(8):1192–1195

[39] Rodriguez KH, Vargas S, Robson C, et al. Pleomorphic adenoma of the parotid gland in children. Int J Pediatr Otorhinolaryngol 2007;71(11):1717–1723

[40] Fu H, Wang J, Wang L, Zhang Z, He Y. Pleomorphic adenoma of the salivary glands in children and adolescents. J Pediatr Surg 2012;47(4):715–719

[41] Chooback N, Shen Y, Jones M, et al. Carcinoma ex pleomorphic adenoma: case report and options for systemic therapy. Curr Oncol 2017;24(3):e251–e254

[42] Yu GY, Li ZL, Ma DQ, Zhang Y. Diagnosis and treatment of epithelial salivary gland tumours in children and adolescents. Br J Oral Maxillofac Surg 2002;40(5):389–392

[43] da Cruz Perez DE, Pires FR, Alves FA, Almeida OP, Kowalski LP. Salivary gland tumors in children and adolescents: a clinicopathologic and immunohistochemical study of fifty-three cases. Int J Pediatr Otorhinolaryngol 2004;68(7):895–902

[44] Choudhary K, Panda S, Beena VT, Rajeev R, Sivakumar R, Krishanan S. Sialoblastoma: A literature review from 1966–2011. Natl J Maxillofac Surg 2013;4(1):13–18

[45] Irace AL, Adil EA, Archer NM, Silvera VM, Perez-Atayde A, Rahbar R. Pediatric sialoblastoma: Evaluation and management. Int J Pediatr Otorhinolaryngol 2016;87:44–49

[46] Luna MA, Batsakis JG, el-Naggar AK. Salivary gland tumors in children. Ann Otol Rhinol Laryngol 1991;100(10):869–871

[47] Hicks J, Flaitz C. Mucoepidermoid carcinoma of salivary glands in children and adolescents: assessment of proliferation markers. Oral Oncol 2000;36(5):454–460

[48] Allan BJ, Tashiro J, Diaz S, Edens J, Younis R, Thaller SR. Malignant tumors of the parotid gland in children: incidence and outcomes. J Craniofac Surg 2013;24(5):1660–1664

[49] Védrine PO, Coffinet L, Temam S, et al. Mucoepidermoid carcinoma of salivary glands in the pediatric age group: 18 clinical

cases, including 11 second malignant neoplasms. Head Neck 2006;28(9):827–833

[50] Rutigliano DN, Meyers P, Ghossein RA, et al. Mucoepidermoid carcinoma as a secondary malignancy in pediatric sarcoma. J Pediatr Surg 2007;42(7):E9–E13

[51] Tugcu D, Akici F, Aydogan G, et al. Mucoepidermoid carcinoma of the parotid gland in childhood survivor of acute lymphoblastic leukemia with need of radiotherapy for treatment and review of the literature. Pediatr Hematol Oncol 2012;29(4):380–385

[52] Spiegel R, Miron D, Sakran W, Horovitz Y. Acute neonatal suppurative parotitis: case reports and review. Pediatr Infect Dis J 2004;23(1):76–78

[53] Özdemir H, Karbuz A, Ciftçi E, Fitöz S, Ince E, Doğru U. Acute neonatal suppurative parotitis: a case report and review of the literature. Int J Infect Dis 2011;15(7):e500–e502

[54] Wentworth AB, Drage LA, Wengenack NL, Wilson JW, Lohse CM. Increased incidence of cutaneous nontuberculous mycobacterial infection, 1980 to 2009: a population-based study. Mayo Clin Proc 2013;88(1):38–45

[55] Gonzalez-Santiago TM, Drage LA. Nontuberculous mycobacteria: skin and soft tissue infections. Dermatol Clin 2015;33(3): 563–577

[56] Carson LA, Bland LA, Cusick LB, et al. Prevalence of nontuberculous mycobacteria in water supplies of hemodialysis centers. Appl Environ Microbiol 1988;54(12):3122–3125

[57] Donohue MJ, Mistry JH, Donohue JM, et al. Increased Frequency of Nontuberculous Mycobacteria Detection at Potable Water Taps within the United States. Environ Sci Technol 2015;49(10):6127–6133

[58] Wolinsky E. Mycobacterial lymphadenitis in children: a prospective study of 105 nontuberculous cases with long-term follow-up. Clin Infect Dis 1995;20(4):954–963

[59] Panesar J, Higgins K, Daya H, Forte V, Allen U. Nontuberculous mycobacterial cervical adenitis: a ten-year retrospective review. Laryngoscope 2003;113(1):149–154

[60] Blyth CC, Best EJ, Jones CA, et al. Nontuberculous mycobacterial infection in children: a prospective national study. Pediatr Infect Dis J 2009;28(9):801–805

[61] Lindeboom JA. Surgical treatment for nontuberculous mycobacterial (NTM) cervicofacial lymphadenitis in children. J Oral Maxillofac Surg 2012;70(2):345–348

[62] Luong A, McClay JE, Jafri HS, Brown O. Antibiotic therapy for nontuberculous mycobacterial cervicofacial lymphadenitis. Laryngoscope 2005;115(10):1746–1751

[63] Lindeboom JA, Kuijper EJ, Bruijnesteijn van Coppenraet ES, Lindeboom R, Prins JM. Surgical excision versus antibiotic treatment for nontuberculous mycobacterial cervicofacial lymphadenitis in children: a multicenter, randomized, controlled trial. Clin Infect Dis 2007;44(8):1057–1064

[64] Varghese BT, Sebastian P, Ramachandran K, Pandey M. Actinomycosis of the parotid masquerading as malignant neoplasm. BMC Cancer 2004;4:7

[65] Sittitrai P, Srivanitchapoom C, Pattarasakulchai T, Lekawanavijit S. Actinomycosis presenting as a parotid tumor. Auris Nasus Larynx 2012;39(2):241–243

[66] Malatskey S, Fradis M, Ben-David J, Podoshin L. Cat-scratch disease of the parotid gland: an often-misdiagnosed entity. Ann Otol Rhinol Laryngol 2000;109(7):679–682

[67] Hollitt A, Buttery J, Carr J, Chan Y, Ditchfield M, Burgner D. Cat scratch disease of the parotid gland. Arch Dis Child 2016; 101(1):63–64

[68] Iacovou E, Vlastarakos PV, Papacharalampous G, Kampessis G, Nikolopoulos TP. Diagnosis and treatment of HIV-associated manifestations in otolaryngology. Infect Dis Rep 2012;4(1):e9

[69] Dave SP, Pernas FG, Roy S. The benign lymphoepithelial cyst and a classification system for lymphocytic parotid gland enlargement in the pediatric HIV population. Laryngoscope 2007;117(1):106–113

[70] Capaccio P, Sigismund PE, Luca N, Marchisio P, Pignataro L. Modern management of juvenile recurrent parotitis. J Laryngol Otol 2012;126(12):1254–1260

[71] Francis CL, Larsen CG. Pediatric sialadenitis. Otolaryngol Clin North Am 2014;47(5):763–778

[72] Nahlieli O, Shacham R, Shlesinger M, Eliav E. Juvenile recurrent parotitis: a new method of diagnosis and treatment. Pediatrics 2004;114(1):9–12

[73] Katz P, Hartl DM, Guerre A. Treatment of juvenile recurrent parotitis. Otolaryngol Clin North Am 2009;42(6):1087–1091

[74] Mandel L, Bijoor R. Imaging (computed tomography, magnetic resonance imaging, ultrasound, sialography) in a case of recurrent parotitis in children. J Oral Maxillofac Surg 2006;64(6): 984–988

[75] Leerdam CM, Martin HC, Isaacs D. Recurrent parotitis of childhood. J Paediatr Child Health 2005;41(12):631–634

[76] Schneider H, Koch M, Künzel J, et al. Juvenile recurrent parotitis: a retrospective comparison of sialendoscopy versus conservative therapy. Laryngoscope 2014;124(2):451–455

[77] Roby BB, Mattingly J, Jensen EL, Gao D, Chan KH. Treatment of juvenile recurrent parotitis of childhood: an analysis of effectiveness. JAMA Otolaryngol Head Neck Surg 2015;141(2):126–129

[78] Iannuzzi MC, Rybicki BA, Teirstein AS. Sarcoidosis. N Engl J Med 2007;357(21):2153–2165

[79] Cimaz R, Casadei A, Rose C, et al. Primary Sjögren syndrome in the paediatric age: a multicentre survey. Eur J Pediatr 2003;162(10):661–665

[80] Baszis K, Toib D, Cooper M, French A, White A. Recurrent parotitis as a presentation of primary pediatric Sjögren syndrome. Pediatrics 2012;129(1):e179–e182

[81] Liang Y, Yang Z, Qin B, Zhong R. Primary Sjogren's syndrome and malignancy risk: a systematic review and meta-analysis. Ann Rheum Dis 2014;73(6):1151–1156

[82] Sigismund PE, Zenk J, Koch M, Schapher M, Rudes M, Iro H. Nearly 3,000 salivary stones: some clinical and epidemiologic aspects. Laryngoscope 2015;125(8):1879–1882

[83] Chung MK, Jeong HS, Ko MH, et al. Pediatric sialolithiasis: what is different from adult sialolithiasis? Int J Pediatr Otorhinolaryngol 2007;71(5):787–791

[84] Capaccio P, Gaffuri M, Pignataro L. Sialendoscopy-assisted transfacial surgical removal of parotid stones. J Craniomaxillofac Surg 2014;42(8):1964–1969

[85] Reid SM, McCutcheon J, Reddihough DS, Johnson H. Prevalence and predictors of drooling in 7- to 14-year-old children with cerebral palsy: a population study. Dev Med Child Neurol 2012;54(11):1032–1036

[86] Shirley WP, Hill JS, Woolley AL, Wiatrak BJ. Success and complications of four-duct ligation for sialorrhea. Int J Pediatr Otorhinolaryngol 2003;67(1):1–6

[87] Chanu NP, Sahni JK, Aneja S, Naglot S. Four-duct ligation in children with drooling. Am J Otolaryngol 2012;33(5):604–607

[88] Khan WU, Islam A, Fu A, et al. Four-Duct Ligation for the Treatment of Sialorrhea in Children. JAMA Otolaryngol Head Neck Surg 2016;142(3):278–283

[89] Stamataki S, Behar P, Brodsky L. Surgical management of drooling: clinical and caregiver satisfaction outcomes. Int J Pediatr Otorhinolaryngol 2008;72(12):1801–1805

[90] Daniel S. Botulinum toxin injection techniques for pediatric sialorrhea. Oper Tech Otolaryngol--Head Neck Surg 2015;26(1):42–49

[91] Lakraj AA, Moghimi N, Jabbari B. Sialorrhea: anatomy, pathophysiology and treatment with emphasis on the role of botulinum toxins. Toxins (Basel) 2013;5(5):1010–1031

[92] Lungren MP, Halula S, Coyne S, Sidell D, Racadio JM, Patel MN. Ultrasound-Guided Botulinum Toxin Type A Salivary Gland Injection in Children for Refractory Sialorrhea: 10-Year Experience at a Large Tertiary Children's Hospital. Pediatr Neurol 2016;54: 70–75

[93] Vashishta R, Nguyen SA, White DR, Gillespie MB. Botulinum toxin for the treatment of sialorrhea: a meta-analysis. Otolaryngol Head Neck Surg 2013;148(2):191–196

[94] Terrell JE, Kileny PR, Yian C, et al. Clinical outcome of continuous facial nerve monitoring during primary parotidectomy. Arch Otolaryngol Head Neck Surg 1997;123(10):1081–1087

[95] Meier JD, Wenig BL, Manders EC, Nenonene EK. Continuous intraoperative facial nerve monitoring in predicting postoperative injury during parotidectomy. Laryngoscope 2006;116(9): 1569–1572

[96] Grosheva M, Klussmann JP, Grimminger C, et al. Electromyographic facial nerve monitoring during parotidectomy for benign lesions does not improve the outcome of postoperative facial nerve function: a prospective two-center trial. Laryngoscope 2009;119 (12):2299–2305

[97] Xie CM, Kubba H. Parotidectomy in children: indications and complications. J Laryngol Otol 2010;124(12):1289–1293

[98] Carter JM, Rastatter JC, Bhushan B, Maddalozzo J. Thirty-Day Perioperative Outcomes in Pediatric Parotidectomy. JAMA Otolaryngol Head Neck Surg 2016;142(8):758–762

9 Parapharyngeal Space Surgery in the Pediatric Population

Aviyah Peri, Dan M. Fliss

Summary

Parapharyngeal space (PPS) pathologies are uncommon in the pediatric population, yet infections and tumors occupying this fibrofatty fascial compartment may be life threatening. The incidence of parapharyngeal abscess is estimated at 1.29–1.49 per 100,000 children. Pediatric primary neoplasms of the PPS make up less than 0.1% of total head and neck cancers. Detailed knowledge of cervical anatomy is essential for accurate diagnosis and treatment, as most lesions that inhabit the PPS actually represent secondary spread from neighboring fascial compartments. High index of suspicion is also required for diagnosis, as clinical presentation is oftentimes insidious and symptoms may overlap with those of other, more frequent, pathologies. Within the PPS, location relative to the stylopharyngeal fascia may affect clinical manifestation. Pre-styloid lesions are more readily apparent, due to intra-oral bulging and trismus, while retro-styloid pathology may be complicated by neurologic and/or vascular damage to the structures traversing this compartment. Although uncommon at presentation, impending risk of airway compromise should be evaluated and addressed at first priority. Medical workup should include full medical history and physical examination, blood work and imaging. While many infections may be treated conservatively using empiric, wide-range, IV antibiotics, surgical excision is the mainstay of treatment for PPS neoplasms. Pus cultures, if obtained for infectious etiology, will most probably reveal polymicrobial bacterial infection. For neoplasms, a tissue sample should be obtained via preoperative FNA and/or intraoperative frozen-section and may alter the course of treatment. Surgical drainage of PPS infections is done via the transcervical approach, or, in selected cases, using a transoral approach. Most PPS tumors are also excised transcervically. Alternative surgical approaches include transmandibular, transparotid, transcervical/transparotid and transoral robotic routs. Surgery should be planned based on tumor anatomy, histology and considering patient-specific characteristics.

Keywords: Parapharyngeal space, deep cervical fasciae, pre-styloid compartment, post-styloid compartment, deep neck infection (DNI), parapharyngeal abscess (PPA), Lemmier syndrome, transcervical approach, transmandibular approach, transparotid approach, transcervical/transparotid approach, transoral (robotic) approach

9.1 Introduction

The PPS is a fibrofatty fascial compartment encapsulating major structures of suprahyoid anatomy. Both infectious and neoplastic pathologies that occupy this space tend to represent secondary spread from neighboring fascial compartments. Knowledge of the intricate anatomy of cervical fasciae and the compartments that they form is thus key to the understanding PPS pathology.

The cervical fasciae traverse between and around organs of the neck, tying them in distinct fascial compartments (▶ Fig. 9.1). The superficial cervical fascia lies directly beneath the dermis. The more complex deep cervical fascia divides into three layers: superficial (investing), middle (pretracheal), and deep (prevertebral).

The subcutaneous tissues of the head and neck, including the platysma muscles, subcutaneous fat and lymph nodes, superficial veins (e.g., the external jugular vein), and neurovascular supply to the skin, are encompassed between the superficial cervical fascia and the superficial (investing) layer of the deep cervical fascia.

The superficial (investing) layer of the deep cervical fascia forms a tube shape around the entire neck circumference. It splits to envelope the trapezius, sternocleidomastoid (SCM), and muscles of facial expression. Its leaflets also surround the submandibular and parotid salivary glands, as well as the muscles of mastication (the masseter, pterygoid, and temporalis muscles), forming the parotid, masticator, and buccal spaces.

The middle (pretracheal) layer of the deep cervical fascia divides into two components: muscular and visceral. The muscular portion encloses the strap muscles (sternohyoid, sternothyroid, and thyrohyoid) and omohyoid muscle. The visceral portion forms the visceral compartment of the neck. It surrounds the pharynx, larynx, trachea, esophagus, thyroid, parathyroids, buccinators, and constrictor muscles of the pharynx. The mucosa lining these structures, lymphoid tissue of Waldeyer's ring (adenoids, tonsils), and minor salivary glands are all included within the visceral compartment.

The deep (prevertebral) layer of the deep cervical fascia surrounds the paraspinous muscles and cervical vertebrae. The prevertebral compartment spans the space between the prevertebral fascia anteriorly and the vertebral bodies and longus-colli muscle posteriorly.

The retropharyngeal space forms between the visceral fascia anteriorly and the prevertebral fascia posteriorly. The alar fascia, a subdivision of the prevertebral fascia, splits the retropharyngeal space into anterior and posterior compartments. The posterior retropharyngeal compartment extends inferiorly to the posterior mediastinum at the level of the diaphragm. It is commonly referred to as the "danger space," signifying the risk for spread of infection through this space from the neck into the mediastinum. These fascial compartments are especially important in cases of infectious-inflammatory disease.

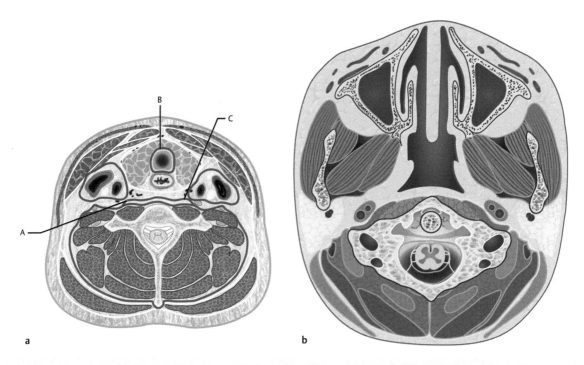

Fig. 9.1 Fasciae and the deep spaces of the neck. **(a)** Infra-hyoid neck. **(b)** Supra-hyoid neck. The parapharyngeal space (PPS) is colored orange, the carotid space within it is colored red. Notice how all three layers of the deep cervical fascia contribute to the formation of the parapharyngeal space. The proximity of the PPS to other seep spaces of the neck is also apparent: masticator space (*purple*), parotid space (*blue*), retropharyngeal space (*magenta*).

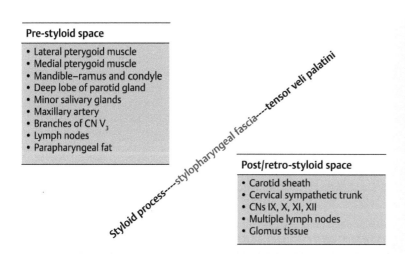

Pre-styloid space

- Lateral pterygoid muscle
- Medial pterygoid muscle
- Mandible–ramus and condyle
- Deep lobe of parotid gland
- Minor salivary glands
- Maxillary artery
- Branches of CN V$_3$
- Lymph nodes
- Parapharyngeal fat

Styloid process---stylopharyngeal fascia----tensor veli palatini

Post/retro-styloid space

- Carotid sheath
- Cervical sympathetic trunk
- CNs IX, X, XI, XII
- Multiple lymph nodes
- Glomus tissue

Fig. 9.2 The parapharyngeal space (PPS) divides into pre-styloid and post-styloid compartments by the fascia running from the styloid process to the tensor veli palatini muscle. The contents of the pre-styloid compartment include the deep lobe of the parotid gland, minor salivary glands, lymph nodes, and parapharyngeal fat. The post-styloid compartment, also known as the carotid space, consists of lymph nodes and glomus tissue and is traversed by major blood vessels and nerves, including the internal carotid artery, internal jugular vein, cranial nerves IX–XII, and the cervical sympathetic chain.

As mentioned above, the PPS, the focus of the current chapter, is yet another fibrofatty fascial compartment within the neck. It has the shape of an inverted teepee, extending from the base of the skull superiorly to the greater cornu of the hyoid bone inferiorly. All three layers of the deep cervical fascia contribute to the formation of the PPS. Its anatomical borders span the nasopharynx and oropharynx medially, the masticator space anterolaterally, the deep lobe of the parotid gland posterolaterally, and the retropharyngeal space posteromedially.

The PPS divides into *pre-styloid* and *post-styloid* compartments by the fascia running from the styloid process to the tensor veli palatini muscle (▶Fig. 9.2). The contents of the pre-styloid compartment include the deep lobe of the parotid gland, minor salivary glands, lymph nodes, and parapharyngeal fat. The post-styloid compartment, also known as the carotid space, consists of lymph nodes and glomus tissue and is traversed by major blood vessels and nerves, including the internal carotid artery, internal jugular vein, cranial nerves IX–XII, and the cervical sympathetic chain.

In pathology, however rare, the PPS may accommodate congenital, infectious, or neoplastic disease. Pathologic processes can inhabit the space via:

- *Direct spread from neighboring compartments:* Primary pathologies of the PPS are rare. As mentioned above, most pathological processes are found to involve the PPS stem, in fact, from adjacent fascial compartments, and are therefore secondary. The central anatomic location of the PPS, surrounded by the peritonsillar, retropharyngeal, submandibular, parotid, and masticator spaces (see ▶ Fig. 9.1), dictates possible routes of direct spread, both for infection and neoplastic processes.
- *Local malformation/transformation:* The diverse, naturally populating, structures within the PPS may give rise to tumors or congenital lesions.
- Distant hematogenous, lymphatic, or perineural seeding.

9.2 Infectious Disease of the PPS

In the pediatric population, parapharyngeal pathology is dominated by infection. Deep neck infections (DNIs) are more common in children than in adults.[1] They may involve the parapharyngeal space (PPDNI), and in some cases, evolve into full-blown parapharyngeal abscess (PPA). In the United States, the incidence of deep neck space infections (including both retropharyngeal and parapharyngeal abscesses) was estimated to be 4.6 per 100,000 children.[2] For PPA specifically, estimated incidence ranged between 1.29 and 1.49 per 100,000 children during the years 2003 to 2012, with skewed tendency toward younger (<5-year-old), male patients.

Unlike in the adult population, where the odontogenic route of infection prevails, pediatric DNIs are commonly acquired through the spread of tonsillitis, pharyngitis, deep cervical lymph-node suppurative adenitis, or hematogenous dissemination. DNIs are notoriously known for their ability to cross the fascial planes and potential spaces of the neck. The submandibular, retropharyngeal, parotid, and masticator spaces all neighbor the PPS and thus serve as potential sources of infection[3] (▶ Fig. 9.1).

Most cases of PPDNI are of bacterial etiology; cultures of aspirated fluid are often polymicrobial. The most commonly isolated microorganisms in pediatric DNI are *Staphylococcus aureus* and group A *Streptococcus*. Anaerobic species include *Fusobacterium*, *Peptostreprococcus*, and *Porphyromonas*.[3]

PPDNIs have a rapidly progressive nature, their complications may be life-threatening, including airway obstruction, infectious internal jugular vein thrombosis (Lemmier syndrome), carotid artery aneurism or rupture, mediastinitis, and sepsis.[3,4] Ipsilateral Horner syndrome and cranial nerve IX–XII palsies might also result from PPDNI involving the post-styloid compartment.[3] The incidence of DNI's life-threatening complications is reported to be 2.2%.[3] Nonetheless, in light of these possible complications, early diagnosis and assertive management are required.

High index of suspicion is crucial for early detection of PPDNI in younger children, because symptoms are not verbalized and clinical signs might be subtle at first, overlapping with other common childhood diseases, such as tonsillitis and lymphadenitis.[4] The most prevalent clinical manifestations of DNI in children are fever (83%), odynophagia (67%), pharyngeal bulging (67%), adenomegaly (53%), and neck mass (40%).[4] Neck pain, torticollis, reduced motion range, dysphagia, trismus, and drooling should also raise suspicion.

PPDNI localized to the pre-styloid compartment will commonly present with fever, neck pain, trismus, and medial displacement of the ipsilateral palatine tonsil. Infections localized to the post-styloid compartment are both more common in children and more difficult to diagnose. Their initial presentation is subtler, and is often devoid of pain, trismus, or obvious swelling; however, the potential for serious complications is significant, due to the richness of vital structures populating the post-styloid compartment.[3]

Respiratory distress is not common at the presentation of PPDNI, but impending risk for airway compromise should always be evaluated and addressed at first priority upon suspicion of DNI. Airway obstruction or edema, suggestive of unstable airway patency, may necessitate prompt intubation or surgical tracheostomy.[3]

Workup should consist of complete history, physical examination, and blood tests. Signs of bacterial infection such as leukocytosis (elevated WBC) and elevated inflammatory markers (such as C-reactive protein) are most commonly evident in blood tests.

Imaging should be carried out in all cases where the suspicion of PPA is high. Imaging, especially computed tomography (CT), is utilized to predict the risk of impending airway and to delineate the presence of abscess or inflammatory collection, its size, and the involvement of other cervical compartments. These findings may crucially affect the decision for surgical intervention as well as surgical approach and extent of surgery.

The mainstays of treatment include: (1) appropriate antibiotic therapy; (2) surgical drainage; and (3) management of complications. There is lack of consensus regarding the role surgery should play in the management of these patients. Advocates of the conservative approach favor an empiric trial of intravenous antibiotics, reserving surgery for cases that fail to clinically improve. Others reckon that a more aggressive approach, with immediate surgical drainage, is justified, given the rapidly progressive nature of DNIs and the risk of hazardous complications. Children with complicated or unstable presentation should with no doubt be treated with immediate surgical drainage. Younger children (<51 months) and children with larger abscesses (>2 cm in diameter) are less likely to sufficiently improve under conservative therapy, and will likely require surgery.[3,4] Airway compromise, complications, septicemia, progressive infection, or the lack of clinical improvement within 48 hours of appropriate empiric intravenous antibiotics are all definite indications for surgery.

Highlights—Infections of the PPS in the pediatric population:
General Characteristics
Demographics
- Estimated incidence: 1.29 and 1.49 cases per 100,000.
- Up to 2.2% life-threatening complications.
- Age: Usually <5 years.
- Male > Female.

Etiology
- Bacterial, polymicrobial:
  - Most prevalent bacteria: *Staphylococcus aureus*, Group A *Streptococcus.*
  - Most prevalent anaerobic bacteria: *Fusobacterium*, *Peptostreprococcus*, and *Porphyromonas.*
- Source:
  - Secondary spread from nearby infection: neighboring cervical fascial compartments, tonsillitis, pharyngitis, suppurative lymphadenitis.
  - Hematogenous spread.

Presentation
(Clinical signs might be subtle at first, especially for post-styloid infections)
- Fever.
- Odynophagia, dysphagia.
- Pharyngeal bulging, medial displacement of the ipsilateral palatine tonsil.
- Adenomegaly.
- Neck mass.
- Neck pain.
- Torticollis, reduced motion range.
- Trismus.
- Drooling.

Possible Major Complications
- Airway obstruction.
- Lemmier syndrome.
- Carotid artery aneurism or rupture.
- Mediastinitis.
- Sepsis.
- Ipsilateral Horner syndrome.
- Cranial nerve IX–XII palsy.

Empiric antibiotic treatment should be administrated in all PPDNI cases and may be adjusted according to culture and sensitivity results when these become available. The empiric regimen should effectively target both aerobic and anaerobic bacteria. An amoxicillin with clavulanic acid preparation, or β-lactamase-resistant antibiotics, such as cefuroxime, imipenem, or meropenem, in combination with an agent that is highly effective against anaerobes, such as clindamycin or metronidazole, is recommended as an empiric treatment.

9.2.1 Preoperative Evaluation

Laboratory workup is essential to the evaluation of PPDNI, regardless of the route of management (i.e., conservative or aggressive). Diagnostic radiological evaluation is essential prior to any drainage attempt.

Blood Workup and Cultures

Blood workup is integral to the assessment of any infectious state. Upon suspicion of PPDNI, blood workup should include a complete blood count with differential count, inflammatory markers (e.g., C-reactive protein), and blood cultures.

Coagulation parameters, electrolytes, and serum glucose level should also be surveyed, in preparation for possible surgical drainage.

Any pus or aspirate obtained from the site of infection should be sent to culture as well. Blood and pus cultures should cover aerobic and anaerobic bacteria. Fungal and acid-fast cultures should also be performed in immunocompromised patients. Cultures for mycobacteria and other atypical agents should be considered in clinically relevant cases.[3]

Imaging Studies

Contrast-enhanced computed tomography (CT) is the imaging procedure of choice in the case of suspected PPA, with 89% accuracy in differentiating between cellulitis and drainable abscess, when combined with clinical examination.[3] Lateral neck radiographs have been used in the past to evaluate for the presence of PPA but have been generally abandoned for the lack of sensitivity compared to the CT modality. Sonography has been reported to have greater accuracy than CT in differentiating drainable abscess from cellulitis; however, this modality is not suitable for the visualization of deeper neck space infections, and the exam quality is largely operator dependent. Magnetic resonance imaging (MRI) usually requires general anesthesia in the pediatric population, and is thus less favored in the PPDNI setting, regardless of its superiority in the delineation of soft tissue. Contrast-enhanced CT is the gold standard for the depiction of jugular vein thrombophlebitis, which is often the first diagnostic clue of a major complication—Lemmier syndrome. Magnetic resonance angiography (MRA) is valuable in the evaluation of vascular complications such as Lemmier syndrome and carotid aneurism or rupture. Sonography may also depict a hyperechoic internal jugular vein thrombus; however, the underlying site of infection is frequently not demonstrated with this modality.

Highlights—Infections of the PPS in the pediatric population.

Workup

Full Medical History

Full Physical Examination

In case impending airway obstruction is suspected, distress causing pharyngeal examination should be avoided or reserved to an OR setting.

Blood Workup

• CBC.
• Inflammatory markers: CRP.
• Bacterial cultures should cover:
  – Aerobic and anaerobic bacteria.
  – Fungal, acid-fast—in immunocompromised.
  – Mycobacteria, atypical agents—selected cases.
• Coagulation parameters.
• Electrolytes.
• Serum glucose level.

Imaging

• Contrast-enhanced CT—imaging is obligatory if drainage is considered.

Pus Cultures

Whenever pus is obtained from aspirate or surgical drainage.

Treatment

Protective Airway

• In case of impending airway obstruction.
• Intubation or surgical tracheostomy.

Appropriate IV Antibiotic Therapy

• Empiric—Amoxicillin+clavulanic-acid/cefuroxime/ imipenem/meropenem + clindamycin/ metronidazole.
• Should be adjusted according to culture results.

Surgical drainage—in selected cases.

Management of Complications

9.2.2 Surgical Technique

Surgical planning must rely on high-quality imaging studies, and should aim to provide good access to all of the involved cervical compartments. High-resolution preoperative CT scan can sufficiently delineate the anatomy, enabling the informed choice of surgical approach.

Access to the PPS may be gained either via an external transcervical approach or through a transoral route (▶Fig. 9.3). Endoscopic transoral techniques for PPA drainage, employing endoscopes and image guidance, have also been described.[3]

The transcervical approach is the most robust. It allows for excellent visualization and control of the major vessels and nerves, suits both pre-styloid and retro-styloid PPAs, and permits the placement of a drain. It is thus the surgical procedure of choice in most cases.

The intraoral approach is appealing for its less extensive nature; however, cases treated with this approach must be chosen carefully. Small, pre-styloid PPAs, that are located medial to the great vessels may be attempted transorally. Intraoral drainage of deeply situated abscesses, which are not directly facing the pharynx or oral cavity, poses risk for neurovascular damage.[3] Moreover, such abscesses might be impossible to fully drain intraorally.

The Transcervical Approach for PPS Surgery

As mentioned above, the transcervical approach is utilized to drain most PPAs, including the more challenging ones, i.e., larger or more deeply situated abscesses.[5]

The patient should be positioned supine on the operating table with his head supported by a soft ring-shaped holder. A slight head-up tilt of the table is preferable to minimize intraoperative bleeding. It is recommended to mark the skin incision on a slightly flexed neck. In this position skin tension is relaxed, allowing identification of the natural skin creases. Incision should be planned to a natural skin crease at Level 2a of the neck,

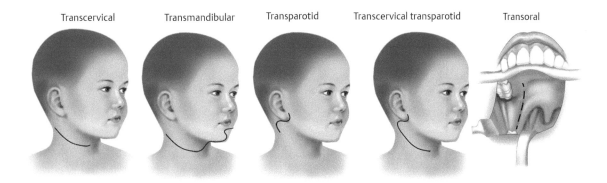

Transcervical   Transmandibular   Transparotid   Transcervical transparotid   Transoral

Fig. 9.3 Surgical incisions that are commonly utilized to gain access to the parapharyngeal space in pediatric patients.

about two fingers below the mandible, to protect against injury to the marginal mandibular branch of the facial nerve (▶Fig. 9.3 and ▶Fig. 9.4a). Finally, a roll should be placed under the patient's shoulders to hyperextend the neck, and the head should be rotated toward the contralateral side.

Skin incision is executed with a #15 blade. Subsequently, delicate electrocautery, using the lowest effective setting, is utilized for subcutaneous and platysmal dissection. Subplatysmal flaps are elevated superiorly, leaving the superficial layer of the deep cervical fascia intact on the submandibular gland. This protects the marginal mandibular branch of the facial nerve, which runs within the fascia superior to the submandibular gland. Dissection then proceeds, using electrocautery, to divide the superficial (investing) layer of the deep cervical fascia along the anterior border of the sternocleidomastoid (SCM) muscle. The superior two-thirds or the SCM are treated first, approaching from its anterior border. Small vessels interconnecting the superficial and deep borders of the SCM are cauterized with bipolar electrocautery. Care is taken to avoid injury to the spinal accessory nerve, as we approach its entry point at the deep aspect of the SCM, which occurs at the junction of the muscle's upper and middle third and lateral to its medial border. Major anatomic structures are now identified and preserved, including the spinal accessory nerve, posterior belly of the digastric muscle, internal jugular vein, common carotid artery and its branches, and the vagus nerve. Dissection continues from below toward the exposed digastric muscle, making a point to identify and preserve

the hypoglossal nerve. The hypoglossal nerve should be visible inferior to the posterior belly of the digastric muscle, superficial to the internal and external branches of the carotid artery, and anterior to the distal part of the internal jugular vein. Anterior branches of the Ansa Cervicalis are also helpful in tracing the nerve.

The abscess is now approached through blunt dissection—a finger is passed deep to the posterior belly of the digastric muscle, dissecting bluntly along the carotid sheath and up to the tip of the styloid (▶Fig. 9.4b). Loculations are thoroughly broken using blunt dissection. Any pus encountered is aspirated, in attempt to achieve adequate drainage. A sample of the aspirate is sent for culture. Finally, the cavity is scooped gently to remove necrotic debris.

Irrigation, using at least 1 L of warm saline, and hemostasis of the wound are carefully executed as indicated. Sufficient hemostasis should be confirmed with adequate blood pressure.

A drain should be left in the surgical bed. Usually, a Penrose drain is placed into the abscess cavity and exits through the incision. A "ghost" stitch may be placed where the Penrose drain exists to reapproximate the skin once the drain is removed. The Penrose itself is sutured to the skin with 4.0 nylon suture. A balled-up super-sponge gauze is placed around the Penrose drain and covered with clear dressing.

The platysma is sutured with absorbable sutures and the skin with 5.0 nylon sutures. Depending on the need for additional drainage, the surgical incision may also be left partially open.

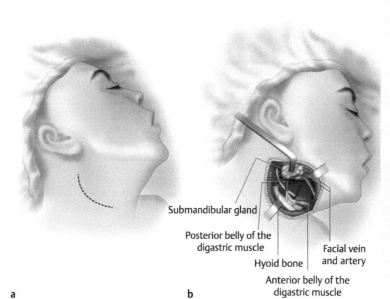

Fig. 9.4 The transcervical approach to parapharyngeal space abscess drainage. **(a)** For a transcervical approach, the surgical incision is through a skin crease at Level 2a, about two finders below the mandible. **(b)** Major anatomic structures are identified and preserved. A finger is passed deep the posterior belly of the digastric muscle and bluntly dissect along the carotid sheath and up to the tip of the styloid, making a point to break any encountered loculations.

Submandibular gland

Posterior belly of the digastric muscle

Hyoid bone

Facial vein and artery

Anterior belly of the digastric muscle

a

b

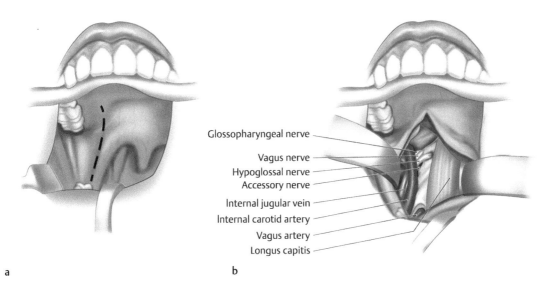

Glossopharyngeal nerve

Vagus nerve

Hypoglossal nerve

Accessory nerve

Internal jugular vein

Internal carotid artery

Vagus artery

Longus capitis

a

b

Fig. 9.5 The transoral approach to parapharyngeal space abscess drainage. **(a)** The abscess is located through inspection and palpation of the oropharynx and lateral pharyngeal wall. Longitudinal incision is then made in the mucosa overlying the abscess. **(b)** Mucosa and pharyngeal constrictors have been incised and reflected medially to allow direct access to the superomedial parapharyngeal space.

The Transoral Approach

Medially situated PPAs in children may be drained transorally (▶ Fig. 9.5). The transoral approach is associated with decreased operative time and shorter hospital stays.[3] Preoperative high-resolution CT scan is essential to ensure that important PPS neurovascular structures reside laterally to the abscess.

Extension of the neck should be achieved using a shoulder roll. A Crowe-Davis mouth gag is carefully inserted into the patient's mouth and expanded. The abscess is located through inspection and palpation of the oropharynx and lateral pharyngeal wall. An 18-gauge needle is then carefully inserted, with constant suction, through the lateral pharyngeal wall and abscess contents are aspirated. Aspirated contents are sent for culture. Longitudinal incision is then made in the mucosa overlying the abscess. A tonsil or a long Kelly clamp is used to dilate the opening, destroy septations, and further drain the abscess. The cavity is then thoroughly irrigated and the incision is left open to allow for further drainage. Finally, the mouth gag is removed.

9.2.3 Postoperative Treatment

Continued intravenous antibiotic treatment is indicated after surgery for PPDNIs. The empiric broad-spectrum regimen may be adjusted upon the establishment of culture results.

If the patient's condition does not improve significantly after surgery with continued antibiotic treatment, repeat CT should be performed to look for residual abscess.

Highlights—Infections of the PPS in the pediatric population.
Surgical Drainage
Definite Indications
- Airway compromise or impending airway.
- Complicated PPA.
- Septicemia.
- Progressive infection or the lack of clinical improvement within 48 hours of appropriate empiric intravenous antibiotics.

Relative Indications
- Younger children (<51 months).
- Large abscesses (>2 cm in diameter).

Surgical Approach
- Transcervical:
  - Suitable for all PPA types.
- Transoral:
  - Associated with decreased operative time and shorter hospital stays.
  - Appropriate for small, pre-styloid PPAs, that are located medial to the great vessels.

9.3 Parapharyngeal Space Tumors in the Pediatric Population

Pediatric primary tumors of the PPS are a rare heterogeneous group, including both malignant and benign lesions.

Infections and congenital lesions are far more prevalent than tumors as primary pathologies of the PPS in the pediatric population.[6] Tumors involving the PPS more commonly represent direct spread through neighboring fascial compartments or metastasis than in-site transformation. As a whole, primary PPS tumors account for no more than 0.5% of all head-and-neck neoplasms, and pediatric cases make up only 0% to 17% of these cases.[7]

Primary tumors may potentially arise from any of the naturally occurring, diverse, tissue types encompassed within the PPS. Indeed, literature review reveals a wide variety of tumor types through pediatric case reports,[7–13] but their exact incidence is difficult to assert due to their scarcity.

The histopathologic landscape of pediatric PPS tumors deviates from that of adult population. Unlike in adult population, most primary PPS tumors found in children are malignant.[6,7,14] While nearly 80% of adult cases are benign, papers reporting on multiple pediatric cases find 56% to 67% of PPS primary tumors to be malignant (▶Fig. 9.6).[6,7,15] Salivary gland tumors and benign paragangliomas, which dominate this compartment in adults, are exceedingly rare in children.[11] Sarcoma, lymphoma, and neurogenic tumors seem to be the most abundant primary malignant histopathologic types, in agreement with pediatric malignant distribution in other head-and-neck sub-sites.[6,7] Soft-tissue sarcomas, specifically rhabdomyosarcomas (▶Fig. 9.6), and neuroblastomas are most prevalent in existing reviews.[6,7] Benign tumors of neurogenic origin, such as neurofibroma, neuroma, and ganglioneuroma, are the most abundant primary benign lesions seen in the PPS of children.[7] Lipomas and congenital malformations, such as cystic hygroma, branchial cyst, and vascular malformations, are also among the more common nonmalignant lesions found at the pediatric PPS.[7] As previously mentioned, nonprimary involvement of the PPS is the prevailing scenario. Metastasis and local advancing nasopharyngeal carcinoma involving the pediatric PPS are well documented.[6]

In a review of 23 pediatric PPS lesions, all treated in one tertiary center,[6] most lesions (74%) were found to be pre-styloid.Clinical presentation of pediatric PPS tumors is variable, most often insidious, and may overlap with more common childhood inflammatory and infectious disease. Painless, slowly growing, neck mass is the most common presenting symptom, along with intraoral swelling.[6] With disease advancement severe symptoms may appear, such as dysphagia, stridor, and cranial nerve palsy (VI or VII). Painless intraoral or neck swelling in children below one year of age should always raise suspicion of malignancy. The same is true for cranial nerve palsy in children of any age.[6]

In certain cases, fever may be a presenting symptom, obscuring the differential diagnosis. Tumor swelling must be differentiated from the more common adenoidal and tonsillar infections as well as from normal lymphoid hypertrophy of adenoidal tissue.[6] Some PPS tumors are discovered completely asymptomatic and anamnesis might be meager, as is oftentimes the case with young children.

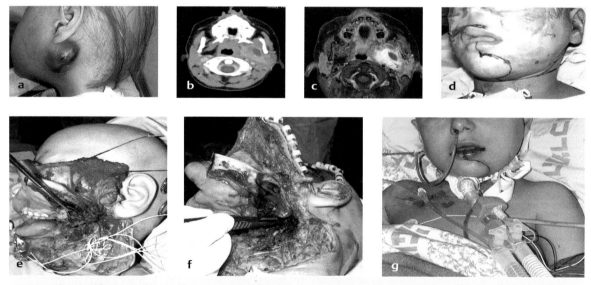

Fig. 9.6 The case of a 5-year-old girl with rhabdomyosarcoma of the parapharyngeal space. Initial chemotherapeutic treatment was administrated abroad, at the girl's birth country. She presented to us after treatment, with obvious massive local recurrence of her disease (a). CT (b) and MRI (c) imaging studies depicted the necrotic tumor in the left parapharyngeal space. A transmandibular approach was indicated, as the tumor was malignant, recurrent, and situated high in the parapharyngeal space. (d) Marking of the planned incision. (e) Intraoperatively. After performing a para-median mandibulectomy, the mandible was deflected upwards to expose the parapharyngeal space. (f) At the end of the surgery, after the removal of the tumor. The forceps indicate the location of the jugular foramen. (g) After surgery, the girl was transferred to the pediatric ICU for initial postoperative recovery.

For this myriad of reasons, most pediatric PPS tumors are already locally advanced upon diagnosis, a fact that negatively affects treatment options and prognosis.[6] High index of suspicion is thus crucial for diagnosis, and prompt evaluation is indicated when suspicion arises.

Highlights—Neoplasms of the PPS in the pediatric population.
General Characteristics
Demographics
- Rare: 0% to 17% of all PPS tumors appear in the pediatric population.
- Exact prevalence of specific pathologic types was not estimated due to scarcity.

Etiology
- Metastasis and local spread from neighboring compartments more frequent than primary tumors.
- Malignant > benign.
- Most abundant malignant types: sarcoma (rhabdomyosarcoma), lymphoma, neurogenic tumors (neuroblastoma).
- Most abundant benign types: Benign neurogenic tumors, lipoma, congenital malformation.
- Pre-styloid > post-styloid.

Presentation
- Often insidious.
- Painless, slowly growing, neck mass.
- Intraoral swelling.
- Dysphagia.
- Stridor.
- Cranial nerve palsy (VI or VII).
- Some tumors are discovered completely asymptomatic.

9.3.1 Preoperative Evaluation and Anesthesia

Blood workup and diagnostic radiological evaluation are essential prior to any PPS involving surgery. Preoperative pathologic investigation of PPS tumors should also be performed where possible.

Blood Workup

Coagulation parameters must be tested in preparation for surgical intervention. Preoperative blood workup should also include: complete blood count with differential count, electrolytes, and serum glucose levels.

Imaging Studies

For the case of PPS tumors, contrast-enhanced CT and/or fat-suppressed MRI of the neck are the imaging procedures of choice[16] (▶Fig. 9.6). With the advent of these techniques, they may provide detailed representation of the lesion and its surrounding anatomy. Radiologic characteristics of the lesion itself, as well as characteristic displacement of fascial planes, may contribute to the differential diagnosis.[6] Precise radiologic delineation of the extent of the lesion and its anatomical relationships is absolutely essential for informed surgical planning. The PPS may accommodate hypervascular lesions, such as paragangliomas, metastatic carcinomas, and hemangiomas. Detection of these lesions prior to attempting biopsy or excision is extremely important and may be life-saving.[6] Visualization of a vascular flow void on MRI is oftentimes sufficient for the diagnosis of hypervascular tumors. MRA may aid in more precise diagnosis.[16] The more common primary PPS malignancies in children: sarcomas, lymphomas, and neurogenic tumors are all hypovascular, and unfortunately share similar radiographic features, making it impossible to confidently radiologically differentiate between them.[7] Lipomas and cysts are hypovascular lesions with distinct CT and MRI appearance, and thus can be usually distinguished on the basis of imaging.[7] Radiologic findings that should raise suspicion of malignancy include: adjacent space invasion, irregular lesion boundaries, multiple pathologic lymph nodes with no evidence of infection, adjacent bony destruction with intracranial extension, and vascular encasement.[6,16] The CT scan may show mild enhancement, and T1-weighted MRI may demonstrate strong postcontrast enhancement.[16]

Tissue Diagnosis

Tumor diagnosis cannot be made certain until it is histopathologically proven. Lack of suspicious clinical and/or radiological signs does not exclude malignancy. Fine needle aspiration cytology (FNAC) should be considered as part of the preoperative workup and may be executed using CT guidance for improved yield and safety. As mentioned above, imaging is obligatory prior to any attempted invasive procedure and FNAC should be avoided altogether in case of suspected paraganglioma or juvenile angiofibroma.[16] Although valuable, FNAC may be nonconclusive in a significant portion of the cases.[6,7] False-positive FNAC results have also been reported.[6] Moreover, FNAC may prove difficult to perform in children due to unsatisfactory cooperation. Thus, in many of the cases, an intraoperative biopsy is performed and the material is sent for frozen section analysis. Intraoperative pathology report may dramatically alter the course of surgery, as surgery will continue if surgical disease is detected but halted in case of malignant lymphoma.[6,7] Definitive diagnosis must always be based on final pathology report performed on the resected lesion.

Highlights—Neoplasms of the PPS in the pediatric population.

Workup
Full Medical History
Full Physical Examination
Blood Workup
- Coagulation parameters.
- CBC.
- Electrolytes.
- Serum glucose level.

Imaging
- Gold standard for anatomic delineation:
  – Contrast-enhanced CT and/or
  – Fat-suppressed MRI.
- Aim to identify vascular lesions:
  – CT: Avid enhancement, delayed washout.
  – MRI: Flow void.
  – MRA.
- Look for signs of malignancy:
  – Irregular lesion boundaries.
  – Adjacent space invasion.
  – Adjacent bony destruction, intracranial extension.
  – Multiple pathologic lymph nodes.
  – Vascular encasement.
  – Mild enhancement on CT.
  – Strong postcontrast enhancement on T1-weighted MRI.

Tissue Diagnosis
- Preoperative FNA:
  – Avoid if vascular lesion is suspected.
  – Perform preoperatively where possible.
- Intraoperative frozen-section:
  – In case tumor type is not certain.
  – May alter surgical course in some cases.
- Definitive diagnosis should always rely on final pathology report.

Treatment
Tumor Resection
Adjunctive Therapy
- Depending on tumor type.
- Chemotherapy and/or radiotherapy.
- Aim to minimize surgical extent, improve ssprognosis, and reduce overall morbidity.

9.3.2 Surgical Technique

Most commonly, external surgical approaches are utilized for the excision of PPS neoplasms.[15,17] These include the transcervical, transmandibular, transparotid, and transcervical/transparotid approaches. ▶ Fig. 9.3 depicts the appropriate skin incisions for the most prevalent surgical approaches.

Selection of the specific approach should be directed by lesion size, location, relation to the major vessels, and assumed gravity.[7,16] Transcervical and transcervical/transmandibular approaches provide relatively wide access to the PPS, allowing for satisfactory resection of even very large tumors.[7] A transmandibular incision might hamper further growth of the still developing pediatric jaw.[15] The transmandibular approach thus entails greater functional and aesthetic morbidity and should preferably be spared from children. Transmandibular surgery may be necessary, however, to achieve tumor-free margins in the resection of large infiltrative malignant tumors of the PPS.[16] Benign tumors that are extremely voluminous or that are situated high at the skull base may also require transmandibular resection.[7] Unfortunately, the anatomical complexity of the PPS, combined with the high-grade advanced nature of most pediatric PPS tumors, implies grave prognosis for infiltrative disease even with meticulous surgical effort.[6,7] Adjunctive chemotherapy and/or radiotherapy should be utilized where possible with aim to minimize surgical extent, improve prognosis, and reduce overall morbidity. Arguably, vital nerves and vessels should be spared where adjunctive therapy is available, even at the expanse of compromising the tumor-free margins.[6]

The Transcervical Approach for PPS Surgery

The majority of pediatric PPS tumors are excised via the transcervical approach[6,7] (▶ Fig. 9.7). This approach is suitable for both pre-styloid and post-styloid lesions. In case the tumor extends from the parotid gland, a transparotid approach should be preferred to protect against facial nerve damage.

The patient should be positioned supine on the operating table with his head supported by a soft ring-shaped holder. A slight head-up tilt of the table is preferable to minimize intraoperative bleeding. It is recommended to mark the skin incision on a slightly flexed neck. In this position skin tension is relaxed, allowing identification of the natural skin creases. Incision should be planned to a natural skin crease about two fingers below the mandible, to protect against injury to the marginal mandibular branch of the facial nerve. Finally, a roll should be placed under the patient's shoulders to hyperextend the neck, and the head should be rotated toward the contralateral side.

Skin incision is executed with a #15 blade. Subsequently, delicate electrocautery, using the lowest effective setting, is utilized for subcutaneous and platysmal dissection. Subplatysmal flaps are elevated superiorly, leaving the superficial layer of the deep cervical fascia intact on the submandibular glad. This protects the marginal mandibular branch of the facial nerve, which runs within the fascia superior to the submandibular

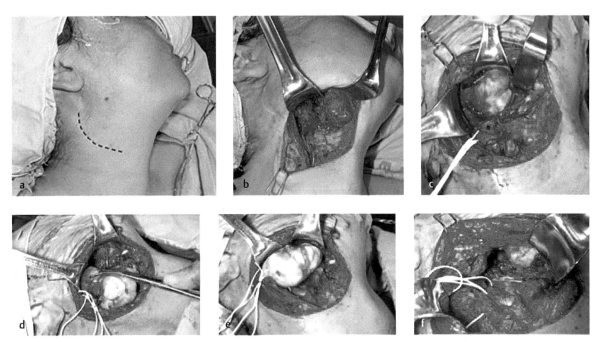

Fig. 9.7 The transcervical approach for parapharyngeal space (PPS) tumor excision. **(a)** Skin incision for the transcervical approach should be made ~2 fingers below the mandible, preferably on a preexisting skin crease. **(b)** The submandibular gland is identified and freed from the surrounding fascia. **(c)** The posterior belly of the digastric muscle is divided and the mylohyoid muscle is retracted anteriorly. **(d)** Blind dissection serves to mobilize the tumor from its surrounding tissue. Small bundles are divided with the use of Hudson or Kelly clamps. **(e)** The tumor is delivered caudally. **(f)** To avoid spillage, care is taken not to compromise the tumor capsule during its delivery.

gland. Dissection then proceeds, using electrocautery, to unwrap the SCM muscle off the superficial layer of the deep cervical fascia. The superior two-thirds or the SCM are treated first, approaching from its anterior border. Small vessels interconnecting the superficial and deep borders of the SCM are cauterized with bipolar electrocautery. Care is taken to avoid injury to the spinal accessory nerve, as we approach its entry point at the deep aspect of the SCM, which occurs at the junction of the muscle's upper and middle third and lateral to its medial border. Major anatomic structures are now identified and preserved, including the spinal accessory nerve, posterior belly of the digastric muscle, internal jugular vein, common carotid artery and its branches, and the vagus nerve. Dissection continues from below toward the exposed digastric muscle, making a point to identify and preserve the hypoglossal nerve. The hypoglossal nerve should be visible inferior to the posterior belly of the digastric muscle, superficial to the internal and external branches of the carotid artery and anterior to the distal part of the internal jugular vein. Anterior branches of the Ansa Cervicalis are also helpful in tracing the nerve. The submandibular gland is identified and dissection continues to free it from its surrounding fascia. The facial artery and vein may be divided to allow better anterior retraction of the submandibular gland. If exposure of the caudal margin of the PPS is required, as in the case of large PPS tumors, the gland may be removed altogether. At this point the lesion, tumor, or abscess should be visible within the PPS, and its relation to the major cranial nerves explored.

The posterior belly of the digastric muscle is divided and the mylohyoid muscle retracted anteriorly. To allow wide approach to the PPS from below, the stylohyoid muscle and stylomandibular ligament may be also divided. Doing so will also reduce the risk of injuring the internal jugular vein at the jugular foramen.

A thin hemostat is preferably used to dissect around the tumor, freeing it from its surrounding tissue without compromising the great vessels and nerves in its proximity. The tumor is then mobilized gently in a blind fashion using finger dissection. Remaining tissue bands are divided using Hudson or Kelly clamps. Care is taken to maintain the integrity of the tumor's capsule to prevent spillage. Finally, the tumor is delivered caudally.

Irrigation, using at least 1 L of warm saline, and hemostasis of the wound are carefully executed as indicated. Sufficient hemostasis should be confirmed with adequate blood pressure. A drain, most commonly of the Jackson-Pratt type, should be left in the surgical bed. The platysma is sutured with absorbable sutures and the skin with 5.0 nylon sutures.

The Transmandibular Approach for Resection of PPS Tumor

The osteotomy entailed in the transmandibular approach (▶ Fig. 9.8) may compromise subsequent normal development of the pediatric jaw, inflicting both functional and aesthetic morbidity. This approach should thus be reserved only for the most challenging of cases, and it

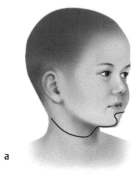

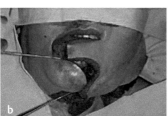

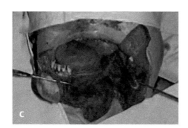

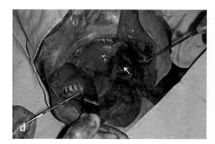

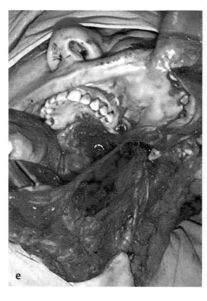

Fig. 9.8 The transmandibular approach for parapharyngeal space (PPS) tumor excision. **(a)** Skin incision for the transmandibular approach. **(b)** The lip incision is performed in the midline, carried around the chin toward the side of the tumor and extended caudally to the level of the cricoid cartilage. **(c)** Once the mandible is split, the ramus on the ipsilateral side is swung laterally. **(d)** The gingivolabial incision is extended toward the anterior pillar of the tonsil, allowing further exposure of the PPS. **(e)** The tumor is excised en-bloc.

is very rarely employed in children. Very large, recurrent, previously resected or highly vascular tumors may necessitate its use. Arguably, the use of adjuvant chemo- or radiotherapy, where possible, may allow for a less stringent approach to extirpation, realizing narrower tumor-free margins and thus permitting a less mutilating surgical approach.[7]

Protective tracheostomy should be executed when employing the transmandibular approach.

A midline lip-split incision is executed, carried around the chin toward the side of the tumor and then caudally to the neck, up to the level of the cricoid cartilage. The neck incision is further extended laterally to the ipsilateral side, with a formal collar neck incision, up to the level of the mastoid bone. The lip-chin incision is deepened to the level of the outer cortex of the mandible. The incision is extended to the gingivolabial sulcus, preserving 0.5 cm of the oral mucosa on the mandible for later suturing. Two to three cm of soft tissue on each side of the planned osteotomy are elevated laterally, taking care not to harm the mental nerve, which enters at the mental foramen.

To minimize free movement of the mandible, two titanium miniplates are prebanded and fixed to the mandible before performing the osteotomy. The first miniplate is fixed at the anterior face of the mandibular cortex. The second is stabilized on the inferior border of the mandible.

The osteotomy is performed in an angled direction, at a paramedian position ipsilateral to the tumor. To minimize bone loss, thin-bladed reciprocal sagittal mechanical saw is utilized. Once the mandible is split, the ramus on the ipsilateral side is swung laterally. To allow further exposure of the PPS, the gingivolabial incision is extended backward toward the anterior pillar of the tonsil. The mylohyoid muscle must be divided to permit lateral retraction of the mandible. After adequate visualization of the PPS is achieved, the tumor is excised en-bloc. Reconstruction usually proceeds with an anterolateral thigh-free flap.

The Transparotid Approach for Resection of PPS Tumor

PPS tumors originating from the parotid gland are exceedingly rare in children, but their presentation may require adjustment of the surgical approach. It is estimated that less than 5% of all parotid gland tumors appear in people younger than 16 years of age.[18] Benign neoplasms are more common than malignant ones for this site, with malignancy rate ranging from 15% to 50% according to different data series.[18,19] Pleomorphic adenoma is the most abundant benign pathology, while mucoepidermoid carcinoma and acinic cell carcinoma are found most frequently among malignant pathologies.[18–20]

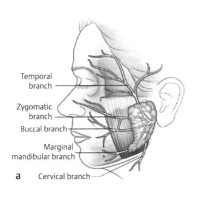

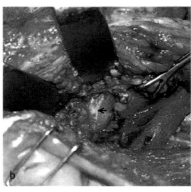

Temporal branch

Zygomatic branch

Buccal branch

Marginal mandibular branch

a   Cervical branch

Fig. 9.9 The transparotid approach for PPS tumor excision. **(a)** Branches of the facial nerve and their course within the parotid gland. **(b)** The facial nerve, exposed during a transparotid surgery.

The transparotid approach (▶ Fig. 9.9) is used for the resection of deep-lobe parotid tumors that extend to the PPS. These lesions typically appear dumbbell-shaped on imaging studies. Preservation of facial nerve function is a primary goal of the resection, as dissection of the parotid tissue around the nerve is required. Muscle relaxants are usually not administered, to allow for nerve monitoring throughout the surgery. The buccal and zygomatic branches are closely monitored by measurement of the electrophysiological signal emitted from the orbicularis oris and orbicularis oculi, respectively. The orbicularis oris electrode should be placed into the commissure of the muscle to also allow for the monitoring of the marginal mandibular branch. Electrodes are inserted prior to draping. Meticulous dissection, which limits bleeds in the surgical field to the bare minimum, positively contributes to the timely and safe identification of nerve branches. Facial movements should be visualized throughout the dissection, and more closely as it approaches the approximate anatomic location of the nerve.

Sterile ophthalmic prep solution is utilized for prepping of the periocular region, including the eyelid, brow area, and cheek. To allow for intraoperative facial monitoring, the face is covered with a transparent adhesive drape sheath.

Surgical access is obtained through a modified Blair incision (▶ Fig. 9.3) using a #15 blade. The incision draws a downward, vertical, preauricular line, starting at the level of the tragus. It then encircles the lobule and drops down, posterior to the helix, along the nuchal hair line. If neck dissection is indicated, the incision is extended medially up to the level of the cricoid cartilage. Subsequent dissection of the subcutaneous tissues is carried out using an electrocautery device at the lowest effective setting. A skin flap is elevated to the superficial musculoaponeurotic system (SMAS) and deep to the subcutaneous fatty tissue. Keeping with this plane lowers the risk for skin perforation and Frey syndrome on the one hand, and tumor spillage on the other hand, as the SMAS makes up the capsule of the parotid gland. The flap is elevated anterior to the edge of the tumor. Care is taken to avoid injury to the distal branches of the facial nerve as they exit the gland. Inferiorly, a subplatysmal flap is elevated, reaching 2 cm below the ramus of the mandible. A small posterior flap is also cautiously elevated, making sure not to injure the anterior wall of the cartilaginous part of the external auditory canal. The anterior border of the SCM muscle is exposed over the mastoid bone. Several Babcock's graspers are placed over the tail of the parotid, and it is then separated from the muscle via anterior retraction. Care is taken to preserve the branches of the greater auricular nerve.

The posterior belly of the digastric muscle is considered a valuable anatomic landmark for facial nerve identification, as the nerve lies deep to the muscle. The posterior belly of the digastric muscle is thus clearly identified. Next, meticulous dissection is performed to release the cartilaginous anterior wall of the external auditory canal from the parotid capsule. Fine hemostats are placed along the posterior border of the tragus, at the tympano-mastoid fissure. As the dissection advances toward the facial nerve, one or two Army-Navy angled retractors are placed at the tympano-mastoid fissure, retracting the posterior edge of the gland anteriorly.

The main trunk of the facial nerve is identified at the confluence of three anatomical landmarks: (1) the mastoid process, (2) the anterior-inferior surface of the cartilaginous wall of the external auditory canal, and (3) the posterior belly of the digastric muscle. A small branch of the stylomandibular artery may occasionally lie superficial to the main trunk of the nerve. In these occasions, the artery should carefully be ligated and divided to maintain the surgical field bloodless.

Dissection continues in a plane superficial to the epineurium of the facial nerve branches. This allows accurate identification of the nerve branches, and complete extirpation of the parotid tissue superficial to the nerve, without its compromise. Fine hemostat and bipolar electrocautery are utilized. First, the main two branches of the nerve, the cervicofacial and zygomaticotemporal, are exposed, and the glandular tissue overlying them is reflected superficially. The dissection continues along the main branches of the nerve, starting with its superior and inferior divisions. The hemostat, held open, is directed superficially along the nerve, while the bipolar electrocautery is used for hemostasis. Stensen duct, if identified, adjacent to the buccal nerve branches, should be divided and tied.

The superficial lobe is left attached at its anterior border, as the surgeon moves to free the deep glandular lobe. Starting from the lower or upper divisions, nerve branches are elevated, using a nerve hook or vessel loop, and meticulously freed circumferentially. Detachment of the nerve from its deep attachments allows for the mobilization of the deep parotid lobe between the main trunk's upper and lower divisions. The tumor is dissected from the fibrofatty tissue at the lateral border of the PPS. The tumor is excised along with the deep parotid lobe. If preserved, the superficial lobe is turned over the facial nerve and sutured in place with a 4.0 Vicryl suture. Absorbable sutures are used to suture the platysma and SMAS. The skin is sutured with 5.0 nylon.

The Transcervical/Transparotid Approach for Resection of PPS Tumor

This combination approach is suitable for deep parotid lobe lesions that extend not only to the PPS but also to the neck (▶ Fig. 9.10). The lower extent of the incision is used to gain excess to the PPS, as usual via the transcervical approach (see section 9.3.2.1, ▶ Fig. 9.3). After the spinal accessory nerve is dissected away from the tumor, a Richardson's retractor is utilized to elevate the posterior belly of the digastric muscle, exposing the tumor in the PPS. The submandibular salivary gland is identified and excised. The digastric muscle is then retracted superiorly or divided.

Next, the great vessels, the internal jugular vein and common carotid artery, are identified and held with vessel loops. The internal jugular vein is divided proximally and the tumor retracted superiorly. The hypoglossal nerve is also identified and carefully separated from the tumor. As the dissection proceeds, the internal and external branches of the carotid artery are identified. The internal jugular vein is divided again, caudally. The tumor is cautiously dissected from the arteries using bipolar electrocautery. The dissection continues along the internal carotid artery. The internal jugular vein is divided again distally and the tumor is completely excised.

Transoral Robotic Surgery

A transoral robotic approach may be used for selected cases of PPS tumors, located anterior to the carotid artery (▶ Fig. 9.11). The robotic transoral approach has been mainly used for PPS pathology in adults, but can be employed in children as well.[3]

The *da Vinci surgical system* (Intuitive Surgical; Sunnyvals, CA) is docked at an angle of approximately 15° to the right of the patient's bed. The patient is placed supine and is nasally intubated. After intubation, the eyes are covered for safety. A McIvor mouth gag or FK retractor is inserted. An 8-mm camera is installed and inserted into the mouth. The robotic arm ipsilateral to the lesion is loaded with a 5-mm monopolar cautery with spatula tip. The contralateral robotic arm is loaded with a 5-mm Maryland dissector. The arms are positioned to put the instrument tips within the endoscope's field of view. To minimize collisions, they are aligned approximately parallel to the optical arm.

A second surgeon assists at the head of the bed with pediatric Yankauer suction, bipolar cautery, and nonrobotic hemoclips.

Using unipolar cautery, an inverted L-shaped incision is made at the lateral aspect of the palatoglossal arch. Deep dissection through the superior constrictor muscle is then performed using unipolar cautery. The tumor is retracted with the Maryland dissector. The PPS is reached via dissection through the superior constrictor and medial to the pterygoid muscles. Dissection extends into the parapharyngeal fat. Monopolar and bipolar electrocautery are utilized for the control of minor arterial bleedings. Circumferential dissection frees the tumor from the surrounding tissue, while keeping its capsule intact. The robotic arms are then turned aside and the tumor is shelled out similar to the transcervical approach. Hemostasis is achieved with bipolar electrocautery, and the wound is thoroughly irrigated. The oropharyngeal flaps are sutured in place with 2.0 Vicryl suture.

9.4 Postoperative Treatment

Prophylactic antibiotic treatment is not indicated after the removal of PPS tumors.

The transmandibular approach requires a temporary, protective tracheostomy. Should the postoperative course be unremarkable, this tracheostomy is removed on the third postoperative day.

The patient is extubated upon the end of surgery and is transferred to the postsurgery care unit to be closely monitored before relocating back to the pediatric ENT/surgical department. For external surgical approaches, care for the surgical wound includes saline rinses three times a day, followed by the application of antibiotic ointment. Drains are removed when the daily fluid accumulation is less than 20 to 30 mL, usually by the third postoperative day. Adequate pain control is essential for successful recovery and should be achieved using the customary postoperative pain relief protocols for the department.

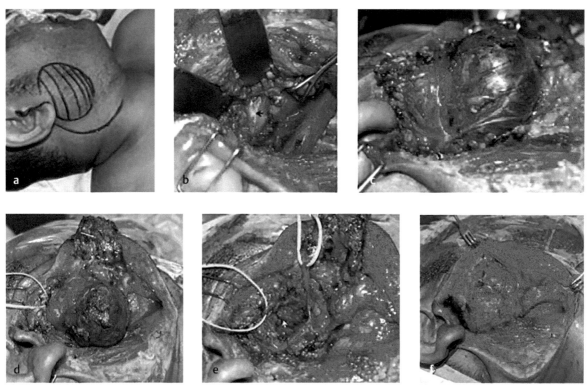

Fig. 9.10 The transcervical transparotid approach for PPS tumor excision. **(a)** The modified Blair skin incision is extended to provide cervical excess. **(b)** One or two Army-Navy angled retractors are placed at the tympanomastoid fissure to retract the posterior edge of the parotid gland anteriorly. **(c)** The facial nerve is meticulously freed circumferentially. **(d)** Freeing the facial nerve from its deep attachments will allow mobilization of the deep lobe between its upper and lower divisions of the main trunk. **(e)** The surgical field after removal of the deep-lobe parotid tumor from the border of the PPS. **(f)** If preserved, the superficial lobe is turned over the facial nerve and sutured in place with a number 4.0 Vicryl.

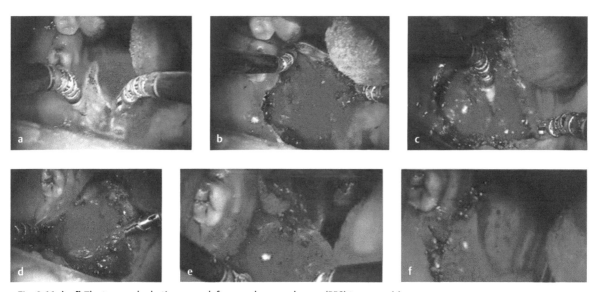

Fig. 9.11 (a–f) The transoral robotic approach for parapharyngeal space (PPS) tumor excision.

Highlights—Neoplasms of the parapharyngeal space in the pediatric population.

Surgical Resection

Surgical Approach

- Transcervical:
  - Most commonly utilized.
  - Allows wide PPS access.
  - Suitable both for pre-styloid and post-styloid lesions.
- Transmandibular:
  - Allows wide PPS access.
  - Entails functional and aesthetic morbidity.
  - Necessary for adequate resection of tumors that are:
    - Very large/voluminous.
    - Infiltrative.
    - Highly vascular.
    - Situated high at the skull-base.
- Transparotid:
  - Utilized for deep-lobe parotid tumors that extend to the PPS.
  - Preservation of facial nerve function is a primary goal.
  - Muscle relaxants not administrated.
- Transcervical/transparotid:
  - Deep parotid lobe lesions that extend to the PPS and to the neck.
- Transoral robotic:
  - Selected cases.
  - Tumor must be located anterior to the carotid artery.

Postoperative Treatment

- Protective tracheostomy removed on POD 3.
- External wound care: saline rinses ×3/day, antibiotic ointment.
- Drains removed at 20 to 30 mL/24 h.
- Adequate pain control.

References

[1] Woods CR, Cash ED, Smith AM, et al. Retropharyngeal and parapharyngeal abscesses among children and adolescents in the United States: epidemiology and management trends, 2003–2012. J Pediatric Infect Dis Soc 2016;5(3):259–268

[2] Adil E, Tarshish Y, Roberson D, Jang J, Licameli G, Kenna M. The public health impact of pediatric deep neck space infections. Otolaryngol Head Neck Surg 2015;153(6):1036–1041

[3] Lawrence R, Bateman N. Controversies in the management of deep neck space infection in children: an evidence-based review. Clin Otolaryngol 2017;42(1):156–163

[4] Côrte FC, Firmino-Machado J, Moura CP, Spratley J, Santos M. Acute pediatric neck infections: outcomes in a seven-year series. Int J Pediatr Otorhinolaryngol 2017;99:128–134

[5] Blumberg JM, Judson BL. Surgical management of parapharyngeal space infections. Oper. Tech. Otolaryngol. Neck Surg. 2014;25:304–309

[6] El Fiky L, Shoukry T, Hamid O. Pediatric parapharyngeal lesions: criteria for malignancy. Int J Pediatr Otorhinolaryngol 2013;77(12):1955–1959

[7] Stárek I, Mihál V, Novák Z, Pospíšilová D, Vomácka J, Vokurka J. Pediatric tumors of the parapharyngeal space: three case reports and a literature review. Int J Pediatr Otorhinolaryngol 2004;68(5):601–606

[8] Zheng Z, Jordan AC, Hackett AM, Chai RL. Pediatric desmoid fibromatosis of the parapharyngeal space: a case report and review of literature. Am J Otolaryngol 2016;37(4):372–375

[9] Hung Y, Huang C-S, Yang L-Y. A huge parapharyngeal space tumor in a child. Ear Nose Throat J 2017;96(4–5):158–159

[10] Garzorz N, Diercks GR, Lin HW, Faquin WC, Romo LV, Hartnick CJ. A case of pediatric parapharyngeal space ganglioneuroma. Ear Nose Throat J 2016;95(4–5):E16–E20

[11] Brigger MTT, Pearson SEE. Management of parapharyngeal minor salivary neoplasms in children: a case report and review. Int J Pediatr Otorhinolaryngol 2006;70(1):143–146

[12] Kaufman MR, Rhee JS, Fliegelman LJ, Costantino PD. Ganglioneuroma of the parapharyngeal space in a pediatric patient. Otolaryngol Head Neck Surg 2001;124(6):702–704

[13] Bruyeer E, Lemmerling M, Poorten VV, Sciot R, Hermans R. Paediatric lipoblastoma in the head and neck: three cases and review of literature. Cancer Imaging 2012;12:484–487

[14] Riffat F, Dwivedi RC, Palme C, Fish B, Jani P. A systematic review of 1143 parapharyngeal space tumors reported over 20 years. Oral Oncol 2014;50(5):421–430

[15] Shlomi B, Chaushu S, Gil Z, Chaushu G, Fliss DM. Effects of the subcranial approach on facial growth and development. Otolaryngol Head Neck Surg 2007;136(1):27–32

[16] Fliss DM, Gil Z. Approaches to the parapharyngeal space. In: Atlas of Surgical Approaches to Paranasal Sinuses and the Skull Base. Berlin: Springer; 2016: 169–188

[17] Yafit D, Horowitz G, Vital I, Locketz G, Fliss DM. An algorithm for treating extracranial head and neck schwannomas. Eur Arch Otorhinolaryngol 2015;272(8):2035–2038

[18] Friedman E, Patiño MO, Udayasankar UK. Imaging of pediatric salivary glands. Neuroimaging Clin N Am 2018;28(2):209–226

[19] Stevens E, Andreasen S, Bjørndal K, Homøe P. Tumors in the parotid are not relatively more often malignant in children than in adults. Int J Pediatr Otorhinolaryngol 2015;79(8):1192–1195

[20] Inaka Y, et al. A study on 21 cases of parotid gland tumors in adolescents. Pract. Oto-Rhino-Laryngol Suppl. 2017;151:50–52

10 Submandibular Gland Excision

Sam J. Daniel

Summary

Submandibular Gland Excision is most commonly performed via a transcervical approach. It is indicated for a number of conditions including refractory recurrent sialadenitis, sialolithiasis not amenable to sialoendoscopy or lithotripsy, salivary gland neoplasms, and debilitating sialorrhea.

This chapter highlights the surgical anatomy, preoperative preparation, surgical approaches, and pearls to avoid intraoperative complications of submandibular gland excision. Safe surgery of the submandibular glands requires clear identification of the digastric and mylohyoid muscles, as well as knowledge of the course of the marginal mandibular, the hypoglossal, the lingual nerves, and the facial artery.

Novel approaches that are gaining in popularity include transoral excision and endoscopic excision. In comparison to the traditional transcervical approach, the transoral route avoids a cervical scar with potential keloid formation, and decreases the risk of injury to the marginal mandibular branch of the facial nerve. This approach also eliminates the risk of leaving ductal stone remnants since the entire duct and papilla are removed.

Keywords: Submandibular glands, calculus, stone, drooling, submandibular tumor, marginal mandibular nerve, hypoglossal nerve, lingual nerve, facial artery, Wharton's duct

10.1 Surgical Anatomy

The submandibular glands are paired major salivary glands containing both serous and mucinous acini. Each gland is composed of a superficial lobe that extends inferior to the posterior half of the body of the mandible, and a deep lobe that hooks around the posterior margin of the mylohyoid entering the oral cavity through a triangular aperture as it lies on the lateral surface of the hyoglossus (▶Fig. 10.1). The superficial lobe, which accounts for the greater portion of the gland, is located in the submandibular triangle, between the anterior belly and the tendon of the digastric muscle. It is bounded superomedially by the mylohyoid muscle, and inferiorly by the investing layer of the deep cervical fascia and platysma. Each submandibular gland drains into an excretory duct, also known as Wharton's duct that emerges from its deep lobe, and courses anteriorly, deep to the mylohyoid muscle and lateral to hyoglossus and genioglossus. It abuts the sublingual gland below the mucosa of the floor of the mouth before opening into an orifice in the sublingual papilla lateral to the lingual frenulum (▶Fig. 10.2). This opening is the narrowest part of the duct and is dilated prior to sialoendoscopy. The submandibular glands are small in young infants and are contiguous to the sublingual glands. They grow rapidly during the first 2 years of life.

During submandibular gland excision the surgeon has to be cognizant of important anatomical relationships of

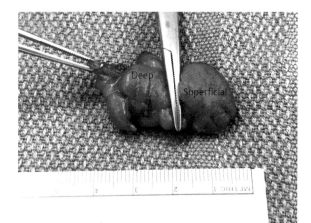

Fig. 10.1 Superficial and deep lobe of a resected submandibular gland. The Clamp is sitting where the mylohyoid was as the gland wraps around its posterior border. The clip is on the ligated Wharton's duct.

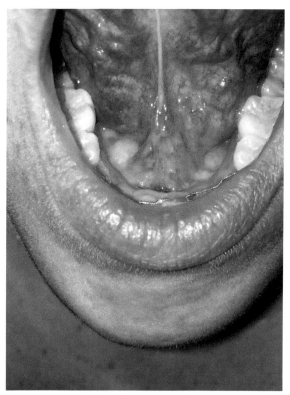

Fig. 10.2 Stone obstructing the anterior duct behind the right papilla.

the lingual nerve, the hypoglossal nerve, and the marginal mandibular branch of the facial nerve (MMN). The latter is the most vulnerable during submandibular gland surgery particularly in young children as it is located higher than in adults often taking a superficial course over the mandible, and portions of it may be exposed due to limited parotid gland development. It usually exits the anteroinferior portion of the parotid gland close to the angle of the mandible and traverses the margin of the mandible in the plane between platysma and the investing layer of deep cervical fascia covering the submandibular gland. When the MMN descends below the border of the mandible, it usually runs superficial to the anterior facial vein and immediately over the superficial lobe of the submandibular gland. Strategies to avoid injuring the marginal mandibular nerve (MMN) include making the incision 2 fingerbreadths inferior and parallel to the body of the mandible, or slightly above the level of the hyoid bone. Another strategy is to ligate the facial vein and retract it cephalad so that the MMN is included in the superior flap and protected.

Posteriorly, the lingual nerve is above the duct, then, as it descends forward, it crosses the lateral side of the duct, passes below the duct winding round its lower border, before crossing it medially and ascending towards the genioglossus. It terminates as several medial branches ascending on the external and superior surface of hyoglossus to provide general somatic afferent innervation to the mucous membrane of the anterior two-thirds of the tongue.

The hypoglossal nerve emerges from behind the posterior belly of the digastric muscle and courses along the floor of the submandibular triangle lying deep to the submandibular gland. It passes forward into the gap between the hyoglossus medially and the myelohyoid laterally and supplies innervation to the intrinsic and extrinsic muscles of the tongue.

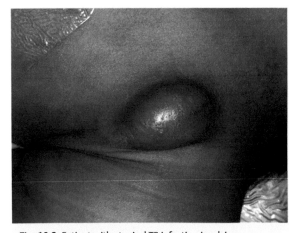

Fig. 10.3 Patient with atypical TB infection involving submandibular area and gland.

10.2 Preoperative Evaluation

A detailed history and physical examination are of utmost help in diagnosing the specific salivary gland disorder. The differential diagnosis includes acute or chronic inflammatory (and/or infectious) conditions, congenital lesions, benign or malignant tumors, vascular malformations, and manifestations of systemic diseases. In a recent retrospective review of 193 patients post submandibular gland excision, 56% had non-neoplastic disorders (sialolithiasis and sialadenitis) while the remaining had a submandibular gland tumor. The most common benign neoplasm was pleomorphic adenoma (27%). Ten percent of tumors were malignant and included adenoid cystic carcinoma, mucoepidermoid carcinoma, and adenocarcinoma.[1]

Important elements on history include the onset, duration, severity, and frequency of the symptoms. Perinatal salivary gland swelling is more likely to be secondary to a congenital lesion such as a lymphatic or vascular malformation. A gradual painless increase in size suggests a neoplasm, especially in older children.[2] An acute onset of pain and swelling, especially with fever, indicates an infectious or inflammatory lesion. Ductal obstruction often presents with intermittent and/or recurrent postprandial swelling. Painless violaceous lesions of the skin are often seen with atypical mycobacteria infections or cat scratch disease (▶Fig. 10.3). A history of trauma suggests ductal injury.

Physical examination should include inspection of the floor of the mouth, as well as bimanual palpation of the gland and duct. The quality of the saliva expressed at the papilla should be inspected for purulence. An enlarged submandibular gland with decreased or absent salivary flow suggests obstruction secondary to a stone or ductal stenosis. In cases of acute infection the patient is prescribed antibiotics and elective surgery is planned at a later date.

Indications for submandibular gland excision are listed in ▶Table 10.1. It is the author's belief that the management of sialolithiasis and ductal pathology should aim for gland-sparing procedures before considering gland excision. Sialoendoscopy is now well established as a minimally invasive and effective

Table 10.1 Potential indications for submandibular gland excision

Symptomatic calculus not amenable to sialoendoscopy or intraoral approach

Chronic sialadenitis with or without sialolithiasis

Suspicion of a neoplasm

A persistent firm submandibular mass of uncertain etiology

Vascular malformation

Sialorrhea with pulmonary aspiration

Chronic or severe sialorrhea

tool for the diagnosis of salivary gland ductal pathology (inflammation, stenosis, stricture), as well as the treatment of sialolithiasis. Despite advances in sialoendoscopy indications remain for gland removal in chronically inflamed gland with recurring episodes of painful swelling whereby conservative treatment options have failed, and symptomatic or recurrent sialadenitis caused by intraparenchymal stones or large stones not amenable to sialoendoscopy and lithotripsy. Gland removal may also be indicated in patients with recurrent calculus formation (▶ Fig. 10.4), intraoperative complications of sialendoscopy, inability to extract the stone during minimally invasive procedures, and residual symptoms despite stone removal. In rare cases acute inflammation transforms into Ludwig's angina with elevation of the floor of the mouth and tongue by the inflammatory phlegmon and tissue edema adjacent to the gland. In these patients, the airway can be protected with fiberoptic intubation.

Bilateral submandibular gland excision combined with bilateral parotid duct ligation is an effective surgical procedure for the treatment of patients with severe sialorrhea or aspiration.[3] A long-term follow-up study reported significant improvement in 87% of patients with no major complications and only 8% experiencing xerostomia.[4] In less severe cases, bilateral submandibular gland excision can be performed without parotid duct ligation to avoid the latter complication.

Several imaging modalities can be helpful preoperatively. While plain X-rays may detect radiopaque stones, they miss radiolucent ones. Ultrasound remains the most helpful test in the pediatric population, because of its non-invasiveness and lack of radiation exposure. Ultrasound can detect up to 90% of stones greater than 2 mm, and can distinguish benign from malignant lesions in the majority of cases.[5,6] Ultrasound can also help differentiate whether masses are intraglandular or extraglandular.[2] CT at times provides complementary information to distinguish gland enlargement from an intraglandular mass versus a mass abutting the gland.

CT and/or MRI are important to assess parapharyngeal extension, deep cervical lymphadenopathies, as well as skull base extension. CT can also be useful for surgical planning in inflammatory conditions such as sialadenitis, ductal stones or stenosis, ranulas, and abscesses. CT is also useful to detect bony erosion in cases of tumors. Preoperative knowledge of the presence of calculi in the duct is important as failure to excise the duct up to the floor of the mouth can result in retained fragments, which can lead to chronic inflammation or recurrent infections.

Despite the ionizing radiation, the CT scan has the advantage of being a short procedure as opposed to MRI. MRI with IV gadolinium contrast remains the test of choice in cases suspicious for an underlying neoplasm and in lesions of the parapharyngeal space as it provides excellent soft tissue detail. Flow voids also assist in determining the nature of vascular malformations. Newer MR techniques can help delineate benign from malignant processes using dynamic contrast or diffusion-weighted methods. A sialogram may reveal narrowing of the duct from scarring and secondary ductal ectasia within the hilum and the gland itself.

While fine needle aspiration biopsy (FNAB) can be very useful in the work-up of suspected neoplasm of the submandibular gland, a negative FNAB is not definitive and the surgeon should still proceed with gland resection for final diagnosis. Also in cases of a malignancy a nodal neck dissection is indicated.

10.3 Surgical Approaches

The traditional approach to excision of the submandibular gland is via the transcervical route. Other approaches include intraoral and endoscopic excision.

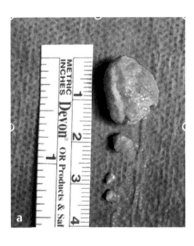
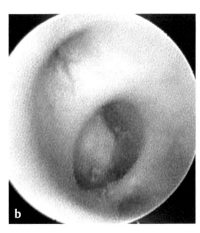

Fig. 10.4 (a, b) Multiple stones in submandibular duct requiring gland excision. Sialoendoscopy was not possible here due to the ductal scarring.

10.3.1 Transcervical Approach

The procedure is performed under general anesthesia with orotracheal intubation. The endotracheal tube is positioned and secured on the contralateral side of the surgery. Paralytic agents are avoided to allow for intraoperative marginal mandibular nerve monitoring. The patient is placed supine with a shoulder roll to allow the neck to be extended, and the head is turned away from the operative side in order to enhance the exposure of the submandibular triangle. The operative field is draped with sterile transparent drapes to allow exposure of the corner of the mouth. In case of a small or retracted submandibular gland, depressing the floor of the mouth with a gloved finger can facilitate its identification.

After adequate infiltration with local anesthesia, a skin incision is performed in a natural skin crease (if possible), approximately two fingerbreadths below the inferior border of the mandible slightly above the level of the hyoid bone. After carrying the incision through subcutaneous tissue and platysma to the underlying investing layer of the deep cervical fascia, skin flaps are elevated to obtain adequate exposure. Dissection is started at the inferior aspect of the submandibular gland and is maintained deep to the investing fascia. The facial vein is isolated, ligated, and elevated in order to protect the marginal mandibular nerve. As the fascia is elevated superiorly, one remains attentive not to go above the border of the mandible as this increases the risk to the marginal mandibular nerve, which usually runs under platysma, in the investing fascia of the submandibular gland.

Once its lateral surface separated from fascia, the anterior portion of the gland is freed from surrounding tissue at the anterior belly of the digastric by incising the fascia over the digastric and reflecting it posteriorly. This reveals the mylohyoid muscle. The latter is demarcated by the direction of its fibers extending from posterosuperior to anteroinferior. Having the mylohyoid muscle in view guarantees that the hypoglossal and lingual nerves are protected, as they lie deep to it. The dissection is then carried posterior to the edge of the mylohyoid muscle. Perforating vessels are ligated to free the overlying part of the submandibular gland, and a right-angled retractor is used to retract the mylohyoid muscle anteriorly off the deep portion of the gland. The anterior portion of the gland, the duct with the closely adherent sublingual gland, and the lingual nerve are then encountered deep to the muscle. The lingual nerve can be seen superiorly extending from deep to the mandible posteriorly and looping close to the anterior portion of the gland, where it gives rise to nerve roots extending into the submandibular ganglion. The nerve ascends superiorly as it extends anteriorly to innervate the anterior aspect of the tongue and floor of the mouth. The nerve must be carefully dissected free and the rootlets incised. Following this, the duct is identified and followed anteriorly. If the patient has a stone in the duct, the surgeon has to ensure that the duct is ligated distal to the stone and the stone is removed. A large vein running along the duct should be ligated separately. It is not uncommon to have salivary tissue along the course of the duct as it exits the gland. This can partially obscure the duct and increases the risk of injury to the hypoglossal nerve. The lingual and hypoglossal nerves must be clearly seen prior to ligating the submandibular ganglion and Wharton's duct.

The hypoglossal nerve can then be seen running along the floor of the triangle, as it emerges from behind the posterior belly of the digastric muscle. Care must be taken to avoid injuring it as it courses along the floor of the submandibular triangle.

Once the anterior portion of the gland has been freed from the lingual nerve and submandibular duct, the remainder of gland is easily detached from the underlying fascial planes over the floor of the submandibular triangle. The gland can then be retracted inferiorly with counter-traction placed on the soft tissue superior to the gland, and the superior aspect of the gland is dissected free from the soft tissue just inferior to the mandible. Care must again be taken to avoid injury to the marginal mandibular nerve as it may be running just lateral and superior to the gland. Either identifying the nerve or maintaining dissection within a plane immediately on the substance of the gland helps to avoid injury.

As the gland is reflected inferiorly, the facial artery can be seen indenting the posterosuperior surface of the gland. It can be divided as it leaves the gland superiorly and then again as it enters the gland inferiorly. In most cases the facial artery can be freed off the gland and branches feeding the gland identified and ligated. Once the gland is freed from the artery, the gland is removed and the entire surgical field is inspected for hemostasis. The wound is irrigated, a Hemovac suction or Penrose drain is inserted, and the wound is closed in layers beginning with the platysma muscle using an absorbable braided suture, followed by subcutaneous closure, and then an absorbable monofilament subcuticular skin closure.

In chronically inflamed glands, dissection may be tedious and bleeding may be an issue; the surgeon can avoid injury to the nerves by identifying them under magnification and carefully preserving them.

An alternative to the technique described above is to start, once the lateral surface of the gland freed from the investing fascia, by ligating the facial artery as it enters the submandibular triangle from deep to the posterior belly of the digastric muscle and freeing the superficial portion of the submandibular gland fully. The mylohyoid muscle can then be retracted, and submandibular gland can then be pedicled on the lingual nerve and Wharton's duct. Then the deep lobe of the gland and duct are excised. This may allow in certain cases better exposure of the lingual nerve and Wharton's duct during dissection of these structures.

10.3.2 Intraoral Approach

All patients should be consented for a possible transcervical approach.

Optimizing the exposure is crucial. If possible, nasal intubation enhances access; otherwise the oral tube is placed on the contralateral side. The surgeon wears a headlight and stands on the contralateral side of the operated gland. A bite block is placed on the surgeon's side to sustain the mouth opening. The surgical assistant can improve the visualization of the floor of the mouth by holding a Weider retractor in order to medialize the lateral surface of the tongue, and a Minnesota retractor to lateralize the cheek and the lower lip. Wharton's duct is cannulated with a salivary duct probe that is secured close to the papilla with a suture ligature. The floor of mouth mucosa is generously infiltrated with Xylocaine and epinephrine, extending from the papilla to the retromolar areas. A superficial mucosal incision is made with a scalpel or a fine-tip needle cautery, encircling the ipsilateral papilla and extending in a linear fashion to the retromolar region. The mucosa is gently elevated using blunt dissection with a Peanut medially toward the tongue and laterally toward the gingiva, unroofing the paralingual space. The exposed sublingual gland is then excised using a combination of blunt dissection and bipolar cautery. Care is taken to preserve the lingual nerve and Wharton's duct, which are separated before delivering the sublingual gland. Once the sublingual gland is removed, Wharton's Duct can be gently tunneled under the lingual nerve and followed to its hilum connecting with the deep lobe of the submandibular gland.[7] The submandibular ganglion is separated from the deep lobe, allowing the lingual nerve to retract away from the field. A combination of blunt and bipolar dissection is used to separate the deep lobe of the submandibular gland from surrounding structures. The posterior free margin of the mylohyoid muscle is retracted antero-laterally allowing visualization of the superficial portion of the submandibular gland. Blunt dissection is used to free the submandibular gland from surrounding structures. The assistant pushes the submandibular gland into the surgical field by applying an external upwards pressure in the submandibular triangle. This elevates the gland in the floor of the mouth and enhances visualization. The submandibular gland continues to be freed from its attachments with blunt dissection. Because of the narrow surgical field, dissection and delivery of the submandibular gland may not always be simple. A good exposure and good lighting of the surgical field are essential. The insertion of an endoscope in the oral cavity during this step or a fiberoptic retractor can enhance visualization. Traction on the gland usually separates the main facial artery from the gland, allowing for the small penetrating vessel branches to be visualized. To prevent severe bleeding during surgery and postoperative hematoma, these should always be cauterized or ligated. In all cases, the surgeon should be prepared to control the bleeding from the facial artery, including the conversion to an open approach.

Once the submandibular gland is extracted, the field is irrigated and examined with bimanual palpation for any residual gland and for the need for hemostasis. The lingual and hypoglossal nerves can be identified in the bed of the surgical field. The intraoral incision is then closed with interrupted 3–0 chromic sutures. A Barton dressing or Veronique support dressing can be used to support the wound and jaw. This will markedly reduce pain and swelling. Most patients can be discharged on a soft diet and a course of antibiotics.

10.3.3 Endoscopic Approach

An endoscope can be introduced through an intraoral incision with excellent visualization of the surgical field. Surgery is conducted as described in the intraoral approach.

A transcervical endoscopic approach has been described in a cadaver model with small incisions placed in the inferior aspect of the neck providing entry for the instruments. Subcutaneous dissection is performed with an inflated balloon prior to insufflation of carbon dioxide.[8]

Finally, the robotic endoscopic approach is under development in a number of centers and could lead in the future to decrease in operative times.

10.3.4 Complications

The two most common undesired side effects of transcervical submandibular excision are the development of a scar at the incision site and injury to the marginal mandibular branch of the facial nerve. The latter is the most frequently damaged nerve in the transcervical approach, with rates ranging from 1 to 7%. This results in impairment of the lower lip depressor function. Temporary marginal mandibular nerve paresis can also happen from nerve stretching during retraction or operative manipulation.

Injury to the lingual nerve may result during division of the submandibular ganglion, in chronic inflammation with an adherent nerve, or if the duct is sectioned without properly freeing the nerve. This can lead to the loss of sensation of the anterior two-thirds of the ipsilateral tongue.

Hypoglossal nerve injury may happen in chronically inflamed glands with an adherent nerve to the medial aspect of the gland or accidentally during bleeding control from the adjacent lingual veins. Injury causes ipsilateral tongue paralysis. If the hypoglossal nerve is accidentally divided, it should be repaired.

Other potential complications include intraoperative hemorrhage from the facial artery, postoperative wound hematoma with secondary airway obstruction, infection and abscess development, retained stones, xerostomia,

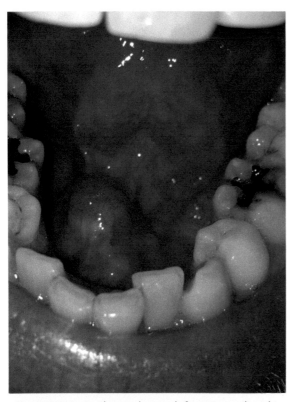

Fig. 10.5 Patient with secondary ranula formation on the right side requiring excision of the sublingual gland.

ranula secondary to sublingual duct injury (▶Fig. 10.5), and chronic inflammation.

The transoral approach eliminates the risk of a neck hypertrophic scar or keloid, decreases the risk of injury to the marginal mandibular nerve, and allows for a full removal of the duct with a decreased risk of retained calculi. Pitfalls of the transoral approach include transient symptoms ranging from pain and numbness to a decrease in tongue mobility and floor of mouth edema.[9]

Postoperative hemorrhage can also lead to significant airway obstruction as a result of swelling of the floor of the mouth and tongue musculature.

10.4 Postoperative Management

Patients are observed overnight to monitor for bleeding or postoperative airway obstruction secondary to swelling. Post transcervical submandibular excision, a Penrose or a suction drain is left in place for 24 to 48 hours.

10.4.1 Pearls to Avoid Intraoperative Complications

- All retraction at the inferior border of the mandible should be done gently to prevent trauma to the marginal mandibular nerve (MMN). The latter is protected by direct identification and subcapsular dissection below the investing layer of deep cervical fascia covering the submandibular gland. Another strategy is to use the Hayes–Martin maneuver involving ligation of the anterior facial vein and superior reflection of the investing fascia below the mandible to preserve the marginal mandibular nerve.
- Facial nerve monitoring with a nerve integrity monitor (NIM) and a use of a nerve stimulator can sometimes be helpful in patients with an inflamed gland.
- Bimanual palpation of Wharton's duct along its course and use of sialoendoscopy when in doubt ensures that all stones have been removed.
- After the gland is freed posteriorly, the hypoglossal nerve should be identified as it courses deep to the vessels, parallel to the submandibular duct. It can also be identified inferior to the posterior belly of the digastric muscle and followed in a posterior-to-anterior direction through the submandibular triangle. Often, it will be identified within the fascia medial to the mylohyoid muscle.
- Once the mylohyoid muscle is retracted anteriorly and the lingual nerve/submandibular ganglion is visualized, the submandibular ganglion and abutting vein are ligated. Wharton's duct is located inferior to the nerve as it exits the anterior aspect of the gland. The duct is ligated as far distally as possible after having well-visualized and protected he lingual nerve and the hypoglossal nerve.
- After the gland is removed, the surgical field is re-evaluated for adequate hemostasis prior to closure. The proximal stump of the facial artery should be double-ligated.

10.5 Highlights

a. Indications
   - Refractory recurrent sialadenitis.
   - Sialolithiasis not amenable to sialoendoscopy or lithotripsy.
   - Salivary gland suspicious lesions or neoplasms.
   - Debilitating sialorrhea.
b. Contraindications
   - Absent submandibular gland (document presence of gland before resection for sialorrhea as gland occasionally absent).
   - Severe bleeding disorder.
   - When available, sialoendoscopy should be performed instead of gland resection in isolated accessible ductal sialolithiasis unless chronic sialadenitis requiring gland removal.
c. Complications
   - Scar at the incision site, hypertrophic scar, keloid.
   - Injury to the marginal mandibular branch of the facial nerve.

- Injury to the lingual nerve (loss of sensation of the anterior two thirds of the ipsilateral tongue).
- Hypoglossal nerve injury.
- Intraoperative hemorrhage.
- Postoperative wound hematoma with secondary airway obstruction.
- Infection and abscess development.
- Retained stones.
- Xerostomia.
- Ranula secondary to sublingual duct injury.
- Chronic inflammation.

d. Special preoperative considerations
- General oral endotracheal intubation if transcervical approach.
- Nasal intubation if intra-oral approach; and all patients should be consented for a possible transcervical approach.
- Antibiotics.
- Paralytic agents are avoided to allow for intraoperative marginal mandibular nerve monitoring.
- Facial nerve monitoring with a nerve integrity monitor (NIM) and a use of a nerve stimulator can sometimes be helpful in patients with an inflamed gland.
- If available, consider sialoendoscopy rather than gland resection in the presence of isolated accessible ductal stones.
- Assess the need for elective neck dissection, in cases of submandibular gland malignancy.
- Preoperative imaging very helpful for planning purposes: Ultrasound can detect up to 90% of stones greater than 2 mm. CT and/ or MRI are important to assess parapharyngeal extension, deep cervical lymphadenopathies, and skull base extension. CT is useful to detect bony erosion in cases of tumors.

e. Special intraoperative considerations
- Most commonly performed via a transcervical approach. Intraoral and endoscopic approaches gaining popularity.
- In case of a small or retracted submandibular gland, depressing the floor of the mouth with a gloved finger can facilitate its identification.
- Clear identification of the digastric and mylohyoid muscles.

- Remaining mindful of the course of the marginal mandibular, the hypoglossal, the lingual nerves.
- Strategies to avoid injuring the marginal mandibular nerve (MMN) include making the incision 2 fingerbreadths inferior and parallel to the body of the mandible, or slightly above the level of the hyoid bone.
- Another strategy is to ligate the facial vein and retract it cephalad so that the MMN is included in the superior flap and protected.
- Be mindful of the facial artery location and free it and/or its branches from the gland.
- If the patient has a stone in the duct, ensure that the duct is ligated distal to the stone and that the stone is removed.

f. Special postoperative considerations
- An overnight hospitalization.
- Hemovac suction or penrose drain is inserted after transcervical approach.

References

[1] Mizrachi A, Bachar G, Unger Y, Hilly O, Fliss DM, Shpitzer T. Submandibular salivary gland tumors: Clinical course and outcome of a 20-year multicenter study. Ear Nose Throat J 2017;96(3):E17–E20

[2] Sam J. Daniel AK. Salivary Gland Disease in Children. In: Marci Lesperance PF, ed. Cummings Pediatric Otolaryngology: Elsevier; 2015:293–308

[3] Daniel SJ. Pediatric sialorrhea: Medical and Surgical Options. In: Hartnick CJ, ed. Sataloff's Comprehensive Textbook of Otolaryngology Head & Neck Surgery. 6: Jaypee; 2016:807–14

[4] Stern Y, Feinmesser R, Collins M, Shott SR, Cotton RT. Bilateral submandibular gland excision with parotid duct ligation for treatment of sialorrhea in children: long-term results. Arch Otolaryngol Head Neck Surg 2002;128(7):801–803

[5] Jäger L, Menauer F, Holzknecht N, Scholz V, Grevers G, Reiser M. Sialolithiasis: MR sialography of the submandibular duct—an alternative to conventional sialography and US? Radiology 2000;216(3):665–671

[6] Gritzmann N. Sonography of the salivary glands. AJR Am J Roentgenol 1989;153(1):161–166

[7] Lee JC, Kao CH, Chang YN, Hsu CH, Lin YS. Intraoral excision of the submandibular gland: how we do it. Clin Otolaryngol 2010;35(5):434–438

[8] Terris DJ, Haus BM, Gourin CG. Endoscopic neck surgery: resection of the submandibular gland in a cadaver model. Laryngoscope 2004;114(3):407–410

[9] Hong KH, Kim YK. Intraoral removal of the submandibular gland: a new surgical approach. Otolaryngol Head Neck Surg 2000;122(6):798–802

11 Pediatric Endoscopic Salivary Gland Surgery

Oded Nahlieli

Summary

In this chapter pediatric salivary gland inflammatory pathology and minimal invasive approach for the treatment of pediatric cases have been discussed in details.

We will review the anatomy, clinical and imaging evaluation, endoscopic and minimal invasive surgery for treatment of children suffering from these pathologies. This chapter includes surgical approaches to pediatric sialolithiasis, juvenile recurrent parotitis, the author's approach to various cases, and rare pathologies that affect children.

Keywords: Pediatric salivary gland pathology, sialolithiasis, obstructive sialadenitis, juvenile recurrent parotitis, sialoendoscopy

11.1 Introduction

Inflammatory salivary gland disease represents more than one-third of the salivary gland pathology in childhood.[1,2] Since salivary gland disorders are infrequently encountered in children, there are relatively few papers in the literature dealing with these problems. In this chapter, we discuss salivary gland inflammatory conditions and salivary gland stones in childhood, their diagnostic methods, and treatment.

11.2 General Anatomical Considerations

By the end of intrauterine life, the salivary glands are well developed and ready to produce saliva at the time of the first breastfeeding.[3] While the anatomy of the salivary glands themselves is similar in children and adults, their topography and shape have some pediatric peculiarities (▶Fig. 11.1a).

In an embryo, the *parotid glands* appear first and are the largest salivary glands weighing from 2 to 3 g in neonates to almost 30 g in adolescents.[3] Each parotid gland is located behind the *mandibular ramus* and in front of the *mastoid process* of the *temporal bone*. The parotid duct and Stensen's duct, is formed from several large interlobular ducts inside the gland. Its orifice can be observed at the parotid papilla, which lies in the *vestibule of the mouth* between the *cheek* and the *gums*. The second superior molar tooth serves as the landmark in older children and adolescents. Moving from the orifice to the gland, the duct passes through the buccinator muscle, takes a steep turn at the border of the masseter muscle, and runs backward along the lateral side of the masseter muscle. In this course, the Stensen's duct is surrounded by the buccal fat pad.[4]

This buccal fat is to be taken into account in pediatric cases. This deep anatomic compartment is situated posterior and lateral to the zygomaticus major muscle that exists as multiple lobes or lobules.[5] It is responsible for the fullness of the cheeks in infants and young children and aids in cushioning and sucking function. The pad is prominent in neonates and infants and is often referred to as the "sucking pad." It represents a special type of tissue that is distinct from subcutaneous fat and serves to line the masticatory space, separating the muscles of mastication from each other, from the zygomatic arch, and from the ramus of the mandible.[6] The mean diameter of the Stensen's duct at four different segments along its length ranges between 0.4 and 0.8 mm in young children and between 0.5 and 1.2 mm in adolescents. There is a narrowing at the middle segment of the duct and the minimum width of the secretory duct is at the ostium.

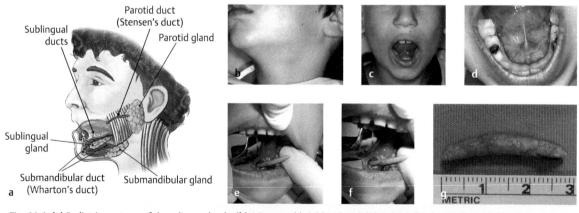

Fig. 11.1 (a) Pediatric anatomy of the salivary glands. **(b)** A 7-year-old child with sialolith in his left submandibular Wharton's duct, note the swelling at the inferior edge of the submandibular region. **(c)** Intraoral view of the same child, note the small sialolith in the anterior part of the Wharton's duct. **(d)** A 5-year-old child with small sialolith in the anterior part of the Wharton's duct. **(e–g)** Removal of 3-cm giant submandibular stone from a 4-year-old child.

Therefore, the diameter of 1 to 1.2 mm should be considered the upper limit for duct endoscopes in case of the Stensen's duct. A discrete lobe of fat within the buccal space, the inferior lobe of the buccal fat, predicts the location of the parotid duct in infants and young children when the second molar cannot be used for this purpose.[7]

The Stensen's duct is located above the inferior lobe of the buccal fat. The facial nerve lies immediately on top of most of these deep fat pads, with the exception of buccal fat. The nerve may actually penetrate buccal fat, as does the duct. However, with proper knowledge of the anatomy of the buccal fat, it can be manipulated with safety. The inferior lobe of the fat is a safe region to manipulate, because the parotid duct travels above this lobe, between the inferior and the middle lobe. Distinguishing the position of this fat pad tells the observer that the Stensen's duct must be located superior to this location. This is another way to identify the position of the parotid duct in addition to using its course toward the second molar. In children, the drainage of saliva from the parotid glands is lateral from the paired ducts.

The *submandibular gland* is located in the anterior cervical region in the submandibular triangle, and its duct, the Wharton's duct, leaves the body of the gland between the mylohyoid, hyoglossus, and genioglossus muscles. The duct opens by a narrow orifice on the summit of a small *papilla* at the side of the *frenulum of the tongue*. The tongue of a child is large relatively to the body proportions. When the tongue is elevated, these orifices are quite visible from both sides of the midline of the underside of it. From the orifice, the Wharton's duct runs into the gland via a gap between the muscles. The main part of the Wharton's duct is surrounded by gland tissue from the submandibular and partly from the sublingual gland. From the orifice, the duct may run deep into the gland either almost horizontally backward, or in a slightly curved semicircle, or obliquely downward and backward. As a rule, it curves around the mylohyoid muscle. That is why as it proceeds from its entrance in the oral cavity deeper, it curves, and in children the size of the angle of this curve varies between 20 and 170 degrees.

In children, the Wharton's duct is 1 to 4 cm long, according to the age. Its diameter ranges between 0.4 and 1.2 mm in various segments.[8] The narrowest duct diameter is identified at the ostium. The practicality of these facts for the endoscopic intervention is obvious. For diagnostic and therapeutic purposes, sialoendoscopes with stone-extraction baskets or forceps and balloon catheters should conform as much as possible to physiological duct widths. While modern sialoendoscopes may be less than 1 mm in diameter, the diameter of 1.2 mm should be considered the upper limit for duct instruments in pediatric cases. The best results for children 10-year-old and older can be achieved when the maximum size of a stone or a stone fragment does not exceed 1.2 mm.

The pathology of the sublingual glands is extremely rare in children. Usually the sublingual duct, the Bartholin's duct, joins the submandibular duct to drain through the sublingual caruncle that is a small papilla near the midline of the floor of the mouth on each side of the lingual frenum. But a variation exists when the Bartholin's duct opens independently near to the orifice of the Wharton's duct. Congenital anatomic variations of the ductal system of the sublingual glands might be a possible cause of ranulas in patients with simple or plunging ranulas, especially in pediatric patients.[9]

11.3 Preoperative Evaluation and Anesthesia

11.3.1 Clinical Evaluation

Accurate history and physical examination are paramount for the clinical presurgical evaluation. Children usually complain of pain and swelling occurring minutes to several hours after meals. The swelling often slowly recedes with time and often the parents and child relate that massage of the gland and/or application of a cold pad relieves the symptoms. The child may have a history of multiple episodes, treated with and responding to antibiotic therapy.

Visualization of submandibular, preauricular, and postauricular regions is the first step in assessing swelling and erythema (▶ Fig. 11.1a).

The next step is the intraoral examination. Oral examination notes the degree of trismus, if any, the state of salivary papillae (Stensen's and Wharton's ducts), the lingual papillary color, the degree of mucosal dehydration, evidence of posterior pharyngeal secretions, tonsillar size and color, and presence of exudates on the tonsils. The tongue depressor can be moved around the upper and lower alveoli, permitting comfortable and complete evaluation of the mucosa, the salivary ducts, gingiva, and dentition. Surgical magnification loops (×2.5–3.5) are very useful to improve visualization of the orifice of Wharton's and Stensen's ducts. The orifice may be red and edematous and may appear as a papilla. Plaques or whitish secretions from the duct may represent an acute infection. Sometimes a small calculus can be found in the orifice; occasionally, the white–yellow color of a stone can be seen through the translucent mucosa (▶ Fig. 11.1b–e).

Bimanual palpation is particularly important when examining the submandibular gland and duct. It helps to differentiate the gland from adjacent lymph nodes, inferior to the gland, and to ascertain the presence of any firm mass in the take-off of the Wharton's duct from the hilum of the gland. For the parotid gland, manual palpation allows the surgeon to determine the consistency of the gland. One should also massage the gland to milk and inspect the saliva. The fingers of the directing hand may be used to milk secretions from both the parotid and the submandibular glands.

11.4 Salivary Imaging

There are a variety of available imaging methods to detect calculi and inflammatory diseases of the salivary glands. In this section we focus on those techniques that are most suitable for children. In general, ultrasonography may be the initial imaging study used for the examination of pediatric salivary gland lesions. Most of them are benign and are well detected with this modality. Ultrasonography may differentiate intraglandular and extraglandular lesions, but additional studies such as color Doppler, computed tomography (CT) scans, cone-beam computed tomography (CBCT), CBCT sialography (if possible), or MRI may be needed as well.[10-13] The best way to assess a lesion is the sialoendoscopic observation.

11.4.1 Submandibular Gland

In the case of infants, parents are often able to assist the child to allow completion of the image taking (▶Fig. 11.2a–d).

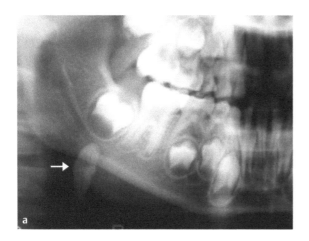
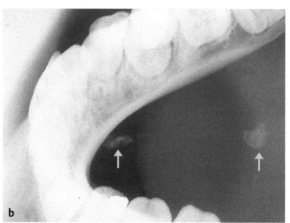
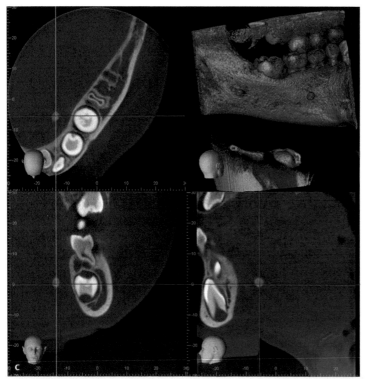
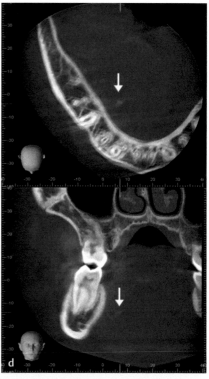

Fig. 11.2 (a) Panorex X-ray reveals (*arrow*) large calculi in a 10-year-old child. **(b)** Occlusal X-ray of a 10-year-old boy demonstrating 2 sialoliths (*yellow arrows*) in the anterior and middle third of the Wharton's duct. **(c)** CBCT scan demonstrating calculus in the anterior part of the right Wharton's duct. **(d)** CBCT demonstrating small sialolith (2 mm) in the middle part of the right submandibular duct of a 11-year-old child (*arrows*). CBCT, cone-beam computed tomography.

Sialography

Sialography in children is often impossible and is reserved, if necessary, for selected cooperative patients. In the past, when there were no alternatives, this technique was accomplished in the operating room. The discomfort during sialography may be reduced by applying topical anesthesia to Wharton's duct papilla and/or by lavaging the gland through the orifice with 2% lidocaine prior to the injection of the water-soluble dye. Sialography provides images of the morphology of the ductal system, and allows the diagnosis of strictures, dilatations, and filling defects. This technique also provides information on glandular function.[14,15]

Ultrasound

High-resolution ultrasound (above 10 MHz) is a good imaging method to assess the submandibular glands in children. It is noninvasive and there is no associated discomfort. It is useful to distinguish the submandibular gland from surrounding lymph nodes and to locate calculi. The portion of the Wharton's duct that leads from the hilum of the gland toward the floor of the mouth, precisely after the penetration of the mylohyoid muscle, is difficult to identify.[16,17]

Computed Tomography

CT scan is especially useful for evaluating inflammatory conditions of the submandibular gland. Sialoliths are readily identified on CT imaging (▶Fig. 11.2c). The

standard images should be 1-mm cuts with three-dimensional (3D) reconstruction. In this way the glands and ducts can be visualized in all planes and stones are less likely to be missed.[18]

11.4.2 Parotid Gland

Most inflammatory conditions of the parotid glands are not a consequence of sialolithiasis. Therefore, the imaging techniques are directed toward documenting changes in the Stensen's duct morphology and size and changes in the substance of the gland. The most effective imaging methods for the inflammatory parotid conditions in childhood are sialography, ultrasound, and sialoendoscopy.

Sialography

This is an excellent imaging technique to demonstrate changes in the parenchyma (sialectasis), small strictures, and dilatations in the main and secondary ducts. As noted for the submandibular gland, discomfort during the dye injection is a limiting factor. Topical anesthesia and Lidocaine 2% lavage may be used but in young children, the procedure requires general anesthesia (▶Fig. 11.3).

Ultrasound

Ultrasound is useful to demonstrate parenchymal changes such as sialectasis and morphologic alterations of the parotid duct. The same advantages for ultrasound noted in the submandibular gland apply for the parotid (▶Fig. 11.4).[19,20]

The parotid gland and duct can also be imaged by CT.

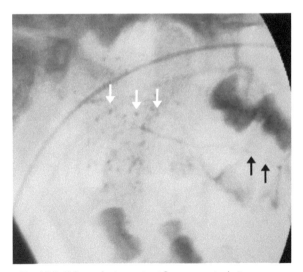

Fig. 11.3 Sialography in constant fluoroscopy technique under general anesthesia demonstrating right parotid gland of a 7-year-old child with JRP-note presentation of stricture in the middle of the Stensen's duct (*black arrows*) and multiple sialectasis (*white arrows*). JRP, juvenile recurrent parotitis.

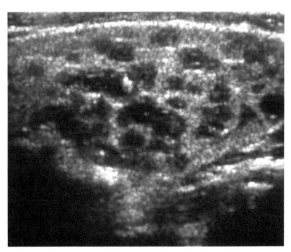

Fig. 11.4 Ultrasound of parotid gland affected with JRP. Note the demonstration of multiple sialectasis. JRP, juvenile recurrent parotitis.

11.4.3 Magnetic Resonance Sialography

An MRI examination is usually performed upfront to exclude tumor and mass effect, but it may also be used to look for other complications. MRI offers benefits of increased soft tissue resolution, which is important in evaluating the soft salivary gland tissues. Although MRI has the advantage of providing improved resolution of salivary tissue structures, it has the disadvantage of higher cost and longer image acquisition times requiring general anesthesia in the pediatric population. The lack of radiation is a major advantage of MRI in pediatric cases.[15,21]

Specifically for the parotid gland, a mass associated with facial nerve symptoms should be evaluated with MRI because it is the only modality that can consistently demonstrate the facial nerve. Findings at MRI allow localization of parotid lesions and may suggest a specific cause.[22] The evaluation of the function of the parotid glands may be also achieved by using an intrinsic susceptibility-weighted MRI method (blood oxygenation level dependent, BOLD-MRI) at 1.5 and 3 T.[23] This modality can detect changes in the parotid glands during gustatory stimulation, consistent with an increase in oxygen consumption during saliva production. The magnetic resonance sialography was reported to be convenient for evaluating parotid gland damage in young patients with Sjögren's syndrome.[14] It can evaluate Stage II approximately III parotid gland damage in juvenile Sjögren's syndrome. However, magnetic resonance sialography may have difficulties in detecting subtle changes in the duct.

11.5 The Thallium Scan for All Salivary Glands

While not widely used, this investigation may be helpful in pediatric cases. Intravenously injected thallium, which is concentrated in the functioning salivary gland tissues, is excreted into the mouth with saliva. This can be used to quantify oral secretions aspirated over time. Images of labeled secretions are obtained with a gamma camera. In normal studies, the label is found in the salivary glands and stomach, with low levels in the oral cavity, pharynx, and esophagus. In children who aspirate oral secretions, label is also seen throughout the lung fields.[24–26]

11.6 Laboratory Data

Laboratory studies are helpful in the diagnosis of viral and bacterial infections as well as noninfectious inflammatory disorders. Complete blood count with differential white blood cell count is helpful in distinguishing viral from bacterial infection. In the former lymphocytosis is often found whereas in the latter leukocytosis. Serum amylase and serum antibody titers are helpful in cases with the acute phase of parotitis. Secretions or drainage from the salivary ducts should be Gram stained and sent for anaerobic and aerobic culture and sensitivity test.

This is especially helpful during the acute stages of sialadenitis. The common aerobic organisms are *Streptococci* and *Staphylococci* in immunocompromised systemically ill children. Common anaerobes include: anaerobic gram-negative bacilli (e.g., pigmented *Prevotella* and *Porphyromonas*); *Fusobacterium* spp.; and *Peptostreptococcus* spp. In addition, *Streptococcus* spp. (including *Streptococcus pneumoniae*) and aerobic and facultative Gram-negative bacilli (including *Escherichia coli*) have been reported. Aerobic and facultative Gram-negative bacilli are often seen in hospitalized patients. Organisms less frequently found are *Haemophilus influenzae, Treponema pallidum, Bartonella henselae*, and *Eikenella corrodens*.[27–29] The parotid gland is the salivary gland most commonly affected by inflammation.

11.7 Sialoendoscopy

The rapid developments in technology in the twenty-first century directed maxillofacial surgeons to develop new methods of treatment by means of noninvasive, minimally invasive, and less invasive interventions. The salivary gland endoscopic and endoscopic assistance techniques, the ductal stretching, and some other intraoral procedures can be applied in pediatric cases as well.

Endoscopes designed for the salivary gland ducts, sialoendoscopes, are produced by various manufacturers (PloyDiagnost GmbH, Germany; Karl Storz, Germany).[30–32] These sialoendoscopes are divided into diagnostic and therapeutic devices. Not all of them are suitable for pediatric practice, but endoscopes with the exterior diameter of 0.65 to 0.9 mm are suitable for observation and irrigation. Semi-rigid optic specifications vary from 3000 to 30,000 pixels.

We believe that good sialoendoscope should contain a telescope with at least 6000-pixel illumination fibers and focal length of 2 to 15 mm and 70 degree field of view. However the best results can be obtained with the 10,000 pixel optic with 120° field of view. Such microendoscopes can change the view field from 0 to 70 degree and further to 120 degree. The diameter of the telescope is usually 0.5 to 0.9 mm. The endoscopes can be either designed with the fixed exterior diameter or have disposable sleeves of various diameters (PloyDiagnost GmbH, Germany) (▶Fig. 11.5a, b).

Endoscopes with the exterior diameter of 0.9 to 1.2 mm can be used for older children and adolescents. The useful

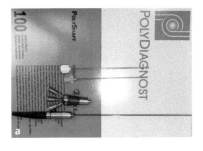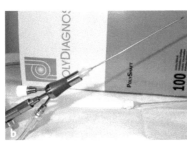

Fig. 11.5 (a) Modular Sialoendoscope (Telescope 0.9 mm 10,000 pixels with handle and disposable 1.1 cannula) (Polydiagnost Ltd Germany). **(b)** Modular Sialoendoscope prepared for surgery.

tools are grasping forceps, basket, grasper, and balloon-like Fogarty or Sialoballoon catheter (AD-TECH-MED Ltd Lublin, Poland), biopsy forceps intracorporeal electrohydraulic lithotripter probes, and Er-YAG and Holmium-YAG laser probes. It is best to work under direct vision, but occasionally in children, it is necessary to work in a semiblind manner because of size constraints of the duct. In this case, the obstruction is identified with the endoscope and then the telescope is removed to make room for the working instrument.[8,33,34]

11.8 Pediatric Anesthesia

In children, the endoscopic salivary gland procedure is done under general anesthesia. It should be remembered that infants have poor respiratory reserves, and respiratory failure is a common sequel to pathology in any other system. Elective surgery should not take place when the patient has an acute intercurrent illness. The sialoendoscopy should be deferred about a month after the last symptoms of respiratory tract infection, croup, or the acute exanthems have subsided, as related adverse events can occur for up to several weeks. Specialized apparatus with low resistance to breathing (less than 30 cmH$_2$O/L per second during quiet breathing) and minimal dead space is necessary for infants. Older children and adolescents are significantly less fragile in this matter.

11.9 Differential Diagnostics with Rare Nonsurgical Conditions

Although rare, the following specific conditions may cause salivary gland infection and swelling or mimic infection in children: *pneomoparotid, atypical mycobacteria, tuberculosis, actinomycosis,* and *acquired immunodeficiency syndrome* (AIDS). Such disorders do not require surgical intervention but endoscopic observation and the above-mentioned sialoendoscopy may be used for differential diagnostic purposes in complicated cases.

Pneumoparotid is a rare condition of the parotid gland in which it is inflated with air as a result of positive air pressure inside the mouth (up to 150 mm Hg). Physical examination reveals parotid enlargement, usually unilateral but also bilateral. Palpation of the affected gland produces crepitus.[35,36] The best imaging technique is CT scan, which will show air in the parotid gland, Stensen's duct, and occasionally in the surrounding tissue.[37] In childhood most of the cases are self-induced but a few are accidental, e.g., blowing up a balloon, aggressive blowing of the nose, inflating a bicycle tire inner tube without a pump, or inveterate gum chewing.

Atypical mycobacteria infections have been identified as an important cause of infection in the head and neck in children.[38] The parotid and submandibular gland can be affected as can the neighboring lymph nodes. The clinical appearance is swelling of the affected gland and sometimes-spontaneous drainage. Diagnosis relies upon culture, histology, chest radiography, and purified protein derivative (PPD).

Tuberculosis of the salivary gland in children can develop primarily or secondary to pulmonary tuberculosis.[39,40] The parotid gland is affected more than the submandibular gland and the clinical picture is a firm swelling sometimes with draining fistula. Diagnostic tests of suspected cases include chest X-ray, (PPD) skin test, and acid fast staining from drainage material and from tissue. It should be remembered that calcification of lymph nodes and sometimes salivary tissue can be identified in tuberculosis and can mimic sialoliths.

Actinomycotic infections can affect the salivary glands, with 10% of actinomycosis orofacial cases being in the salivary glands.[39] The infection can be acute or chronic and in most of the cases the only method to distinguish this specific infection from other forms of sialadenitis is culture.

Speaking of AIDS, children infected with human immunodeficiency virus (HIV) develop salivary gland enlargement in 18% of cases.[41,42] Parotid gland enlargement is typically an early manifestation in the HIV-positive patient and should alert healthcare professionals to the likelihood of HIV infection.[41] Fine needle aspiration cytology investigation (FNAC) of the parotid gland is required to confirm the diagnosis. The surgical operation may be required in cases when the parotid enlargement results from benign lymphoepithelial cysts.[43] The prognosis of children with salivary gland enlargement is poor only 5.4 years.

11.10 Surgical Technique

There are three possible techniques for introducing the endoscope into the ductal lumen:

1. Introduction into the natural orifice after dilatation with a lacrimal duct probe.
2. Ductal cutdown involves surgical dissection and exposure of the anterior portion of the duct using loop magnification. The duct is then incised longitudinally to allow the intraluminal insertion of the endoscope. If there are any difficulties in introducing the endoscope in the anterior part (e.g., stricture, too narrow ductal lumen), it may be necessary to expose the duct more posteriorly to arrive at a location where the diameter will accommodate the endoscope.
3. Usage of the sialolithotomy opening. The endoscope can be inserted through the same opening in the salivary duct where the stone was extracted.

11.10.1 Irrigation

Irrigation is crucial in every endoscopy procedure. The cavity must be filled with fluid to allow free movement of the instrument and the area needs to be lavaged to permit good visualization. Isotonic saline is the fluid of choice. An intravenous bag containing isotonic saline is connected to the irrigation port and the endoscope is moved forward accompanied by a gentle flow of saline. In adults, 2% lidocaine is also injected through this port, resulting in the anesthesia of the entire ductal system and it might be possible in some adolescent cases. But generally in pediatric cases the general anesthesia is the choice.

11.10.2 Sialoendoscopic Sialolithotomy

The following methods are available for removal of stones:
- Intraductal approach.
- Extraductal approach (endoscopic-assisted surgery).

Intraductal Approach

The intraductal approach is a pure endoscopic technique. The extraductal approach involves endoscopically assisted techniques.[34,44–46]

When a sialolith is encountered, its diameter is estimated and the method of choice for its removal is selected from two *intraductal sialolithotomy* possibilities:

1. Removal of a stone in one piece with the help of grasping forceps, wire baskets, or hydrostatic pressure posterior to the stone.
2. Combined use of an extracorporeal shock wave lithotripter (ESWL) and endoscopic removal.

The primary goal is to remove the calculus in one piece.

The following approaches are available in cases when the extraductal technique is chosen.[33,44,47,48,49]
- Intraoral techniques: These techniques can be used for the submandibular, sublingual, and parotid stones (▶ Fig. 11.6a–f).
- Extraoral technique: This technique is exclusively used for impacted parotid stones.

Extraductal Approach (Endoscopic-Assisted Surgery)

Transoral/intraoral surgical approaches with or without endoscopic assistance are mainly used for removal of the salivary stones located in the ducts, including giant sialoliths.

This technique can be applied for removal of hiloparenchymal submandibular calculi as well. Since endoscopy became a commonly used minimally invasive technique, surgeons realized that endoscopic surgery is unable to overcome large posterior sialoliths that are connected to the ductal walls or located in the posterior part of the salivary ducts. Nahlieli published his ductal stretching technique (endoscopic-assisted surgery) in 2007, dissecting the Wharton's duct for safe and easy exploration and removal of hilar submandibular stones.

The leading arguments for endoscopy-assisted intraoral surgery are the size and the position of the calculus and/or the presence of a stricture associated with the calculus. Another important factor is the presence of multiple calculi and the diameter of the duct. Thus, the performing surgeons should choose their approach not because of advantages and disadvantages of the preferred technique but because of the dimensions and localization of the sialoliths. The dissection technique can be performed without endoscopy. The pinpoint technique also can be performed without endoscopy in cases when a large, well-palpable sialolith is located in the main duct itself.

The surgeons, however, appreciate the endoscopy during surgery for the exact location of the stone and

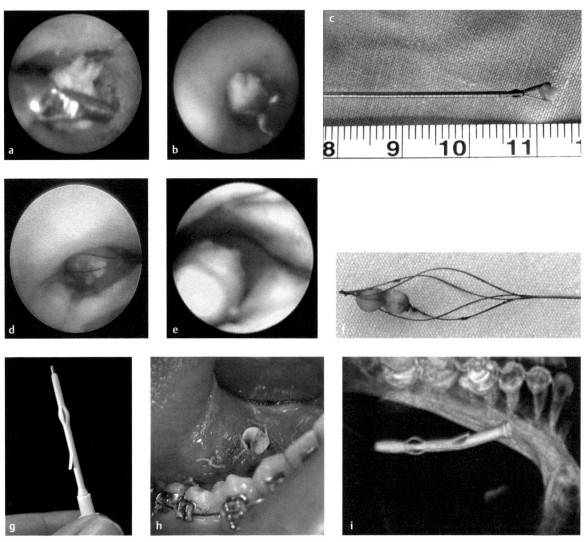

Fig. 11.6 **(a, b)** Mini forceps grasper removal of stone from the submandibular hilum. **(c)** The sialolith on the prong of the mini forceps grasper after its removal. **(d, e)** Basket retrieval of sialolith from the Stensen's duct. **(f)** Two sialoliths after removal with 4 wires basket. **(g)** The polymeric Sialostent (Sialodrain). **(h)** The polymeric Sialostent (sialodrain) is inside the Wharton's duct. **(i)** Cone-beam computed tomography (CBCT) of Sialodrain (Sialostent). Note the flaps and basket holding the stent. CBCT, cone-beam computed tomography.

following the removal of the stone for direct visualization and assessment of pathologic changes in the salivary duct system (strictures) and the detection of additional stones.

Following every endoscopic surgical intervention sialostent (sialodrain) is essential to prevent obstruction of the affected gland (AD-TECH-MED Ltd Lublin, Poland) (▶ Fig. 11.6g–i).

Extraoral Approach to Parotid Stones

This approach is exclusively reserved for removal of parotid stones in the middle posterior and hilar part of the parotid duct, which cannot be removed via intraductal approach, and also for removal of intraparenchymal stones. Identification of the stones can be performed either by sialoendoscopic technique or by ultrasound technique. The endoscopic approach is indicated when there is a possibility to introduce the endoscope into the duct.

Sialoendoscopic technique: The stone is located with the help of an insertion of the sialoendoscope into the Stensen's duct, identification of the stone on the endoscope monitor, and with the aid of the transillumination effect on the outer skin. The surgeon marks the exact location on the skin. The same technique is used during the surgery for final location of the stone.

Ultrasound technique: When insertion of the endoscope is impossible or in cases with intraparenchymal stones the only diagnostic method is to use high-resolution ultrasound and to locate the stone with the aid of biopsy marker.

There are two options to explore and to remove the stone: via face lift approach and by direct incision. The author prefers the first option due to the better esthetic results. The second option can be used in older patients when there are prominent skin creases (▶Fig. 11.7a–g).

Extracorporeal Shock-Wave Lithotripsy

In general, the ESWL is a reliable, effective, and safe technique.[50] Three sessions of 1000 low-energy extracorporeal shock wave (0.09 mJ/mm^2) treatment per patient were administered with 1-month interval between each session. No sedation is needed (▶Fig. 11.8). No specific

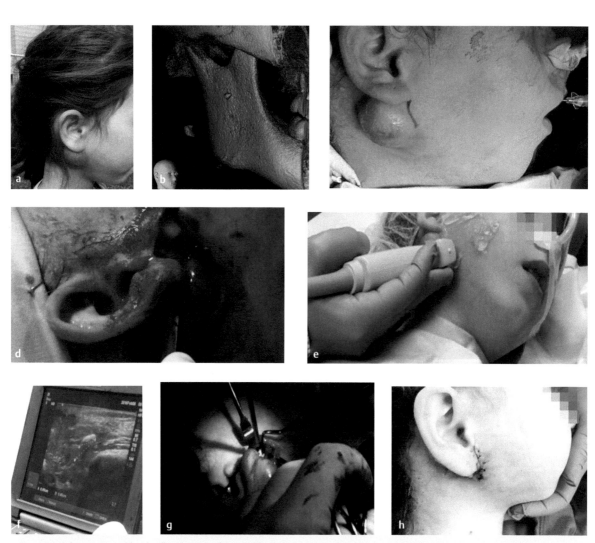

Fig. 11.7 (a) An 8-year-old girl suffered 2 years from swelling of her right parotid gland. Note the sialocele presented in the parotid tail. **(b)** 3D cone-beam CT of the same girl demonstrated 2 stones in the parotid duct and the posterior part of the parotid gland. **(c)** The sialoendoscope inside the parotid duct for the removal of the first ductal stone. **(d)** The transilluminator effect helps to locate and to remove the first stone. **(e, f)** Locating the second stone intraoperative with US. **(g)** Removal of the stone via rhytidectomy approach. **(h)** The patient 1 week after surgery.

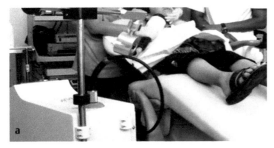 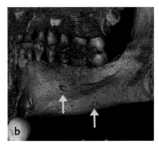 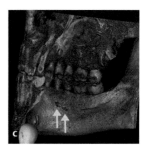

Fig. 11.8 **(a)** Extracorporeal Shock Wave Lithotripsy (low energy) for right submandibular hilar stone (7-year-old child). **(b)** 3D cone-beam computed tomography (CBCT) demonstrating 2 stones in the submandibular duct first in the anterior part of the duct and the second in the posterior part (*yellow arrows*). **(c)** 3D CBCT following 3 sessions of ESWL demonstrating the deep stone migrates near the anterior stone (*yellow arrows*).

ESWL-related side effects were detected. Disconnecting the outer cortex of the stone during/after lithotripsy and the positive effect on scar tissue provides a possibility for saliva leakage to the oral cavity bypassing the affected stone.

11.11 Combination of ESWL and Sialoendoscopic Approach

The ESWL + the intraductal or extraductal endoscopic treatment of sialolithiasis is a highly effective surgical method of eliminating/removal of salivary stones, especially of deeply located stones and in advanced sialolithiasis cases. It has broader applications in comparison with pure ESWL but careful selection of patients is important for this technique to achieve sound results.

The selection of patients with the submandibular gland calculi is as follows:
- A small (<5 mm) stone in secondary ducts or intraparenchymal stone.
- A small (<5 mm) fixed stone in the main duct or in the hilus region.
- A medium-to-large (>5 mm) hilar or intraglandular stone attached to the surrounding tissue—immobile or difficult to palpate.

For the parotid duct and gland calculi, every stone located in the middle third part of the duct and posteriorly is considered as an advanced and complicated case. The combination of ESWL and sialoendoscopic approach is specifically indicated for such cases.

The treatment starts with an application of the ESWL (see above). Following the results of ESWL being assessed by CBCT, CT, and ultrasonography variations for further management of a patient are possible.

Thus, three types of treatment can be performed following the ESWL:
1. The ESWL as a solo treatment.
2. The ESWL + intraductal endoscopic approach (the pure endoscopy).
3. The ESWL + endoscopic-assisted extraductal approach.

The third method is a stretching procedure for the submandibular stones or extraoral approach for the parotid stones.[50] The second and the third methods can be used in cases when a salivary stone was not eliminated by the lithotripsy alone.

The endoscopic removal of the stones after the ESWL procedures is easier and less complicated due to disconnection of the stone from the surrounding ductal tissue that seems to be the major positive effect of the ESWL. We believe that this combined lithotripsy-endoscopy approach might help to overcome the various sizes and locations of the stones and most of the obstruction pathologies as it involves multiple techniques and technologies: the pure endoscopy, the endoscopic-assistance technique, and the ESWL, which could be combined in a treatment of the same patient. The implementations of these three methods mainly rely not on the advantages of each method but rather on careful diagnostic evaluation of the size, location, and number of sialoliths. The ESWL + the intraductal or extraductal endoscopic treatment might lead to effective management of most of the obstruction and inflammatory conditions of the salivary glands.

11.12 The Author's Approaches to Various Cases

In this section I will describe my way to treat sialolithiasis of the major salivary glands.

Approach 1: If the stones are located in the anterior third part of the Wharton's or Stensen's duct, the surgery will include:
- Incision.
- Extraction of a calculus.
- Endoscopic exploration.
- Sialostent insertion.

Approach 2: If the stones are located in the middle third part of the Wharton's duct, the surgery will include:
- Ductal dissection and exploration.
- Stone removal.

- Endoscopic exploration.
- Sialostent insertion.

Approach 3: If mobile stone/stones are found in the hilum of the Wharton's duct, the approach depends on the stone diameter. The surgical procedure includes:

- Endoscopic removal of the calculus.
- Extraductal removal of the calculus via stretching procedure.
- Endoscopic exploration.
- Sialostent insertion.

All advanced sialolithiasis cases should be treated according to the protocol of combined ESWLtripsy with sialoendoscopic approach.

11.12.1 Surgical Approach to Specific Disorders

Juvenile Recurrent Parotitis (JRP)

When the diagnosis of JRP is established, the disease can be treated by endoscopic means (▶ Fig. 11.9a, b). At the diagnostic stage the endoscopic technique can confirm histopathologic inspection of the diseased gland. These examinations reveal a lymphocytic infiltrate that tends to form lymphoid follicles, and small ductal dilatations. These intraductal cyst-like dilatations are demonstrated clearly by sialography, and are called sialectasis or sialectasia. Sialectasis is usually present in the asymptomatic contralateral gland as well.[51,52] These sialographic changes remain unaltered in adult life. Ultrasonographic examinations demonstrate multiple small hypoechogenic areas and punctate calcifications, corresponding to the sialectasis demonstrated by sialography.[53]

If sialoendoscopy was chosen as the main treatment, the endoscope firstly should be used to examine the main duct and secondary ducts as possible (age limitations). Through the endoscope, the gland is to be thoroughly lavaged with 30 to 60 cc of normal saline, according to the age of a patient (▶ Fig. 11.10a–c).

The duct system is dilated with saline under pressure, and when necessary, with a balloon. Following the lavage and the dilatation, hydrocortisone can be injected into the duct system, and dosage, according to the age of a patient, should exceed 100 mg anyway. The patients can

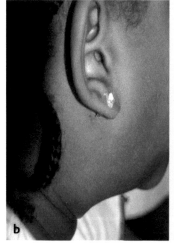

Fig. 11.9 (a, b) An 8-year-old girl with right parotid swelling due to juvenile recurrent parotitis.

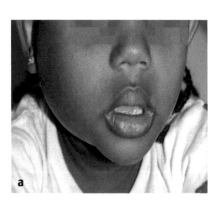

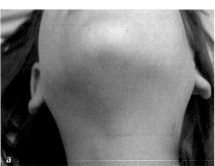
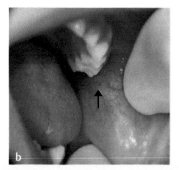
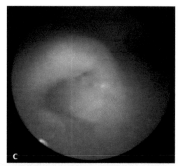

Fig. 11.10 (a) A 6-year-old girl suffering from JRP. Note bilateral swelling. This girl suffered *30 attacks* of swelling episodes *during 1 year*. **(b)** Close-up of Stensen's duct of the 6-year-old girl. Note the wide opening of the orifice. **(c)** Endoscopic picture of the Stensen's duct wide opening of JRP patient. JRP, juvenile recurrent parotitis.

be treated with amoxicillin-clavulanic acid, clindamycin, or similar antibiotics for one week, along with frequent massage of the glands.[54,55]

In between episodes, a regimen of massage, encouragement of fluid intake, application of heat, use of chewing gum or sour candy, and sialogogues has been advocated. Intermittent duct probing and dilatation as well as overfilled sialograms have also been recommended.[53] Other treatment methods mentioned in the literature include duct ligation to produce glandular atrophy, parotidectomy, and tympanic neurectomy.[54,56]

The recurrent swelling of the gland is possible. In the first few hours following the procedure bilateral swelling of the parotid glands can be noticed due to the irrigation. The swelling usually resolved spontaneously within 12 hours after the procedure (▶Fig. 11.11 and ▶Fig. 11.12).

Obstructive Sialadenitis and Sialolithiasis

In children, salivary gland calculi are uncommon. Yet, sialadenitis in the pediatric population accounts for up to 10% of all salivary gland disease.[57] A review of the English literature revealed sporadic cases of sialolithiasis of the submandibular gland in children ages 3 weeks to 15 years.[58-67] According to the literature it is assumed that 3% of all sialolithiasis cases are in children.[68]

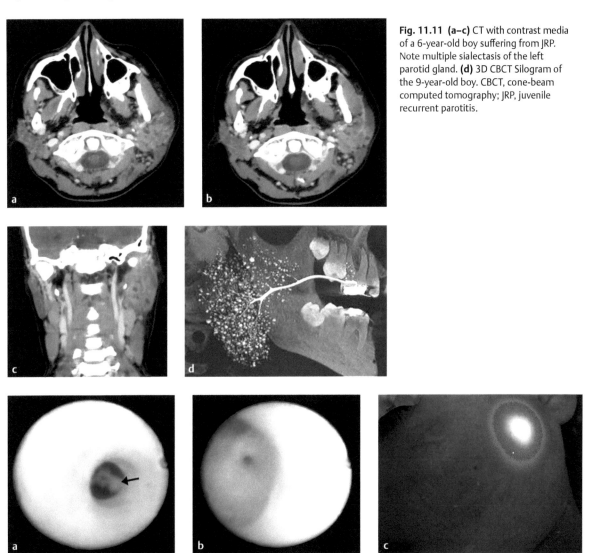

Fig. 11.11 (a–c) CT with contrast media of a 6-year-old boy suffering from JRP. Note multiple sialectasis of the left parotid gland. **(d)** 3D CBCT Silogram of the 9-year-old boy. CBCT, cone-beam computed tomography; JRP, juvenile recurrent parotitis.

Fig. 11.12 (a) Endoscopic appearance of a 5-year-old child diagnosed with JRP. Note white avascular appearance of the duct and a cloudy plaque (*arrow*). **(b)** Endoscopic appearance of the same child near the hilum of the gland. **(c)** Intraoperative figure demonstrating endoscope inside the gland. Note transillumination effect. It helps to locate the site of the endoscope tip. JRP, juvenile recurrent parotitis.

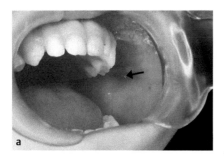
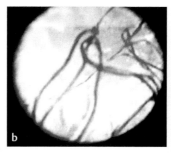

Fig. 11.13 **(a)** A 5-year-old child with a hair follicle in the right Stensen's duct (*black arrow*). **(b)** Endoscopic view of the hair follicle inside the parotid duct. **(c)** The hair follicle after its removal. Notice the stone formation around the hair follicle. **(d)** Endoscopic view following retrieval of sialolith—note the formation of intraductal evagination.

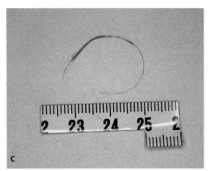
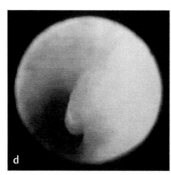

11.12.2 Location Statistics

Eighty to 81% of stones are located in the submandibular duct system (53% hilar/proximal, 37% distal, 10% intraparenchymal).

Nineteen to 20% are parotid stones (83% in Stensen's duct, 17% intraparenchymal).[60,61]

Sialography is reserved only for cooperative patients. Younger children should be under general anesthesia, and adolescents can remain under local anesthesia. Cases of parotid sialolithiasis are well detected in the Stensen's duct. Submandibular sialolithiasis can be associated with foreign bodies, with a hair follicle, and with a particle of plant (Phytobezoar) (▶Fig. 11.13a–d). In most of the cases the calculi are visible as radiopaque objects on radiographic film. If it is impossible to perform precise imaging due to the young age of the patients, the calculus could be clinically diagnosed in the anterior part of the duct. The prognosis is good with minimal chances of recurrence of the disease.

Sialolithiasis is a relatively common condition in adults but is rarely found in children.[58,62,69] Nevertheless it must be included in the differential diagnosis of facial swelling and intermittent pain in youngsters. The main complaint is unilateral swelling. Historically, authors suspected that congenital anomalies and foreign bodies were the etiologic factors for most cases of sialolithiasis.[70,71] Endoscopic findings support this hypothesis.[72] Finally, another striking phenomenon is the predominance of males in the reported series of sialolithiasis.[59–61] There is no current explanation for this.

Submandibular sialadenitis without obstruction of the gland is a very rare condition in childhood. Most of the submandibular infections in children are caused

and associated with obstruction of Wharton's duct.[2] Nonobstructive inflammatory disease is a diagnosis of exclusion using all the diagnostic modalities discussed previously. The treatment in the acute phase is hydration and antibiotic treatment. The most common organisms are *Streptococcus viridians*. Care must be taken not to confuse submandibular gland infections with submandibular space infection or lymphadenitis of dental origin.[30,73]

In conclusion, pediatric sialolithiasis is a well-known but uncommon problem. Sialendoscopy is a promising new technique for its management. The procedure is minimally invasive and preliminary results suggest that excision of the gland can be avoided in most cases.

11.12.3 Acute Suppurative Parotitis

A special entity is acute neonatal suppurative parotitis, which is a very rare condition; only 138 cases have so far been reported in the literature, and known risk factors are, prematurely, malnutrition and dehydration.[74] Physical examination reveals tender swelling involving both the pre- and postauricular regions and extending to the mandibular angle. The skin is erythematous and tender. Stensen's papilla is usually enlarged and purulent material can often be expressed from the duct spontaneously or after massaging the gland. *Staphylococcus aureus* is the most common organism cultured from the gland, but in rare cases *E. coli* and *Pseudomonas* have been isolated (▶Fig. 11.14a, b).[75]

The treatment is aggressive management of the associated illness, rehydration, and antibiotic therapy. While no surgical management is needed, this disorder

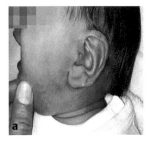
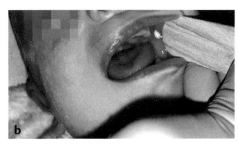

Fig. 11.14 (a, b) A 2-week-old baby with acute suppurative parotitis. Note the swelling of the left parotid region and the pus from the left Stensen's duct.

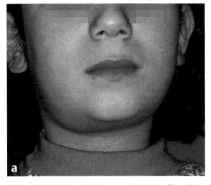
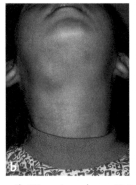
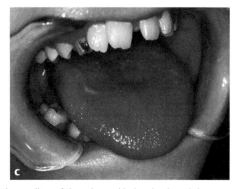

Fig. 11.15 (a–c) A 7-year-old girl suffers from Juvenile Sjögren's syndrome. Note the swelling of the submandibular glands and the dryness of the tongue and mouth.

must be taken into account in differential diagnosis with other salivary diseases. If recovery is delayed, the endoscopic observation of the affected gland is possible.

11.13 The Sjögren's Syndrome

The Sjögren's syndrome is a chronic inflammatory disease of the exocrine glands with a broad range of extraglandular manifestation. Symptoms of dry mouth, xerostomia, keratoconjunctivitis sicca, and dry eyes are common signs of the Sjögren's syndrome.[76]

On presurgical clinical examination, while milking the parotid glands, salivary secretion can be accompanied by plaques that are of high gelatin-like viscosity. Rarely pus can be seen coming out of glands. Ultrasound examination may reveal multiple hypoechogenic areas in the glands' parenchyma. In the majority of cases, the sialogram demonstrates parenchymatic sialectasis and strictures of the Stenson's duct. The sialogram and sialo-CT may also demonstrate sialoceles of the Stenson's duct in addition to a sever stricture. The combination of the Sjögren's syndrome with calculi is possible and X-rays aimed to the glandular region may demonstrate sialoliths in the ducts and/or in the hilum of the gland. In such cases sialolithotomy (retrieval of the sialoliths) may be needed (▶ Fig. 11.15a–c).[77]

For majority of patients, the treatment consists of parotid sialoendoscopy with thorough rinsing, and Stenson's duct dilatation using hydrostatic pressure and high pressure balloon as needed. Hydrocortisone 30 to 100 mg (according to the age of a patient) can be injected through direct vision into the duct. Rarely parotid sialoendoscopy may detect that the Stenson's duct ends abruptly in a cull de sac in the middle third of it. For such cases, hydrostatic pressure can be applied, and hydrocortisone can be injected directly into this fibrotic obstruction through the endoscope. In all cases, the plaques should be washed out, and strictures dilated.[77]

11.13.1 Postoperative Treatment

The postoperative treatment can be divided into general postoperative management and specific management in cases when postoperative complications occurred.

General Postoperative Management

All patients are to be treated postoperatively with antibiotics that are to be selected in type and dosage according to the age of a patient for 7 days. Imaging of the affected gland—panorex oclusal and oclusal oblique—is usually performed on the same day of surgery. Hydration after the procedure is needed, drinking more than 0.5 to 2 L of water a day (according to the age of a patient) without sialogogues or spicy food. Follow-up following the surgical procedure is usually set at 1, 3, 6, 12, and 24 months but may vary according to physician's preferences.

Specific Management

There are several types of specific complications following sialendoscopic procedures, namely avulsion of the duct, strictures, gland swelling, salivary fistulas and perforations (false rout), traumatic ranulas, and lingual nerve paresthesia. Of them, avulsion of the duct and perforations are usually detected during the surgical operation. The rest should be managed as a part of postoperative treatment.

Some measures are to be taken already at the end of surgery. Following endoscopy, a temporary polymeric stent (sialodrain, sialostent) in the diameter of the inner part of the duct can be introduced into the duct and kept in place.

The stent insertion helps to avoid kinks. The next step is to correct the unfavorable angle of the duct that is one of the main causes for the formation of sialoliths. The aim of this procedure is to prevent recurrence of new stones. Ideally, a 2-week period of retention is most desirable. Its purpose is to prevent obstruction of the ductal lumen by postoperative edema and to allow any particles of calculus to be washed out by the saliva and to act as a stent in an attempt to reduce the possibility of stenosis. Ductal marsupialization, consisting of suturing the incised ductal margins to the overlying incised mucosal margins, can act as a supplement to provide added insurance of retaining the ductal opening.[50]

Strictures of the duct are the main complication pathology following sialendoscopic procedures. The treatment of the stricture in the orifice area could be performed with dilator and irrigation of the duct with hydrocortisone. Treatment of strictures in the other parts of the ductal system is the same as for primary strictures, i.e., mainly by high-pressure sialoballoon, but extreme cautiousness is needed in cases of little children. Postoperative *gland swelling* occurs when the main goal of the minimally invasive surgery was achieved, i.e., the gland was preserved. Excessive swelling following sialendoscopy is usually due to obstruction of the main duct, peroration of the duct, or excessive irrigation.[30,73] Swelling can be prevented or treated by insertion of sialodrain, administering of dexamethasone intraoperatively and postoperatively in doses according to the age of a patient, massage of the affected gland, and hydration. Formation of *ranula* can occur in patients following submandibular sialendoscopy. The treatment of ranula is relatively simple and consists of unroofing or marsupialization and insertion of iodoform gauze with vicryl sutures for 2 weeks (▶ Fig. 11.16). In most of the cases, this procedure will solve the problem. In some cases, the second attempt of marsupialization might be needed. If the *lingual nerve* is damaged, steroid treatment should be administered immediately after the correct diagnosis; surgical treatment is possible according to the lingual nerve damage guidelines.[50]

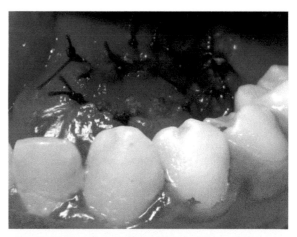

Fig. 11.16 Marsupialization and suturing of the ranula lining to the oral mucosa with 4/0 vicryl suture.

11.14 Highlights

a. Indications
   - Juvenile recurrent parotitis.
   - Sialolithiasis (calculi in the gland).
   - Obstructive sialadenitis.
   - Evidence of ductal dilatation or stenosis on sialography or ultrasound.
   - Recurrent episodes of major salivary gland swelling without obvious cause.
   - Foreign bodies (rare).
b. Contraindications
   - Benign and malignant tumors of the gland.
c. Complications
   - The avulsion of the salivary duct.
   - Secondary strictures.
   - The gland swelling.
   - Salivary fistulas and perforations (false rout).
   - Traumatic ranulas.
   - The lingual nerve paresthesia.
d. Special preoperative considerations
   - Decide: minimally invasive endoscopic approach vs. standard surgery.
   - Inspect the size of the natural orifice of the duct.
   - Choose the appropriate endoscope, consider the age of a patient.
   - Choose the right instrument: basket, forceps.
e. Special intraoperative considerations
   - Irrigation is crucial in every endoscopy procedure.
   - Estimate the diameter of the calculus.
   - Choose the strategy: intraductal vs. extraductal procedure.
f. Special postoperative considerations
   - Consider a temporary polymeric stent in the duct.
   - Consider massage of the gland very cautiously.

References

[1] Welch KJ, Trump DS. The salivary glands. In: Mustard WT et al, eds. Pediatric Surgery. Chicago, IL: Year Book Medical; 2007

[2] Kaban LB, Mulliken JB, Murray JE. Sialadenitis in childhood. Am J Surg 1978;135(4):570–576

[3] Dudek RW. Embryology. 5th ed. Philadelphia, PA: Lippincott Williams & Wilkins; 2011: 30:150

[4] Agur AMR, Dalley AF II. Grant's Atlas of Anatomy. 12th ed. Philadelphia, PA: Lippincott Williams & Wilkins; 2011: 662

[5] Zhang HM, Yan YP, Qi KM, Wang JQ, Liu ZF. Anatomical structure of the buccal fat pad and its clinical adaptations. Plast Reconstr Surg 2002;109(7):2509–2518, discussion 2519–2520

[6] Schmidlin J, Prüfer F, Gürtler N, Ritz N. Buccal fat pad herniation in an infant. J Pediatr 2016;173:263

[7] Kim JT, Naidu S, Kim YH. The buccal fat: a convenient and effective autologous option to prevent Frey syndrome and for facial contouring following parotidectomy. Plast Reconstr Surg 2010;125(6):1706–1709

[8] Bruch JM, Setlur J. Pediatric sialendoscopy. Adv Otorhinolaryngol 2012;73:149–152

[9] Zhang B, Yang Z, Zhang RM, et al. Are the patients with anatomic variation of the sublingual/Wharton's duct system predisposed to ranula formation? Int J Pediatr Otorhinolaryngol 2016;83:69–73

[10] Salerno S, Giordano J, La Tona G, De Grazia E, Barresi B, Lo Casto A. Pediatric sialolithiasis distinctive characteristic in radiological imaging. Minerva Stomatol 2011;60(9):435–441

[11] Sodhi KS, Saxena AK, Khandelwal N. Pediatric salivary gland imaging: comments on pictorial essay by Boyd et al. Pediatr Radiol 2010;40(5):785–, author reply 786

[12] Gadodia A, Seith A, Sharma R. Pediatric salivary gland imaging. Pediatr Radiol 2009;39(12):1380–1381, author reply 1382

[13] Yepes JF, Booe MR, Sanders BJ, et al. Pediatric Phantom Dosimetry of Kodak 9000 Cone-beam Computed Tomography. Pediatr Dent 2017;39(3):229–232

[14] Tomiita M, Ueda T, Nagata H, et al. Usefulness of magnetic resonance sialography in patients with juvenile Sjögren's syndrome. Clin Exp Rheumatol 2005;23(4):540–544

[15] Kelly TG, Faulkes SV, Pierre SK, et al. Imaging submandibular pathology in the paediatric patient. Clin Radiol 2015;70(7):774–786

[16] Rooks VJ, Cable BB. Head and neck ultrasound in the pediatric population. Otolaryngol Clin North Am 2010;43(6):1255–1266, vi–vii

[17] Koch A, Schick B, Bozzato A. Today's importance of ultrasound in ENT Rev Laryngol Otol Rhinol (Bord) 2015;136(2):51–59

[18] Brown RE, Harave S. Diagnostic imaging of benign and malignant neck masses in children: a pictorial review. Quant Imaging Med Surg 2016;6(5):591–604

[19] Gungor G, Yurttutan N, Bilal N, et al. Evaluation of parotid glands with real-time ultrasound elastography in children. J Ultrasound Med 2016;35(3):611–615

[20] Sodhi KS, Bartlett M, Prabhu NK. Role of high resolution ultrasound in parotid lesions in children. Int J Pediatr Otorhinolaryngol 2011;75(11):1353–1358

[21] Boyd ZT, Goud AR, Lowe LH, Shao L. Pediatric salivary gland imaging. Pediatr Radiol 2009;39(7):710–722

[22] Lowe LH, Stokes LS, Johnson JE, et al. Swelling at the angle of the mandible: imaging of the pediatric parotid gland and periparotid region. Radiographics 2001;21(5):1211–1227

[23] Simon-Zoula SC, Boesch C, De Keyzer F, Thoeny HC. Functional imaging of the parotid glands using blood oxygenation level dependent (BOLD)-MRI at 1.5T and 3T. J Magn Reson Imaging 2008;27(1):43–48

[24] Nagata S, Jin YF, Yoshizato K, et al. Early uptake and continuous accumulation of thallium-201 chloride in a benign mixed tumor of soft tissue: case report. Diagn Pathol 2010;5:34

[25] Arbab AS, Koizumi K, Toyama K, et al. Various imaging modalities for the detection of salivary gland lesions: the advantages of 201Tl SPET. Nucl Med Commun 2000;21(3):277–284

[26] Arbab AS, Koizumi K, Hiraike S, Toyama K, Arai T, Araki T. Will thallium-201 replace gallium-67 in salivary gland scintigraphy? J Nucl Med 1996;37(11):1819–1823

[27] Brook I. The bacteriology of salivary gland infections. Oral Maxillofac Surg Clin North Am 2009;21(3):269–274

[28] Komatsuzawa H, Ouhara K, Kawai T, et al. Susceptibility of periodontopathogenic and cariogenic bacteria to defensins and potential therapeutic use of defensins in oral diseases. Curr Pharm Des 2007;13(30):3084–3095

[29] Beck G, Puchelle E, Laroche D, Mougel D, Sadoul P. Quantitative bacteriology of sputum collected by a simple technic limiting salivary contamination Bull Eur Physiopathol Respir 1982;18(6):885–892

[30] Nahlieli O, Eliav E, Hasson O, Zagury A, Baruchin AM. Pediatric sialolithiasis. Oral Surg Oral Med Oral Pathol Oral Radiol Endod 2000;90(6):709–712

[31] Faure F, Querin S, Dulguerov P, Froehlich P, Disant F, Marchal F. Pediatric salivary gland obstructive swelling: sialendoscopic approach. Laryngoscope 2007;117(8):1364–1367

[32] Faure F, Froehlich P, Marchal F. Paediatric sialendoscopy. Curr Opin Otolaryngol Head Neck Surg 2008;16(1):60–63

[33] Martins-Carvalho C, Plouin-Gaudon I, Quenin S, et al. Pediatric sialendoscopy: a 5-year experience at a single institution. Arch Otolaryngol Head Neck Surg 2010;136(1):33–36

[34] Jabbour N, Tibesar R, Lander T, Sidman J. Sialendoscopy in children. Int J Pediatr Otorhinolaryngol 2010;74(4):347–350

[35] Yamazaki H, Kojima R, Nakanishi Y, Kaneko A. A case of early pneumoparotid presenting with oral noises. J Oral Maxillofac Surg 2018;76(1):67–69

[36] Cabello M, Macías E, Fernández-Flórez A, Martínez-Martínez M, Cobo J, de Carlos F. Pneumoparotid associated with a mandibular advancement device for obstructive sleep apnea. Sleep Med 2015;16(8):1011–1013

[37] Bhat V, Kuppuswamy M, Santosh Kumar DG, Bhat V, Karthik GA. Pneumoparotid in "puffed cheek" computed tomography: incidence and relation to oropharyngeal conditions. Br J Oral Maxillofac Surg 2015;53(3):239–243

[38] Jervis PN, Lee JA, Bull PD. Management of non-tuberculous mycobacterial peri-sialadenitis in children: the Sheffield otolaryngology experience. Clin Otolaryngol Allied Sci 2001;26(3):243–248

[39] Rice DH. Chronic inflammatory disorders of the salivary glands. Otolaryngol Clin North Am 1999;32(5):813–818

[40] Mert A, Ozaras R, Bilir M, et al. Primary tuberculosis of the parotid gland. Int J Infect Dis 2000;4(4):229–230

[41] Ebrahim S, Singh B, Ramklass SS. HIV-associated salivary gland enlargement: a clinical review. SADJ 2014;69(9):400–403

[42] Pinto A, De Rossi SS. Salivary gland disease in pediatric HIV patients: an update. J Dent Child (Chic) 2004;71(1):33–37

[43] Piyasatukit N, Awsakulsutthi S, Kintarak J. Benign lymphoepithelial cyst of parotid glands in HIV-positive patient. J Med Assoc Thai 2015;98(Suppl 3):S141–S145

[44] Hackett AM, Baranano CF, Reed M, Duvvuri U, Smith RJ, Mehta D. Sialoendoscopy for the treatment of pediatric salivary gland disorders. Arch Otolaryngol Head Neck Surg 2012;138(10):912–915

[45] Nguyen AM, Francis CL, Larsen CG. Salivary endoscopy in a pediatric patient with HLA-B27 seropositivity and recurrent submandibular sialadenitis. Int J Pediatr Otorhinolaryngol 2013;77(6):1045–1047

[46] Semensohn R, Spektor Z, Kay DJ, Archilla AS, Mandell DL. Pediatric sialendoscopy: initial experience in a pediatric otolaryngology group practice. Laryngoscope 2015;125(2):480–484

[47] Wu CB, Xi H, Zhang LM, Zhou Q. Sialendoscopy-assisted treatment of trauma to Stensen's duct: technical note. Br J Oral Maxillofac Surg 2015;53(1):102–103

[48] Rosbe KW, Milev D, Chang JL. Effectiveness and costs of sialendoscopy in pediatric patients with salivary gland disorders. Laryngoscope 2015;125(12):2805–2809

[49] Su CH, Lee KS, Hsu JH, et al. Pediatric sialendoscopy in Asians: a preliminary report. J Pediatr Surg 2016;51(10):1684–1687

[50] Nahlieli O. Advanced sialoendoscopy techniques, rare findings, and complications. Otolaryngol Clin North Am 2009;42(6):1053–1072

[51] Ramakrishna J, Strychowsky J, Gupta M, Sommer DD. Sialendoscopy for the management of juvenile recurrent parotitis: a systematic review and meta-analysis. Laryngoscope 2015;125(6):1472–1479

[52] Canzi P, Occhini A, Pagella F, Marchal F, Benazzo M. Sialendoscopy in juvenile recurrent parotitis: a review of the literature. Acta Otorhinolaryngol Ital 2013;33(6):367–373

[53] Capaccio P, Sigismund PE, Luca N, Marchisio P, Pignataro L. Modern management of juvenile recurrent parotitis. J Laryngol Otol 2012;126(12):1254–1260

[54] Nahlieli O, Shacham R, Shlesinger M, Eliav E. Juvenile recurrent parotitis: a new method of diagnosis and treatment. Pediatrics 2004;114(1):9–12

[55] Shacham R, Droma EB, London D, Bar T, Nahlieli O. Long-term experience with endoscopic diagnosis and treatment of juvenile recurrent parotitis. J Oral Maxillofac Surg 2009;67(1):162–167

[56] Roby BB, Mattingly J, Jensen EL, Gao D, Chan KH. Treatment of juvenile recurrent parotitis of childhood: an analysis of effectiveness. JAMA Otolaryngol Head Neck Surg 2015;141(2):126–129

[57] Francis CL, Larsen CG. Pediatric sialadenitis. Otolaryngol Clin North Am 2014;47(5):763–778

[58] Myer C, Cotton RT. Salivary gland disease in children: a review. Part 1: Acquired non-neoplastic disease. Clin Pediatr (Phila) 1986;25(6):314–322

[59] Bodner L, Fliss DM. Parotid and submandibular calculi in children. Int J Pediatr Otorhinolaryngol 1995;31(1):35–42

[60] Steiner M, Gould AR, Kushner GM, Weber R, Pesto A. Sialolithiasis of the submandibular gland in an 8-year-old child. Oral Surg Oral Med Oral Pathol Oral Radiol Endod 1997;83(2):188

[61] Sugiura N, Kubo I, Negoro M, et al. A case of sialolithiasis in a two-year-old girl Shoni Shikagaku Zasshi 1990;28(3):741–746

[62] Zou ZJ, Wang SL, Zhu JR, Wu QG, Yu SF. Chronic obstructive parotitis: report of ninety-two cases. Oral Surg Oral Med Oral Pathol 1992;73(4):434–440

[63] McCullom C III, Lee CY, Blaustein DI. Sialolithiasis in an 8-year-old child: case report. Pediatr Dent 1991;13(4):231–233

[64] Reuther J, Hausamen JE. Submaxillary salivary calculus in children (author's transl) Klin Padiatr 1976;188(3):285–288

[65] Di Felice R, Lombardi T. Submandibular sialolithiasis with concurrent sialoadenitis in a child. J Clin Pediatr Dent 1995;20(1):57–59

[66] Shinohara Y, Hiromatsu T, Nagata Y, Uchida A, Nakashima T, Kikuta T. Sialolithiasis in children: report of four cases. Dentomaxillofac Radiol 1996;25(1):48–50

[67] Won SJ, Lee E, Kim HJ, Oh HK, Jeong HS. Pediatric sialolithiasis is not related to oral or oropharyngeal infection: a population-based case control study using the Korean National Health Insurance Database. Int J Pediatr Otorhinolaryngol 2017;97:150–153

[68] Ogden MA, Rosbe KW, Chang JL. Pediatric sialendoscopy indications and outcomes. Curr Opin Otolaryngol Head Neck Surg 2016;24(6):529–535

[69] Nahlieli O, Nakar LH, Nazarian Y, Turner MD. Sialoendoscopy: a new approach to salivary gland obstructive pathology. J Am Dent Assoc 2006;137(10):1394–1400

[70] Sigismund PE, Zenk J, Koch M, Schapher M, Rudes M, Iro H. Nearly 3,000 salivary stones: some clinical and epidemiologic aspects. Laryngoscope 2015;125(8):1879–1882

[71] Nahlieli O, Baruchin AM. Endoscopic technique for the diagnosis and treatment of obstructive salivary gland diseases. J Oral Maxillofac Surg 1999;57(12):1394–1401, discussion 1401–1402

[72] Kaban LB. Salivary gland disease. In: Kaban LB, ed. Pediatric Oral and Maxillofacial Surgery. Philadelphia, PA: W.B. Saunders; 1990:34–52

[73] Nahlieli O. Endoscopic surgery of the salivary glands. Alpha Omegan 2009;102(2):55–60

[74] Isfaoun Z, Radouani MA, Azzaoui S, Knouni H, Aguenaou H, Barkat A. Acute neonatal suppurative parotiditis: about three clinical cases and review of the literature Pan Afr Med J 2016;24:286

[75] Tian X, Eldadah M, Cheng W. Neonatal suppurative parotitis: two cases. Pediatr Infect Dis J 2016;35(7):823–824

[76] Talal N. What is Sjögren's syndrome and why is it important? J Rheumatol Suppl 2000;61(suppl 61):1–3

[77] Shacham R, Puterman MB, Ohana N, Nahlieli O. Endoscopic treatment of salivary glands affected by autoimmune diseases. J Oral Maxillofac Surg 2011;69(2):476–481

Suggested Readings

Gillespie MB, Walvekar RR, Schaitkin BM, Eisele DW, Eds. Gland-Preserving Salivary Surgery: A Problem-Based Approach. Berlin and New York: Springer; 2017

Greer RO, Marx RE, Said S, Prok LD. Pediatric Head and Neck Pathology. Cambridge: Cambridge University Press; 2017

Hunter JG, Spight DH. Atlas of Minimally Invasive Surgical Operations (Medical/Dentistry). New York: McGraw-Hill Education; 2018

Nahlieli O. Minimally Invasive Oral and Maxillofacial Surgery. Springer-Verlag Berlin Heidelberg; 2018

Nahlieli O, Iro H, McGurk M, Zenk J. Modern Management Preserving the Salivary Glands. Herzeliya: Isradon; 2006

Tucker AS, Miletich I, Eds. Salivary Glands: Development, Adaptations and Disease: 14 (Frontiers of Oral Biology). Basel and London: Karger; 2010

12 Salivary Gland Ductal Diversion, Botulinum Toxin Injection, and Salivary Ductal Ligation

Sam J. Daniel

Summary

Salivary gland ductal diversion or relocation, salivary ductal ligation, and botulinum toxin injection in the salivary glands are effective strategies in the treatment of drooling or sialorrhea. The latter is mostly caused by the inability of the patient to control oral secretions rather than by an increased production of saliva. Patients may suffer from anterior drooling, posterior drooling, or both. Anterior drooling is defined as saliva spilling from the mouth. This can lead to social rejection, isolation, poor hygiene, and an increased burden of care on the family. In patients with posterior drooling, saliva spills through the oropharynx and into the hypopharynx with potentially serious medical complications including chronic aspiration and chronic lung disease. Viewed by some as a cosmetic issue, drooling may lead to serious medical complications such as choking, pneumonia, feeding issues, skin infections and speech problems.[1]

While nonsurgical treatment options exist for sialorrhea, including rehabilitation (oral motor and behavior therapy) and medication (anti-cholinergic), tailored surgical options give rapid long-lasting results especially in patients with moderate or severe anterior drooling who failed conservative approaches and those with posterior drooling. Also many patients benefit from a combination of different treatment modalities.

This chapter highlights the surgical anatomy, preoperative preparation, technical details, and pearls to avoid intraoperative complications of submandibular gland ductal relocation or diversion, Wharton and Stenson's ductal ligation, and botulinum toxin injection in the salivary glands.

Keywords: Salivary gland ductal diversion, salivary duct relocation, salivary ductal ligation, botulinum toxin injection, submandibular glands, parotid glands, drooling, sialorrhea, technique, complications

12.1 Pathophysiology of Drooling and Surgical Anatomy

The parotid and submandibular glands are paired major salivary glands responsible for most of the salivary output in the oral cavity (▶Fig. 12.1). The rest of the saliva is produced by the sublingual glands and minor glands located mainly in the palatine and oral mucosa. Between 0.5 and 1.5 L of saliva are secreted daily in children.[2] Saliva is composed of mostly water (99%), and contains electrolytes, proteins, and enzymes. Secretions from the parotid glands are mostly serous in nature with high water content and lower mucin content, while submandibular gland secretions are more viscous with mixed mucous and serous saliva. The submandibular glands produce most of the resting salivary secretions, while the parotids are responsible for the bulk of stimulated saliva during feeding. Drooling is considered pathological

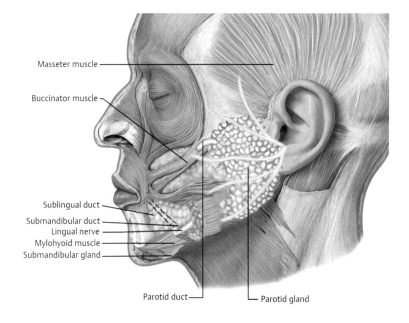

Fig. 12.1 Anatomy of the parotid and submandibular glands. Caption showing the relationship of the lingual nerve and the submandibular duct.

Masseter muscle

Buccinator muscle

Sublingual duct
Submandibular duct
Lingual nerve
Mylohyoid muscle
Submandibular gland

Parotid duct

Parotid gland

if it persists after the age of 4 years in healthy children with normal development.[1,3] It is typically caused by the inability of the patient to control oral secretions rather by an increased production of saliva[1] and is more commonly seen in patients with neurological disorders. Patients may suffer from anterior drooling, posterior drooling, or both. Anterior drooling is defined as saliva spilling from the mouth. This can lead to social rejection, isolation, poor hygiene, and an increased burden of care on the family. In patients with posterior drooling, saliva spills through the oropharynx into the hypopharynx, with potentially serious medical complications including chronic aspiration and progressive lung disease.

The parotid and submandibular salivary glands do not differ in size in children with or without drooling.[4] The parotid is the largest major salivary gland. It lies between the external auditory canal, the ramus of the mandible, and the mastoid tip, and it is separated from the submandibular gland by the stylomandibular ligament. The parotid is artificially divided by the facial nerve into a deep and a superficial lobe. The submandibular gland is composed of a larger superficial lobe located in the submandibular triangle between the anterior belly and the tendon of the digastric muscle, and a smaller deep lobe that hooks around the posterior margin of the mylohyoid entering the oral cavity through a triangular aperture as it lies on the lateral surface of the hyoglossus.

Both submandibular and parotid glands are formed by an aggregate of multiple secretory units composed of acini and ducts. Saliva produced by the secretory cells of the acini passes through intercalated, intralobular, and excretory ducts, before collecting in Stensen's and Wharton's ducts, which are the main excretory ducts of the parotid and the submandibular, respectively. Stensen's duct is 4 to 7 cm in length, and about 0.5 to 1.4 mm in diameter.[5] It arises from the anterior border of the parotid gland, runs superficial to the masseter muscle parallel to and below the zygoma, then turns sharply, pierces the buccinator, and enters the oral cavity opposite the second upper molar. Some patients have accessory parotid glands located at variable distances from the main gland along the duct.[6] Wharton's duct emerges from the deep lobe of the submandibular gland and courses anteriorly, deep to the mylohyoid muscle and lateral to hyoglossus and genioglossus. It runs medial to the sublingual gland before opening into an orifice in the sublingual papilla lateral to the lingual frenulum. Wharton's duct is 5 cm long, and has a mean diameter ranging between 0.5 and 1.5 mm.[5] During submandibular duct relocation or diversion as well as ductal ligation, the surgeon has to be cognizant of important anatomical relationships of the lingual nerve vis-à-vis the duct (▶Fig. 12.1). The lingual nerve starts superior to the submandibular duct and then, as it descends forward, it crosses the lateral side of the duct, passes below the duct winding round its lower border, before crossing it medially and ascending toward the genioglossus proceeding antero-medially to terminate

as medial branches providing general somatic afferent innervation to the anterior two-thirds of the tongue. The hypoglossal nerve emerges from behind the posterior belly of the digastric muscle and courses along the floor of the submandibular triangle lying deep to the submandibular gland. It passes forward into the gap between the hyoglossus medially and the myelohyoid laterally and supplies innervation to the intrinsic and extrinsic muscles of the tongue.

Salivary flow is controlled by the autonomic nervous system. The parotid glands receive parasympathetic secretomotor innervation from fibers arising in the inferior salivatory nucleus. These fibers travel with the glossopharyngeal nerve, leave it as Jacobson's nerve passing through the middle ear space in the tympanic plexus, and then exit the temporal bone as the lesser petrosal nerve. The latter leaves the middle cranial fossa through the foramen ovale, where preganglionic fibers synapse in the otic ganglion. The postganglionic fibers travel with the auriculotemporal nerve to supply the parotids.

The submandibular and sublingual glands receive innervation from preganglionic fibers originating in the superior salivatory nucleus. These fibers leave the brainstem as the nervus intermedius to join the facial nerve, and then leave it with the chorda tympani in the mastoid segment, through the middle ear, and petrotympanic fissure to the infratemporal fossa. They are then carried by the lingual nerve before they synapse in the submandibular ganglion. Postganglionic fibers innervate the submandibular and sublingual glands. This parasympathetic postganglionic cholinergic innervation leads to the secretion of large amounts of low-protein, serous saliva. Sympathetic innervation of the glands happens via preganglionic nerves in the thoracic segments T1–T3, which synapse in the superior cervical ganglion. Postganglionic sympathetic innervation is through the external carotid plexus, with postganglionic neurons releasing norepinephrine. Sympathetic stimulation causes the secretion of a small amount of high protein thicker saliva.

12.2 Mechanism of Action of Botulinum Toxin

Botulinum toxin is thought to inhibit the release of presynaptic acetylcholine at the neuroglandular junction leading to reduction of salivary secretion. The toxin has a heavy and a light chain. The former attaches to proteins on the surface of axon terminals, allowing toxin uptake into neurons by endocytosis. The light chain has protease activity. Type A toxin degrades a synaptosomal-associated protein (SNAP-25) preventing neurosecretory vesicles from docking with the nerve synapse plasma membrane and from releasing their neurotransmitters leading to chemical parasympathetic denervation of the gland. The latter occurs 48 to 72 hours following the injection and lasts on average for 3 to 6 months.[7,8] This explains why patients require repeated injections for drooling control.[9–11] Botulinum Toxin B binds to another presynaptic receptor protein called vesicle-associated membrane protein (VAMP) with similar effects.[12] Botulinum toxin use for the treatment of sialorrhea is still considered off-label. There are currently three botulinum toxin A products and one botulinum toxin B that have been used clinically for sialorrhea in various centers. These are onabotulinumtoxin A (BOTOX, Allergan Inc., Irvine, CA, USA), incobotulinumtoxin A (Xeomin, Merz Pharma Ltd, Germany), abobotulinumtoxin A (Dysport, Ipsen Ltd, UK), and rimabotulinumtoxin B (Botulinum Toxin B, Myobloc, Solstice Neurosciences, San Francisco, CA).[13] These are not identical and should not be considered interchangeable as they differ in molecular structure, and/or manufacturing processes.[14] One unit of Botox is comparable to one unit of Xeomin, to about 3 to 4 units of Dysport, and to 20 to 30 units of Myobloc (in certain publications).[15] These conversion ratios should be used with caution and vary in the literature and according to indications.

12.3 Preoperative Evaluation

12.3.1 Clinical Evaluation

A majority of patients referred for anterior drooling under the age of 4 years benefit from a conservative approach and improve over time. Knowledge of the underlying etiology and the progress or evolution of the patient's condition is essential prior to offering surgical treatment. It is very important to review all the medications of the patient as certain antipsychotics, sedatives, and cholinergic agonists can increase salivation.[16,17] Also in many patients with developmental delay, there could be a slower progress in oral motor function that can persist until the age of 6 years.

In view of the diverse etiologies of drooling and the limitations of approaches relying on a single-treatment modality, the author has founded a multi-disciplinary Saliva Management Clinic, described elsewhere.[1] An interdisciplinary approach to children with sialorrhea, whereby each patient is offered a number of rehabilitative, medical, and surgical options based on a consensus recommendation of the team ensures that patients get access to the options that best suit their needs.

When assessing patients referred for surgery, it is essential to evaluate if their drooling is anterior, posterior, or mixed. This guides the surgeon as to the best treatment modality for the patient. For example salivary duct relocation should never be performed in posterior drooling, as it will only worsen the problem. Symptoms of posterior drooling include congested breathing, coughing, gagging, a wet voice, and at times, penetration into the airway, and aspiration pneumonia.[18,19] All patients should undergo a flexible upper airway endoscopy to detect adenoid hypertrophy, airway obstruction, laryngeal pooling, and laryngeal penetration or aspiration. This assessment can also help in predicting a difficult intubation. The oral cavity should be examined for gingivitis, dental caries, and occlusion issues. The face should be examined for peri-oral erythema. The head and body posture should also be assessed as well as the efficiency of swallowing and the overall nutritional status. The lungs should be auscultated.

The severity of the drooling problem and its impact on the patient and family also helps the treating physician select the most appropriate treatment. Tools to quantify this include weighing oral rolls or bibs, counting the number of bib changes per day, the Teacher's Drooling Scale, the Drooling Frequency and Severity Scale, the Visual Analogue Scale (VAS), and the Drooling Impact Scale.[20–23] The Drooling Quotient (DQ) can be calculated by determining, for every interval of 15 seconds, the presence or absence of drooling over a 10-minute period. Drooling episodes are counted in the 40 observations made, and the drooling score is calculated as percentage. Traditionally, it is done when the child is resting and another time during activities. DQ can be difficult to measure in non-cooperative patients.[21] Our group concurs with others that the DQ calculated over 5 minutes during which the child is engaged in an activity to be equivalent to the 10 minutes score as an accurate representative measure of anterior drooling.[24] Specific questions should be asked to detect any effect of drooling on self-esteem, social interaction, quality of life, and burden of care.[1]

Our group has developed a tool, Daniel drooling impact score (DDIS) scale that helps us document and quantify an impact score for the drooling on the patient and their family (▶Table 12.1). DDIS is based on the severity as well as the medical and social effects of drooling. This score has helped us guide the recommendations of therapeutic options based on the severity of the impact. The postoperative score also assists us in evaluating the effect of surgery on the quality of life and health of our patients.

12.3.2 Anesthetic Considerations

Patients with impaired communication skills may be agitated and distressed. In our experience, parental presence at anesthesia induction greatly decreases the level of anxiety of these children and the need for premedication. A potentially difficult intubation should be detected prior and adequate equipment made available accordingly. Anesthesia has to be planned with the comorbidities in mind. This includes optimizing the pulmonary condition in patients with lung disease as a result of chronic aspiration, using rapid sequence induction in patients with reflux, using active warming measures in patients with neuromuscular conditions that put them at risk for hypothermia, being mindful of the interaction of epileptic disorders and their treatment.[25] Many surgical candidates

Table 12.1 Daniel drooling impact score (DDIS); based on a window of 1 month prior to the visit

Quantity				/30
1. How often does your child drool?				
1	2	3	4	5
Never	On occasion	Not every day	A few times a day	Constantly
2. How severe is your child's drooling?				
1	2	3	4	5
No drooling	Lips are wet	Chin is wet	Clothes are wet	Environment is wet
3. How often do you have to change your child's bibs and/or clothes due to drooling?				
1	2	3	4	5
None	Once a day	2–3 times a day	4–5 times a day	> 6 times a day
4. How often do you have to wipe your child's mouth?				
1	2	3	4	5
Never	1–3 times a day	4–6 times a day	7–10 times a day	>10 times a day
5. How often do you have to change sheets, pillow cases and furniture covers because of your child's drooling?				
1	2	3	4	5
Never	Once in a while	Once a week	A few times a week	Every day
6. How often do the objects (toys/books/communication devices) require cleaning due to your child's drooling?				
1	2	3	4	5
Never	Once in a while	Once a week	A few times a week	Every day
Impact on caregiver/family				/30
1. Does your child's drooling bother you?				
1	2	3	4	5
Not at all	A little	Moderately	Quite a bit	A great deal
2. Does your child's drooling affect you as a caregiver?				
1	2	3	4	5
Not at all	A little	Moderately	Quite a bit	A great deal
3. Does your child's drooling affect your family's life?				
1	2	3	4	5
Not at all	A little	Moderately	Quite a bit	A great deal
4. Are you bothered by the smell of your child's saliva?				
1	2	3	4	5
not at all	A little	Moderately	Quite a bit	A great deal
5. Does your child's drooling affect his/her interaction with siblings and extended family?				
1	2	3	4	5
Not at all	A little	Moderately	Quite a bit	A great deal
6. Does your child's drooling have an impact on your financial situation?				
1	2	3	4	5
Not at all	A little	Moderately	Quite a bit	A great deal
Impact on child				/40
1. Does your child's drooling affect his/her self-esteem?				
1	2	3	4	5
Not at all	A little	Moderately	Quite a bit	A great deal
2. Does your child's drooling affect his/her interactions with friends, peers, at school and/or with the community at large?				
1	2	3	4	5
Not at all	A little	Moderately	Quite a bit	A great deal

Table 12.1 (*Continued*) Daniel drooling impact score (DDIS); based on a window of 1 month prior to the visit

3. Does your child's drooling limit his/her participation in activities outside the home (ex. restaurants, parks, travel)?

1	2	3	4	5
Not at all	A little	Moderately	Quite a bit	A great deal

4. What is the degree of skin irritation (face/neck) caused by excess saliva?

1	2	3	4	5
None	Sometimes red	Often red	Always red	Skin breakdown

5. How often does your child choke on or aspirate his saliva?

1	2	3	4	5
Never	Rarely	Sometimes	Often	Always

6. How often is there noisy breathing or "gurgling" caused by excess saliva?

1	2	3	4	5
Never	Once/week to few times a week	Once a day	Often times in a day	Always

7. How often does your child have bad breath (halitosis)?

1	2	3	4	5
Never	Rarely	Sometimes	Often	Always

8. In the past year, how often was you child hospitalized because of excess secretions / salivary aspiration / aspiration pneumonia?

1	2	3	4	5
Never	Once	Twice	3 times	4 and more

TOTAL SCORE				/100

(21–40: Mild impact; 40–60: Moderate impact; 60–80: Severe impact; 80–100 extremely severe impact/debilitating).

have an associated neurological condition, such as cerebral palsy (CP). In patients on valproic acid for epilepsy concerns had been raised in the past on potential effects on coagulation and postoperative bleeding, but a recent study failed to show an impairment of hemostasis when it is maintained within the therapeutic range.[26] In patients with a vagal nerve stimulator, arrangements should be taken prior to surgery for the preoperative deactivation of the device. When and if possible, it can be helpful to avoid using anticholinergic agents that dry up secretions as it can make identification of the salivary ducts more challenging.

12.4 Other Investigations

The radionuclide salivagram is sensitive and specific for detecting pulmonary aspiration of saliva.[27,28] In a study of children with cerebral palsy comparing three imaging modalities for aspiration, the salivagram was the most frequently positive, followed by barium videofluoroscopy, and a milk scan study was the least helpful.

Although not standard of care, the author recommends performing salivary gland ultrasonography prior to salivary gland surgery or botulinum toxin injection in order to detect individual anatomical variations as some patients can have unilateral agenesis of the parotid and/or submandibular glands.[29,30]

12.5 Treatment Options for Sialorrhea

Several treatment options are available to manage children with sialorrhea, including rehabilitative therapies such as oral motor and behavior therapy, pharmacotherapy, botulinum toxin injection into the salivary glands, and surgery. A combination of treatments such as glycopyrolate and botulinum toxin injection can be more effective for some patients than a single modality. Ancillary procedures that can help decrease drooling and could be performed prior to or in conjunction with salivary surgery include tonsillectomy +/- adenoidectomy, turbinate reduction, tongue reduction, and craniofacial or orthodontic surgery.

12.6 Surgical Options

Surgery is generally considered in patients who fail conservative interventions including rehabilitation and pharmacotherapy, patients with severe to profuse anterior drooling that are older than 6 years (DDIS over 60), patients with posterior drooling, and patients requiring chronic and frequent care to manage secretions. Surgical options for drooling can be classified into procedures that divert saliva into the oropharynx and those that reduce the quantity of saliva.[31] The former is contraindicated in posterior drooling. Patients with pulmonary aspirationand those with severe drooling benefit from bilateral submandibular gland excisions and parotid gland duct ligation.

Salivary diversion procedures include submandibular duct rerouting and parotid duct rerouting. Salivary reduction procedures include submandibular gland excision, ductal ligation, botulinum toxin injection in the salivary glands, and tympanic neurectomy. Our approach is to discuss with the family the pros and cons of all procedures that could benefit the child and decide jointly on the best-individualized therapy, factoring in the impact of drooling on the child and family (DDIS). It is important to ensure a close follow-up with a dentist in all patients undergoing surgery for drooling or botulinum toxin injection due to the potentially increased postoperative risk of dental caries.[32,33]

12.7 Operative Techniques

12.7.1 Salivary Diversion Procedures

Submandibular Duct Relocation with Sublingual Gland Excision (SDRSGE)

See ▸ Fig. 12.2, ▸ Fig. 12.3, ▸ Fig. 12.4, ▸ Fig. 12.5, ▸ Fig. 12.6. This procedure is to be avoided in any patient with aspiration problems. The technique consists of freeing the submandibular ducts from the papilla anteriorly until

the level of their entry into the submandibular gland at the hilum, being careful not to injure the lingual nerve that double crosses the duct[34] (▸ Fig. 12.1). The sublingual

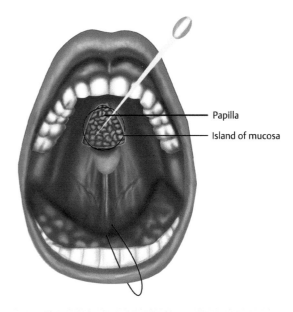

Fig. 12.2 The tongue is sutured to the palate to enhance exposure. A probe is inserted in the submandibular duct opening, After infiltrating the floor of the mouth anterior and posterior to the submandibular papillae, an elliptical incision is made around both papillae creating an island of mucosa.

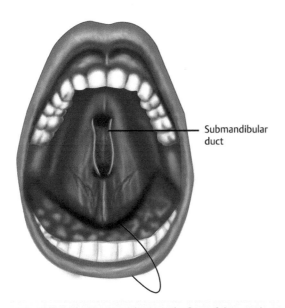

Fig. 12.3 An incision is made along the floor of the mouth for exposure. Ducts are then freed from surrounding tissues by blunt dissection until reaching the anterior border of the submandibular glands. The anterior mucosal island is kept intact and is sutured temporarily to the tongue to protect the ducts.

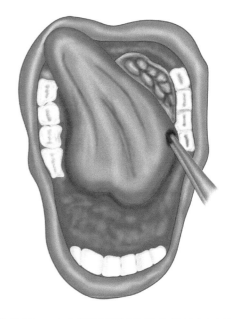

Fig. 12.4 Once the sublingual gland is mobilized off the myelohyoid and genioglossus by blunt dissection and excised, a submucosal tunnel is then developed between the incision and the tonsillar fossa using a closed Kelly clamp.

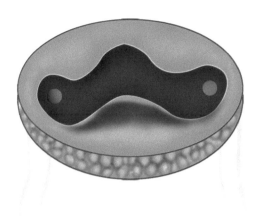

Fig. 12.5 Sutures holding the mucosal island to the tongue are cut and the island is split in the middle, separating the left and right submandibular ducts.

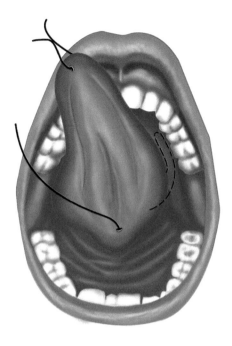

Fig. 12.6 A catheter is passed from the tonsillar fossa into the operative field. The divided island is sutured to the catheter and pulled into the tonsillar fossa. The trajectory is highlighted with a dashed line. Each duct is sutured to the posterior aspect of the anterior tonsillar pillar with two to three simple absorbable suture.

gland is mobilized and excised. A submucosal tunnel is created from the anterior face of the submandibular gland to the tonsillar fossa. A tonsillectomy is performed, if the patient has large tonsils. The submandibular ducts are pulled through this tunnel and sutured in the tonsil fossa.

Wearing a headlight and magnifying loupes greatly improve visualization. Exposure is of paramount importance and can be facilitated by placing a self-retaining retractor to keep the mouth open and suturing the tongue tip to the soft palate. The patient is placed in a reverse trendelenburg position and the surgeon sits at the head of the operating table. After infiltrating the floor of the mouth anterior and posterior to the submandibular papillae, an elliptical incision is made around both papillae creating an island of mucosa. Each duct is identified by grasping the posterior border of the island and pulling it towards the lower dentition and dissecting laterally from the midline under the border of the mucosal island. Ducts are then freed from surrounding tissues by blunt dissection until reaching the anterior border of the submandibular glands. Care is taken not to injure the lingual nerve, as it is crossing Wharton's duct.

An incision is made along the floor of the mouth and the anterior sublingual gland is mobilized off the inner mandible with blunt dissection. A clamp is placed on the sublingual gland, which is then mobilized off the myelohyoid and genioglossus by blunt dissection. Bipolar is used to cauterize feeding vessels. Care is taken to avoid the large veins deep to the lingual nerve and close to the tongue. Once the sublingual gland is removed, a submucosal tunnel is then developed between the incision and the tonsillar fossa created using a closed Kelly clamp. The latter is then used to pull a red rubber or a suction catheter from the tonsillar fossa into the operative field. The mucosal island containing the submandibular papillae is divided in the midline. The divided island is sutured to the catheter and pulled into the tonsillar fossa. Once the ducts are pulled into the fossa, the sutures are cut on the catheters and a Boyle Davis mouth gag is inserted. Each duct is sutured to the posterior aspect of the anterior tonsillar pillar with two to three simple absorbable sutures. The floor of the mouth is also closed with simple, interrupted, absorbable sutures.

The author believes that the addition of sublingual gland excision to submandibular duct relocation (SDR) decreases the likelihood of ranula formation and improves the drooling control.[31] In a large study by Crysdale, no ranula occurred in the group of patients undergoing sublingual gland excision in addition to SDR as compared to over 8% incidence of ranulas in the SDR alone group. Also the secondary surgery rate for persistent drooling was higher in the SDR group. In a prospective study of cerebral palsy children with moderate to severe drooling who did not respond to rehabilitation therapies, 86% had an improvement in the postoperative severity and frequency of drooling with bilateral submandibular duct transposition and sublingual gland excision.[35]

Patients are hospitalized postoperatively for airway and bleeding monitoring as well as pain control. Good intravenous hydration is important to prevent dehydration in some patients. Prophylactic antibiotics are also recommended. Advantages to this procedure include the absence of facial scar and less risk of xerostomia. Drawbacks include an increased risk of aspiration and longer hospitalization. Also some question whether the efficacy of this procedure is merely secondary to ductal blockage from kinking during its repositioning into the tonsillar fossa.

Parotid Duct Relocation

Parotid duct diversion is used in some centers, mostly in conjunction with SDR for the control of sialorrhea.[36] While advantages include the lack of facial scar, parotid duct relocation has fallen out of favor due to the risks of ductal obstruction, chronic parotitis, sialocele formation, and facial nerve palsy.

12.7.2 Salivary Reduction Procedures

Bilateral Submandibular Gland Excision and Parotid Duct Ligation

Bilateral submandibular gland excision combined with bilateral parotid duct ligation is an effective surgical procedure for the treatment of chronic sialorrhea in children.[37,38] It has been shown to reduce the frequency of lower respiratory tract infections, the need for suctioning, and the rate of hospitalization for pneumonias in children with cerebral palsy.[37] A long-term follow-up study reported significant improvement or arrest of drooling in 87% of patients.[39] There were no major complications; 8% of patients experienced xerostomia and 2% reported an increase in dental caries.[39] Other potential complications include hypertrophic scar, risk of injury to the marginal mandibular, lingual, and hypoglossal nerves, sialocele, and parotitis. For the surgical technique of submandibular gland excision, the reader is referred to Chapter 10.

Duct Ligation

Ligation of Wharton's and/or Stenson's ducts is a well-established treatment modality for the management of sialorrhea. A study in a rabbit model demonstrated reduction in the size of the parotid glands post ductal ligation due to acinar atrophy, and apoptosis of both acinar and ductal cells.[40] Studies have reported on outcomes of various combinations of salivary gland ductal ligations including only the submandibular ducts, only the parotid ducts, two submandibular and one parotid duct, or all four ducts.[41–46] While several studies have reported a significant reduction in drooling, long-term results analyzed in some studies have been less encouraging.[45] The author favors four-duct ligation as it appears more effective in

the long-term in patients with severe sialorrhea due to recannulation in some cases. This technique may not be feasible in some patients with severe retrognatia that limits access or in certain cases with ductal scarring, for example, from chronic cheek biting at the level of Stenson's duct, leading to failure to cannulate the duct at the beginning of the procedure.

Wearing a headlight and magnifying loupes greatly improves visualization. Exposure is also of paramount importance and can be facilitated by suturing the tongue tip to the soft palate and placing a self-retaining retractor or a bite block that keeps the mouth open.

Parotid Duct Ligation

The procedure begins by cannulation of the duct with a salivary or lacrimal probe. After mucosal infiltration of the tissue anterior to the duct opening with a local anesthetic agent and epinephrine, an elliptical incision is placed 5 mm anterior to the duct orifice. Following dissection and identification of the duct close to its orifice, a small curved Lahey or Mixter clamp is inserted around the duct. The ductal probe is then removed, and surgical clips or ligatures of nonabsorbable ligation sutures are applied. The buccal mucosa incision is closed with interrupted absorbable sutures (▶Fig. 12.7, ▶Fig. 12.8, ▶Fig. 12.9, and ▶Fig. 12.10).

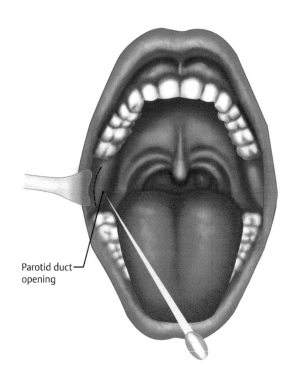

Parotid duct opening

Fig. 12.7 Parotid duct ligation begins by cannulation of the duct with a salivary probe. An elliptical incision is placed 5 mm anterior to the duct orifice.

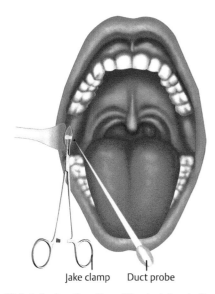

Jake clamp   Duct probe

Fig. 12.8 Following dissection of the duct close to its orifice, a small curved Lahey or Jake clamp is inserted around the duct.

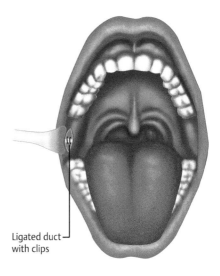

Ligated duct with clips

Fig. 12.9 The probe is removed, and surgical clips or ligatures of nonabsorbable ligation sutures are applied around the duct.

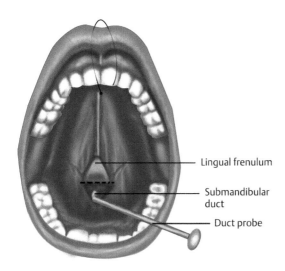

Lingual frenulum

Submandibular duct

Duct probe

Fig. 12.10 Wharton's ducts are cannulated with a larimal probe.

12.7.3 Submandibular Duct Ligation

Wharton's ducts are first cannulated with a larimal or salivary probe. After mucosal infiltration with a local anesthetic agent and epinephrine, a small mucosal incision is made approximately 1 cm behind the papillae. The duct is identified by pulling the anterior edge of the incision toward the lower dentition and gently dissecting laterally from the midline with a Jake forceps.

Once identified, the duct is freed from surrounding tissue with sharp scissor dissection. A small curved Lahey or Mixter clamp is placed around the duct and clips or nonabsorbable suture ligatures are applied after removing the ductal probe. The incision in the floor of the mouth is closed with simple interrupted absorbable sutures making sure not to injure the duct to avoid fistulization.

In most cases, duct ligations are done in same day ambulatory surgical setting. Swelling of the parotid or submandibular gland can occur in the immediate postoperative period. Patients may also need to be admitted for various reasons related to comorbidities.

Advantages of this technique include the absence of facial scars and the rapidity of the surgery. Complications include xerostomia, increased saliva thickness or viscosity, sialocele, ranula, sialadenitis, transient tongue edema, and fistula formation.[41,43,46] Postoperatively, there is usually a transient swelling that usually subsides over the following 1 to 2 weeks. Prophylactic postoperative antibiotics are recommended (▶Fig. 12.11, ▶Fig. 12.12, ▶Fig. 12.13, and ▶Fig. 12.14).

Tympanic Neurectomy

Tympanic plexus neurectomy with or without chorda tympani section can be a useful option in the management of drooling.[47] This can be achieved by raising the tympanic membrane through an ear canal approach and cutting the tympanic plexus located just anterior to the round window niche of the middle ear or vaporizing it with laser.[48] In some cases the chorda tympani is also sectioned. Advantages of this technique include its relatively

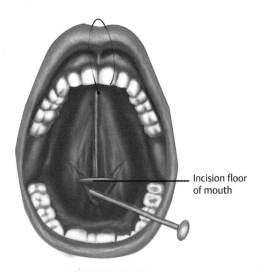

Fig. 12.11 A small mucosal incision is made approximately 1 cm behind the papillae.

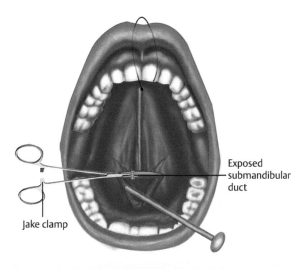

Fig. 12.12 Once the duct is freed from surrounding tissue, a small curved Lahey or a Jake clamp is placed around the duct.

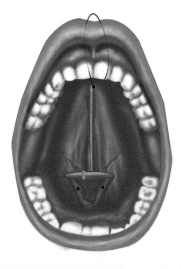

Fig. 12.13 Nonabsorbable suture ligatures are applied after removing the ductal probe.

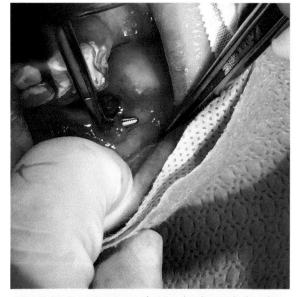

Fig. 12.14 Operative picture showing the clips applied on the duct prior to mucosal incision closure.

low morbidity. However it has had varying reported success rates, ranging from 25 to 87%.[31,49,50] Complications include tympanic membrane perforation, taste disturbance, and recurrence on long-term follow-up.[31]

12.8 Botulinum Toxin Injection in the Salivary Glands

Of the various types of botulinum toxin used for drooling management in children, onabotulinumtoxin A (OBTXA) remains the most commonly utilized. The frozen toxin is reconstituted with 0.9% sterile saline solution and diluted to the desired dosage. To date there is no consensus as to the dosage as well as which salivary glands should be injected in order to obtain the most optimal reduction in drooling. A review of the literature reveals multiple variations in terms of dosage and delivery techniques. Several studies describe injections to either the paired parotid or submandibular glands alone, whereas most authors recommend injecting both submandibular and parotid glands bilaterally,[51] with a low risk of xerostomia. One study reported a higher rate of nonrespondents to BoNTs treatment when only the submandibular glands were injected.[52] The parotid gland is usually injected in two or three places and the submandibular gland in one to three places.[53] Racette found a poor correlation between the dose adjusted for body weight in adults and the reduction of saliva production, suggesting that dose response is independent of body weight.[54]

Based on the author's practice, which encompasses one of the largest world series of botulinum toxin injection for sialorrhea, it is recommended to tailor the dosage to each individual patient with a total dose range of 1 to 5.5 units of onabotulinumtoxin A per kg distributed into two to four glands.[55] In patients injected for the first time, the author starts with a small dose and gradually increases it over time depending on the response. The maximum dose irrespective of the weight was of 250 units and was given in one patient. When using higher doses and in some fragile patients one has to be mindful of potentially serious adverse effects including dysphagia and aspiration pneumonia. A clinical trial was even aborted due to these side effects.[56] Of importance, the potency differs amongst various botulinum toxin preparations. Studies using rimabotulinum toxin B have reported a total dose of 1500 to 5000 units of botulinum toxin B.[57] A small number of patients may become nonresponders after many years of successful injections and in our experience 10% of children do not respond to onabotulinumtoxin A injection.[1]

While general anesthesia is still commonly used for ultrasound-guided injection of botulinum toxin into the salivary glands,[13] our group pioneered this treatment as a regular outpatient clinic procedure performed with topical anesthesia using the local anesthetics tetracaine hydrochloride gel 4% or EMLA (eutectic mixture of local analgesics, Shaumburg, IL) cream.[1,55] General anesthesia may be necessary in uncooperative or severely agitated patients.

Injection using anatomic landmarks and manual palpation, ultrasound guidance, and electromyography (EMG) guidance are three different botulinum toxin injection techniques. Preference for one technique depends on the expertise of the treating team and available resources.

- *Using anatomic landmarks and manual palpation*:
  Although easy to perform, this technique is not recommended by the author as it does not detect anatomical variants such as gland agenesis,[30] as well as venous or lymphatic abnormalities. For parotid injections, the skin inferior to the tragus is lifted, creating a cavity. A 21-gauge needle is inserted and advanced anteriorly until the tip is at the anterior border of the masseter. Aspiration is performed prior to injection in order to make sure vessels are avoided. Once confirmed, the injection is done slowly until the needle is close to the posterior edge of the mandibular ramus. For submandibular gland injection, the patient is placed in decubitus position with the head turned to the contralateral side. The injection needle is placed 0.5 cm anterior, and 1 to 1.5 cm inferior to the level of the palpated facial artery and advanced within the substance of the gland to a depth of 1.5 to 2.0 cm. Aspiration is always performed prior to injection. In cases of difficulty

palpating the gland, intraoral counter pressure can be useful in patients under anesthesia and in cooperative older patients.
- *Ultrasound guidance*: In the opinion of the author, when available, ultrasound guidance is safer than manual palpation. It assures that the botulinum toxin is delivered in the parenchyma of the gland while avoiding injecting into blood vessels or muscles as this may lead to dysphagia and weakness of swallow and mastication.[58] Both the parotid and the submandibular glands can be very well appreciated with the ultrasound. While the injection needle may not be always visualized, the motion of adjacent tissue can be clearly observed. The normal parotid is seen via ultrasound as a homogeneous echo texture that is similar to the thyroid gland. While the facial nerve is usually not identified, the retromandibular vein can be a useful landmark as the nerve follows an arc immediately lateral to the retromandibular vein and postero-lateral to the ramus of the mandible. The deep parotid lobe is only partially visible because of interference from the mandibular ramus.[59] For submandibular gland (SMG) visualization, the ultrasound is usually placed in a transverse view, where the SMG has an oval to triangular shape. The larger part of the gland is superficial to the mylohyoid and a smaller and deeper lobe wraps around the posterior border of the muscle. The facial artery loops through the gland's posterior portion, and the submandibular duct is not visible by ultrasound unless dilated. After turning the head of the patient opposite to the site to be injected, the needle is introduced into the deep aspect of the gland and aspiration is done to ensure that the needle is not in a vessel. As botulinum toxin is injected its diffusion is visualized in real time, the needle is withdrawn slowly stopping during withdrawal to inject small amount of the toxin. When the needle is close to the surface, the needle is angled anteriomedially (AM) and advanced within the superficial lobe. Repeated injections can be done using the described technique.[60] The parotid gland is usually injected over two or three tracts and the submandibular gland in one to three passes.[53]
- *Electromyography (EMG) guidance:* This technique is not as widely used as ultrasound guidance. It is useful to avoid intramuscular injection, therefore preventing the potential risk of worsening dysphagia or aspiration.[61] An electromyography needle is attached to the syringe filled with botulinum toxin and ground and reference electrodes are installed in the neck. The absence of motor unit potentials confirms the correct placement of the injecting needle in the glandular tissue.

Our experience confirms the safety of this treatment when injected in a guided fashion. A review of 1200 injections in our prospectively collected database revealed no deaths and no major morbidities related to botulinum toxin A injection in our clinic.[1] We believe this is the result of using guided injections, a smaller volume of injected fluid, and the smallest effective dosage. None of our patients have required a feeding tube for dysphagia post-injection unlike many other series in the literature. However, 10% of patients did not respond to the treatment, even after having increased the dosage.[1] Common side effects include tenderness, erythema at the injection site, and increased saliva thickness. Complications reported in the literature include dysphagia, weakened motor control of the head, and aspiration pneumonia.[62] These uncommon side effects are presumably caused by diffusion of the toxin into the surrounding neck muscles, or inadvertent injection into these muscles. Other reported side effects include local injuries of vessels or branches of the facial nerve.[53] Many of the complications reported were caused by the general anesthesia administered during the procedure rather than the injection per se.[10] Patients are seen 6 weeks to 2 months after the first injection and subsequent follow-up visits can be spaced out longer as recurrent injection give longer lasting effects.[52]

12.9 Conclusion

Effective procedures for the treatment of drooling or sialorrhea include techniques to divert the saliva such as duct relocation and others to reduce the amount of saliva such as salivary ductal ligation, submandibular gland excision, and botulinum toxin injection in the salivary glands.

Documenting the physical and psychosocial impact on the child and caregivers is crucial in order to recommend the appropriate treatment strategy and to establish a baseline in order to monitor long-term success.

12.10 Highlights

a. Indications
   - Patients who fail conservative interventions including rehabilitation and pharmacotherapy.
   - Patients with severe to profuse anterior drooling that are older than 6 years.
   - Patients with posterior drooling at risk of pulmonary aspiration.
   - Patients requiring chronic and frequent care to manage secretions.
   - An interdisciplinary team approach to children with sialorrhea, whereby each patient is offered a number of rehabilitative, medical, and surgical options based on a consensus recommendation can be valuable.
b. Contraindications
   - Healthy patients under age 4 years with anterior drooling and who are likely to improve spontaneously.

   - Salivary duct relocation should never be performed in posterior drooling, as it will only worsen the problem.
c. Complications
   - Xerostomia.
   - Increase in dental caries.
   - Hypertrophic scar, risk of injury to the marginal mandibular, lingual, and hypoglossal nerves in submandibular gland excision.
   - Ranula, risk of aspiration, in submandibular gland relocation.
   - sialocele, parotitis, sialadenitis, recurrence, weakness of the buccal branch of the facial, lingual nerve injury, ranula, in ductal ligation.
   - Tympanic membrane perforation, taste disturbance, and recurrence, in tympanic neurectomy.
   - Dysphagia, weakened motor control of the head, local diffusion, in botulinum toxin injection.
d. Special preoperative considerations
   - The radionuclide salivagram is sensitive and specific for detecting pulmonary aspiration of saliva.
   - General Endotracheal Anesthesia; nasal intubation can be helpful in intra-oral surgery.
   - Optimizing the pulmonary condition in patients with lung disease as a result of chronic aspiration.
   - Using rapid sequence induction in patients with reflux.
   - Documenting the impact of drooling on the child and the family using a validated scale (such as the DDIS).
e. Special intraoperative considerations
   - Using active warming measures in patients with neuromuscular conditions that put them at risk for hypothermia.
   - Facial nerve monitoring in submandibular gland excision.
   - Using good exposure, headlight, and magnification, for ductal ligation and relocation.
f. Special postoperative considerations
   - An overnight hospitalization depending on co-morbid conditions.
   - Antibiotics.
   - Long-term follow-up to monitor for relapse.

References

[1] Daniel SJ. Multidisciplinary management of sialorrhea in children. Laryngoscope 2012;122(Suppl 4):S67–S68
[2] Navazesh M, Kumar SK; University of Southern California School of Dentistry. Measuring salivary flow: challenges and opportunities. J Am Dent Assoc 2008;139(Suppl):35S–40S
[3] Senner JE, Logemann J, Zecker S, Gaebler-Spira D. Drooling, saliva production, and swallowing in cerebral palsy. Dev Med Child Neurol 2004;46(12):801–806
[4] Cardona I, Saint-Martin C, Daniel SJ. Salivary glands of healthy children versus sialorrhea children, is there an anatomical difference? An ultrasonographic biometry. Int J Pediatr Otorhinolaryngol 2015;79(5):644–647

[5] Zenk J, Hosemann WG, Iro H. Diameters of the main excretory ducts of the adult human submandibular and parotid gland: a histologic study. Oral Surg Oral Med Oral Pathol Oral Radiol Endod 1998;85(5):576–580

[6] Horsburgh A, Massoud TF. The salivary ducts of Wharton and Stenson: analysis of normal variant sialographic morphometry and a historical review. Ann Anat 2013;195(3):238–242

[7] Benson J, Daugherty KK. Botulinum toxin A in the treatment of sialorrhea. Ann Pharmacother 2007;41(1):79–85

[8] Lim M, Mace A, Nouraei SA, Sandhu G. Botulinum toxin in the management of sialorrhoea: a systematic review. Clin Otolaryngol 2006;31(4):267–272

[9] Hay N, Penn C. Botox(®) to reduce drooling in a paediatric population with neurological impairments: a Phase I study. Int J Lang Commun Disord 2011;46(5):550–563

[10] Khan WU, Campisi P, Nadarajah S, et al. Botulinum toxin A for treatment of sialorrhea in children: an effective, minimally invasive approach. Arch Otolaryngol Head Neck Surg 2011;137(4):339–344

[11] Schroeder AS, Kling T, Huss K, et al. Botulinum toxin type A and B for the reduction of hypersalivation in children with neurological disorders: a focus on effectiveness and therapy adherence. Neuropediatrics 2012;43(1):27–36

[12] Guntinas-Lichius O. Injection of botulinum toxin type B for the treatment of otolaryngology patients with secondary treatment failure of botulinum toxin type A. Laryngoscope 2003;113(4):743–745

[13] Lakraj AA, Moghimi N, Jabbari B. Sialorrhea: anatomy, pathophysiology and treatment with emphasis on the role of botulinum toxins. Toxins (Basel) 2013;5(5):1010–1031

[14] Heinen F, Molenaers G, Fairhurst C, et al. European consensus table 2006 on botulinum toxin for children with cerebral palsy. Eur J Paediatr Neurol 2006;10(5–6):215–225

[15] Fuster Torres MA, Berini Aytés L, Gay Escoda C. Salivary gland application of botulinum toxin for the treatment of sialorrhea. Med Oral Patol Oral Cir Bucal 2007;12(7):E511–E517

[16] Freudenreich O. Drug-induced sialorrhea. Drugs Today (Barc) 2005;41(6):411–418

[17] Drug-induced sialorrhoea and excessive saliva accumulation. Prescrire Int 2009;18(101):119–121

[18] Jongerius PH, van Hulst K, van den Hoogen FJ, Rotteveel JJ. The treatment of posterior drooling by botulinum toxin in a child with cerebral palsy. J Pediatr Gastroenterol Nutr 2005;41(3):351–353

[19] Daniel SJ. Alternative to tracheotomy in a newborn with CHARGE association. Arch Otolaryngol Head Neck Surg 2008;134(3):322–323

[20] George KS, Kiani H, Witherow H. Effectiveness of botulinum toxin B in the treatment of drooling. Br J Oral Maxillofac Surg 2013;51(8):783–785

[21] Reid SM, Johnson HM, Reddihough DS. The Drooling Impact Scale: a measure of the impact of drooling in children with developmental disabilities. Dev Med Child Neurol 2010;52(2):e23–e28

[22] Thomas-Stonell N, Greenberg J. Three treatment approaches and clinical factors in the reduction of drooling. Dysphagia 1988;3(2):73–78

[23] Camp-Bruno JA, Winsberg BG, Green-Parsons AR, Abrams JP. Efficacy of benztropine therapy for drooling. Dev Med Child Neurol 1989;31(3):309–319

[24] van Hulst K, Lindeboom R, van der Burg J, Jongerius P. Accurate assessment of drooling severity with the 5-minute drooling quotient in children with developmental disabilities. Dev Med Child Neurol 2012;54(12):1121–1126

[25] Kofke WA. Anesthetic management of the patient with epilepsy or prior seizures. Curr Opin Anaesthesiol 2010;23(3):391–399

[26] Zighetti ML, Fontana G, Lussana F, et al. Effects of chronic administration of valproic acid to epileptic patients on coagulation tests and primary hemostasis. Epilepsia 2015;56(1):e49–e52

[27] Kang Y, Chun MH, Lee SJ. Evaluation of salivary aspiration in brain-injured patients with tracheostomy. Ann Rehabil Med 2013;37(1):96–102

[28] Heyman S, Respondek M. Detection of pulmonary aspiration in children by radionuclide "salivagram". J Nucl Med 1989;30(5):697–699

[29] Yan Z, Ding N, Liu X, Hua H. Congenital agenesis of all major salivary glands and absence of unilateral lacrimal puncta: a case report and review of the literature. Acta Otolaryngol 2012;132(6):671–675

[30] Daniel SJ, Blaser S, Forte V. Unilateral agenesis of the parotid gland: an unusual entity. Int J Pediatr Otorhinolaryngol 2003;67(4):395–397

[31] Daniel SJ. Controversies in the management of pediatric sialorrhea. Curr Otorhinolaryngol Rep 2015;3:1–8

[32] Pitak-Arnnop P. Dental health care for drooling patients: personal comments. Clin Otolaryngol 2014;39(2):131–132

[33] Ferraz Dos Santos B, Dabbagh B, Daniel SJ, Schwartz S. Association of onabotulinum toxin A treatment with salivary pH and dental caries of neurologically impaired children with sialorrhea. Int J Paediatr Dent 2015

[34] Crysdale WS, White A. Submandibular duct relocation for drooling: a 10-year experience with 194 patients. Otolaryngol Head Neck Surg 1989;101(1):87–92

[35] Chakravarti A, Gupta R, Garg S, Aneja S. Bilateral submandibular duct transposition with sublingual gland excision for cerebral palsy children with drooling. Indian J Pediatr 2014;81(6):623–624

[36] Ozgenel GY, Ozcan M. Bilateral parotid-duct diversion using autologous vein grafts for the management of chronic drooling in cerebral palsy. Br J Plast Surg 2002;55(6):490–493

[37] Manrique D, do Brasil OdeO, Ramos H. Drooling: analysis and evaluation of 31 children who underwent bilateral submandibular gland excision and parotid duct ligation. Rev Bras Otorrinolaringol (Engl Ed) 2007;73(1):40–44

[38] Gallagher TQ, Hartnick CJ. Bilateral submandibular gland excision and parotid duct ligation. Adv Otorhinolaryngol 2012;73:70–75

[39] Stern Y, Feinmesser R, Collins M, Shott SR, Cotton RT. Bilateral submandibular gland excision with parotid duct ligation for treatment of sialorrhea in children: long-term results. Arch Otolaryngol Head Neck Surg 2002;128(7):801–803

[40] Maria OM, Maria SM, Redman RS, et al. Effects of double ligation of Stensen's duct on the rabbit parotid gland. Biotech Histochem 2014;89(3):181–198

[41] Chanu NP, Sahni JK, Aneja S, Naglot S. Four-duct ligation in children with drooling. Am J Otolaryngol 2012;33(5):604–607

[42] Klem C, Mair EA. Four-duct ligation: a simple and effective treatment for chronic aspiration from sialorrhea. Arch Otolaryngol Head Neck Surg 1999;125(7):796–800

[43] Shirley WP, Hill JS, Woolley AL, Wiatrak BJ. Success and complications of four-duct ligation for sialorrhea. Int J Pediatr Otorhinolaryngol 2003;67(1):1–6

[44] Heywood RL, Cochrane LA, Hartley BE. Parotid duct ligation for treatment of drooling in children with neurological impairment. J Laryngol Otol 2009;123(9):997–1001

[45] Martin TJ, Conley SF. Long-term efficacy of intra-oral surgery for sialorrhea. Otolaryngol Head Neck Surg 2007;137(1):54–58

[46] Scheffer AR, Bosch KJ, van Hulst K, van den Hoogen FJ. Salivary duct ligation for anterior and posterior drooling: our experience in twenty-one children. Clin Otolaryngol 2013;38(5):425–429

[47] Thomas RL. Tympanic neurectomy and chorda tympani section. Aust N Z J Surg 1980;50(4):352–355

[48] Daube D, et al. Management of chronic sialorrhea with argon laser chorda tympani and tympanic plexus neurectomy. Oper Tech Otolaryngol—Head Neck Surg 1995;6:241–244

[49] Shott SR, Myer CM III, Cotton RT. Surgical management of sialorrhea. Otolaryngol Head Neck Surg 1989;101(1):47–50

[50] Parisier SC, Blitzer A, Binder WJ, Friedman WF, Marovitz WF. Evaluation of tympanic neurectomy and chorda tympanectomy surgery. Otolaryngology 1978;86(2):ORL308–ORL321

[51] Suskind DL, Tilton A. Clinical study of botulinum-A toxin in the treatment of sialorrhea in children with cerebral palsy. Laryngoscope 2002;112(1):73–81

[52] Bhayani MK, Suskind DL. The use of botulinum toxin in patients with sialorrhea. Oper Tech Otolaryngol—Head Neck Surg 2008;19:243–247

[53] Scully C, Limeres J, Gleeson M, Tomás I, Diz P. Drooling. J Oral Pathol Med 2009;38(4):321–327

[54] Racette BA, Good L, Sagitto S, Perlmutter JS. Botulinum toxin B reduces sialorrhea in parkinsonism. Mov Disord 2003;18 (9):1059–1061

[55] Daniel SJ. Pediatric sialorrhea: medical and surgical options. In: Hartnick CJ, ed. Sataloff's Comprehensive Textbook of Otolaryngology Head & Neck Surgery. Jaypee; 2016:807–814

[56] Nordgarden H, Østerhus I, Møystad A, et al. Drooling: are botulinum toxin injections into the major salivary glands a good treatment option? J Child Neurol 2012;27(4):458–464

[57] Vashishta R, Nguyen SA, White DR, Gillespie MB. Botulinum toxin for the treatment of sialorrhea: a meta-analysis. Otolaryngol Head Neck Surg 2013;148(2):191–196

[58] Schroeder AS, Berweck S, Lee SH, Heinen F. Botulinum toxin treatment of children with cerebral palsy: a short review of different injection techniques. Neurotox Res 2006;9(2–3):189–196

[59] Orloff LA, Hwang HS, Jecker P. The role of ultrasound in the diagnosis and management of salivary disease. Oper Tech Otolaryngol—Head Neck Surg 2009;20:136–144

[60] Gok G, Cox N, Bajwa J, Christodoulou D, Moody A, Howlett DC. Ultrasound-guided injection of botulinum toxin A into the submandibular gland in children and young adults with sialorrhoea. Br J Oral Maxillofac Surg 2013;51(3):231–233

[61] Jackson CE, Gronseth G, Rosenfeld J, et al; Muscle Study Group. Randomized double-blind study of botulinum toxin type B for sialorrhea in ALS patients. Muscle Nerve 2009;39(2):137–143

[62] Chan KH, Liang C, Wilson P, Higgins D, Allen GC. Long-term safety and efficacy data on botulinum toxin type A: an injection for sialorrhea. JAMA Otolaryngol Head Neck Surg 2013;139(2):134–138

13 Thyroglossal Duct Cyst Excision

Oshri Wasserzug, Ari DeRowe, Dan M. Fliss

Summary

Thyroglossal duct cyst (TGDC) is the most common congenital malformation of the neck, usually diagnosed in children. TGDC usually presents as an asymptomatic, painless, mobile neck mass located anterior to the hyoid bone. The differential diagnosis includes dermoid cysts, branchial cleft cysts and lymphadenopathy. TGDC carcinoma is very rare in children. The treatment of TGDC is surgical excision, which includes excision of the cyst, the duct and the middle portion of the hyoid bone, as well as resection of a cuff of lingual musculature. An ultrasound of the neck is performed before the surgery in order to confirm the presence of an orthotopic thyroid gland. Recurrence is the most common postoperative complication, which range between 5.2 to 33%.

Keywords: Neck mass, midline, ultrasound, Sistrunk procedure, hyoid, tract, recurrence

13.1 Introduction

TGDC is the most common congenital malformation of the neck.[1] It is usually diagnosed in children, but it may occur at any age.[2] TGDCs form as a result of failure of the thyroglossal duct to obliterate during the embryonic period.

Thyroid development is usually completed by the end of the eighth week of gestation, and the thyroglossal duct involutes between the 8th and 10th week of gestation. If viable epithelium persists somewhere along the path of the thyroglossal duct, TGDC may form. Hence, TGDC can appear anywhere from the foramen cecum to the level of the thyroid gland.[3,4] Most commonly the tract is located anterior to the hyoid bone,[5] but it may be located posterior to the hyoid bone in up to 30% of the patients.[6]

TGDC usually presents as an asymptomatic, painless, mobile neck mass that move superiorly upon swallowing.[7,8] TGDCs most commonly appear in the midline. Less than 1% are located off the midline.[3,4]

Shah and colleagues[9] classified the location of TGDC into four subdivisions:
1. Intralingual.
2. Suprahyoid/submental.
3. Thyrohyoid.
4. Suprasternal.

It is usually located just above or below the hyoid bone, but up to one-third of the cases may present in the lower cervical regions or in the submental space.

The differential diagnosis includes: Dermoid cysts, branchial cleft cysts, lymphadenopathy, lymphatic malformations, lipomas, hemangiomas, ectopic thyroid gland, and sebaceous cysts. TGDC carcinoma is very rare in children, and is reported to occur in less than 1% of TGDCs in adults.[10,11]

Although usually asymptomatic, TGDC may present with acute suppurative infection—swelling, erythema of the skin, pain, and spontaneous drainage of pus. Surgery is deferred in these cases, and a course of antibiotics should be administered first. Surgery should be performed 6 weeks after resolution of the infection. The lingual subtype may cause upper airway obstruction, dysphagia, odynophagia, and even stridor.

The radiologic criteria for differentiating TGDC from other midline cervical masses is based on the presence of cystic or ductular structures.[12] Recently, Choy et al[13] reported of additional features that can differentiate TGDC from dermoid cysts. TGDC were significantly more likely than dermoid cysts to have an irregular shape, ill-defined margins, attachment to the hyoid bone, an intramuscular location, multilocularity, heterogeneous internal echogenicity, and longitudinal extension into the tongue base.[13]

Because of the high risk for recurrent infections and the possibility (although rare, approaching 1%) of malignancy, the treatment of TGDC is surgical excision.

Traditionally, excision of a TGDC included simple excision of the cyst and the duct. In 1893, Schlange[14] reported of excision of the cyst, the duct, and the middle portion of the hyoid bone, based on his knowledge in embryology. In 1920, Sistrunk[15] reported of a new technique, which included also resection of a cuff of lingual musculature. This procedure, named after him as "the Sistrunk procedure," is still recognized as the most effective surgical treatment of TGDC, due to its low rate of recurrence.[2] Several authors reported of variants of the Sistrunk procedure, basically suggesting wider dissections, removal of more tongue base tissue or central neck dissection.[16]

Although uncommon, when the TGDC is located low in the neck, a stepladder approach with at least two separate horizontal incisions is required in order to be able to complete the dissection all the way to the hyoid bone and the deep lingual musculature.[17]

13.2 Preoperative Evaluation and Anesthesia

An ultrasound of the neck mass is performed before the surgery for two reasons. First, in order to confirm the presence of a normal, orthotopic thyroid gland, which is of utmost importance. Second, recent studies report that it may be possible to differentiate between TGDC and dermoid cysts located in the midline.[18] Computerized tomography of the neck is unnecessary.

If there is no orthotopic thyroid gland, thyroid function tests should be performed and the child should be referred to endocrinologist. The lack of an orthotopic thyroid gland may not change the decision to operate but is highly important because the child may have to take thyroid hormones for the rest of his life, and this matter should be discussed with the parents when informed consent is obtained.

13.3 Surgical Technique—Sistrunk Procedure

- A shoulder roll should be used to enhance the exposure of the neck mass and to ease the procedure.
- A transverse cervical skin incision is outlined in the midline, immediately inferior to the neck mass (▶Fig. 13.1).
- The incision site is infiltrated with Lidocadren.
- The incision is carried out through the platysma muscle, taking care not to violate the cyst itself. If the cyst is violated, meticulous dissection encompassing its wall should be undertaken.
- Subplatysmal skin flaps are elevated, superiorly to the level of the hyoid bone and inferiorly to the level of the cricothyroid muscle.
- The strap muscles are divided in the midline and dissection deep to the lower pole of the cyst is performed (▶Fig. 13.2).
- The trachea and the thyroid notch are identified to assist in orientation.
- The cyst is dissected off the surrounding tissues up to the hyoid bone. It should not be separated from the hyoid bone.
- An incision is made along the superior border of the hyoid bone (▶Fig. 13.3). An Allis clamp is used to grasp the hyoid bone, and the contents of the posterior hyoid space are dissected off the surrounding tissues. In cases of revision TGDC excision, a more aggressive

central neck dissection is undertaken to make sure that no tract or cyst remnants are left behind.
- The muscles attached to the midportion of the hyoid bone are dissected off, and Mayo or Liston scissors are used to cut the midportion of the hyoid bone (▶Fig. 13.4). Transecting the hyoid bone at the level of the lesser cornu medial to the anterior belly of the digastric muscle will avoid damage to the hypoglossal nerve.
- If the tract continues superiorly, it is dissected free along with a cuff of tongue musculature.
- A gloved finger is inserted into the mouth to palpate the tongue and tongue base to estimate the depth of the dissection in order to prevent violation of the oropharynx. (▶Fig. 13.5).
- The cyst is removed along with the tract, the midportion of the hyoid bone, and a cuff of tongue musculature.
- Hemostasis is performed and the wound is irrigated with sterile saline solution.
- A passive Penrose drain is left in the surgical field and the strap muscles are reapproximated using 4–0 Vicryl sutures (▶Fig. 13.6).
- The skin is closed in two layers using 4–0 Vicryl for the subdermis and 5–0 Monocril for the dermis.

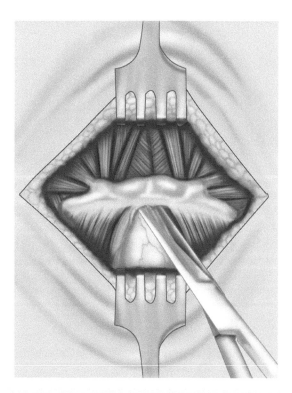

Fig. 13.2 Division of the strap muscles in the midline and exposure of the cyst.

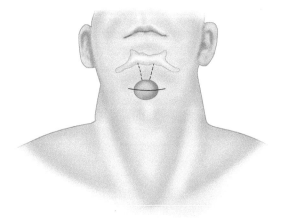

Fig. 13.1 Incision site for Sistrunk procedure.

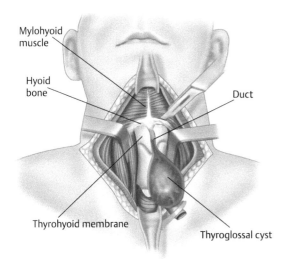

Fig. 13.3 An incision is made along the superior border of the hyoid bone.

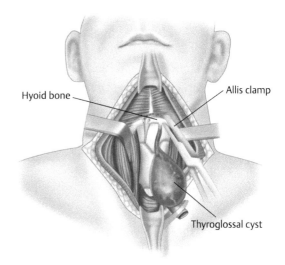

Fig. 13.4 Mayo or Liston scissors are used to cut the midportion of the hyoid bone

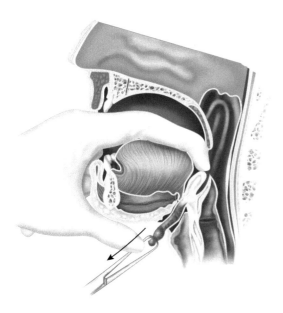

Fig. 13.5 A gloved finger is inserted into the mouth to palpate the tongue and tongue base.

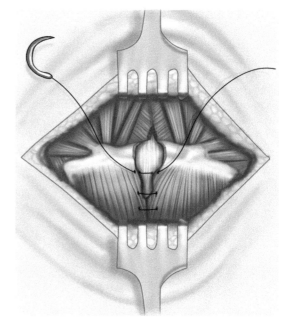

Fig. 13.6 Reapproximation of the strap muscles.

13.4 Surgical Technique—Revision

- Excision of the previous skin incision and fistula.
- Elevation of subplatysmal skin flaps.
- Dissection of the TGDC remnant with a wide cuff of normal tissue. Some surgeons perform central neck dissection.
- Removal of 1 cm of tissue surrounding the foramen cecum.

13.5 Postoperative Treatment

Antibiotics are not routinely administered. However, if an active infection is identified during the surgery, antibiotics are administered postoperatively.

The child is observed overnight because possible postoperative complications include airway compromise and cervical hematoma.

13.6 Complications

- Recurrence is the most common postoperative complication. When the Sistrunk procedure or one of its modifications are used, recurrence rates range between 5.2 and 33%.[19,20,21]
- Hematoma, which may require surgical drainage if the lingual artery is damaged.
- Wound infection.
- Seroma.
- Stitch abscess.
- Wound dehiscence.
- Hypoglossal nerve paralysis.
- Laryngotracheal injury and resultant airway compromise if the trachea or larynx is mistakenly identified as the hyoid bone. For that reason, the author believes that identification of the thyroid notch is a mandatory step in the Sistrunk procedure.
- Hypothyroidism, if no orthotopic thyroid gland exists.

13.7 Highlights

- TGDC has a 1% potential of malignancy, and hence the diagnosis of a TGDC mandates its surgical excision.
- Preoperative ultrasound confirming the presence of an orthotopic thyroid gland should be undertaken before the surgery.
- Recurrence rates range between 5% and 33%.
- Without removal of the midportion of the hyoid bone, recurrence rates may be greater than 50%.
- In cases of recurrence, a more aggressive tissue removal at the base of tongue should be performed.

References

[1] Santiago W, Rybak LP, Bass RM. Thyroglossal duct cyst of the tongue. J Otolaryngol 1985;14(4):261–264

[2] Maddalozzo J, Venkatesan TK, Gupta P. Complications associated with the Sistrunk procedure. Laryngoscope 2001;111(1):119–123

[3] Guarisco JL. Congenital head and neck masses in infants and children. Part I. Ear Nose Throat J 1991;70(1):40–47

[4] Guarisco JL. Congenital head and neck masses in infants and children. Part II. Ear Nose Throat J 1991;70(2):75–82

[5] Ellis PD, van Nostrand AW. The applied anatomy of thyroglossal tract remnants. Laryngoscope 1977;87(5 Pt 1):765–770

[6] Chandra RK, Maddalozzo J, Kovarik P. Histological characterization of the thyroglossal tract: implications for surgical management. Laryngoscope 2001;111(6):1002–1005

[7] Lin ST, Tseng FY, Hsu CJ, Yeh TH, Chen YS. Thyroglossal duct cyst: a comparison between children and adults. Am J Otolaryngol 2008;29(2):83–87

[8] Prasad KC, Dannana NK, Prasad SC. Thyroglossal duct cyst: an unusual presentation. Ear Nose Throat J 2006;85(7):454–456

[9] Shah R, Gow K, Sobol SE. Outcome of thyroglossal duct cyst excision is independent of presenting age or symptomatology. Int J Pediatr Otorhinolaryngol 2007;71(11):1731–1735

[10] Motamed M, McGlashan JA. Thyroglossal duct carcinoma. Curr Opin Otolaryngol Head Neck Surg 2004;12(2):106–109

[11] Torcivia A, Polliand C, Ziol M, Dufour F, Champault G, Barrat C. Papillary carcinoma of the thyroglossal duct cyst: report of two cases. Rom J Morphol Embryol 2010;51(4):775–777

[12] Lee DH, Jung SH, Yoon TM, Lee JK, Joo YE, Lim SC. Preoperative computed tomography of suspected thyroglossal duct cysts in children under 10-years-of-age. Int J Pediatr Otorhinolaryngol 2013;77(1):45–48

[13] Choi HI, Choi YH, Cheon JE, Kim WS, Kim IO. Ultrasonographic features differentiating thyroglossal duct cysts from dermoid cysts. Ultrasonography 2018;37(1):71–77

[14] Schlange H. Ueber die fistula colli congenita. Arch Klin Chir 1893;46:390–392

[15] Sistrunk WE. The surgical treatment of cysts of the thyroglossal tract. Ann Surg 1920;71(2):121–122, 2

[16] Hewitt K, Pysher T, Park A. Management of thyroglossal duct cysts after failed Sistrunk procedure. Laryngoscope 2007;117(4):756–758

[17] Oomen KP, Modi VK, Maddalozzo J. Thyroglossal duct cyst and ectopic thyroid: surgical management. Otolaryngol Clin North Am 2015;48(1):15–27

[18] Oyewumi M, Inarejos E, Greer ML, et al. Ultrasound to differentiate thyroglossal duct cysts and dermoid cysts in children. Laryngoscope 2015;125(4):998–1003

[19] Lin ST, Tseng FY, Hsu CJ, Yeh TH, Chen YS. Thyroglossal duct cyst: a comparison between children and adults. Am J Otolaryngol 2008;29(2):83–87

[20] Davenport M. ABC of general surgery in children: lumps and swellings of the head and neck. BMJ 1996;312(7027):368–371

[21] Swaid AI, Al-Ammar AY. Management of thyroglossal duct cyst. Open Otorhinolaryngol J 2008;2:26–28

14 Branchial Cleft Anomalies, Sinuses, and Cysts

Oshri Wasserzug, Ari DeRowe, Dan M. Fliss

Summary

Branchial cleft anomalies are the most common congenital lateral neck pathologies in children. These lesions can occur as a sinus, a fistula or a cyst. First branchial cleft anomalies comprise 5 to 25% of all branchial anomalies, and are a duplication of the external ear canal. They are divided into 2 types, according to the location and the histology.

Second branchial anomalies are the most common, comprising 40 to 95% of all branchial anomalies. They usually present as a painless neck mass, an acute enlargement following upper respiratory tract infection or as a draining pit.

Pyriform fossa anomalies (formerly third and fourth branchial cleft anomalies) are relatively rare. Third branchial cleft sinus usually presents as recurrent thyroid infection or abscess. Fourth branchial cleft anomaly can present either asneonatal neck mass or as recurrent deep neck infection or suppurative thyroiditis. While the treatment of fourth branchial cleft anomaly is endoscopic cauterization, thedefinitive treatment of first, second, and third branchial cleft anomalies is surgical excision.

Keywords: Branchial, sinus, fistula, cyst, tract, neck mass, infection, surgical resection, endoscopic cauterization

14.1 Introduction

Branchial cleft anomalies are the most common congenital lateral neck pathologies in children. These lesions can occur as a sinus (connecting the skin or the pharynx to a blind pouch in the neck), a fistula (an open tract connecting the skin to the pharynx), or a cyst (if there is no connection to the skin or to the pharynx).

The branchial arches appear from the fourth to the seventh gestational weeks. They are located on the supero-lateral aspect of the fetus, and are composed of mesoderm. The arches are separated by external clefts and internal pouches. Each arch develops into a nerve, a blood vessel, and a muscle bundle. Incomplete obliteration of the clefts or grooves between the arches causes a variety of anomalies.

This chapter will focus on the surgical resection of these anomalies. Complete explanation of the normal and pathological developmental process of these structures is beyond the scope of this chapter and hence will not be discussed.

14.2 First Branchial Cleft Anomalies

First branchial cleft anomalies comprise 5 to 25% of all branchial anomalies.[1,2] These anomalies were divided by Work[3] into two types, according to the location and the histology (▶Fig. 14.1a).

Type I first branchial cleft anomalies are less common and considered to be a duplication of the membranous external auditory canal (EAC). It courses parallel to the EAC, supero-lateral to the facial nerve, and terminates either in the cartilaginous–bony junction or in the middle ear cavity, attached to the umbo or to the malleus (▶Fig. 14.1a). Once infected, they drain either to the pre-auricular region, in the post-auricular region, or inferior to the lobule.[4]

Type II cysts are more common. They are considered to be duplications of both the cartilaginous and bony EAC. The tract is located lateral or medial to the facial nerve (▶Fig. 14.1b). Once infected, it presents as otorrhea in the EAC or as a draining pit in the angle of the mandible. Of note, type II cysts may present as cysts in the parotid gland, mimicking a primary parotid mass.[4]

Work type I lesions characteristically occur in young children, presenting as a cystic lesion obstructing the external auditory canal, as a draining pit in the external ear canal or as recurrent infections.

Work type II lesions characteristically occur in older children. They present similarly to type I but can also present as a draining pit in the neck, near the angle of the mandible.

Acute infection should be treated with antibiotics that cover *S. Aureus*, methicillin-resistant *S. aureus,* and upper respiratory tract anaerobes, and incision and drainage may be necessary if an abscess is formed. Surgical removal is indicated shortly after the resolution of the acute infection.

14.2.1 Preoperative Evaluation and Anesthesia

A CT scan with contrast should be performed prior to the surgery. MRI typically demonstrates low T1 signal and high T2 signal, and can be of help in visualizing the parotid gland and its relation to the lesion. The risk of potential facial nerve injury should be discussed with the patient and family.

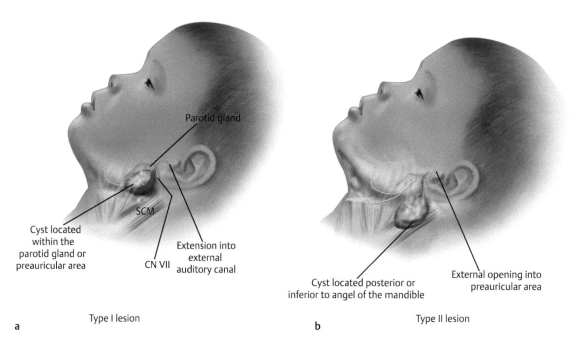

Fig. 14.1 (a, b) First branchial cleft cyst types I and II location. SCM, sternocleidomastoid muscle; CN VII, seventh carnial nerve.

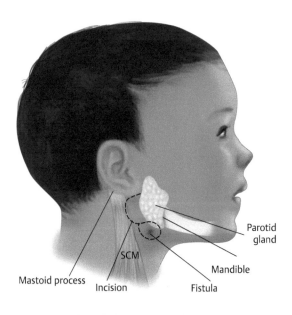

Fig. 14.2 A pre-auricular incision that extends behind the ear and incorporates the fistulous tract in the neck. SCM, sternocleidomastoid muscle.

The anesthesiologist should be informed that the child must not be paralyzed throughout the procedure, in order to enable the surgeon to identify and stimulate the branches of the facial nerve. A nerve integrity monitor should be used.

The neck is extended and the head is rotated to the opposite side.

The face and the upper area of the neck should not be covered with sheets but draped, in order to allow visualization of the mouth angle and the corner of the eye.

14.2.2 Surgical Technique

- A pre-auricular incision that extends behind the ear and incorporates the fistulous tract in the neck is created (▶ Fig. 14.2). A flap is raised to expose the parotid gland, and the fistulous tract is identified and dissected free from the surrounding tissue.
- The facial nerve stem is identified according to the same landmarks used in adults (▶ Fig. 14.3).
- In young children, the nerve is located further laterally, and because the mastoid tip is not fully developed, the nerve can appear more superficial than might be expected.
- Dissection along the fistulous area should be continued. It may lead to a cartilaginous tube containing dermal elements, which should all be resected.
- The fistula usually passes medial to the facial nerve stem and its branches, ending either directly in the external ear canal or in a cartilaginous structure adjacent to the ear canal. This structure should be dissected and excised. Of note, the dissection may leave a defect in the external ear canal which can either be closed primarily or left for secondary healing.
- The dissection continues deep to the facial nerve (▶ Fig. 14.4). Small branches of the superficial temporal artery should be identified and ligated.
- A passive or an active drain is placed in the surgical field, according to the amount of dissection performed.

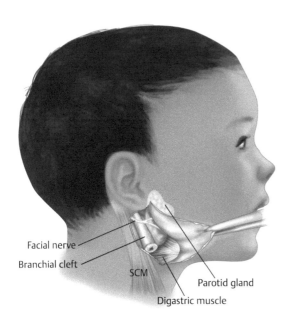

Fig. 14.3 Identification of the facial nerve. SCM, sternocleidomastoid muscle.

The skin flaps are sutured using 4–0 Vicryl for the subcutaneous tissue and a 5–0 Monocryl for the skin.
- A pressure dressing is applied to the wound for 24 hours.

Of note, simple excision of the lesion without facial nerve identification may be suitable for excision of uninfected type I lesions. A nerve integrity monitor should be used in these cases.

14.2.3 Postoperative Treatment

Antibiotics are not routinely administered. If an active infection is identified during the surgery, antibiotics are administered postoperatively. The drain is left in place for 1 to 3 days, depending on the amount of drainage. The child is observed overnight because possible postoperative complications include facial or cervical hematoma.[1]

14.2.4 Complications

- Facial nerve palsy or paralysis.
- Wound infection.
- Wound dehiscence.
- Seroma.
- Hematoma.
- External auditory canal stenosis.

14.3 Second Branchial Cleft Anomalies

Second branchial anomalies are the most common branchial anomalies (40–95%)]. They are located along the anterior border of the sternocleidomastoid muscle.[5,6]

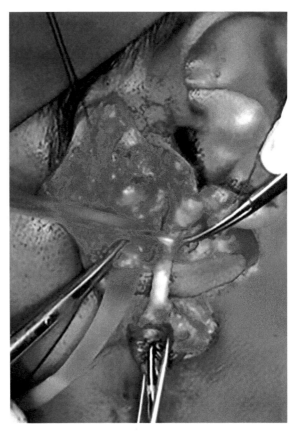

Fig. 14.4 Dissection deep to the facial nerve.

They occur more commonly on the right side and cysts are more common than sinuses or fistulas. Second branchial anomalies can be a manifestation of branchiootorenal (BOR) syndrome, and hence it should be ruled out in children with a family history of similar lesions and children with bilateral lesions. These children should undergo both hearing examination and renal US.

It usually presents as a painless neck mass, an acute enlargement following upper respiratory tract infection or as a draining pit.

Imaging is unnecessary for second branchial cleft sinuses. CT with contrast will demonstrate a homogenous cyst with rim enhancement.

Second branchial cleft fistula starts its course anterior to the SCM and traverses between the external and the internal carotid arteries. Cysts are usually located deep to the platysma and the facial nerve. They are closely related to the glossopharyngeal nerve (CN IX) (▶ Fig. 14.5) which lies medially. The course continues medial to the posterior belly of the digastric muscle, to end in the tonsillar fossa.

Acute infection should be treated with antibiotics that cover *S. Aureus*, methicillin-resistant *S. aureus,* and upper respiratory tract anaerobes, and incision and drainage may be necessary if an abscess is formed.

As a rule of thumb, these lesions are better excised at young age, because in older children these operations may require a stepladder incision in order to perform complete excision of the tract.

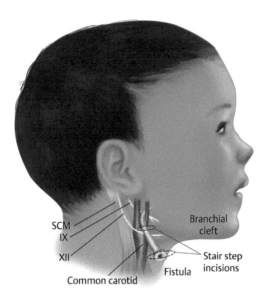

Fig. 14.5 Anatomical relations of the second branchial cleft fistula. SCM, sternocleidomastoid muscle; IX, ninth cranial nerve (glossopharyngeal); XII, twelfth cranial nerve (hypoglossal).

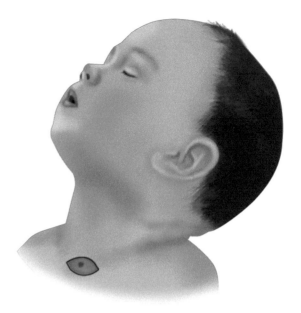

Fig. 14.6 An elliptical incision is performed around the opening of the fistula.

Lacrimal probes and Fogarty catheter are used to cannulate the tract to ease the identification of the tract through its dissection. Methylene blue can also be used to demonstrate the tract.

14.3.2 Surgical Technique

- A lacrimal probe or a Fogarty catheter is inserted into the tract slowly and gently, not to create a false root.
- Diluted methylene blue solution is injected through the probe or the catheter.
- An elliptical incision is performed along skin tension lines around the opening of the fistula (▶ Fig. 14.6).
- The tract is identified and dissected off the adjacent tissues.
- In most cases, adequate retraction enables good exposure of the whole tract. In some cases, the tract is too long and cannot be reached through a single skin incision.
- In these cases, a stepladder incision is required in order to reach the deepest part of the tract (▶ Fig. 14.7). A Mosquito is passed along the tract to its edge and a second skin incision is made above it.
- The tract is pulled through this skin incision and the dissection continues further (▶ Fig. 14.8), taking care not to penetrate the pharyngeal mucosa.
- A clip is applied to the distal part (stump) of the tract which is then excised and sent for definitive pathology (▶ Fig. 14.9).

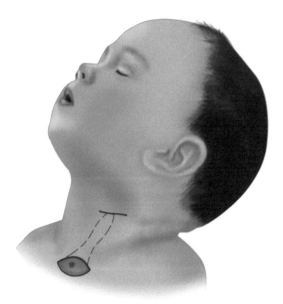

Fig. 14.7 A stepladder incision is created by passing a hemostat along the dissected fistula tract.

14.3.1 Preoperative Evaluation and Anesthesia

The child should not be paralyzed throughout the procedure.

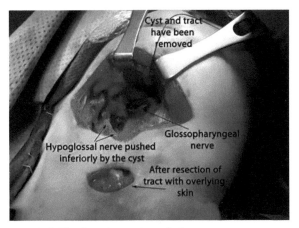

Fig. 14.8 The dissection continues further.

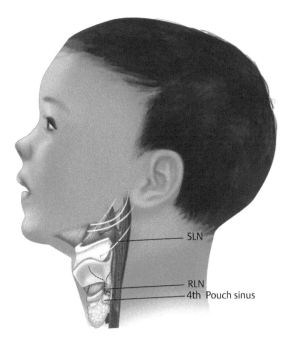

Fig. 14.10 Fourth branchial pouch sinus originating in the rostral end of the pyriform fossa. RLN, recurrent laryngeal nerve; SLN, superior laryngeal nerve.

- A Penrose drain is left in the surgical field, depending on the extensiveness of the dissection and the amount of bleeding during the procedure. Vicryl sutures are used to close the subcutaneous tissue and Monocryl sutures are used to close the skin incision. Compression dressing is used for 24 hours.

14.3.3 Postoperative Treatment

If no signs of infection exist, antibiotics are not required. The child is discharged the next day.

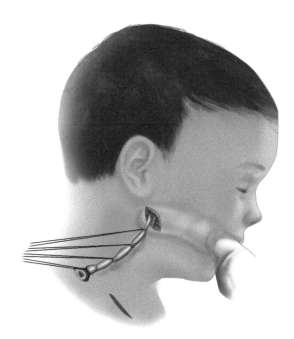

Fig. 14.9 Excision of the tract.

14.3.4 Complications

- Mandibular branch nerve palsy.
- Wound infection.
- Seroma.
- Hematoma.

14.4 Pyriform Fossa Anomalies (Formerly Third and Fourth Branchial Cleft Anomalies)

These lesions are relatively rare, comprising between 2 and 8% of branchial cleft anomalies.[7,8] These lesions are mostly sinuses and not fistulas. Differentiation between a third and fourth branchial pouch sinus can only be made by surgical confirmation of the anatomical course.

The *third* branchial cleft sinus usually presents as recurrent thyroid infection or abscess. It originates in the rostral end of the pyriform fossa, where it can be visualized, and passes cranial to the superior laryngeal nerve (SLN). Then it turns inferiorly between the vagus nerve and the common carotid artery, and ends lateral to the thyroid gland[9] (▶ Fig. 14.10).

The *fourth* branchial pouch sinus is the most uncommon of all branchial cleft anomalies comprising 1 to 4% of all branchial cleft anomalies.[10] It has two characteristic clinical presentations:

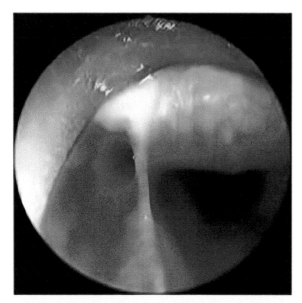

Fig. 14.11 The sinus tract opening at the pyriform apex is identified.

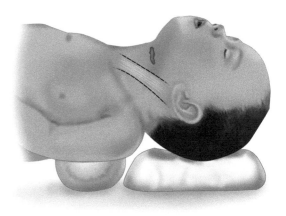

Fig. 14.12 Skin incision for fourth branchial pouch sinus.

- Neonatal neck mass: a neonate presents with a lateral neck cyst or abscess associated with actual or impending airway compromise. The mass mimics a cystic hygroma, and may contain air or increase in size during crying or Valsalva.[11,12]
- Recurrent deep neck infection or suppurative thyroiditis: a child, adolescent, or occasionally an adult presents with recurrent deep neck abscess or suppurative thyroiditis, despite several attempts at drainage or neck exploration.[13,14]

These lesions originate in the hypopharynx behind the thyroid ala, and descend caudal to the SLN and cranial to the recurrent laryngeal nerve (RLN), to end in the thyroid gland or the paratracheal region.[9] They occur on the left side of the neck in 95 to 97% of the cases.[15,16]

14.4.1 Preoperative Evaluation and Anesthesia

The diagnosis can be confirmed by barium swallow, a CT scan, MRI, or in a direct laryngoscopy.[17]

If a neck abscess is present, I&D is the treatment of choice. However, these lesions recur in 89 to 94% of the time, and hence a definitive treatment should follow.[9,13]

Definitive surgical treatment can be performed either endoscopically or through an open tract excision, with or without a hemithyroidectomy. Each of these methods will be discussed separately.

14.4.2 Surgical Technique

Endoscopic Treatment of a Fourth Branchial Cleft Anomalies

Endoscopic cauterization of a fourth branchial cleft anomaly can be performed either by electrocauterization using bipolar or monopolar diathermy, by chemocauterization using trichloroacetic acid, or by application of silver nitrate or fibrin glue.

- The smallest possible endotracheal tube should be used in order to allow for good exposure of the pyriform sinus.
- Teeth guard is inserted, followed by a Lindholm laryngoscope, which is inserted in a manner that elevates the larynx anteriorly and superiorly to better expose the pyriform sinus.
- The sinus tract opening at the pyriform apex is identified (▶ Fig. 14.11). An insulated laryngeal diathermy is inserted superficially into the mucosal layer at the tract opening and the tract is cauterized at low power.

Open Transcervical Excision

- Skin incision is made along the anterior border of the ipsilateral sternocleidomastoid muscle from the superior edge of the thyroid cartilage to the level of the cricoid cartilage (▶ Fig. 14.12).
- The posterior aspect of the lateral thyroid cartilage is exposed by lateral retraction of the SCM muscle.
- In cases where the tract exits from the thyrohyoid membrane superior to the SLN, identification of the pyriform fossa is unnecessary because it is characteristic of a third pouch sinus. The tract is tied and dissected in a retrograde fashion.

- In cases where no tract is apparent close to the thyrohyoid membrane, the diagnosis of a fourth branchial cleft anomaly is confirmed and the pyriform fossa should be exposed: a vertical incision is made along the posterior margin of the lateral thyroid cartilage and inferior cornu down to and through the perichondrium.
- The inferior constrictor is dissected posteriorly, very close to the cartilage, while elevating the perichondrium on the posterior aspect and on the medial side enough to detach the inferior constrictor muscle.
- The posterior edge of the thyroid ala is retracted anteriorly and the joint between the inferior thyroid cornu and the cricoid cartilage is separated as close to the inferior cornu as possible, taking care not to harm the RLN.
- A strip of posterior thyroid ala is resected, exposing the underlying pyriform sinus. In most cases a 1-cm strip suffices. The tract is then ligated from its origin at the pyriform apex.
- The pharyngeal connection must be ligated promptly, as failure to do so may result in recurrence. The tract is resected in a retrograde fashion including the fistula opening at the skin (in cases of a fistula).

14.4.3 Postoperative Treatment

- Soft diet is recommended for 24 hours following endoscopic cauterization.
- Antibiotic treatment is unnecessary.
- When open surgery is undertaken, a passive drain should be left in the surgical field.

14.4.4 Complications

- The RLN can be injured not only during open surgery but also during endoscopic cauterization in the pyriform fossa, causing unilateral vocal cord palsy.
- Wound infection.
- Seroma.
- Hematoma.

14.5 Highlights

- Branchial cleft anomalies are the most common congenital lateral neck pathologies in children.
- First branchial cleft anomalies comprise 5 to 25% of all branchial anomalies and are a duplication of the external ear canal.
- Second branchial anomalies are the most common branchial anomalies, comprising 40 to 95% of all branchial anomalies. It usually presents as a painless neck mass, an acute enlargement following upper respiratory tract infection or as a draining pit.
- Second branchial anomalies can be a manifestation of branchiootorenal (BOR) syndrome.

- These lesions are better excised at young age, because in older children these operations may require a stepladder incisions.
- Pyriform fossa anomalies (formerly third and fourth branchial cleft anomalies) are relatively rare, comprising between 2 to 8% of branchial cleft anomalies.
- Third branchial cleft sinus usually presents as recurrent thyroid infection or abscess.
- Fourth branchial cleft anomaly can present either asneonatal neck mass or as recurrent deep neck infection or suppurative thyroiditis.
- Thetreatment of first, second and third branchial cleft anomalies is surgical excision, whereas the treatment of fourth branchial cleft anomaly is endoscopic cauterization.

References

[1] Bajaj Y, Ifeacho S, Tweedie D, et al. Branchial anomalies in children. Int J Pediatr Otorhinolaryngol 2011;75(8):1020–1023

[2] Liberman M, Kay S, Emil S, et al. Ten years of experience with third and fourth branchial remnants. J Pediatr Surg 2002;37(5): 685–690

[3] Work WP. Newer concepts of first branchial cleft defects. Laryngoscope 1972;82(9):1581–1593

[4] Liu W, Chen M, Hao J, Yang Y, Zhang J, Ni X. The treatment for the first branchial cleft anomalies in children. Eur Arch Otorhinolaryngol 2017;274(9):3465–3470

[5] Al-Mufarrej F, Stoddard D, Bite U. Branchial arch anomalies: Recurrence, malignant degeneration and operative complications. Int J Pediatr Otorhinolaryngol 2017;97:24–29

[6] Ford GR, Balakrishnan A, Evans JN, Bailey CM. Branchial cleft and pouch anomalies. J Laryngol Otol 1992;106(2):137–143

[7] James A, Stewart C, Warrick P, Tzifa C, Forte V. Branchial sinus of the pyriform fossa: reappraisal of third and fourth branchial anomalies. Laryngoscope 2007;117(11):1920–1924

[8] Neff L, Kirse D, Pranikoff T. An unusual presentation of a fourth pharyngeal arch (branchial cleft) sinus. J Pediatr Surg 2009;44(3):626–629

[9] Rosenfeld RM, Biller HF. Fourth branchial pouch sinus: diagnosis and treatment. Otolaryngol Head Neck Surg 1991;105(1):44–50

[10] Watson GJ, Nichani JR, Rothera MP, Bruce IA. Case series: endoscopic management of fourth branchial arch anomalies. Int J Pediatr Otorhinolaryngol 2013;77(5):766–769

[11] Takai SI, Miyauchi A, Matsuzuka F, Kuma K, Kosaki G. Internal fistula as a route of infection in acute suppurative thyroiditis. Lancet 1979;1(8119):751–752

[12] Lee FP. Occult congenital pyriform sinus fistula causing recurrent left lower neck abscess. Head Neck 1999;21(7):671–676

[13] Nicollas R, Ducroz V, Garabédian EN, Triglia JM. Fourth branchial pouch anomalies: a study of six cases and review of the literature. Int J Pediatr Otorhinolaryngol 1998;44(1):5–10

[14] Taylor WE Jr, Myer CM III, Hays LL, Cotton RT. Acute suppurative thyroiditis in children. Laryngoscope 1982;92(11):1269–1273

[15] Godin MS, Kearns DB, Pransky SM, Seid AB, Wilson DB. Fourth branchial pouch sinus: principles of diagnosis and management. Laryngoscope 1990;100(2 Pt 1):174–178

[16] Shugar MA, Healy GB. The fourth branchial cleft anomaly. Head Neck Surg 1980;3(1):72–75

[17] Garrel R, Jouzdani E, Gardiner Q, et al. Fourth branchial pouch sinus: from diagnosis to treatment. Otolaryngol Head Neck Surg 2006;134(1):157–163

15 Preauricular Anomalies

Lindsey Moses, Max M. April

Summary

A preauricular pit is a benign congenital malformation of the preauricular soft tissues that may be accompanied by a sinus tract or subcutaneous cyst. In a minority of cases, the presence of a preauricular anomaly may be associated with a multiple congenital anomaly syndrome. Most preauricular anomalies are asymptomatic, however approximately 25% of patients will experience an infection at some point after which excision of the pit and associated cyst/sinus tract is indicated. Excision is best performed under general anesthesia during a period of quiescence following infection. The supra-auricular approach offers a lower recurrence rate that simple cyst excision and is the preferred technique. Dissection along the helical cartilage ensures that the sinus tract will not be violated, and a cuff of cartilage can be safely taken along with the soft tissues if needed. Skin can be closed primarily and Dermabond used to create a water-tight seal. Postoperatively, Tylenol and Motrin are sufficient for pain control and antibiotics are not needed. Risks associated with the procedure are low and consist primarily of minor wound complications.

Keywords: Preauricular pit, congenital anomaly

15.1 Introduction

The preauricular pit is a benign congenital malformation of the preauricular soft tissues first described by Heusinger in 1864.[1-3] It is most frequently noted during routine physical exam and appears as a small pit close to the anterior margin of the ascending portion of the helix (▶ Fig. 15.1). The sinus pit may represent the full extent of the deformity or the beginning of a tortuous sinus tract,

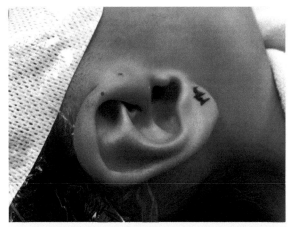

Fig. 15.1 Preauricular pit after injection of local anesthesia.

an adjacent subcutaneous cyst may also be present.[4,5] The most accepted theory is that the development of a preauricular sinus is due to incomplete or defective fusion of the six hillocks of His during the development of the external ear during the sixth week of gestation.[1-6] The majority are asymptomatic; however, they can become infected and present with pain, swelling, erythema, discharge, or abscess formation in approximately 25% of patients.[2] Surgical excision is indicated after an episode of symptomatic infection and should be performed during a period of quiescence. The incidence of preauricular sinuses varies among populations and is estimated to be 0.1% to 0.9% among Western populations, 4% to 6% in Asians and up to 10% in some regions of Africa.[5] Greater than 50% of cases are unilateral and sporadic. Bilateral cases are more likely to be inherited by incomplete autosomal dominance with reduced penetrance.[1]

The initial surgical technique used for excision was the simple sinectomy, in which an elliptical incision is made around the pit and the sinus tract is followed and excised. Due to the variation in sinus tracts and small ramifications that may be present, this technique resulted in a high recurrence rate likely secondary to incomplete excision. In 1990 Prasad described the supra-auricular approach in which the incision is extended postauricularly and all subcutaneous tissues between the temporalis fascia and cartilage of the helix are removed en bloc without dissection of the sinus tract.[7] He reported a recurrence rate of 42% with simple sinectomy and only 5% with the supra-auricular approach. Further studies have shown similar results; Lam et al reported in 2001 a recurrence rate of 32% with simple sinectomy versus 3.7% with the supra-auricular approach.[6] A meta-analysis by El-Anwar looking at all published series of preauricular cases since 2001 showed a recurrence rate of 8.1% with simple sinectomy and 1.2% with supra-auricular approach, a smaller yet statistically significant difference.[3]

15.2 Preoperative Evaluation and Anesthesia

Preauricular sinus pits are most often an isolated congenital malformation requiring no further workup. However, like many other malformations related to the ear, the incidence of renal anomalies in patients with preauricular sinus pits is higher than that in the general population.[1] Guidelines developed by Wang et al in 2001 state that a patient with isolated preauricular pit(s) accompanied by any one of the following should undergo renal ultrasound to aid in the diagnosis of a multiple congenital anomaly syndrome: maternal history of gestational diabetes, family history of deafness, branchial cleft sinus or cyst, another malformation or dysmorphic feature of the face, limbs, heart, or gastrointestinal system.[8] In all other cases, renal ultrasound is not recommended.

Surgery is indicated only in cases of symptomatic infection and should be performed after complete resolution of infection or drainage from the sinus. Preoperative clearance should be obtained from a pediatrician.

Excision can be performed under local or general anesthesia, although superior results with lower recurrence rates have been shown when general anesthesia was used.[1,2,5] This is likely due to patient intolerance and potential distortion of tissues from infiltration of local anesthesia around the areas of dissection.[1] We recommend the procedure be performed under general anesthesia in all cases unless contraindicated by patient factors.

15.3 Surgical Technique

An ear wick is placed in the external auditory canal and the patient is prepped and draped in a sterile fashion (▶Fig. 15.2). Using a 15-blade, an elliptical incision is made around the pit and extended superiorly then posteriorly around the ear to complete the supra-auricular incision.

The Colorado tip bovie is then used to dissect down to cartilage at the supra-auricular apex of the incision. Once helical cartilage is identified, dissection is carried forward in this plane (▶Fig. 15.3 and ▶Fig. 15.4). By maintaining contact with cartilage, which serves as the posterior border of the sinus tract, you avoid the potential hazard of violating the cyst and risking recurrence (▶Fig. 15.5 and

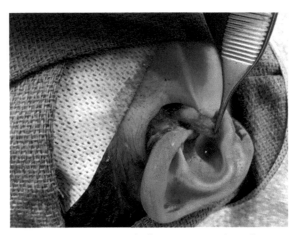

Fig. 15.3 Starting posteriorly, dissection is carried out along helical cartilage until the back wall of the cyst is encountered.

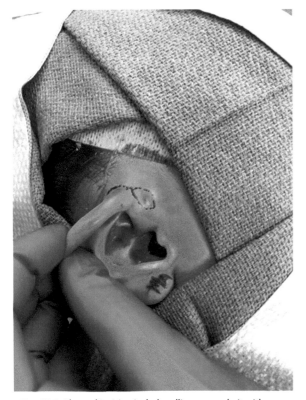

Fig. 15.2 Planned incision includes ellipse around pit with supra-auricular extension.

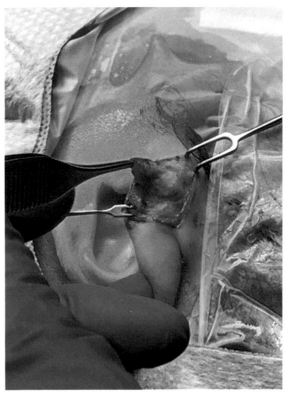

Fig. 15.4 Supra-auricular incision and dissection to posterior limit of sinus tract.

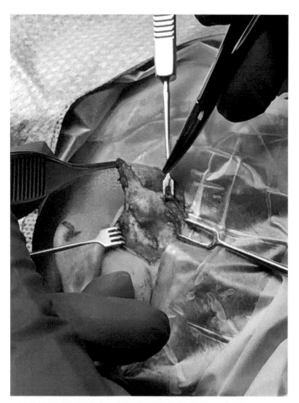

Fig. 15.5 Dissection continuing along helical cartilage.

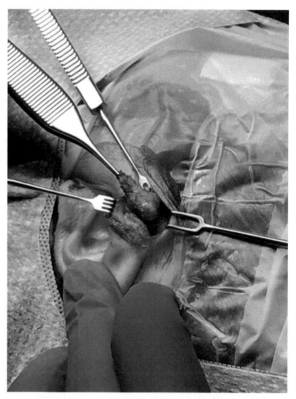

Fig. 15.6 Soft tissues surrounding sinus tract included in the specimen to ensure complete resection and reduce the risk of recurrence.

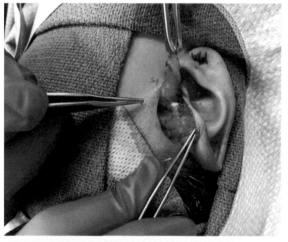

Fig. 15.7 Dissection continues anteriorly, an Allis clamp is used to retract the ellipse of skin.

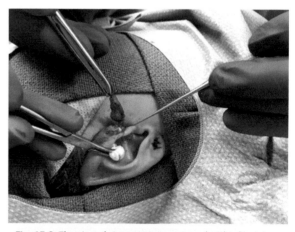

Fig. 15.8 The pit and sinus tract are removed with adjacent soft tissues and a small rim of helical cartilage.

▶Fig. 15.6). Single prong retractors can be used to lift up the elliptical island of skin while the subcutaneous tissues superficial to the temporalis fascia are dissected and removed with the specimen (▶Fig. 15.7). A small segment of cartilage can be excised where the sinus tract is adherent if needed (▶Fig. 15.8, ▶Fig. 15.9, and ▶Fig. 15.10). It is important to take care not to "button-hole" through the skin during dissection of the anterior portion of the cyst

where there may be very little soft tissue between the skin and sinus tract. Once the sinus pit, tract, and cyst have been excised en bloc with adjacent soft tissues, the surgical bed is irrigated and hemostasis achieved (▶Fig. 15.11 and ▶Fig. 15.12). Drain placement is not needed in the majority of cases. Dead space is closed with deep vicryl sutures (▶Fig. 15.13) and the skin is closed with either a running subcuticular monocryl or

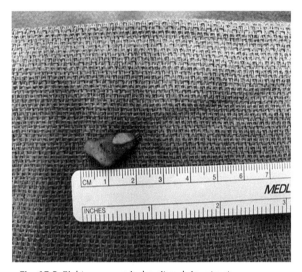

Fig. 15.9 Right ear preauricular pit and sinus tract.

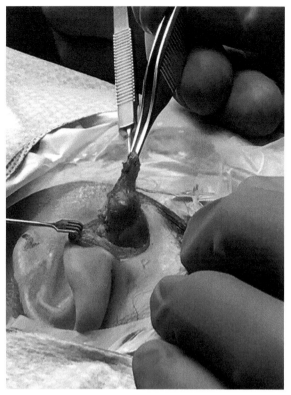

Fig. 15.10 Rim of helical cartilage taken with specimen.

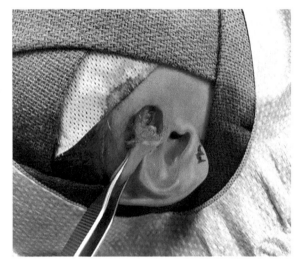

Fig. 15.11 Surgical cavity following removal of specimen.

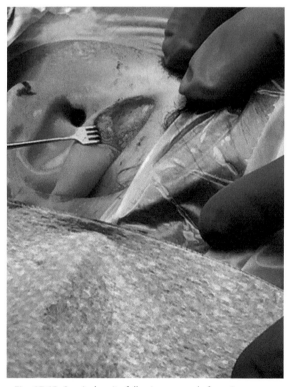

Fig. 15.12 Surgical cavity following removal of specimen.

simple interrupted sutures using fast absorbing plain gut (▶Fig. 15.14). Dermabond is placed over the incision to create a water-tight barrier (▶Fig. 15.15 and ▶Fig. 15.16).

15.4 Postoperative Treatment

Patients are instructed to keep the surgical site clean and avoid touching or rubbing it. They may shower or wash their hair and face, as the Dermabond provides a water tight barrier but should not take baths or submerge their head under water. Tylenol and Motrin usually provide adequate pain control. Antibiotics are not given unless there was concern for residual infection or inflamed tissues during the procedure.

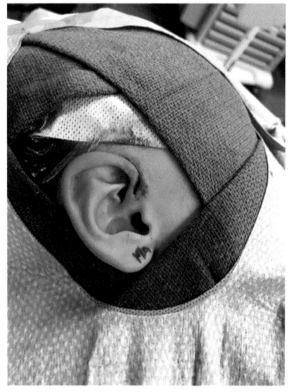

Fig. 15.13 Dead space closed with 4–0 vicryl suture.

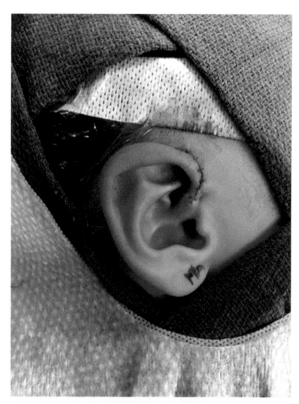

Fig. 15.14 Skin closed with 5–0 fast gut interrupted sutures.

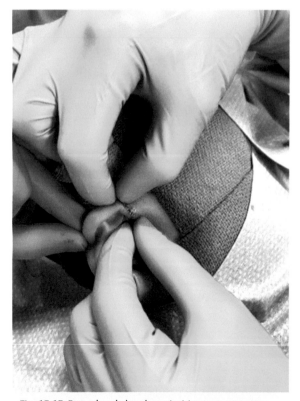

Fig. 15.15 Dermabond placed over incision to create water tight seal.

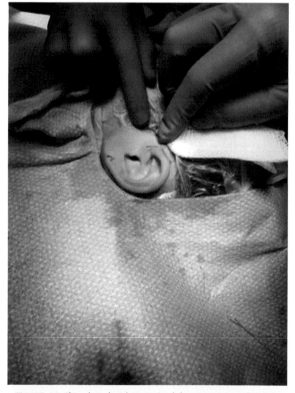

Fig. 15.16 Skin closed with 4–0 vicryl deep sutures and 5–0 monocryl subcuticular suture.

15.5 Highlights

a. Indications
 – Prior symptomatic infection of preauricular sinus.
b. Contraindications
 – Active infection of preauricular sinus.
c. Complications
 – Recurrence of sinus tract.
 – Wound infection.
 – Hematoma or seroma.
d. Special preoperative considerations
 – Presence of another malformation or dysmorphic feature of the face, limbs, heart, or gastrointestinal system may be an indication of a multiple congenital anomaly syndrome prompting the need for further workup, including possible renal ultrasound.
e. Special intraoperative considerations
 – Must resect the entire sinus tract to prevent recurrence, best achieved with the supra-auricular approach and resection of a small cuff of helical cartilage with the specimen.
f. Special postoperative considerations
 – Routine postoperative instructions should be given (i.e., do not submerge incision in water, use Tylenol or Motrin for pain, limit strenuous activity until follow-up).

References

[1] Kumar Chowdary KV, Sateesh Chandra N, Karthik Madesh R. Preauricular sinus: a novel approach. Indian J Otolaryngol Head Neck Surg 2013;65(3):234–236
[2] Gan EC, Anicete R, Tan HKK, Balakrishnan A. Preauricular sinuses in the pediatric population: techniques and recurrence rates. Int J Pediatr Otorhinolaryngol 2013;77(3):372–378
[3] El-Anwar MW, ElAassar AS. Supra-auricular versus sinusectomy approaches for preauricular sinuses. Int Arch Otorhinolaryngol 2016;20(4):390–393
[4] Bruijnzeel H, van den Aardweg MT, Grolman W, Stegeman I, van der Veen EL. A systematic review on the surgical outcome of preauricular sinus excision techniques. Laryngoscope 2016; 126(7):1535–1544
[5] Leopardi G, Chiarella G, Conti S, Cassandro E. Surgical treatment of recurring preauricular sinus: supra-auricular approach. Acta Otorhinolaryngol Ital 2008;28(6):302–305
[6] Lam HC, Soo G, Wormald PJ, Van Hasselt CA. Excision of the preauricular sinus: a comparison of two surgical techniques. Laryngoscope 2001;111(2):317–319
[7] Prasad S, Grundfast K, Milmoe G. Management of congenital preauricular pit and sinus tract in children. Laryngoscope 1990; 100(3):320–321
[8] Wang RY, Earl DL, Ruder RO, Graham JM Jr. Syndromic ear anomalies and renal ultrasounds. Pediatrics 2001;108(2):E32

16 Surgery for Lymphatic Vascular Malformations

Sonia Kumar, Ben Hartley

Summary

Vascular anomalies encompass a huge range of pediatric conditions and are broadly classified as vascular malformations or hemangiomas. They are defined by their individual morphology and growth rate and are in rare cases part of a global syndrome. Hemangiomas are largely treated medically, surgery is reserved for lesions resistant to medical therapy or those causing a significant functional deficit. Vascular malformations may be treated with sclerotherapy or surgery depending on size, anatomical site, and morphology. While both medical and surgical therapy has its advantages, the risk of damage to surrounding neuromuscular structures with each individual case should be weighed up. In experienced hands, resection of lesions in low risk areas can offer removal of the disease, improved cosmesis, restoration of function, and minimal risk to surrounding neurovasular structures.

Keywords: Vascular malformation, hemangioma, cystic hygroma, venous malformation, sclerotherapy

16.1 Introduction

Vascular anomalies encompass a wide range of pediatric head and neck lesions. They are commonly classified according to the Mulliken and Glowacki classification system, which divides them into two broad categories, vascular malformations and hemangiomas (▶Table 16.1).

Table 16.1 Classification of vascular anomalies

Vascular malformations	Hemangiomas
Slow flow: • Capillary malformations • Venous malformations • Lymphatic malformations	Infantile hemangiomas
Fast flow: • Arterial malformation • Arteriovenous fistula • Arteriovenous malformation	Congenital hemangiomas: • RICH rapidly involuting hemangiomas • NICH non-involuting hemangiomas • PICH partially involuting hemangiomas
Complex-combined	Kaposiform hemangioendothelioma (with or without Kasabach–Merritt syndrome)
	Spindle cell hemangioendothelioma (with or without Kasabach–Merritt syndrome)
	Other rare hemangioendothelioma, e.g., epithelioid, composite, retiform, polymorphous
	Dermatologic acquired vascular tumors, e.g., pyogenic granuloma, targetoid hemangioma

The former are classified according to the morphology of the dominant vasculature and the flow rate. Slow flow lesions include capillary, lymphatic, and venous malformations. These are commonly mixed, i.e., venolymphatic malformations. Fast flow lesions include arterial and arteriovenous malformations. Unlike hemangiomas, vascular malformations are characterized by normal growth and normal turnover of endothelial cells. They grow commensurately with the child. Hemangiomas, often known as "birthmarks" are flat or absent at birth. They exhibit three stages of development, a period of rapid endothelial proliferation shortly after birth, followed by regression, and eventually complete involution. In this chapter we aim to describe the surgical approach and preoperative considerations to lymphatic disease of the head and neck and give the reader an overview of this complex and challenging disease process.

16.2 Hemangiomas

Infantile hemangiomas are the most common and present shortly after birth as red or bluish macules. They grow rapidly from 6 weeks of age and their proliferative phase is between 6 and 12 months followed by regression. The rate of involution is approximately 10% per year. Complete involution can occur but may also leave stigmata such as redundant skin, fibro-fatty tissue, or telangiectasia. The treatment of hemangiomas is dependent on the site and size of the lesion. For example, a skin lesion may cause anything from a minor cosmetic defect to a compressive or restrictive effect on the eye, ear, or airways. Large hemangiomas may lead to congestive cardiac failure and subglottic hemangiomas present as worsening stridor and increasing respiratory compromise. Congenital hemangiomas are less common and are present and fully formed at birth. They either undergo rapid involution within 12 to 18 months or no involution.

The treatment of hemangiomas has therefore always been based on the functional impact. Prior to 2008, treatment of these lesions involved the use of high-dose corticosteroids or lasers or surgery. Propranolol is now used for the majority of lesions as it was accidently discovered to cause involution of hemangiomas. Whilst most children do not experience side effects, patients are monitored for bronchospasm, hypoglycemia, bradycardia, and hypotension. If the lesion is sensitive to propranolol, involution occurs fairly quickly and the duration of treatment is dependent on the size and site of the lesion. Small subsets of hemangiomas that are resistant to propranolol or causing a significant functional defect require laser, endoscopic, or open excision alongside corticosteroid treatment.

16.3 Vascular Malformations

Lymphatic malformations, often known as cystic hygromas, consist of several dilated lymphatic channels lined by a single layer of epithelium and have an incidence of 1 in 5000 at birth. They form a collection of thin-walled cysts that vary in size and architecture. Macrocystic disease, where the malformation compromises one or a few very large cysts, may invade large spaces, causing compression and displacement of surrounding structures such as the pharynx, airway, or esophagus (▶Fig. 16.1 and ▶Fig. 16.2). Microcystic disease is formed of multiple tiny cysts clustered together, which, in the head and neck region, can invade other structures, (e.g., parotid gland). Lymphatic malformations may also be categorized as mixed lesions such as venous-lymphatic malformations.

Lymphatic malformation may present at birth or may become apparent during childhood as a result of minor trauma, inflammation, or infection. Large malformations may be evident on prenatal scans (▶Fig. 16.3) and if preventing normal delivery may require an EXIT procedure (ex utero intrapartum treatment) to secure the airway. Commonly lymphatic malformations involve levels II–IV in the neck but may extend superiorly to the floor of the mouth and tongue or infiltrate the larynx affecting the voice and airway. Lesions involving the tongue may lead to tongue protrusion (▶Fig. 16.4). This, in turn, causes ulceration and bleeding and interferes with feeding and speech.

Venous malformations appear as a soft bluish compressible swelling commonly in the skin and subcutaneous tissue, sometimes infiltrating skeletal muscle. They grow with the child and often have a rapid enlargement during trauma and puberty. Surgical excision can be challenging with a high risk of massive hemorrhage. Capillary malformations, colloquially known as "port-wine stain," are abnormally dilated capillaries in the superficial dermis. Present from birth, the color deepens in adulthood and may be associated with Sturge–Weber syndrome. Surgery

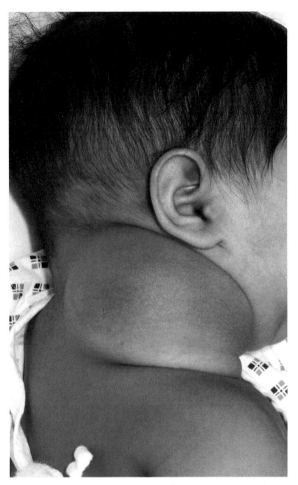

Fig. 16.1 Macrocystic lymphatic malformation in a 2-month-old child causing restriction of arm movement.

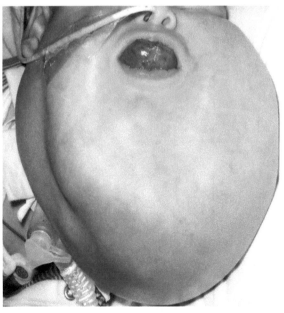

Fig. 16.3 Microcystic disease in a newborn identified prenatally and requiring a tracheostomy at birth.

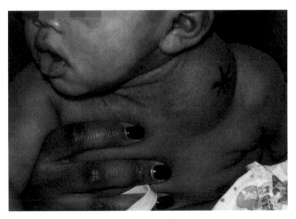

Fig. 16.2 Macrocystic lymphatic malformation in a 2-month-old child causing restriction of arm movement and swallowing difficulties due to pharyngeal compression.

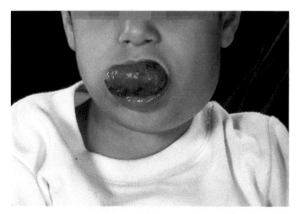

Fig. 16.4 Macroglossia due to lymphatic malformation of the oral cavity and tongue.

for such lesions mostly involved the use of the pulsed-dye laser to achieve lightening of the lesion and rarely surgical excision with skin grating has been undertaken.

16.4 Surgery for Neck Disease

As mentioned, lymphatic malformations may present with a variety of clinical symptoms. For example, large cervical lesions detected in utero may constitute an airway emergency upon birth and are therefore delivered via EXIT procedures. However, smaller lesions may cause only a cosmetic defect. Mostly lymphatic malformations of the head and neck may cause varying degrees of impairment of the airway, swallowing, voice, and movement, and therefore surgery aims to address this.

16.5 Preoperative Investigations

An ultrasound (US) of the lesion will delineate a solid or cystic tumor, but cross-sectional imaging is essential for diagnosis and surgical planning. A contrast-enhanced MRI scan will delineate and characterize the disease and its extent, and differentiate not only hemangioma, lymphatic, or venous disease but also microcystic and macrocystic lymphatic malformations. A preoperative microlaryngoscopy and bronchoscopy may be required if there is concern regarding the airway.

16.6 Preoperative Considerations

Three options still exist for these lesions: watchful waiting, sclerotherapy, and surgery. While the former are beyond the remit of this chapter, it is worth noting that these are extremely viable options and may be used

in conjunction with surgery at varying points through the natural history of the disease. Advantages of surgical resection are that it has the potential to completely eradicate the disease and confer a lifelong cure. However, factors that influence the decision for surgery are the anatomical site of the malformation and whether it is micro- or macrocystic disease. In high-risk sites, e.g., within the parotid gland or deep neck space malformations, a balance between the comorbidity of surgery and likelihood of temporary or permanent damage to nervous and vascular structures should be weighed up against the risk of sclerotherapy. In experienced surgical hands, low-risk sites such as the neck and oral cavity, the likelihood of permanent injury to nerves and complications from surgery are low. In general, macrocystic lymphatic disease confers the best prognosis whichever treatment modality is chosen and therefore the decision may be influenced by local experience and expertise.

The decision to offer surgery is based on the individual case. The two ends of the spectrum in relation to head and neck lymphatic malformations include the child with a single macrocystic lesion of the neck (the commonest clinical scenario) and the child with more extensive cervicofacial microcystic or mixed disease of the head and neck. The former has the best prognosis with surgery, often enabling the patient to be disease-free with one operation. Sclerotherapy may also be successful, although it may take several treatments. Post sclerotherapy there is usually a degree of swelling immediately after each treatment, which eventually settles. Extensive microcystic disease, however, responds poorly to sclerotherapy, and surgical resection is often technically challenging. Due to its nature, surgical resection is usually only partial or incomplete; post-surgery there is often swelling of the site due to disruption of lymphatic drainage, and the excretion of lymphatic fluid from the residual disease. A multimodality treatment approach to microcystic or mixed disease would therefore always be advisable.

16.7 Contraindications and Risks

The only absolute contraindication to surgery is medical instability and unsuitability for general anesthesia. Surgery may be delayed in patients who are very young, have acutely infected malformations, or have other significant medical comorbidity, but this should be balanced against the symptoms from the mass.

Depending on the site of the mass, the patient and family should be adequately counseled for the risk to cranial nerves and vascular structures. Postoperative lymphedema and swelling should also be mentioned, especially if microcystic disease may require compression bandaging or further resection at a later stage.

16.8 Anesthesia

General anesthesia is required and neuromuscular blockade should be avoided so intraoperative neural monitoring can take place, (e.g., facial nerve monitoring). Local anesthetic infiltration with adrenaline prior to incision may reduce bleeding and allow hydrodissection. Antibiotics at induction are given especially when dealing with microcystic disease.

16.9 Operative Technique

- Once anesthetized, the relevant nerve monitors should be attached to the patient. Often monitoring of the marginal mandibular nerve is essential.
- The patients should be positioned supine, with the head tilted away from the operative side and full exposure of the operative site (▶Fig. 16.5).
- The surgical incision should be centered over the malformation with adequate access to its superior and inferior extent. This will be determined by the size of the lesion and should ideally be placed in current or future skin creases to ensure adequate cosmesis (▶Fig. 16.6).
- If there is airway compromise the patient may already have a tracheostomy placed, but if there is airway concern a tracheostomy should be placed at the beginning of the procedure with careful thought about the position of the incision in relation to the stoma and postoperative care of the tracheostomy, ties, and Velcro tapes.
- Subplatysmal flaps are raised superior and inferior to the disease. The marginal mandibular nerve should be avoided during this procedure and may be actively identified at this point (▶Fig. 16.7 and ▶Fig. 16.8).
- The flaps are either retracted manually, using sutures or via elasticated retractors, (e.g., Lone star retractors).
- The cystic lesion is identified, and careful and gentle dissection in the plane over the cyst takes place. Care must be taken to identify all neurovascular structures in the vicinity that may be adherent to the cystic

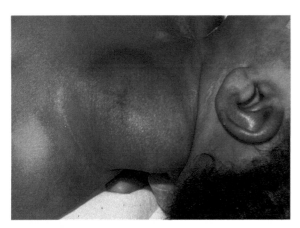

Fig. 16.5 Preoperative positioning.

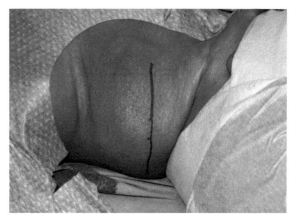

Fig. 16.6 Large incision marked over cyst to ensure adequate exposure.

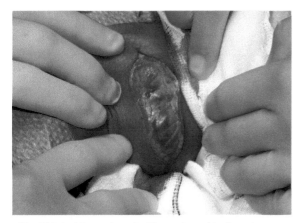

Fig. 16.7 Incision on to cyst with care to avoid adherent or closely related neurovascular structures.

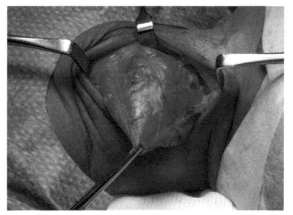

Fig. 16.8 Subplatysmal flaps raised and retracted to expose the malformation.

capsule. Vascular slings can be used to protect nerves and maneuver them during the dissection. They are also used to gain control of large vessels. Intraoperative neural monitoring can be used to also identify various nerves (▶Fig. 16.9 and ▶Fig. 16.10).

- In macrocystic disease the plane between normal tissue and the cyst is often quite well delineated and a surgical swab may be used to sweep the tissues and surgical planes apart while causing minimal trauma (▶Fig. 16.11).
- Ideally the cyst would be excised in entirety but if very large may need to be decompressed using a needle and syringe prior to the start of excision or during surgery.
- Dissection should continue from different angles until the cyst is free. If there are difficulties in the dissection, the operating surgeon should always consider incomplete resection (▶Fig. 16.12 and ▶Fig. 16.13).

- The aim of surgery is to restore the function and incomplete resection will in most cases accomplish this. Permanent iatrogenic neurovascular damage can cause significant morbidity while residual disease is often asymptomatic.
- Microvascular disease is more challenging as there is no single lesion in which to follow. The microcystic disease should be debulked from all angles, paying careful attention to avoid neurovascular damage (▶Fig. 16.14 and ▶Fig. 16.15).
- A surgical drain should be placed prior to closure of the incision, especially if a large volume of tissue has been excised. If microcystic disease has been debulked, the residual tissue will continue to leak and therefore a drain will be required.
- Closure is usually straightforward, but if a large volume of disease has been resected, it may be

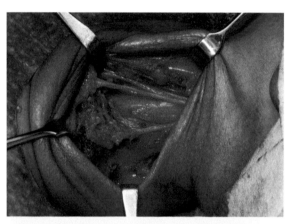

Fig. 16.9 Identification and dissection of cervical nerves.

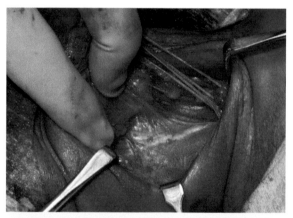

Fig. 16.10 Identification of jugular vein medial to the malformation.

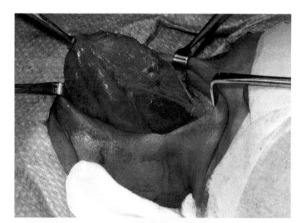

Fig. 16.11 Dissection and retraction from multiple angles to excise the malformation.

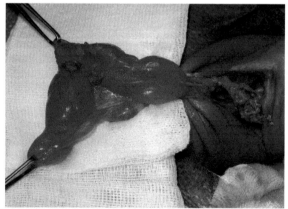

Fig. 16.12 Macrocystic malformation comprising multiple large cysts.

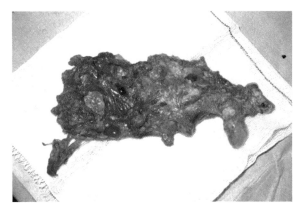

Fig. 16.13 Microvascular specimen.

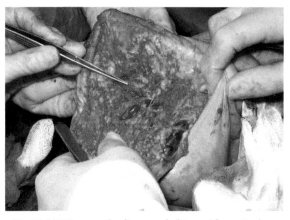

Fig. 16.14 Microvascular disease; subplatysmal flaps raised dissection up to mandible for wide exposure.

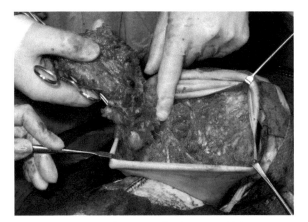

Fig. 16.15 Excision of microvascular disease, multiple cysts in specimen.

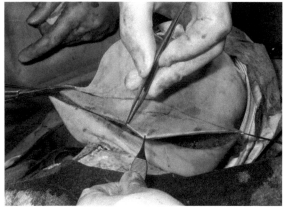

Fig. 16.16 Excess skin during closure; excess excised.

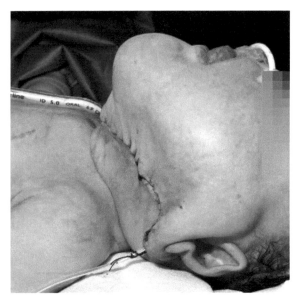

Fig. 16.17 Wound closure after skin excision.

necessary to excise excess or redundant skin (▶ Fig. 16.16), being careful not to make the closure too tight (▶ Fig. 16.17).

16.10 Postoperative Management

The surgical drain should stay in place for 24 to 48 hours, longer if draining significant lymphatic fluid or if there is postoperative swelling (▶ Fig. 16.18). Postoperative antibiotics may be required if there is evidence of infection at the time of surgery or if there is a prolonged use of the drain. In the immediate to early period, the patient should be monitored for significant lymphedema, especially in microcystic disease or if there is incomplete resection. In most cases this will settle spontaneously, some may require compression bandaging. If they are significantly symptomatic then needle aspiration of the fluid or in rare cases surgical drainage may be needed but should be

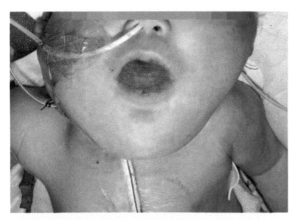

Fig. 16.18 Postoperative nasogastric tube, surgical drain. Postoperative appearance compared with ▶ Fig. 16.3 shows massive debulking of lesion, contouring of the mandible and cosmetic facial appearance.

avoided where possible to allow natural resorption and redistribution or lymphatic pathways. If a tracheostomy is sighted for airway compromise, this should be left in situ with the airway reassessed at a later date once healing has taken place.

16.11 Evidence-based Management

A review of 118 children who were treated for a cervicofacial lymphatic malformation by the senior author (Dr. Ben Hartley), 53 had surgical excision as the primary treatment modality, and approximately half only required one procedure. Eighty percent of these patients had complete or near-complete resolution and of these most had macrocystic disease. Of the 20% that had a partial response only one had pure macrocystic disease, four underwent sclerotherapy, and the rest further surgical or laser excision. Patients that had disease localized only to the neck all had a complete or near-complete response after primary surgery, and 97% of those with pure macrocystic disease had a complete or near-complete response. Only minor complications were described in this group, such as infection and lymphedema; there were no permanent nerve palsies.

16.12 Lymphatic Malformations of the Tongue and Floor of Mouth

Lymphatic malformations of the oral cavity tend to be microcystic in nature and most commonly involve the anterior tongue. In some cases this may extend to the floor of the mouth and further into the neck and invade other cervical structures. Surgery again will be based on symptoms such as airway compromise, ability to feed, and cosmesis. Some large malformations may cause tongue protrusion, ulceration, and bleeding, and affect growth of the maxilla, mandible, palate, and teeth. Lesions of the tongue can be fully or partially resected, anterior lesions may be amenable to a wedge resection, and surface ulcerative lesions may be resurfaced using a Coblator. Those involving the floor of the mouth may also be resected but care should be taken to isolate and retract the submandibular ducts at the start of the procedure.

16.13 Highlights

a. Indications
 - Airway compromise.
 - Inability to feed/failure to thrive.
 - Impact on voice.
 - Impairment of movement of neck or upper limbs.
b. Contraindications
 - Medical instability and therefore unsuitable for general anesthesia.
c. Complications
 - Postoperative lymphoedema.
 - Reaccumulation of microcystic disease and further surgery.
 - Damage to cranial nerves or vascular structures.
 - Superficial or deeper neck space infections.
 - Cosmetic deformity/scar.
d. Special preoperative considerations
 - Preoperative MRI scan to delineate anatomy of lesion and proximity to head and neck structures/vasculature/cranial nerves.
 - Preoperative microlaryngoscopy and bronchoscopy if there are symptoms of airway compromise.
 - Consider need for preoperative tracheostomy.
 - Consider macrocystic versus microcystic disease and the role of sclerotherapy.
e. Special intraoperative considerations
 - Cranial nerve monitoring.
 - Intraoperative antibiotics.
 - Balance complete resection versus risk to adjacent structures.
f. Special postoperative considerations
 - Overnight hospitalization.
 - Postoperative surgical drain.
 - Immediate or prolonged postoperative compression bandaging.

17 Cervical Lymph Node Biopsy in Children

Barak Ringel, Gadi Fishman

Summary

Palpable cervical lymphadenopathy is a very common referral cause in children. It is mostly of an inflammatory/benign etiology. The clinician should be suspicious but he/she should also remain safe and use timely and cost-effective methods in lymphadenopathy evaluation. Open cervical lymph node biopsy will enable the establishment of an accurate histopathological diagnosis when other means are inconclusive.

Keywords: Pediatric, cervical lymphadenopathy, biopsy, children

17.1 Introduction

Palpable cervical lymphadenopathy is very common in children; therefore, much thought must be given to the justification of carrying out a surgical biopsy with its associated risks of complications and comorbidities. There are currently no evidence-based guidelines for conducting such biopsies in the evaluation of pediatric neck lumps.[1,2]

The lymphatic system is a major component of the immune system. It consists of lymphatic fluid, lymphatic vessels, lymph nodes, spleen, tonsils, adenoid, Peyer patches, and the thymus. Along these channels reside approximately 600 lymph nodes, with about 300 of them located in the neck (▶Fig. 17.1). Exposure to immune challenge mediates a proliferation process leading to lymph node activation and enlargement.[3,4]

Lymphadenopathy is defined as a disease of the lymph nodes in which they are abnormal in size, number, or consistency. Lymph node enlargement is due to either proliferation of normal cells or infiltration by abnormal cells. There are five broad etiologic categories of lymph node enlargement:

1. Immune response to infective agents (e.g., bacteria, viruses, fungi).
2. Inflammatory cells in infections involving a lymph node(s).
3. Localized neoplastic proliferation of lymphocytes or macrophages (e.g., leukemia, lymphoma).
4. Infiltration of neoplastic cells carried to the node by lymphatic or blood circulation (metastasis).
5. Infiltration of macrophages filled with metabolite deposits (e.g., storage disorders).[5–7]

A lump is most often randomly discovered by a parent, a caregiver, or a pediatrician. The major challenge is to

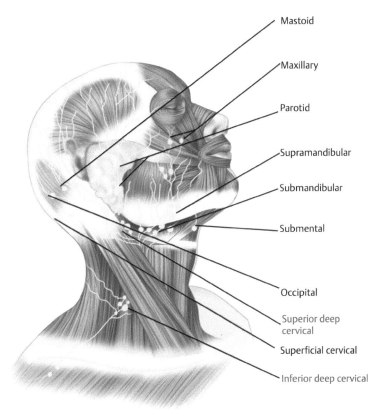

Fig. 17.1 Lymph node groups in the neck.

Mastoid

Maxillary

Parotid

Supramandibular

Submandibular

Submental

Occipital

Superior deep cervical

Superficial cervical

Inferior deep cervical

Table 17.1 Differential diagnosis of pediatric neck masses

Congenital	Branchial cleft cyst Thyroglossal duct cysts Lymphatic malformations Lymphangiomas Hemangiomas Teratomas Dermoid cysts Laryngoceles Thymic cysts Vascular malformations
Acquired	Viral lymphadenopathy (e.g., EBV, CMV, Rubella, Measles) Bacterial lymphadenopathy (e.g., staphylococci, strep-tococci, cat scratch disease, brucellosis, mycobacterial infection) Fungal infections Parasitic/protozoan Noninfectious inflammatory disorders (e.g., Kawasaki disease, sinus histiocytosis, sarcoidosis, systemic lupus erythematosus) Sialadenitis/sialolithiasis Drug-induced lymphadenopathies Hypersensitivity Storage diseases
Benign neoplasms	Lipomas Thyroid adenomas Neurofibromas Benign salivary neoplasms
Malignant neoplasms	Lymphomas Leukemias Rhabdomyosarcomas Thyroid carcinomas Salivary gland malignancies Nasopharyngeal carcinomas Neuroblastomas

differentiate between a benign and a pathologic process. The differential diagnosis of pediatric neck lumps is detailed in ▶ Table 17.1. There are differences in therapeutic approaches to pediatric lymph adenopathy from that of adult lymph adenopathy since the former is such a common cause for referral and made mostly on the basis of a benign/inflammatory etiology. The clinician should relieve the parent's and child's fear of malignancy while being suspicious enough but still being safe, timely, and cost-effective. Open cervical lymph node biopsy will enable the establishment of an accurate histopathological diagnosis when other means are inconclusive.[8–10]

17.2 Preoperative and Anesthesia Considerations

A thorough stepwise approach that includes in-depth history acquisition, physical examination, laboratory examinations, and preoperative imaging studies is mandatory for planning treatment, for contributing to the establishment of a likely etiology, and in order to avoid carrying out unnecessary tests. However, an excisional biopsy is unavoidable when the diagnosis is uncertain or there is need for further characterization, especially when there is suspicion of a potential malignancy.

17.2.1 History

The medical history should focus upon the duration of symptoms, the presence and nature of any systemic signs (e.g., fever, malaise, weight loss, night sweats), recent infections, local or adjacent pain, local trauma, exposure to animals, immunosuppression, and sexual behavior (adolescents). Previous antibiotic treatment should be reviewed for reason and type.[11,12]

17.2.2 Physical Examination

The physical examination should be thorough and focus upon the enlarged lymph nodes. Benign nodes are differentiated from malignant nodes by their being soft, mobile, tender, and smaller than 1 cm. Malignant nodes tend to be non-tender, firm, and fixed. Other features of note are signs of inflammation, skin involvement, and trauma. The location of the lymph nodes is also significant. Localized lymphadenopathy usually results from a localized abnormality that had originated in its drainage pathway, and might be inflamed, infected, or misleading congenital neck mass. The most worrisome regional lymph adenopathy in terms of malignancy is in the supraclavicular area. Generalized lymphadenopathy is more suggestive of a systemic disease (viral infections, malignancies, tuberculosis, autoimmune diseases, and drug exposure).[7,13]

17.2.3 Laboratory Studies

A complete blood count with differential, blood chemistry (including serum lactate dehydrogenase levels), and selected serologic tests (e.g., Epstein-Barr virus, cytomegalovirus, Bartonella bacteria) further contribute to establishing the diagnosis.[14,15]

17.2.4 Imaging Studies

Chest radiography may be helpful in identifying sources of infection, in defining hilar and mediastinal adenopathy, and, in some cases, in providing preoperative assessment relevant to the anesthesiologist. Ultrasonography (US) is a widely available, noninvasive, quickly performed radiographic test with no exposure to radiation. It is very useful in defining the nature and architecture of a lymph node for establishing its etiology. US is also useful in the operating room for identifying and marking the exact location of the lymph node for the purpose of determining the site for the incision. Computed tomography (CT) is helpful in defining deep lymph nodes, as well as in characterizing their nature and likelihood of malignancy.

Due to the high level of radiation exposure, CT is usually not performed routinely for pediatric patients but rather reserved for specific cases. 18F-fluorodeoxyglucose positron emission tomography ([18F]FDG-PET) or integrated PET-CTs are applied for staging Hodgkin's and non-Hodgkin's lymphomas. The high rate of false-positive results for inflammatory processes as well as the high level of radiation exposure precludes its use before a histopathological diagnosis has been made.[16-19]

17.2.5 Needle Biopsy

The use of fine-needle aspiration (FNA) is very widespread for defining neck masses in adults, due to the fact that it is an office-based, rapidly executed, and simple procedure, with no need for general anesthesia. It is associated with low morbidity and high cost-effectiveness. FNA often requires sedation in most pediatric patients for whom it is less useful than adults. Although its specificity is high (~92–100%), it sensitivity is uncertain (67–100%), and it may not rule out the need for excisional tissue biopsy. Core-needle biopsy (FNB) techniques under US or CT guidance allow the sampling of more tissue while maintaining its architecture, but they are still controversial for the same reasons as those for performing FNA in children.[20-24]

17.2.6 Final Presurgical Preparations

All children scheduled for operation are evaluated preoperatively by a pediatric otolaryngologist or head and neck surgeon, by a pediatric hematologist, and by an anesthesiologist. Routine complete blood count and coagulation function tests are carried out to assess bleeding tendencies. Surgery can be performed either under general anesthesia for younger children or under conscious sedation for adolescents. It is not recommended to administer muscle relaxants during general anesthesia in order to allow continuous monitoring of the relevant cranial nerves. Routine administration of prophylactic antibiotics in clean operations is also not recommended.

17.3 Surgical Technique for Lymph Node Biopsy of Level III

An example of the surgical techniques for biopsy of level III lymph node have been discussed below. ▶ Fig. 17.2 demonstrates the various neck levels and ▶ Table 17.2 details the important structures for each level.

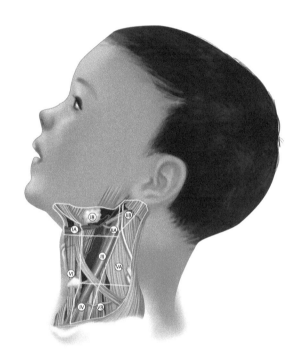

Fig. 17.2 Levels of the neck.

Table 17.2 Important structures in the neck according to neck level

Neck level	Nerves	Blood vessels	Other
I	Marginal branch of the facial, lingual branch of the trigeminal, hypoglossal, submandibular ganglion	Facial vessels	
II	Vagus and accessory	Internal jugular vein, internal + external carotid arteries	
III	Vagus, sympathetic trunk	Internal jugular vein, common carotid artery, superior thyroid vessels	
IV	Vagus, cervical plexus, brachial plexus, phrenic	Internal jugular vein Common carotid artery	Thoracic duct/lymphatic duct
V	Accessory, brachial plexus, cervical plexus	Transverse cervical artery External jugular vein	
VI	Recurrent laryngeal	Common carotid artery, subclavian vessels, innominate artery, inferior thyroid vessels	Parathyroid blood supply

17.3.1 Skin Incision

The patient is placed on the operating table in a supine position. The head is stabilized with a soft donut holder and the operating table is then elevated at an angle with the head up in order to minimize bleeding. The surgical access is planned through the shortest possible transverse neck incision (▶Fig. 17.3). The incision is usually located one finger breadth under the mandible, extending from the anterior border of the sternocleidomastoid muscle 2 cm anteriorly. It is preferably placed along a transverse skin crest. The incision should be panned in such a way that it can be extended for a neck dissection if necessary without making a separate incision. Marking of the incision is performed with the neck slightly flexed in order to identify the lines of relaxed skin tension. A US-guided mark can be made on the skin when the target lymph node is not prominent.

After marking the site of the incision, a roll is placed under the child's shoulders in order to hyperextend the neck, and the head is rotated toward the side contralateral to the node. This position moves the lymphatic content of the neck anteromedial and cephalad, and facilitates the dissection. The patient is then prepped and draped in standard surgical fashion.

17.3.2 Elevation of Subplatysmal Flaps

The skin is incised with a number 15 blade or a Colorado monopolar electrocautery needle (Stryker), after which dissection of the subcutaneous tissue and the platysma is carried out by electrocauterization at the lowest effective setting. Subplatysmal flaps are elevated superiorly and

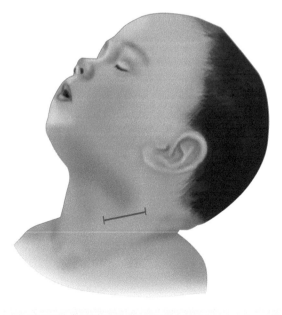

Fig. 17.3 Skin incision.

inferiorly and the skin flaps are elevated with skin hooks or fish hooks.

The location of the target lymph node should be palpated.

17.3.3 Dissection along the Lymph Node in Level III

The sternocleidomastoid muscle is retracted posteriorly with a Richardson retractor, separating it from the superficial layer of the deep cervical fascia (▶Fig. 17.4). The enlarged node should be identified by palpation along the jugular chain. The dissection and the separation of the node from the adjacent soft tissue and the preservation of the external jugular vein and greater auricular nerve must be meticulous.

The specimen is submitted to the pathology laboratory for analysis (▶Fig. 17.5). The wound is irrigated copiously and carefully inspected, and hemostasis is performed if indicated. A Valsalva maneuver can be performed by keeping a positive ventilation pressure for several seconds in order to force bleeding of bleeders. Surgicel or Woundclot dressings may be left in the surgical bed for hemostasis. A Hemovac or Polyvac 7 drain is left when the surgical bed is relatively large, but no drain is required if the surgical bed is small. The platysma is sutured with absorbable stitches and the skin is closed with 5–0 Monocryl stitches/skin glue (Dermabond).

17.4 Postoperative Treatment

After undergoing the surgery, the patient is extubated and immediately transferred to the post-surgery care unit before being transferred to the ward. The wound is kept clean by rinsing with saline three times a day. The drains are removed either 3 days after the operation or when the collected fluid is less than 20–30 mL in 24 hours. Prophylactic antibiotic treatment is not indicated in the postoperative period. For pain control, the patients are treated with nonsteroidal anti-inflammatory drugs (peroral syr. Ibuprofen 10 mg/kg or paracetamol 10 mg/kg max. 3 times per day) if the patient asks for them or if the nurses consider it necessary. Stitches should be removed 1 week after the surgery.

17.5 Highlights

a. Indications
   - >2 cm lymph cervical lymph node persists over 4 weeks.
   - Supraclavicular lymph node.
   - Post FNA/FNB for suspicious lymph node—in order to achieve architecture and define oncologic treatment.
   - Undiagnosed neck lump.
b. Contraindications
   - Known etiology with a benign self-limiting course.
   - Involvement of related structures (relative)

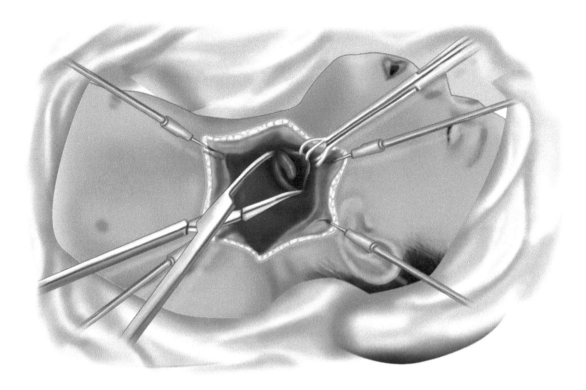

Fig. 17.4 Posterior retraction of the sternocleidomastoid muscle and identification of the enlarged lymph node.

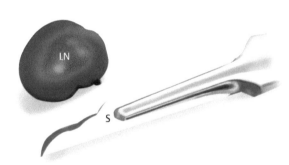

Fig. 17.5 Excised lymph node.

c. Complications
   - Bleeding.
   - Seroma.
   - Chyle leak.
   - Wound infection.
   - Nerve neuropraxia/nerve neuropraxia/axonotmesis/neurotmesis.
   - Anesthesia risks.
d. Special preoperative considerations
   - Stepwise comprehensive evaluation.
   - Ultrasound guided incision marking to minimize scar size.

e. Special intraoperative considerations
   - Operation is performed without relaxation for cranial nerve monitoring. Consider nerve monitoring.
   - Early identification and preservation of relevant nerves and blood vessels.
   - Proper surgical technique and careful hemostasis during and after surgery diminish the risk of bleeding.
   - Valsalva maneuver may be used to identify bleeding vessels.
   - Drainage placement.
   - Meticulous suturing for aesthetic scar formation.
f. Special postoperative considerations
   - Identify complications as early as possible.
   - Bleeding in this area can lead to an imminent airway obstruction. Open and evacuate the wound at the bedside if airway obstruction occurs.

References

[1] Herzog LW, Herzog MD. Prevalence of lymphadenopathy of the head and neck in infants and children. Clin Pediatr (Phila) 1983;22(7):485–487
[2] Bamji M, Stone RK, Kaul A, Usmani G, Schachter FF, Wasserman E. Palpable lymph nodes in healthy newborns and infants. Pediatrics 1986;78(4):573–575

[3] Trotter HA. The surgical anatomy of the lymphatics of the head and neck. Ann Otol Rhinol Laryngol 1930;39:384–397

[4] H R. Lymphatic System of the Head and Neck. Ann Arbor, MI: Edwards Brother; 1938

[5] Knight PJ, Mulne AF, Vassy LE. When is lymph node biopsy indicated in children with enlarged peripheral nodes? Pediatrics 1982;69(4):391–396

[6] Segal GH, Perkins SL, Kjeldsberg CR. Benign lymphadenopathies in children and adolescents. Semin Diagn Pathol 1995;12(4):288–302

[7] Ghirardelli ML, Jemos V, Gobbi PG. Diagnostic approach to lymph node enlargement. Haematologica 1999;84(3):242–247

[8] Slap GB, Connor JL, Wigton RS, Schwartz JS. Validation of a model to identify young patients for lymph node biopsy. JAMA 1986;255(20):2768–2773

[9] Torsiglieri AJ Jr, Tom LWC, Ross AJ III, Wetmore RF, Handler SD, Potsic WP. Pediatric neck masses: guidelines for evaluation. Int J Pediatr Otorhinolaryngol 1988;16(3):199–210

[10] Moore SW, Schneider JW, Schaaf HS. Diagnostic aspects of cervical lymphadenopathy in children in the developing world: a study of 1,877 surgical specimens. Pediatr Surg Int 2003;19(4):240–244

[11] Oguz A, Karadeniz C, Temel EA, Citak EC, Okur FV. Evaluation of peripheral lymphadenopathy in children. Pediatr Hematol Oncol 2006;23(7):549–561

12] Papadopouli E, Michailidi E, Papadopoulou E, Paspalaki P, Vlahakis I, Kalmanti M. Cervical lymphadenopathy in childhood epidemiology and management. Pediatr Hematol Oncol 2009;26(6):454–460

[13] Soldes OS, Younger JG, Hirschl RB. Predictors of malignancy in childhood peripheral lymphadenopathy. J Pediatr Surg 1999; 34(10):1447–1452

[14] Leung AKC, Robson WLM. Childhood cervical lymphadenopathy. J Pediatr Health Care 2004;18(1):3–7

[15] Locke R, Comfort R, Kubba H. When does an enlarged cervical lymph node in a child need excision? A systematic review. Int J Pediatr Otorhinolaryngol 2014;78(3):393–401

[16] Papakonstantinou O, Bakantaki A, Paspalaki P, Charoulakis N, Gourtsoyiannis N. High-resolution and color Doppler ultrasonography of cervical lymphadenopathy in children. Acta Radiol 2001; 42(5):470–476

[17] Restrepo R, Oneto J, Lopez K, Kukreja K. Head and neck lymph nodes in children: the spectrum from normal to abnormal. Pediatr Radiol 2009;39(8):836–846

[18] Robson CD. Imaging of head and neck neoplasms in children. Pediatr Radiol 2010;40(4):499–509

[19] Payabvash S, Meric K, Cayci Z. Differentiation of benign from malignant cervical lymph nodes in patients with head and neck cancer using PET/CT imaging. Clin Imaging 2016;40(1):101–105

[20] Kardos TF, Maygarden SJ, Blumberg AK, Wakely PE Jr, Frable WJ. Fine needle aspiration biopsy in the management of children and young adults with peripheral lymphadenopathy. Cancer 1989;63(4):703–707

[21] Sklair-Levy M, Amir G, Spectre G, et al. Image-guided cutting-edge-needle biopsy of peripheral lymph nodes and superficial masses for the diagnosis of lymphoma. J Comput Assist Tomogr 2005;29(3):369–372

[22] Rapkiewicz A, Thuy Le B, Simsir A, Cangiarella J, Levine P. Spectrum of head and neck lesions diagnosed by fine-needle aspiration cytology in the pediatric population. Cancer 2007; 111(4):242–251

[23] Anne S, Teot LA, Mandell DL. Fine needle aspiration biopsy: role in diagnosis of pediatric head and neck masses. Int J Pediatr Otorhinolaryngol 2008;72(10):1547–1553

[24] Annam V, Kulkarni MH, Puranik RB. Clinicopathologic profile of significant cervical lymphadenopathy in children aged 1–12 years. Acta Cytol 2009;53(2):174–178

18 Pediatric Maxillectomy

Gilad Horowitz, Anton Warshavsky, Ahmad Safadi, Avraham Abergel, Dan M. Fliss

Summary

Tumors involving the maxillary sinus are uncommon in the pediatric population. Since aesthetics and the developing cranium are a major concern in children, endoscopic approaches are usually favored. With that being said, endoscopic approaches may be insufficient for tumor resection and open approaches are therefore indicated. This chapter will summarize and review the various open approaches for performing maxillectomies in the pediatric population.

Keywords: Pediatric, maxillectomy, incisions, approach

18.1 Introduction

Tumors of the pediatric maxillofacial skeleton are a rare clinical entity with a broad differential diagnosis.[1-3] Tumors may be classified by origin as being either odontogenic or non-odontogenic or malignant or benign.[4] Odontogenic tumors arise from quiescent tooth-forming tissues of the jaws and are most commonly located within the bones of the jaw (central odontogenic tumor), though occasionally they may arise in surrounding soft tissue (peripheral odontogenic tumor).[4] The etiology of these tumors remains unknown, and they vary widely in their level of aggression.[4] Non-odontogenic tumors encompass a wide range of pathologic conditions and may arise from mesenchymal tissue within the jaw or from the osseous tissue of the jaw.[5] No matter the origin, prompt identification and treatment of jaw tumors is critical because some tumors may be either locally destructive or malignant.[4,6]

The past few decades have shown slow progression from open surgeries to lesser invasive surgery—all in the name of facial esthetics. The initial progress has been the shift from open maxillectomies to facial degloving and the other large step forward was made possible with the advances in endoscopic surgery. Since many tumors are benign, the concept of a non–"En-bloc" resection is feasible and acceptable. Recently, data published from several groups regarding base of skull malignant tumors have shown that a "piecemeal" resection is an acceptable oncologic solution, without compromising survival results.[7-10]

This chapter is meant to represent and review the various maxillectomies performed nowadays.

18.2 Surgical Approach to Pediatric Maxillectomy

In an open maxillectomy a lateral rhinotomy incision (▶Fig. 18.1) is commonly used to gain access to the maxillary sinus.[11] If the lesion involves the hard palate, this procedure can be extended to include a lip split also known as a Weber-Ferguson incision (▶Fig. 18.2).

If there is any difficulty with exposure or if the lesion is located laterally or posteriorly, it is vital to extend the approach to allow better access to the tumor. More complete exposure of the maxilla is obtained by extending the incisions below the lower eyelid. The inferior orbital extension is possible in either a subciliary crease, a midciliary plain, or in an inferior ciliary plain, also known as Diffenbach incision. Another extension of the Lateral Rhinotomy/Weber-Ferguson incision is a Lynch incision that will allow an open approach to the ethmoid sinuses.

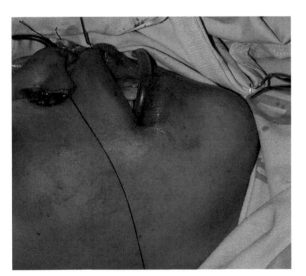

Fig. 18.1 Lateral rhinotomy.

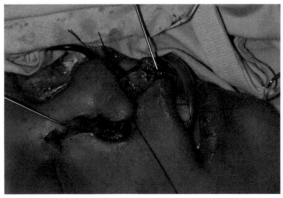

Fig. 18.2 Weber-Ferguson incision.

The lateral rhinotomy incision extends along the lateral border of the nose, approximately half a cm from the dorsum of the nose. It starts cephalad, medial to the medial canthus and extends down through the skin crest bordering the nasal ala. It is continued toward the philtrum. Following the skin incision, the dissection continues up to the level of the nasal bone and medial buttress of the maxilla. Skin flaps are elevated medially and laterally to the level of the periosteum (▶Fig. 18.3) with the aid of a freer elevator and electrocautery. Care is taken not to injure the infraorbital nerve, which will be piercing the anterior maxillary wall approximately 1 cm below the infraorbital rim (▶Fig. 18.4 and ▶Fig. 18.5). The flaps can be developed to the level of the maxillary tuberosity (laterally), the upper gingiva (inferiorly), the frontal sinus and infraorbital rim (superiorly), and to the pyriform aperture and nasal septum (medially). The flaps are held with hooks.

The osteotomies along the anterior and medial walls of the maxilla are now performed with a motorized reciprocating saw (▶Fig. 18.6).

The lines of the osteotomies are inferior border of the fossa canina, above the dental roots; superiorly, the orbit; laterally, the malar eminence; and medially the nasal cavity In children, the inferior line is higher than usual, since the second line of teeth does not erupt yet. The medial and part of the anterior wall of the maxilla is now retracted anteriorly with a Babcock's grasper and the tumor is freed from its attachments with a Mayo scissors and freer elevator. If necessary, the rest of the tissue is extirpated with a Kerrison Rongeur. Hemostasis is performed with 50% hydrogen peroxide and 4 × 4 gauze sponge. The cavity is inspected and hemostasis is completed with bipolar electrocautery. In most cases, branches of the sphenopalatine artery can be identified at the posterior wall of the maxilla, lateral and superior to the choana. These are clamped with medium size clip to prevent further bleeding.

The intraoral mucosal cuts on the palate are made and the periosteum is elevated and bony cuts are made with an oscillating saw. Consistent with disease removal, the incision should be made as far posteriorly in the palate as possible to spare the premaxilla. The premaxilla preserves facial contours and enhances support and stability of the prosthesis. The orbital rim is spared if the orbital contents have not been invaded. The pterygoid plates and the soft tissues of the pterygo-maxillary space are resected or spared according to sound oncological basis but may be resected in an extended maxillectomy.

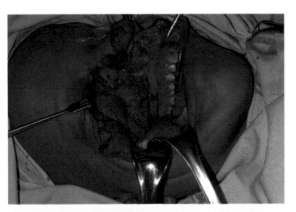

Fig. 18.3 Elevation of skin flaps.

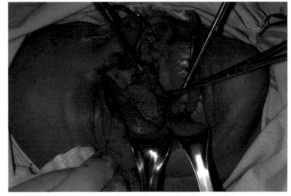

Fig. 18.4 Continuation of dissection.

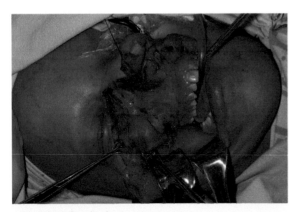

Fig. 18.5 Infraorbital nerve.

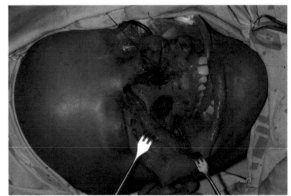

Fig. 18.6 Osteotomies.

Reconstruction of the surgical defect is achieved with an obturator, soft-tissue free flaps, or bony flaps in case of a large bony defect. We will usually prefer a Scapular-free flap based on the angular branch (tip) of the scapula to reconstruct the maxillary sinus.

Obviously, an intraoral procedure should be considered if the extent of disease is limited and the tumor can be resected with sound oncological principles. Although postoperative healing of a superior cheek flap tends to heal beautifully (▶ Fig. 18.7), it adds to postoperative disfigurement and decreases oral opening.

When the initial incision is made through a tooth socket or diastema, extreme care should be taken to remove the involved permanent tooth buds.

Open approaches to the Maxillary sinus may be combined with a subcranial approach to the base of skull as dictated by surgical needs.[12] Previous published literature has shown that extirpation of skull base tumors by use of conventional surgical techniques is feasible and safe among infants and children.[13] The long-term cosmetic effect of the subcranial approach is negligible.[14] A comprehensive algorithm for anterior skull base reconstruction after oncological resections was previously described.[15,16]

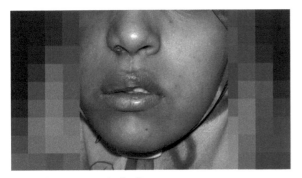

Fig. 18.7 Postoperative healing.

18.2.1 Midfacial Degloving

The procedure used was previously described by Maniglia et al[17] and by Howard and Lund.[18]

The procedure begins with infiltration of 1% Lidocaine and 1:200,000 Adrenaline to the nasal septum, intercartilaginous and sublabial in the area of the columella, and the anterior alveolar process of the maxilla. A sublabial incision is made in the alveolar process of the maxilla about 4 to 6 mm above the teeth from first molar to first molar. This incision can be extended even further back to the third molars if a larger exposure is needed. Bilateral intercartilaginous incisions between the upper and lower lateral cartilages are then made, with full transfixion between the septum and columella. These incisions are extended in order to meet across the floor of the nose permitting elevation of the soft tissues of the dorsum of the nose. Finally, bilateral pyriform aperture incisions are performed to allow the skin and soft tissues of the middle third of the face to be degloved completely. The entire midfacial skin is stripped from the dorsum of the nose and anterior wall of maxilla (▶ Fig. 18.8).

Elevation of the maxillary periosteum and the soft tissues of the cheek allow exposure and preservation of the infraorbital nerves (▶ Fig. 18.9). The elevation is continued till the level of glabella superiorly and medial canthus laterally. The bony nasal pyramid and the attached upper lateral cartilages are exposed completely. Two rubber drains (Penrose type) are passed through the nose and upper lip and are used to retract the midfacial flap along with the upper lip.

Osteotomies are then performed according to the surgical plan. In case of a medial maxillectomy, the procedure begins with removal of the anterior wall of the maxillary sinus (previously described by P. Mallur and G. Har-El).[19] This is best achieved with Kerrison-Rongeurs with bone removal starting inferomedially and continuing superomedially toward the ethmoid air cells and superolaterally

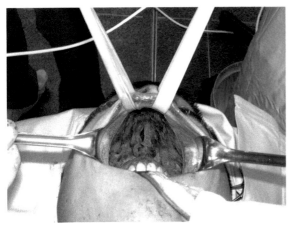

Fig. 18.8 Midfacial degloving: retraction of midfacial flap.

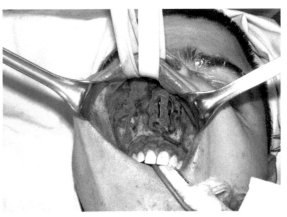

Fig. 18.9 Midfacial degloving: preservation of the infraorbital nerve.

toward the zygomatic arch. Care must be taken to protect and preserve the infraorbital nerve. This is best done by leaving a narrow bony ledge around the infraorbital foramen (▶ Fig. 18.9). Once this is performed, the nasolacrimal sac and duct are addressed. This can be managed by simple transection at the level of the orbital rim, with or without stenting. A cut is made along the nasal bone from the pyriform aperture to the glabella and connected to a posteriorly directed cut along or below and parallel to the frontoethmoidal suture line. The posterior extent of this frontoethmoidal cut is then connected to an oblique cut ending at the orbital rim, medial to the infraorbital foramen. Medial osteotomies are made along the floor of the nasal cavity, separating the lateral nasal wall. Soft-tissue cuts follow each bony osteotomy, freeing the specimen stepwise. The final cut is made with curved osteotomies or heavy curved scissors, freeing the specimen from the posterolateral nasal wall and ascending process of the palatine bone.

This invariably exposes a bleeding sphenopalatine artery, which can be ligated directly.

Alternatively, this can be addressed by ligating the internal maxillary artery in the pterygopalatine fossa after removing the ascending process of the palatine bone. Special consideration can be given to other anatomical areas once the medial maxillectomy is complete. Orbital contents are exposed and the optic nerve may be exposed through systematic drill out toward the optic foramen. The pterygopalatine fossa, infratemporal fossa, and middle cranial fossa skull base can similarly be exposed by removing the posterior and lateral maxilla. Anterior sphenoidotomy can give wide access to the sella turcica and carotid artery. The anterior cranial base can be exposed through middle turbinate excision, though conventional literature supports need for frontal craniotomy or subfrontal approach for "En-bloc" removal of neoplasms encroaching or involving the anterior cranial base.

Traditional limitations for the MFD in accessing the frontal sinus can be overcome by performing ethmoidectomy first and then by detaching the medial canthal tendon to provide additional superiorly based soft-tissue retraction. This maneuver allows complete exposure of the frontal sinus by removing its floor in a posterior-to-anterior direction, starting at the frontal outflow tract. Though rarely needed, an additional exposure can be obtained by removing the anterior frontal sinus wall in an inferomedial-to-superolateral direction. At the conclusion of the extirpative procedure, the maxillectomy cavity is packed with Vaseline gauze strips. Meticulous attention is paid to the previously mentioned intranasal and sublabial incisions. The intranasal incisions are closed with fine absorbable sutures with attention to proper alignment, projection, and rotation (▶ Fig. 18.10). The sublabial incisions can be closed with 3–0 absorbable sutures.

As in open approaches, a combined approach to the base of skull is also feasible. In the classical case of JNAs, a midfacial degloving (▶ Fig. 18.11) can be combined with a subcranial approach effectively for intracranial extensions of this tumor.[20,21]

18.2.2 Combined Approach

See ▶ Fig. 18.12, ▶ Fig. 18.13, ▶ Fig. 18.14, ▶ Fig. 18.15, ▶ Fig. 18.16, and ▶ Fig. 18.17.

18.2.3 Hemi–degloving

See ▶ Fig. 18.18, ▶ Fig. 18.19, and ▶ Fig. 18.20.

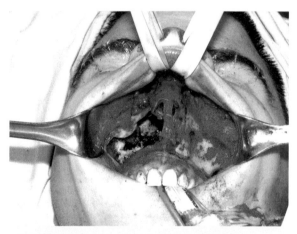

Fig. 18.10 Midfacial degloving: osteotomy of anterior maxillary wall with preservation of the infraorbital nerve be leaving a bony ledge.

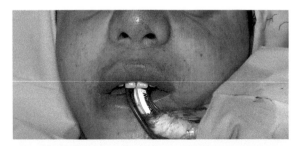

Fig. 18.11 Midfacial degloving: closure of the flaps.

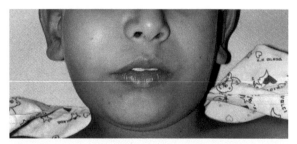

Fig. 18.12 Preoperative picture.

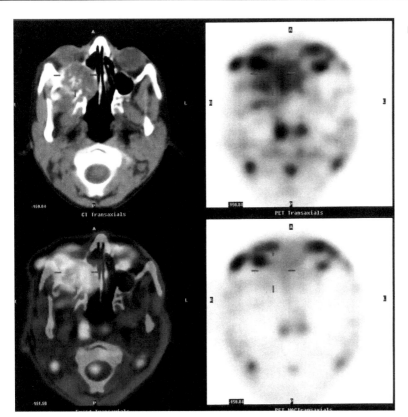

Fig. 18.13 Preoperative PET-CT.

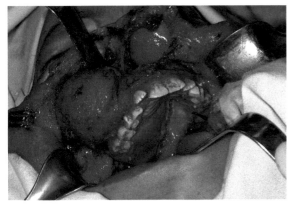

Fig. 18.14 Weber-Ferguson incision with palatal incision.

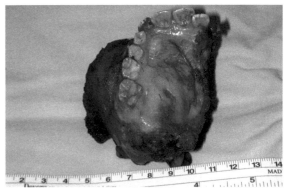

Fig. 18.15 Resected specimen.

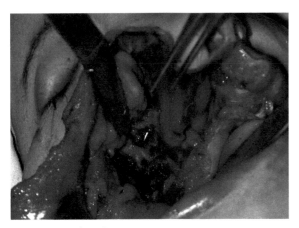

Fig. 18.16 Defect after resection.

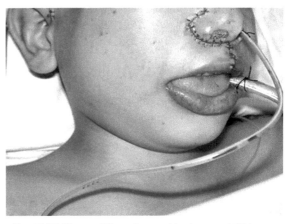

Fig. 18.17 Closure of flaps after combined approach Weber-Ferguson + infratemporal.

18.3 Endoscopic Maxillectomy

With continued advances in endoscopic techniques, a substantial number of open surgeries have been supplanted by endonasal procedures.[22] These approaches have expanded considerably to encompass progressively larger, more complex lesions. This paradigm shift has been clearly demonstrated in surgical approaches to the maxillary sinus, where open medial maxillectomy has given way to endoscopic approaches.[22] The

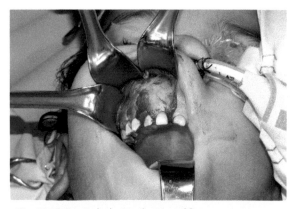

Fig. 18.18 Hemi–degloving elevation of flaps.

technique described herein involves En-bloc resection of the entire lateral nasal wall, along with the tumor. General endotracheal anesthesia is used. Topical intranasal decongestion is achieved with 2% oxymetazoline–soaked neurosurgical pledgets. Lidocaine 1% with 1:100,000 epinephrine is injected intranasally along the inferior meatal wall, into the turbinates, and along the maxillary crest up to the attachment of the middle turbinate. Initial incision is made along the superior resection margin, which includes ethmoid sinuses. The middle turbinate is resected using a back biter and followed with bipolar cautery. Using a Freer elevator, dissection is carried just inferior to the fovea ethmoidalis up to the sphenoid rostrum. The ethmoid arteries are identified and cauterized with bipolar cautery along the way. This frees the specimen superiorly. Inferior incision is carried out at the inferior meatus. The mucosa is incised with the unipolar electrocautery at the junction of the lateral wall with the floor of the nose. Inferior meatotomy is performed at the anterior end of the meatus. Using a straight osteotome, inferior meatal wall is osteotomized up to the posterior wall of the maxillary sinus. The anterior margin of resection includes a cut made from the anterior attachment of the middle turbinate to the lateral nasal wall downward inferiorly to include not only the uncinate

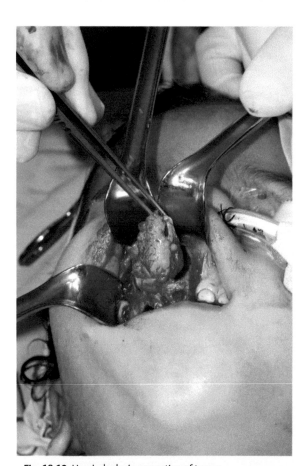

Fig. 18.19 Hemi–degloving resection of tumor.

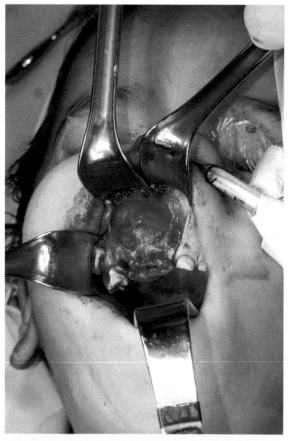

Fig. 18.20 Hemi–degloving postresection surgical space.

process but also the frontal process of the maxilla containing the nasolacrimal canal and duct. This incision is continued anterior to the inferior turbinate head to connect to the inferior meatotomy cuts. Following elevation of the soft tissue, anterior osteotomy is made along the frontal process of the maxilla into the maxillary sinus. This osteotomy is anterior to the nasolacrimal canal. Following osteotomy, the nasolacrimal duct, as it descends from the lacrimal sac, is divided with the endoscopic scissors and included in the specimen. The lateral wall is mobilized medially with progressive dissection allowing entry into the maxillary sinus. Likewise, any tumor in the sinus is mobilized with the lateral nasal wall medially. If there is significant lateral extension of the tumor within the sinus that prevents exposure, its piecemeal removal may be required to allow further work. At this point, the dissection is within the maxillary sinus. Posterior cuts are made using a Freer elevator through the maxillary sinus, just posterior to the maxillary ostium at its junction with the orbit. With progressive dissection, the entire specimen is pended on the sphenopalatine artery. The sphenopalatine artery is clipped, cauterized, and cut. The posterior attachment of the inferior turbinate is cut with curved endoscopic scissors, and the lateral wall along with the tumor is removed. The remaining mucosa of the ethmoid sinuses superiorly and laterally is removed for margin control. Likewise, margins can be taken from the maxillary sinus. Using 30° and 70° Endoscopes, the entire lining of the superior, lateral, inferior, and anterior walls of the maxillary sinus can be visualized and mucosa can be removed to clear a potential multicentric disease. However, this may not be necessary if there is no involvement of the maxillary sinus. If necessary, the bony walls of the maxillary sinus may be drilled. Likewise, the lamina papyracea and the adjacent medial wall of the orbit may be removed. The anterior wall of the sphenoid sinus can easily be resected if necessary. A dacryocystorhinostomy is then performed, and a lacrimal stent is placed and kept for 3 months.

A modification of the "En-bloc" resection may utilize the versatility of an endoscopic approach and tailored for tumor removal. For tumors limited to the medial maxillary wall, resection of the inferior turbinate and medial wall is indicated, whereas the nasolacrimal duct can be preserved or included in the resection as needed. In cases with lateral or anterior extension, the medial maxillectomy can be extended anteriorly up to the piriform aperture or anteromedially to the infraorbital foramen. This procedure is known as an endoscopic Denker's or a Sturmann-Canfield procedure. This is done by first exposing the frontal process of the maxilla along the piriform aperture, just anterior to the anterior head of the inferior turbinate using monopolar cautery. A subperiosteal elevation of the soft tissue off the anterior wall of the maxilla follows until identifying the infraorbital foramen. An osteotome is then utilized to cut the anterior wall of

the maxilla laterally as needed and superiorly up to the infraorbital fissure under the soft tissue. This allows a wide angle of visualization and control of the anterior, lateral, and inferior walls of the maxillary sinus. Similarly, ethmoidectomy and sphenoidectomy can be performed according to the tumors extent.

18.4 Highlights

- Surgical resection of pediatric maxillary sinus pathology has evolved from open to endoscopic approaches.
- Open approaches still remain the gold standard for extirpation for the extirpation of tumors especially in the developing countries where cutting edge technology and expertise are lacking.
- Surgeons operating in this anatomical location should be able to perform both endoscopic and open approaches.
- All surgical approach must take into consideration the developing pediatric craniofacial skeleton.
- It seems that maxillary sinus osteotomies have negligible cosmetic and functional effect on the growing facial skeleton.

References

[1] Perry KS, Tkaczuk AT, Caccamese JF Jr, Ord RA, Pereira KD. Tumors of the pediatric maxillofacial skeleton: a 20-year clinical study. JAMA Otolaryngol Head Neck Surg 2015;141(1):40–44
[2] Aregbesola SB, Ugboko VI, Akinwande JA, Arole GF, Fagade OO. Orofacial tumours in suburban Nigerian children and adolescents. Br J Oral Maxillofac Surg 2005;43(3):226–231
[3] Sato M, Tanaka N, Sato T, Amagasa T. Oral and maxillofacial tumours in children: a review. Br J Oral Maxillofac Surg 1997;35(2):92–95
[4] Mamabolo M, Noffke C, Raubenheimer E. Odontogenic tumours manifesting in the first two decades of life in a rural African population sample: a 26 year retrospective analysis. Dentomaxillofac Radiol 2011;40(6):331–337
[5] McCarthy EF. Fibro-osseous lesions of the maxillofacial bones. Head Neck Pathol 2013;7(1):5–10
[6] Zhang J, Gu Z, Jiang L, et al. Ameloblastoma in children and adolescents. Br J Oral Maxillofac Surg 2010;48(7):549–554
[7] Lund V, Howard DJ, Wei WI. Endoscopic resection of malignant tumors of the nose and sinuses. Am J Rhinol 2007;21(1):89–94
[8] Nicolai P, Battaglia P, Bignami M, et al. Endoscopic surgery for malignant tumors of the sinonasal tract and adjacent skull base: a 10-year experience. Am J Rhinol 2008;22(3):308–316
[9] Snyderman CH, Carrau RL, Kassam AB, et al. Endoscopic skull base surgery: principles of endonasal oncological surgery. J Surg Oncol 2008;97(8):658–664
[10] Hanna E, DeMonte F, Ibrahim S, Roberts D, Levine N, Kupferman M. Endoscopic resection of sinonasal cancers with and without craniotomy: oncologic results. Arch Otolaryngol Head Neck Surg 2009;135(12):1219–1224
[11] Fliss DM, Gil Z. Atlas of surgical approaches to paranasal sinuses and the skull base. Springer; 2016:109–137
[12] Fliss DM, Abergel A, Cavel O, Margalit N, Gil Z. Combined subcranial approaches for excision of complex anterior skull base tumors. Arch Otolaryngol Head Neck Surg 2007;133(9):888–896
[13] Gil Z, Constantini S, Spektor S, et al. Skull base approaches in the pediatric population. Head Neck 2005;27(8):682–689
[14] Shlomi B, Chaushu S, Gil Z, Chaushu G, Fliss DM. Effects of the subcranial approach on facial growth and development. Otolaryngol Head Neck Surg 2007;136(1):27–32

[15] Gil Z, Abergel A, Leider-Trejo L, et al. A comprehensive algorithm for anterior skull base reconstruction after oncological resections. Skull Base 2007;17(1):25–37

[16] Duek I, Pener-Tessler A, Yanko-Arzi R, et al. Skull base reconstruction in the pediatric patient. J Neurol Surg B Skull Base 2018;79(1):81–90

[17] Maniglia AJ. Indications and techniques of midfacial degloving: a 15-year experience. Arch Otolaryngol Head Neck Surg 1986; 112(7):750–752

[18] Howard DJ, Lund VJ. The midfacial degloving approach to sinonasal disease. J Laryngol Otol 1992;106(12):1059–1062

[19] de Souza C. Atlas of Head & Neck Surgery. JP Medical Ltd; 2013

[20] Fliss DM, Zucker G, Amir A, Gatot A. The combined subcranial and midfacial degloving technique for tumor resection: report of three cases. J Oral Maxillofac Surg 2000;58(1): 106–110

[21] Margalit N, Wasserzug O, De-Row A, Abergel A, Fliss DM, Gil Z. Surgical treatment of juvenile nasopharyngeal angiofibroma with intracranial extension: clinical article. J Neurosurg Pediatr 2009;4(2):113–117

[22] Lee JT, Suh JD, Carrau RL, Chu MW, Chiu AG. Endoscopic Denker's approach for resection of lesions involving the anteroinferior maxillary sinus and infratemporal fossa. Laryngoscope 2017;127(3):556–560

19 Vagal Nerve Stimulation

Oded Ben-Ari, Gilad Horowitz, Itzhak Fried, Dan M. Fliss

Summary

Vagal nerve stimulation (VNS) is indicated in cases of epilepsy which are refractory to medical treatment. Under general anesthesia, a left cervical incision is made to expose the vagus nerve. Electrodes are then placed over the nerve and connected to a generator which is inserted to a subclavicular skin pocket. The procedure is safe, well tolerated and effective.

Keywords: Vagal nerve stimulation, VNS, epilepsy, intractable seizures, seizure control

19.1 Introduction

Approximately one-third of all patients with epilepsy will suffer from refractory seizures despite optimal antiepileptic drug therapy, or they will experience unacceptable side effects of their medications.[1] In July 1997, the US Food and Drug Administration (FDA) approved the use of intermittent stimulation of the left vagal nerve "… as adjunctive therapy in reducing the frequency of seizures in adults and adolescents over 12 years of age with partial onset seizures which are refractory to antiepileptic medications."[1] Since then, VNS has been used as an effective treatment for medically intractable seizures. The elaboration of indications to include children younger than 12 years has gained popularity during the past decade, with mounting evidence demonstrating the procedure as being safe and effective.[2–5] Coykendall et al.[6] concluded that VNS treatment is safe in young children, with a reported efficacy surpassing 50% in reducing frequency of attacks. The procedure is well tolerated and was reported to carry a low complication rate.[7] There is as yet no consensus regarding the mechanism of action of VNS, but it most probably acts at multiple sites.[8] Alternating synchronization and de-synchronization of electrical activity may reflect the mechanism of action of VNS in achieving seizure control.[9]

19.2 Preoperative Evaluation and Anesthesia

Preoperative antibiotics are administered (first-generation cephalosporins) intravenously. A short-acting muscle relaxant is used for the procedure. General endotracheal anesthesia is performed. The patient is placed in the supine position. A shoulder roll is placed to allow for head extension. The patient's head is turned to the right and the surgical field is scrubbed and draped (▶Fig. 19.1).

19.3 Surgical Technique

A small horizontal left neck incision is performed, half way between the mastoid and the clavicle above the anterior border of the sternocleidomastoid muscle (▶Fig. 19.2). The left carotid sheath is exposed. The vagus nerve is located within the carotid sheath. A segment of 3 cm from the vagus nerve is exposed below the branching of the cervical cardiac nerves and above the branching of the recurrent laryngeal nerve (▶Fig. 19.3). The exposed nerve should be handled with care and may be raised with a vessel loop (▶Fig. 19.4). Three electrodes are then placed on the exposed segment of the vagus nerve. A strain relief loop is made to allow for lead movement that will not result in pulling of electrodes or the generator. Two silastic tie-downs, using

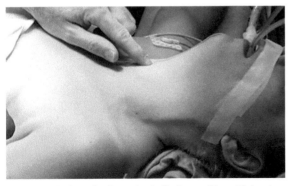

Fig. 19.1 Endotracheal anesthesia. Supine position with head extension.

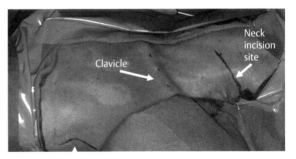

Fig. 19.2 Draping and locations of left horizontal cervical and subclavicular incisions.

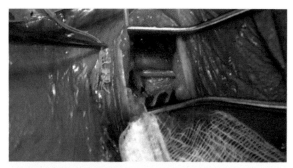

Fig. 19.3 Left carotid sheath with a 3 cm segment of exposed vagus nerve.

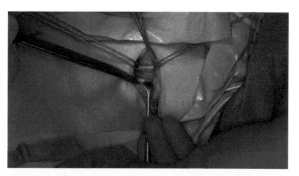

Fig. 19.4 The vagus nerve is raised with vessel loops.

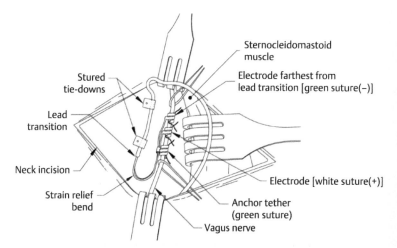

Sternocleidomastoid muscle

Electrode farthest from lead transition [green suture(–)]

Stured tie-downs

Lead transition

Neck incision

Strain relief bend

Electrode [white suture(+)]

Anchor tether (green suture)

Vagus nerve

Fig. 19.5 Placement of electrodes on vagus with a strain relief loop and tie-down sutures.

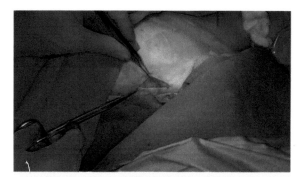

Fig. 19.6 Incision for chest subclavicular pocket and creation of a sub-cutaneous tunnel to the neck.

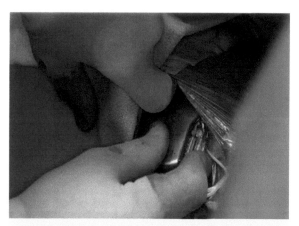

Fig. 19.7 Generator is inserted to the subclavicular pocket.

a nonabsorbable suture, are made to secure the strain relief loop to the cervical fascia (▶Fig. 19.5). A chest sub-cutaneous pocket is created in the thorax just below the clavicle (▶Fig. 19.6). The generator is inserted to this pocket and secured using a nonabsorbable suture to the fascia (▶Fig. 19.7). The lead connecting the generator to the electrode runs through a subcutaneous tunnel connecting the two.

19.4 Postoperative Treatment

A short overnight hospitalization is usually required during which the patient is observed for complications. The generator is activated by a neurologist only 2 to 4 weeks following the surgical procedure.

19.5 Highlights

a. Indications
   - Adjunctive therapy in seizures refractory to antiepileptic medications.
   - To reduce the frequency of seizures in partial onset epilepsy.
b. Contraindications
   - One vagus nerve.
   - Hoarseness.
   - Heart arrhythmias.
   - Lung or breathing disorder.
   - Vasovagal syncope.
c. Complications
   - Skin infection.
   - Hoarseness or change of voice.
   - Coughing.
   - Laryngospasm.
   - Vocal cord paralysis.
   - Nausea and vomiting.
   - Implant infection.
   - Heart rate changes.
d. Special preoperative considerations
   - General endotracheal anesthesia.
   - Antibiotics and short-acting relaxants.
e. Special intraoperative considerations
   - Cervical incision to expose vagus nerve.
   - Placing of electrodes on the nerve.
   - Creating a subclavicular skin pocket for the generator.
   - Skin tunnel for the lead connecting the generator to the electrode.
f. Special postoperative considerations
   - An overnight hospitalization.
   - Activation of generator after 2 to 4 weeks.

References

[1] Milby AH, Halpern CH, Baltuch GH. Vagus nerve stimulation in the treatment of refractory epilepsy. Neurotherapeutics 2009;6(2):228–237

[2] Patwardhan RV, Stong B, Bebin EM, Mathisen J, Grabb PA. Efficacy of vagal nerve stimulation in children with medically refractory epilepsy. Neurosurgery 2000;47(6):1353–1357, discussion 1357–1358

[3] Saneto RP, Sotero de Menezes MA, Ojemann JG, et al. Vagus nerve stimulation for intractable seizures in children. Pediatr Neurol 2006;35(5):323–326

[4] Alexopoulos AV, Kotagal P, Loddenkemper T, Hammel J, Bingaman WE. Long-term results with vagus nerve stimulation in children with pharmacoresistant epilepsy. Seizure 2006;15(7):491–503

[5] Helmers SL, Wheless JW, Frost M, et al. Vagus nerve stimulation therapy in pediatric patients with refractory epilepsy: a retrospective study. J Child Neurol 2001;16(11):843–848

[6] Coykendall DS, Gauderer MW, Blouin RR, Morales A. Vagus nerve stimulation for the management of seizures in children: an 8-year experience. J Pediatr Surg 2010;45(7):1479–1483

[7] Horowitz G, Amit M, Fried I, et al. Vagal nerve stimulation for refractory epilepsy: the surgical procedure and complications in 100 implantations by a single medical center. Eur Arch Otorhinolaryngol 2013;270(1):355–358

[8] Mapstone TB Vagus nerve stimulation: current concepts Neurosurg Focus 2008;25:E9

[9] Koo B. EEG changes with vagus nerve stimulation. J Clin Neurophysiol 2001;18(5):434–441

20 Pediatric Hypoglossal Nerve Stimulation

Gillian R. Diercks, Christopher Hartnick

Summary

Hypoglossal nerve stimulation is a new technology used to treat refractory cases of obstructive sleep apnea (OSA) in appropriately selected adult patients. Use of the stimulator in pediatric patients is limited to research investigations currently, but initial studies suggest this technology may be useful for alleviating upper airway obstruction in adolescents and young adults with Down syndrome who have persistent OSA after adenotonsillectomy. Here we outline the general principles and considerations for hypoglossal nerve stimulator implantation, as well as discuss surgical modifications to allow for implantation in pediatric patients.

Keywords: Hypoglossal nerve stimulator, obstructive sleep apnea, Down syndrome

20.1 Introduction

Hypoglossal nerve stimulator implantation is an emerging technology for treatment of OSA. The stimulator is an implantable device that senses respiratory variation and delivers electrical impulses to anterior branches of the hypoglossal nerve during inspiration. Stimulation of the genioglossus and geniohyoid muscles results in protrusion of the tongue base, which alleviates nocturnal upper airway obstruction in patients who respond to therapy (▶ Fig. 20.1).

Initial studies published in 2001[1] demonstrated that nerve stimulator therapy reduced the apnea hypopnea index (AHI) in both rapid-eye movement (REM) and non-REM sleep by over 50% as well as reduced oxygen desaturations in adults with severe OSA. Additional trials performed randomized, controlled therapy withdrawal in patients who responded to stimulation and noted that with therapy non-use, AHI increased significantly, as did oxygen desaturations.[2] Thirty-six month follow-up data suggests that nerve stimulation is well tolerated, with up to 81% of patients reporting daily use. In addition, patients with follow-up polysomnography data at 36 months continued to demonstrate significant reductions in AHI (>50%) compared to baseline measurements.[3] The hypoglossal nerve stimulator (Inspire Medical Systems®) is currently approved by the United States Food and Drug Administration (FDA) for implantation in adults age 22 years or older with moderate-to-severe OSA (15≥ AHI ≤65 events/hour) who cannot tolerate or have failed to improve with positive airway pressure therapy and who are without concentric airway collapse at the level of the soft palate. Moreover, eligible subjects should have a central apnea index that accounts for ≤25% of the total AHI on baseline polysomnography.

While the device is only approved for commercial use in adult patients, an investigational device exemption was granted by the FDA for study of this technology in adolescent and young adult patients, aged

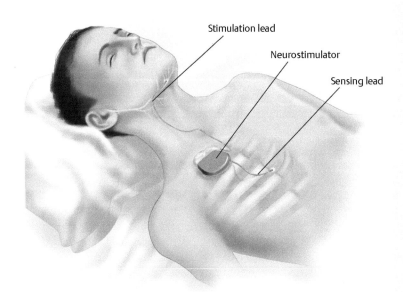

Fig. 20.1 The hypoglossal nerve stimulator is an implantable device with a pacemaker-like impulse generator that receives input about respiratory variation from a pleural sensing lead placed between the intercostal muscles. An electrical impulse then stimulates medial branches of the hypoglossal nerve that result in genioglossus activation and tongue protrusion.

Stimulation lead

Neurostimulator

Sensing lead

10 to 22 years, with Down syndrome (DS) and refractory severe OSA after tonsillectomy and adenoidectomy (T&A) who are nonresponders or nonadherent with positive airway pressure therapy. Patients with DS have an increased risk of OSA in comparison to the general pediatric population (30–80% vs. 2–5.7%), in part due to their unique anatomic and physiologic differences that include decreased muscular tone, macroglossia, maxillary hypoplasia, and lingual tonsil hypertrophy. Up to 67% of children with DS and OSA will have persistent upper airway obstruction after T&A. Initial pilot studies of hypoglossal nerve stimulator implantation in the pediatric DS population demonstrate excellent device adherence and tolerance, quality of life improvement, and a significant (>50%) reduction in AHI at 6 to 12-month follow-up.[4,5] With further investigation, we anticipate the device will be approved for use in adolescents and young adults with Down syndrome, and perhaps other special populations as well.

This chapter outlines necessary preoperative investigations, as well as provides step by step guidance on how hypoglossal nerve stimulator implantation is performed in children. We also highlight several modifications to surgical technique that facilitate stimulator placement in smaller patients.

20.2 Preoperative Evaluation and Anesthesia

As with adult patients, successful hypoglossal nerve stimulator implantation begins with appropriate patient selection. In adult patients, prior T&A, lingual tonsillectomy, uvulopalatoplasty, tongue base reduction, and other surgical procedures to reduce the burden of disease are not needed prior to implantation; however, documentation of a patient's inability to tolerate or failure to respond to positive airway pressure therapy is required. In children and adolescents, because adenotonsillectomy is a first-line therapy for treatment of OSA, surgical removal of the adenoids and both tonsils should be performed prior to considering hypoglossal nerve stimulator implantation. For children with persistent severe OSA (10 ≥ AHI ≤50 events/hour) after adenotonsillectomy, attempts at treatment of residual disease with noninvasive positive airway pressure therapy should be performed. Nerve stimulator implantation may be considered in children who do not respond to or cannot tolerate therapy. All children being considered for implantation should undergo full-night diagnostic polysomnography scored using AASM pediatric criteria within 6 months of planned implantation surgery. Baseline measurements allow for inclusion of children with severe OSA who have ≤25% contribution by central apnea or mixed events to the total AHI. Height and weight measurements should also be obtained so that children with significant obesity, which may be a contributing factor to their persistent disease, are excluded. In adult patients, a body mass index (BMI) >32 kg/m^2 has been associated with a failure to respond to therapy, though a cut-off has not yet been established in children. In children, BMI percentiles calculated through the centers for disease control (CDC) BMI-for-age growth chart are often utilized by the pediatric community. We have utilized the 95th percentile for children under the age of 18 as a cut-off for inclusion in our investigational trials.[5]

All candidates should have a thorough examination of the facial bones, nasal cavity, oral cavity, and oropharynx to assess for anatomic factors that could be contributing to airway obstruction and easily corrected. All children should also have a baseline tongue exam to document tongue size, resting position, and hypoglossal nerve function. All candidates should also be screened for behavioral and communication issues that would preclude participation with treatment; in our experience children should be able to communicate and localize any sources of discomfort with their caregivers.

Studies of the hypoglossal nerve stimulator in adult patients suggest that patients with circumferential airway collapse at the level of the velopharynx are less likely to respond to therapy. Therefore, a drug-induced sleep endoscopy (DISE) is required in order to evaluate patterns of obstruction including at the levels of the soft palate, oropharynx, hypopharynx, and larynx. Technique for DISE is beyond the scope of this chapter, but a team approach is critical to the success of this evaluation. During the procedure, the child is sedated using propofol and/or dexmedetomidine until adequate sedation is achieved to initiate obstructive events, which the anesthesiologist should allow to continue during evaluation. The surgeon should be a skilled endoscopist and evaluate and categorize patterns of collapse in the upper airway. Collapse should be evaluated both before and after a jaw thrust maneuver. We have found it useful to utilize the VOTE classification scheme[6] to record and communicate airway findings in a systematic way. Patients without circumferential collapse at soft palate can be considered for implantation.

Beyond anatomic and behavioral considerations, the patient's medical history must be taken into account to optimize patient selection as well. For example, surgery should be deferred, or at least delayed, in children with active cardiopulmonary disease that will require further thoracic surgical procedures which might disrupt the impulse generator or associated electrodes. With the advent of new generations of the device which are MRI compatible for imaging of the head, abdomen, and extremities, disease processes such as cholesteatoma that could require serial MRI imaging are no longer absolute contraindications to implantation. However, the need for future imaging, particularly of the thorax, should be a consideration because current devices are not compatible with MRI imaging of the chest.

Prior to implantation, a full discussion of the risks and benefits of implantation should be conducted. Patients should be aware of the risks of surgery, including long-term risks of device extrusion or the need for device explantation. Patients and their families must also be informed that the impulse generator battery will need to be replaced after approximately 10 years, and that further surgery will be required to do so. Particularly for the pediatric population, it should be clear that long term data is lacking to determine if device settings will remain stable over time. It should be emphasized that in order for the device to be effective, the patient and/or family will need to activate it each night with a remote control device. Finally, patients and their families should be aware that at least annual follow-up will be required to assess surgical wounds and device functioning.

Once the decision has been made to proceed with surgical implantation, the surgical team and equipment should be assembled. Two of each component of the hypoglossal nerve stimulator, including the sensing lead, stimulation lead, and impulse generator, must be available so that backup hardware can be used if needed. At our institution, a separate nerve monitoring team is utilized during hypoglossal nerve stimulator cases to perform Electromyographic (EMG) monitoring of the hypoglossal nerve during nerve dissection and cuff placement, as well as system validation after implantation is completed.

Because EMG monitoring of the genioglossus and hyo-styloglossus musculature is performed during nerve dissection and cuff placement, the patient's tongue motion should not be restricted. Therefore, a nasotracheal tube is preferred to an orotracheal tube. Long-term paralytics should be avoided to facilitate nerve stimulation. Particularly in children with Down syndrome, care should be taken in patient positioning to prevent unnecessary neck manipulation and minimize neck extension due to the risk of atlantoaxial instability.

20.3 Surgical Technique

20.3.1 Incision Placement and Preparation

Classically, the stimulator has been placed through three incisions in the right neck and chest: one in the anterior submental region, one inferior to the clavicle over the pectoralis major muscle, and one in the fourth to sixth intercostal region. A 4-cm transverse submental incision should be marked more anterior than the typical incision used for a submandibular approach at the level of or slightly above the hyoid bone, approximately 0.5 cm from the midline. A second incision, approximately 4 to 5 cm, should be marked 3 fingerbreadths below the clavicle over the pectoralis muscle and the approximate outline of the impulse generator should be marked extending inferior from this incision to identify the extent of pocket dissection. Finally, a 5-cm incision should be marked over the fourth to sixth intercostal space for pleural sensing lead placement. We have found that the intercostal incision is best placed anteriorly, inferior to the nipple line, to aid in identification of the costochondral junction where the internal and external intercostal margin is best identified to facilitate the plane of dissection. In younger children with a small thorax, we have described placement of the impulse generator and pleural sensing lead through a single incision rather than two separate incisions, to reduce the risk of impulse generator extrusion. In these smaller children, we have also described lateral positioning, rather than medial positioning, of the pleural sensing lead to reduce the risk of cardiac interference[7] (▶Fig. 20.2).

The incisions should be injected with local anesthetic.

20.3.2 EMG Monitoring

We prefer to place electrodes for EMG monitoring of the tongue musculature after the neck incisions have been marked to minimize patient movement that could

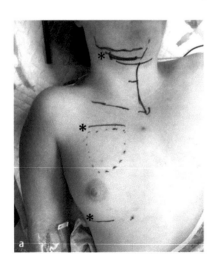
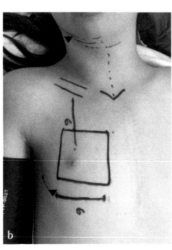

Fig. 20.2 Three-incision approach **(a)** and two-incision approach **(b)**. In the three-incision approach, submental, subclavicular, and intercostal incisions (demarcated with the "*") are used. In the two-incision approach (each incision is identified by the *arrowhead*), a submental incision is used to place the stimulator lead, and the impulse generator and pleural sensing lead are placed through the same subcostal incision.

displace the monitoring electrodes. Prass-paired 18-mm electrodes are used. The tongue is grasped with a gauze and pulled anterolaterally to expose the ventrolateral surface and floor of mouth. The first, exclusion, channel is placed into the hyo-styloglossus along the ventrolateral aspect of the right tongue 5 cm posterior to the tongue tip, taking care to keep the electrode needles superficial in a submucosal plane. The second, inclusion, channel is placed into the genioglossus muscle by angling the electrode into the floor of the mouth to the right of the frenulum, approximately 5 cm posterior to the anterior tongue (▶ Fig. 20.3 and ▶ Fig. 20.4). Care should be taken to avoid trauma to the submandibular ducts. Redundant lead length should be created prior to securing leads with a tegaderm to allow for tongue mobility without electrode displacement. A dental roll can be placed between the molars to maintain an open mouth position to prevent electrode migration and also facilitate tongue mobility during stimulation (▶ Fig. 20.4). Monitoring of the marginal mandibular branch of the facial nerve can also be considered but is not critical as the submandibular dissection is performed superior and anterior to the nerve.

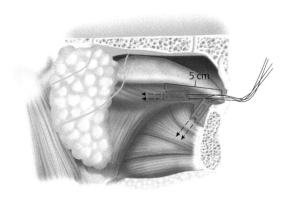

● Inclusion channel: genioglossus

● Exclusion channel: hyo-styloglossus

Fig. 20.3 Electromyographic (EMG) potential monitoring lead placement demonstrating electrode needle vectors into the ventrolateral tongue (hyo-styloglossus) and floor of mouth (genioglossus).

20.3.3 Preparation

The skin is prepared using betadine antiseptic solution. The surgical field is then draped using sterile towels followed by loban dressing inferior to the mandible. A translucent sterile drape is then placed superiorly to allow for visualization of the tongue and electrodes. Additional sterile drapes are applied. Intravenous antibiotics are administered prior to incision.

20.3.4 Sensing Lead Placement

Hypoglossal nerve dissection and placement of the sensing lead are then performed. A No. 15 blade is used to make an incision which is carried through the skin, subcutaneous tissue, and platysma. Subplatysmal flaps are then developed superiorly and inferiorly. The anterior belly of the digastric muscle is identified and dissection is carried inferiorly until the digastric tendon is identified and skeletonized. Two vessel loops are then placed around the tendon to allow for anteroinferior retraction. Fascial bands around anteroinferior aspect of the submandibular gland are incised to allow for improved retraction of the gland. Richardson retractors are particularly useful for retraction. The posterior border of the myohyoid muscle is skeletonized as well, which facilitates retraction of the muscle anteriorly to expose the floor of mouth and anterior branches of the hypoglossal nerve during dissection (▶ Fig. 20.5). A fine dissector and bipolar cautery are then used to dissect anteriorly and divide fascia overlying the hypoglossal nerve. Delicate ranine veins should be identified and divided to prevent bleeding in the surgical field. As dissection is carried anteriorly, lateral branches of the nerve extending to the styloglossus and hyoglossus musculature should be identified for exclusion. As dissection is carried anteriorly, medial branches to the genioglossus and geniohyoid should be identified for inclusion (▶ Fig. 20.6). The main branch point at which lateral and medial branches occur should be noted, and EMG monitoring should be used to assess for any exclusion nerve fibers with a late branch point. Once late branches have been excluded, a right-angle dissection can be used to dissect circumferentially around the nerve to create a tunnel underneath the nerve, through which an additional vessel loop can be used to facilitate

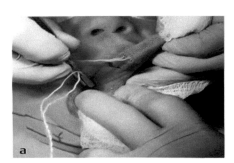

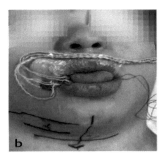

Fig. 20.4 Example of intraoperative EMG lead placement. Note anterolateral leave placement is in a submucosal, superficial plane **(a)**. Leads should have some redundancy to allow for tongue movement during the case **(b)**.

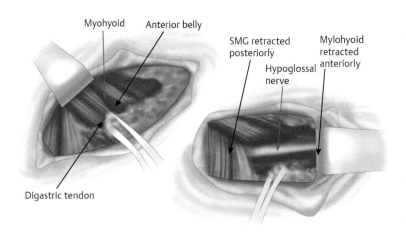

Myohyoid Anterior belly

SMG retracted
posteriorly

Mylohyoid
retracted
anteriorly

Hypoglossal
nerve

Digastric tendon

a

b

Fig. 20.5 Anatomic landmarks, including the myohyoid, anterior belly of the digastric and submandibular gland, are identified **(a)** and retracted **(b)** to expose the main trunk of the hypoglossal nerve.

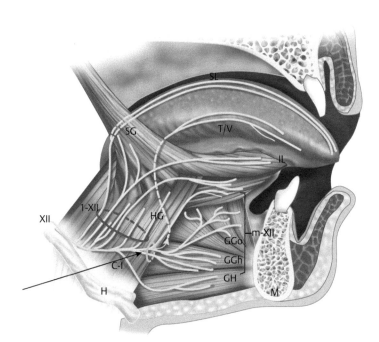

Fig. 20.6 As the hypoglossal nerve is dissected anteriorly, lateral branches to the hyo-styloglossus muscles should be identified and excluded. More medial branches extending to the genioglossus should be included in the stimulator cuff. The C-1 branch to the geniohyoid, if identified, can be included in the cuff as well.

identification of inclusion branches and provide gentle retraction (▶ Fig. 20.7). Fascial bands approximately 1 cm anterior to the branchpoint are then divided circumferentially to facilitate placement of the stimulation electrode silicone cuff around the nerve without resistance.

Angled forceps are used to unfurl and expose the anterior corner of the outer silicone flap of the stimulation electrode cuff. A right-angle dissector is then passed under the inclusion branches of the nerve and the vessel loop is removed. The exposed corner of the cuff is then grasped with the dissector, and the outer flap is carefully unfurled advanced under the nerve. As the flap is advanced, the angled forceps are used to carefully elevate the posterior

aspect of the shorter, inner flap of the electrode cuff to facilitate cuff placement around the ventral and inferior aspect of the nerve. The outer flap is then released and positioned over the shorter, inner flap. Care is taken to ensure all inclusion branches are in good contact with the cuff. Sterile saline is then instilled between the nerve and the inner flap of the cuff with an angiocath (▶ Fig. 20.8).

The electrode is then passed under the digastric tendon and anchored to the ventral aspect of the tendon with permanent suture.

The wound is then irrigated with sterile saline and bacitracin solution. Hemostasis is verified. Excess lead is then placed into submandibular pocket and a sterile gauze is used to protect the lead and keep the wound clean.

20.3.5 Impulse Generator Pocket Placement

A No. 15 blade is used to incise the skin and dermis at the subclavicular incision. Monopolar cautery is then used to extend the incision through subcutaneous fat and soft tissue until fascia superficial to the pectoralis major is identified. A pocket overlying this fascia is then created using blunt dissection, taking care to maintain a pocket small enough to accommodate the impulse generator and excess lead length only; over enlargement of the pocket may result in impulse generator migration. The wound is

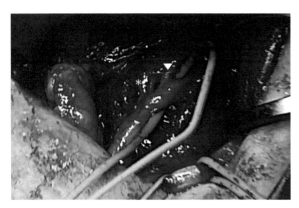

Fig. 20.7 Hypoglossal nerve dissection demonstrating the main trunk of the nerve, lateral branches (*), late lateral branch point (*arrow head*) and medial branches for inclusion in the stimulation cuff (surrounded by vessel loop). Two other vessel loops are depicted at the bottom of the image retracting the digastric tendon.

then inspected and hemostasis is verified. The wound is irrigated with antiseptic solution and packed.

20.3.6 Sensing Lead Placement

As noted above, we have found that a more anterior intercostal incision, which allows for identification of the costochondral junction, can be useful in helping to identify the borders of the internal and external intercostal muscles to facilitate lead placement in the plane between them. The premarked incision site is incised with a No. 15 blade and subcutaneous tissues are divided until the fifth intercostal space and ribs are identified. Identification of the costochondral junction can aid in identifying the plane of dissection. We have found that a small malleable retractor can be used to develop the intercostal plane in an atraumatic fashion. As the plane is dissected, care should be taken to maintain position parallel and along the superior aspect of the rib to avoid injury to the neurovascular bundle. The pleural sensing lead is then grasped with a dissector, with the sensing component facing the pleura, and advanced into the intercostal tunnel (▶ Fig. 20.9). Classically, the plane between the intercostal muscles is identified and the pleural sensing lead is advanced medially. In smaller children, however, medial placement of the sensing lead could lead to artifact secondary to cardiac motion. In these cases, the plane between the intercostal muscles can be developed and the lead can be advanced laterally. We have found that pleural sensing is not compromised with lateral placement[7] (▶ Fig. 20.10). Fixed and moveable anchors of the lead are then secured to the chest

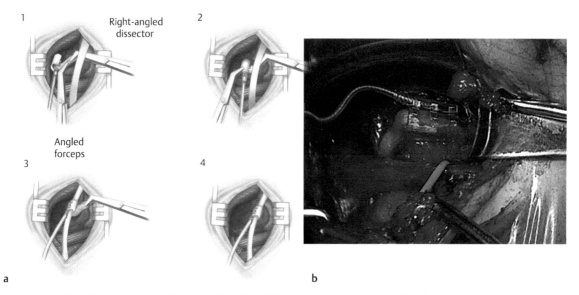

Fig. 20.8 (a, b) Cuff placement around the medial branches of the hypoglossal nerve requires that the longer, outer flap be unfurled and passed underneath the nerve as the shorter, inner cuff is carefully advanced over the ventral and inferior aspects of the nerve. The outer flap is then carefully positioned over the inner cuff.

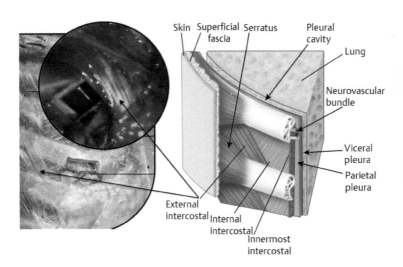

Fig. 20.9 Demonstrates orientation of the internal and external intercostal muscles and the plane of dissection in which to advance the pleural sensing lead.

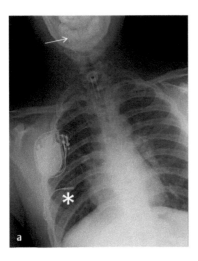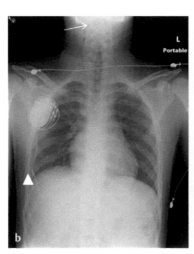

Fig. 20.10 Postoperative posterior–anterior radiograph demonstrating the pleural sensing lead positioned medially (**a**, demarcated by "*") and the pleural sensing lead positioned laterally (**b**, demarcated by the *triangle*). In both images, the stimulator cuff is visible in the submental area and identified with the *arrow*.

wall using permanent suture, taking care to leave a small amount of excess lead between the two to relive any strain created by chest wall movement. Hemostasis is verified and the wound is irrigated.

20.3.7 Lead Tunneling

Wound packing is removed. A tunneling device is then used to pass the stimulation and sensing leads subcutaneously into the pocket created for the impulse generator over the pectoralis major muscle. The device manufacturer provides a disposable tunneling tool, though we have found the tool difficult to manipulate and pass through soft tissue. We have found that commercially available subcutaneous tunneling and delivery tools, such as those used for vascular surgical procedures, allow for more accurate and rapid tunnel placement. As subcutaneous tunnels are created, care should be taken to avoid superficial planes that might result in increased risk of lead palpation or extrusion. In addition, vascular

structures, such as the external jugular vein, should be noted prior to tunneling and avoided.

20.3.8 Impulse Generator Placement

The impulse generator is then brought into the field. The stimulation and sensing leads are then connected to their respective ports on the impulse generator device and secured by tightening screws within each port. Care should be taken not to grasp the lead tips with surgical instruments. Excess lead length is then wrapped around the dorsal aspect of the device. This positioning helps to protect the leads from injury once the impulse generator and excess lead length are placed into the impulse generator pocket over the pectoralis major muscle. The impulse generator is then suspended onto pectoralis major fascia in two different vectors using permanent suture passed through a suture hole on the device. This maneuver is necessary to minimize the risk of impulse generator migration over time (►Fig. 20.11).

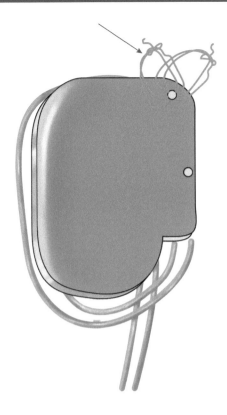

Fig. 20.11 Excess lead length is carefully looped behind the impulse generator as it is placed into the pocket created superficial to the pectoralis major fascia. The impulse generator is suspended from the pectoralis fascia using two permanent sutures placed in different vectors.

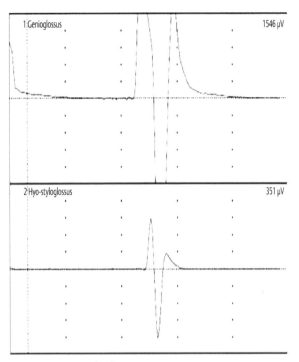

Fig. 20.12 Example of intraoperative system interrogation at 0.4 V stimulation demonstrating minimal exclusion branch stimulation (351 µV) in comparison to inclusion branch activation (1546 µV).

20.3.9 Device Testing

The submandibular incision is gently reexplored to confirm that the cuff has not become dislodged from the nerve during lead tunneling and connection to the impulse generator. The telemetry device is then placed through a sterile sleeve and passed onto the surgical field and placed over the impulse generator. Voltage is gradually increased to verify tongue protrusion and activation of the genioglossus on EMG monitoring, as well as quiescence of the hyo-styloglossus muscle that has been excluded (▶Fig. 20.12). Pleural sensing is also verified. The device is turned back to 0.0 V and turned off.

20.3.10 Wound Closure

All packing is removed. The wounds are reinspected to verify hemostasis. Each incision is then closed in a multilayer fashion. In children we favor a subcuticular closure with an absorbable suture. Drains are not required. The skin is cleaned and surgical tape is applied to the incisions. A pressure dressing is then applied to each incision site.

20.3.11 Postoperative Treatment

A portable two-view (AP and lateral) radiograph should be performed to document device placement immediately after surgery. This not only helps to evaluate for pneumothorax, which is a potential postoperative complication if the pleura was violated during intercostal dissection and sensing lead placement, but can also serve as a reference for future imaging that might be performed to assess for device migration (▶Fig. 20.10).

Children are placed in a sling postoperatively to prevent arm abduction, which in the initial healing phase may result in impulse generator motion and development of a chest wall seroma. Arm abduction past a 45-degree angle is discouraged for the first month after surgery.

All children are admitted postoperatively overnight for monitoring, particularly given their history of severe OSA. Nonsteroidal anti-inflammatories should be avoided to reduce the risk of postoperative bleeding. In our experience, surgery is well tolerated and discomfort can often be managed with acetaminophen alone. Most children are discharged the first postoperative day. Postoperative antibiotics are not necessary if sterile technique is maintained during the surgery and the child does not manipulate the incisions postoperatively.

Postoperative follow-up is planned 1 to 2 weeks after surgery to evaluate the appearance of the surgical sites.

The hypoglossal nerve stimulator is not activated until 1 month after implantation to allow for complete wound healing. Voltage is then increased and the device is titrated. In our initial investigational trials, titrations have been performed during an overnight polysomnogram on the day of activation then 2, 6, and 12 months after surgery and children have not been provided with a range of voltage settings to use at home. As more children are implanted, this schedule may change and voltage ranges, rather than fixed voltage, may be explored.

20.4 Highlights

a. Indications
   - Currently not FDA approved for use in patients <22 years of age; pediatric use is currently investigational.
   - Adults >22 years of age.
   - Moderate-to-severe OSA; 15 ≤AHI ≤65 events/hour (adult criteria) and ≤25% of AHI secondary to central events.
   - Inability to tolerate or poor compliance with positive airway pressure therapy.
   - No concentric collapse of the airway at the level of the soft palate.
b. Contraindications
   - Currently not FDA approved for use in patients <22 years of age; pediatric use is currently investigational.
   - Central or mixed apnea responsible for greater than 25% of the observed AHI.
   - Concentric airway collapse at the level of the soft palate.
   - Patients with neurologic dysfunction and poor control of the upper airway musculature.
   - Patients who are unable to operate the remote control used to activate the device nightly.
   - Patients with a short life expectancy.
   - Patients who are pregnant or plan to become pregnant.
   - Patients who have preexisting medical conditions that require MRI imaging (with the new generation of the device, extrathoracic including extremity and cranial MRI are permitted).
c. Complications
   - Permanent or temporary marginal mandibular nerve and hypoglossal nerve weakness, tongue movement changes resulting in change in speech or swallowing.
   - Pneumothorax.
   - Wound related: infection, scarring, bleeding, hematoma or seroma formation, pain.
   - Device related: allergy or reaction to implanted device or materials, erosion of implant into surrounding tissue or extrusion, migration or fracture of device components, failure to stimulate or need for progressive increase in voltage, battery failure and need for replacement or explantation of device, damage to device secondary to MRI or surgical procedures.
d. Special preoperative considerations
   - Careful patient selection including evaluation of preexisting medical conditions and anatomy.
   - Verification that patient is CPAP intolerant or nonadherent.
   - Preoperative polysomnography to verify patient meets AHI criteria for quality and severity of OSA.
   - Drug-induced sleep endoscopy required to assess patterns of upper airway collapse.
   - Patient ability to participate in therapy with appropriate communication skills, and ability of patient or caregiver to utilize remote control to activate device.
e. Special intraoperative considerations
   - Avoidance of long-acting paralytics.
   - Use of EMG monitoring of the genioglossus and stylo-hyoglossus muscles to help identify inclusion of medial nerve branches in the stimulation pathway.
   - Verify exclusion of any late branchpoints to the stylo-hyoglossus muscles.
   - Consider size of patient when determining whether to utilize a two- vs. three-incision approach and medial vs. lateral advancement of the pleural sensing lead.
   - Gentle manipulation of hardware to prevent damage to the impulse generator and lead components.
   - Secure each component to prevent displacement over time.
f. Special postoperative considerations
   - Postoperative radiographic imaging obtained to rule out pneumothorax and document initial device position in the neck and thorax.
   - Pressure dressing placement.
   - Avoidance of right arm abduction past 45 degrees for 1 month.

References

[1] Schwartz AR, Bennett ML, Smith PL, et al. Therapeutic electrical stimulation of the hypoglossal nerve in obstructive sleep apnea. Arch Otolaryngol Head Neck Surg 2001;127(10):1216–1223

[2] Strollo PJ Jr, Soose RJ, Maurer JT, et al; STAR Trial Group. Upper-airway stimulation for obstructive sleep apnea. N Engl J Med 2014;370(2):139–149

[3] Woodson BT, Soose RJ, Gillespie MB, et al; STAR Trial Investigators. Three-year outcomes of cranial nerve stimulation for obstructive sleep apnea: the STAR trial. Otolaryngol Head Neck Surg 2016;154(1):181–188

[4] Diercks GR, Keamy D, Kinane TB, et al. Hypoglossal nerve stimulator implantation in an adolescent with Down syndrome and sleep apnea. Pediatrics 2016;137(5):e20153663

[5] Diercks GR, Wentland C, Keamy D, et al. Hypoglossal nerve stimulation in adolescents with Down syndrome

and sleep apnea. JAMA Otolaryngol Head Neck Surg 2017; In press

[6] Holenhorst W, Ravesloot MJL, Kezirian EJ, DeVries N. Drug-induced sleep endoscopy in adults with sleep disordered breathing: technique and the VOTE classification system. Head Neck Surg 2012;23:11–18

[7] Bowe SN, Diercks GR, Hartnick CJ. Modified surgical approach to hypoglossal nerve stimulator implantation in the pediatric population. Laryngoscope 2017;doi:10.1002/lary.26808

21 Lingual Tonsillectomy

Sanjay R. Parikh, Craig Miller

Summary

First line therapy for obstructive sleep apnea in patients with findings of tonsillar hypertrophy remains adenotonsillectomy. In patients with persistent signs and symptoms following adenotonsillectomy or clinically small tonsils, other sites of obstruction may need to be addressed. Lingual tonsillectomy is a procedure that can ameliorate obstruction at the tongue base during sleep in the appropriate patient. This chapter outlines assessment, indications, and technique for lingual tonsillectomy in pediatric patients.

Keywords: Lingual tonsillectomy, obstructive sleep apnea, drug-induced sleep endoscopy

21.1 Introduction

Obstructive sleep apnea (OSA) affects 1 to 4% of the US pediatric population.[1] Traditionally, adenotonsillectomy is the first-line treatment for sleep-disordered breathing or polysomnographic-proven OSA. Although effective, studies have shown that more than 20% of children will have persistent OSA after adenotonsillectomy. Many patients with persistent OSA following T&A have identified risk factors such as obesity, craniofacial anomalies, trisomy 21, and other syndromes with associated hypotonia. In addition, it has been demonstrated that children with OSA have a larger degree of cervical lymph node hypertrophy that extends beyond adenotonsillar hypertrophy.[2] Management of children with persistent OSA following is challenging and varies widely by practitioner. Initial interventions and management strategies include weight loss, CPAP, medical treatment (i.e., nasal steroids), and revision sleep surgery.

Choice of second-stage surgery for children with residual OSA following T&A is based on a number of modalities to assess for the site(s) of obstruction. Lateral, soft tissue neck X-ray may be used to assess for adenoid regrowth. CT, MRI, and cine-MRI have been used to assess for lingual tonsillar hypertrophy or palatal involvement. Awake nasendoscopy may be helpful in assessing the presence of lingual tonsillar hypertrophy or base of tongue collapse; however, this may not be helpful in obtaining an accurate assessment in pediatric populations. Drug-induced sleep endoscopy (DISE) is a novel diagnostic tool to assess upper airway obstruction in a pharmaceutically induced sleep state. DISE enables the surgeon to perform a real-time assessment of sites of obstruction to allow for guided interventions accordingly. Studies have demonstrated that airway obstruction sending during DISE correlates with AHI and O2 nadir in children.[3] At our institution, we utilize a validated scale to assess DISE, known as the Chan–Parikh scale.[4] This scale assesses five

levels of obstruction and grades each on a 4-point scale for minimum and maximum obstruction. The five levels are the adenoid, velum, lateral pharyngeal wall, tongue base, and supraglottis.

21.2 Indications for Surgery

When a child continues to have symptoms of OSA following adenotonsillectomy or in children with small tonsils and adenoids,[5] DISE-directed surgery can be employed to identify sites of obstruction and intervene appropriately. Several studies have demonstrated that lingual tonsil hypertrophy is the most common anatomic cause of persistent OSA in children after previous adenotonsillectomy.[6–8] Lingual tonsillar hypertrophy has been demonstrated using a number of modalities including Cine MRI, CT, and DISE.[9,10] When identified by DISE, lingual tonsillar hypertrophy can be managed with a lingual tonsillectomy using a number of techniques. Below we describe our standard surgical technique for a patient undergoing DISE-directed surgery with the findings of lingual tonsillar hypertrophy.

21.3 Surgical Technique

Prior to surgery, patients are seen with their family or caregivers and full history and physical examination is carried out, identifying risk factors and potential sites of obstruction. Most patients that are candidates for lingual tonsillectomy have previously undergone T&A or have been found to have small tonsils on physical exam. A discussion of management options is held, including observation, conservative interventions as described above (weight loss, CPAP, etc.), and surgical intervention. Without imaging findings of lingual tonsillar hypertrophy preoperatively, management then proceeds with a discussion of the role of drug-induced sleep endoscopy in identifying sites of obstruction and possible surgical interventions based on findings, including revision adenoidectomy, lingual tonsillectomy, or supraglottoplasty. Risks specific for lingual tonsillectomy include bleeding, damage to the lingual vessels and nerves, pain, scarring, need for revision procedure, and damage to surrounding structures. Informed consent is signed and operative scheduling is initiated.

The patient is brought to the operating room and an IV is placed, typically after induction anesthesia with an inhaled anesthetic. At our institution, drug-induced sleep is initiated with a propofol infusion. Other institutions may favor the use of dexmedetomidine. It is vital to have good communication with the anesthesia provider so that there is mutual understanding of the goals and plan for flexible laryngoscopy and bronchoscopy, as well as contingency plans based on possible findings.

Once a steady plane of anesthesia has been reached, such that the patient is breathing spontaneously, but will not react to the scope being passed, DISE is initiated with evaluation of each of the five subsites in the scoring system, as well as the trachea and proximal bronchi. ▸Fig. 21.1 demonstrates technique for performing a sleep endoscopy. In patients with identified lingual tonsil hypertrophy, the scope is withdrawn and the patient is nasally intubated to allow for adequate access of the surgical site. ▸Fig. 21.2 demonstrates varying degrees of lingual tonsil obstruction observed during DISE. This is graded using a validated grading scale, Chan–Parikh, from 0 to 3.

Using either a Lindholm laryngoscope or a McIvor mouth gag, the lingual tonsils are exposed and a 30-degree Hopkins rod is used for visualization. The patient is placed in suspension either utilizing the Mayo stand if using a McIvor or using the Lewy arm and suspension table for a laryngoscope (▸Fig. 21.3 and ▸Fig. 21.4). In our institution, a Coblator ProCise wand on the ablate setting is applied to the lingual tonsillar tissue in order to debulk

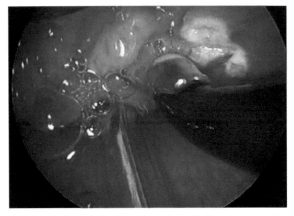

Fig. 21.3 Endoscopic view of lingual tonsillar hypertrophy with mouth gag in place.

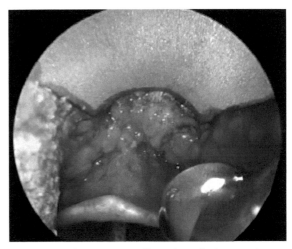

Fig. 21.4 Endoscopic image of lingual tonsillar hypertrophy with laryngoscope in place.

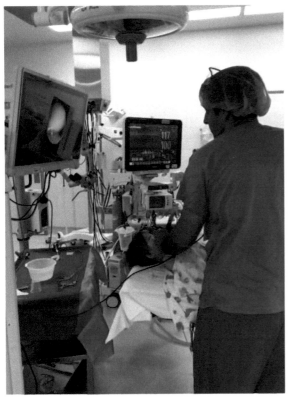

Fig. 21.1 Technique for performing drug-induced sleep endoscopy in the operating room.

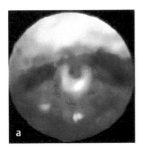
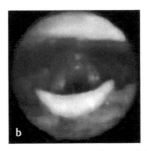
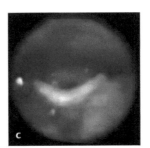
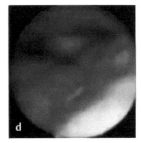

Fig. 21.2 Nasendoscopic view of tongue with varying degree of obstruction. **(a)** 0. **(b)** 1. **(c)** 2. **(d)** 3. Grading of each image is based on the validated Chan–Parikh grading scale.

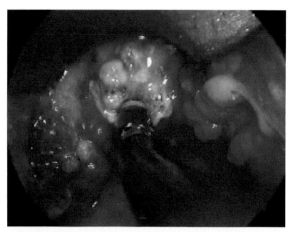

Fig. 21.5 Technique for debulking of lingual tonsil tissue using a Coblator.

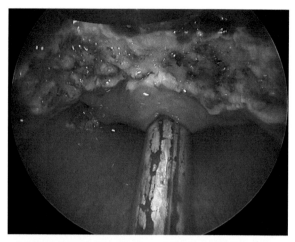

Fig. 21.6 Debulked tonsillar tissue following coblation.

down to the underlying muscle, taking care not to injure the muscle or disrupt the glossoepiglottic ligament, which lies at the midline at the base of the lingual portion of the epiglottis. Dissection is carried laterally being cognizant that the tonsillar tissue is more scarce at the lateral aspects of the base of the tongue than at the midline (▶Fig. 21.5 and ▶Fig. 21.6).

Dissection is carried out until all lymphoid tissue has been debulked and hemostasis has been achieved. The patient is taken out of suspension and the mouth gag or laryngoscope is removed. The patient is returned to the anesthesia team and extubated when stable.

21.4 Avoiding Complications

Lingual tonsillectomy can be a fairly straightforward and safe operation; however, a number of precautions should be employed to ensure optimal patient outcomes. For safety and in order to prevent injury to the facial skin and eyes, a head wrap is placed using towels and a penetrating towel clamp, much as someone would use for a traditional tonsillectomy. In regard to surgical technique, it is important to debulk only tonsillar tissue and not the underlying musculature. When only the tonsillar tissue is removed with minimal collateral damage to surrounding tissues, recovery is quick and relatively painless. However, if the intrinsic tongue muscles are affected, recovery may be prolonged with increased need for opioid medication that is already a concern in patients with obstructive sleep apnea. When using the Coblator for dissection, proper technique can prevent unwanted injury to surrounding structures. The use of the Coblator may be challenging and requires a learning curve for optimal utility. The surgeon should ensure adequate irrigation to avoid plugging

and clogging of the device. In order to avoid damage to deep tissues, the Coblator should be used in a feathering motion over the tissue rather than a deep plunging movement. Consistent movement over tissue, rather than holding the device over a single location is also beneficial in preventing clogging of the tubing. It is also important for the surgeon to be cognizant of the duration of surgery and the amount of time the patient is in suspension. Postoperative tongue paresthesia and numbness can make recovery more difficult and may also lead to swelling that can affect respiratory status.

Perioperatively, patients are administered airway dosed steroids, typically dexamethasone at 0.5 mg/kg with maximum dose of 8 mg. This not only ameliorates potential airway swelling, but can improve pain control, oral intake immediately postoperatively, and present nausea and vomiting.

21.5 Postoperative Care

Patients are typically admitted postoperatively for pain control and to ensure adequate oral intake. Risk of postoperative hemorrhage is lower than that of traditional tonsillectomy patients and therefore postoperative use of ketorolac and NSAIDs is encouraged. In order to assure adequate basal pain control, patients are prescribed acetaminophen and ibuprofen alternating doses every 3 hours with oxycodone for breakthrough pain.

Most patients are discharged on postoperative day 1; however, some may require a prolonged hospital stay if there is hesitancy to eat during the initial postoperative period. Patients are usually recommended a soft, cool, bland diet following surgery to make swallowing easier and less painful.

21.6 Highlights

a. Indications
   - Refractory OSA following adenotonsillectomy.
   - Obstructive sleep apnea in a child with small palatine tonsils and no evidence of adenoid hypertrophy.
   - Visualized lingual tonsillar hypertrophy or obstruction on flexible laryngoscopy, drug-induced sleep endoscopy, cine-MRI, or CT scan.
b. Contraindications
   - Significant bleeding diasthesis or history of such (relative contraindication).
   - Untreated adenoid or palatine tonsillar obstruction.
c. Complications
   - Bleeding (both intraoperative and postoperative).
   - Damage to the lingual vessels and nerves.
   - Pain.
   - Scarring.
   - Need for revision procedure.
   - Dmage to surrounding structures (lips, teeth, gums, or tongue).
d. Special preoperative considerations
   - General endotracheal anesthesia.
   - Surgeon preference for prophylactic antibiotics.
   - Airway steroid dosing (0.5–1 mg/kg of dexamethasone IV).
e. Special intraoperative considerations
   - Head wrap to protect face and eyes.
   - Tooth guard if using laryngoscope for exposure.
   - Care to avoid lingual vessels and nerves, as well as glossoepiglottic ligament.
   - Feathering motion of Coblator to prevent clogging.
f. Special postoperative considerations
   - Pain control to encourage early PO intake.
   - Low bleeding risk so encourage NSAIDs if appropriate.
   - Judicious use of opioids to avoid excess postoperative somnolence and obstruction.
   - Continued steroid administration for 24 hours postoperative.
   - Soft, cool, bland diet following surgery.

References

[1] Rivero A, Durr M. Lingual tonsillectomy for pediatric persistent obstructive sleep apnea: a systematic review and meta-analysis. Otolaryngol Head Neck Surg 2017;157(6):940–947

[2] Parikh SR, Sadoughi B, Sin S, Willen S, Nandalike K, Arens R. Deep cervical lymph node hypertrophy: a new paradigm in the understanding of pediatric obstructive sleep apnea. Laryngoscope 2013;123(8):2043–2049

[3] Dahl JP, Miller C, Purcell PL, et al. Airway obstruction during drug-induced sleep endoscopy correlates with apnea-hypopnea index and oxygen nadir in children. Otolaryngol Head Neck Surg 2016;155(4):676–680

[4] Chan DK, Liming BJ, Horn DL, Parikh SR. A new scoring system for upper airway pediatric sleep endoscopy. JAMA Otolaryngol Head Neck Surg 2014;140(7):595–602

[5] Miller C, Purcell PL, Dahl JP, et al. Clinically small tonsils are typically not obstructive in children during drug-induced sleep endoscopy. Laryngoscope 2017;127(8):1943–1949

[6] Durr ML, Meyer AK, Kezirian EJ, Rosbe KW. Drug-induced sleep endoscopy in persistent pediatric sleep-disordered breathing after adenotonsillectomy. Arch Otolaryngol Head Neck Surg 2012;138(7):638–643

[7] Steinhart H, Kuhn-Lohmann J, Gewalt K, Constantinidis J, Mertzlufft F, Iro H. Upper airway collapsibility in habitual snorers and sleep apneics: evaluation with drug-induced sleep endoscopy. Acta Otolaryngol 2000;120(8):990–994

[8] Rabelo FA, Braga A, Küpper DS, et al. Propofol-induced sleep: polysomnographic evaluation of patients with obstructive sleep apnea and controls. Otolaryngol Head Neck Surg 2010;142(2):218–224

[9] Abdel-Aziz M, Ibrahim N, Ahmed A, El-Hamamsy M, Abdel-Khalik MI, El-Hoshy H. Lingual tonsils hypertrophy; a cause of obstructive sleep apnea in children after adenotonsillectomy: operative problems and management. Int J Pediatr Otorhinolaryngol 2011;75(9):1127–1131

[10] Prosser JD, Shott SR, Rodriguez O, Simakajornboon N, Meinzen-Derr J, Ishman SL. Polysomnographic outcomes following lingual tonsillectomy for persistent obstructive sleep apnea in Down syndrome. Laryngoscope 2017;127(2):520–524

22 Tonsillectomy and Adenoidectomy

Marisa Earley, Max M. April

Summary

This chapter serves to review pertinent anatomy, surgical technique, and perioperative considerations for both intracapsular and extracapsular tonsillectomy and for adenoidectomy.

Keywords: Tonsillectomy, intracapsular tonsillectomy, adenoidectomy, obstructive sleep apnea

22.1 Introduction

Tonsillectomy and adenoidectomy (T&A) is one of the most common procedures performed in pediatric patients. These procedures may be performed alone or in combination. Adenoidectomy may be considered for many different indications including nasal obstruction, recurrent or chronic rhinosinusitis, chronic otitis media with effusion, hyponasal voice, mouth breathing, and to effect change on dentofacial development. T&A was often recommended for infectious reasons (recurrent tonsillopharyngitis and streptococcal tonsillitis) but with increased availability of oral antibiotics in liquid form, the number of children undergoing T&A began to decrease in the 1980s. With the decline in frequency of performing T&A for infectious causes, a new diagnosis began to emerge as a surgical indication, obstructive sleep apnea (OSA). OSA from adenotonsillar hypertrophy was first reported in 1987. Tonsil surgery has undergone change, and the concept of partial tonsillectomy, tonsillotomy, subcapsular tonsillectomy, or intracapsular tonsillectomy has been recommended over the past 20 years.

Advances in technology have provided otolaryngologists with multiple options for instrumentation to perform both techniques of tonsillectomy and adenoidectomy. Adenoidectomy can be performed with curettage, suction electro cautery, a microdebrider, and coblation. Complete tonsillectomy can be performed with cold dissection, electrocautery, coblation, plasma blade, lasers, microbipolar dissection, and other techniques. Partial tonsillectomy has evolved from removing enough tonsil tissue to the level of the tonsil pillars to a more thorough dissection removing most of the tonsil tissue (intracapsular tonsillectomy) and may be performed with a microdebrider, coblator, or laser.

22.2 Preoperative Evaluation and Anesthesia

A preoperative bleeding questionnaire (▶Fig. 22.1) is used to determine whether blood work is necessary prior to surgery. If the questionnaire is positive, then a complete blood count (CBC) with platelet count and coagulation studies including a partial thromboplastin time (PTT) and prothrombin time (PT) are ordered. If the preoperative questionnaire is negative, then blood work may not be necessary.

When evaluating a child for OSA, the history and physical exam are paramount. If the exam matches the history in an otherwise healthy patient, then a sleep study may not be necessary. Indications for polysomnography include children that are obese, those with craniofacial abnormalities, children with Down syndrome, children under the age of 2, or those in which the examination does not match the history. In addition, there are situations where the parents desire a formal sleep study to confirm the diagnosis prior to contemplating surgery.

In children with Down syndrome, a C-spine X-ray to evaluate the atlanto-occipital area prior to surgery is important to prevent injury.

Communication with the anesthesia team is imperative. Narcotic usage intraoperatively and postoperatively in children with obstructive sleep apnea needs to be considered with extreme caution. Methods to prevent intraoperative airway fires should be implemented with the oxygen percentage throughout the surgical procedure below 29% if electrocautery is used. Dexamethasone (0.5–1.0 mg/kg, up to 10–12 mg/dose) is given once the intravenous has been started. Antibiotics are rarely indicated with exceptions for an acute infection, Quinsy tonsillectomy, or in children with pediatric autoimmune and neuropsychiatric disorders associated with streptococcal infection (PANDAS).

22.3 Surgical Technique

22.3.1 Adenoidectomy

- Various techniques are available to perform this surgery; we will discuss suction Bovie ablation here followed by powered microdebrider adenoidectomy.
- Patient is placed under general anesthesia and after intubation, the endotracheal tube (ETT) is secured in midline to lower lip when tonsillectomy is also performed (▶Fig. 22.2).
- When adenoidectomy is performed alone or in combination with turbinate surgery, a laryngeal mask airway (LMA) may be used (▶Fig. 22.3).
- Topical oxymetazoline is placed in each nasal cavity to decrease nasal congestion prior to placing the red rubber catheters (▶Fig. 22.4).
- Place the patient in the Rose position with a shoulder roll to extend the neck and a head drape with blue surgical towel to protect the face and eyes (▶Fig. 22.5).

PATIENT'S NAME: _____ DATE OF BIRTH: _____
MOTHER'S FIRST NAME: _____ FATHER'S FIRST NAME: _____

I.   PERSONAL HISTORY:

Y   N   1. Has the patient ever had surgery, stitches for trauma or a broken nose?
Y   N   2. If YES, did the patient experience <u>excessive bleeding</u> during or after the procedure?
              What was the procedure? _____
Y   N   3. Does the patient bruise easily, compared to normal?
Y   N   4. If the patient is a male, was there <u>excessive bleeding</u> after circumcision?
Y   N   5. Has the patient had frequent nosebleeds?
Y   N   6. Has the patient bled excessively after tooth extractions, wisdom tooth surgery or with loss of baby teeth?
Y   N   7. Is the patient taking any of the following?   A) Aspirin   Y   N
                                                                      B) Ibuprofen products   Y   N
                                                                         (ie: Motrin, Advil, etc)
                                                                      C) Antihistamines   Y   N
Y   N   8. Is there any history of heavy menstrual periods?

II.   FAMILY HISTORY:

Y   N   1. Are there women in your family (mother, sister, aunt, grandmother..) who have <u>heavy monthly periods requiring</u>
              <u>either iron therapy or transfusions?</u>
Y   N   2. Is there anyone in the family with a history of <u>frequent nosebleeds</u> judged to be <u>severe or requiring transfusions?</u>
Y   N   3. Is there anyone in your family who bled <u>heavily</u> after tooth extraction, wisdom tooth surgery, or loss of baby teeth?
Y   N   4. Has anyone in your family required a blood transfusion? Who? _____
              Reason: _____
Y   N   5. Has anyone in the family been called a "free bleeder"?
Y   N   6. Has anyone in your family every bled excessively after tonsil surgery, childbirth or other surgery?
Y   N   7. Is there anyone in your faintly with blood disorder such a Hemophilia, Von Willebrand disease, lower platelets or
              ITP?
              Who? _____
              Diagnosis? _____
Y   N   8. Is there any history of heavy ineustiiial periods?

III. ACTION PLAN:

1. If ALL answers to the above questions are NO, obtain CBC and PLATELETS only.
2. If Part I. Questions 2 answer is YES, and all the other answers are NO, obtain CBC, PLATELETS, PT & PTT only.
   * The <u>patient must stop aspirin 2 weeks prior to surgery and Ibuprofen products 2 days prior to surgery</u>*
3. If answers in <u>any item in Part II is YES</u>, discuss work-up with pediatric hematologist before ordering blood studies.
4. If answers to ANY of the othe questions (except Part I, Question &) are YES, obtain a HEMATOLOGY CLEARANCE
   & discuss results with hematologist.

PATIENT/GUARDIAN'S SIGNATURE: _____ DATE:_____
I've reviewed this medical information with the patient. Physician's signature: _____ DATE: _____

Fig. 22.1 Preoperative questionnaire to assess for bleeding risk.

- Visualize adenoid tissue with angled mirror; define limits of adenoid tissue and avoid injury to torus tubarius bilaterally and vomer superiorly (▶ Fig. 22.6).
- Bend suction Bovie cautery with gentle ~90 degree curve 2 to 3 cm from distal tip.
- Setting between 30 and 35 watts.
- Bury tip of suction cautery in tissue and coagulate until tissue turns white and ablates away.

- Begin at choana and continue inferiorly.
- Alternatively, the microdebrider with the RADenoid 40 blade may be used to remove adenoid tissue. It is set to 1,500 rpm on oscillating mode. Additional exposure is obtained with gentle retraction of the left clamp with your fourth finger further elevating the soft palate (▶ Fig. 22.7). Always be aware of the angle of the nasopharynx when using the debrider (▶ Fig. 22.8).

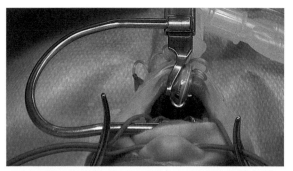

Fig. 22.2 Proper insertion of mouth gag demonstrating tongue and endotracheal tube centered at the midline of the gag. Red rubber catheters are inserted and secured loosely extraorally.

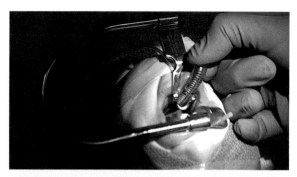

Fig. 22.3 When using an laryngeal mask airway (LMA) for adenoidectomy, upon insertion of the mouth gag the LMA often need to be pulled back gently to allow for proper air movement.

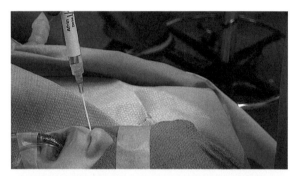

Fig. 22.4 Topical oxymetazoline is placed into each nostril.

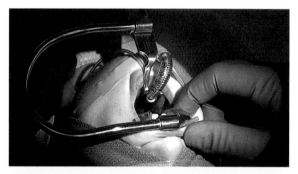

Fig. 22.5 Protection of the eyes and face with proper drapes.

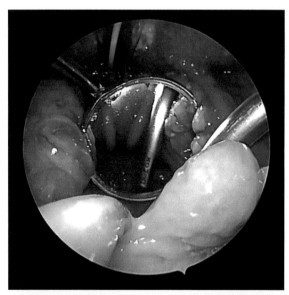

Fig. 22.6 An angled mirror is used to visualize the adenoid with two red rubber catheters retracting the soft palate.

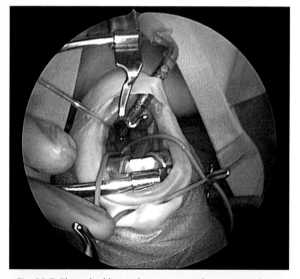

Fig. 22.7 The red rubber catheters are gently retracting the soft palate but with the fourth finger the left Kelly clamp is retracted more temporarily to provide better visualization for the procedure.

Assure the dissection inferiorly is not too deep, especially in the lateral aspect where there can be excessive bleeding. An advantage of using the microdebrider is to be able to leave an inferior ledge of adenoid tissue to reduce postoperative velopharyngeal incompetence.

When removing the microdebider blade from the oral cavity, cover the opening of the blade with the mirror to avoid suction damage to the uvula and soft palate (▶Fig. 22.9). After microdebriding adenoid

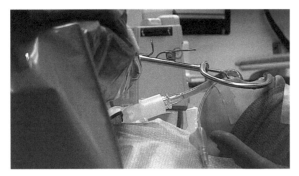

Fig. 22.8 Always look at the angle the patient is in to ensure the dissection with the microdebrider blade is not too deep when removing tissue inferiorly.

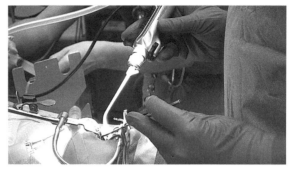

Fig. 22.9 The mirror is used to cover the opening of the microdebrider blade when removing it, to reduce the possibility of a suction injury to oral cavity structures especially the uvula.

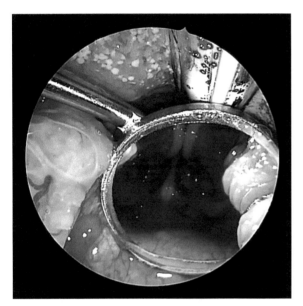

Fig. 22.10 One year after adenoidectomy. Notice the complete removal and healed nasopharynx.

tissue, pack the nasopharynx with one to two tonsil sponges soaked in oxymetazoline. Suction cautery on low setting of 20 watts to obtain hemostasis. Here is an example of a nasopharynx a year after microdebrider adenoidectomy (▶ Fig. 22.10).

22.3.2 Complete Tonsillectomy

- Patient is placed under general anesthesia, and after intubation, the endotracheal tube (ETT) is secured in midline to lower lip.
- There are multiple techniques available including monopolar cautery (**Video 22.1**), Coblation, PEAK plasma blade (**Video 22.2**), harmonic scalpel and lasers.
- Place the patient in the Rose position with a shoulder roll to extend the neck and a head drape with blue surgical towel to protect the face and eyes.

- Insert mouth gag transorally with care to avoid injury to lips, teeth, tongue, and pharynx. Be sure to keep ETT midline.
- Secure mouth gag to mayo stand.
- Instill 0.5 mL of topical oxymetazoline into each nasal passage to improve nasal patency in the postoperative period and reduce bleeding from adenoidectomy (▶ Fig. 22.4).
- Inspect the uvula and palpate the soft for a submucosal cleft as well as adenoid hypertrophy and ability to contact posterior pharynx.
  - If there is a submucosal cleft, bifid uvula, or a short soft palate (that does not contact the posterior pharyngeal wall), consider a superior adenoidectomy,[1] which leaves an inferior ledge of adenoid tissue in place to decrease risk of velopharyngeal insufficiency (VPI) postoperatively.
- Place red rubber catheters transnasally and secure extraorally. Do not secure them tightly to reduce palatal and uvular edema (▶ Fig. 22.5).
- Grasp mid-to-superior pole of tonsil with an Allis clamp and apply inferomedial traction to create tension.
- Incise anterior tonsillar pillar with spatula tip Bovie electrocautery from midtonsil moving superiorly in curvilinear manner, continuing incision medially at superiormost aspect of tonsil.
  - Use the lowest setting to reduce thermal damage (12–15 watts).
  - Use Bovie tip to bluntly dissect and find peritonsillar space and plane of dissection.
  - Other instruments that can be used include coblation, plasma blade, or harmonic scalpel.
- Adjust traction on tonsil and regrab if needed to expose relatively avascular loose areolar tissue plane of dissection and continue cautery dissection with care to apply cautery gently to tissue so as not to create significant char.
- Dissect tonsil from tonsillar fossa and posterior pillar.

- Transect inferiorly in a controlled manner to avoid avulsing tonsil from inferiormost aspect.
- Obtain hemostasis of tonsillar fossa and cauterize large vessels with suction Bovie. Using a foot pedal control will reduce incidental thermal damage to the normal structures of the soft palate and uvula.
- Perform in identical manner on contralateral side. Release the mouth gag at end of case and then resuspend to confirm complete hemostasis.

22.3.3 Powered Intracapsular Tonsillectomy and Adenoidectomy

- See (Video 22.3a, b).
- Patient is placed under general anesthesia and after intubation, the endotracheal tube (ETT) is secured in midline to lower lip.
- Place the patient in the Rose position with a shoulder roll to extend the neck and a head drape with blue surgical towel to protect the face and eyes.
- The microdebrider with RADenoid 40 blade set to 1,500 rpm on oscillating mode is used.
- Retract anterior tonsillar pillar with Hurd retractor.

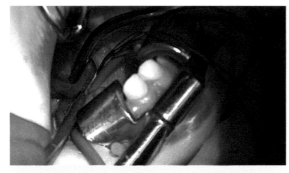

Fig. 22.11 The curved microdebrider blade is positioned at the apex of the left tonsil as the uvula is retracted with the coated Hurd elevator. It is imperative to begin the dissection at the superior most portion of the tonsil.

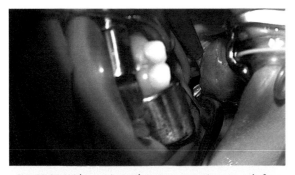

Fig. 22.12 With experience the more aggressive removal of left tonsil tissue. The Hurd elevator is placed posterior to the left tonsil, thereby reducing blood flow and bleeding, but this retraction can make it easier to dissect too deep.

- Starting location at superior aspect in the apex of the tonsillar fossa (▶Fig. 22.11).
- Protect posterior pillar with the blunt end of the debrider blade.
- For trainees or in initial experience using the same hand as the side that is being operated on to hold the debrider is more conservative and safer—reducing the dissection going too deep.
- With increased experience using the opposite hand to the tonsil that you are dissecting allows for more aggressive removal of tonsil tissue (▶Fig. 22.12).
- As lymphoid tissue is removed, there is a color change and the tissue no longer is lymphoid as one approaches the inside portion of the capsule.
- Hemostasis is achieved with suction Bovie electrocautery on a low setting of 15 to 20 watts. Cauterize the lower ¾ of the tonsillar fossa first, leaving the superior ¼ of the fossa until after red rubber catheters are removed.
- Next remove the nasopharyngeal packing if present due to completion of adenoidectomy with microdebrider prior to starting tonsillectomy, and cauterize the nasopharynx.
- When the nasopharynx is dry, remove the red rubber catheters. This gives better exposure to the superior portion of the tonsillar fossa.
- Use a foot pedal for the suction cautery. This allows the surgeon to cauterize superiorly in the tonsil fossa without the suction port covered, reducing the possibility of thermal damage to the uvula.
- Use the suction cautery to make the tonsil fossa and the nasopharynx smooth which reduces potential reformation of cryptic areas in the future (▶Fig. 22.13).

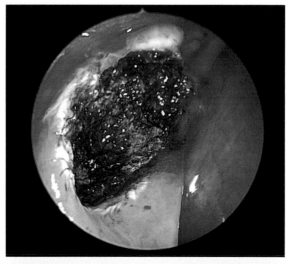

Fig. 22.13 The suction cautery is used to ensure hemostasis and smooth the area. Note that the superior poles of the tonsillar fossa are cauterized without the red rubber catheters in place to improve exposure and reduce the potential damage to the anterior and posterior pillars.

- The nasopharynx and oropharynx are irrigated with iced saline, which reduces postoperative discomfort.[2]
- Prior to extubation in operating room, one may suction stomach contents with a Salem sump tube and place oral airway yourself if one is desired by anesthesia team.

22.4 Postoperative Treatment

Overnight admission if indicated for those with severe sleep apnea (Apnea Hypopnea Index >10 or oxygen nadir <80%), craniofacial abnormalities, bleeding disorder, age less than 2, or underlying medical conditions that warrant admission.

Duration for monitoring in PACU if discharging home can differ based on whether intracapsular technique or complete tonsillectomy has been performed.[3]

Postoperative pain control is of utmost importance.[4] Acetaminophen (15 mg/kg/dose q 6 hours with maximum dose of 75 mg/kg/day) and ibuprofen (10 mg/kg/dose q 6 hours with maximum of 400–600 mg/dose) are alternated postoperatively. Many surgeons also consider a narcotic such as oxycodone 0.1–0.15 mg/kg/dose q 6 hours prn severe or breakthrough pain.

If complete tonsillectomy is performed, then soft diet and limited physical activity are recommended for 2 weeks.

If intracapsular tonsillectomy is performed, diet is more liberal and there is little restriction on activity. Even more important that diet is emphasis on adequate hydration post-operatively. Due to pain, may children may have decreased oral intake, but hydration status is critical for recovery and to reduce the risk of post-tonsillectomy hemorrhage. Parents should be encouraged to return to emergency department if they cannot keep their child adequately hydrated or pain adequately controlled at home.

22.5 Highlights

a. Indications
  - OSA.
  - Sleep disordered breathing.
  - Recurrent tonsillitis or pharyngitis ('Paradise criteria').
  - Dysphagia.
  - Periodic fever syndrome associated with aphthous stomatitis, pharyngitis, and cervical adenitis (PFAPA).
  - PANDAS.
  - Rule out malignancy.
  - Lymphoproliferative disorder.
  - Asymmetric tonsils.
  - Tonsiloliths.
    ○ Consider complete tonsillectomy for endophytic tonsils and intracapsular tonsillectomy for exophytic tonsils.

b. Contraindications
  - Submucosal cleft palate.
  - Untreated bleeding disorder.
  - Relative contraindication: recent upper respiratory infection.
  - Trismus.

c. Complications
  - Hemorrhage (primary or delayed).
  - Dehydration.
  - VPI.
  - Injury to lips (commissure), teeth, tongue or pharynx.
  - Voice change.
  - Oropharyngeal stenosis.
  - Altered sense of taste.
  - Postoperative obesity.
    ○ Secondary to change in sense of taste as well as decrease in calories burned while breathing if patient had OSA or sleep disordered breathing preoperatively.
  - Nontraumatic atlantoaxial subluxation (Grisel syndrome).
  - Postobstructive pulmonary edema.
  - Airway fire.

d. Special preoperative considerations
  - Indication for preoperative blood work based on questionnaire.
  - Down syndrome and C-spine assessment.

e. Special intraoperative considerations
  - May consider using flexible LMA for adenoidectomy instead of ETT.
  - Ensure proper positioning, instrumentation, and settings.
  - Risk of airway fire: keep oxygen below 29%.
  - Accidental extubation during procedure by surgeon.
  - Poor ventilation due to mouth gag positioning.

f. Special postoperative considerations
  - Pain control.
  - Minimize narcotic use in obese patients or OSA patients.
  - Codeine has black box warning for use in pediatric patients undergoing adenotonsillectomy.

References

[1] Kakani RS, Callan ND, April MM. Superior adenoidectomy in children with palatal abnormalities. Ear Nose Throat J 2000;79(4):300–, 303–305

[2] Shin JM, Byun JY, Baek BJ, Lee JY. Effect of cold-water cooling of tonsillar fossa and pharyngeal mucosa on post-tonsillectomy pain. Am J Otolaryngol 2014;35(3):353–356

[3] Stucken EZ, Grunstein E, Haddad J Jr, et al. Factors contributing to cost in partial versus total tonsillectomy. Laryngoscope 2013;123(11):2868–2872

[4] Tan GX, Tunkel DE. Control of pain after tonsillectomy in children: a review. JAMA Otolaryngol Head Neck Surg 2017;143(9):937–942

Suggested Readings

Chang DT, Zemek A, Koltai PJ. Comparison of treatment outcomes between intracapsular and total tonsillectomy for pediatric obstructive sleep apnea. Int J Pediatr Otorhinolaryngol 2016; 91:15–18

Rubinstein BJ, Derkay CS. Rethinking surgical technique and priorities for pediatric tonsillectomy. Am J Otolaryngol 2017;38(2): 233–236

Vicini C, Eesa M, Hendawy E, et al. Powered intracapsular tonsillotomy vs. conventional extracapsular tonsillectomy for pediatric OSA: a retrospective study about efficacy, complications and quality of life. Int J Pediatr Otorhinolaryngol 2015;79(7):1106–1110

Koshkareva YA, Cohen M, Gaughan JP, Callanan V, Szeremeta W. Utility of preoperative hematologic screening for pediatric adenotonsillectomy. Ear Nose Throat J 2012;91(8):346–356

Mukhatiyar P, Nandalike K, Cohen HW, et al. Intracapsular and extracapsular tonsillectomy and adenoidectomy in pediatric obstructive sleep apnea. JAMA Otolaryngol Head Neck Surg 2016;142(1):25–31

Kim JS, Kwon SH, Lee EJ, Yoon YJ. Can Intracapsular tonsillectomy be an alternative to classical Tonsillectomy? A meta-analysis. Otolaryngol Head Neck Surg 2017;157(2):178–189

Walton J, Ebner Y, Stewart MG, April MM. Systematic review of randomized controlled trials comparing intracapsular tonsillectomy with total tonsillectomy in a pediatric population. Arch Otolaryngol Head Neck Surg 2012;138(3):243–249

23 Pediatric Transoral Robotic Surgery

Gabriel Gomez, Carlton J. Zdanski

Summary

Pediatric transoral robotic surgery has advantages over traditional endoscopic or open approaches as shown in this text. A wide variety of aerodigestive tract pathology is amenable to treatment via the robotic approach with full potential of the technology yet to demonstrated by future advances and experience.

Keywords: Transoral robotic surgery, pediatric transoral robotic surgery, laryngeal cleft, laryngoplasty

23.1 Introduction

Transoral robotic surgery (TORS) made its debut in the otolaryngology literature in 2005. As early as 2007, pediatric specific publications had appeared.[1] The potential advantages of TORS over other techniques includes improved 3D visualization of difficult to access sites, increased surgical agility and precision in tight anatomical spaces, decreased morbidity by avoiding external incisions, and reduced surgical time in certain cases. TORS also offers an opportunity for a supervising surgeon to offer real-time and on-screen guidance to the operating surgeon as demonstrated in this chapter. The main potential disadvantages of TORS relate to the expense of the equipment and the specialized training required of the surgeon and operative staff. Lack of tactile feedback for the surgeon working at the operating console and the addition of robot positioning time are also cited as potential disadvantages. In the authors' experience, lack of haptics does not outweigh the other advantages and time spent on setup becomes negligible with proficiency. It is interesting to note that whereas adult TORS is often applied to malignant lesions, pediatric cases are most often directed toward benign congenital or acquired lesions of the aerodigestive tract. Some of the most commonly cited indications include laryngeal cleft repair, laryngoplasty, tongue base reduction, and pharyngeal stenosis or other benign lesions such as saccular cyst or lymphangiomas. Several authors have reported on the safety and efficacy of pediatric TORS while also reporting a very low incidence of conversion to traditional techniques.[2,3] These experiences make the application of robotics in pediatric head and neck surgery an innovation whose full potential is yet be seen. This chapter is intended to provide an overview of pediatric transoral surgery and should not be used as a substitute to formal robotic training and proctored cases as required by some facilities.

23.2 Preoperative Evaluation and Anesthesia

The preoperative assessment of robotic cases is similar to that of any head and neck procedure, with emphasis on reviewing previous operative reports detailing ease of transoral exposure and visualization of the different subsites. Imaging studies should be thoroughly reviewed. Communication with operating room staff and anesthesia providers is done before the patient is brought to the robotic operating theater. The patient is placed in supine position with enough space underneath the head of bed in order to accommodate placement of the robot's base underneath the operating table. Depending on the operative table, this may require the patient's head to be placed on the "foot side" of the table or simply rotating the head of the bed 90 degrees (▶ Fig. 23.1).

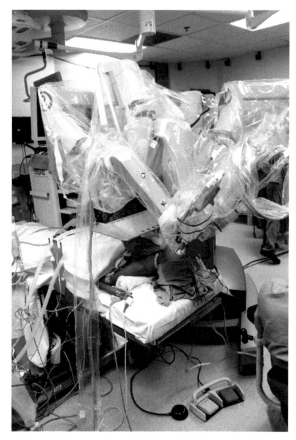

Fig. 23.1 The operative table is turned 90 degrees to allow space for the robotic base and the bedside assistant.

Anesthesia under spontaneous respiration with a native airway is requested for the initiation of procedures. We generally request that an experienced pediatric anesthesia provider perform a direct laryngoscopy and apply 2% lidocaine to the larynx in preparation for a planning endoscopy by the surgeon. After the airway is evaluated and secured to the team's satisfaction, neuromuscular paralysis for the length of time the robot is docked near the patient should be strongly considered. We typically administer intraoperative dexamethasone in non-tracheostomy-dependent children to reduce airway edema that occurs with surgery.

23.3 Exposure, Setup, and Instrumentation

After induction of anesthesia, the operating table is turned 90 degrees toward the surgeons to optimize access to the airway. The surgeon performs a video direct laryngoscopy and bronchoscopy and secures the airway as described below. We use a custom maxillary tooth guard that is rapidly molded for the patient utilizing Aquaplast (Medline, Mundelein, IL). Exposure is individualized based on the child's airway and the lesion in question. In neonates, it is possible to forgo use of a retractor or to employ a simple tongue stitch. In others, a McIvor oropharyngeal retractor with a flat tongue blade suspended onto a mustard stand will provide adequate exposure as distal as the larynx and proximal trachea (▶ Fig. 23.2). Given size limitations, the commonly used FK Retractor is used only for older, larger children. The robot's base is docked underneath the patient's head with the help of an assistant to ensure the patient is protected at all times. The articulating arms are positioned intraorally with either a 30-degree anterior facing telescope or a 0-degree telescope depending on which gives

the best exposure with the least interference with the robotic arms (▶ Fig. 23.3). A bedside, robotics trained surgeon is assigned to provide additional instrumentation (i.e., suction, cautery, assistance with suturing) and directly oversee the patient's airway and safety during the procedure (▶ Fig. 23.4).

The airway can be secured through a variety of ways for pediatric robotic cases. The patient can be intubated either transnasally or transorally. The endotracheal tube can be tucked underneath the tongue blade for improved access to the posterior larynx as will be shown below. Standard laser safety precautions including a laser safe endotracheal tube and fraction of inspired oxygen less than 40% are utilized to reduce the risk of airway fire. A preexisting tracheostomy tube naturally simplifies management of the airway; however, the tube must be exchanged with either a laser safe tube or a metallic tracheostomy tube for laser cases. If an air leak occurs around the ventilation tube or tracheostomy tube we routinely pack the area of the subglottis with moist pledgets. A silicone catheter may also be placed in the pharynx and attached to suction to help prevent scope fogging.

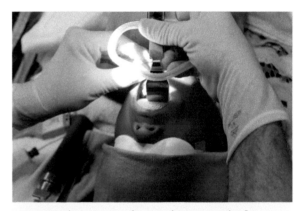

Fig. 23.2 The McIvor oropharyngeal retractor with a flat tongue blade is inserted for exposure. Note the maxillary dental guard in place. Eyes are padded for safety.

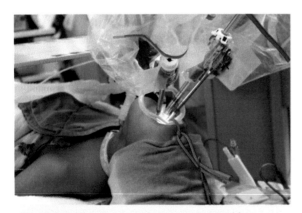

Fig. 23.3 Robotic arms and telescope are positioned intraorally. A silicone catheter was utilized for soft palate retraction in this case. A silicone catheter may also be placed in the pharynx and attached to suction to help prevent scope fogging.

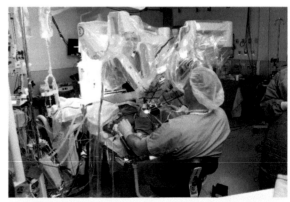

Fig. 23.4 The bedside surgeon ensures patient is protected while the robotic surgeon works at the robotic console (not pictured here).

In addition to pledget safety sutures, optical forceps are prepared in case the pledgets become dislodged into the lower airway. A carbon dioxide (CO_2) laser delivered via fiber is our preference for cases requiring laser, although the robotic cautery arm may be employed for hemostatic dissection as well.

23.4 Select Cases in Pediatric Robotic Surgery

23.4.1 Laryngeal Cleft Repair

A laryngeal cleft (LC) is a congenital defect of the posterior larynx with a wide spectrum of anatomical presentations. Patient symptoms may similarly vary from asymptomatic to oral feeding intolerance due to aspiration in severe cases. The Benjamin and Inglis classification system is the most commonly used grading scheme.[4] Grades 1 and 2 are defects that have traditionally been considered as amenable to repair via a transoral technique (▶ Fig. 23.5). The technique involves application of sutures to close the cleft within the tight confines of a pediatric endolarynx. For this reason, we have found the added agility and visualization of TORS to be useful in these cases.

The patient is setup in a similar fashion as previously described with a McIvor retractor and laser safe tube.

We begin by creating raw opposing surfaces by excising either side of the cleft with a CO_2 laser deployed via a fiber sheath manipulated with a robotic needle driver. The robotic Maryland retractor or needle driver on the non-laser robotic arm is used to provide traction to facilitate dissection (▶ Fig. 23.6). The cleft is then closed in three layers with dissolvable sutures (▶ Fig. 23.7 and ▶ Fig. 23.8). Postoperatively, the patient is extubated and allowed to resume regular oral intake after appropriate recovery from anesthesia. A follow-up modified barium swallow study is typically performed 3 to 4 weeks later as an outpatient. The patient is typically observed overnight in a monitored bed prior to discharge home.

23.4.2 Supraglottoplasty: Epiglottopexy

While supraglottoplasty is an operation mostly described in the context of congenital laryngomalacia in infants, the authors have found it applicable in the treatment of pediatric obstructive sleep apnea in carefully selected patients as has been previously described.[5,6] We have also found this operation useful as an adjunct in tracheostomy-dependent patients with multilevel obstruction

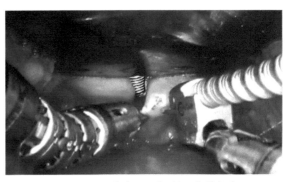

Fig. 23.6 Retraction with the needle driver (left) facilitates CO_2 laser incisions. The laser fiber is manipulated via a robotic needle driver with laser fiber attachment (right). The endotracheal tube is placed underneath the tongue blade for improved visualization of the posterior larynx.

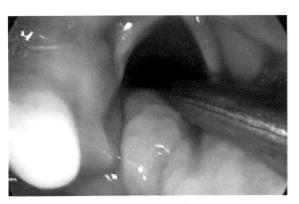

Fig. 23.5 A Type 2 cleft is demonstrated prior to repair.

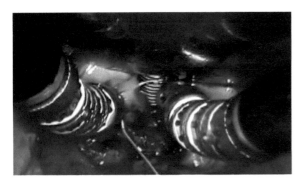

Fig. 23.7 Robotic arms are utilized to suture the laryngeal cleft defect.

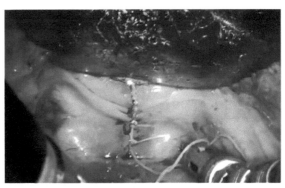

Fig. 23.8 Layered closure is completed.

when seeking airway optimization prior to decannulation. Dysphagia and aspiration after epiglottopexy are rare as shown on a prior pediatric review of such cases.[7] Patients may benefit from swallow evaluations and therapy but almost always accommodate to become safe for oral diets.

Flexible airway endoscopy in the office and/or drug-induced sleep endoscopy (DISE) are useful in identifying sites of airway obstruction. Setup is performed as previously described, with particular attention to exposing the tongue base and epiglottis. The 30-degree angled scope can often be helpful in visualizing this area. Using the robotic electrocautery arm, the tongue base is denuded in the submucosal plane in midline area. This is done to create a raw surface for epiglottopexy, but concomitant lingual tonsillectomy can also be performed. After the initial incision, a free edge of tissue is created for the robotic Maryland retractor or needle driver to grasp for retraction. Similarly, the mucosa on the vallecular surface of the epiglottis can be denuded. These tasks may also be completed with the laser. The two raw surfaces are coapted with sutures to pexy the epiglottis to the base of tongue using the robotic needle drivers. The patient is extubated and monitored appropriately (▶Fig. 23.9 and ▶Fig. 23.10).

23.4.3 Expansion Laryngotracheoplasty with a Posterior Cricoid Graft

Endoscopic laryngotracheal reconstruction with expansion of the posterior glottis and subglottic airway is a well-known tool in the armamentarium of the pediatric otolaryngologist to treat posterior glottic stenosis and bilateral vocal cord paralysis (▶Fig. 23.11).[8] Traditionally, this procedure involves harvesting a costal rib cartilage segment which is carved and inserted into the posterior cricoid plate after the surgeon has performed an endoscopic posterior cricoid split. The inserted graft allows the cricoid to be expanded and is normally held in place by the locking design of the graft without sutures, since placement of sutures has proven to be a difficult task. The robot facilitates suture placement in this area if necessary.

Rather than using an operative laryngoscope with a narrow view and manual microlaryngeal instruments, use of the robot takes full advantage of the oral aperture. Patients are suspended with a McIvor retractor and the robotic arms introduced directly into the pharynx. A 30-degree forward facing robotic telescope is usually used, but the 0-degree telescope may provide adequate or superior visualization and working space. A vocal cord spreader can be initially used but should be removed if fitting the graft without suturing (▶Fig. 23.12). The CO_2

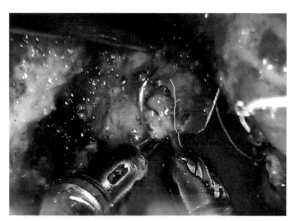

Fig. 23.9 The denuded lingual surface of the epiglottis is coapted to the base of tongue. Note the *blue line* demonstrating the bedside surgeon's on-screen instructions to robotic surgeon.

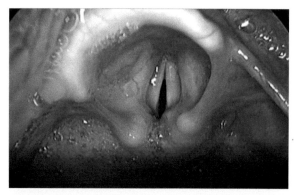

Fig. 23.11 Patient with bilateral vocal cord paralysis just prior to robotic laryngotracheal reconstruction via posterior cricoid costal cartilage graft.

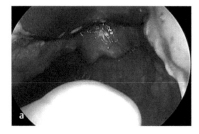
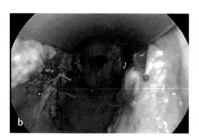

Fig. 23.10 Before **(a)** and after **(b)** photos of the same patient from ▶Fig. 23.9. Note improved oropharyngeal and supraglottic airway.

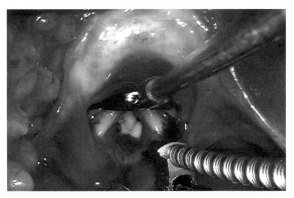

Fig. 23.12 A vocal cord spreader is utilized to improve visualization of the posterior cricoid.

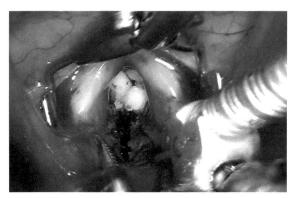

Fig. 23.13 The posterior cricoid is split with the CO_2 laser.

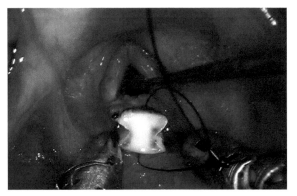

Fig. 23.14 Vocal cord spreader is removed and the previously carved rib graft brought into the field.

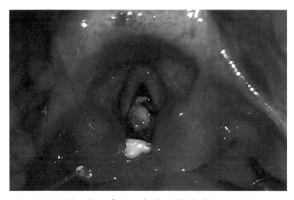

Fig. 23.15 The rib graft is pushed and locked into position with the assistance of the robotic arms. Note the newly widened posterior larynx.

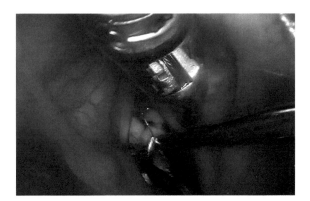

Fig. 23.16 The rib graft can be sutured via the robotic arms. Pledgets can be seen distally in the airway to pack the air leak around the preexisting tracheostomy tube.

laser or a cold knife incision is used to split the posterior cricoid plate in the midline until a release is noted, taking care to avoid injury to the esophagus posteriorly (▶ Fig. 23.13). The previously harvested and carved rib cartilage is inset among the cricoid split with the help of the robotic arms (▶ Fig. 23.14 and ▶ Fig. 23.15). If needed, the graft can now be sutured into place. Dissolvable sutures on a small tapered needle are ideal (▶ Fig. 23.16). In patients without an existent tracheostomy, a naso-tracheal tube can be placed at the end for 3 to 5 days postoperatively. In those with tracheostomy, a T-tube or stent may be placed as appropriate or a naso-tracheal tube may be placed and the patient decannulated. Alternatively, a native airway without stent or endotracheal tube can be considered postoperatively if the graft is sutured in place. We have found that if the graft is not to be sutured in place, the use of the robot in this procedure may only provide an advantage in those few children with a posterior larynx which is very difficult to expose.

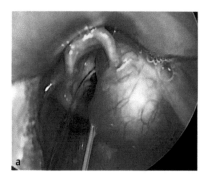
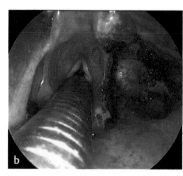

Fig. 23.17 Pre-excision **(a)** and post-excision **(b)** of a saccular cyst. Laser safe tube **(b)**.

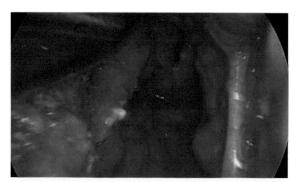

Fig. 23.18 Lymphatic malformation involving the left pharynx and larynx. The true vocal cords are difficult to visualize upon direct laryngoscopy.

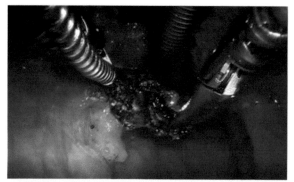

Fig. 23.19 Mucosal incision is made to create a free edge which is utilized for retraction.

23.4.4 Laryngeal Cyst Excision

Saccular cyst and vallecular cyst are uncommon lesions that can cause significant respiratory distress and feeding difficulties in children. Simple endoscopic aspiration has been reported to have an unacceptably high rate of recurrence. Other surgical approaches have been described, such as marsupialization, laser ablation, and endoscopic or open excision.[9] The robotic approach is particularly well suited for excision, since it allows for improved visualization and added surgical maneuverability.

The airway can typically be secured via traditional or endoscopically assisted orotracheal intubation techniques. The lesion can also be decompressed if necessary prior to securing the airway or prior to excision. In neonates, obtaining a laser-safe endotracheal tube of the appropriate size can be a significant challenge. After setup, the lesion is grasped with the robotic Maryland retractor or needle driver. The bedside surgeon may also facilitate in retraction of the lesion. A laser incision is made along the medial surface where these cysts are usually abutting the larynx. The lesion is then dissected using a combination of laser and blunt dissection preserving as much piriform sinus mucosa as possible. It is not uncommon for the cyst to decompress its fluid contents during dissection, making retraction more manageable. The cyst capsule should still be removed en bloc whenever possible. We have

successfully utilized TORS to safely excise saccular neonates as young as day of life 14 and as small as 2.8 kg (▶Fig. 23.17).

23.4.5 Pharyngeal Lymphatic Malformation Excision

Lymphatic malformations are lesions made up of ectatic lymphatic channels and are frequently present at birth. Large malformations in the head and neck can be disfiguring or compromise the airway and swallowing. Large symptomatic lesions can be treated via injections of sclerosing agents or surgical excision.[10] Lesions will typically grow commensurately with the patient and in some cases prevent tracheostomy or gastrostomy tube removal until adequately treated. We have found the robotic approach to be a valuable tool in addressing the pharyngeal and tongue-based components of the lesions. This approach has proved an adjunct to external approaches for large lesions. Surgical goals for children with lymphatic malformations are removing as much disease as possible to provide symptomatic relief, improve cosmesis, and avoid injury to vital neurovascular structures. Negative margins of resection are not necessarily needed to achieve these goals. Preoperative imaging and clearly defined, realistic surgical goals are important when planning.

After robotic setup, a mucosal incision is made on the lesion to create a free edge to grasp (▶Fig. 23.18 and ▶Fig. 23.19). The laser allows for adequate hemostasis while dissecting within the malformation. Robotic electrocautery may also be employed. The lesion can then be grasped with the Maryland retractor or by the bedside assistant. The grasped segment can then be dissected off of the pharyngeal wall or tongue base along the plane of the pharyngeal constrictor or tongue musculature. Dissection across a segment of the lymphatic malformation may be unavoidable as these lesions often obscure normal tissue planes or encompass critical structures. Special attention to the location of the great vessels should be made on preoperative imaging. Any uninvolved mucosa should be preserved and the surgeon should prevent circumferential raw surfaces of the pharynx or larynx to prevent stenosis (▶Fig. 23.20).

23.4.6 Scar Band Lysis and Flaps

Pharyngeal stenosis of the pediatric aerodigestive tract is a challenging problem that can occur secondary to prior interventions such as head and neck irradiation, adenotonsillectomy, other pharyngeal surgery, or caustic ingestion (▶Fig. 23.21). Prior authors have described techniques to address these cases via radial incisions, dilations, skin grafts, local flaps, and free flaps.[11,12] TORS can significantly improve the ability to perform these

operations. We use local flaps whenever possible versus excision in order to follow the principle of mucosal preservation.

After the airway is evaluated and secured and the robot is docked, we will typically perform a z-plasty scar-releasing technique whenever possible. The scar is incised with the CO_2 laser or sharply. For sharp dissection, robotic scissors may be employed or the bedside surgeon may assist. We believe this sharp dissection decreases the collateral damage caused by laser and decreases additional cicatricial healing (▶Fig. 23.22, ▶Fig. 23.23, and ▶Fig. 23.24).

23.5 Postoperative Treatment

More rapid recovery may be seen for those patients able to avoid open, transcervical approaches. With experience, the added agility of the robot has allowed for quicker transoral

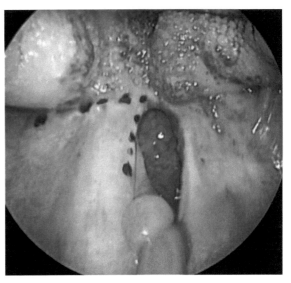
Fig. 23.21 Oropharyngeal stenosis with planned flap demarcated. A silicone tube retracts the soft palate.

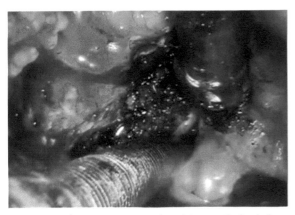
Fig. 23.20 The resection was continued down to the level of the vocal cords to improve the airway.

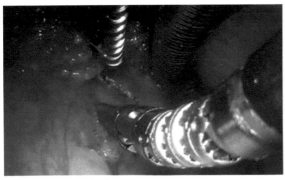
Fig. 23.22 Mucosal incision made with CO_2 laser.

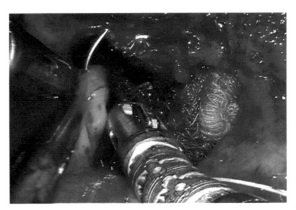
Fig. 23.23 Oropharyngeal flaps are sutured with the robotic arms.

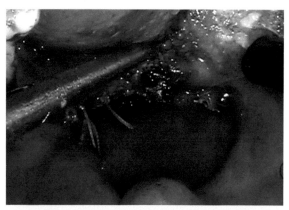

Fig. 23.24 Oropharyngeal stenosis after lysis of scar and flap transposition. An improved oropharyngeal airway is noted.

operations, saving anesthesia time. Nonetheless, the overall same postoperative considerations exist after robotic surgery as with traditional endoscopic and open approaches. The cases in this text show that a wide variety of pediatric head and neck procedures can be performed with robotic assistance with potential advantages for patients.

23.6 Highlights

a. Indications
   – Benign congenital, malignant or acquired lesions of the aerodigestive tract.
   – Transoral oral surgical procedures that require improved visualization and surgical agility in tight anatomical spaces.
b. Contraindications
   – Inadequate transoral exposure.
c. Complications
   – Considerations including airway loss and airway fire.
d. Special preoperative considerations
   – Communication with operating room staff and anesthesia providers is done before the patient is brought to the robotic operating theater.
   – Review of previous operative reports detailing ease of transoral exposure and visualization of the different subsites.
   – Appropriate robotic training by surgeons and operating room staff.

e. Special intraoperative considerations
   – Begin procedure with endoscopic evaluation of the airway.
   – Proper patient and bed positioning for robotic docking.
   – Second robotics trained surgeon for bedside assistance when available.
   – Laser safe endotracheal tube and laser precautions.
   – Plan for possible conversion to open approach.
f. Special postoperative considerations
   – Faster recovery occurs with transoral surgery compared to open approaches.
   – Similar considerations to traditional transoral head and neck surgery.

References

[1] Rahbar RR. Archives of otolaryngology–head & neck surgery: robotic surgery in the pediatric airway: application and safety. American Medical Association; 2007;133:46

[2] Ferrell JK, Roy S, Karni RJ, Yuksel S. Applications for transoral robotic surgery in the pediatric airway. Laryngoscope 2014;124(11):2630–2635

[3] Zdanski CJ, Austin GK, Walsh JM, et al. Transoral robotic surgery for upper airway pathology in the pediatric population. Laryngoscope 2017;127(1):247–251

[4] Benjamin B, Inglis A. Minor congenital laryngeal clefts: diagnosis and classification. Ann Otol Rhinol Laryngol 1989;98(6):417–420

[5] Chan DK, Truong MT, Koltai PJ. Supraglottoplasty for occult laryngomalacia to improve obstructive sleep apnea syndrome. Arch Otolaryngol Head Neck Surg 2012;138(1):50–54

[6] Revell SM, Clark WD. Late-onset laryngomalacia: a cause of pediatric obstructive sleep apnea. Int J Pediatr Otorhinolaryngol 2011;75(2):231–238

[7] Werner JA, Lippert BM, Dünne AA, Ankermann T, Folz BJ, Seyberth H. Epiglottopexy for the treatment of severe laryngomalacia. Eur Arch Otorhinolaryngol 2002;259(9):459–464

[8] Dahl JP, Purcell PL, Parikh SR, Inglis AF Jr. Endoscopic posterior cricoid split with costal cartilage graft: a fifteen-year experience. Laryngoscope 2017;127(1):252–257

[9] Truong MT, Messner AH. Evaluation and Management of the Pediatric Airway: Cummings Pediatric Otolaryngology. Philadelphia, PA: Elsevier; 2015

[10] Hoff SR, Rastatter JC, Richter GT. Head and neck vascular lesions. Otolaryngol Clin North Am 2015;48(1):29–45

[11] McLaughlin KE, Jacobs IN, Todd NW, Gussack GS, Carlson G. Management of nasopharyngeal and oropharyngeal stenosis in children. Laryngoscope 1997;107(10):1322–1331

[12] Prisman E, Miles BA, Genden EM. Prevention and management of treatment-induced pharyngo-oesophageal stricture. Lancet Oncol 2013;14(9):e380–e386

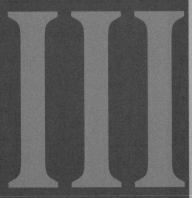

Section III

Skull Base and Craniofacial

III

24 Management of Periorbital Abscess

Narin N. Carmel Neiderman, Dan M. Fliss, Oshri Wasserzug, Gadi Fishman, Avraham Abergel

Summary

Orbital complication are the most common complications of sinusitis in children. The clinical severity ranges from periorbital cellulitis to sub-periosteal abscess and orbital abscess. The latter may also further exacerbate onto intracranial disorders. The microbiology of orbital cellulitis and abscess reflects the underlying sinus involvement and pathology. The management can vary from conservative 48-72 hours antibiotic trial to immediate surgical drainage. Surgical intervention should be considered depending on the patient's ophtalmogoical assessment and systemic inflammatory condition. Imaging studies are of critical importance in defining the extent and nature of orbital inflammation, determining appropriate management and defining surgical approach. Contrast-enhanced computed tomography (CT) has long been the imaging study of choice to evaluate patients with acute sinusitis and suspected orbital involvement. When surgery is indicated, the majority of cases can be treated endoscopicaly. Open approaches should be reserved for cases which difficult to approach endoscopically such as lateral or superior abscesses.

Keywords: Orbital cellulitis, subperiosteal abscess, orbital complications of sinusitis, orbital abscess

24.1 Prevalence and Pathophysiology of Periorbital and Orbital Complications of Sinusitis

Orbital cellulitis, subperiosteal abscess, and orbital abscess are the common complications of sinusitis in children. The latter may also further exacerbate onto intracranial disorders such as brain abscess, subdural empyema, meningitis, facial osteomyelitis, and thrombosis of the cavernous sinus and cortical vein.[1]

The orbit is susceptible to contiguous spread of infection from the sinuses as it is surrounded by sinuses on three sides. Children are particularly susceptible for infection spread because of their thinner bony septa and sinus wall, greater porosity of bones, open suture lines, and larger vascular foramina. The main anatomical landmark in the assessment and diagnosis of orbital cellulitis is the **orbital septum** (▶ Fig. 24.1), a fascial extension of the orbital rim periosteum extending to the tarsal plates of the upper and lower eyelids.

Periorbital cellulitis (preseptal cellulitis) is usually caused by trauma to the eyelid, for example, insect bite, or bacteremia[2] and usually does not result from sinusitis

and complicate to a sequel of orbital complications.[3] **Orbital cellulitis** (postseptal cellulitis) is an invasive bacterial infection of the *postseptal* tissues of the eye. The most common underlying factor for the development of orbital cellulitis is presiding acute ethmoid sinusitis[4,5] and up to 76% of cases of orbital cellulitis occur as a complication of acute sinusitis.[6]

Bagheri et al found that sinusitis was the most common cause in 53.8% of patients with orbital (postseptal) cellulitis, and in only 24.1% of preseptal cellulitis patients. Hence, surgical intervention was less common in periorbital cellulitis and was required in 14.8% of cases in comparison to 48.7% needed in orbital cellulitis.[7] Interestingly, orbital infections secondary to sinusitis are being reported to be 85% to 95% preseptal cellulites and 5% to 15% postseptal infections[8] such as subperiosteal abscess (SPA) (15%) and orbital abscess (less than 1%).[9] However, these rates vary between different series worldwide. For example, Kinis et al presented a series of complicated sinusitis patients with a rate of 42.3% of subperiosteal abscess and 50% preseptal cellulitis.

Depending on the severity of the presentation, eye findings may vary from soft, nontender eyelid edema to marked erythema, proptosis, chemosis, ophthalmoplegia, and decreased visual acuity.[5] Interestingly, while underlying sinusitis may be the cause of majority of cases of orbital cellulitis, orbital complication may be the first and only presenting sign of sinus disease.[1] The appearance of a proptotic eye with periorbital swelling usually arise the suspicion of an infection, caused by not only acute sinusitis but also bacteremia and facial infections, nasal foreign body, a fungal infection, dacryocystitis etc. If sufficient septic clinical characteristics are not available, the differential diagnosis should include other infectious sources such as hemorrhagic cyst, pseudoaneurysm of orbital bones, a cranio-orbital cerebrospinal fluid leak, Langerhans cell histiocytosis, hemorrhagic infarct of orbital bones, orbital myositis, an aneurysmal bone cyst, ossifying fibromatrauma, and iatrogenic causes. In sinus tumors, many primary tumors (i.e., rhabdomyosarcoma or retinoblastoma) and metastasis (i.e., neuroblastoma) may be misdiagnosed as infections.

As for the pathophysiology of infectious spread, the orbit is separated from the ethmoid cells and maxillary sinus by the lamina papyracea which has congenital bony dehiscence. Infections can spread directly by penetration of the lamina or through the dehiscence. Infection may also extend directly by traversing through the anterior and posterior ethmoid foraminas. Moreover, the ophthalmic venous system has no valves, meaning the extensive venous and lymphatic communication between the sinuses and the surrounding structures enables retrograde thrombophlebitis and further spread of the

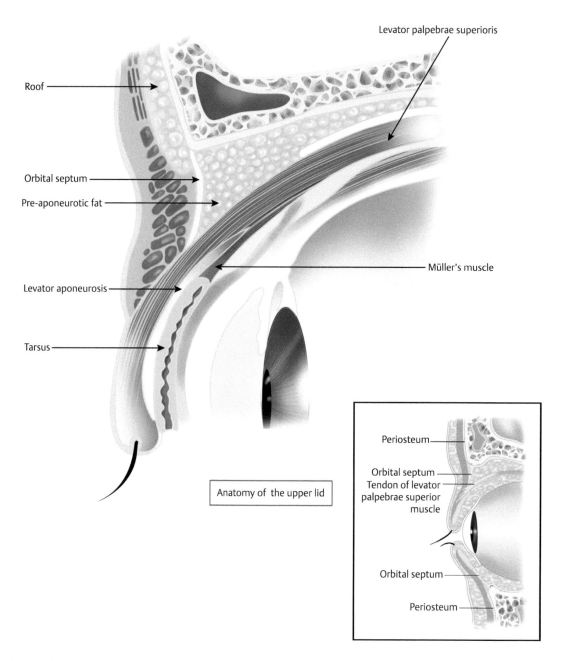

Roof

Orbital septum

Pre-aponeurotic fat

Levator aponeurosis

Tarsus

Levator palpebrae superioris

Müller's muscle

Anatomy of the upper lid

Periosteum

Orbital septum
Tendon of levator palpebrae superior muscle

Orbital septum

Periosteum

Fig. 24.1 Anatomy of the orbita and main anatomical landmarks.

infection.[10] Orbital infection may also occur via foreign body contamination or systemic hematogenous seeding, though these routes are thought to be far less common than direct local spread.[11]

Orbital cellulitis may further complicate into **orbital SPA**, a process in which pus is collected between the bony orbita frame and the periorbita. SPA most commonly arises from a complication of acute sinusitis. It is a relatively rare complication, occurring in 1% to 6% of cases.[11] **Intracranial extensions** are even more rare, and may

lead to potentially life-threatening conditions such as brain abscess, epidural empyema, and sinus vein thrombosis. They may occur directly, through necrotic areas of osteomyelitis in the posterior wall of the frontal sinus or by retrograde thrombophlebitis through the intracranial valveless venous system that interconnects the intracranial venous system with the sinus mucosal vasculature. Pediatric population is more vulnerable to CNS complications, due to the immature arachnoid[10] (▶ Fig. 24.1 and ▶ Fig. 24.2).

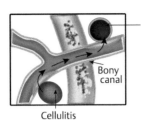

Contamination through vein wall

Bony canal

Cellulitis

Retrograde thrombophlebitis

Fig. 24.2 Trends of spread.

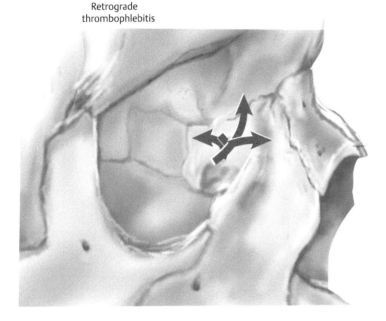

24.2 Classification

Hubert was the first to embark on scientific classification of orbital complications following sinusitis, based on the anatomy of the orbit, progression of infection, responsiveness to treatment, and general prognosis.[12] This classification system was renovated by Chandler,[13] who recognized the orbital septum, anatomical landmark, dividing the orbit into preseptal and postseptal sites. The orbital septum is a fascial extension of the orbital rim periosteum extending to the tarsal plates of the upper and lower eyelids. Chandler's classification describes the signs and symptoms of involvement of different regions of the orbit and does not imply a chronologic progression of symptoms.

Chandler grouped his patients under five categories (see ▶ Table 24.1 and ▶ Fig. 24.4).

Schramm further modified Chandler's classification, focusing on patients with preseptal cellulitis with chemosis as a separate entity. Schramm suggested to consider these patients as a separate entity as they do not consistently improve with antibiotics and surgery needs to be advocated.[15] Chandler's classification was also modified by Moloney who divided orbital complications into preseptal and postseptal complications.[16] Moreover, a recent suggestion by Le et al. was to add computed tomography characteristics such as presence of bony destruction and size of SPA (>3.8 mL) to the original Chandler criteria[17] (▶ Fig. 24.3).

24.3 Microbiology of Orbital Complications Associated with Sinusitis

The microbiology of orbital cellulitis and abscess reflects the underlying sinus involvement and pathology. Common organisms are *Streptococcus pneumoniae*, *Moracella catarrhalis*, haemophilus species, *Staphylococcus aureus*, group A streptococcus and upper respiratory anaerobes such as Peptostreptococcus, Fusobacterium, and Bacteroides.[4,5,10] Historically, *Haemophilus influenzae* cases were common, such as meningitis and bacteremia,[18] but with the introduction of *H. influenzae* type B vaccine in 1985 its incidence sharply declined.[19,20] Nowadays, *Staphylococcus* and *Streptococcus* are the most common pathogens found in the current series.[4,21]

In the recent years, community-acquired methicillin-resistant *Staphylococcus aureus* (MRSA) is a rising concern as a cause of head-and-neck infections. Bedwell et al report that the incidence of MRSA varies from 23% to 72%

Table 24.1 Chandler's classification

Group	Pathophysiology	Physical examination/initial presentation
Group I—Preseptal cellulitis— caused by restricted venous drainage	• Inflammatory edema present anterior to orbital septum, restricting venous drainage of ethmoidal vessels. Inflammation doesn't involve postseptal structures • Spread of the infection is limited to the orbit by the orbital septum and the tarsal plate	• Edema and erythema of the eyelid, no tenderness • No chemosis, Extraocular muscle movement limitations and vision impairment • Proptosis may be present to a mild degree • May present signs and symptoms of sinusitis
Group II—Orbital cellulitis	• Edema, bacterial infiltration of the adipose tissue and inflammation of orbital contents • Posterior to the septum without abscess formation	• Proptosis of varying degree • Reduced ocular mobility • Chemosis is usually present • Loss of vision is very rare
Group III—Subperiosteal abscess (SPA)	• Develops in space between the orbital bony wall and periorbita. May take place in the periosteum of the ethmoid, frontal, and maxillary bone. Orbital contents may be displaced in an inferior (frontal origin) or lateral (ethmoidal origin) direction due to the mass effect of accumulating pus	• Chemosis and proptosis are usually present • Decreased ocular mobility and loss of vision is rare • Vision is usually normal but can become impaired
Group IV—Orbital abscess	• A purulent collection in the orbital soft tissues behind the globe, could be caused due to relentless progression of orbital cellulitis or rupture of orbital abscess • Associated with inflammatory edema, purulence, and fat necrosis	Commonly seen: • Severe chemosis • Severe proptosis • Complete ophthalmoplegia (involvement of CN II, III, IV, V, and VI) • Loss of vision (increased intraocular pressure causing retinal artery occlusion or optic neuritis) • Displacement of the globe forward, or downward and outward
Group V—Cavernous sinus thrombosis	• Retrograde phlebitis extending to the cavernous sinus • Possible because of the absence of valves in the orbital veins that communicate with the cavernous sinus • Life-threatening complication that may clinically deteriorate with the development of meningitis, toxicity, and sepsis. The rate of blindness and death is up to 20%[14]	• Bilateral ocular signs: spread of orbital cellulitis and visual loss to the contralateral eye • Rapid progression of chemosis and limitation of extraocular muscle motility • Severe retinal venous engorgement • Fever • Headache • Photophobia • Proptosis • Ophthalmoplegia • Loss of vision • Orbital pain • Severe loss of visual acuity • Cranial nerve palsies involving III, IV, V1, V2, and VI are common

Abbreviation: CN, cranial nerves.

in the United States.[5,22] Mckinley et al reported that up to 73% of *Staphylococcus* species found and isolated in their cohort were actually MRSA, and the latter was the next most common pathogen (36% of all cultures obtained in this study).

When the sinusitis spreads to the orbital region from the maxillary sinuses, it may also be associated with odontogenic infections in pediatric population. Typical organisms may include alpha-hemolytic streptococci, microaerophilic streptococci, and more rarely, *Streptococcus pyogenes* and *S. aureus*. In anaerobic organisms, gram-negative bacilli *Peptostreptococcus* spp., *Fusobacterium* spp., and *Propionibacterium acnes* were found.[23]

Tissue and pus cultures may be obtained from various sites. The yield of different culture sites was examined and the most yielded cultures were obtained intraoperatively from the orbital and sinus abscess. Sinus aspirate and nasal swabs had a yield of 81% and 83%, and blood culture yield was very low at 7%.[21]

Intravenous antibiotic therapy should not only cover common pathogens but also penetrate central nervous system, in order to reduce the risk of intracranial complications. After obtaining microbiology culture, proper treatment should be done according to the culture results. Several protocols for empiric treatment are available in the literature: Bedwell et al suggest combining Clindamycin with third-generation cephalosporin with

Fig. 24.3 (a, b) Chandler's classification, coronal and sagittal sections.

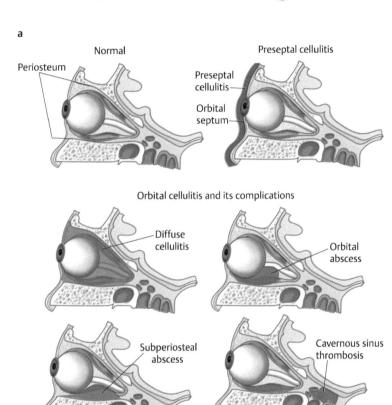

A B C D E

a

Normal

Periosteum

Preseptal cellulitis

Preseptal cellulitis

Orbital septum

Orbital cellulitis and its complications

Diffuse cellulitis

Orbital abscess

Subperiosteal abscess

Cavernous sinus thrombosis

b

good CNS penetration such as cefotaxime, ceftriaxone, or cefuroxime.

The conversion to oral antibiotics takes place when the clinical examination returns to the basal state. In nonsurgical cases, amoxicillin with clavulanic acid or clindamycin is prescribed for 14 days. In surgical cases, culture-directed antibiotic is used.[5] In some series amoxicillin is used as oral therapy in up to 40% of cases, while cefuroxime in 13% of cases only.[21] Although histopathological characteristics, osteitis, and even osteomyelitis signs are present in the specimen of the excised ethmoid bone of surgical patients, a long-term course of therapy is not usually required.[9]

Cannon et al provided preliminary data regarding oral antibiotic treatment for postseptal cellulitis; however, this treatment is still experimental and does not obviate the need for hospitalization for close monitoring.[24]

As for other complementary treatments, nasal vasoconstriction with oxymetazoline, although a controversial treatment, is also sometimes applied.[5] Corticosteroid usage, especially when central nervous system is involved, is also noncommon and controversial. They can retard the encapsulation, increase necrosis, and reduce antibiotic penetration into the abscess. However, these treatments may also have a positive effect by reducing cerebral edema,[10] and they may aid in the treatment of the adjacent sinusitis. These are also hypothesized to suppress and control the exuberant inflammatory response and prevent further spillage to the subperiosteal space. Yen et al showed no significant difference in the number of patients with SPAs requiring surgery with addition of steroids in comparison to patients who did not receive steroids.[25]

24.4 Imaging Role in the Management of Orbital Complications of Sinusitis

Imaging studies are of critical importance in defining the extent and nature of orbital inflammation and determining appropriate management.[5] Contrast-enhanced computed tomography (CT) has long been the imaging study of choice to evaluate patients with acute sinusitis and suspected orbital involvement, due to distinct anatomic bony resolution and rapid scanning.[26] The classic ST appearance of an SPA is a convex low-density lesion with an enhancing rim next to the medial orbital wall. Presence of low density or air within the area is suggestive of abscess formation.[27] Moreover, CT helps in utilizing the intraoperative image-guided systems, which are particularly useful in revision cases or cases with challenging anatomy. CT scans may be significant in achieving definitive diagnosis of SPAs. For example, Fanella et al report that CT scan revealed subperiosteal abscess in 31.5% of orbital cellulitis cases, and 25% of these patients underwent immediate surgery based on the initial CT scan findings. Also, 36.4% of the children who underwent CT had to undergo repeat CT assessment after initiation of ABX protocol. It was found that these children/the latter eventually required surgical intervention,[4] thereby raising the question as to when the clinical accurate timing is to perform the CT scan in the patients' assessment. However, data regarding the optimum timing is scarce.

The role of magnetic resonance imaging (MRI) is being explored as a low radiation alternative to CT scans in pediatric population. MRI was traditionally used as a tool for delineating intracranial complications of orbital cellulitis, including the cavernous sinus. It was found to be more sensitive than CT (97% vs. 87%) in identifying intracranial complications, but its ability in identifying abscesses and sinus disease was not examined in this study.[28] Also, MRI value in identifying orbital abscess has not been established in the current literature. The poor bony resolution is a major pitfall of the MRI as a diagnostic tool. Moreover, it may require

sedation in younger children. Bedwell et al suggest that MRI should be considered when there is concern for intracranial involvement or when a child's clinical picture does not match the CT findings.[5] MRI utilizing diffusion-weighted imaging (DWI) is also being examined as a possible tool to detect abscess without contrast administration and relatively rapid acquisition time. It was shown to increase diagnostic certainty in a series of 10 patients with orbital cellulitis or abscesses (▶ Fig. 24.4).

24.5 Systemic Antibiotic Treatment vs. Surgery—When to Treat Conservatively?

Patients with mild inflammatory eyelid edema or preseptal cellulitis (Chandler's class 1) can be treated with a trial of oral antibiotics and decongestants. However, close supervision and follow-up is mandatory. If postseptal involvement (Chandler's classes 2–5) is suspected or has developed, intravenous antibiotics and hospitalization is mandatory.

While the surgical management evolved from external drainage to endoscopic approaches, the decision about when to surgically drain versus conservative systemic antibiotics (ABX) has remained controversial. In the earlier decades, an abscess was an absolute indication for surgical management; however, in the recent two decades, orbital SPA in children is not considered an absolute indication for immediate surgical intervention, and consideration of a 48 IV antibiotic trial is common.

Garcia and Harris were first (and only) to define prospective criteria for medical versus surgical intervention among patients with radiographically suspected SPAs. Their prospective study found a 93% response rate in patients selected under the age of 9, with medial to small SPA of nondental origin, without optic nerve compromise, gas in abscess space, frontal sinusitis, or evidence of chronic sinusitis.[29] On the contrary, in retrospective studies, such as Rahbar et al's series, when no preselection of patients was applied, some series showed that only 26%

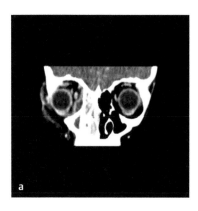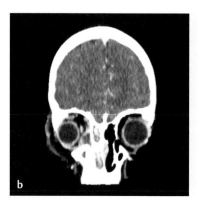

Fig. 24.4 (a, b) Demonstrative coronal sections from a CT scan of a patient with SPC.

of patients were treated with ABX alone, without any surgical intervention.[27]

It is common practice nowadays that patients presenting with septic/toxic appearance and advanced ophthalmologic findings such as impaired visual acuity, elevated IOP, ophthalmoplegia, proptosis >5 mm, or with large abscesses (width >10 mm) are best treated surgically.[5,30] However, multiple series demonstrated that patients with a less fulminant presentation (e.g., small-to-moderate sized abscess, mild-to-moderate chemosis, proptosis, and limited eye motion) may improve with conservative management, including intravenous antibiotics, nasal saline lavage, topical decongestants, with frequent ophthalmologic monitoring.[9,11,27,29,31]

Many studies tried to predict the need for early surgical intervention. However, there is no consensus on what presenting ocular criteria predict the success of medical management. The degree of proptosis, severity of restricted gaze, elevated IOP, and decreased visual acuity have been reported alone or in combination as predictors of success of medical management.[9,32,33] ► Table 24.2 lists the parameters that were commonly found significantly different between antibiotic and surgically treated patients in our literature review.

Table 24.2 Literature review of significant clinical characteristics distinguishing between operated and antibiotic successfully treated pediatric patients for SPAs

Significant characteristic (SX vs. ABX)	Study
Abscess size/volume	Bedwell and Bauman 2011[5] Rahbar et al 2001[27] Ryan et al 2009[9] Todman and Enzer 2011[34] Oxford and McClay 2006[31] Tabarino et al 2015[35] Friling et al 2014[36] Le et al 2014[17]
Age	Bedwell and Bauman 2011[5] Ryan et al 2009[9] Friling et al 2014[36] Fanella et al 2011[4]
Degree of proptosis	Rahbar et al 2001[27] Oxford and McClay 2006[31] Tabarino et al 2015[35] Friling et al 2014[36]
Temperature	Ryan et al 2009[9]
Chemosis	Oxford and McClay 2006[31]
Elevated intraocular pressure	Oxford and McClay 2006[31]
Restriction of extraocular movements	Oxford and McClay 2006[31]
Exophthalmos	Tabarino et al 2015[35]
Severe eye pain	Friling et al 2014[36]
CRP levels	Friling et al 2014[36]
Bony destruction in CT scan	Le et al 2014[17]

There is some evidence that older patients are less likely to be adequately treated with medications alone. In some series, age was not found to be a predictor of ABX failure alone[27,31] while in others[9] it was shown as significant in the success of conservative treatment. The latter was explained by a different bacteriologic profile of the older children (>9 years), polymicrobial infections, leading to a higher increase in failures. Comparatively, smaller sinus ostia and a more developed frontal sinus were cited as age-related factors, increasing the risk of complex anaerobic infections and intracranial extension.[29,37] Moreover, older patients are managed surgically more than younger patients in some series.[9,38] However, according to current literature, age should not be a contraindication to a trial of conservative management, and in some cohorts up to two-thirds of the cohort is successfully treated medically among pediatric patients between ages 10 and 15.[5]

Frontal sinusitis is considered to be an indication for surgery[34] due to its unique anatomy leading to an increased rate of intracranial complications.[39] Superior collections are more likely frontal sinus derived. In the presence of superior abscess, the diploic system of the frontal bone is more likely to be compromised by infection, putting the child at risk for intracranial dissemination through retrograde thrombophlebitis.[40] Taubenslag et al[40] compared cases with ipsilateral frontal sinusitis to ones without in a cohort under the age of 9, and showed that patients with frontal sinusitis had a higher incidence of nonmedial SPA compared to those without frontal sinus involvement, yet a majority of SPAs in the frontal sinusitis group were located medially. All patients with superior or superomedial SPA underwent early surgical intervention. Ninety-three percent in the frontal sinusitis cohort with medial SPAs were managed successfully with medical therapy alone, while all children with frontal sinusitis associated with superior or superomedial SPA were treated surgically. Their study suggests that frontal sinusitis as a surgical criterion should be invoked in younger children only if the frontal sinus is clearly the source of an SPA.

All patients must be monitored closely with serial ophthalmologic examinations, and any deterioration should lead to timely drainage. Presence of fever[4] or leukocytosis upon admission failed to predict the need for surgical drainage, but worsening of these parameters or failure to defervesce after 48 hours of ABX treatment also indicates re-imaging.[5] Failure to improve after 48 hours likely reflects treatment failure and should prompt consideration for surgical intervention.[30]

24.6 Endoscopic versus Open Surgical Approach

Despite the described sensitivity of the different imaging modalities, the surgical procedure is also of an exploratory nature. It is commonly performed within 24 hours of admission or after IV antibiotics treatment failure, within 48 hours.[3] The main aims of surgery are drainage of abscess and treatment of the underlying sinusitis. Surgical procedure may be external or endoscopic, or a combined approach, according to the abscess location. Sinusotomy and orbitotomy are the more common procedures and their prevalence rates in the different series are 52% and 39%, respectively.[21] However, the surgical procedure may include sinus irrigation, sinusotomy, antrostomy and drainage, orbitotomy, and even craniotomy and drainage, depending on the extensiveness of the disease.

The commonly used open approach for medial subperiosteal and orbital abscesses is lynch incision, combined with external ethmoidectomy.

The first five cases treated successfully via intranasal endoscopic approach were reported by Manning in 1993.[41] He presented a technique including ethmoidectomy and maxillary antrostomy with limited opening of the lamina papyracea to allow evacuation of purulent material. This approach is very common and is highly used for its efficacy and safety for the drainage of medial SPAs.

Endoscopic sinus surgery is relatively safe but has been implicated in seeding, rather than preventing, intracranial infection.[11] Minor surgical complications range from symptomatic adhesions to nasolacrimal duct stenosis, while major complications can include hemorrhage, orbital complications such as hematoma, vision loss, and diplopia, as well as skull base complications such as cerebrospinal fluid leakage. Major complications may occur in up to 2% of patients. The main advantage of the open approach is providing a direct access to medial subperiostial abscess (SPOA). However, the cutaneous incision made perpendicular to relaxed skin tension lines may result in cosmetic complications such as webbing. Recent techniques including transnasal endoscopic surgery and transcaruncular approach provide access to medial abscesses without cosmetic morbidity.[31] Moreover, the endoscopic approach was associated with inferior morbidity and shorter hospital stay.[42,43]

As for the extent of endoscopic surgery, Froehlich et al described the minimal endoscopic approach for the treatment of periosteal abscess stating that the only anterior ethmoidotomy and opening the anterior portion of the papyracea is sufficient to the drainage of the abscess.[44] However, Sciarretta et al showed that the minimalistic method described was not sufficient for all cases, and some may necessitate the opening of the posterior portion of the lamina papyracea after a complete ethmoidotomy to obtain the drainage, because of the anterior portion opening was not sufficient.[43]

Despite the increasing popularity of endoscopic surgery, open approaches are still limitedly used, mainly in cases of restrictive anatomy with wide infection, making endoscopic manipulation impossible. Another possible indication for open approach is osteomyelitis of the frontal bone.[45] Moreover, while medial abscesses are facilitated to drain via endoscopic approach, superior and lateral orbital abscesses usually require external approach.[46] Kayhan et al report that the use of external drainage of the SPOA is needed in 6 of 10 patients: for four superiorly located abscesses and two failures of transnasal endoscopic management.[46] Tanna further reported similar rates in a cohort of 13 patients: 29% of patients underwent combined surgical approach and 38% of patients underwent open approach only.[47] In the eight patients who underwent open surgery, the abscess had superolateral extension and extraocular muscle involvement was more extensive. However, no difference was found in temperature, leukocyte count, age, and duration of symptoms[47] (▶ Fig. 24.5 and ▶ Fig. 24.6).

24.7 Highlights

a. Indications
   - Orbital cellulitis, subperiosteal abscess, and orbital abscess are common complications of sinusitis in children.
   - 24 to 48 hours of intravenous antibiotics may be considered in SPA.
b. Indication for surgery
   - Septic/toxic appearance.
   - Advanced ophthalmologic findings such as impaired visual acuity, elevated IOP, ophthalmoplegia, proptosis >5 mm.
   - Large abscesses (width >10 mm) are best treated surgically.
   - No improvement on IV AB after 48 to 72 hours.
c. Complications
   - Cavernous sinus thrombosis.
   - Loss of vision.
   - Cranial nerve palsies (ophthalmoplegia).
d. Special preoperative considerations
   - Younger patients respond better to conservative treatment.
   - Septic children need special anesthetic consideration.
   - Small diameter endoscopes for narrower nasal cavities.
   - Surgery in acute bacterial infection of the sinus is related with bleeding condition.
   - Navigation system should be considered.
e. Special intraoperative considerations
   - Endoscopic versus open approach:
     o Open approaches are still limitedly used nowadays.
     o Restrictive anatomy with wide infection.
     o Superior and lateral orbital abscesses may require external approach.
     o Failures of transnasal endoscopic management.
     o Extraocular muscle involvement.
   - Multidisciplinary team:
     o Intracranial involvement.
     o Ophthalmologic involvement.
     o Anesthesiology team.
     o Infectious disease unit.

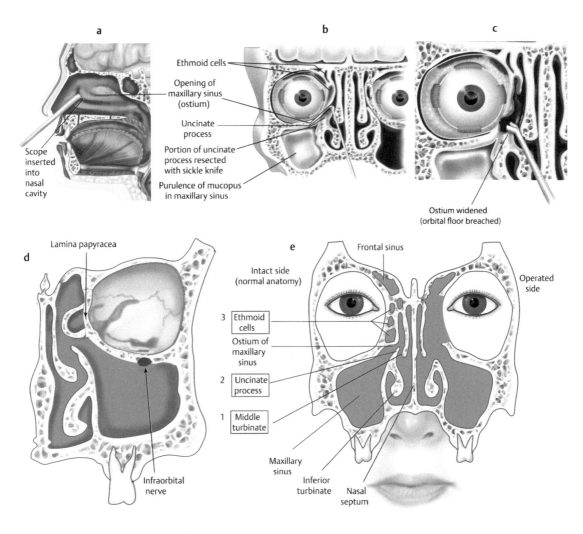

Fig. 24.5 (a–e) Endoscopic approach to the orbita via lamina propreocea.

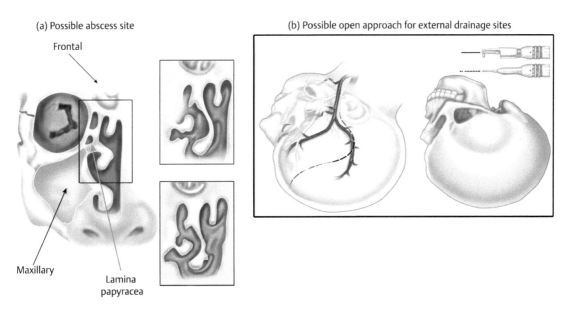

Fig. 24.6 Different surgical approaches. (a) Endoscopic approach. (b) Possible open approach for external drainage.

f. Special postoperative considerations
- Prolonged antibiotic treatment should be considered in intracranial involvement and bony involvement.

References

[1] Brook I, Friedman EM, Rodriguez WJ, Controni G. Complications of sinusitis in children. Pediatrics 1980;66(4):568–572

[2] Rubinstein JB, Handler SD. Orbital and periorbital cellulitis in children. Head Neck Surg 1982;5(1):15–21

[3] Skedros DG, Haddad J Jr, Bluestone CD, Curtin HD. Subperiosteal orbital abscess in children: diagnosis, microbiology, and management. Laryngoscope 1993;103(1 Pt 1):28–32

[4] Fanella S, Singer A, Embree J. Presentation and management of pediatric orbital cellulitis. Can J Infect Dis Med Microbiol 2011;22(3):97–100

[5] Bedwell J, Bauman NM. Management of pediatric orbital cellulitis and abscess. Curr Opin Otolaryngol Head Neck Surg 2011;19(6):467–473

[6] Israele V, Nelson JD. Periorbital and orbital cellulitis. Pediatr Infect Dis J 1987;6(4):404–410

[7] Bagheri A, Tavakoli M, Aletaha M, Salour H, Ghaderpanah M. Orbital and preseptal cellulitis: a 10-year survey of hospitalized patients in a tertiary eye hospital in Iran. Int Ophthalmol 2012;32(4):361–367

[8] Smith TF, O'Day D, Wright PF. Clinical implications of preseptal (periorbital) cellulitis in childhood. Pediatrics 1978;62(6):1006–1009

[9] Ryan JT, Preciado DA, Bauman N, et al. Management of pediatric orbital cellulitis in patients with radiographic findings of subperiosteal abscess. Otolaryngol Head Neck Surg 2009;140(6):907–911

[10] Brook I. Microbiology and antimicrobial treatment of orbital and intracranial complications of sinusitis in children and their management. Int J Pediatr Otorhinolaryngol 2009;73(9):1183–1186

[11] Souliere CR Jr, Antoine GA, Martin MP, Blumberg AI, Isaacson G. Selective non-surgical management of subperiosteal abscess of the orbit: computerized tomography and clinical course as indication for surgical drainage. Int J Pediatr Otorhinolaryngol 1990;19(2):109–119

[12] Hubert L. Orbital infections due to nasal sinusitis. NY State J Med 1937;37:1559–1564

[13] Chandler JR, Langenbrunner DJ, Stevens ER. The pathogenesis of orbital complications in acute sinusitis. Laryngoscope 1970;80(9):1414–1428

[14] Patt BS, Manning SC. Blindness resulting from orbital complications of sinusitis. Otolaryngol Head Neck Surg 1991;104(6):789–795

[15] Schramm VL, Myers EN, Kennerdell JS. Orbital complications of acute sinusitis: evaluation, management, and outcome. Otolaryngology 1978;86(2):ORL221–ORL230

[16] Moloney J, Badham N, McRae A. The acute orbit. Preseptal (periorbital) cellulitis, subperiosteal abscess and orbital cellulitis due to sinusitis. J Laryngol 1987

[17] Le TD, Liu ES, Adatia FA, Buncic JR, Blaser S. The effect of adding orbital computed tomography findings to the Chandler criteria for classifying pediatric orbital cellulitis in predicting which patients will require surgical intervention. J AAPOS 2014;18(3):271–277

[18] Donahue SP, Schwartz G. Preseptal and orbital cellulitis in childhood. A changing microbiologic spectrum. Ophthalmology 1998;105(10):1902–1905, discussion 1905–1906

[19] Barone SR, Aiuto LT. Periorbital and orbital cellulitis in the Haemophilus influenzae vaccine era. J Pediatr Ophthalmol Strabismus 1997;34(5):293–296

[20] Ambati BK, Ambati J, Azar N, Stratton L, Schmidt EV. Periorbital and orbital cellulitis before and after the advent of Haemophilus influenzae type B vaccination. Ophthalmology 2000;107(8):1450–1453

[21] McKinley SH, Yen MT, Miller AM, Yen KG. Microbiology of pediatric orbital cellulitis. Am J Ophthalmol 2007;144(4):497–501

[22] Liao S, Durand ML, Cunningham MJ. Sinogenic orbital and subperiosteal abscesses: microbiology and methicillin-resistant Staphylococcus aureus incidence. Otolaryngol Head Neck Surg 2010;143(3):392–396

[23] Brook I. Microbiology of acute sinusitis of odontogenic origin presenting with periorbital cellulitis in children. Ann Otol Rhinol Laryngol 2007;116(5):386–388

[24] Cannon PS, Mc Keag D, Radford R, Ataullah S, Leatherbarrow B. Our experience using primary oral antibiotics in the management of orbital cellulitis in a tertiary referral centre. Eye (Lond) 2009;23(3):612–615

[25] Yen MT, Yen KG. Effect of corticosteroids in the acute management of pediatric orbital cellulitis with subperiosteal abscess. Ophthal Plast Reconstr Surg 2005;21(5):363–366, discussion 366–367

[26] White JB, Parikh SR. Early experience with image guidance in endoscopic transnasal drainage of periorbital abscesses. J Otolaryngol 2005;34(1):63–65

[27] Rahbar R, Robson CD, Petersen RA, et al. Management of orbital subperiosteal abscess in children. Arch Otolaryngol Head Neck Surg 2001;127(3):281–286

[28] Younis RT, Anand VK, Davidson B. The role of computed tomography and magnetic resonance imaging in patients with sinusitis with complications. Laryngoscope 2002;112(2):224–229

[29] Garcia GH, Harris GJ. Criteria for nonsurgical management of subperiosteal abscess of the orbit: analysis of outcomes 1988–1998. Ophthalmology 2000;107(8):1454–1456, discussion 1457–1458

[30] Bedwell JR, Choi SS. Medical versus surgical management of pediatric orbital subperiosteal abscesses. Laryngoscope 2013;123(10):2337–2338

[31] Oxford LE, McClay J. Medical and surgical management of subperiosteal orbital abscess secondary to acute sinusitis in children. Int J Pediatr Otorhinolaryngol 2006;70(11):1853–1861

[32] Coenraad S, Buwalda J. Surgical or medical management of subperiosteal orbital abscess in children: a critical appraisal of the literature. Rhinology 2009;47(1):18–23

[33] Brown CL, Graham SM, Griffin MC, et al. Pediatric medial subperiosteal orbital abscess: medical management where possible. Am J Rhinol 2004;18(5):321–327

[34] Todman MS, Enzer YR. Medical management versus surgical intervention of pediatric orbital cellulitis: the importance of subperiosteal abscess volume as a new criterion. Ophthal Plast Reconstr Surg 2011;27(4):255–259

[35] Tabarino F, Elmaleh-Bergès M, Quesnel S, Lorrot M, Van Den Abbeele T, Teissier N. Subperiosteal orbital abscess: volumetric criteria for surgical drainage. Int J Pediatr Otorhinolaryngol 2015;79(2):131–135

[36] Friling R, Garty B-Z, Kornreich L, et al. Medical and Surgical Management of Orbital Cellulitis in Children. Folia Med (Plovdiv) 2014;56(4):253–258

[37] Harris GJ. Age as a factor in the bacteriology and response to treatment of subperiosteal abscess of the orbit. Trans Am Ophthalmol Soc 1993;91:441–516

[38] Siedek V, Kremer A, Betz CS, Tschiesner U, Berghaus A, Leunig A. Management of orbital complications due to rhinosinusitis. Eur Arch Otorhinolaryngol 2010;267(12):1881–1886

[39] Hakim HE, Malik AC, Aronyk K, Ledi E, Bhargava R. The prevalence of intracranial complications in pediatric frontal sinusitis. Int J Pediatr Otorhinolaryngol 2006;70(8):1383–1387

[40] Taubenslag KJ, Chelnis JG, Mawn LA. Management of frontal sinusitis-associated subperiosteal abscess in children less than 9 years of age. J AAPOS 2016;20(6):527–531.e1

[41] Manning SC. Endoscopic management of medial subperiosteal orbital abscess. Arch Otolaryngol Head Neck Surg 1993;119(7):789–791

[42] Arjmand EM, Lusk RP, Muntz HR. Pediatric sinusitis and sub-periosteal orbital abscess formation: diagnosis and treatment. Otolaryngol Head Neck Surg 1993;109(5):886–894

[43] Sciarretta V, Macrì G, Farneti P, Tenti G, Bordonaro C, Pasquini E. Endoscopic surgery for the treatment of pediatric subperiosteal orbital abscess: a report of 10 cases. Int J Pediatr Otorhinolaryngol 2009;73(12):1669–1672

[44] Froehlich P, Pransky SM, Fontaine P, Stearns G, Morgon A. Minimal endoscopic approach to subperiosteal orbital abscess. Arch Otolaryngol Head Neck Surg 1997;123(3):280–282

[45] Marshall AH, Jones NS. Osteomyelitis of the frontal bone secondary to frontal sinusitis. J Laryngol Otol 2000;114(12): 944–946

[46] Kayhan FT, Sayin I, Yazici ZM, Erdur O. Management of orbital subperiosteal abscess. J Craniofac Surg 2010;21(4): 1114–1117

[47] Tanna N, Preciado DA, Clary MS, Choi SS. Surgical treatment of subperiosteal orbital abscess. Arch Otolaryngol Head Neck Surg 2008;134(7):764–767

25 Orbital Surgery for Tumors

Shay Keren, Igal Leibovitch

Summary

A variety of tumors, both benign and malignant, can be found in the orbit of the pediatric patient. This chapter elaborates on the different tumors in terms of diagnosis and treatment as on the various different surgical approaches that can be used in treating these tumors.

Keywords: Tumors, orbit, surgery, approach

25.1 Introduction

Orbital tumors in children are quite rare. Most tumors are benign, mainly cysts;[1] however, malignant and life-threatening tumors[2] can also occur. In this chapter we discuss the common orbital tumors as well as the possible surgical management options.

25.1.1 Benign Tumors

Orbital Cysts

Orbital cysts are the most common benign tumors in the pediatric population. Such cysts can be primary or secondary, congenital or acquired, and may have diverse etiologies such as post-surgical, traumatic, inflammatory, or idiopathic.[1]

Dermoid and epidermoid cysts are the most common benign cysts in the orbit. These are choristomas that originate from aberrant ectodermal tissue and are located between two suture lines of the skull that close during embryonic development. Approximately 50% of dermoids involving the head are found in or adjacent to the orbit, either in the supero-temporal or, less commonly, in the supero-nasal aspect of the orbit.[1] These lesions are usually superficial but may also be deep in the orbit. Surgical removal is the treatment of choice, usually held after the age of 1 year. During surgery, care should be given for a complete removal of the cyst without capsule rupture which might lead to local inflammatory response (▶ Fig. 25.1).

Lacrimal duct cysts are cystic lesions that arise from the lacrimal duct epithelium. They appear as a mass in the lacrimal fossa. Caution is required during surgery to avoid damage to the lacrimal duct. Using intra-lesional dye such as indocyanine green allows complete resection of the cyst with its capsule.[3]

Vascular Lesions

Vascular orbital lesions are classified according to pathogenesis, histopathology, and hemodynamic properties. The primary classification is according to the flow within the tumor. High flow malformations contain arterial aneurysm, arteriovenous fistula, and arteriovenous malformation (varices). These lesions usually mandate therapy using invasive radiology with coiling or sclerosing agents. Lesions classified as low flow can be further classified as simple lesions, including venous malformations such as cavernous hemangioma and capillary hemangioma, and lymphatic malformations, such as lymphangioma, which can be macrocystic, microcystic, or mixed. There are also combined lesions, some venous dominant and some lymphatic dominant.[4,5]

Capillary hemangioma is the most common pediatric vascular lesion, usually presents early in life with decreased vision, limited ocular motility, proptosis, or cosmetic disfiguration. Management of capillary hemangiomas changed dramatically with the use of systemic beta blockers, making surgery less common in these tumors today and is reserved to non-responsive tumors, or cases with severe cosmetic disfiguration (▶ Fig. 25.2).[6]

Lymphangioma is a type of low-flow malformation, rarely pure lymphatic, but on most occasions mixed with a venous component. Most cases can be managed conservatively with only follow-up. In cases of cosmetic or medical indication, treatment should be held.[5,7] Treatment of such lesions is challenging and consists of excision and drainage of the lesion with the use of sclerosing agents to allow hemostasis.

In most cases only partial resection is achieved, and recurrence is common.[4]

Tumors of Neural Origin

Optic nerve tumors in the pediatric population are different from adults both clinically and histopathologically.

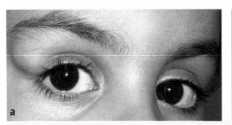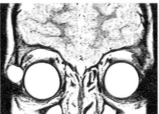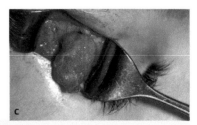

Fig. 25.1 **(a)** A 2-year-old girl with a dermoid cyst on the supero-lateral aspect of the right orbit. **(b)** A coronal CT scan showing a discrete, round, cyst. **(c)** An intraoperative view of the dermoid cyst exposed through a lateral eyelid crease incision.

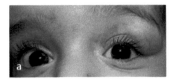
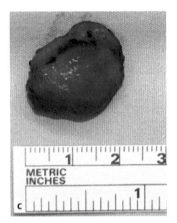
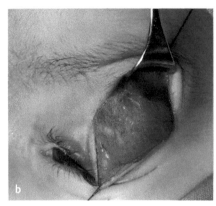
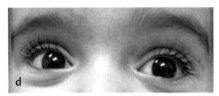

Fig. 25.2 **(a)** A 1.5-year-old boy with a capillary hemangioma on the superolateral aspect of the left orbit. **(b)** An intraoperative view of the hemangioma as seen through a lateral upper crease incision. **(c)** The tumor has been completely excised with surrounding capsule. **(d)** A postoperative view.

Optic nerve glioma is the most common optic nerve tumor in children (~4% of all orbital tumors). It usually presents at the age of 4 to 5 years. More than half of patients have neurofibromatosis type 1 (NF1). Usually no treatment is required due to the slow growing nature of the tumor. In cases of CNS or chiasmatic involvement, radiation therapy should be initiated. Surgery is reserved for anterior tumors that impair vision or cause a cosmetically significant proptosis.[8]

Other benign tumor of a neural origin, also frequently found in the pediatric population, is plexiform neurofibroma. This tumor is common in NF1 patients and is usually located on the temporal side of the upper eyelid, causing an S-shaped lid. These tumors may cause the S-shape upper eyelid and ptosis that may lead to amblyopia. In such cases surgical treatment is indicated promptly. A surgical approach combining ptosis repair with tumor debulking and upper eyelid reconstruction may result in a significant cosmetic and functional improvement, however, tumor recurrence in common.[9]

Schwannoma is an uncommon tumor in the orbit, especially in children, originating from the myelin-producing Schwann cells. They involve mostly sensory nerves as V1 and V2 but can also involve motor nerves and the globe itself. Treatment of such tumors is usually surgical with recent reports advocating adjacent radiotherapy.[10]

Osseous Lesions

Benign osseous lesions may also present in the pediatric population. These include fibrous dysplasia and juvenile ossifying fibroma. These lesions can present as a mass with osseous expansion (e.g., fibrous dysplasia) or as a lytic and sclerotic lesion (e.g., juvenile ossifying fibroma). Fibrous dysplasia is an abnormal growth of immature fibro-osseous tissue in the bone marrow, replacing the normal osteoblasts. It is slow growing and usually requires no treatment unless pressing the optic nerve or causing severe proptosis. Juvenile ossifying fibroma is a yellow-white mass filled with cystic spaces. The treatment of choice is surgical excision.[11] Some tumors may secondarily involve the orbital bones such as dermoid and epidermoid cysts and leukemia.[9]

Osteoma is a benign, slow growing tumor originating from any bone. It commonly arises from the paranasal sinuses and is usually asymptomatic. It appears as sclerotic, dense, well-defined mass. Surgical intervention is required to alleviate pressure on important orbital structures or to improve cosmetic appearance.[12]

Langerhans cell histiocytosis (LCH) is a spectrum of three syndromes in which immature dendritic cells of bone marrow origin proliferate. Eosinophilic granuloma, one of these syndromes, is common in children younger than 4 years, and is the most common expression of LCH in the orbit. It causes proptosis, ptosis, or an enlargement of the palpebral fissure. It most often occurs in the supratemporal frontal bone, where bone marrow is abundant. LCH causes an osteolytic, yellow-colored, hemorrhagic lesion. Treatment consists of surgical excision and sometimes chemotherapy. The other two syndromes, Lettere–Siwe disease and Hand–Schuller–Christian disease rarely affect the orbit (▶ Fig. 25.3).[11]

25.1.2 Malignant Lesions

Rhabdomyosarcoma is the most common malignant orbital tumor in children and accounts for about 5% of tumors. It is a mesenchymal soft-tissue tumor, and its orbital presentation accounts for approximately 25 to 35% of head and neck rhabdomyosarcoma and around 10% of all rhabdomyosarcoma. The orbit may also be involved by spread of mesenchymal tumors from the nasopharynx, pterygopalatine fossa, or paranasal sinuses.[7] Orbital

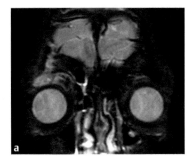
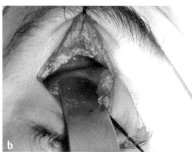

Fig. 25.3 (a) A coronal MRI of a 15-year-old boy with a right orbit superior eosinophilic granuloma. **(b)** A superior eyelid crease incision used to explore and excise the tumor.

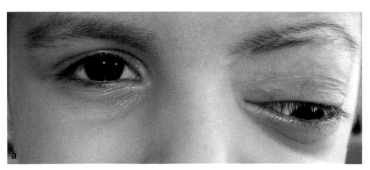
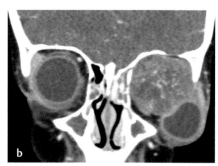

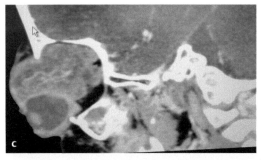
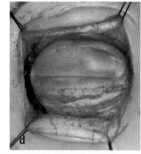
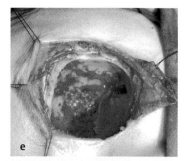

Fig. 25.4 (a) A 4-year-old girl with rapidly progressive development of proptosis and infero-lateral displacement of the globe. **(b)** A coronal CT scan showing the displaced globe and a tumor occupying the orbit. **(c)** A sagittal CT scan showing the relation between the tumor and the globe. **(d)** Exenteration surgery showing deep dissection which allows separation of orbital content from the orbital walls. **(e)** The exenterated orbit with no content.

rhabdomyosarcoma arises most frequently adjacent to the extraocular muscles.[13] It usually occurs in the superior part of the orbit and causes rapidly progressive proptosis with globe displacement and possible motility restriction. About 85% of all orbital rhabdomyosarcoma are of the embryonal type which has a 5-year survival rate (5YSR) of approximately 95%. Other types are the alveolar which is a more aggressive type with a 75% 5 year survival rate and an affinity for the inferior orbit, and the pleomorphic and butteroid types which are much less common in the orbit.[14]

Therapy nowadays consists of systemic chemotherapy with local external-beam radiation therapy. Surgical intervention has remained mainly for tissue diagnosis and for the treatment of repeated tumors after failure of conservative treatments. In some cases, exenteration may be usually required (▶ Fig. 25.4).[14,15]

Retinoblastoma, an intraocular malignant tumor, may spread through the optic nerve into the intracranial optic tracts and the subarachnoid space.[8] Only 2% has extraocular invasion including scleral, extrascleral, and optic nerve. The presence of orbital retinoblastoma is indicative of an advanced disease, appears around the age of 3 years, usually with proptosis (70–85%), redness, swelling, and pain. Diagnosis includes imaging and total-body scanning for metastases. Vast changes in the detection of such tumors along with genetic consultation have improved survival to 88–93%. Current treatment regimens, after systemic evaluation for metastases, include the use of systemic or local chemotherapy (including intra-arterial melphalan) and local external beam radiation.[16] In cases of massive orbital involvement, exenteration may be required.

Osseous malignant tumors in children include osteosarcoma, chondrosarcoma, and Ewing sarcoma. Osteosarcoma

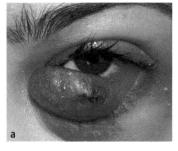
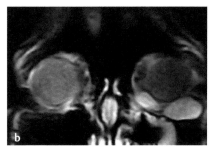
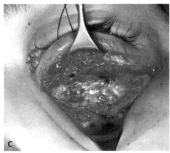
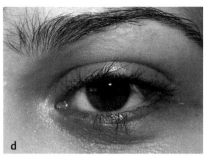

Fig. 25.5 **(a)** A 17-year-old girl with a mass in the lower conjunctiva suspected to be Ewing sarcoma. **(b)** A coronal CT scan showing the hyperdense mass inferior to the globe. **(c)** A sub-ciliary approach allows for separation of the tumor. **(d)** A postoperative view of an almost invisible scar.

induces bone destruction and osteoid production. Treatment consists of surgical excision and chemotherapy.[11] Ewing sarcoma is the second most frequent, extraorbital tumor to involve the orbit. It is usually located in long bones and treatment is by surgery, chemotherapy, and radiation (▶ Fig. 25.5).

Orbital metastases are quite rare and usually indicate neuroblastoma elsewhere in the body. Neuroblastoma includes metastases to the orbit in 28 to 33% of patients. It usually involves soft tissue and can lead to proptosis but the main site of involvement is the orbital bone.[17] Other malignant tumors found in the orbit in pediatric populations are leukemia, which can be intra- or extraocular, and to a less extent, lymphoma.

Pediatric lesions may involve any part of the orbit and the clinical work-up in conjunction with complete history and appropriate imaging, as specified in the next section, dictate the surgical approach for treatment of these lesions (▶ Table 25.1).

25.2 Preoperative Evaluation and Anesthesia

A comprehensive history is essential in the diagnosis of an orbital lesion in a child. The information acquired through questioning the patient or the parents may be crucial in establishing the correct diagnosis and may dictate the urgency of surgical or pharmacological treatment. In cases of an acquired lesion, it is important to know the progression rate of the lesion, as a fast growing lesion may indicate malignancy (e.g., rhabdomyosarcoma) and dictate earlier intervention. Inquiries regarding the dynamic behavior of the lesion may support diagnosis such as

Table 25.1 Classification to benign and malignant orbital tumors

	Benign	Malignant
Cystic	Dermoid	
	Epidermoid	
	Lacrimal duct epithelial cyst	
Vascular	Capillary hemangioma	
	Lymphatic malformation	
	Varices (venous malformation)	
	Arterio-venous malformation	
	Lymphatic-venous malformation	
Neural	Optic nerve glioma	Neuroblastoma
	Optic nerve sheath meningioma	Retinoblastoma (extraocular extension)
	Schwannoma	
	Plexiform neurofibroma	
Osseus	Fibrous dysplasia	Osteosarcoma
	Juvenile ossifying fibroma	Chondrosarcoma
	Osteoma	Ewing sarcoma
	Langerhans cell histiocytoma	Rhabdomyosarcoma
	Osteoblastoma	
Hematology		Leukemia
		Lymphoma

changes during Valsalva (venous lesions), changes after upper respiratory tract infection (lymphangioma), etc.

A complete physical evaluation by a pediatrician is essential to rule out systemic involvement, or find a primary tumor that can be a source for metastases. Examples are optic nerve glioma in NF1, leukemia, lymphoma, neuroblastoma, Ewing sarcoma, etc.

A complete ophthalmic examination should include:

- Best corrected visual acuity should be assessed for any changes such as a hyperopic shift in cases of external globe compression.
- External evaluation for the presence of a palpable mass, proptosis, exophthalmos, globe displacement, and ptosis. The use of warm's view and an upper lid crease symmetry assessment can help detect such changes. The use of Hertel or Naugle exophthalmometers to objectively measure the degree of proptosis may help not only identify changes but also measure progression rate.
- Pupillary reaction to light and afferent pupillary reaction must be examined for determining optic nerve involvement. Ocular movements should also be tested to find out any involvement of one or more of the extraocular muscles.
- Complete ocular examination of the anterior and posterior segment using the slit lamp may reveal signs associated with orbital lesions such as Lisch nodules associated with NF1 and optic nerve glioma, retinoblastoma that might have spread to the orbit, optic nerve head edema or pallor, choroidal folds indicating pressure on the globe and other clues as for the primary pathology.

Imaging must be acquired for all patients to help diagnose the lesion and assess its location, size, involvement of structures, intracranial extension, etc.

- CT is a suitable first option of imaging for most lesions, and has great value, but in a cost of high level of radiation. CT is particularly efficient for osseous lesion or assessing bone remodeling or absorption, and calcification in non-osseous tumors.
- MRI is superior to CT in displaying soft-tissue lesions, especially in the orbital apex, and intracranial extension. It involves no radiation, but doesn't exhibit well osseous lesions and bone lysis or remodeling. MRI should be considered when vascular lesions are suspected since it demonstrates the vessels, flow, or lack of it, and blood products in different stages of degradation.[18]
- Orbital imaging must always include the use of contrast, and coronal, axial, and sagittal sections for allowing better location of the lesion and involvement of adjacent tissue.
- US carried away by a skillful physician may be useful in further characterizing anterior tumors.

In many cases of pediatric orbital lesions, the diagnosis can be made by a complete clinical evaluation and imaging studies. Surgical intervention is warranted in two cases: sampling the lesion for pathologic and cytologic examination, and excision of a lesion. Almost all surgical interventions in children are done under general anesthesia.

25.3 Surgical Approach

25.3.1 Surgical Planning

The orbit is a rather small (30 mL) space with many vital structures: the globe, muscles, nerves, and blood vessels. It can be divided into different surgical planes, each with its unique approaches, structures, and risks.

The preoperative evaluation including imaging is essential to decide the exact location and size of the lesion and to assess the extent of involvement of adjacent structure, hence helping the surgeon decide the surgical plane to be dissected and the approach to be taken. Preoperative evaluation should also include setting specific goals for surgery whether curative, diagnostic, or only cosmetic. Previous treatments, surgical or otherwise, to the orbit are also important in surgical planning due to scar tissue and adhesion expected in the non-naïve orbit, which may alter normal anatomy.

The surgical approach should be efficient but also cosmetically acceptable. The surgeon should always rely on the facial structure to plan as small and hidden incisions as possible.

25.3.2 Orbital Surgical Planes

The orbit can be divided into 5 surgical planes:

1. Subperiosteal space: A potential space between the orbital bones and the periorbita.
2. Extraconal space: The peripheral space lying between the outer periorbita and the inner muscle cone and inter-muscular fascia.
3. Intraconal space: An inner space lying between the outer muscle cone and the inner optic nerve.
4. Sub-tenon space (episcleral): An inner space located between the globe and the tenon's capsule.
5. Subarachnoid space: The space that lies between the optic nerve and the optic nerve sheath.

In addition to the aforementioned planes, cystic lesion such as dermoid cysts may be located superficially; thus, only a skin incision is required, without actually entering the orbit.[19]

An orbital lesion may involve more than one plane; therefore, a combination of surgical approaches through the same incision or through several incisions is required.

The axial location of a lesion is also important in surgery planning. An anterior lesion, usually in the anterior half of the orbit, can usually be approached by an anterior approach, whether superior or inferior, without the removal of orbital bones. For posterior lesions, orbital bone removal may be required, though an anterior approach can sometimes be used, depending on tumor size, location, and other structures' involvement.

Superior Approach

The supero-anterior part of the orbit is the most common location of orbital lesions like hemangiomas, bony tumors, mucoceles, and dermoids. In superior orbital dissection, the supraorbital and supratrochlear vessels should be avoided as well as the levator muscle and the lacrimal gland. In most cases of superior approach surgeries, no bones are removed. In some deeper lesions, the superior orbital rim may be removed to allow better exposure. Usually the superolateral rim can be excised without entering the intracranial space. If done medially, the frontal sinus may be entered. Upon closure, care should be taken to avoid incarceration of sinus mucosa.

An upper crease incision is usually the approach of choice. This incision may be widened as needed and it usually leaves an acceptable well-hidden scar. It can be carried away in several variations, central, lateral, or medial, based on the location of the tumor. This approach allows access to the superior orbital rim and its periosteum. After a skin incision, soft-tissue dissection should be carried away to expose the orbital rim in a supero-posterior fashion. The dissection should be made anteriorly to the septum without opening it until reaching the point where the septum is held by the orbital rim at the arcus marginalis. After proper exposure, the periosteum may be elevated. This approach allows access to the extraconal space or to the intraconal space by reflecting the levator aponeurosis or by a vertical incision through it. The upper eyelid crease incision, if made more medially between the superior and medial rectus muscles, through the intermuscular fascia, allows access to the optic nerve for biopsy or fenestration. A more upper, sub-brow incision may allow access for superior tumors with

an acceptable cosmetic result (▶Fig. 25.6, ▶Fig. 25.1c, ▶Fig. 25.2b, and ▶Fig. 25.3b).

More internal planes such as the sub-tenon, intraconal, or extraconal spaces may be accessed through a superior conjunctival incision, well-hidden under the superior eyelid. In such approach, special care should be given to the Muller and levator muscles to prevent future ptosis (▶Fig. 25.6).

The vertical eyelid splitting approach, used to access the same planes as the transconjunctival incision, includes the vertical splitting of the levator muscle among other structures. Meticulous closure of the incision should be carried away to prevent ptosis or retraction. Special attention should be given to closure of the tarsal plate and the levator muscle to prevent postoperative ptosis (▶Fig. 25.6).

Two more superior approaches exist to allow access to the superior orbit, the sub-brow, and trans-cranial (coronal) approaches. These incisions are less cosmetically acceptable and are used when other approaches cannot be used. Sometimes bone removal may also be required (▶Fig. 25.6).

Inferior Approach

The inferior approach gives good access to tumors located in the inferior half of the orbit. As for the superior approach, there is a transcutaneous approach and a transconjunctival approach. In both cases the addition of an inferior orbital rim bone removal may assist in widening the exposed surgical field, mainly to reach deep inferior located lesion. Special care should be given in such cases to the inferior orbital neurovascular bundle.

The transcutaneous approach includes a subcilliary incision that produces a cosmetic acceptable scar. The incision is usually made around 2 to 3 mm below the lid margin (eyelash line) in a crease or stress line, with a soft-tissue dissection below the level of the orbicularis oculi (much like in the superior approach) to expose the inferior septum to its origin in the inferior orbital rim. With rim exposure, several planes can be accessed. The subperiosteal plane can be accessed by elevating the

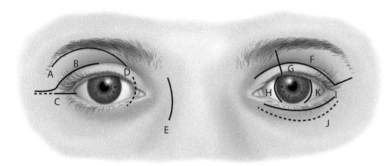

Fig. 25.6 Superior approach. (A) Sub-brow incision. (B) Eyelid crease lateral incision. (C) lateral canthal (canthotomy and canthiolysis) incision. (D) Trans-caruncal incision. (E) Frontoethmoidal (Lynch) incision. (F) Upper eyelid crease. (G) Vertical eyelid split incision. (H) Medical bulbar conjunctival incision. (I) Sub-ciliary incision. (J) Inferior trans-cunjunctival incision. (K) lateral bulbar conjunctival incision.

periosteum. The extraconal plane may be accessed by opening the septum. This approach was neglected due to the obvious advantages of the conjunctival approach. In times of severe conjunctival pathology such as ocular cicatricial pemphigoid this approach may be used (▶ Fig. 25.6, ▶ Fig. 25.7, and ▶ Fig. 25.5c).

The transconjunctival approach is the preferred approach by surgeons nowadays, mainly because it provides good exposure and no visible scars. It also avoids eyelid retraction or the rounding of the lateral canthus, seen in a cutaneous approach. An incision made in the inferior conjunctiva, either below the tarsal plate or in the inferior fornix, along with the inferior eyelid retractors, exposes the extraconal plane. In cases of large or more lateral located lesions, a lateral canthotomy and cantholysis may help with visualization and tumor excision. The eyelid should be retracted using a DesMarres retractor to avoid damage to the septum and skin. Elevation of the periosteum at the arcus marginalis may provide access to the intraconal plane (▶ Fig. 25.6 and ▶ Fig. 25.8).

Another approach to reach the intraconal space is with a conjunctival incision over the globe with retraction of the inferior rectus muscle. This approach, as in the superior globe, may also provide access to the sub-tenon space.

Medial Approach

The medial aspect of the orbit is extremely packed with important structures. Careful dissection with understanding of the orbital anatomy can prevent damage to the medial canthal tendon, the lacrimal apparatus, the trochlea and superior oblique tendon and muscle, the inferior oblique muscle as well as nerves and blood vessels.

A transconjunctival approach may give access to the sub-tenon or extraconal planes. Detachment and reflection of the medial rectus muscle may allow access to medial intraconal lesions, as well as the anterior optic nerve for biopsy, fenestration, or adjacent tumor

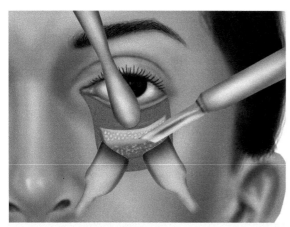

Fig. 25.7 Sub-ciliary cutaneous incision.

resection. When accessing the intraconal space for an optic nerve biopsy, care should be given to separate the orbital fat and adventitial fascia. The latter carries the ciliary arteries. The central retinal artery is also located in the surgical field and should be looked for and avoided to prevent instant, irreversible blindness. The conjunctival incision may be located near the caruncle, or in a more medial fashion near the limbus. Expansion of the conjunctival incision to the superior or inferior fornix may help widen exposure (▶ Fig. 25.6 and ▶ Fig. 25.9).

An incision made in the posterior third of the caruncle (trans-caruncular approach) allows access to the

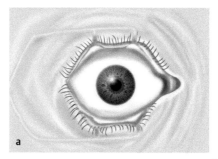

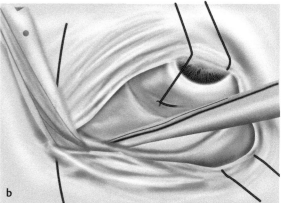

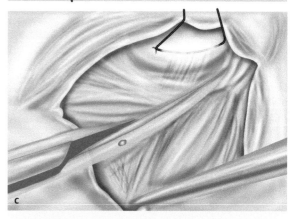

Fig. 25.8 "Swinging eyelid" inferior orbitotomy. (a) Speculum over the eyelids to allow conjunctival access. (b) Lateral canthotomy and cantholysis to release the lower eyelid. (c) Conjunctival incision inferior to the tarsal plate or in the inferior fornix to access the inferior orbit.

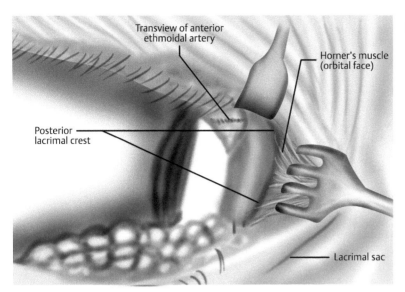

Fig. 25.9 Transcaruncle incision.

Transview of anterior ethmoidal artery

Horner's muscle (orbital face)

Posterior lacrimal crest

Lacrimal sac

subperiosteal plane. The dissection is located posterior to the orbital septum and Horner's muscle (originating at the posterior lacrimal crest and joining the orbicularis sphincter), thus avoiding damage to the lacrimal sac. This approach is preferable cosmetically but holds a greater risk of lacrimal apparatus damage (▶ Fig. 25.6).

Lateral Approach

The lateral approach is different in children mainly due to the fact that the pediatric orbit is shallower than in adults and lateral bone removal is rarely needed. This approach is used mainly for extensive lacrimal gland tumors, optic nerve tumors, or apex tumors. It allows direct visualization of the superolateral and inferolateral extraconal space and the entire intraconal space (▶ Fig. 25.6).

The main incision used is a combination of a superior lid crease or inferior transconjunctival incision, in a more lateral location, along with lateral canthotomy and cantholysis. This approach allows access to the orbital rim and the selection of periosteal elevation for subperiosteal plane, or dissection of the septum to allow access to the intraconal plane and the optic nerve. If the subperiosteum is incised, incision is then continued posteriorly in a T shape. The globe and temporalis are retracted and the rim is sawed at the fronto-zygomatico suture and below the zygomatic arch. The amount of bone to be sawed posteriorly is at the discretion of the surgeon. This approach may necessitate, at times, the detachment and reflection of the lateral rectus muscle. The removal of orbital bone is rarely employed in children but in rare cases it may be done. At the end of surgery, the bony part may be sewed back using drill holes made in advance. Miniplates can also be used (▶ Fig. 25.10).

In this approach, usually when accessing the intraconal plane, special care should be made to avoid damage to the ciliary ganglion located temporally to the optic nerve.

A transconjunctival approach may also be used when accessing not only the sub-tenon but also the extraconal plane.

25.3.3 Exenteration

This surgical approach is quite radical and appropriate for tumor invading the entire globe, those with no visual prognosis and those with high level of malignancy. Exenteration includes the removal of all orbital content including the peri-orbita. The adnexal tissue may remain or may be excised, depending on the tumor location and involvement. Usually adjuvant therapy is indicated. The most frequent cause of exenteration in children is rhabdomyosarcoma as elaborated in Chapter 1 (▶ Fig. 25.4e).

25.4 Postoperative Treatment

The postoperative treatment of a child can be divided into two sections: local treatment of the surgical wound and systemic management.

25.4.1 Local Treatment

After surgical removal of an orbital tumor, the surgical wound should be treated with local ointment, usually a combination of corticosteroids and antibiotics. An application 3 to 4 times a day is usually sufficient in preventing wound infection. Bed head should be elevated to reduce postoperative edema. Ice packing may also be used for this purpose. The wound should be examined on postoperative day 1 and usually after 1 week and 1 month. In cases of local infection, with or without systemic fever, the surgical wound should be revised, systemic antibiotics may be initiated according to surgeons' discretion and in rare cases a revision surgery should be held with

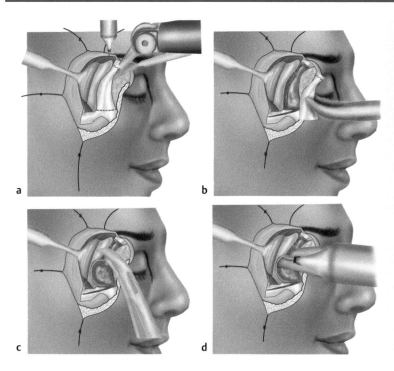

Fig. 25.10 (a) A lateral incision with exposure of the orbital rim. Two incisions are made using and oscillating saw on an upper and lower points of the rim. **(b)** The orbital rim is removed. **(c)** Incision in the periorbita to allow access to intraconal space. **(d)** Intraconal space is accessible.

wound opening, debridement of necrotic tissue, antibiotic wash, and closure of the site.

In selected cases, a drainage silicone tube is left to ensure meticulous drainage of all fluid from the surgical site and prevent local edema and compression on adjacent structures. The drainage device should be checked at least once every 8 hours. Quantity and quality of the fluid should be recorded.

Visual acuity and pupil reaction to light should be recorded periodically, preferably every 12 to 24 hours to detect early signs of optic nerve compression due to edema or hemorrhage and the development of an orbital compartment syndrome.

25.4.2 Systemic Management

Systemic management should be dictated by the type of surgery (incisional or excisional biopsy), type of lesion (benign or malignant), surgical result (complete vs. incomplete excision), and additional clinical tests and imaging results.

Pending pathological results of the specimen, further treatment should, on occasions, be held. In cases of malignant tumors, an oncologic consultation is mandatory with total body imaging for the detection of a primary tumor (in cases of orbital metastasis) or distance metastasis. Adjuvant chemotherapy or radiation treatment may be required.

Clinical follow-up with recording of orbital status such as Hertel measurements, visual acuity, etc., should be held with prolonging intervals in cases of improvement. Repeated orbital imaging is also essential for detecting partly removed lesions or recurrence. Repeated photography of the patient and the comparison to preoperative photographs can help follow improvement.

25.4.3 Complications and Management

- Vision loss is the most serious complication. It can result from direct damage to the optic nerve, damage to the arteries supplying the optic nerve, edema compressing the nerve or arteries, or bleeding in the orbit causing tight orbit. The latter is an emergency and necessitates prompt canthotomy and cantholysis to relieve pressure.
- CSF leak is quite rare and may be seen in medial or lateral orbitotomies. In cases of a mild leak, conservative management is advised. In cases of a severe leak, sealing the location with dura, fat, synthetic glue, or periosteum may be beneficial.
- Diplopia may occur when damage was done to one of the extraocular muscles or to the nerve or artery supplying a muscle. Some cases may be static and necessitate strabismus surgery, although most cases improve over time.
- Eyelid malposition such as ptosis, retraction, ectropion, or entropion may be caused by surgery. If persistent, surgical correction should be carried out.
- Lacrimal apparatus damage may cause tearing. In selected cases DCR is warranted and in others the use of a Jones tube.

25.5 Highlights

a. Indications
   - Tissue diagnosis for an undetermined orbital mass.
   - Suspected malignancy.

- Vision threatening tumor:
  - Compressive optic neuropathy.
  - Exophthalmos with corneal exposure.
- Ocular motility dysfunction.
- Cosmetic disfigurement.
b. Complications
- Vision loss due to compressive, ischemic, or direct damage to the optic nerve.
- Diplopia due to injury to the extraocular muscles.
- Lacrimal apparatus damage.
- Fistula to the sinuses.
- CSF leak.
- Eyelid malposition.
c. Special preoperative considerations
- Patients' age and general condition.
- Tumor size and location.
- Systemic involvement and prognosis.
- Cosmesis.
d. Special intraoperative considerations
- Avoidance of orbital structures including blood vessels, nerves, and other organs.
- Optimal exposure.
- Meticulous hemostasis.
- Maximal tumor removal when needed.
- Postoperative cosmesis.
e. Special postoperative considerations
- Monitoring of vision.
- Monitoring of optic nerve function.
- Monitoring of ocular motility.

References

[1] Shields JA, Shields CL. Orbital cysts of childhood: classification, clinical features, and management. Surv Ophthalmol 2004;49(3):281–299

[2] Browning MB, Camitta BM. The surgeon's role in pediatric orbital malignancies: an oncologist's perspective. Ophthal Plast Reconstr Surg 2003;19(5):340–344.10.1097/01.IOP.0000087072. 85558.90

[3] Keren S, Dotan G, Leibovitch L, Selva D, Leibovitch I. Indocyanine green assisted removal of orbital lacrimal duct cysts in children. J Ophthalmol 2015;2015:130215 10.1155/2015/130215

[4] Rootman J, Heran MKS, Graeb DA. Vascular malformations of the orbit: classification and the role of imaging in diagnosis and treatment strategies. Ophthal Plast Reconstr Surg 2014;30(2):91–104 10.1097/IOP.0000000000000122

[5] Bilaniuk LT. Vascular lesions of the orbit in children. Neuroimaging Clin N Am 2005;15(1):107–120 10.1016/j.nic.2005.03.001

[6] Garza G, Fay A, Rubin PA. Treatment of pediatric vascular lesions of the eyelid and orbit. Int Ophthalmol Clin 2001;41(4):43–55 http://www.ncbi.nlm.nih.gov/pubmed/11698737

[7] Chung EM, Smirniotopoulos JG, Specht CS, Schroeder JW, Cube R. From the archives of the AFIP: pediatric orbit tumors and tumorlike lesions: nonosseous lesions of the extraocular orbit. Radiographics 2007;27(6):1777–1799 10.1148/rg.276075138

[8] Chung EM, Specht CS, Schroeder JW. From the archives of the AFIP: Pediatric orbit tumors and tumorlike lesions: neuroepithelial lesions of the ocular globe and optic nerve. Radiographics 2007;27(4):1159–1186 10.1148/rg.274075014

[9] Keren S, Dotan G, Ben-Cnaan R, Leibovitch L, Leibovitch I. A combined one-stage surgical approach of orbital tumor debulking, lid reconstruction, and ptosis repair in children with orbitotemporal neurofibromatosis. J Plast Reconstr Aesthet Surg 2017;70(3):336–340 10.1016/j.bjps.2016.10.015

[10] Sweeney AR, Gupta D, Keene CD, et al. Orbital peripheral nerve sheath tumors. Surv Ophthalmol 2017;62(1):43–57 10.1016/j.survophthal.2016.08.002

[11] Chung EM, Murphey MD, Specht CS, Cube R, Smirniotopoulos JG. From the Archives of the AFIP. Pediatric orbit tumors and tumorlike lesions: osseous lesions of the orbit. Radiographics 2008;28(4):1193–1214 10.1148/rg.284085013

[12] Wei LA, Ramey NA, Durairaj VD, et al. Orbital osteoma: clinical features and management options. Ophthal Plast Reconstr Surg 2014;30(2):168–174 10.1097/IOP.0000000000000039

[13] Boutroux H, Levy C, Mosseri V, et al. Long-term evaluation of orbital rhabdomyosarcoma in children. Clin Exp Ophthalmol 2015;43(1):12–19 10.1111/ceo.12370

[14] Karcioglu ZA, Hadjistilianou D, Rozans M, DeFrancesco S. Orbital rhabdomyosarcoma. Cancer Contr 2004;11(5):328–333

[15] Boutroux H, Cellier C, Mosseri V, et al. Orbital rhabdomyosarcoma in children: a favorable primary suitable for a less-invasive treatment strategy. J Pediatr Hematol Oncol 2014;36(8):605–612 10.1097/MPH.0000000000000245

[16] Honavar SG, Manjandavida FP, Reddy VAP. Orbital retinoblastoma: An update. Indian J Ophthalmol 2017;65(6):435–442 10.4103/ijo.IJO_352_15

[17] Harreld JH, Bratton EM, Federico SM, et al. Orbital metastasis is associated with decreased survival in stage M neuroblastoma. Pediatr Blood Cancer 2016;63(4):627–633 10.1002/pbc.25847

[18] Gorospe L, Royo A, Berrocal T, García-Raya P, Moreno P, Abelairas J. Imaging of orbital disorders in pediatric patients. Eur Radiol 2003;13(8):2012–2026 10.1007/s00330-002-1738-y

[19] Leibovitch I, Goldberg RA. The approach to orbital surgery. In: Principles and practice of ophthalmology, 3rd edition. Albert DM, Jakobiec FA (eds). Volume 3, section 12, chapter 227, pages: 2897-2901

26 Endoscopic Sinus Surgery in Children for Benign Lesions

Shahaf Shilo, Dan M. Fliss, Avraham Abergel

Summary

Sinonasal tract and the skull base lesions in the pediatric population are rare and include a wide range of pathologies that originate from mesenchymal, neural, notochordal, vascular, and rarely, epithelial tissue. Although mostly benign, these lesions can grow to exert a mass effect and cause significant morbidity, thus requiring excision in most cases. Surgery of benign lesions in pediatric patients should be with maximal preservation of normal anatomy and critical neurological, neurovascular, and endocrine structures. Thus, endoscopic endonasal approach (EEA) is the optimal modality of treatment for sinonasal and skull base lesions in the pediatric population due to its minimally invasive nature. This chapter focuses on the endoscopic management of benign sinonasal and skull base lesions in children, and reviews the considerations unique to the pediatric population, the principal benign pathologies, the structure of the preoperative evaluation, and surgical techniques.

Keywords: Endoscopic endonasal surgery, pediatric patients, benign lesions, midline lesions

26.1 Introduction

Surgery of the sinonasal tract and skull base is a challenging task at any age. The skull base and the paranasal sinuses are characterized by a small and intricate anatomy situated in proximity to critical neurological and vascular structures. The challenge in accessing pathologic processes in these locations is even more pronounced in the pediatric population.

Once dominated solely by open approaches,[1,2] the modern field of sinonasal and skull base surgery is rapidly incorporating endoscopic techniques. Over the past decades, the role of the EEA has been constantly expanding to encompass a broader range of pathologies, pushing the limits of endonasal access toward more distant skull base locations in the coronal and sagittal planes. Although EEA was initially employed for adult sinonasal and skull base surgery, it has been adapted over time for use in pediatric patients as well, and its feasibility and safety in children have been established.[3,4,5] Furthermore, EEA is particularly advantageous in pediatric patients due to its minimally invasive nature compared to open approaches, providing direct access and optimal visualization without neural or vascular manipulation, thereby limiting the therapeutic sequelae of cosmetic deformity and functional deficiencies.

Pediatric lesions of the sinonasal tract and the skull base are rare and include a wide range of pathologies that originate from mesenchymal, neural, notochordal, vascular, and rarely, epithelial tissue. Although mostly benign, these lesions can grow to exert a mass effect and cause significant morbidity, thus requiring excision in most cases. In addition, pediatric skull base lesions commonly occur in the midline, making EEA the optimal modality of treatment.

This chapter focuses on the endoscopic management of benign sinonasal and skull base lesions in children, and reviews the considerations unique to the pediatric population, the principal benign pathologies, the structure of the preoperative evaluation, and surgical techniques.

26.2 Limitations and Special Considerations

The general principles of endonasal endoscopic surgery in the pediatric population correspond to those of adults; however, some critically important differences must be carefully considered. Since the sinonasal and skull base anatomy in children is dynamic, the surgeon encounters diverse stages of development, depending on the age of the patient. Furthermore, sinonasal and skull base lesions, especially those that are congenital, may distort the normal developing anatomy. An understanding of the surgical anatomy is imperative for safe surgical planning.

The age-dependent development and pneumatization patterns of the paranasal sinuses are critical issues to consider in EEA in children. Both the ethmoid and maxillary sinuses are present at birth. The maxillary sinuses expand between ages 0–3 and 6–12 years, and reach full adult size around age 18 years (►Fig. 26.1a). The ethmoid sinuses progressively develop in an anterior-to-posterior fashion until approximately age 12 years. The frontal sinus begins its development last, and becomes radiographically evident during the third year of life. It reaches the frontal bone only at age 5 years, and continues to expand throughout adulthood (►Fig. 26.1b). The sphenoid sinus is a structure of primary importance in endoscopic skull base surgery. It begins pneumatization at its anteroinferior aspect after age 2 years, and slowly proceeds posteriorly and superiorly throughout the first 10 to 15 years of life to aerate the sellae last (►Fig. 26.1c). The sphenoid anterior wall is fully pneumatized at age 6 to 7 years, but the clivus begins pneumatization after age 10 years.[6]

Another potential limiting factor in endoscopic approaches in pediatric patients is the size of the pyriform aperture,

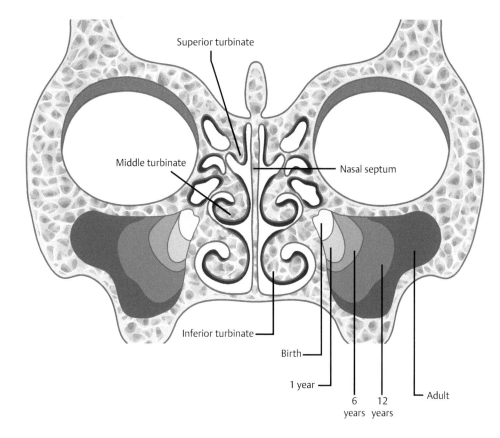

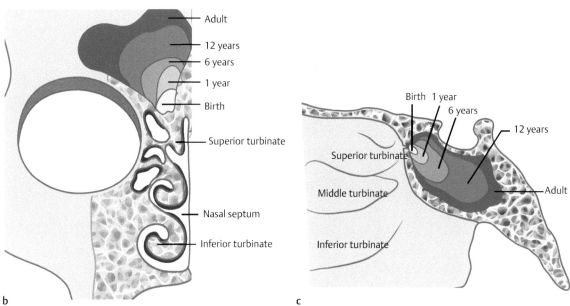

Fig. 26.1 (a) Maxillary sinus development. **(b)** Frontal sinus development. **(c)** Sphenoid sinus development.

which is significantly smaller in children under age 7 years compared with adults. However, it is considered to be an anatomic constraint only in the youngest patients (i.e., under 2 years old).[7] The intercarotid distance is an anatomic parameter that also must be considered, especially in cases of a non-pneumatized sphenoid sinus. It is known to be significantly narrower at the level of the cavernous sinus in patients up to 6 to 7 years old compared with adults, whereas at the level of the superior clivus no significant difference between children and adults was found.[7] The extent of the sphenoid sinus pneumatization, the size of the pyriform aperture, and the intercarotid distance limitations do not pose a contraindication for EEA in children, and can be safely overcome by an experienced team and with the use of an intraoperative navigation system.

Craniofacial growth is another aspect unique to sinonasal and skull base surgery in the pediatric population.[8] Ossification of the skull base occurs throughout the first two decades of life, concluding with the fusion of the spheno-occipital synchondrosis, one of the primary skull base growth centers, between ages 12 and 16 years.[9] Disruption of the craniofacial growth center or tooth buds can have a long-term impact on subsequent development and may result in facial asymmetry and injury to permanent dentition. In contrast to traditional external approaches, EEA is believed to minimize the effect of surgery on facial growth, although long-term data are still lacking. Therefore, it is mostly recommended to preserve the normal anatomy as much as possible, especially in cases of benign lesions.

26.3 Preoperative Evaluation

A multidisciplinary collaborative team consisting of otolaryngologists, maxillofacial surgeons, neurosurgeons, pediatricians, and radiologists is required for the evaluation and treatment planning in any type of skull base lesion in children. An ophthalmologic evaluation is also necessary whenever the lesion is in proximity to the orbit or the optic nerve. However, a smaller team may be sufficient for purely intranasal benign lesions.

The clinical presentation of sinonasal and skull base lesions varies for each lesion and is dependent upon its location, extent, and compression on adjacent structures. Some lesions may present at birth, whereas others present later during childhood or adolescence. Clinical manifestations of sinonasal lesions include nasal obstruction, respiratory distress, rhinorrhea, or epistaxis. Lesions with skull base and intracranial involvement may present with a visible mass or facial deformity, headaches, visual disturbances, cranial nerve palsy, focal neurological deficiencies, seizures, and endocrinopathy if the sellar region is involved. Skull base defects with respiratory mucosa and intracranial communication may lead to recurrent meningitis.

A complete history, including the onset and progression of symptoms, is essential. The physical examination should include a thorough head and neck exam and a neurologic function assessment, although it can be challenging in young children due to their inability to cooperate. Nasal endoscopy is an essential part of the physical examination, but it may be limited in small children.

Preoperative imaging should consist of both computed tomography (CT) and magnetic resonance imaging (MRI)

to provide complementary information critical for diagnosis, assessment of the lesion extent, and surgical planning. CT demonstrates bone anatomy, sinus size, and degree of pneumatization, whereas MRI better demonstrates the characteristics of the lesion and the surrounding soft tissue. Pediatric patients often require sedation during the MRI scan in order to obtain adequate images. A fine-cut CT angiography allows evaluation of the vasculature within and adjacent to the lesion, and it is used for intraoperative surgical navigation, often merged with MRI scan. The lack of sinus pneumatization in smaller children conceals the usual intraoperative anatomical landmarks, thus increasing the dependence on a navigation system. Angiography may be used for evaluation and preoperative embolization of highly vascular lesions.

A biopsy from the lesion should be considered only after a comprehensive review of imaging findings, and involved risks, such as bleeding from vascular lesions, or CSF leak and intracranial infection in cases of intracranial connection, must be evaluated beforehand. Some lesions do not require a biopsy and can be correctly diagnosed by imaging and clinical examinations. If a tissue diagnosis is indicated, the procedure should be done in the operating room.

26.4 Congenital Midline Lesions

Congenital midline nasal masses are rare benign lesions. Approximately 60% of them are dermoid cysts, while the others are gliomas or encephaloceles. Encephaloceles are discussed in Chapter 33.

26.4.1 Nasal Dermoid Cyst

Nasal dermoid cyst is the most common midline congenital nasal lesion. It is a benign tumor composed of ectoderm and mesoderm, and comprises approximately 4 to 12% of all head and neck dermoid cysts.[10] Nasal dermoid cysts usually presents at birth or in early childhood as a midline mass that may be located anywhere from the base of the columella, along the nasal dorsum, to the nasoglabellar region (▶Fig. 26.2). It may cause a cosmetic deformity of the nose, resulting in nasal broadening that often appears similar to hypertelorism.

Dermoid cyst is a noncompressible and nonpulsatile mass that does not transilluminate. It does not enlarge when the patient cries, and it has a negative Furstenberg sign (no enlargement with compression of the jugular veins). Nasal dermoid cyst can present with a cutaneous pit that secretes sebaceous material and may become intermittently infected (▶Fig. 26.3). Hair protruding through a cutaneous pit over the nasal dorsum is pathognomonic for a nasal dermoid cyst.

Intracranial extension through the anterior skull base is reported to occur in 5% to 45% of the cases, and it is

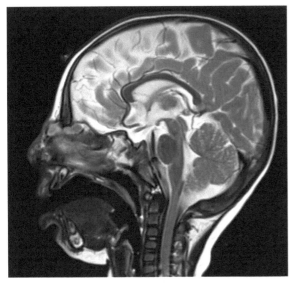

Fig. 26.2 Sagittal T2-weighted preoperative MRI scan of a 1.5-year-old female demonstrating a dermoid cyst and its tract.

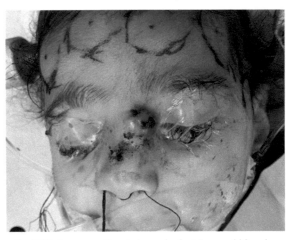

Fig. 26.3 A preoperative photograph of a 1.5-year-old female demonstrating a nasal pit of an infected dermoid cyst.

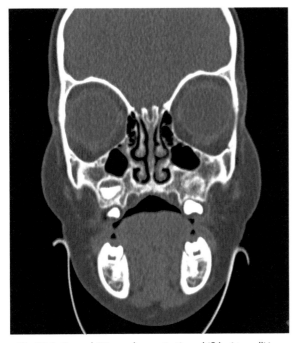

Fig. 26.4 Coronal CT scan demonstrating a bifid crista galli in a 2.5-year-old female with dermoid cyst.

usually located at the foramen cecum or crista galli.[11] Although the great majority remains extradural, intradural extensions with involvement of brain parenchyma have also been reported.

MRI and CT studies provide complementary information and both contribute in making the diagnosis, determining the extent of the lesion and planning the surgery. Since dermoid cyst is a nonenhancing lesion, it can be distinguished from the enhancing nasal mucosa and other lesions, such as teratomas and hemangiomas, with the use of contrast material. The demonstration of a bifid crista galli and enlarged foramen cecum on a CT scan is suggestive of intracranial involvement (▶ Fig. 26.4); however, these findings are not pathognomonic. MRI is preferred in delineating soft tissue and determining whether there is intracranial extension.[12] Complete surgical resection is imperative since recurrence rates of 50 to 100% are reported when the cyst or its sinus tract have not been completely resected.[13]

26.4.2 Glioma

Nasal glioma is a benign congenital lesion of the craniofacial region composed of heterotropic mature neuroglial tissue. It is believed to be derived from either a nasal encephalocele which has lost its intracranial connection or from entrapped neuroectodermal tissue after the closure of the skull base. Nasal gliomas are present at birth, but may be identified only later in life, depending upon their size and location. Gliomas may manifest extranasally (60%), intranasally (30%), or both (10%).[14] Extranasal gliomas are typically located in the region of the glabella, but they can also extend down to the nasal tip. Intranasal gliomas are most frequently located in the nasal cavity, but they have been found in other locations, such as the nasopharynx and the pterygopalatine fossa. Within the nasal cavity, they usually arise from the lateral wall adjacent to the middle turbinate, and less frequently from the nasal septum.[15] Intranasal gliomas may present with nasal obstruction and respiratory distress. Nasal gliomas are firm, noncompressible masses, and, in contrast to encephaloceles, they are nonpulsatile, they do not expand with crying or straining, and they are negative on the Furstenberg test.

Nasal gliomas have a fibrous stalk extending toward the base of skull with an underlying bony defect in 10 to 25% of cases. MRI is used to evaluate whether there is an intracranial connection. Surgical excision should be performed as early as possible to minimize the risks of complications, such as distortion of the nasal anatomy. Total resection that includes the stalk is imperative not only to decrease recurrence rates (4–10%), but also to minimize the risks of CSF leak and subsequent meningitis.[16] Extranasal gliomas are usually managed by external approaches, while intranasal gliomas are increasingly managed by transnasal endoscopic approach.

26.5 Middle Skull Base Lesions

26.5.1 Pituitary Adenoma

Pituitary adenomas are relatively rare in the pediatric population, representing 3% of all intracranial neoplasms in children. In comparison to adults, pituitary adenomas in children are more predominantly functional, with prolactinomas being the most frequent adenoma subtype, followed by adrenocorticotropin hormone (ACTH)- and growth hormone (GH)-secreting adenomas. Other secreting adenoma subtypes and nonfunctioning adenomas are much less common, and account for only 3 to 6% of all pituitary tumors in children.[17]

Clinical manifestations are usually related to the hormone secreted by the functioning adenoma. Prolactinomas mostly present during puberty with amenorrhea, and less commonly with growth arrest, delayed puberty, or galactorrhea in males. ACTH-secreting adenomas usually present at the onset of puberty, and may manifest as growth arrest, Cushingoid appearance, weight gain, hypertension, hyperglycemia, and psychiatric changes. GH-secreting tumors often present in prepubertal children and infants with precipitous growth, acromegaly, or headaches. Symptoms related to a mass effect, such as visual disturbances and focal neurologic signs, may also be present; however, they are more typical of nonfunctioning macroadenomas that dominate adult disease.[18]

Surgical resection is indicated for most pituitary adenomas, with the goals of surgery being total resection with preservation of endocrine and CNS function. Prolactinoma can be managed medically.

26.5.2 Craniopharyngioma

Craniopharyngioma is the most common benign sellar/parasellar tumor in the pediatric population, accounting for 50% of all pediatric sellar tumors (▶Fig. 26.5). They are thought to arise from epithelial remnants of Rathke's pouch, and the adamantinomatous subtype is most often seen in pediatric patients. Craniopharyngiomas contain cystic and solid components, and are generally slow-growing tumors that manifest insidiously as they enlarge. Although they are histologically benign, their location close to critical neurovascular and endocrine

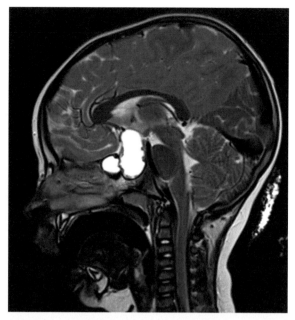

Fig. 26.5 Sagittal T2-weighted preoperative MRI scan of a 4-year-old male with craniopharyngioma.

structures can cause significant morbidity. Presenting signs and symptoms are usually related to a mass effect, and they include neurological disturbances, such as headache and visual field defects (classically bitemporal hemianopia), and manifestations of endocrine deficiency, such as diabetes insipidus, growth retardation, precocious puberty, poor school performance, and obesity.[19]

The goal of treatment is gross total resection, when possible, while preserving neurologic and endocrine functions. Tumor debulking to reduce a mass effect followed by radiotherapy is an alternative approach used for large lesions with hypothalamic involvement. Craniopharyngiomas may be resected through open, endoscopic, or combined open-endoscopic approaches, depending upon the characteristics of the lesion and the patient, as well as the experience and preference of the surgical team. The appropriate endoscopic approach is chosen according to the location of the lesion with respect to the pituitary stalk (pre/trans/retro infundibular).[20]

Long-term surveillance with serial imaging is required following treatment of craniopharyngioma. Recurrence rates are approximately 20% even after gross total resection, and mostly occur 3 to 4 years following surgery.[21]

26.5.3 Rathke's Cleft Cyst

Rathke's cleft cyst is a benign epithelium-lined non-neoplastic cyst in the sellar and suprasellar regions, thought to be a remnant of the Rathke's pouch. It is usually asymptomatic and often discovered incidentally. Rathke's cleft cyst must be differentiated from craniopharyngioma and cystic pituitary adenoma, although imaging findings are often inconclusive. A radiological finding of a small nonenhancing intracystic nodule is thought to be pathognomonic.[22]

Management of incidentally discovered Rathke's cleft cyst is usually conservative, consisting of sequential imaging. Treatment is indicated if interval growth is demonstrated or the patient becomes symptomatic. Characteristic symptoms in pediatric patients are headaches, visual loss, and endocrine insufficiency. Treatment includes cyst floor fenestration and drainage, with maximal pituitary gland preservation.

26.6 Other Sinonasal and Skull Base Lesions

26.6.1 Schwannoma

Benign peripheral nerve sheath tumors generally include schwannomas and neurofibromas. Between 25 and 45% of these tumors occur in the head and neck region, and only 4% of them arise within the sinonasal tract.[23] Schwannomas of the nasal cavity and paranasal sinuses have been postulated to arise from the ophthalmic or maxillary divisions of the trigeminal nerve, or from autonomic nerves within the nasal mucosa. They are grossly well-circumscribed, round or lobulated, slow-growing masses, and, unlike their counterparts in other anatomic locations, schwannomas in sinonasal location frequently lack a perineurial capsule. Most schwannomas are solitary, whereas multiple tumors may be associated with neurofibromatosis type 2.

The most commonly involved sites are the ethmoidal sinus and the nasal cavity, followed by the other paranasal sinuses and the nasal septum. Less frequently, schwannomas may also involve the anterior skull base, and are often referred to as subfrontal, olfactory, or olfactory groove schwannomas when they arise from the intracranial compartment. Since the olfactory nerve is unmyelinated, the origin of these tumors is still debatable.[24] Gross total resection is curative, and recurrence rates are low. However, since schwannomas are benign lesions with a growth rate of 1 mm/year, active observation might be a prudent therapeutic alternative for asymptomatic lesions.

26.6.2 Neurofibroma

Neurofibroma is very uncommon in the sinonasal tract, with only few reported cases in the literature. It develops from Schwann cells and perineurites, and is blended with fibroblastic cells. Solitary sinonasal neurofibromas are usually sporadic; however, multiple tumors or sinonasal plexiform neurofibroma may be associated with neurofibromatosis type 1.[25] The tumor is firm, glistening, with a

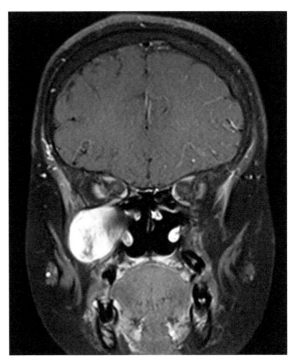

Fig. 26.6 Coronal T1-weighted preoperative MRI scan demonstrating right infratemporal fossa neurofibroma.

grey-tan color, and found in a submucosal location with an intact surface epithelium (▶ Fig. 26.6).

26.6.3 Hemangioma

Hemangiomas are the most common tumor of infancy, and most frequently involve the head and neck region. Although most hemangiomas arise in the skin and subcutaneous tissue, they may also be found in the sinonasal tract. Presenting symptoms include unilateral nasal obstruction and epistaxis, and the presence of a blue-red mass on nasal inspection. Imaging studies including MRI are obtained to distinguish it from other possible pathologies. Hemangiomas can be treated medically, whereas endoscopic surgical excision, sometimes combined with preoperative embolization to prevent bleeding, is reserved for refractory lesions.

26.6.4 Papilloma

Inverted papilloma of the sinonasal tract is a benign tumor derived from epithelial tissue (Schneiderian epithelium). It is a relatively common benign sinonasal lesion in adults, but exceedingly rare in children. The etiology of inverted papilloma is still controversial, but human papillomavirus and Epstein–Barr virus have been implicated in its development.[26,27] Inverted papilloma typically presents as an isolated, unilateral polypoid mass arising in the middle meatus or along the lateral nasal wall, or, less frequently, in the septum and nasal vestibule.

Associated squamous cell carcinoma arising in the same area of the inverted papilloma is present in 5 to 7% of cases;[28,29] however, malignant disease is more common among adults.

Imaging studies should include a CT scan, which may demonstrate bony changes associated with the lesion and assess the extent of invasion into the maxillary and ethmoid sinuses. Orbit involvement and intracranial extension should be evaluated as well. MRI can distinguish the lesion from thickened mucosa, secretions, and mucoceles.

Endonasal endoscopic surgery has become the standard of care for inverted papillomas. The lesion is completely debulked, and the underlying bone is drilled with a diamond bur to eliminate deep-reaching infiltration. Recurrence rates for endoscopic surgery are approximately 12 to 14%.[28,29]

26.6.5 Juvenile Nasopharyngeal Angiofibroma

Juvenile nasopharyngeal angiofibromas are discussed separately in Chapter 27.

26.7 Surgical Technique

The procedure is performed under general anesthesia with the patient in a supine position on the operating room table with the head resting on a padded support and fixated in a neutral position with a slight rotation to the right, using a pediatric Mayfield head clamp. Both surgeons stand to the right of the patient, and the monitor is positioned on the left side of the patient's head. Neuro-navigation system and endoscopic Doppler ultrasound probe are set up.

Perioperative antibiotics that include second-generation cephalosporin are administered. Patients undergoing pituitary surgery receive a perioperative single dose of hydrocortisone (100 mg).

The nasal cavity is decongested with topical application of 1% lidocaine and adrenaline (10:1) solution–soaked pledgets into both nares, and infiltrated with 2% lidocaine and adrenaline (1:100,000) solution. The nose, upper lip, and both nares are scrubbed with 4% iodine solution. The left thigh or the periumbilical area is scrubbed and draped if harvesting of fascia lata or periumbilical fat is expected to be required for reconstruction. A lumbar drain is placed in cases where the third ventricle is involved.

The target lesion can be removed through one or both nostrils, depending upon its location and extent. A uni-nostril approach can better preserve normal anatomy, but it can limit the maneuverability and number of instruments that are being used simultaneously. As such, that approach is generally reserved for small sinonasal and anterior skull base lesions. A bi-nostril approach

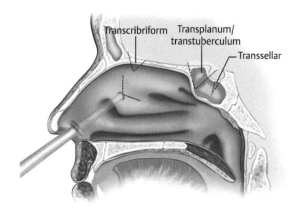

Fig. 26.7 Endoscopic approaches to the midline skull base: transcribriform, transplanum/transtuberculum, transsellar.

allows the use of four hands technique, and is selected for more extensive lesions as well as in lesions that require a transsphenoidal or a transclival approach, especially in pediatric patients where the nasal cavities are narrow. As noted earlier, a small pyriform aperture may be an anatomically limiting factor in young children, and the use of a pediatric 2.7 mm endoscope for the initial steps of the surgery can overcome that problem.

The goal of treatment for most benign lesions in pediatric patients is generally total resection in order to reduce the tumor recurrence rates and improve outcomes. The appropriate endoscopic approach is chosen based on the location and origin of the lesion. Endoscopic approaches to the midline skull base are demonstrated in ▸ Fig. 26.7. Once the lesion has been successfully accessed and is properly visualized, it is progressively debulked to achieve a minimal remnant around the lesion's origin. Next, resection of the remaining tumor stem with small margins is performed. In contrast to malignant lesions, where each of the involved compartments must be approached and resected with clear oncologic margins, surgery of benign lesions should be as minimally invasive as possible, with maximal preservation of normal anatomy. Furthermore, preservation of critical neurological, neurovascular, and endocrine structures' function is of prime importance, and may compromise the extent of resection if necessary.

26.8 Surgical Approaches

26.8.1 Transnasal Approach

The transnasal approach does not traverse any sinuses, and essentially keeps the septum and the middle turbinate as the boundaries. It is used for purely intranasal lesions, and may also serve as a corridor directly to the cribriform plate and olfactory groove superiorly, and to the clivus and odontoid through the choana inferiorly.

26.8.2 Sagittal Plane

Endoscopic Transseptal Approach for Dermoid Cyst

Methylene blue is injected into the pit in order to demonstrate the tract of the dermoid cyst during the surgery. The anterior septal mucosa in the left nostril is incised and elevated, and with the use of 0° endoscope, a sub-perichondrium dissection is performed in order to create a tunnel from the nasal cavity floor toward the antero-superior nasal septum (▶ Fig. 26.8). The septal cartilage is gently disconnected from the perpendicular plate and pushed to the right, and the antero-superior portion of the nasal septum is resected in order to widen the working space. The cyst is identified and its contents are emptied while preserving the integrity of the walls. The cyst walls are dissected away from the surrounding bony structures and the foramen cecum. In cases of intracranial involvement, the dissection is continued superiorly following its intracranial extension until its insertion in the falx cerebri is identified and removed. The use of microscissors or other cutting instruments may be necessary if the cyst is tightly attached to the dura, with the possible risk of a CSF leak. The remnants in the insertion area are cauterized with bipolar coagulation to reduce the risk of recurrence.

Next, the dermoid cyst tract is followed rostrally in a retrograde fashion using an angled endoscope (70°). The tract is resected along the septum with a small backbiter punch and dissected away from the periosteum of the nasal bones and the glabella. The tract is resected up to its subcutaneous portion. In order to guide the surgeon and to mark the subcutaneous portion of the tract, a high-gauge intravenous catheter is inserted through

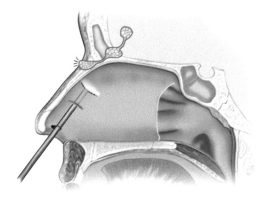

Fig. 26.8 Transseptal endoscopic approach to nasal dermoid cyst. A sub-perichondrium dissection is performed in order to create a tunnel from the nasal cavity floor toward the antero-superior nasal septum.

the pit, and its tip can be visualized by the endoscope, thereby indicating the anterior boundary of the endoscopic resection.

The next step is the removal of the fistula opening on the nasal dorsum, if present, along with its tract remnant. A minimal midline vertical incision around the pit is performed, and the fistulous tract remnant is followed and removed under endoscopic control to ensure complete resection.

In cases of a CSF leak, the defect is covered with Tacho-Sil, and mucoperiosteum from the resected portion of nasal septum is positioned on the exposed bone and dural surface to contain the CSF leak and seal the defect. Nasal packing is kept in place for 2 to 3 days.

Transsphenoidal Approach

The sphenoid sinus provides the most versatile endoscopic corridor to the skull base. The transsphenoidal approach can be used to reach the sella posterosuperiorly, the tuberculum sellae and planum sphenoidale superiorly, the cavernous sinus laterally, and the superior third of the clivus posteroinferiorly.

In the transsphenoidal approach, a 0 degree endoscope is introduced transnasally and positioned superiorly at 12 o'clock below the nasal valve. The right and left middle turbinates are lateralized in order to expand the nasal corridor. Although the initial approach in the pediatric population involves preservation of the normal nasal anatomy as much as possible, removal of the right or even both middle turbinates is almost always necessary to allow a wider exposure of the posterior nasal septum, vomer, and sphenoid ostium. The right sphenoid ostium is identified medial to the superior turbinate and enlarged in a circumferential fashion using a Kerrison punch in order to form a wide right sphenoidotomy. The variable, age-dependent, sphenoid sinus pneumatization needs to be taken into account when drilling into the bone. In addition, drilling into immature vascularized bone may necessitate careful hemostasis. A right posterior ethmoidectomy is performed in a posterior-to-anterior direction in order to create a wide working space.

Next, a nasoseptal flap is elevated from the left septum according to the following steps. First, the left sphenoid ostium is identified through the left nostril. Adjacent to the level of the left sphenoidal ostium, a longitudinal incision of the septal mucosa is performed in a posterior-to-anterior direction until the anterior end of the inferior turbinate is reached. From this point, the incision is continued downwards in a vertical fashion, all the way to the nasal floor. The flap is elevated inferolaterally using a Freer elevator and placed along the nasal cavity floor. A neurosurgical patty is used to protect the flap. After the nasoseptal flap has been prepared, a left wide sphenoidotomy is performed.

The mucosa over the right posterior septum is resected, and 1 to 2 centimeters of the posterior vomer bone is removed through the right nostril. The removed part of the vomer bone can be preserved for later reconstruction. At this point, a bi-nostril technique can be implemented by introducing the endoscope and suction through the right nostril and the dissecting instruments through the left nostril.

A complete sphenoidotomy is accomplished along with drilling of the sphenoid rostrum and extension of the lateral margins of the sphenoidotomy to the level of the medial pterygoid plates. The septa inside the sphenoid sinus are drilled and their attachments to the planum and the optic and carotid prominences are carefully removed. Resection of the mucosa that lines the sinus is performed in order to achieve hemostasis, to facilitate the identification of surgical landmarks, if possible, and to promote the adherence of the nasoseptal flap to the bare bone following the reconstruction. Eventually, the cavity of the sphenoid sinus is exposed between the two carotid prominences posterolaterally, between the two orbital apices anterolaterally, and from the planum superiorly to the clivus inferiorly. The medial and lateral opticocarotid recesses are identified as well. However, since the sphenoid sinus is not yet pneumatized in younger children, identification of surgical landmarks may not be feasible, and the anatomic orientation mainly relies upon the navigation system.

Transsellar Approach

Using the transsphenoidal corridor, the transsellar approach is most suitable for intrasellar lesions with minimal or no suprasellar extension. Common lesions in this location in the pediatric population include pituitary adenomas, intrasellar craniopharyngiomas, and Rathke's cleft cysts. Following the steps described earlier, the floor of the sphenoid sinus is drilled back to the level of the clivus in order to enhance the rostral-caudal trajectory into the suprasellar and retrosellar space. The sellar floor is removed with bone punchers or a microdrill to an extent dictated by the specific pathological process, and the dura is incised (▶Fig. 26.9). The inferior and the superior intercavernous sinuses may bleed upon dural incision and require hemostasis. The tumor is debulked with curettes or with two suction devices, and sellar reconstruction is performed to create a watertight seal.

Transplanum/Transtuberculum Approach

This approach uses the transsphenoidal corridor to reach the suprasellar cistern without violating the sella. The anterior aspect of the planum sphenoidale is adequately exposed by removing the posterior ethmoid sinus

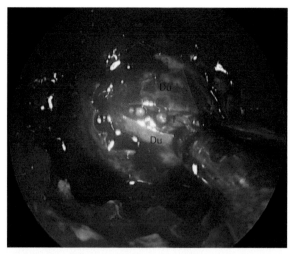

Fig. 26.9 Transsellar approach for craniopharyngioma resection. The dura mater (Du) has been incised and opened, and the tumor (T) has been resected.

septations laterally until the lamina papyracea. The planum sphenoidale is drilled in a rostral–caudal direction to remove the bone. The rostral portion of the sella can be opened as well if a combined transsellar approach is required.

Transcribriform Approach

The transcribriform approach allows the resection of sinonasal lesions involving the anterior skull base, encephaloceles/meningoceles, olfactory groove meningiomas, and olfactory schwannomas. In this approach, the anterior limit of the transtuberculum/transplanum approach is extended to the level of the crista galli and, if necessary, to the frontal sinus as well. Olfaction is almost universally damaged.

The first step is performing a bilateral middle turbinate resection to the level of the skull base followed by complete bilateral ethmoidectomy and sphenoidotomy, thus enabling a large exposure of the medial orbital walls and skull base. Since oncological margins are not required in benign lesions, the lamina papyracea is preserved unless additional lateral exposure is necessary. A frontal sinusotomy is usually required to access the back wall of the frontal sinus, but its extent and laterality vary according to the extent of disease and the exposure required. The size of the frontal sinus varies, depending on the patient's age, and it needs to be considered as well. Optional procedures are Draf III or endoscopic Lothrop, Draf IIA, or Draf IIB procedures. In cases for which a large dural resection is needed, a Draf III procedure is required to enable crista galli removal, which facilitates resection and reconstruction. The posterior nasal septum attachment to the ventral skull base is resected, and the anterior and posterior ethmoidal arteries are identified, coagulated, and transected medial to the lamina papyracea, contributing to tumor devascularization. Prior to drilling, soft tissues overlying the cribriform plates are cauterized with bipolar electrocautery and removed to expose the bone. The frontoethmoidal recess is identified, and the skull base is drilled in a rostral–caudal direction. After bilateral removal of the cribriform plate, the crista galli is drilled until it is eggshell thin and fractured. Eventually, the boundaries of the exposure are the frontal sinuses anteriorly, the planum sphenoidale posteriorly, and the lamina papyracea laterally. In cases of intradural involvement, the exposed dura is coagulated and incised separately on each side of the falx cerebri, while preserving the midline part. The tumor is debulked from each side to expose the free edge of the falx cerebri bilaterally, followed by coagulation of the falx cerebri and its feeding vessels that arise from the falcine arteries. The falx is then transected to create a single intradural working cavity, after which the tumor is debulked.

26.8.3 Coronal Plane

Transmaxillary Approach

This approach allows resection of lesions in the medial maxillary wall, exposure of the maxillary antrum, and creation of a corridor for the retromaxillary space, pterygopalatine fossa, and infratemporal fossa. Common lesions in these locations in the pediatric population include juvenile nasopharyngeal angiofibromas and schwannomas. The surgical approach to juvenile nasopharyngeal angiofibromas is discussed separately in Chapter 28.

The first step is the removal of the middle turbinate ipsilateral to the lesion side with microscissors or a through-cut, preferably without a prior bipolar cauterization of the turbinate since it may damage the olfactory nerves

and cause anosmia. The uncinate process is removed and the maxillary sinus ostium is enlarged by means of a backbiter. The inferior turbinate is fractured by using a Freer. Care must be taken not to injure the sphenopalatine artery posteriorly and the nasolacrimal duct anteriorly while performing an antrostomy. The maxillary sinus can now be fully inspected.

A complete medial maxillectomy may be required when an approach to the maxillary sinus floor and the masticatory space is indicated. A long mucosal incision at the nasal cavity floor is performed by a monopolar electrocautery in order to delineate the lower border of the resection. The nasal floor mucosa is elevated by a Freer dissector to expose the inferior meatus. An osteotomy of the inferior portion of the medial maxillary wall is performed, and the inferior turbinate is resected.

When an approach to the retromaxillary space or to the infratemporal fossa is indicated, a wide sphenoidectomy is performed first in order to delineate the borders of resection, specifically, the choana and the sphenoid sinus on the medial side, and the maxillary antrum and the orbit on the lateral side. The posterior wall of the maxillary sinus is the anterior wall of the pterygopalatine fossa, which contains the vidian nerve and artery, the pterygopalatine ganglion and its branches (the infraorbital and palatine nerves), and the maxillary nerve and artery and its branches (the descending palatine and the sphenopalatine arteries).

The retromaxillary space and pterygopalatine fossa are approached by drilling along the posterior wall of the maxillary sinus (▶ Fig. 26.10). If a nasoseptal flap reconstruction is not expected, the sphenopalatine artery is identified at the medial border of the maxillary sinus and clamped at its exit from the sphenopalatine foramen with an endoscopic silver clip. The sphenopalatine foramen is enlarged and a high-speed drill is used to remove the orbital process of the palatine bone along with the posterior maxillary sinus wall, from the palatine bone vertical process medially to the lateral maxillary sinus wall laterally, in order to expose the pterygopalatine fossa.

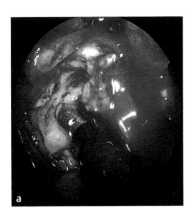
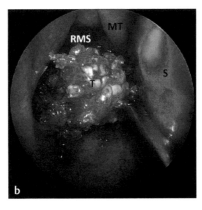

Fig. 26.10 (a) Transmaxillary approach. The photograph demonstrates drilling along the right posterior wall of the maxillary sinus to reach the infratemporal fossa. **(b)** Neurofibroma resection from the infratemporal fossa. The photograph demonstrates pulling out the tumor (T) from the retromaxillary space (RMS). Middle turbinate (MT), septum (S).

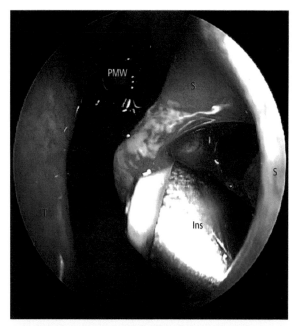

Fig. 26.11 Introduction of an instrument (Ins) via the contralateral nostril and through a vertical septal (S) incision to allow a more lateral access to the retromaxillary space. Inferior turbinate (IT), posterior maxillary wall (PMW).

The infratemporal fossa can be reached by further drilling laterally along the posterior and lateral walls, and through the pterygomaxillary fissure. Introducing the endoscope and instruments via the contralateral nostril and through a vertical incision in the septal cartilage allows a further lateral access to the retromaxillary space (▶ Fig. 26.11). We do not recommend Denker's approach in pediatric patients due to its esthetic and developmental consequences.

26.9 Highlights

a. Special preoperative considerations
   - Age-dependent sinus development and pneumatization.
   - Intercarotid distance.
   - Size of pyriform aperture.
   - A multidisciplinary collaborative team.
   - Neurologic, ophthalmologic, and endocrine function assessment, according to the location of the lesion.
b. Special intraoperative considerations
   - Experienced endoscopic endonasal skull base team.
   - Intraoperative navigation system.
   - The surgical approach is chosen according to the anatomic location of the lesion—sagittal plane for midline lesions, coronal plane for maxillary and retromaxillary lesions.

- The tumor should be debulked in order to reach its stem.
- Surgery of benign lesions should be as minimally invasive as possible, with maximal preservation of normal anatomy.
- Avoiding disruption of craniofacial growth center and tooth buds.
- Preservation of critical neurological, neurovascular, and endocrine structures function is of prime importance, and may compromise the extent of resection if necessary.
c. Special postoperative considerations
   - Follow-up consisting of clinical examination and periodic imaging.
   - Treatment of recurrence depends on size, growth rates, location, and patient symptoms.

26.10 Acknowledgment

Esther Eshkol, the institutional medical and scientific copyeditor, is thanked for editorial assistance.

References

[1] Gil Z, Constantini S, Spektor S, et al. Skull base approaches in the pediatric population. Head Neck 2005;27(8):682–689

[2] Horowitz G, Amit M, Ben-Ari O, et al. Cranialization of the frontal sinus for secondary mucocele prevention following open surgery for benign frontal lesions. PLoS One 2013; 8(12):e83820

[3] Kassam A, Thomas AJ, Snyderman C, et al. Fully endoscopic expanded endonasal approach treating skull base lesions in pediatric patients. J Neurosurg 2007;106(2, Suppl):75–86

[4] Chivukula S, Koutourousiou M, Snyderman CH, Fernandez-Miranda JC, Gardner PA, Tyler-Kabara EC. Endoscopic endonasal skull base surgery in the pediatric population. J Neurosurg Pediatr 2013;11(3):227–241

[5] Locatelli D, Rampa F, Acchiardi I, Bignami M, Pistochini A, Castelnuovo P. Endoscopic endonasal approaches to anterior skull base defects in pediatric patients. Childs Nerv Syst 2006; 22(11):1411–1418

[6] Rastatter JC, Snyderman CH, Gardner PA, Alden TD, Tyler-Kabara E. Endoscopic endonasal surgery for sinonasal and skull base lesions in the pediatric population. Otolaryngol Clin North Am 2015;48(1):79–99

[7] Tatreau JR, Patel MR, Shah RN, et al. Anatomical considerations for endoscopic endonasal skull base surgery in pediatric patients. Laryngoscope 2010;120(9):1730–1737

[8] Shlomi B, Chaushu S, Gil Z, Chaushu G, Fliss DM. Effects of the subcranial approach on facial growth and development. Otolaryngol Head Neck Surg 2007;136(1):27–32

[9] Gruber DP, Brockmeyer D. Pediatric skull base surgery. 1. Embryology and developmental anatomy. Pediatr Neurosurg 2003;38(1):2–8

[10] Sessions RB. Nasal dermal sinuses—new concepts and explanations. Laryngoscope 1982;92(8 Pt 2, Suppl 29):1–28

[11] Rahbar R, Shah P, Mulliken JB, et al. The presentation and management of nasal dermoid: a 30-year experience. Arch Otolaryngol Head Neck Surg 2003;129(4):464–471

[12] Zapata S, Kearns DB. Nasal dermoids. Curr Opin Otolaryngol Head Neck Surg 2006;14(6):406–411

[13] Bloom DC, Carvalho DS, Dory C, Brewster DF, Wickersham JK, Kearns DB. Imaging and surgical approach of nasal dermoids. Int J Pediatr Otorhinolaryngol 2002;62(2):111–122

[14] Penner CR, Thompson L. Nasal glial heterotopia: a clinicopathologic and immunophenotypic analysis of 10 cases with a review of the literature. Ann Diagn Pathol 2003;7(6):354–359

[15] Rahbar R, Resto VA, Robson CD, et al. Nasal glioma and encephalocele: diagnosis and management. Laryngoscope 2003;113(12):2069–2077

[16] Ajose-Popoola O, Lin HW, Silvera VM, et al. Nasal glioma: prenatal diagnosis and multidisciplinary surgical approach. Skull Base Rep 2011;1(2):83–88

[17] Mindermann T, Wilson CB. Pediatric pituitary adenomas. Neurosurgery 1995;36(2):259–268, discussion 269

[18] Perry A, Graffeo CS, Marcellino C, Pollock BE, Wetjen NM, Meyer FB. Pediatric pituitary adenoma: case series, review of the literature, and a skull base treatment paradigm. J Neurol Surg B Skull Base 2018;79(1):91–114

[19] Fernandez-Miranda JC, Gardner PA, Snyderman CH, et al. Craniopharyngioma: a pathologic, clinical, and surgical review. Head Neck 2012;34(7):1036–1044

[20] Kassam AB, Gardner PA, Snyderman CH, Carrau RL, Mintz AH, Prevedello DM. Expanded endonasal approach, a fully endoscopic transnasal approach for the resection of midline suprasellar craniopharyngiomas: a new classification based on the infundibulum. J Neurosurg 2008;108(4):715–728

[21] Elliott RE, Hsieh K, Hochm T, Belitskaya-Levy I, Wisoff J, Wisoff JH. Efficacy and safety of radical resection of primary and recurrent craniopharyngiomas in 86 children. J Neurosurg Pediatr 2010;5(1):30–48

[22] Byun WM, Kim OL, Kim D. MR imaging findings of Rathke's cleft cysts: significance of intracystic nodules. AJNR Am J Neuroradiol 2000;21(3):485–488

[23] Hillstrom RP, Zarbo RJ, Jacobs JR. Nerve sheath tumors of the paranasal sinuses: electron microscopy and histopathologic diagnosis. Otolaryngol Head Neck Surg 1990;102(3):257–263

[24] Sunaryo PL, Svider PF, Husain Q, Choudhry OJ, Eloy JA, Liu JK. Schwannomas of the sinonasal tract and anterior skull base: a systematic review of 94 cases. Am J Rhinol Allergy 2014;28(1):39–49

[25] Azani AB, Bishop JA, Thompson LD. Sinonasal tract neurofibroma: a clinicopathologic series of 12 cases with a review of the literature. Head Neck Pathol 2015;9(3):323–333

[26] Buchwald C, Franzmann MB, Jacobsen GK, Lindeberg H. Human papillomavirus (HPV) in sinonasal papillomas: a study of 78 cases using in situ hybridization and polymerase chain reaction. Laryngoscope 1995;105(1):66–71

[27] Macdonald MR, Le KT, Freeman J, Hui MF, Cheung RK, Dosch HM. A majority of inverted sinonasal papillomas carries Epstein-Barr virus genomes. Cancer 1995;75(9):2307–2312

[28] Busquets JM, Hwang PH. Endoscopic resection of sinonasal inverted papilloma: a meta-analysis. Otolaryngol Head Neck Surg 2006;134(3):476–482

[29] Goudakos JK, Blioskas S, Nikolaou A, Vlachtsis K, Karkos P, Markou KD. Endoscopic resection of sinonasal inverted papilloma: systematic review and meta-analysis. Am J Rhinol Allergy 2018;32(3):167–174

27 Endoscopic Treatment of Juvenile Angiofibroma: Surgical Technique

Ahmad Safadi, Alberto Schreiber, Dan M. Fliss, Piero Nicolai

Summary

Endoscopic approach for the resection of juvenile angiofibroma (JA) has become the mainstay of treatment of this lesion, and more advanced lesions are being managed by a pure endoscopic approach. In this chapter, we present the endoscopic endonasal approach for JA in a step by step manner.

Keywords: Juvenile angiofibroma, endoscopic, skull base, surgical technique

27.1 Introduction

JA is a rare vascular lesion of the nasopharynx and nasal cavity. It affects young male adolescents mainly between 9 and 19 years old.[1] JA is a highly vascular tumor composed of a proliferating and irregular vascular component within a fibrous stroma. JA originates from the upper portion of the sphenopalatine foramen where the sphenoid process of the palatine bone meets the sphenoid bone and vomer (▶Fig. 27.1).

Although benign, JA has a local invasive and destructive behavior, and has the tendency to spread not only through minor resistance areas, but also through fissures and sutures and even by direct invasion of cancellous bone.

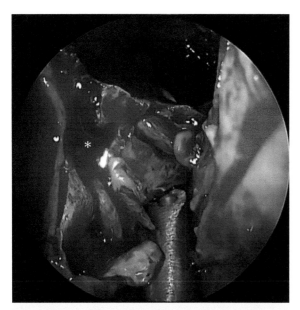

Fig. 27.1 Intraoperative endoscopic view of the right nasal fossa showing the junction between the sphenoid process of palatine bone (indicated by the suction tip) and anterior wall of sphenoid sinus. Asterisk indicates the sphenopalatine foramen.

JA follows a characteristic pattern of spread, which distinguishes it from other vascular lesions of the pediatric skull base. From its origin in the sphenopalatine foramen, JA spreads to the nasal cavity and nasopharynx in a submucosal and subperiosteal plane. Laterally it usually spreads anterior to the pterygoid plates and involves the pterygopalatine fossa (PPF) in more than 70% of cases.[2] Filling the PPF, the lesion anteriorly displaces the posterior maxillary wall, and in extreme cases the maxillary sinus is obliterated. Posteriorly, the tumor remodels and erode the pterygoid plates and may reach the pterygoid fossa. Laterally, the tumor spreads through the pterygomaxillary fissure to the infratemporal fossa (ITF). Superiorly JA spreads through the inferior orbital fissure (IOF) to involve the orbit and through the superior orbital fissure (SOF) and foramen rotundum it reaches the cavernous sinus. The sphenoid sinus can be involved by a submucosal spread of the tumor from the nasopharynx as well as through erosion and expansion of the vidian canal. A posterolateral route of extension is less common, and consists of tumor spread from the nasopharynx to the pharyngeal recess, and laterally to the pterygoid fossa posterior to the medial pterygoid plate or through erosion of the medial pterygoid plate. From the pterygoid fossa JA may progress to the parapharyngeal space laterally, while superior extension will involve the foramen lacerum and carotid canal. Bony involvement by JA can have one of three patterns: erosion, remodeling, and direct cancellous bone invasion. JA spreads through fissures and foramens by means of expansion, thinning, and remodeling of the involved bones, and has a tendency to erode and involve cancellous bone, most typical in the clivus and pterygoid base. Large tumors with extensive infratemporal spread may also destruct the greater sphenoid wing. Intracranial extension occurs in 10% to 20% of cases, while intradural extension is very rare[3] (Box 27.1).

> ### Box 27.1 Juvenile angiofibroma pattern of spread
>
> - JA originate from the sphenopalatine foramen
> - In more the 70% involve the PPF
> - Vidian canal and cancellous bone invasion are typical findings
> - 10–20% IC extension, extradurally

Surgical treatment of JA is challenging due to the young age of the patients, the complexity of skull base anatomy, and the rich vascularity of the lesion. Many external approaches have been used for surgical excision of JA, including transpalatal, Le Fort I osteotomies, lateral rhinotomy, midfacial degloving, facial translocation, anterior craniofacial and lateral infratemporal/subtemporal approaches. Each approach has its own advantage over the other according to tumor extent. Midfacial degloving has been widely adopted due to avoidance of facial scars. However, external approaches usually involve extensive osteotomies which are associated with increased blood loss, and may interfere with the normal facial growth of the adolescent patient. Since Kamel[4] first introduced the endoscopic endonasal approach for resection of JA, this approach gained increasing popularity and was recently adopted in large centers for advanced tumors.[5-11] The endoscopic approach has many advantages over external transfacial approaches, which include the avoidance of facial incisions, osteotomies, and bone plating, which do not expose young patients to the risk of craniofacial alterations. In addition, the magnified field of view and angled view "behind the corner" may be associated with more complete inspection of the resection cavity and shorter hospitalization time. In this chapter, we present the endoscopic endonasal approach for JA in a step by step manner.

27.2 Diagnosis and Preoperative Management

JA is often suspected when a young male boy presents with nasal obstruction and epistaxis. Nasal endoscopy commonly shows a hypervascularized lobulated mass with a smooth surface typically bulging behind the tail of the middle turbinate, obstructing the choana or completely filling the nasal fossa (▶Fig. 27.2).

Diagnosis is made by the typical clinical and imaging findings, while tissue biopsy is unnecessary and may lead to brisk hemorrhage. At imaging, JA appears as a highly vascularized and expansile lesion centered on the PPF in both contrast-enhanced computerized tomography (CT) and gadolinium-enhanced magnetic resonance imaging (MRI). CT and MRI are complementary in the diagnosis of JA, as

CT emphasizes skull base bony involvement while MRI is superior in the demonstration of intracranial, orbital, and cavernous sinus invasion. On both T1- and T2-weighted, unenhanced MRI, the lesion shows flow-void spotty signals, due to enlarged blood vessels. The typical pattern of spread of JA and the typical bony changes associated with this lesion as well as its rich vascularity distinguish this lesion from other lesions that may involve the skull base, and obviate the risk of tissue sampling (▶Fig. 27.3).

Staging is most commonly according to Andrews[12] or Radkowski's[13] staging systems. Recently, Snyderman et al[15] proposed the UPMC staging system, emphasizing the role of residual tumor vascularization by the ICA following embolization and the route of intracranial extension (medial or lateral to ICA and cavernous sinus) as the most important factors for determining the feasibility of endoscopic resection and the risk of residual or recurrent tumor. ▶Table 27.1 shows the staging systems most commonly highlighted in the literature.

Preoperative embolization is usually considered for all cases of JA except for very small lesions. Embolization is done through a transarterial approach (TAE). This technique uses small particle material (PVA—polyvinyl alcohol, microspheres, ...) that is introduced by a superselective catheterization of the feeding vessels. In advanced JA lesions, a blood supply from the ICA branches should be sought, as embolization in these feeders is discouraged, as it may result in neurologic complications due to particle dislodgement to the central nervous system. Embolization should be done close to the scheduled operation, usually within 24 to 72 hours before the surgery, as collateral blood supply may develop and reduce the efficacy of embolization (Box 27.2).

> **Box 27.2 Preoperative embolization**
>
> - Transarterial embolization should be done 24–72 hours before surgical intervention
> - Embolization is discouraged in cases with significant ICA blood supply

27.3 Indications and Contraindications for Endoscopic Endonasal Approach

Endoscopic treatment of advanced JA with extensive skull base and ITF involvement should only be practiced in highly specialized centers, with surgeons experienced in endoscopic approaches as well as adequate and dedicated equipment and support of interventional radiology, neurosurgery, and intensive care unit. External approaches should be considered in JAs with large invasion of the skull base, extensive vascular feeders from

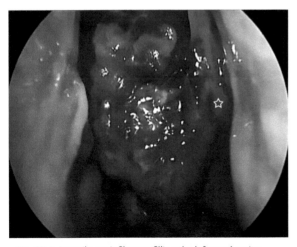

Fig. 27.2 Juvenile angiofibroma filling the left nasal cavity, pushing the middle turbinate *(yellow star)* laterally.

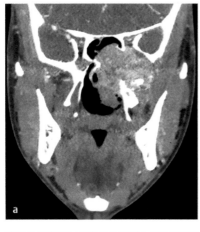
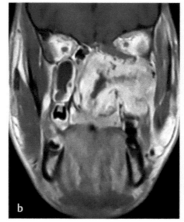
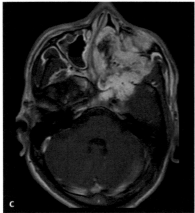
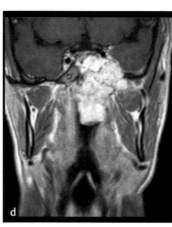

Fig. 27.3 Juvenile angiofibroma in a 15-year-old male. **(a)** Contrast-enhanced CT, coronal plane, showing involvement of the pterygopalatine and infratemporal fossae with remodeling of the IOF, and destruction of the pterygoid plates. **(b)** Gad-enhanced T1-weighted MRI, coronal plane, showing extensive infratemporal fossa involvement; notice the hour-glass appearance of tumor due to extension through the pterygomaxillary fissure. **(c)** T2-weighted axial MRI showing involvement of the greater wing of sphenoid bone; the tumor juxtaposes the clival internal carotid artery. Notice the dark spots presenting signal voids. **(d)** Gad-enhanced T1-weighted MRI, coronal plane, showing intracranial extradural involvement.

Table 27.1 Staging systems most commonly adopted in the literature

Andrews et al[12]	
I	Limited to the nasopharynx and nasal cavity. Bone destruction negligible or limited to the sphenopalatine foramen
II	Invading the pterygopalatine fossa or the maxillary, ethmoid, or sphenoid sinus with bone destruction
III	• Invading the infratemporal fossa or orbital region without intracranial involvement • Invading the infratemporal fossa or orbit with intracranial extradural (parasellar) involvement
IV	• Intracranial intradural without infiltration of the cavernous sinus, pituitary fossa, or optic chiasm • Intracranial intradural with infiltration of the cavernous sinus, pituitary fossa, or optic chiasm
Radkowski et al[13]	
I	• Limited to posterior nares and/or nasopharyngeal vault • Involving the posterior nares and/or nasopharyngeal vault with involvement of at least one paranasal sinus
II	• Minimal lateral extension into the pterygopalatine fossa • Full occupation of pterygopalatine fossa with or without superior erosion orbital bones • Extension into the infratemporal fossa or extension posterior to the pterygoid plates
III	• Erosion of skull base (middle cranial fossa/base of pterygoids)—minimal intracranial extension • Extensive intracranial extension with or without extension into the cavernous sinus
Snyderman et al[15]	
I	No significant extension beyond the site of origin and remaining medial to the midpoint of the pterygopalatinefossa
II	Extension to the paranasal sinuses and lateral to the midpoint of the pterygopalatinefossa
III	Locally advanced with skull base erosion or extension to additional extracranial spaces, including orbit and infratemporal fossa, no residual vascularity following embolization
IV	Skull base erosion, orbit, infratemporal fossa Residual vascularity
V	Intracranial extension, residual vascularity M: Medial extension L: Lateral extension

the ICA, or critical encasement of ICA. The possibility of a combined endoscopic and external approach should also be considered. Advanced JAs, especially those with residual vascularity from ICA after embolization, can show massive intraoperative bleeding with a considerable increase in surgical risk and need for intraoperative transfusion. In such a situation, it is wise to consider a multistage treatment, a possibility that should be preoperatively discussed with the patient. Another strategy for very advanced JAs with critical intracranial extension and unacceptable surgical hazard is to endoscopically resect the extracranial portion intentionally leaving residual disease and subsequently evaluate for "wait and see" monitoring or surgical treatment based on the rate of growth as demonstrated radiologically. The management of residual tumors involving critical areas or neurovascular structures (i.e., ICA, optic nerve, cavernous sinus, dura, cerebral arteries) should always be carefully discussed, considering the need for external approaches due to the impact that adhesions could have on the possibility to perform a safe dissection (Box 27.3).

> **Box 27.3 Management of advanced juvenile angiofibroma**
>
> - Advanced JA should only be managed in highly specialized centers
> - Residual tumor in critical areas can be followed because of high risk for neurovascular structures
> - Spontaneous resolution may occur

27.4 Surgical Settings

The surgery is performed under general anesthesia, oral endotracheal intubation is done, and the ventilating tube is fixed to the left side of the mouth and aliened to the left side of the patient. As surgery may last long, it is recommended to monitor the patient's blood pressure, pulse rate, and urine output using arterial line and urine catheter. Total intravenous anesthesia (TIVA), using continuous infusion of propofol, is preferable to gas anesthesia, such as isoflurane and sevoflurane, as TIVA causes less vasodilation. Beta blockers and clonidine can be used in addition to propofol to maintain low and stable mean blood pressure and pulse rate. The child should be warmed and the temperature monitored using a rectal thermometer. The patient is set supine, with the head in neutral position (neither flexed nor extended) slightly tilted to the left and rotated to the right. The operating table is tilted to 30-degree anti-Trendelenburg. This is recommended to facilitate venous return and reduce blood loss. An electromagnetic navigation system, easy to handle and obviating the need for head fixation, is also used to provide the intraoperative orientation. The nose then is prepared by neurosurgical cottoned patties soaked in adrenaline-amethocaine solution (1 mL of adrenaline 1:1,000 and 9 mL of amethocaine 2%), the eye closed with transparent dressing, and preoperative antibiotics, usually second-generation cephalosporin is given. The surgeon and scrub nurse stand to the right side of the patient and the assistant surgeon near the patient's head or on his left side. The monitor is aligned to the left side of the patient's head (▶Fig. 27.4).

27.5 Surgical Instrumentation

The following surgical equipment should be available in the operative room for endoscopic treatment of JA:
- Endoscopic skull base set including angled and miniaturized instruments.
- Powered endoscopic-angled blades and burs.
- Angled endoscopes with HD camera.
- Laser or monopolar electrocautery with malleable tip.
- Hemostatic agents (absorbable gelatin powder, sponge oxidized regenerated cellulose, microfibrillar collagen, or fibrin or synthetic sealants).
- Navigation system.
- Endoscopic ultrasonic Doppler probe.
- Endoscopic bipolar cautery.

27.6 Surgical Technique

The resection of large lesions can rarely be achieved in a single bloc and it is preferable to disassemble the JA in piecemeal modality (▶Video 27.1). Usually, bulky JAs can be divided in nasal-nasopharyngeal, sphenoethmoidal, and infratemporal-PPF portions, which are connected together on the pterygoid base. Prior to resection of the nasal-nasopharyngeal portion, it is recommended to achieve a good exposure of the surgical field by first completing an ethmoidectomy, sphenoidotomy, middle turbinectomy, and a large middle antrostomy extended posteriorly to expose the sphenopalatine foramen. Whenever needed, medial maxillectomy can

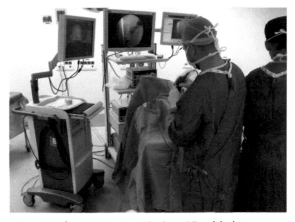

Fig. 27.4 The patient is set supine in anti-Trendelenburg position. Electromagnetic navigation system is set up. The surgeon and nurse stand on the right side of the patient and the assistant surgeon (not shown) near the patient's head or on his left side. The monitor is aligned to the left side of the patient's head.

be done by removing the posterior two-thirds of the inferior turbinate and medial maxillary sinus wall, just distal to the opening of the Hasner valve in the inferior meatus. This can be extended anteriorly by sectioning the lacrimal duct at the inferior limit of the lacrimal sac or also removing the medial part of the anterior maxillary wall with type D endoscopic medial maxillectomy.[14] The fovea ethmoidalis, planum sphenoidale, and lamina papyracea are exposed by completing ethmoidectomy and gentle subperiosteal dissection of the lesion using suction-dissection instrument. By following subperiosteal dissection posteriorly, the opticocarotid recess can usually be exposed and used as a crucial anatomic landmark. The posterior third of nasal septum is now removed to expose the nasopharyngeal portion of the lesion and enable the assistant surgeon to keep clean the surgical field and pull the lesion.

The three portions are now disassembled on the level of the sphenopalatine foramen and choana, using a monopolar electrocautery or LASER (▶Fig. 27.5).

Bleeding at this stage depends mainly on the success of preoperative embolization; however, using a monopolar or LASER helps in reducing blood loss. The soft palate is protected during the operation by passing two rubber catheters that are passed around the soft and hard palate and tied externally above the upper lip. In this way the soft palate is protected by downward retraction while enlarging the nasopharyngeal area.

The first cut is done on the level of posterior end of maxillary antrostomy and curved to the upper edge of choana, proceeding to the depth of the lesion while maintaining downward and backward traction (toward the nasopharynx) by the assistant surgeon. At the level of nasopharyngeal roof, the lesion is usually strictly adherent as it spreads submucosally and invades the sphenoid floor, and should be strongly tracted downward from the clivus. If nasal nasopharyngeal portion is too big to be extracted transnasally, it can be pushed down in the oropharynx and pulled transorally. By first removing the nasal-nasopharyngeal portion, the surgeon gains space to manage the other involved areas.

At this point, it is recommended to proceed to ITF dissection in order to early control the lesion blood supply. This is achieved by incising the periosteum after removal of the posterior maxillary wall. It is noteworthy that the maxillary periosteum can be easily confused with the surface of the JA, leading the surgeon along the wrong surgical plane of dissection. Careful dissection is achieved by continuous gentle traction of the lesion and dissection of soft tissue and fat of the ITF from the lesion surface (▶Fig. 27.6).

Even far lateral projections of JA that extend to the infratemporal/temporal fossa can usually be extracted in this way, as the lesion never invades soft tissues. If the lesion extends to involve the buccal space, this portion should be gently pulled backward with the help of simultaneous pressure through the oral cavity. In addition, care should be taken to identify and spare the infraorbital nerve, which can be displaced by the lesion. In some cases the nerve is sharply dissected from the tumor surface (▶Video 27.2 and ▶Fig. 27.6). The dissection plane into the PPF lies behind the palatine nerves; therefore, the nerves can be

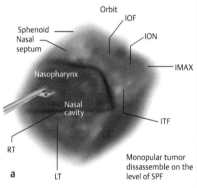
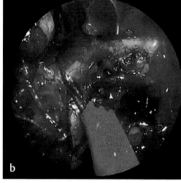

Fig. 27.5 (a) Illustration showing tumor piecemeal resection converging on the SPF and choana. Resection of the nasal portion. (b) Intraoperative image showing monopolar cut on the level of SPF. IMAX, internal maxillary artery; IOF, inferior orbital fissure; ION, infraorbital nerve; ITF infratemporal fossa; SPF, sphenopalatine foramen.

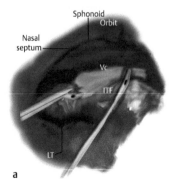
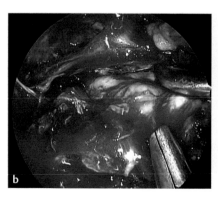

Fig. 27.6 (a) Illustration showing tumor disassembling at the level of sphenopalatine foramen and choana. Resection of ITF portion. (b) Intraoperative image showing dissection of tumor from the ION. ION, infraorbital nerve; ITF infratemporal fossa; VC, vidian canal.

preserved only in lesions with a small lateral extension. The maxillary artery runs from lateral to medial between the two heads of the lateral pterygoid muscle and is usually identified easily during soft-tissue dissection off the tumor. The artery should be clipped early in order to reduce intraoperative bleeding and prevent its accidental damage during the dissection. The ITF portion is brought medially and cut on the level of the pterygoid base.

At this moment, the foramen rotundum and vidian canal are identified. The sphenoethmoid portion is brought inferolaterally by submucosal dissection from the sphenoid walls and cut on the level of pterygoid base. Care should be taken to protect the opticocarotid recess and lateral sphenoid wall, as the optic nerve and carotid canal are often dehiscent (▶Fig. 27.7).

After removal of these three portions, the "root" of the lesion should be managed, which usually invades the vidian canal and can extend to IOF, clivus, and cavernous sinus. Since JA has the tendency to invade the vidian canal and basisphenoid an extensive drilling of these areas is crucial to avoid recurrence. The vidian canal is usually expanded by the lesion, and should be emptied by gentle traction and drilling of the bony walls. The nerve is usually sacrificed; however, rarely the patient complains on dry eye. Just lateral and superior to the vidian canal, the foramen rotundum is identified, and the maxillary nerve is identified and followed to the IOF which should be cleared from tumor invasion (▶Fig. 27.8). Drilling of the basisphenoid (the sphenoid floor and sphenoid portion

of clivus), vidian canal, and pterygoid root, as well as all bony areas involved by the lesion, is crucial in order to clean all microscopic nests of the lesion that may not be visible.

The cavernous sinus can be involved through the IOF and then orbital apex and SOF involvement, or following the maxillary nerve. JA does not commonly show tight adhesions with adjacent neurovascular structures and can usually be safely pulled from the cavernous sinus. This step should be kept last as it is associated with brisk bleeding from the cavernous sinus, which is easily controlled by infusion of hemostatic powder such as Surgiflo (Ethicon US, LLC) to the cavernous sinus and pressing with neurosurgical patty for 3 minutes. The dissection of JA from ICA should be cautiously performed with the help of small cottonoids to avoid any direct traumatic pressure on the vessel. The use of intraoperative navigation and Doppler is mandatory to precisely identify the artery and avoid its injury (▶Fig. 27.9). Until the operation is completed, the presence of an interventional radiologist in the hospital who can manage uncontrolled ICA bleeding is another precautionary measure that should be considered. Residual lesions in critical areas such as the cavernous sinus may be followed rather than aggressively approached, as they can remain asymptomatic or even spontaneously regress. If the ICA is exposed during the resection, it could be covered with a vascularized tissue such as a pedicled buccal fat (▶Fig. 27.10).

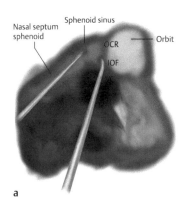
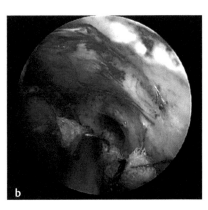

Fig. 27.7 (a) Illustration showing tumor disassembling at the level of sphenopalatine foramen and choana. Resection of sphenoid portion. **(b)** Intraoperative image showing subperiosteal dissection and opticocarotid recess (OCR). IOF, inferior orbital fissure; VC, vidian canal.

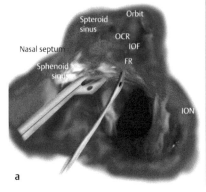
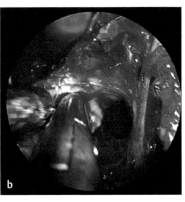

Fig. 27.8 (a) Illustration showing tumor disassembling at the level of sphenopalatine foramen and choana. Vidian canal, inferior orbital fissure, and pterygoid base dissection. **(b)** Intraoperative image showing removal of tumor from the enlarged vidian canal. FR, foramen rotundum; IOF, inferior orbital fissure; OCR, opticocarotid recess.

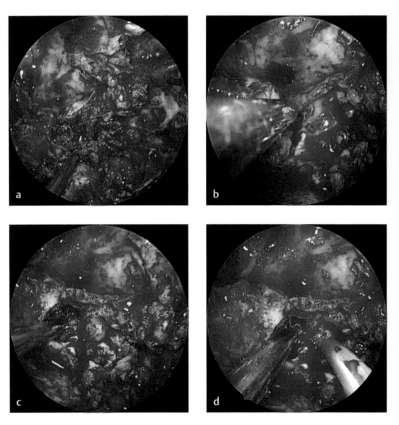

Fig. 27.9 **(a)** Extensive clival involvement by JA. **(b)** Tumor (T) extracted from cancellous bone. **(c)** Clival portion of internal carotid artery (ICA) is exposed and preserved after tumor clearance. This was done by following the vidian nerve (VN) and confirmed by Doppler probe **(d)**.

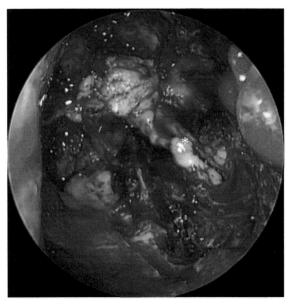

Fig. 27.10 The exposed ICA was covered by pedicled fat (*asterisk*) pulled from the buccal fat pad.

Intracranial extension is present in 10% to 20% of advanced lesion; however, dural invasion is very rare.[3] This fact translates into the need to combine gentle movements of tumor traction and dissection from critical structures (i.e., ICA, cavernous sinus, dura).

Before the end of the surgical procedure, all the possible routes of JA spread should be carefully checked to avoid any possible residue. One possibility is the pterygoid fossa (between the medial and lateral pterygoid plates) which may be involved due to tumor erosion of the pterygoid process of the sphenoid bone. The tumor may also spread posterior to the pterygoid plates to involve the upper parapharyngeal space. In this case, the inferior turbinate and the medial wall of the maxillary sinus should be resected to the floor of the nasal cavity to optimize exposure.

Light packing is placed in the nasal cavities for 24 to 48 hours and a third-generation cephalosporin is administered until nasal packing is removed. Cleaning of the surgical cavity is performed under endoscopic control to remove clots and fibrin, and the patient is instructed to perform daily irrigations of the sinonasal cavity with saline solution to moisten secretions and minimize crust formation.

27.6.1 Bleeding Control

This is mainly achieved by preoperative embolization which is done 24 to 48 hours before surgery. Early detection and control of the maxillary artery and other feeding vessels reduce intraoperative bleeding. Even in cases of feeding vessels from the ICA, which are not amenable to embolization, these tributaries can be coagulated.

A subperiosteal plane of dissection should be followed to minimize bleeding, as well as the use of a monopolarelectrocautery or diode laser is mandatory to minimize bleeding during tumor disassembling. Hemostatic materials should be used to control venous bleeding from the cavernous sinus, pterygoid plexus, and basilar plexus. Hemostasis is also achieved by continuous irrigation with warm water (40–45°C). For resection of large JAs, when extensive bleeding is encountered, staging of the operation with delayed resection of the skull base component should be considered to allow patients to recover, equilibrate blood volume, and correct hemorrhage-induced coagulopathies before addressing the residual part of the lesion.

Imaging surveillance after surgery is always required because persistences or recurrences are typically localized submucosally, and inaccessible to endoscopic evaluation. Moreover, postoperative MRI within 72 hours after surgery has shown to be effective in differentiating vascularized nodules of persistence in the early postoperative period. Imaging should be performed every 6 to 8 months for at least 3 years after surgery. Persistent JAs, either intentionally unresected due to unacceptable surgical hazard or detected by routine follow-up scans, require close surveillance with contrast-enhanced MRI to assess its possible growth before establishing that treatment is actually required.

27.7 Highlights

- Diagnosis is made by contrast enhanced imaging showing a vascular lesion with a typical pattern of spread.
- Preoperative embolization is recommended for all cases of JA except the very small ones.
- Endoscopic treatment of advanced JA with extensive skull base and ITF involvement should only be practiced in highly specialized centers.
- For advanced JA with residual vascularity after embolization, a staged procedure may be considered.
- Residual tumor in critical skull base sites can be managed by a "wait and see" strategy.
- En bloc resection is rarely feasible, and tumor disassembly around the PPF is the principal of endoscopic approach.

- Vidian foramen and pterygoid base should always been drilled to prevent recurrence.
- Embolization, subperiosteal dissection, and early vascular control are critical for bleeding control.

References

[1] Lund VJ, Stammberger H, Nicolai P, et al; European Rhinologic Society Advisory Board on Endoscopic Techniques in the Management of Nose, Paranasal Sinus and Skull Base Tumours. European position paper on endoscopic management of tumours of the nose, paranasal sinuses and skull base. Rhinol Suppl 2010;22(22):1–143

[2] Szymańska A, Szymański M, Czekajska-Chehab E, Szczerbo-Trojanowska M. Two types of lateral extension in juvenile nasopharyngeal angiofibroma: diagnostic and therapeutic management. Eur Arch Otorhinolaryngol 2015;272(1):159–166

[3] Danesi G, Panciera DT, Harvey RJ, Agostinis C. Juvenile nasopharyngeal angiofibroma: evaluation and surgical management of advanced disease. Otolaryngol Head Neck Surg 2008;138(5):581–586

[4] Kamel RH. Transnasal endoscopic surgery in juvenile nasopharyngeal angiofibroma. J Laryngol Otol 1996;110(10):962–968

[5] Onerci TM, Yücel OT, Oğretmenoğlu O. Endoscopic surgery in treatment of juvenile nasopharyngeal angiofibroma. Int J Pediatr Otorhinolaryngol 2003;67(11):1219–1225

[6] Wormald PJ, Van Hasselt A. Endoscopic removal of juvenile angiofibromas. Otolaryngol Head Neck Surg 2003;129(6):684–691

[7] Hackman T, Snyderman CH, Carrau R, Vescan A, Kassam A. Juvenile nasopharyngeal angiofibroma: the expanded endonasal approach. Am J Rhinol Allergy 2009;23(1):95–99

[8] Nicolai P, Villaret AB, Farina D, et al. Endoscopic surgery for juvenile angiofibroma: a critical review of indications after 46 cases. Am J Rhinol Allergy 2010;24(2):e67–e72

[9] Cloutier T, Pons Y, Blancal JP, et al. Juvenile nasopharyngeal angiofibroma: does the external approach still make sense? Otolaryngol Head Neck Surg 2012;147(5):958–963

[10] Huang Y, Liu Z, Wang J, Sun X, Yang L, Wang D. Surgical management of juvenile nasopharyngeal angiofibroma: analysis of 162 cases from 1995 to 2012. Laryngoscope 2014;124(8):1942–1946

[11] Langdon C, Herman P, Verillaud B, et al. Expanded endoscopic endonasal surgery for advanced stage juvenile angiofibromas: a retrospective multi-center study. Rhinology 2016;54(3):239–246

[12] Andrews JC, Fisch U, Valavanis A, Aeppli U, Makek MS. The surgical management of extensive nasopharyngeal angiofibromas with the infratemporal fossa approach. Laryngoscope 1989;99(4):429–437

[13] Radkowski D, McGill T, Healy GB, Ohlms L, Jones DT. Angiofibroma: changes in staging and treatment. Arch Otolaryngol Head Neck Surg 1996;122(2):122–129

[14] Schreiber A, Ferrari M, Rampinelli V, et al. Modular endoscopic medial maxillectomies: quantitative analysis of surgical exposure in a preclinical setting. World Neurosurg 2017;100:44–55

[15] Snyderman CH, Pant H, Carrau RL, Gardner P. A new endoscopic staging system for angiofibromas. Arch Otolaryngol Head Neck Surg 2010;136(6):588–594

28 Juvenile Angiofibroma with Intracranial Extension

Philippe Lavigne, Carl H. Snyderman, Paul A. Gardner

Summary

Advanced juvenile angiofibromas (JAs) are challenging tumors to treat surgically due to the involvement of skull base structures and vascularity derived from the intracranial circulation. Tumor infiltration of the pterygoid base and the pterygoid canal allows development of blood supply from branches of the internal carotid artery (ICA). Large tumors may surround the petrous and cavernous segments of the ICA and increase the risk of vascular injury during surgery.

With proper planning, large JAs with intracranial extension can be managed using endoscopic techniques. The biggest challenges are bleeding from tumor vessels derived from the intracranial circulation. The The University of Pittsburgh Medical Center (UPMC) staging system is useful in planning a surgical strategy based on the degree of residual vascularity and the route of intracranial extension. A staged approach with excision of vascular territories of the tumor allows safe resection with minimal morbidity. There is a higher risk of residual tumor with advanced JA with skull base involvement, but not all patients require further surgery. Radiation therapy can be avoided with a comprehensive surgical strategy.

Keywords: Juvenile angiofibroma, cranial base surgery, endoscopic endonasal surgery, advanced stage juvenile angiofibroma

28.1 Introduction

Juvenile angiofibromas (JA) are challenging tumors to treat surgically because of their vascularity and anatomical location. They likely originate from remnants of the first branchial arch artery and some authors consider them to be vascular malformations.[1,2] Traditionally, JAs are classified as benign tumors with locally aggressive features. They arise from the lateral basisphenoid and extend through foramina and fissures: (1) the sphenopalatine foramen into the nasopharynx and paranasal sinuses, (2) the pterygomaxillary fissure into the infratemporal fossa, and (3) the infraorbital fissure into the orbit. JAs have the potential for skull base erosion and intracranial extension, as seen in 10 to 20% of cases.[3] True dural invasion is rare and the tumor will usually have a well-circumscribed pushing border. Tumors that extend medial to the orbital apex can erode the bone of the planum sphenoidale to gain access to the anterior cranial fossa. JA can also extend to the middle cranial fossa through the inferior orbital fissure, orbital apex, and superior orbital fissure.

Recent advances in endoscopic endonasal surgery (EES) now allow surgeons to resect advanced JAs. A growing body of evidence supports purely endoscopic and endoscopic-assisted approaches. Case series and systematic reviews demonstrate favorable rates of residual and recurrent disease with reduced morbidity (►Table 28.1).[4–6]

28.2 Preoperative Evaluation and Anesthesia

Evaluation of tumor extension and staging is mandatory for optimal surgical planning. Computed tomography (CT) and magnetic resonance imaging (MRI) are both essential to assess tumor extension and can be used for intraoperative image guidance. Imaging should be obtained prior to angiographic embolization as embolized tumor segments are more challenging to delineate. CT is superior for identification of bony landmarks and remodeling and destruction of bone. Characteristic findings include anterior bowing of the posterior wall of the maxillary sinus (Holman–Miller sign) and tumor infiltration of the pterygoid base.[7,8] CT angiogram is useful for intraoperative navigation of the internal carotid artery (ICA). MRI is better for assessing soft tissues and intracranial

Table 28.1 Available multicenter and systematic reviews on the endoscopic approach for JAs

Study	Year	Design	Study groups	Conclusion
Langdon et al[4]	2016	Multicenter retrospective review	Endoscopic approach (74) for stage IIIA and IIIB	Average blood loss 1279.7 mL Residual: 33.3% (18/54) (16 observed and stable, 1 adjuvant radiation therapy, 1 revision surgery and radiation therapy)
Khoueir et al	2013	Systematic review	821 cases, all endoscopic	Average blood loss 564 mL Complication rate 9.3% Residual 7.7% Recurrence 10%
Boghani et al[6]	2013	Systematic review	Individual patient data: 158 endoscopic, 15 combined, 172 open	Average blood loss: Endoscopic 544.0 mL (20–2000 mL) vs. open 1579.5 (350–10,000 mL) When controlled for tumor stage, recurrence rates in endoscopic group are at least as good as open

extension. On MRI, JAs appear isointense to hyperintense on T1- and T2-weighted sequences. Flow voids related to small high-flow vessels supplying the tumor can be seen. There is intense enhancement following administration of gadolinium contrast.

Angiography is used to identify vascular contributions to the tumor. Combined with embolization, it reduces blood loss that improves visualization and tumor resection. It is commonly performed 24 to 48 h before the surgery.[8] In advanced JAs, both external carotid artery (ECA) and ICA can supply feeding vessels to the tumor. Bilateral vascular supply is also common in advanced tumors.[9] Residual vascularization from the ICA following embolization of ECA branches is predictive of increased operative blood loss.[10] Although feeders from the ICA can be embolized, the risk of complications (stroke, visual loss, facial paralysis, carotid dissection) is significant and its routine use is not recommended.[11–14] Preoperative balloon occlusion testing of the ICA may be considered with extensive tumors that encase the ICA, especially in surgical or radiation failures where risk of vessel injury is higher. This will assess the adequacy of the collateral circulation and the feasibility of carotid sacrifice, if necessary.

UPMC staging system (▶Table 28.2 and ▶Fig. 28.1) accounts for tumor vascularity derived from intracranial circulation and the route of intracranial extension.[10,15] Compared to previous staging systems, the UPMC staging system demonstrates stronger correlation with intraoperative blood loss, need for multiple surgeries (staged), and residual or recurrent tumor.

Advanced JAs demand special anesthetic consideration. Prior adjuvant radiation therapy, angiographic embolization, or surgical dissection of the masticatory space

Table 28.2 UPMC staging system

Stage	Staging criteria
I	Nasal cavity, medial PPF No residual vascularity
II	Paranasal sinuses, lateral PPF No residual vascularity
III	Skull base, orbit, infratemporal fossa No residual vascularity
IV	Skull base, orbit, infratemporal fossa With residual vascularity
V	Intracranial extension: medial; lateral With residual vascularity

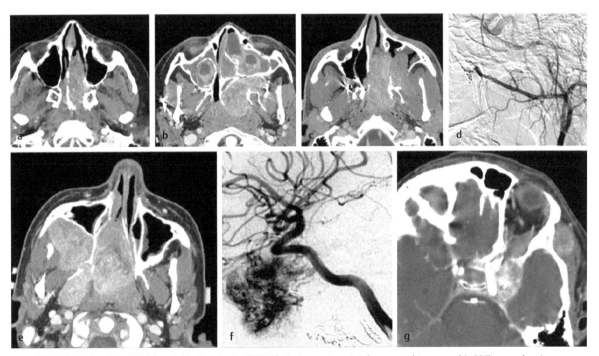

Fig. 28.1 The University of Pittsburgh Medical Center (UPMC) staging system: Axial computed tomographic (CT) scans showing tumor confined to the left nasal cavity and medial pterygopalatine fossa (UPMC stage I) **(a)** and tumor involving left lateral pterygopalatine fossa (UPMC stage II) **(b)**. Figure panels c and d are from the same patient in whom the axial CT scan **(c)** shows tumor involving the left infratemporal fossa and an angiogram **(d)** shows no residual vascularity after embolization of the external carotid artery tributaries (UPMC stage III). Figure panels e and f are from the same patient in whom the axial CT scan **(e)** shows tumor involving the infratemporal fossa and angiogram **(f)** with residual vascularity from the internal carotid artery after embolization of the external carotid artery tributaries (UPMC stage IV). Figure panel **(g)** is an axial CT scan showing tumor lateral to the cavernous internal carotid artery (UPMC stage VL). (Reproduced with permission of Snyderman CH, Pant H, Carrau RL, et al. A new endoscopic staging system for angiofibromas. *Arch Otolaryngol Head Neck Surg.* 2010;136:588–594.)

can result in difficult intubation due to trismus.[16] Large tumors may displace the soft palate inferiorly or extend to the oropharynx. With intracranial extension, increased intracranial pressure (ICP) may be present.[17] Measures to be considered in this setting are: smooth induction of anesthesia, invasive monitoring of blood pressure, and promotion of moderate hyperventilation. Invasive hemodynamic monitoring will provide safe hypotensive anesthesia and guide intravascular replacement strategies, if needed. In EES for advanced JAs, the average blood loss is more than 1000 mL.[4] In a patient population with low intravascular volume, excessive blood loss with consumption, dilution, and dysfunction of clotting factors and platelets can result in intraoperative coagulopathy.[18] Monitoring with thromboelastometry and early replacement of clotting factors are part of the management.[19] Restrictive transfusion strategies have been proposed to reduce the potential for transfusion-related complications (at Hb of 7–8 g/dL).[20] However, a strict transfusion threshold is difficult to recommend as this decision depends on many factors such as patient comorbidities and ongoing surgical variables.[18] Staging of surgery should be considered for large UPMC stage IV/V tumors if blood loss is excessive (50–100% of total blood volume), especially if significant tumor remains.

In patients where there is risk of ICA injury, neurophysiologic monitoring of cortical function (somatosensory-evoked potentials) is performed to detect global brain ischemia. Cranial nerves with motor function (III, IV, VI, and V_3) can be monitored with electromyography (EMG). EMG aids in detection and protection of nerves with dissection and provides prognostic information for recovery.[21]

28.3 Surgical Technique

The primary goal of surgery is complete tumor resection with preservation of major neurovascular structures. Secondary goals are to minimize morbidity and avoid the need for radiation therapy in this young patient population.[22] The general surgical strategy consists of wide multi-corridor access to the tumor, identifying anatomical landmarks, dissection around the periphery of the tumor to define its limits, and minimizing tumor manipulation until necessary. In advanced JAs with multiple feeding vessels, the tumor can be divided into vascular territories. Each segment is addressed sequentially to facilitate control of blood loss and to allow staging of the surgery if needed. The intracranial component is left for last (see ▶ Video 28.1).

- The patient is positioned supine in reverse Trendelenburg position with >15° elevation. This reduces venous pressure that lessens mucosal and tumor bleeding. The head is rotated toward the surgeons and secured in place with a pediatric Mayfield head holder. For very young patients, the head is

also supported on a cushioned ring. The navigation system is registered, and needle electrodes for neurophysiological monitoring are placed. After the eyes are secured with occlusive adhesive tape, the face is prepped with 10% povidone-iodine solution and the nasal cavity is decongested with oxymetazoline (0.05%) soaked cottonoids. Perioperative antibiotic prophylaxis with a third-generation cephalosporin with cerebrospinal fluid (CSF) penetration is administered in cases at risk for intradural exposure; otherwise, a second-generation cephalosporin is administered.

- A multicorridor approach is developed to facilitate identification of landmarks and extracapsular tumor dissection. A unilateral or bilateral Caldwell–Luc approach (anterior maxillotomy) provides lateral exposure of the masticator space and additional room for instrumentation. The posterior maxillary wall is removed to expose the pterygopalatine fossa (PPF) and establish a lateral limit for the JAs. The infraorbital nerve is identified along the roof of the maxillary sinus (▶ Fig. 28.2).

- A wide endonasal corridor is developed to facilitate binarial team surgery: bilateral ethmoidectomies, sphenoidotomies, and posterior septectomy are performed without violation of the tumor. The ethmoid corridor provides access to the superior surface of the tumor with separation of the tumor from the anterior cranial base. The medial wall of the orbit is exposed.

- On the dominant side of the tumor, an endoscopic medial maxillectomy is performed. In combination with the anterior maxillotomy, an endoscopic medial maxillectomy augments lateral access to the tumor in the PPF and infratemporal fossa. Tumor dissection typically begins in the PPF with dissection of soft tissues from the tumor capsule in a medial to lateral direction. With large tumors, it is often difficult to identify and preserve the descending palatine branch

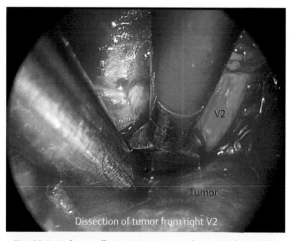

Fig. 28.2 Right maxillotomy view: tumor dissection from right infraorbital nerve (V2).

of the maxillary nerve superficial to the tumor. The lateral margin of the tumor is dissected from the pterygoid muscles and the embolized internal maxillary artery is transected. Portions of the tumor that extend inferiorly behind the maxilla can be delivered with careful traction; this is facilitated by transoral finger palpation of the tumor posterior to the maxillary tuberosity.

- Wide access through the anterior maxillary wall in combination with nasal endoscopy facilitates the use of a bayonet-style bipolar electrocautery forceps and Harmonic scalpel. As the tumor is dissected, large segments of tumor are transected with the Harmonic scalpel and removed to create more working space and improve visualization (▶ Fig. 28.3). For large bilateral tumors, this dissection is completed on each side.
- Attention is then directed to the sphenoid sinus with separation of tumor from the planum sphenoidale and identification of key landmarks: optic canals, optic-carotid recess, parasellar ICA, and sella (▶ Fig. 28.4). If

the sinus is filled with tumor, dissection starts on the side with least vascular involvement. Generally, tumor is dissected in a superior to inferior and medial to lateral direction with careful extracapsular dissection of tumor from the bone and dura (▶ Fig. 28.5). The optic nerve is identified first followed by the cavernous and paraclival segments of the ICA (▶ Fig. 28.6). Venous bleeding can be managed with flowable Gelfoam (Surgifoam) or similar hemostatic agents.

- Tumor extension to the Meckel's cave region and orbital apex is dissected next. The pterygoid canal is an important landmark in this area for the petrous and lacerum segments of the ICA (▶ Fig. 28.7).[23] Furthermore, the vidian artery is often a major source of vascularity due to tumor infiltration of the pterygoid base surrounding the pterygoid canal. As dissection proceeds, arterial feeders to the tumor (including the vidian artery) must be individually localized and cauterized with endoscopic bipolar electrocautery. The pterygoid base must be drilled to remove all remnants of tumor and prevent recurrence (▶ Fig. 28.8).[24]
- Residual tumor along the inferior orbital fissure and orbital apex is dissected with preservation of the second division of the trigeminal nerve. A combined

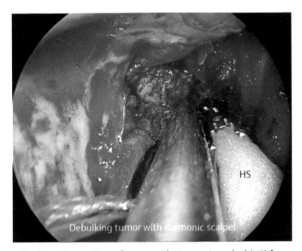

Fig. 28.3 Transection of tumor with Harmonic scalpel (HS) for initial tumor (T) debulking.

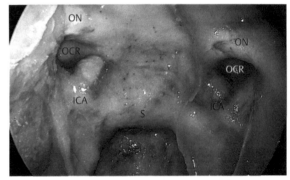

Fig. 28.4 Anatomical specimen demonstrating key landmarks: optic nerve (ON), lateral optic-carotid recess (OCR), parasellar ICA (ICA), sella (S).

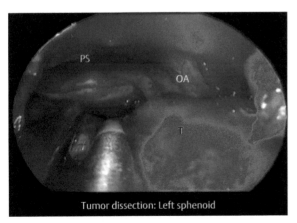

Fig. 28.5 Extracapsular dissection of tumor (T) in left sphenoid sinus: planum sphenoidale (PS), orbital apex (OA).

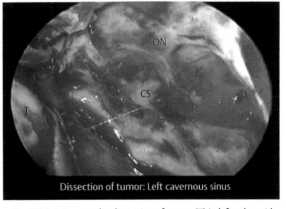

Fig. 28.6 Extracapsular dissection of tumor (T) in left sphenoid sinus: optic nerve (ON), cavernous sinus (CS).

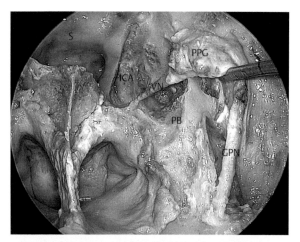

Fig. 28.7 Left anatomical dissection demonstrating the relation between the pterygopalatine ganglion (PPG), greater palatine nerve (GPN), Vidian nerve (VN), paraclival internal carotid artery (ICA), pterygoid base (PB) partially drilled, sella (S).

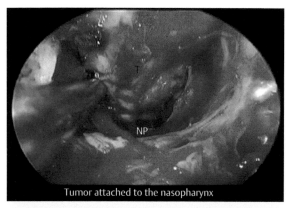

Tumor attached to the nasopharynx

Fig. 28.9 Tumor (T) infiltration of the nasopharynx (NP).

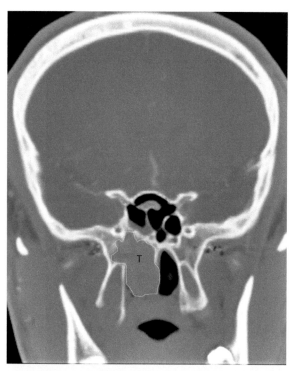

Fig. 28.8 Tumor (T) involvement of the right base of pterygoid and pterygoid canal (tumor outline).

endonasal and transmaxillary approach may provide the best access. Tumor growing through the inferior orbital fissure may gain access to the middle cranial fossa via the superior orbital fissure. The tumor is followed lateral to the orbital apex and dissected from the dura of the middle cranial fossa and from the lateral aspect of the cavernous sinus.

- Delivery of the resected tumor requires separation from the nasopharyngeal mucosa. Needle-tip electrocautery is used to incise the mucosa inferior to the tumor and establish a plane of dissection deep to the tumor at the clival surface (▶ Fig. 28.9).
- If dura is not transected during tumor dissection, no reconstruction of the surgical defect is needed. Adipose tissue graft can be used to fill an exposed middle fossa defect or cover an exposed ICA. The surgical field is coated with fibrin glue and gelfoam. Nasal tampons (Merocel) may be placed for additional hemostasis. If the need for a vascularized flap is anticipated, a nasoseptal flap should be elevated from the contralateral septum at the origin of the surgery.

28.3.1 Staging of Surgery

Advanced JAs with ICA vascular contribution are at risk for significant blood loss. The risk of coagulopathy is increased when the operative blood loss exceeds the patients intravascular volume.[25] Reduced body temperature and blood pH lower than 7.2 are also major contributors to coagulopathy. A predetermined blood loss limit should be set with the anesthesia team. It is generally recommended that after the loss of half of the patient's intravascular volume, surgeons should prepare to terminate the procedure. The time to achieve complete hemostasis with cauterization of bleeding sites should not be underestimated and can result in significant additional blood loss. Nasal packing with Merocel tampons or similar packing are used. Optimal timing of the next stage depends on the physiological recovery of the patient. This decision should involve the surgical, anesthesia, and intensive care unit teams. Some tumors require multiple stages to achieve complete resection.

28.3.2 Outcomes

Prior review of our experience at the University of Pittsburgh Medical Center (UPMC) identified 12 advanced JAs with intracranial involvement (UPMC stage IV and V). Six had prior surgical treatment. All patients had preoperative angiography and embolization of contributions of the ECA to tumor vasculature. A staged surgery was performed in 50% of cases. Complete tumor resection was achieved in 7 patients (58%), and gross total resection (>90%) in the other cases. With an average follow-up of 29 months, 2 patients (17%) required further endoscopic resection for growth of residual disease. Postoperative complications were seen in 6 patients: four cases of transient VI nerve palsy, one unilateral blindness secondary to central retinal artery occlusion 2 days following surgery (possibly related to vasospasm) and one intraoperative ICA sacrifice due to injury (no neurologic sequelae).

A recently published multicenter retrospective review of 74 Radkowski stage IIIA (71.9%) and IIIB (28.1%) tumors found similar outcomes.[4] Seventy-one patients underwent preoperative embolization of ECA contributors. The average operative blood loss was 1280 mL, and was correlated to the number of involved subsites. At an average 37.9 months of follow-up, residual disease was found in 33% of cases. Three patients had further therapy: one had radiosurgery, one radiotherapy, and one surgery. All others were observed, with no growth after an average of 35.6 months. Postoperative complications were seen in 5 patients: one hemorrhage, two trigeminal (V2) paresthesias, one transient VI nerve palsy, and one palatal insufficiency.

28.4 Postoperative Treatment

Most investigators recommend follow-up with nasal endoscopy and MRI for at least 5 years postoperatively.[3] Tumor recurrence is most likely due to incomplete resection of the primary tumor and usually occurs within 6 to 36 months.[8] It is associated with increased number of involved subsites, and is reduced by drilling the basisphenoid and base of pterygoids.[3,4,26,27] The management of recurrence depends on the size, growth, location, and patient symptoms. A second endoscopic surgery is the recommended option when the likelihood of complete tumor resection is high, and the risk of morbidity is low.[5,28] Ardehali et al. found no difference in recurrence rate when utilizing the endoscopic approach for primary (6/31) and revision surgery (3/16).[29] When complete resection of recurrent disease is impossible or high risk (cavernous sinus, ICA, intracranial), a wait and see policy can be adopted.[3,30] Adjuvant stereotactic radiosurgery or fractionated radiation therapy have both been described in small series, but their use is controversial in this young patient population.

28.5 Highlights

a. Indications
   - Early stage JA.
   - Advanced stage JA with anterior and middle cranial fossa extension.
   - Localized recurrent disease.
b. Contraindications
   - Severe medical comorbidities.
   - Refusal of blood product transfusion (relative contraindication).
   - Residual disease in challenging locations (cavernous sinus, intracranial, orbital apex) (relative contraindication).
c. Complications
   - Blood loss and transfusion.
   - Vascular injury.
   - Cranial nerve injury.
   - Brain manipulation.
   - CSF leak.
d. Special preoperative considerations
   - Angiography and angioembolization.
   - University of Pittsburgh Medical Center (UPMC) tumor staging.
   - Ophthalmologic consultation.
e. Special intraoperative considerations
   - Neurophysiologic monitoring.
   - Experienced endoscopic endonasal skull base team.
   - Blood loss and coagulopathy management.
   - Staged intervention if blood loss greater than half of intra-vascular volume.
f. Special postoperative considerations
   - Endoscopic + imaging follow-up for minimum of 5 years.
   - Treatment of recurrence depends on size, growth rates, location, and patient symptoms.

References

[1] Starlinger V, Wendler O, Gramann M, Schick B. Laminin expression in juvenile angiofibroma indicates vessel's early developmental stage. Acta Otolaryngol 2007;127(12):1310–1315

[2] Schick B, Plinkert PK, Prescher A. Aetiology of angiofibromas: reflection on their specific vascular component. [article in German] Laryngorhinootologie 2002;81(4):280–284

[3] Nicolai P, Berlucchi M, Tomenzoli D, et al. Endoscopic surgery for juvenile angiofibroma: when and how. Laryngoscope 2003;113(5):775–782

[4] Langdon C, Herman P, Verillaud B, et al. Expanded endoscopic endonasal surgery for advanced stage juvenile angiofibromas: a retrospective multi-center study. Rhinology 2016;54(3):239–246

[5] Leong SC. A systematic review of surgical outcomes for advanced juvenile nasopharyngeal angiofibroma with intracranial involvement. Laryngoscope 2013;123(5):1125–1131

[6] Boghani Z, Husain Q, Kanumuri VV, et al. Juvenile nasopharyngeal angiofibroma: a systematic review and comparison of endoscopic, endoscopic-assisted, and open resection in 1047 cases. Laryngoscope 2013;123(4):859–869

[7] López F, Triantafyllou A, Snyderman CH, et al. Nasal juvenile angiofibroma: current perspectives with emphasis on management. Head Neck 2017;39(5):1033–1045

[8] Rodriguez DP, Orscheln ES, Koch BL. Masses of the nose, nasal cavity, and nasopharynx in children. Radiographics 2017;37(6):1704–1730

[9] Overdevest JB, Amans MR, Zaki P, Pletcher SD, El-Sayed IH. Patterns of vascularization and surgical morbidity in juvenile nasopharyngeal angiofibroma: a case series, systematic review, and meta-analysis. Head Neck 2018;40(2):428–443

[10] Snyderman CH, Pant H, Carrau RL, Gardner P. A new endoscopic staging system for angiofibromas. Arch Otolaryngol Head Neck Surg 2010;136(6):588–594

[11] Borghei P, Baradaranfar MH, Borghei SH, Sokhandon F. Transnasal endoscopic resection of juvenile nasopharyngeal angiofibroma without preoperative embolization. Ear Nose Throat J 2006;85(11):740–743, 746

[12] Janakiram N, Sharma SB, Panicker VB, Srinivas CV. A drastic aftermath of embolisation in juvenile nasopharyngeal angiofibroma. Indian J Otolaryngol Head Neck Surg 2016;68(4):540–543

[13] Janakiram TN, Sharma SB, Panicker VB. Endoscopic excision of non-embolized juvenile nasopharyngeal angiofibroma: our technique. Indian J Otolaryngol Head Neck Surg 2016;68(3):263–269

[14] Ramezani A, Haghighatkhah H, Moghadasi H, Taheri MS, Parsafar H. A case of central retinal artery occlusion following embolization procedure for juvenile nasopharyngeal angiofibroma. Indian J Ophthalmol 2010;58(5):419–421

[15] Snyderman CH, Pant H. Endoscopic management of vascular sinonasal tumors, including angiofibroma. Otolaryngol Clin North Am 2016;49(3):791–807

[16] Li JR, Qian J, Shan XZ, Wang L. Evaluation of the effectiveness of preoperative embolization in surgery for nasopharyngeal angiofibroma. Eur Arch Otorhinolaryngol 1998;255(8):430–432

[17] Goma H. Anesthetic considerations of brain tumor surgery. In: Abujamra AL, ed. Diagnostic Techniques and Surgical Management of Brain Tumors. Rijeka, Croatia: In Tech; 2011

[18] Vincent JL. Indications for blood transfusions: too complex to base on a single number? Ann Intern Med 2012;157(1):71–72

[19] Schöchl H, Nienaber U, Hofer G, et al. Goal-directed coagulation management of major trauma patients using thromboelastometry (ROTEM)-guided administration of fibrinogen concentrate and prothrombin complex concentrate. Crit Care 2010;14(2):R55

[20] Hébert PC, Wells G, Blajchman MA, et al. A multicenter, randomized, controlled clinical trial of transfusion requirements in critical care. Transfusion Requirements in Critical Care Investigators, Canadian Critical Care Trials Group. N Engl J Med 1999;340(6):409–417

[21] Domenick Sridharan N, Chaer RA, Thirumala PD, et al. Somatosensory evoked potentials and electroencephalography during carotid endarterectomy predict late stroke but not death. Ann Vasc Surg 2017;38:105–112

[22] Dubey SP, Schick B, eds. Juvenile Angiofibroma. Cham, Switzerland: Springer; 2017

[23] Vescan AD, Snyderman CH, Carrau RL, et al. Vidian canal: analysis and relationship to the internal carotid artery. Laryngoscope 2007;117(8):1338–1342

[24] Howard DJ, Lloyd G, Lund V. Recurrence and its avoidance in juvenile angiofibroma. Laryngoscope 2001;111(9):1509–1511

[25] Paluszkiewicz P, Mayzner-Zawadzka E, Baranowski W, et al; Association for Severe Bleeding Care. Recommendations for the management of trauma or surgery-related massive blood loss. Pol Przegl Chir 2011;83(8):465–476

[26] Nicolai P, Villaret AB, Farina D, et al. Endoscopic surgery for juvenile angiofibroma: a critical review of indications after 46 cases. Am J Rhinol Allergy 2010;24(2):e67–e72

[27] Lund VJ, Stammberger H, Nicolai P, et al; European Rhinologic Society Advisory Board on endoscopic techniques in the management of nose, paranasal sinus and skull base tumours. European Position Paper on endoscopic management of tumours of the nose, paranasal sinuses and skull base. Rhinol Suppl 2010;22:1–143

[28] Hackman T, Snyderman CH, Carrau R, Vescan A, Kassam A. Juvenile nasopharyngeal angiofibroma: the expanded endonasal approach. Am J Rhinol Allergy 2009;23(1):95–99

[29] Ardehali MM, Samimi Ardestani SH, Yazdani N, Goodarzi H, Bastaninejad S. Endoscopic approach for excision of juvenile nasopharyngeal angiofibroma: complications and outcomes. Am J Otolaryngol 2010;31(5):343–349

[30] Onerci TM, Yücel OT, Oğretmenoğlu O. Endoscopic surgery in treatment of juvenile nasopharyngeal angiofibroma. Int J Pediatr Otorhinolaryngol 2003;67(11):1219–1225

Suggested Reading

Khoueir N, Nicolas N, Rohayem Z, Haddad A, Abou Hamad W. Exclusive endoscopic resection of juvenile nasopharyngeal angiofibroma: a systematic review of the literature. *Otolaryngol Head Neck Surg.* 2014;150:350–358

29 Expanded Endonasal Approaches for Treatment of Malignancy in Children

Meghan Wilson, Carl H. Snyderman, Paul A. Gardner, Elizabeth C. Tyler-Kabara

Summary

In the pediatric population, malignant tumors of the skull base are rare. Sarcoma (rhabdomyosarcoma, osteosarcoma, chondrosarcoma, Ewing sarcoma), chordoma, lymphoma, olfactory neuroblastoma, and germinoma have all been documented at the skull base in pediatric patients. Comprehensive multidisciplinary evaluation is essential for both diagnosis and management of these patients. Endoscopic endonasal surgery (EES) of the skull base provides access in sagittal and coronal planes and enhances the role of surgical management for these pathologies. Sinonasal malignancies that involve the anterior cranial base require a transfrontal/transcribriform/transplanum approach to the anterior cranial fossa. Reconstruction may be accomplished with a nasoseptal flap or extracranial pericranial flap. Skull base tumors such as chordomas and chondrosarcomas require a transclival approach to the posterior cranial fossa. Reconstruction is multilayer including fascia, fat, and a vascularized flap. Postoperative diversion of cerebrospinal fluid with a lumbar drain decreases the risk of a cerebrospinal fluid leak. Excellent oncologic outcomes can be achieved with acceptable morbidity when EES is incorporated into a multidisciplinary treatment plan.

Keywords: Endoscopic endonasal surgery, transcribriform approach, transclival approach chordoma, chondrosarcoma, sarcoma, Ewing sarcoma, olfactory neuroblastoma

29.1 Introduction

Endoscopic endonasal surgery (EES) of the skull base includes the entire ventral skull base in sagittal and coronal planes. These approaches are well established as surgical options for adult patients and are increasingly applied to pediatric patients with skull base tumors. Multiple studies have shown that these approaches are safe and effective in the pediatric population.[1–6] Open craniofacial surgery in children can potentially disrupt growth centers of the craniofacial skeleton and result in facial asymmetry. It is therefore important to consider endoscopic endonasal approaches when feasible based on patient and tumor characteristics.

In the sagittal plane, endoscopic endonasal approaches extend from the frontal sinus to the craniovertebral junction.[1] Access to the anterior cranial base is provided by transfrontal, transcribriform, and transplanum approaches.[7,8] They can be combined to achieve a complete resection of the anterior cranial base for sinonasal malignancy, equivalent to a craniofacial resection. The transsellar approach can be combined with transclival and transodontoid approaches to provide access to the posterior cranial fossa for malignancies of the skull base and nasopharynx.[9,10] The main considerations in pediatric EES are the constraints of the developing skull and facial skeleton and small size of patients. As described in this chapter, special considerations are required in the evaluation and treatment of pediatric patients.

EES can be used for both benign and malignant pathology, with the text of this chapter focusing on considerations with malignant tumors. Pediatric skull base malignancies are uncommon and comprise multiple pathologies.[6,11] Sarcoma (rhabdomyosarcoma, osteosarcoma, chondrosarcoma, Ewing sarcoma), chordoma, lymphoma, olfactory neuroblastoma, and germinoma have all been documented at the skull base in pediatric patients. Comprehensive multidisciplinary evaluation is essential for both diagnosis and management of these patients. In many cases, surgical resection or surgical debulking is necessary. In some cases, initial treatment with chemotherapy and/or external beam radiation therapy is the best course. A brief description of each tumor type is provided below.

29.1.1 Chordoma

Chordomas originate from the embryonic notochord and present in the midline clival region. They are typically slow-growing tumors that exhibit local invasion, though some tend to grow more aggressively in children.[12] While originating in the clivus, intradural extension is possible. The mainstay of treatment is surgical resection followed by postoperative radiotherapy. While complete resection is best, tumor involvement of vital neurovascular structures may limit resectability. Chordomas of the craniovertebral junction are often more aggressive and gross total resection is more difficult to achieve.

29.1.2 Chondrosarcoma

Chondrosarcomas present with similar symptoms as chordomas as they are also typically in the clival region, though they originate and grow in a paramedian position (petroclival synchondrosis). Chondrosarcomas can be subdivided into classic, mesenchymal, and dedifferentiated types, with the mesenchymal and dedifferentiated types showing more aggressive growth. Prognosis is closely related to histologic grade.[13]

29.1.3 Sarcomas

Rhabdomyosarcoma is the most common sarcoma in the pediatric population and can occur even in the very young. Alveolar and embryonal subtypes are the most common at the skull base. Smaller tumors, lower stage and young age have been shown to have improved prognosis.[14] Parameningeal rhabdomyosarcomas are most commonly treated initially using aggressive chemotherapy with surgery reserved for persistent disease after completion of chemotherapy regimen.[15] If after chemotherapy, the tumor remains unresectable or resection margins are positive, radiation therapy is administered.

Osteosarcoma is an aggressive malignancy of mesenchymal cell origin. Most cases of pediatric osteosarcoma arise in the limbs, but craniofacial osteosarcomas at the skull base have been reported as well.[16] Prior radiation therapy is a risk factor for development. Most but not all cases of osteosarcoma are associated with elevations in alkaline phosphatase levels. Complete resection is preferred, though chemotherapy is often needed initially to shrink the tumor to a size amenable to resection. Dural involvement, even in the absence of signs on imaging, is common. Radiation-induced sarcomas are particularly difficult to manage and surgery often plays a more prominent role in treatment of these tumors.[15]

29.1.4 Ewing Sarcoma

Ewing sarcoma is a primitive tumor of neuro-ectodermal origin and can involve the pediatric skull base. Ewing sarcoma is responsive to aggressive chemotherapy. The role of surgery is limited to resection of residual disease following chemotherapy. Radiotherapy is reserved for those patients with no response to chemotherapy or residual disease following surgery.[17]

29.1.5 Olfactory Neuroblastoma

Much less common in children than adults, olfactory neuroblastoma, also known as esthesioneuroblastoma, is a neuroectodermal neoplasm. It arises in the basal layer of the olfactory epithelium and frequently has both intranasal and intracranial components. The most commonly used staging system is the Modified Kadish staging system.[18] Stage A is tumor limited to the nasal cavity, Stage B defines tumor in the nasal cavity and sinuses, Stage C is tumor extending outside the sinonasal cavity, and Stage D includes distant spread of disease. While there is limited data regarding the outcome of pediatric olfactory neuroblastoma, in adult studies, 5-year disease-specific survival rates following treatment range from 92% in low-grade tumors (limited to nasal cavity and sinuses) to 50% in high-grade tumors (intracranial and metastatic disease).[19] In general, surgical resection with negative margins is the primary treatment of choice. In larger tumors and those with adverse histologic features,

adjuvant radiation therapy is recommended. In cases where the tumor has extended into brain parenchyma or into the orbit, neoadjuvant chemotherapy followed by surgery or radiation therapy may be considered to improve outcome and decrease morbidity. In young pediatric patients, olfactory neuroblastomas are aggressive tumors but respond well to chemotherapy.[20,21]

29.1.6 Germinoma

Germinomas are rare tumors affecting children and young adults. They arise from intracranial midline germ cells (totipotent cells), commonly in intrasellar and suprasellar locations. Dissemination of primary intracranial germinomas through the cerebrospinal fluid (CSF) is common, spreading through both the ventricular system and the subarachnoid space.[22] It is essential to image the entire brain and spine to evaluate for additional disease. Germinomas are chemo- and radio-sensitive; therefore, total resection is not essential.[22] Histologic diagnosis is necessary and can often be achieved through an endoscopic endonasal approach.

29.1.7 Lymphoma

Primary lymphoma at the skull base is very rare. In pediatric patients, both Burkitt's lymphoma and non-Hodgkin's lymphoma have been reported in the skull base.[23-25] In most of these case reports, the presenting symptom was related to cavernous sinus involvement. Tissue is necessary for diagnosis but treatment is primarily chemotherapy.

29.2 Preoperative Evaluation

A full head and neck exam and neurologic exam are prudent in all patients. In young children this can be challenging due to the inability to follow commands to test neurologic function. However, with diligent examination, it can often be accomplished. For example, eye movements can be assessed by visual tracking of a toy or interesting object. Careful attention to reactions to touch sensation can help determine sensory nerve function. Facial movement is evident if the patient is crying. If the tumor is in proximity to the orbit or optic nerve, an ophthalmology evaluation is prudent. Nasal endoscopy can provide useful information and a limited examination is well tolerated by most patients, even infants. Biopsy of a nasal mass is generally not attempted in an office setting due to discomfort and risk of bleeding.

Both computed tomography (CT) and magnetic resonance imaging (MRI) are essential in the evaluation of children with skull base malignancy. Sedation is often needed to obtain high-quality images, particularly for MRI. Consideration of these needs (including discussions with the pediatric radiologist and anesthesiologist) will enable good images to be obtained the first time. Both CT and MRI should be configured to work with an intraoperative image guidance system. If treatment will involve primary chemotherapy and/or radiation, it is still important to obtain high-quality imaging prior to treatment to have knowledge of pre-treatment tumor boundaries. If a tumor appears highly vascular, angiography with possible embolization just prior to surgery may reduce intraoperative blood loss and improve visualization. In tumors encasing the internal carotid artery, preoperative balloon occlusion testing should be considered.

Treatment planning includes careful review of preoperative imaging. Development and pneumatization of the sinuses is dependent on the age of the patient.[26–28] The frontal sinuses are the last to develop and are often aplastic on one side. Incomplete pneumatization of the sphenoid sinus (conchal or pre-sellar pattern) obscures key anatomical landmarks (optic nerves and carotid arteries) and necessitates careful drilling with increased reliance on image-based navigation. If any adjunctive transmaxillary approach is being considered, carefully note the position of permanent tooth buds; the surgical corridor is limited and there is risk of injury to permanent dentition.

In cases of malignant tumors, patients and their guardians should have a full discussion of treatment options not only with the surgical team but also with a pediatric hematologist-oncologist for consideration of all medical implications and treatments of the cancer diagnosis. It is highly advised that cases are discussed in a multidisciplinary tumor board format with providers knowledgeable in medical, surgical, interventional treatment as well as rehabilitation specific to pediatric patients.

29.3 Perioperative Management

All patients should be at least typed and screened. For infants and small children, blood should be readily available, due to their smaller total blood volume and limited reserve with hemorrhage. Similarly, good intravenous access is necessary. If only small bore intravenous lines are possible due to patient size, multiple lines should be placed. Expected blood loss and resuscitation needs should be discussed with the anesthesia team prior to surgery and throughout the case.

Preoperative antibiotics should be administered prior to the start of the surgical procedure. If intradural resection is planned, the use of antibiotics with good CSF penetration is recommended. Children have thinner skin and are at higher risk of pressure ulceration; therefore, all pressure points should be carefully padded. Children, particularly infants, are highly susceptible to hypothermia and adequate warming should be maintained.

The patient is placed in the supine position and the head is fixated with a pediatric Mayfield head clamp with additional support for the head using a padded

horse-shoe attachment. Fixation of the head facilitates extension and rotation of the head to a more ergonomic surgical position and prevents any movement during critical parts of the surgical dissection.

Neuromonitoring should be used when tumor is in proximity to neurovascular structures and/or cranial nerves.[29] Somatosensory-evoked potentials monitor cortical brain function and provide a measure of global ischemia. Electromyography of motor cranial nerves can be performed to aid in identification and prevention of injury.[29] In these cases, paralysis should be avoided. If significant intradural dissection is anticipated, CSF diversion through a lumbar drain should be discussed. Spinal drains are usually placed at completion of the surgery.

29.4 Surgical Technique

29.4.1 Anterior Cranial Fossa: Transfrontal/Transcribriform/Transplanum Approach

Sinonasal malignancies often involve the bone of the anterior cranial base and may extend to the dura. The goal of surgery is to remove all bone surrounding the tumor and remove the layers of the cranial base that are involved by tumor (▶ Fig. 29.1). For a prototypical skull base malignancy such as an olfactory neuroblastoma, this usually includes resection of the bone, dura, and olfactory bulbs and tracts on one or both sides.

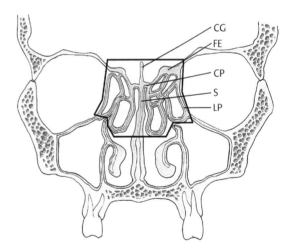

Fig. 29.1 The margins of resection for a sinonasal malignancy with skull base involvement (e.g., olfactory neuroblastoma) include the ethmoid sinuses, superior nasal septum (S), medial walls of the orbit, roof of the ethmoid sinuses (FE), cribriform plates (CP), crista galli (CG), posterior table of frontal sinus, planum sphenoidale, dura and olfactory bulbs and tracts. Periorbita is resected if the lamina papyracea (LP) is involved. The skull base resection may be extended to include the roof of the orbit.

- If the tumor is large, debulking of the tumor is performed to establish the extent of the tumor and provide visualization of surrounding landmarks. Bipolar electrocautery of the tumor surface provides hemostasis.
- Bilateral complete ethmoidectomies and sphenoidotomies are performed and mucosa is stripped from the skull base to expose the bony margins. The middle turbinates are resected to the plane of the skull base without violation of the dura.
- On the side of the tumor, the lamina papyracea is removed to the plane of the skull base to establish a lateral margin (►Fig. 29.2). If there is tumor invasion of the bone, the periorbital may be resected for an additional margin.
- The anterior and posterior ethmoidal arteries are identified on the orbital side of the bone, cauterized with bipolar electrocautery, and transected. The orbital periosteum is elevated from the orbital roof to provide additional exposure if there is lateral extension of the tumor along the skull base or dura (►Fig. 29.3).
- On the side opposite the tumor, the lateral margin of resection is the roof of the ethmoid sinus unless the tumor crosses the midline.
- The nasal septum is transected inferior to the tumor from the nasion to the posterior edge of the septum. If there is no invasion of the nasal septum, a nasoseptal flap can be elevated on the side contralateral to the tumor. A frozen section of the septal mucosa margin on the side of the tumor is performed.
- A Draf 3 frontal sinusotomy is performed with drilling of the crista galli in the midline to expose the posterior table of the frontal sinus (►Fig. 29.4).
- The optic canals are identified posteriorly and the bone of the planum sphenoidale is thinned with a drill (4 mm coarse diamond bit) anterior to the optic canals.

- The roof of the ethmoids is thinned with the drill to expose the dura beyond the margins of resection (►Fig. 29.2 and ►Fig. 29.5). This may include the orbital roof on the side of the tumor.
- Periosteum is elevated from the crista galli which is drilled in an anterior to posterior direction. It is not necessary to remove the entire crista galli. The bone of the posterior table of the frontal sinus is drilled to establish a margin anterior to the tumor and the cribriform plate.

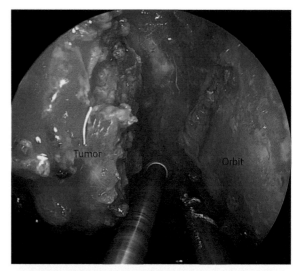

Fig. 29.2 After the tumor is debulked, the medial wall of the orbit (lamina papyracea) on the side of the tumor is removed and the anterior and posterior ethmoid arteries are sacrificed. The bone of the fovea ethmoidalis (roof of ethmoid) is drilled to expose the dura lateral to the tumor.

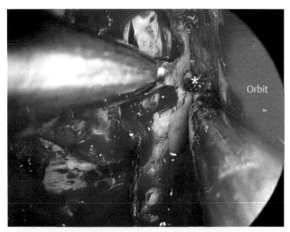

Fig. 29.3 Following transection of the ethmoidal arteries (*asterisk*), the periorbita is elevated from the orbital roof to provide access to the skull base beyond the ethmoid bone.

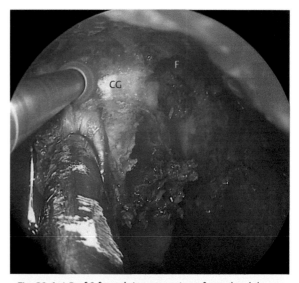

Fig. 29.4 A Draf-3 frontal sinusotomy is performed and the crista galli (CG) and posterior walls of the frontal sinuses (F) are drilled to expose dura anterior to the tumor.

- All bone is elevated from the skull base to expose the dura (▶Fig. 29.6). The cribriform plates can be fractured at the midline.
- Epidural dissection of the dura from the bone is performed circumferentially to facilitate resection of dural margins later in the procedure.
- The dura is incised laterally (roof of ethmoid or orbit), and the incisions are extended with microscissors, taking care not to injure underlying cortical vessels (▶Fig. 29.7).
- Anteriorly, the falx is cauterized and transected with microscissors in an anterior-to-posterior direction to the free edge of the falx (▶Fig. 29.8). This releases the specimen anteriorly.
- The olfactory bulbs and tracts are dissected free from the frontal lobes and remain attached to the dural specimen. If tumor is adherent, a subpial dissection of tumor from the surface of the brain is performed (▶Fig. 29.9).
- The posterior dural cut at the planum sphenoidale includes the dura and olfactory tracts.
- The entire dural specimen is removed en bloc and oriented for pathology.

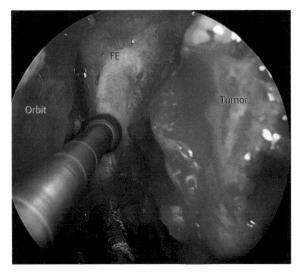

Fig. 29.5 The bone is drilled circumferentially around the tumor to expose the dura. On the side opposite the tumor, the lateral margin may be the fovea ethmoidalis (FE) if the tumor does not cross the midline.

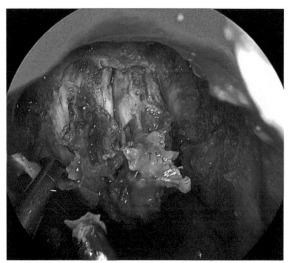

Fig. 29.6 The bone is peeled from the underlying dura to fully expose the margins of tumor (T) invasion.

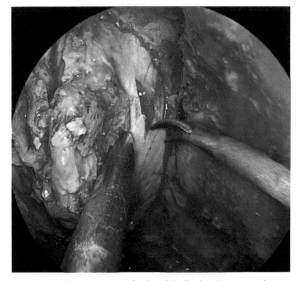

Fig. 29.7 The tumor (T) is further debulked and cauterized. The dura is incised laterally and the incision is extended anteriorly and posteriorly, avoiding injury to cortical vessels.

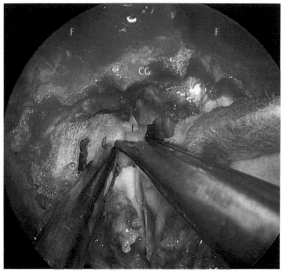

Fig. 29.8 After the lateral dural cuts have been made, the anterior dural cut is made with transection of the falx (f) in the midline. CG, crista galli; F, frontal sinuses.

- Circumferential dural margins are excised for frozen section analysis (▶Fig. 29.10). If necessary, additional bone can be removed from the orbital roof to extend the lateral margin. Additional margins are taken from the olfactory tracts (▶Fig. 29.11).
- The dural defect (▶Fig. 29.12) is reconstructed with an inlay fascial graft, onlay fascial graft tucked in an epidural plane, and a vascularized flap (nasoseptal flap or extracranial pericranial flap) that covers all exposed dura and bone surrounding the dural defect (▶Fig. 29.13). Fascial grafts may be cadaveric or autologous fascia lata.

29.4.2 Posterior Cranial Fossa: Transclival Approach

Malignant neoplasms involving the soft tissues of the nasopharynx cannot be dissected from the surface of the clivus without removal of the outer cortical bone. If periosteum is involved, the outer cortical bone is drilled. Malignant tumors that arise from the bone (chordoma, chondrosarcoma) require removal of bone to the underlying dura. If there is dural invasion, dural resection is indicated. The anatomy of the transclival approach is shown in ▶Fig. 29.14.

- A nasoseptal flap is elevated if there is no tumor involvement of the vascular pedicle. The mucosa from the nasal floor and inferior meatus is included to create a wider flap for a horizontal orientation.
- Bilateral sphenoidotomies are performed with removal of the sphenoid rostrum and complete detachment of the posterior nasal septum.

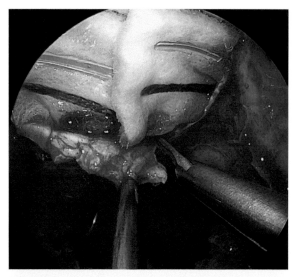

Fig. 29.10 After removal of the primary specimen, the posterior dural margin (shown here) is excised to confirm microscopically complete removal of the tumor.

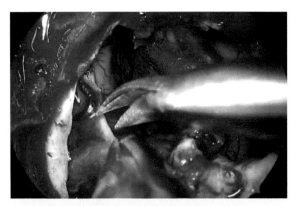

Fig. 29.9 Along with the olfactory bulbs and tracts, the tumor-involved dura is dissected from the surface of the brain. If necessary, a subpial dissection can be performed.

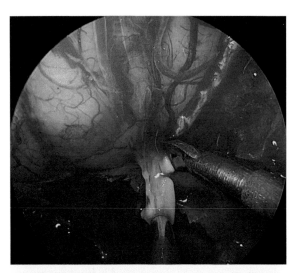

Fig. 29.11 The olfactory tract margins are also assessed for microscopic residual tumor.

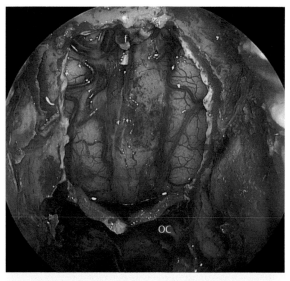

Fig. 29.12 The final dural defect extends from the frontal sinus to the planum and from orbit to orbit. OC, optic canal; f, falx.

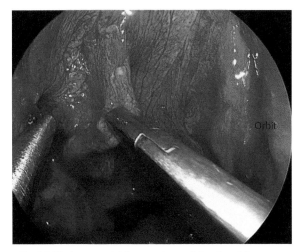

Fig. 29.13 A nasoseptal flap or extracranial pericranial flap (shown here) overlaps the dural and bone margins of the defect. If the periorbita is excised, the pericranial flap can also be used to reconstruct the orbit.

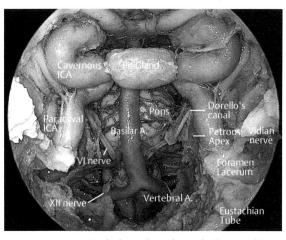

Fig. 29.14 Anatomical relationships of transclival approach to posterior cranial fossa. A, artery; Pit: pituitary; ICA, internal carotid artery.

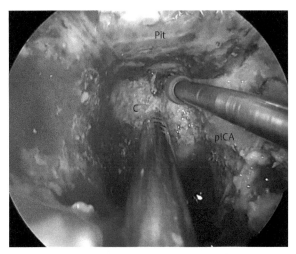

Fig. 29.15 The dura over the pituitary gland (Pit) has been exposed. The bone of the mid-clivus (C) is drilled between the paraclival internal carotid arteries (pICA).

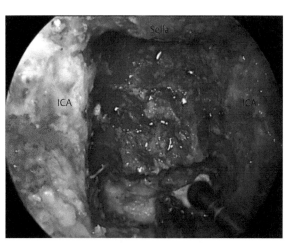

Fig. 29.16 The bone of the middle and lower clivus is removed to the underlying dura. ICA: internal carotid artery.

- Mucosa is stripped from the sphenoid sinus and bony landmarks (sella, optic canals, paraclival ICAs) are identified.
- The mucosa of the nasopharynx and underlying longus capitis muscles are excised using needle-tip electrocautery to expose the lower clivus from the floor of the sphenoid sinus to the inferior margin of the tumor.
- The floor of the sphenoid sinus and middle clivus are drilled (4 mm extended, coarse diamond drill bit) between the paraclival ICAs (▶ Fig. 29.15). The lower clivus is drilled with the paraclival ICAs in view.
- Removal of tumor and tumor-involved bone continues to the inner cortex of the clivus overlying the posterior cranial fossa (▶ Fig. 29.16).

- The bone deep to the paraclival ICAs (medial petrous apex) is drilled to establish a lateral limit of resection (▶ Fig. 29.17). Nerve stimulation (electromyography) with neurophysiological monitoring is performed to aid in identification of the abducens nerve in Dorello's canal.
- If more lateral exposure is needed, the paraclival ICAs are mobilized by thinning the overlying bone with the drill and lifting off the bone with the footplate of a Kerrison rongeur. An alternative approach is the contralateral transmaxillary approach if there is extensive tumor involvement of the petrous apex.[30]
- If tumor involves the superior clivus, a pituitary transposition can be performed by opening the cavernous sinus on each side (▶ Fig. 29.18).[31] The inferior hypophyseal artery is cauterized and the pituitary gland is elevated to provide access to the posterior

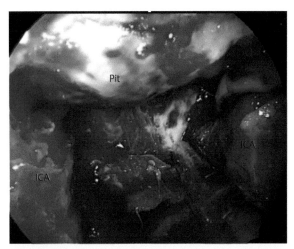

Fig. 29.17 A nerve stimulator is used to localize the abducens nerve which is interdural as it passes into Dorello's canal. Dorello's canal is typically at the junction of the lower 2/3 and upper 1/3 of the paraclival internal carotid artery (pICA). Pit, pituitary.

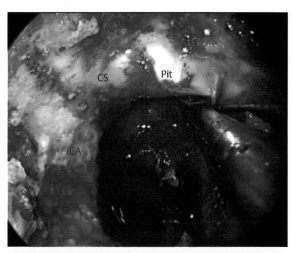

Fig. 29.18 Access to the upper clivus requires transposition of the pituitary gland (Pit). The dura of the cavernous sinus (CS) is incised to release the attachments of the gland so that it can be transposed. The inferior hypophyseal branch of the internal carotid artery (ICA) is sacrificed on one or both sides.

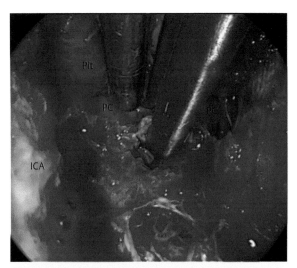

Fig. 29.19 Once the pituitary gland (Pit) is transposed, the dorsum sella is divided with a bone rongeur and the posterior clinoids (PC) are removed. Caution is advised to avoid injury to the internal carotid artery (ICA).

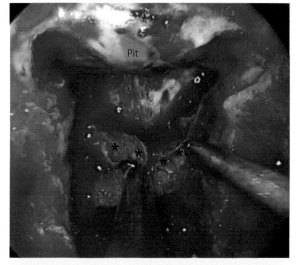

Fig. 29.20 Chordomas spread within the interdural space. The outer (periosteal) layer of dura is stripped (*asterisks*) to expose the interdural space. Pit, pituitary.

clinoids (▶Fig. 29.19). The superior clivus is divided in the midline with a bone rongeur and each posterior clinoid is removed separately in order to avoid injury to the parasellar ICA.

- Tumor-involved bone and the inner cortex of the clivus are removed to expose the dura.
- The outer (periosteal) layer of the dura is stripped to remove tumor between the two layers of dura, expose the inner/meningeal layer, and control the basilar venous plexus (▶Fig. 29.20). Hemostatic material

(Surgifoam, Floseal) is injected between the dural layers into the venous plexus to achieve hemostasis.

- The inner layer of dura is excised if it is invaded by tumor (▶Fig. 29.21).
- Reconstruction of the defect includes an inlay fascial graft, onlay fascial graft with wide coverage of the surrounding bone, adipose tissue graft to fill the clival defect, and transposition of the nasoseptal flap (oriented horizontally) to cover the fascial and fat grafts (▶Fig. 29.22, ▶Fig. 29.23, and ▶Fig. 29.24).

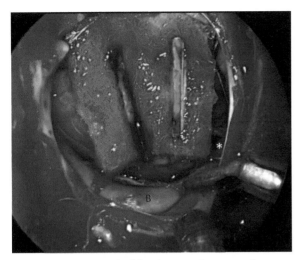

Fig. 29.21 Tumor-involved dura is resected to expose the neurovascular structures of the posterior cranial fossa. B, basilar artery; *, abducens nerve.

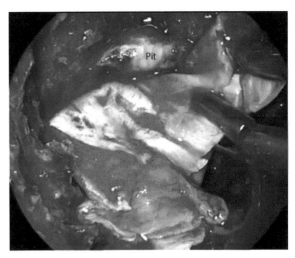

Fig. 29.22 Following placement of an inlay fascial graft, the dural defect is covered with a fascia lata graft. Pit, pituitary.

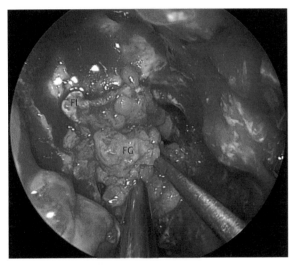

Fig. 29.23 In order to prevent herniation of the brainstem, a fat graft (FG) fills the clival recess superficial to the fascia lata (FL) graft.

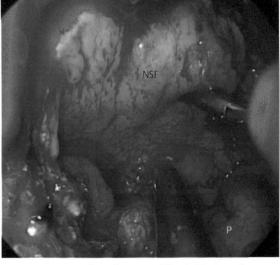

Fig. 29.24 A vascularized nasoseptal flap (NSF) covers the entire defect. P; vascular pedicle of flap.

29.5 Postoperative Management

Monitoring of the patient in an Intensive Care Unit is recommended postoperatively. Pediatric intensive care unit specialized physicians offer support and guidance in the management of these patients. Ideally, patients should be extubated in the operating room prior to transfer unless there are concerns about the airway or patient compliance. The extent of neurologic evaluation possible will depend on the age of the child. If too young to follow commands, planned postoperative imaging should be considered in most cases within 24 hours.

Patients should be monitored for epistaxis and all nasal bleeding carefully evaluated. If any nasal packing is used, this should be monitored as well. Keep in mind, neonates are obligate nasal breathers and nasal packing can result in respiratory distress. Strings attached to nasal packing may be trimmed to prevent removal by patients.

Following operative recovery, adjuvant treatment and a plan for further imaging should be discussed in a multidisciplinary fashion. With regards to imaging, CT and other forms of ionizing radiation deserve special consideration in children, particularly those patients who will require multiple surveillance scans for years to come. The team must balance ordering scans necessary for monitoring without exposing the child to unnecessary excess radiation.

29.6 Outcomes

Outcomes data in pediatric patients is very limited due to the rare nature of these tumors. At the University of Pittsburgh, two series of pediatric patients who underwent EES for skull base lesions (both benign and malignant) have been described.[5,6] The surgery was successful in all cases approaching tumors at the cribriform, planum, sella, and clivus. In the 10 patients with chordoma, gross total resection was achieved in 50% with near-total resection in the others.[6] Those with near-total resection were limited by tumor involvement of critical neurovascular structures such as the ICA or cavernous sinus. This rate of gross total resection is on the high end of what is published in the adult literature. Cases with residual chordoma were followed by adjuvant proton beam irradiation. In this small series, recurrence was 30%, well in line with recurrence rates in adult studies.

29.7 Complications

In published case series, major complications are infrequent.[5,6] CSF leak with risk of meningitis is the most frequent complication, especially for clival defects.[17] Diagnosis of a CSF leak can be difficult in pediatric patients due to decreased reporting of symptoms.[32] Drainage of CSF into the pharynx may precipitate a nocturnal cough. Endoscopic repair with placement of a lumbar spinal drain is recommended to minimize the risk of infectious complications. Herniation of the brainstem is a rare complication associated with large clival defects and can be prevented by performing a 4-layer reconstruction including inlay fascia, onlay fascia, adipose tissue, and vascularized flap.[33]

Cranial nerve palsies are very rare. Anterior cranial base resection is associated with loss of olfaction; diplopia from an abducens nerve palsy is most frequent with transclival approaches. Manipulation of the pituitary gland with superior transclival approaches can result in diabetes insipidus. Epistaxis is rare; severe bleeding is usually associated with branches of the sphenopalatine artery but the possibility of a pseudo-aneurysm from the ICA should always be considered.

29.8 Highlights

a. Indications for surgery
   - Anterior cranial base: sinonasal malignancy (olfactory neuroblastoma).
   - Posterior cranial fossa (clivus): malignant bone tumors (chordoma, chondrosarcoma).

b. Contraindications for surgery
   - Advanced stage tumors (brain, orbit, ICA, cavernous sinus).
   - Sarcomas: chemotherapy with surgical salvage.

c. Special preoperative considerations
   - Tumor staging.
   - Multidisciplinary planning.

d. Special intraoperative considerations
   - Neurophysiologic monitoring.
   - Experienced endoscopic endonasal skull base team.

e. Complications
   - Blood loss and transfusion.
   - Vascular injury.
   - Cranial nerve injury.
   - Brain manipulation.
   - CSF leak.

f. Special postoperative considerations
   - Early detection and management of CSF leak.

References

[1] Kassam A, Thomas AJ, Snyderman C, et al. Fully endoscopic expanded endonasal approach treating skull base lesions in pediatric patients. J Neurosurg 2007;106(2, Suppl):75–86

[2] Chivukula S, Koutourousiou M, Snyderman CH, Fernandez-Miranda JC, Gardner PA, Tyler-Kabara EC. Endoscopic endonasal skull base surgery in the pediatric population. J Neurosurg Pediatr 2013;11(3):227–241

[3] Quon JL, Hwang PH, Edwards MS. Transnasal endoscopic approach for pediatric skull base tumors: a case series. Neurosurgery 2016;63(Suppl 1):179

[4] Munson PD, Moore EJ. Pediatric endoscopic skull base surgery. Curr Opin Otolaryngol Head Neck Surg 2010;18(6):571–576

[5] Banu MA, Rathman A, Patel KS, et al. Corridor-based endonasal endoscopic surgery for pediatric skull base pathology with detailed radioanatomic measurements. Neurosurgery 2014;10(Suppl 2):273–293, discussion 293

[6] LoPresti MA, Sellin JN, DeMonte F. Developmental considerations in pediatric skull base surgery. J Neurol Surg B Skull Base 2018;79(1):3–12

[7] Gardner PA, Snyderman CH. Endonasal transcribriform approach to the anterior cranial fossa. In: Snyderman CH, Gardner PA, eds. Master Techniques in Otolaryngology—Head and Neck Surgery: Skull Base Surgery Volume. Philadelphia, PA: Wolters Kluwer; 2015:123–130

[8] Casiano RR. Endonasal resection of the anterior cranial base. In: Snyderman CH, Gardner PA, eds. Master Techniques in Otolaryngology—Head and Neck Surgery: Skull Base Surgery Volume. Philadelphia, PA: Wolters Kluwer; 2015:173–183

[9] Gardner PA, Snyderman CH. Transclival approach to the middle and lower clivus. In: Snyderman CH, Gardner PA, eds. Master Techniques in Otolaryngology—Head and Neck Surgery: Skull Base Surgery Volume. Philadelphia, PA:Wolters Kluwer; 2015:365–372

[10] Snyderman CH, Gardner PA, Tormenti MJ, Fernandez-Miranda JC. Sella and beyond: approaches to the clivus and posterior fossa, petrous apex, and cavernous sinus. In: Georgalas C, Fokkens WJ, eds. Rhinology and Skull Base Surgery. Stuttgart, Germany: Thieme; 2013:758–771

[11] Tsai EC, Santoreneos S, Rutka JT. Tumors of the skull base in children: review of tumor types and management strategies. Neurosurg Focus 2002;12(5):e1

[12] Fernandez-Miranda JC, Gardner PA, Snyderman CH, et al. Clival chordomas: a pathological, surgical, and radiotherapeutic review. Head Neck 2014;36(6):892–906

[13] Bohman LE, Koch M, Bailey RL, Alonso-Basanta M, Lee JY. Skull base chordoma and chondrosarcoma: influence of clinical and

demographic factors on prognosis: a SEER analysis. World Neurosurg 2014;82(5):806–814

[14] Unsal AA, Chung SY, Unsal AB, Baredes S, Eloy JA. A population-based analysis of survival for sinonasal rhabdomyosarcoma. Otolaryngol Head Neck Surg 2017;157(1):142–149

[15] Deneuve S, Teissier N, Jouffroy T, et al. Skull base surgery for pediatric parameningeal sarcomas. Head Neck 2012;34(8):1057–1063

[16] Hadley C, Gressot LV, Patel AJ, et al. Osteosarcoma of the cranial vault and skull base in pediatric patients. J Neurosurg Pediatr 2014;13(4):380–387

[17] Iatrou I, Theologie-Lygidakis N, Schoinohoriti O, Tzermpos F, Mylonas AI. Ewing's sarcoma of the maxillofacial region in Greek children: report of 6 cases and literature review. J Craniomaxillofac Surg 2018;46(2):213–221

[18] Kadish S, Goodman M, Wang CC. Olfactory neuroblastoma: a clinical analysis of 17 cases. Cancer 1976;37(3):1571–1576

[19] Tajudeen BA, Arshi A, Suh JD, St John M, Wang MB. Importance of tumor grade in esthesioneuroblastoma survival: a population-based analysis. JAMA Otolaryngol Head Neck Surg 2014;140(12):1124–1129

[20] El Kababri M, Habrand JL, Valteau-Couanet D, Gaspar N, Dufour C, Oberlin O. Esthesioneuroblastoma in children and adolescent: experience on 11 cases with literature review. J Pediatr Hematol Oncol 2017;36(2):91–95

[21] Bisogno G, Soloni P, Conte M, et al. Esthesioneuroblastoma in pediatric and adolescent age. A report from the TREP project in cooperation with the Italian Neuroblastoma and Soft Tissue Sarcoma Committees. BMC Cancer 2012;12:117

[22] Douglas-Akinwande AC, Mourad AA, Pradhan K, Hattab EM. Primary intracranial germinoma presenting as a central skull base lesion. AJNR Am J Neuroradiol 2006;27(2):270–273

[23] Aronson PL, Reilly A, Paessler M, Kersun LS. Burkitt lymphoma involving the clivus. J Pediatr Hematol Oncol 2008;30(4):320–321

[24] Ceyhan M, Erdem G, Kanra G, Kaya S, Onerci M. Lymphoma with bilateral cavernous sinus involvement in early childhood. Pediatr Neurol 1994;10(1):67–69

[25] Choi HK, Cheon JE, Kim IO, et al. Central skull base lymphoma in children: MR and CT features. Pediatr Radiol 2008;38(8):863–867

[26] Wilson M, Snyderman C. Endoscopic management of developmental anomalies of the skull base. J Neurol Surg B Skull Base 2018;79(1):13–20

[27] Rastatter JC, Snyderman CH, Gardner PA, Alden TD, Tyler-Kabara E. Endoscopic endonasal surgery for sinonasal and skull base lesions in the pediatric population. Otolaryngol Clin North Am 2015;48(1):79–99

[28] Gump WC. Endoscopic endonasal repair of congenital defects of the anterior skull base: developmental considerations and surgical outcomes. J Neurol Surg B Skull Base 2015;76(4):291–295

[29] Elangovan C, Singh SP, Gardner P, et al. Intraoperative neurophysiological monitoring during endoscopic endonasal surgery for pediatric skull base tumors. J Neurosurg Pediatr 2016;17(2):147–155

[30] Patel CR, Wang EW, Fernandez-Miranda JC, Gardner PA, Snyderman CH. Contralateral transmaxillary corridor: an augmented endoscopic approach to the petrous apex. J Neurosurg 2017;1–9. Epub ahead of print

[31] Gardner PA, Snyderman CH. Endoscopic endonasal pituitary transposition approach to the superior clivus. In: Snyderman CH, Gardner PA, eds. Master Techniques in Otolaryngology—Head and Neck Surgery: Skull Base Surgery Volume. Philadelphia, PA: Wolters Kluwer; 2015:357–364

[32] Stapleton AL, Tyler-Kabara EC, Gardner PA, Snyderman CH, Wang EW. Risk factors for cerebrospinal fluid leak in pediatric patients undergoing endoscopic endonasal skull base surgery. Int J Pediatr Otorhinolaryngol 2017;93:163–166

[33] Koutourousiou M, Filho FV, Costacou T, et al. Pontine encephalocele and abnormalities of the posterior fossa following transclival endoscopic endonasal surgery. J Neurosurg 2014;121(2):359–366

Suggested Readings

Pant H, Snyderman CH, Tyler-Kabara EC, et al. Pediatric skull base surgery. In: Bluestone CD, Simons JP, Healy GB, et al., eds. *Bluestone and Stool's Pediatric Otolaryngology, 5th Edition*. Shelton, CT: PMPH-USA; 2014:1919–1942.

Rastatter JC, Snyderman CH, Gardner PA, Alden TD, Tyler-Kabara E. Endoscopic endonasal surgery for sinonasal and skull base lesions in the pediatric population. *Otolaryngol Clin North Am.* 2015; 48:79–99.

30 Open Approaches to the Anterior Skull Base in Children

Oshri Wasserzug, Ari DeRowe, Barak Ringel, Dan M. Fliss

Summary

The wide variety, nature, and extent of pediatric skull base lesions along with its rarity entail customization of the appropriate surgical approach for its extirpation. Also, the anatomical differences, anticipated craniofacial growth, and the significant overall psychosocial effect compared to adults pose a much more difficult therapeutic challenge.

This chapter will review the different open approaches to the anterior skull base while discussing their advantages and disadvantages.

Keywords: Pediatric, skull base surgery, craniofacial surgery, open approaches

30.1 Introduction

Skull base lesions in children and adolescents are rare, and comprise only 6.4% of all skull base surgery.[1] It includes a wide range of pathological conditions originating from neural, mesenchymal, notochordal, and epithelial origin.[2] Anterior skull base lesions dominate, averaging slightly more than 50% of the cases.[3]

There are several differences between cranial base lesions and tumors in adults and in children. First, the types of tumors, their biological behavior, and oncologic management vary between adults and children.[4] Second, anatomic differences in children may influence the choice of surgical approach.[3,5,6] Third, in addition to the different anatomy, the surgeon should also consider the growth centers in children, trying to avoid damage to these important structures.[7]

In sharp contradiction to the adult population, the most common lesions of the anterior skull base in the pediatric population are congenital lesions: encephaloceles and fibrous dysplasias. Nevertheless, malignant tumors, of which sarcomas are the most frequent, are not uncommon in children.

Although endoscopic skull base surgery in children is gaining popularity in developed countries, in many cases open surgery is still required. In addition, in developing countries, which accounts for more than 80% of the world's population, limited access to expensive equipment precludes the use of endoscopic surgery.

The open approaches that are used most frequently for surgical resection of anterior skull base tumors are the transfacial/transmaxillary, subcranial, and subfrontal. Reconstruction of anterior skull base defects is discussed in a separate chapter in this book.

With this large armamentarium of surgical approaches, tailoring the most suitable approach to a specific lesion in regard to its nature, location, and extent is of utmost importance.

In this chapter we review the literature on the current role of open approaches to the anterior skull base in children.

The following approaches are currently applied for surgical extirpation of anterior skull base tumors in children: (1) subfrontal, (2) subcranial, (3) transfacial/transmaxillary, (4) combined subcranial–transfacial approach, (5) combined subcranial–midfacial degloving, and (6) combined subcranial–transorbital.[1,3,4,8–15]

The approaches that are used most widely for surgical resection of anterior skull base tumors are the transfacial/transmaxillary, subcranial, and subfrontal approaches.[3–5]

30.2 Bilateral/Unilateral Subfrontal Approach

This approach is primarily used for tumors of the anterior skull base with intracranial involvement. It has the advantage of minimizing brain retraction due to wider exposure of the floor of the anterior cranial fossa.

30.2.1 Surgical Technique

- The patient is placed supine with his head held in a Mayfield headholder.
- The skin is cut posterior to the frontal hairline from one zygoma to the other (▶ Fig. 30.1), and the scalp flap and the pericranial flap are reflected anteriorly (▶ Fig. 30.2).

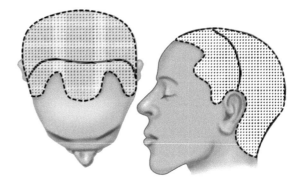

Fig. 30.1 The bicoronal incision line. The skin is cut posterior to the frontal hairline from one zygoma to the other.

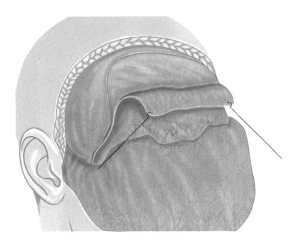

Fig. 30.2 The scalp flap is raised and separated from the pericranium. The pericranium is dissected as a pedicled flap in continuity with the periorbit.

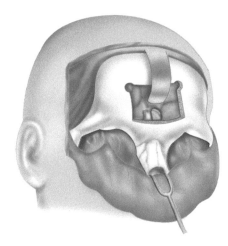

Fig. 30.3 Craniotomy is performed involving both the anterior and posterior tables of the frontal sinuses.

30.3 The Subcranial Approach

The subcranial approach is the most widely used approach to the anterior skull base in our institution.

The main advantage of the subcranial approach is wide exposure of the anterior skull base from below, providing superb access to the sphenoethmoidal, clival, nasal, and orbital regions. Another advantage is minimal manipulation of the frontal lobe and the avoidance of facial scars.

30.3.1 Surgical Technique

- A skin incision is made 2 cm behind the hairline with its lateral border being the supra-auricular area and a bicoronal flap is raised in a supraperiostal plane.
- The flap is raised anteriorly beyond the glabella and the supraorbital ridges (▶Fig. 30.4). The periosteum is elevated from the nasal bones, exposing the nasal tip medially and the lacrimal crests laterally (▶Fig. 30.5).

The dissection is then continued superficial to the temporalis fascia laterally, and the supraorbital nerve, vein, and artery are dissected from the supraorbital notch.

- Exposure of the roofs and the medial and lateral walls of both orbits is done and the anterior ethmoidal arteries are clipped. The periosteum overlying the nasal bones is dissected. The bicoronal flap is then reflected forward over the face and held in position with fishhooks.[16]
- The next step is osteotomy of the anterior or the anterior and posterior walls of the frontal sinus, the proximal segment of the nasal bone, and part of the medial wall of the orbit (▶Fig. 30.6). Miniplates are applied to enable precise repositioning of the bony fragments at the end of the surgery. A type A (▶Fig. 30.6) osteotomy signifies osteotomy of the

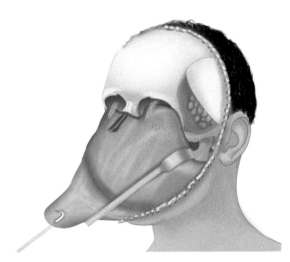

Fig. 30.4 The flap is raised anteriorly beyond the glabella and the supraorbital ridges.

- Craniotomy is performed involving both the anterior and posterior tables of the frontal sinuses[16] (▶Fig. 30.3). If an obliteration of the frontal sinus is performed, the pericranial flap is used after meticulous removal of all visible mucosa.
- In cases in which cranialization is carried out, the posterior wall of the frontal sinus is drilled out and the anterior wall osteotomized segment is repositioned in its original location. When the tumor extends more inferiorly into the orbits and the cribriform area, nasal osteotomies are performed along the mid-portion of the nasal bones and along the naso-lacrimal suture line.
- The dura is dissected off the bone and then orbital osteotomies are done, i.e., the roof and lateral wall of each orbit are removed. By that stage, the tumor is widely exposed and extirpated.

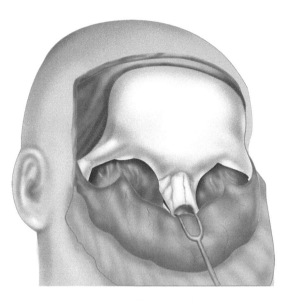

Fig. 30.5 The periosteum is elevated from the nasal bones, exposing the nasal tip medially and the lacrimal crests laterally.

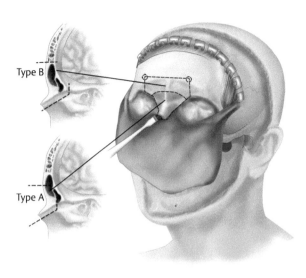

Fig. 30.6 Type A osteotomy leaves the posterior wall of the frontal sinus intact, whereas type B osteotomy includes the posterior wall.

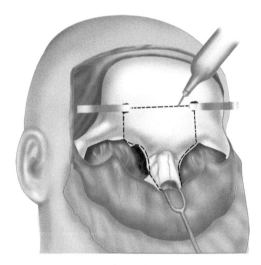

Fig. 30.7 Two burr holes mark the upper lateral limits of the naso-fronto-orbital segment in type B osteotomy.

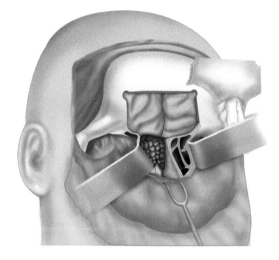

Fig. 30.8 The fronto-naso-orbital segment is extracted.

anterior frontal sinus wall and nasal bone that are removed en-bloc. A type B osteotomy signifies drilling burr holes (▶ Fig. 30.7), after which the posterior frontal sinus wall is resected.

- The fronto-naso-orbital segment is then extracted (▶ Fig. 30.8) and stored in saline. Bilateral sphenoidotomy and bilateral ethmoidectomy ensues, and by that time the tumor is fully exposed and oncological resection can be undertaken.
- Reconstruction begins with the dura, which can be repaired primarily with sutures or using fascia. The fascia is placed in two layers—the first layer is tucked under the dura, and the second layer is aligned to cover the lower surface of the ethmoidal roof and the sphenoidal area (▶ Fig. 30.9).
- In order to reduce telecanthus, two threads are guided through the medial canthal ligament and driven underneath the fronto-naso-orbital segment to the contralateral anterior frontal sinus wall and fixed to the plates.
- The bony fronto-naso-orbital segment is then repositioned and fixed with titanium miniplates in its original anatomical place (▶ Fig. 30.10).

• ▶ Fig. 30.11 depicts the subcranial cavity post-subcranial excision of a pediatric sarcoma. The naso-fronto-orbital segment has been elevated. On the right, the superior, medial, and inferior walls of the orbit have been reconstructed with 3D titanium mesh.

Reconstruction for the subcranial part of the operation is performed identical to the repair of a subcranial defect while the maxilla can be reconstructed either with an obturator or a bony free flap (e.g., scapula or fibula).

30.4 Subcranial–Transfacial Approach

Anterior skull base tumors involving the lateral, anterior, or posterior maxillary walls or the alveolar bone can be exposed and extirpated via a combined subcranial–transfacial approach.[4,5] The transfacial approach includes a Weber–Fergusson incision and maxillectomy (▶ Fig. 30.12a, b). This approach enables wide exposure of the superior and inferior margins of the tumor and its complete en-bloc resection including the maxilla and skull base.

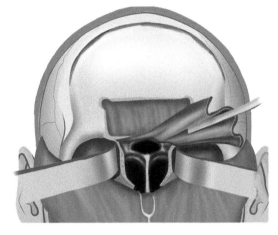

Fig. 30.9 The fascia is placed in two layers—the first layer is tucked under the dura, and the second layer is aligned to cover the lower surface of the ethmoidal roof and the sphenoidal area.

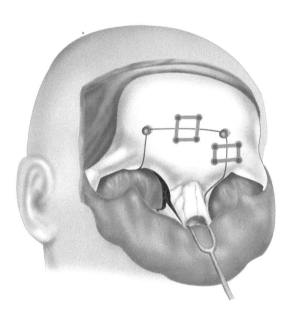

Fig. 30.10 The bony fronto-naso-orbital segment is then repositioned and fixed with titanium miniplates in its original anatomical position.

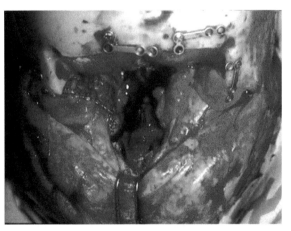

Fig. 30.11 The subcranial cavity post excision of a pediatric sarcoma. The naso-fronto-orbital segment has been elevated. On the right, the superior, medial, and inferior walls of the orbit have been reconstructed with 3D titanium mesh.

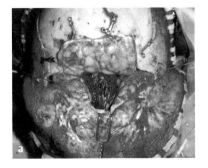

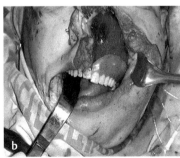

Fig. 30.12 (a, b) A bicoronal and Weber–Ferguson incisions enabled adequate exposure of the surgical field. The skull base was reconstructed using fascia lata. The soft tissue defect was reconstructed with rectus abdominis free flap and an obturator was used to reconstruct the hard palate.

▶Fig. 30.12 (a and b) depicts the combined subcranial–transfacial approach. In this case a maxillectomy has been performed and the subcranial and maxillary defect has been reconstructed with a soft tissue free flap (rectus abdominis) and a prefabricated obturator.

30.5 Midfacial Degloving Approach

The midfacial degloving approach is suitable for small tumors of the anterior skull base which do not invade the superior craniofacial skeleton or skull base but extends inferior and lateral to the midface.[4,9,16]

Its main advantage is cosmetic, as it leaves no scars on the face.

30.5.1 Surgical Technique

- An incision is made at the gingivobuccal sulcus 0.5 cm above the teeth from the first molar on one side to the first molar on the other side (▶Fig. 30.13).
- Transfixion incision is made (▶Fig. 30.14) and connected bilaterally with a complete intercartilagenous incision that separates the lower lateral cartilage from the upper lateral cartilage. The intercartilagenous incision is continued caudomedially through the periosteum of the nasal floor and pyriform aperture.
- The nasal skeleton is being undermined (▶Fig. 30.15), and release and elevation of the soft tissue overlying the maxilla and laterally till the tuberosity and superiorly till the orbital wall ("degloving") follows (▶Fig. 30.16). Care should be taken not to injure the infraorbital nerve.
- The maxillary walls involved are osteotomized on one or two sides, and the tumor is removed after completion of the osteotomies (▶Fig. 30.17).

▶Fig. 30.18 (a and b) show midfacial degloving followed by anterior, medial, and lateral maxillectomy. Care should be taken to avoid injury to the infraorbital nerve.

30.6 The Combined Subcranial–Midfacial Degloving Approach

In tumors of the anterior skull base with caudal extension into the lower and posterior craniofacial planes, the subcranial approach may not provide an adequate exposure.

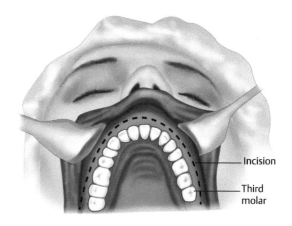

Fig. 30.13 An incision is made at the gingivobuccal sulcus from the first molar on one side to the first molar on the other side.

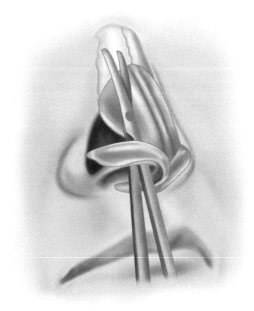

Fig. 30.15 The nasal skeleton is being undermined.

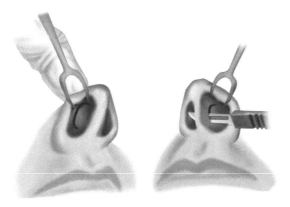

Fig. 30.14 An intercartilaginous incision and a full transfixion incision.

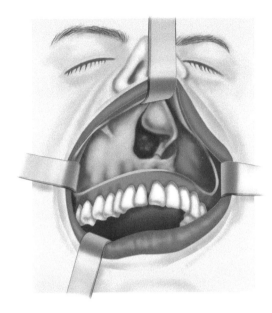

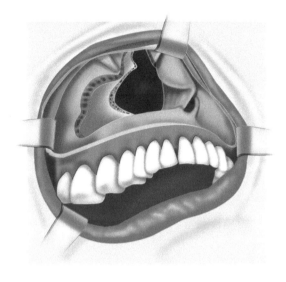

Fig. 30.16 Elevation of the soft tissue overlying the maxilla and laterally till the tuberosity and superiorly till the orbital wall.

Fig. 30.17 The maxillary walls involved are osteotomized on one or two sides, and the tumor is removed after completion of the osteotomies.

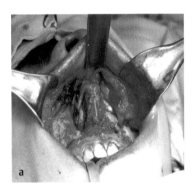

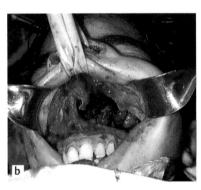

Fig. 30.18 Midfacial degloving **(a)** followed by anterior, medial, and lateral maxillectomy **(b)**.

In these cases the combined subcranial and midfacial degloving technique may be required.[4,9,16]

Upon completion of the subcranial approach with resection of the upper part of the tumor, the midfacial degloving technique follows. Lidocadrain is infiltrated in the gingivobuccal sulcus, the collumella, and the intercartilaginous area. A gingivobuccal incision is done down to the periosteum. The soft tissues overlying the maxilla are raised with preservation of the infraorbital nerves and vessels. Intercartilaginous incisions are made and are continued into a full transfixion incision around the nasal vestibule. Lateral retraction of the soft tissues exposes the maxilla further and enables antrotomy. By that time the tumor should be completely accessible both from its superior and lower extensions.

30.7 The Subcranial–Transorbital Approach

A combined subcranial–transorbital approach is used for tumors that penetrate the bony orbit and infiltrate the orbital content and the anterior skull base.[9,15,17] The subcranial approach is performed as described, followed by orbital exanteration. The eyelids can be spared if there is no tumor involvement, allowing for a better cosmetic result and insertion of an orbital implant in the future. If the tumor extends to the maxilla, a combined subcranial–transorbital–transfacial approach with total maxillectomy should be performed. The defects created by this combined surgical approach are usually reconstructed by a free flap.

30.8 Subcranial–Le Fort I Approach

This approach is used to resect large tumors originating in the clivus with intracranial extension.

The combined subcranial–Le Fort I approach enables wide exposure of the lesion from the cribriform plate to the inferior part of the clivus.[11] Upon completion of the subcranial approach, an osteotomy and down-fracture of the alveolus are performed via a gingivobuccal incision. A partial maxillectomy follows, making the inferior aspect of the tumor and its extension to the nasal cavity and clival region accessible. Specifically, we use the subcranial approach, which provides excellent exposure of the tumor and its circumference for anterior skull base tumors that involved the sphenoid clivus. Most surgeons choose a combination of the subcranial approach with a Le Fort I down-fracture osteotomy when the tumor extends from the anterior skull base inferoposteriorly to involve the lower part of the clivus.

30.8.1 Reconstruction

Anterior skull base defects require reconstruction in order to provide a barrier between the intracranial compartment and the nasal and paranasal cavities.

The type of reconstruction depends on the location, the size, the extent, and the function of the defect, which can be estimated based on preoperative imaging studies and eventually dictated by the intraoperative findings.[16]

The general principles of anterior skull base reconstruction in adults are also applicable to children. However, because children are more likely to suffer from soft tissue sarcomas than adults, the surgical defect is often relatively large and can cause significant aesthetic, psychological, and functional problem. In addition, the effect on facial growth and development should be taken into account. Hence, minimizing developmental and aesthetic complications is of utmost importance.

Whenever possible, primary closure of the dura should be undertaken. When primary closure is not feasible, locoregional flaps should be used. When the defect is small, temporalis fascia which is in the surgical field may be sufficient. When the defect is larger, double layer fascia lata sheath is used to repair the dura. The fascia is inserted under the dura and sutured, trying to achieve watertight closure. In order to protect against CSF leak, fibrin glue is applied to the external layer.[12]

Soft tissue free flaps are the mainstay of treatment for large, three-dimensional defects or defects involving more than one region of the skull base. This method provides soft tissue which is reliable, well vascularized, can cover mucosa, skin, and bone, and can obliterate dead space.

Reconstruction with free flap should also be performed[18,19] in cases of preoperative radiation therapy, osteoradionecrosis, huge median defect, failed anterior skull base reconstruction, or multiple previous surgeries.

Due to its possible influence on facial skeleton growth, bony flaps are used only in adolescents who have reached skeletal maturity.

Reconstruction of the medial orbital wall is undertaken in cases in which complete removal of this segment is mandatory or if the periorbit is excised. Fascia lata sling, split calvarial bone graft, or a titanium mesh covered with pericranium may be used.

30.9 Highlights

a. Indications
   - Subfrontal approach: Tumors of the anterior skull base with intracranial involvement (minimizing brain retraction).
   - Subcranial–transfacial approach: Anterior skull base tumors involving the lateral, anterior or posterior maxillary walls (wide exposure, en bloc resection including the maxilla and skull base).
   - Midfacial degloving approach: Small tumors of the inferior or lateral anterior skull base which do not invade the superior skull base (cosmetic advantage).
   - Subcranial–midfacial degloving approach: Tumors of the anterior skull base with caudal extension into the lower and posterior craniofacial planes.
   - Subcranial–transorbital approach: Tumors that penetrate the bony orbit and infiltrate the orbital content and the anterior skull base.
   - Subcranial–Le Fort I approach: Large tumors originating in the clivus with intracranial extension.
b. Contraindications
   - When endoscopic approach is inaccessible, tailoring the most suitable approach to a specific lesion (nature, location and extent).
c. Complications
   - Wound: infection, dehiscence, seroma, fistula, osteoradinecrosis.
   - CNS: CSF leak, meningitis, pneumocephalus, hemorrhage, seizures.
   - Orbital: globe injury, optic nerve injury, muscles injury, ectropion, telecanthus, ptosis, diplopia, epiphora, enophthalmos.
d. Special preoperative considerations
   - Antibiotics and short acting relaxants.
   - A multidisciplinary team effort.
   - Imaging studies for tumor staging.
   - Consider angiography.
e. Special intraoperative considerations
   - Consider insertion of a lumbar drainage.
   - Avoid shaving the patient's head.

– Form craniotomy segment as small as possible.
– Ensure a tight dural seal to prevent CSF leak.
– Consider vascularized locoregional/free flap for reconstruction.

References

[1] Gil Z, Patel SG, Cantu G, et al; International Collaborative Study Group. Outcome of craniofacial surgery in children and adolescents with malignant tumors involving the skull base: an international collaborative study. Head Neck 2009;31(3):308–317

[2] Kassam A, Thomas AJ, Snyderman C, et al. Fully endoscopic expanded endonasal approach treating skull base lesions in pediatric patients. J Neurosurg 2007;106(2, Suppl):75–86

[3] Mandonnet E, Kolb F, Tran Ba Huy P, George B. Spectrum of skull base tumors in children and adolescents: a series of 42 patients and review of the literature. Childs Nerv Syst 2008;24(6):699–706

[4] Gil Z, Constantini S, Spektor S, et al. Skull base approaches in the pediatric population. Head Neck 2005;27(8):682–689

[5] Brockmeyer D, Gruber DP, Haller J, Shelton C, Walker ML. Pediatric skull base surgery: experience and outcomes in 55 patients. Pediatr Neurosurg 2003;38(1):9–15

[6] Stapleton AL, Tyler-Kabara EC, Gardner PA, Snyderman CH, Wang EW. Risk factors for cerebrospinal fluid leak in pediatric patients undergoing endoscopic endonasal skull base surgery. Int J Pediatr Otorhinolaryngol 2017;93:163–166

[7] Shlomi B, Chaushu S, Gil Z, Chaushu G, Fliss DM. Effects of the subcranial approach on facial growth and development. Otolaryngol Head Neck Surg 2007;136(1):27–32

[8] Youssef CA, Smotherman CR, Kraemer DF, Aldana PR. Predicting the limits of the endoscopic endonasal approach in children: a radiological anatomical study. J Neurosurg Pediatr 2016;17(4):510–515

[9] Fliss DM, Zucker G, Amir A, Gatot A. The combined subcranial and midfacial degloving technique for tumor resection: report of three cases. J Oral Maxillofac Surg 2000;58(1):106–110

[10] Rastatter JC, Snyderman CH, Gardner PA, Alden TD, Tyler-Kabara E. Endoscopic endonasal surgery for sinonasal and skull base lesions in the pediatric population. Otolaryngol Clin North Am 2015;48(1):79–99

[11] Lewark TM, Allen GC, Chowdhury K, Chan KH. Le Fort I osteotomy and skull base tumors: a pediatric experience. Arch Otolaryngol Head Neck Surg 2000;126(8):1004–1008

[12] Fishman G, Fliss DM, Benjamin S, et al. Multidisciplinary surgical approach for cerebrospinal fluid leak in children with complex head trauma. Childs Nerv Syst 2009;25(8):915–923

[13] Gao X, Zhang R, Mao Y, Wang Y. Childhood and juvenile meningiomas. Childs Nerv Syst 2009;25(12):1571–1580

[14] Hassler W, Zentner J. Pterional approach for surgical treatment of olfactory groove meningiomas. Neurosurgery 1989;25(6): 942–945, discussion 945–947

[15] Wasserzug O, DeRowe A, Ringel B, Fishman G, Fliss DM. Open approaches to the anterior skull base in children: review of the literature. J Neurol Surg B Skull Base 2018;79(1):42–46

[16] Fliss DM, Abergel A, Cavel O, Margalit N, Gil Z. Combined subcranial approaches for excision of complex anterior skull base tumors. Arch Otolaryngol Head Neck Surg 2007;133(9):888–896

[17] Fliss DM, Zucker G, Amir A, Gatot A, Cohen JT, Spektor S. The subcranial approach for anterior skull base tumors. Oper Tech Otolaryngol—Head Neck Surg 2000;11:238–253

[18] Li Z, Li H, Wang S, Zhao J, Cao Y. Pediatric SBM:. clinical features and surgical outcomes. J Child Neurol 2016;31(14): 1523–1527

[19] Turazzi S, Cristofori L, Gambin R, Bricolo A. The pterional approach for the microsurgical removal of olfactory groove meningiomas. Neurosurgery 1999;45(4):821–825, discussion 825–826

31 Surgical Approach to the Lateral Skull Base

Omer J. Ungar, Dan M. Fliss, Yahav Oron

Summary

The infratemporal fossa–middle cranial fossa approach gives wide access to all of the subcranial tissues that underlie the middle fossa floor. Ugo Fisch of Zurich, designed the infratemporal fossa approach and first presented it in 1977. It forms the basis for all the accesses to the lateral and inferolateral skull base that have been developed since. The procedure described in this chapter is closely similar to Schramm and Sekhar's operation, with some modifications. The primary consideration in this chapter is the presence of a tumor, but patients who require lateral skull base surgery present with a wide variety of disease processes. A thorough preoperative evaluation is crucial for a successful operation. The surgical procedure includes the following steps: extensive preparation; incision (anterior or posterior); external auditory canal obliteration; internal carotid artery and internal jugular vein exposure; temporalis muscle elevation; zygomatic ostectomy; mandibular condylectomy; exposure of the subtemporal trapezoid muscle; otologic exposure; craniotomy; carotid dissection and eustachian tube removal; cavernous sinus resection; dura and brain resection; and reconstruction.

Keywords: Lateral skull base surgery, infratemporal fossa, middle cranial fossa, surgical approach

31.1 Introduction

Probably the most difficult and complex of all the pathways in skull base surgery is the infratemporal fossa–middle cranial fossa approach. It is also the most versatile, giving access not only to all of the subcranial tissues that underlie the middle fossa floor from the zygoma to the nasopharynx, but also to the contents of the middle cranial fossa from the lesser sphenoid wing to the tentorium, including the petrous ridge and cavernous sinus (▶Fig. 31.1). The clivus will be widely exposed and cutting the tentorium can expose the upper brain stem.

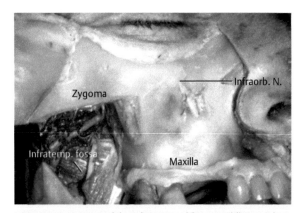

Fig. 31.1 Anatomy of the infratemporal fossa–middle cranial fossa.

Considerable credit must be given to the originators of this operation. Ugo Fisch of Zurich designed the infratemporal fossa approach and first presented it in 1977.[1] It forms the basis for all the accesses to the lateral and inferolateral skull base that have been developed since.[2] The first well-coordinated intracranial and extracranial approach to this region was designed by Victor Schramm[3] and Laligam Sekhar. They modified Fisch's design and created an excellent simultaneous exposure of the intracranial and extracranial aspects of the middle fossa through a small but strategically placed craniotomy. The removal of this bony barrier improved maneuverability in both the intracranial and extracranial compartments. The procedure described in this chapter is closely similar to Schramm and Sekhar's operation, with some modifications.

Patients who require resection of malignant disease using the middle fossa skull base approach usually have a more extensive lesion than those who need anterior fossa skull base surgery. They often require longer periods of time in the intensive care unit and a more prolonged hospital stay. The keystone structures that are responsible for many of the problems arising from this surgery are the cavernous sinus and the internal carotid artery (ICA). Resection of either or both structures may leave the patient with substantial deficits. In cases of malignancy, the entire sinus often needs to be removed, creating an immobile and sometimes insensate eye with ptosis of the upper lid. The cornea, therefore, is extremely prone to injury, not only from trauma but also from sympathetic dystrophy secondary to autonomic denervation. If the original tumor is an extension from a lesion in the paranasal sinuses, the orbit will usually be exenterated and those sequelae would not be issue. Management of the carotid is still inconclusive, but arterial invasion usually mandates resection in cases of malignancy and grafting rather than sacrifice, even in the presence of a negative balloon test occlusion (BTO) and a favorable single-photon emission computed tomography (SPECT) scan. It should be noted that resection of the cavernous ICA and the cavernous sinus in the setting of malignancy, especially squamous cell carcinoma, remains highly controversial.

31.2 Preoperative Evaluation and Anesthesia

Patients who require lateral skull base surgery present with a wide variety of disease processes. The primary consideration in this chapter is the presence of a tumor. A tumor may be benign or malignant and may originate either intracranially from dura or calvarial bone or extracranially from the numerous soft tissues that occupy the subcranial area. Most common among the intracranial neoplasms that extend extracranially are meningioma, chordoma, chondroma, and chondrosarcoma. Among the extracranial tumors that extend intracranially are schwannoma (often of the trigeminal nerve), parotid tumors (both benign and malignant, especially from the deep lobe), and squamous cell carcinomas from the paranasal sinuses, nasopharynx, and temporal bone. Metastatic deposits in lymph nodes from any head and neck site, but more often from the nasopharynx or paranasal sinuses, may erode through the middle fossa skull base. Rarely, metastases from distant sites may present as a pathologic node at the skull base. A rather curious inflammatory lesion that may present as a skull base neoplasm both in symptomatology and in radiographic appearance is a variant of Tolosa–Hunt syndrome.

Unfortunately, the presenting symptoms of lesions in this area are often subtle. Many patients complain of pain only in the region of the infratemporal fossa, ear, or behind the eye. This symptom is often passed off as myofascial dysfunction or "temporomandibular joint" (TMJ) syndrome. Trismus secondary to pterygoid muscle invasion or direct involvement of the mandibular branch of the trigeminal nerve may likewise be misdiagnosed. Any patient with a history of carcinoma of the nasopharynx or oropharynx must be considered with a high index of suspicion when presenting with pain in the infratemporal fossa.

Special attention should be focused on the patient with oropharyngeal carcinoma who, after the standard therapy of composite resection and postoperative radiation therapy, presents with pain deep in the infratemporal fossa, especially if the pain is new. There is often little to find on physical examination other than an occasional increase in trismus. Because the inferior alveolar nerve had been sacrificed in the initial resection, the only remaining sensory nerve from V3 is the auriculotemporal, which may also have been injured at surgery. Such patients should undergo magnetic resonance imaging (MRI). Because of the anatomic distortions created by past surgery and radiation, it is often difficult to distinguish fibrosis and edema from tumor, even with gadolinium contrast. Serial MRIs at 6-week to 3-month intervals are often the only means by which a diagnosis can be made. Unfortunately, valuable time may be lost as the tumor continues to grow and is constantly at risk of metastasizing. Analysis by positron emission tomography (PET) scanning may be of considerable assistance. Symptoms of carcinoma of the temporal bone may range from subtle to obvious. Painful otorrhea unresponsive to vigorous local therapy is highly suspicious of carcinoma.

As in temporal bone carcinoma, malignancies in the infratemporal fossa, especially parotid gland carcinomas, may present with a facial nerve paralysis. Recurrent carcinoma or tumors of the deep lobe often involve the facial nerve. Paresis or complete paralysis of the entire nerve, indicating main trunk invasion, is usually the rule.

Extension of tumor through the foramen ovale along the third division of the trigeminal nerve can produce numbness over its sensory distribution and, by spreading through the gasserian ganglion, hypesthesia of both the first and second divisions of the trigeminal nerve. This manifests itself initially as numbness over the chin and lower face and then advances to numbness over the midface, especially the area innervated by the infraorbital nerve with V2 involvement and the forehead and cornea with V1 involvement. Extension into the cavernous sinus is imminent once the tumor has reached the gasserian ganglion in Meckel's cave, and paralysis of the oculomotor, trochlear, and abducens nerves often follows, resulting in ptosis and ophthalmoplegia.

Tumor extension directly from the nasopharynx usually follows the foramen lacerum. The subsequent invasion of the cavernous sinus commonly produces abducens nerve paralysis with a lateral rectus palsy. Invasion of the lateral wall of the sinus results in affliction of cranial nerves III and IV, and eventually involvement of V2, V3, and the optic nerve with extension superiorly.

Invasion of the carotid artery is usually asymptomatic. The tumor is rarely so advanced as to completely occlude the vessel but, were that to occur, a stroke may ensue. This is possible even with reduced flow in a patient with already compromised cerebral circulation.

Involvement of temporal dura commonly produces unremitting, intense headache. Because much of the temporal lobe is "silent," brain invasion provides little in the way of differentiating signs and symptoms.

Lower cranial nerves may be affected when there is metastatic spread to high internal jugular, parapharyngeal, or retropharyngeal lymph nodes. Extracapsular tumor spread from those nodes may erode skull base bone and invade the jugular foramen, producing symptoms secondary to affliction of cranial nerves IX, X, XI, and XII (the latter with spread to the adjacent hypoglossal canal). The cervical sympathetic may be involved, producing Horner's syndrome. Clinical investigation of these patients, after a thorough head and neck and neurologic examination, includes a thorough general medical assessment. If a tumor is deemed operable, two other medical conditions preclude an attempt at infratemporal fossa–middle cranial fossa excision. The first is the presence of distant metastasis and the second is general lack of medical fitness, such as that from extensive physiologic aging, severe cardiovascular disease, poorly controlled diabetes, or incipient renal or hepatic failure, all of which are contraindications to that surgery. A final contraindication to surgery is lack of patient commitment. Some natural reluctance to undergo such an extensive procedure is anticipated, but a tendency toward resistance on the part of the patient, coupled with overzealous enthusiasm on the part of family or friends, should be carefully assessed as well.

MRI with gadolinium contrast and, if indicated, fat suppression should be complemented by fine-cut computed tomography scanning through the skull base. The coronal plane is most helpful in clearly outlining carotid involvement and cavernous sinus invasion. Bony detail is best delineated with computed tomography, and soft tissue invasion by MRI. Gadolinium contrast is extremely helpful in differentiating tumor from adjacent soft tissue, especially in recurrent or persistent disease. A word of warning regarding these studies: there are false-negative and false-positive scans, and those studies do not always accurately delineate the extent of tumor, tending to minimize or exaggerate the true dimensions.

There are many methods of evaluating the patency of the circle of Willis but, more importantly, the surgeon must assess the amount of blood flow from the collateral circulation if the ICA on the tumor side is removed. The gold standard has been BTO of the ICA using radioactive xenon to provide a calculation of cerebral blood flow before and after temporary occlusion. Xenon studies are notoriously difficult to perform because of frequent fluctuations in gas concentrations and problems with the measuring equipment. The determination of cerebral blood flow SPECT with technetium-99m hexamethylpropyleneamine oxime contrast has been proven to be much more practical.

The PET scan is the investigative tool most recently incorporated into the armamentarium. Because of the avidity of tumor cells for glucose, the patient is given a non-metabolizing, radioactive, fluoridated analogue after which the PET scans are carried out. As with all skull base tumor patients, there must be extensive discussion between the patient and the head and neck surgeon, the neurosurgeon, and the plastic surgeon. It is important for the patient to understand the arduousness of the procedure, what functions will be lost, what cosmetic deformities will result, and what other treatment options exist. Skull base surgery often remains the only chance for cure for malignant tumors. The surgeon must be realistic—not overly enthusiastic, but encouraging—when discussing options with these often desperate patients.

The usage of paralytic agents during anesthesia should enable proper monitoring of the cranial nerves. Perioperative antibiotics should be administered.

31.3 Surgical Technique

31.3.1 Preparation

A Mayfield horseshoe head rest is used for ease of surgical access unless the neurosurgeon insists upon fixation pins. Central venous pressure and arterial lines are usually placed, and cranial nerve monitoring devices are inserted. Electroencephalography electrodes are sutured or stapled to the scalp to monitor cerebral electrical activity in cases of possible ICA sacrifice.

An extensive surgical preparation is usually necessary, including a scrub of the entire face, head, neck, and anterior chest.[3,4] The abdomen is also prepared if a rectus abdominis flap is to be used as a vascularized free tissue transfer for reconstruction. Both legs are often scrubbed in anticipation of the possible harvest of a lateral thigh-free flap, split-thickness skin, fascia lata, or saphenous vein grafts.

31.3.2 Incision

There are two standard types of skin incision,[5–8] depending upon the location of the lesion (▶ Fig. 31.2). The incision for parotidectomy extends in a curvilinear fashion from the vertex of the skull, in front of the ear in a preauricular crease, and under the lobule of the ear, then curves forward in the upper neck, resembling a modified Blair incision (▶ Fig. 31.2a). The posterior incision for more anteriorly located lesions, such as deep-lobe parotid tumors, lesions invading the foramen ovale, or nasopharyngeal carcinoma, starts 2 to 4 cm behind the ear, similar to the incision described by Fisch, and extends into the neck toward the hyoid (▶ Fig. 31.2b). Posterior incisions are used for lesions such as temporal bone carcinomas, extensive glomus jugulare tumors, and clival chordomas A lazy-S incision is subtended into the neck if a neck dissection is planned to accompany the procedure.

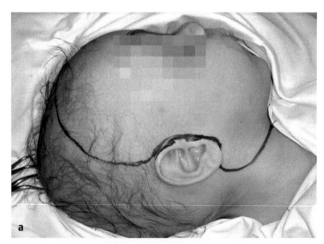
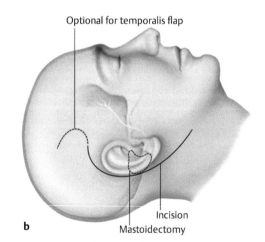

Optional for temporalis flap

Incision

Mastoidectomy

a

b

Fig. 31.2 (a) Anterior skin incision. **(b)** Posterior skin incision.

The scalp incision extends to the level of the pericranium[5] (▶ Fig. 31.3 and ▶ Fig. 31.4). The temporalis muscle is identified as the flap is formed. The superficial and deep temporalis fascia are incised in a semilunar manner to include the frontal branch of the facial nerve, which emerges approximately 1.5 cm in front of the auricle and arches into the frontalis muscle approximately 2 to 2.5 cm above the brow.[6] This maneuver protects the nerve from injury.

The cervicofacial portion of the incision proceeds superficially to the platysma and superficial muscular aponeurotic system fascia in a plane similar to that in a superficial plane face lift. It continues forward anteriorly from the angle of the mandible to the lateral orbital rim. When using this anterior incision, a decision whether to cut across the external auditory canal (EAC) is made, usually predicated on the necessity of exposing the ICA. In contrast, the posterior incision always cuts across the canal because carotid exposure is usually necessary.

31.3.3 External Auditory Canal Obliteration

Exposure of the petrous portion of the ICA will be required in most instances of both anterior and posterior incisions. This is best facilitated by exposing and later obliterating the eustachian tube. A decision regarding the elimination of the middle ear cleft and the EAC or the preservation of a non-ventilated middle ear cleft and the permanent instillation of a ventilating tube is often difficult. For ease of management and fewer complications, there is little question that obliteration is the treatment of choice. However, maintenance of the integrity of the middle ear and EAC and the use of a ventilating tube is preferable in patients for whom the preservation of hearing is a consideration as well as in young patients.

If the EAC is to be obliterated, it is best done at this juncture. The obliteration technique described by Fisch is easy to perform and has predictable results. This is certainly the technique of choice in patients with nasopharyngeal carcinoma or in those with failed radiation therapy.

31.3.4 Internal Carotid Artery and Internal Jugular Vein Exposure

The internal jugular vein (IJV) and ICA are identified and dissected superiorly as close as possible to the skull base foramina through which they pass.[6-8] Care is taken to avoid injury to cranial nerves IX through XII during the dissection. Soft rubber catheters are placed around the IJV and ICA for later control of bleeding, if necessary. The upper end of this dissection may need to be postponed until the mandibular condylectomy has been completed. The ICA will eventually need to be exposed in order to visualize the fibrous ring and the entrance of the artery into the skull at the carotid foramen. Similarly, the IJV will need to be dissected up to the jugular foramen.

31.3.5 Temporalis Muscle Elevation

The temporalis muscle body is exposed in its entirety[5-9] (▶ Fig. 31.5). It may serve as the reconstructive flap that separates the middle cranial fossa from the upper aerodigestive tract. Maintaining its viability is essential, and integral to that is an understanding of its blood supply. The superior supply from the superficial temporal artery and branches of the postauricular artery is unavoidably eliminated during the muscle elevation. The integrity of the inferior supply through the deep temporal branches is maintained with great care. These deep branches emerge from the internal maxillary artery both directly posteriorly and anteriorly to the foramen ovale. The posterior

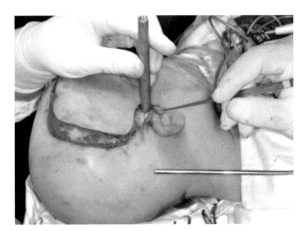

Fig. 31.3 Scalp incision.

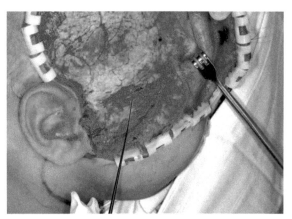

Fig. 31.4 Scalp incision.

artery exits the internal maxillary artery just anterior to its emergence from under the neck of the mandible. The anterior deep temporal artery leaves the internal maxillary artery just before its disappearance into the pterygomaxillary fissure. Indiscriminate cautery in this area in an attempt to achieve hemostasis of the prolific bleeding often encountered from the pterygoid plexus of veins may compromise the anterior deep temporal artery. The use of bipolar cautery is advised.

The temporalis muscle is elevated in its entirety, usually with a 2-cm cuff of pericranium (▶Fig. 31.6). Careful elevation with a broad, flat elevator, like the von Langenbeck device helps to maintain the integrity of the muscle. The muscle is elevated along the calvarium as it curves from a vertical to an oblique plane. Further dissection for exposure of the deep inferior part of the infratemporal fossa is impeded by the presence of the zygomatic arch.

Infiltration of the temporalis muscle may be observed at this point in highly invasive tumors. The muscle must then become part of the resection. If tumor involvement is suspected by preoperative studies, the pericranium adjacent to the muscle is preserved if it is oncologically sound.

31.3.6 Zygomatic Ostectomy

The zygomatic arch, including a part of the body and the orbital process, is removed in one piece in order to completely expose the infratemporal fossa[7] (▶Fig. 31.7a–c). Incision of the periosteum is followed by a subperiosteal elevation from directly in front of the articular process to the posterior part of the malar eminence, superiorly around the lateral orbital rim, and immediately adjacent to the lateral orbital wall. Care is taken to avoid perforating the periorbita and to gently protect it with a malleable retractor during subsequent drilling. Drill holes are placed in the arch and the orbital rim in anticipation of placing miniplates for later reconstruction.

A fine-blade power saw is used to cut across the posterior arch just anterior to the articular eminence. The sagittal saw then cuts across the lateral orbital rim above the zygomaticofrontal suture at an approximate depth of 2 to 4 mm until the thin lateral orbital wall is encountered. This cut is extended down the lateral orbital wall just inside the rim until the inferior orbital fissure has been reached. The final cut is through the posterior portion

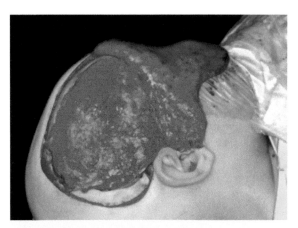

Fig. 31.5 Temporalis muscle exposure.

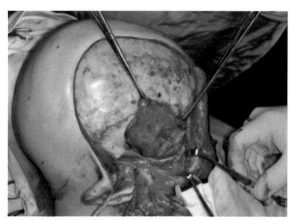

Fig. 31.6 Temporalis muscle elevation.

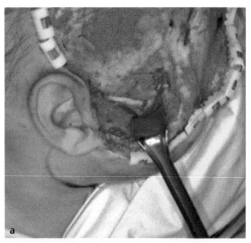
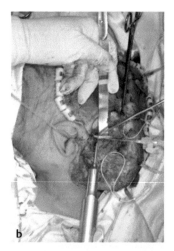
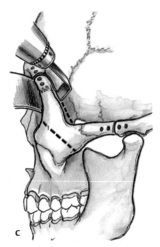

Fig. 31.7 (a–c) Zygomatic osteotomy.

of the zygomatic body, from the beginning of the malar eminence to the inferior orbital fissure. The last vestiges of soft tissue are removed from their attachments to the zygoma, and the bone is removed and stored in a saline-soaked sponge until the reconstructive phase.

31.3.7 Mandibular Condylectomy

A mandibular condylectomy is the last step in removing impediments to the deep infratemporal fossa.[5-7] Some controversy surrounds the management of the condylar process and the TMJ during this procedure. In the opinion of some surgeons, an incision of the TMJ and inferior retraction of the meniscus and condylar head provide adequate exposure and preserve joint integrity. There have, however, been some reports of stiffness, pain, and TMJ dysfunction resulting from this technique.

Key to the removal of the condyle is avoiding severance of the internal maxillary artery that runs deep to the condylar neck. Protection of this vessel is vital because its destruction will devascularize the temporalis muscle. The secret to its preservation is a subperiosteal dissection.

Some of the insertion of the lateral pterygoid muscle that penetrates the anterior surface of the TMJ capsule is dissected away by cauterization. The periosteum is incised along the anterior and lateral aspects of the condylar head by going through the temporomandibular ligament and the TMJ capsule. Sharp dissection with an elevator, such as the Obwegeser device, allows dissection around the mandibular neck. A malleable retractor is placed deep within the mandibular neck and a cutting tool is used to transect it just below the condyle. Removal of the condyle is completed by dissecting the remaining soft tissue attachments on the deep and posterior surface of the TMJ. Both the condyle and the meniscus are removed. This exposes the glenoid fossa and opens an access for the dissection of the subcranial part of the middle cranial fossa floor.

31.3.8 Exposure of the Subtemporal Trapezoid Muscle

With the removal of the zygomatic arch and the condyle, the temporalis muscle can now be dissected down to its insertion on the coronoid process and anterior surface of the mandibular ramus.[9,10] As this dissection continues and the muscle is carefully retracted inferiorly, exposure of the undersurface of the sphenoid and temporal bones is gradually achieved. The glenoid fossa is cleared of residual soft tissue in order to expose the anteromedial aspect of the fossa, which leads to the sphenoid spine. The middle meningeal artery, which is the posteromedial target of the dissection at this point, is deep and anterior to the sphenoid spine. A few millimeters anterior to it is the foramen ovale and the emergence of cranial nerve V3, the second medial target structure. Soft tissue dissection from the lateral orbital wall inferiorly leads to the

origin of the pterygoid plates, the superior surfaces of the pterygoid muscles, and the pterygoid venous plexus.

A line that connects the articular eminence to the hamulus of the medial pterygoid plate, from there to the occipital condyle and then to the mastoid process and back to the eminence, will form a trapezoid. All of the important neurovascular structures relevant to the middle fossa skull base are contained within that shape. The two target structures for the inferomedial extent of the craniotomy, namely, the foramen spinosum and foramen ovale, are seen when a direct line is made anteriorly from the anteromedial extremity of the glenoid fossa.[6]

At this point, if there is any doubt about an intracranial spread of tumor up the mandibular branch of the trigeminal nerve, it should be sampled for biopsy. If subcranial tumor is found to be present, the bone around the foramen ovale is drilled away and the nerve is exposed at the level of the middle fossa dura on the floor of Meckel's cave. The nerve is amputated at this point and sent for frozen-section histologic analysis. If the result is positive for tumor spread, the craniotomy proceeds, beginning with the otologic exposure.

31.3.9 Otologic Exposure

The auricle is retracted posteriorly after the EAC has been transected at the bony–cartilaginous junction. There are often a few millimeters of thick canal skin with some remnants of conchal cartilage that need to be excised into the bony EAC. If the ear is planned to be obliterated, less care needs to be exercised in excising this skin because the entire remaining medial canal skin as well as the tympanic membrane will be removed. The operating microscope is brought in for the next phase.

An anterior tympanomeatal flap is constructed when the middle ear is to be preserved. The flap is cut through two incisions in the canal skin at approximately 6 and 12 o'clock and connected laterally. The inferior incision is carried to the annulus and the superior incision is approximately 2 mm short of the notch of Rivinus. The skin sleeve is dissected down the anterior canal wall to the tympanic annulus from the hypotympanic level up to the anterior mallear fold. The skin is elevated over the bone of the scutum and is reflected posteriorly to promote flap mobilization. The annulus is prized from its sulcus, and the anterior hypotympanum and the entire protympanum are exposed. The tympanomeatal flap is reflected posteriorly to provide full exposure of the tympanic portion of the eustachian tube and the hemicanal of the tensor tympani muscle above it.

Two bony incisions in the EAC are constructed. The superior one starts at the squamosal part of the temporal bone directly above the EAC at 12 o'clock. The cut progresses through the bone until the temporal bone dura is exposed for a few millimeters and the floor of the middle fossa is reached. A drill cut is directed from this point to the anterior part of the epitympanum to the mallear head. It is even better to angle this cut such that it goes through posterior zygomatic root cells, missing the malleus altogether. The exposed anterior mallear ligaments are cut, and the bur is carried over the hemicanal of the tensor tympani, taking great care to remain anterior to the cochleariform process and thus avoiding the facial nerve. The hemicanal is transected and a deep groove made in the superior wall of the protympanum.

Inferiorly, a bur cut is made in the EAC bone, going through the tympanic bone into the glenoid fossa. The cut proceeds medially down the canal and into the inferior aspect of the protympanum at about 7 o'clock. The tympanic annulus is transected at this point, and a fissure is again made in the protympanum but less deep than the superior one in order to avoid injuring the ICA. The subsequent craniotomy cuts will merge with these incisions in the temporal bone.

31.3.10 Craniotomy

The key to the exposure of the middle fossa and its immediate subcranial structures is an L-shaped craniotomy that has a vertical component comprised of the greater wing of the sphenoid and squamosal aspects of the temporal bone, and a short horizontal component that ends at the foramen ovale and foramen spinosum[5–9] (▶Fig. 31.8a, b). Often a modest-sized craniotomy provides adequate exposure. The size is usually determined by intracranial tumor extent.

Initially, it is advisable to perform the inferior part of the craniotomy, only a part of which exposes dura. A switch from the otologic round bur to the Midas Rex B5 attachment increases the speed at which these inferior bony cuts can be made. A through-and-through incision is made through the anterior EAC bone into and through the glenoid fossa plate. The complete full-thickness incision stops at the level of the tympanic annulus. This bony incision extends into the mesotympanum from the annulus to the inferior protympanum at a depth of approximately 2 to 3 mm. A similar incision of the same depth is made in the glenoid fossa and extended from the annulus to the foramen spinosum. Too deep a cut will endanger the ICA. The middle meningeal artery is clipped or coagulated with a bipolar cautery. The foramen spinosum is connected to the posterior lip of the foramen ovale. The dura is exposed by this incision from the foramen spinosum anteriorly. Venous extensions of the cavernous sinus may sometimes supply the foraminal portion of V3. Inadvertent rupture of these vessels often occurs during the bony cuts and even during the soft tissue extension. The bleeding usually stops with bipolar cautery. Anteriorly, this incision is extended horizontally until the cutting tool reaches just above the insertion of the pterygoid plates. This point marks the beginning of the vertical course of the craniotomy. It will proceed superiorly in the anterior reach of the infratemporal fossa.

With the near-completion of the inferior portion of the craniotomy, the superior part over the greater sphenoid wing and squamosal temporal bone is initiated. The extent of the craniotomy depends mainly upon the degree of invasion of the temporal lobe dura. Often, only the dura of the floor of the middle fossa is involved, whereupon no more than a limited craniotomy will be required.

A bur hole is made at or inferior to the pterion[5,6,9] with the M5 bur of the Midas Rex or a standard craniotome. Dural elevation permits the introduction of the footed handpiece, and the craniotomy proceeds in a posterior superior loop, ending at the dural exposure at the top of the otologic incision superior to the EAC. The handpiece is removed, reinserted into the bur hole, and directed inferiorly to the previously made cut above the pterygoid plates.

The dura is carefully elevated at the periphery of the bone cuts, with special attention paid to its brittleness in the elderly. A broad elevator is used to dissect the dura from the superior craniotomy incision to the middle fossa floor. A gentle prying motion is used to fracture the craniotomy bone flap through the previously drilled faults in the temporal bone. The fracture will be through the lateral wall of the bony eustachian tube. This is a crucial maneuver. The open eustachian tube reveals the bulge of the ICA canal in its medial wall. The bony wall is sometimes dehiscent and carotid pulsations can be visualized through the tubal mucosa. This relationship is the vital key to the safe dissection of the carotid artery. At this point, the vertical portion of the artery is bending into the horizontal part.

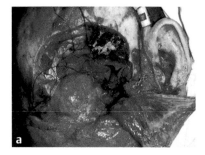
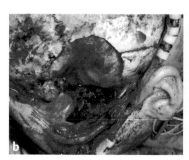

Fig. 31.8 (a, b) Craniotomy.

The cut through the foramen ovale reveals the mandibular branch of the trigeminal nerve as it approximates the dura that invests it.[6]

31.3.11 Carotid Dissection and Eustachian Tube Resection

Two principal structures complicate middle fossa surgery: the ICA and the cavernous sinus. The ICA is exposed as much as is necessary to resect the entire tumor.[7,8,10] Once identified in the medial wall of the bony eustachian tube, the vertical portion of the artery is uncovered by beginning at the fibrous ring at the carotid foramen and working superiorly to the tube. The carotid canal is progressively exposed by removing bone first laterally, then anteriorly, posteriorly, and even medially when required.

The bony eustachian tube is now removed with the drill, gradually exposing the ICA. The artery often parallels the tube for a short distance, but then the tube angles inferiorly and away from the vessels. The bony tube quickly gives way to cartilage because the latter comprises two-thirds of its length. The cartilage is a little more difficult to drill, but it is excised as far as is necessary to expose the artery. In nasopharyngeal carcinoma and other tumors with tubal involvement, the entire cartilaginous tube is usually excised and the bone in which it nestles is removed wide of all tumor invasion. This approach is especially suited to nasopharyngeal carcinoma resection because the entire eustachian tube, the origins of the palatal muscles, and all adjacent bone can be widely resected, a feature that is not possible in all other approaches to nasopharyngeal malignancy. This is the most direct and by far the safest surgical method for this disease. The artery lies under a very thin layer of bone on the middle fossa floor where the bone is often dehiscent in spots. In its more medial course, it underlies the gasserian ganglion, which may need to be sacrificed if carotid involvement by tumor extends that far.

The bony removal continues under microscopic control up to the foramen lacerum. The ICA then resumes a vertical course through the middle fossa floor into the cavernous sinus. It is now fully freed (when required by tumor involvement) from the fibrous ring to the foramen lacerum. Any middle fossa floor invaded by tumor is resected. The tough periosteal lining of the carotid canal provides a firm barrier to the penetration of even the most aggressive tumors.

Decisions regarding carotid artery management are still controversial and center around two main features: The first is the biology of the tumor in question, and the second involves the anatomic site of invasion. For the most part, benign tumors and low-grade malignancies tend to have pushing rather than infiltrating borders. The acinic cell and adenoid cystic carcinomas tend to be quite infiltrative extracranially, but are a pushing, less aggressive type of tumor intracranially. Squamous cell carcinomas and malignant melanomas, on the other hand, are more locally aggressive. The anatomic location along the course of the carotid also determines the extent of resection. The fibrous ring at the entrance to the skull base is very dense and thick, providing a protective barrier to the penetration of even squamous cell carcinoma. The ring can sometimes be dissected to the arterial media and the tumor can be encompassed. The petrous course of the carotid also has a configuration that resists tumor penetration. The inner surface of the canal is lined with periosteum. A loose connective tissue containing a few small nutrient blood vessels connects the periosteum to the denser collagenous tissue comprising the arterial adventitia, followed by the arterial media and intima. The vessel is suspended within the canal and possesses three barriers for the tumor to breach before actual arterial invasion takes place.

The cavernous carotid has very thin connective tissue on most of its wall. The medial wall is plastered to the cavernous sinus dura and is intimately related to the intracranial side of the lateral wall of the sphenoid sinus. Spread of tumor to the main body of the cavernous sinus usually leads to carotid invasion. The arterial wall is thin and easily penetrated by tumor. The safety of ICA excision in its cranial course without the placement of a graft is very much open to question. If the artery must be excised, the current wisdom is to use an interposition graft. The saphenous vein is probably the best graft material, although synthetics may also be used. Once the artery is removed, the graft is placed quickly while the patient is under barbiturate coma. The patient is heparinized during graft placement, then reversed with protamine once all leaks have been sealed. Clamp time is kept to a minimum.

The carotid resection and graft are done under microscopic control. All preliminary steps, such as vascular sutures, instruments, and alternative graft materials, must be readily at hand before clamping of the vessel. It must also be ensured that there is adequate exposure at the distal and proximal ends of the artery, leaving room to clamp and then excise the vessel with an adequate cuff for suturing. This is facilitated by total mobilization of the artery from the cervical part to the cavernous portion. Once both anastomoses are completed, the clamps are removed, the leaks are sutured, and Gelfoam patches soaked in thrombin are placed around the suture lines.

31.3.12 Cavernous Sinus Resection

A cavernous sinus resection often precedes the management of the carotid artery. The artery is freed from its canal, and the cavernous sinus is resected if tumor persists beyond the petrous part. Small outpouchings of the sinus project along the three branches of the trigeminal nerve as they enter their foramina. In addition, there are numerous connections to other veins and dural sinuses. Minimal invasion at these sites can limit the amount of the sinus that can be removed. Frozen-section examination of these margins is critical.

Major invasion of the sinus tends to compress the venous structures within, and dissection proceeds rather easily until the invasive edge is reached. The profuse hemorrhage characteristic of this structure is then encountered. Both the soft tissue component of the sinus and the adjacent bone must be removed.

Due to its complicated anatomy, cavernous dissection is done in a slow and methodical manner under an operating microscope. Because of its propensity for brisk hemorrhage, the cavernous sinus must be removed piecemeal. Once the relatively avascular areas of frank tumor involvement have been excised, the sinus that still possesses microscopic residua is systematically removed. Bleeding is often profuse and problematic. After a small area of sinus is cleared, thrombin-soaked Gelfoam pledgets are placed and held over that area with a cottonoid, and an adjacent area of the sinus is then removed. Liberal use of a bipolar cautery and hemostatic gauze aid in hemorrhage control. Each grossly normal piece of tissue that is removed is submitted for frozen-section analysis. In this way, little by little, the entire cavernous sinus is removed. Removal of the carotid artery is still controversial. If a decision is made to remove this vessel, the lateral wall of the sphenoid sinus, a portion of the middle fossa floor, a portion of the petrous tip, and occasionally the bone surrounding the superior orbital fissure are removed. Hemostasis is required at the basilar plexus, the superior petrosal sinus, the circular sinus, ophthalmic veins, and the vein of Vesalius. In addition, two or more cerebral veins that also enter the sinus may require hemorrhage control.

31.3.13 Dura and Brain Resection

Dural invasion varies from minimal involvement at the neural and vascular foramina at the sites of entry into the intracranial space to widespread involvement characteristic of recurrent tumors after full-course radiation therapy. The dura is sometimes replaced almost entirely by tumor tissue. A cuff of 5 to 10 mm of grossly healthy dura is excised and the periphery is examined by frozen-section analysis. Grossly normal dura often has tumor extensions and requires further resection as dictated by the pathologist's report.

Certain limitations to resection are imposed by vital central structures and the restrictions of certain reconstructive options. In the middle fossa, the two major structures that impede further dural excision are the vein of Labbe and the superior sagittal sinus. The vein of Labbe, or inferior anastomotic cerebral vein, drains into the lateral sinus at variable distances from the sigmoid sinus. If the superior anastomotic vein of Trolard is not patent or has a small caliber, the vein of Labbe will be the only vein draining the entire ipsilateral cerebral hemisphere and sacrificing it would then result in a massive infarction and often death. Cerebral venography may establish the venous drainage pattern in those patients in whom the vein of Labbe is in jeopardy.

The superior sagittal sinus can usually be safely obliterated in the anterior fossa from the anterior fossa floor up to the coronal suture. The middle fossa component cannot be ligated because it will lead to quadriplegia and often death in most instances. Fortunately, few skull base tumors extend that far.

The second dural restriction concerns the potential for dural reconstruction and the provision of a watertight seal. In parallel with an increase of dural resection along the clivus and under the brainstem, there is a progressive increase in the difficulty in obtaining a sound dural closure. A cerebrospinal fluid (CSF) leak at this site is an opening to the nasopharynx, which possesses one of the highest concentrations of pathogenic bacteria in the entire upper aerodigestive tract. Tissue glue helps, but the adhesive strength of most fibrin glues is lost in about one week. A suture line is superior both in strength and duration.

Brain resection is controversial. Much of the reluctance to perform it is a reflection of the neurosurgical experience with primary brain tumors. Most of these lesions are multifocal in character, with a large primary site and multiple scattered satellite lesions. A sufficient margin of healthy, uninvolved tissue that is completely free of tumor involvement is often not feasible without causing serious neurologic side effects. Upper aerodigestive tract carcinomas have a more pushing type of edge and can be excised with a narrower resection margin.

Silent areas of the brain, such as the frontal lobes and the anterior part of the temporal lobes, can be sacrificed with impunity. Speech may be at risk of impairment as the more posterior aspect of the temporal lobe is reached, especially on the dominant side. Local control can be achieved with brain resection in a high percentage of patients. Meningeal carcinomatosis is a distinctly rare event.

31.3.14 Reconstruction

The key procedure in reconstruction is separating the intracranial cavity from the upper aerodigestive tract with a watertight seal whenever possible. Infection will not only produce meningitis or, worse, an abscess, but it may cause spontaneous rupture of the ICA. An arterial graft is particularly vulnerable to such exposure. Either a fascia lata graft, a temporalis fascia graft, or an allograft is used to patch resected dura. Careful suturing, especially on the inferior aspects above the clivus, is essential. The closure may be augmented with tissue glue.

The next layer comprises muscle. If the temporalis muscle is preserved, it is placed under and across the craniotomy site. The pericranial cuff is sutured to the basipharyngeal fascia of the nasopharynx. In this way, the potential dead space left by resected soft tissues under the sphenoid bone can be obliterated. The integrity of the muscle is carefully ensured before this step.

Other myogenous or musculocutaneous flaps can be used if the temporalis flap has questionable viability. The sternocleidomastoid muscle has been used when the resection has not progressed too far medially from the foramen ovale because it is too short to reach the nasopharynx. Care must be taken to preserve its blood supply from the occipital artery. A cuff of clavicular periosteum helps hold the sutures.

The lateral thigh-free flap is the frequently used one in our institution. Its advantages include tolerable donor-site morbidity, with the ability to harvest it simultaneously with the tumor resection. It also provides suitable amounts of skin, tissue volume, and length of vascular pedicle. Another useful flap is the rectus abdominis myogenous free flap which can provide fresh vascularized tissue and greatly enhance healing. Although facial asymmetry is often created by the muscle bulk, revision at a later date can produce a good cosmetic result. The rectus abdominis flap is usually pedicled on the deep inferior epigastric artery and vein and sewn into the external carotid artery and IJV. The donor site is reinforced with Marlex mesh when it is below the arcuate line. The anterior rectus sheath remnants are approximated when possible, and the skin usually closed primarily. The flap is inserted so that the muscle extends into the resected nasopharynx and secured as best as possible onto the pharyngobasilar fascia. It is vital to ensure that an adequate paddle of soft tissue is interposed between the dural repair, the exposed ICA, and the upper aerodigestive tract. A skin paddle is sometimes required to line the pharynx when it is extensively resected. Whenever possible, muscle is carried superiorly into the infratemporal fossa to aid in compensating for the cosmetic defect caused by the absence or atrophy of the temporalis muscle.

The skin paddle is checked frequently in the first 36 postoperative hours for viability and the pedicle is monitored with Doppler ultrasonography. This is a vigorous flap that usually has excellent vessels of large caliber, and flap failure is rare.

The zygoma and the craniotomy bone flaps are returned and secured with miniplates (▶ Fig. 31.9). The inferior aspect of the L-shaped craniotomy flap is often partially missing because of bone erosion by tumor and subsequent osseous resection to ensure tumor-free

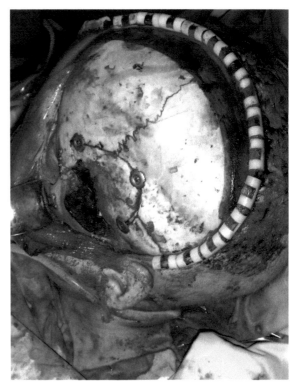

Fig. 31.9 Reconstruction.

margins. The muscle flap fills in the dead space and adds support.

Skin closure is then carried out and the wound is drained with a closed system of suction drainage. Careful attention is paid to removing all eustachian tube remnants before wound closure. A ventilating tube is placed if the middle ear space is planned to be maintained. If the ear is to be ablated, all middle ear mucosa and ossicles are removed as are the tympanic membrane and residual canal skin. A mastoidectomy is performed, with the usual precautions taken to protect the facial nerve.

31.4 Postoperative Treatment

Extubation is performed after the surgery, and the patient is transferred to the critical care unit. CT scan is performed in the case of an intracranial resection, to rule out pneumocephalus or bleeding. Wound rinsing is performed and an antibiotic ointment is applied after each rinsing for 10 days. The drains are removed when the fluid measures less than 20 mL in 24 h or 3 days after the operation. Broad-spectrum antibiotics should be started preoperatively and continued until the packing is removed. The tracheostomy and nasogastric tube are discontinued as soon as the airway is no longer jeopardized and oral alimentation can ensue. In order to reduce the chance of an increase in the intracranial pressure, stool softeners are given. Pain should be controlled adequately.

31.5 Highlights

- Probably the most difficult and complex of all the pathways in skull base surgery is the infratemporal fossa–middle cranial fossa approach.
- It is the most versatile, giving access not only to all of the subcranial tissues that underlie the middle fossa floor and to the contents of the middle cranial fossa from the lesser sphenoid wing to the tentorium, including the petrous ridge and cavernous sinus.
- Patients who require lateral skull base surgery present with a wide variety of disease processes.
- The key to the exposure of the middle fossa and its immediate subcranial structures is an L-shaped craniotomy.
- The key procedure in reconstruction is separating the intracranial cavity from the upper aerodigestive tract with a watertight seal whenever possible.

References

[1] Fisch U, Pillsbury HC. Infratemporal fossa approach to lesions in the temporal bone and base of the skull. Arch Otolaryngol 1979;105(2):99–107

[2] Duek I, Pener-Tessler A, Yanko-Arzi R, et al. Skull base reconstruction in the pediatric patient. J Neurol Surg B Skull Base 2018;79(1):81–90

[3] Fliss DM, Gill Z. Atlas of Surgical Approaches to Paranasal Sinuses and the Skull Base. Berlin: Springer; 2016

[4] Fliss DM, Gill Z. Atlas of Head and Neck Surgery. New Delhi: Jaypee; 2016

[5] Sekhar LN, Schramm VL Jr, Jones NF. Subtemporal-preauricular infratemporal fossa approach to large lateral and posterior cranial base neoplasms. J Neurosurg 1987;67(4):488–499

[6] Samii M, Draf W. Surgery of the Skull Base: An Interdisciplinary Approach. Springer Science & Business Media; 2012

[7] Lang J. Skull Base and Related Structures: Atlas of Clinical Anatomy. Schattauer Verlag; 2001

[8] Han DY, Cousins VC, Wang GJ, et al. Lateral Skull Base Surgery. In Stereo Operative Atlas of Micro Ear Surgery. Singapore: Springer; 2017:223–281

[9] Krespi YP. Lateral skull base surgery for cancer. Laryngoscope 1989;99(5):514–524

[10] Fisch U. Infratemporal fossa approach to tumours of the temporal bone and base of the skull. J Laryngol Otol 1978;92(11):949–967

32 Lateral Skull Base Surgery in a Pediatric Population

Golda Grinblat, Abdelkader Taibah, Alessandra Russo, Mario Sanna, Gianluca Piras

Summary

Pediatric lateral skull base (LSB) surgery and procedures are rare and only a few series dealing with this subject are available in literature. Pathology that involves the deep parts of the LSB not only causes functional disturbances that can be devastating in children but also makes extirpation of such tumors a challenging proposition. Being one of the most experienced centers for the treatment of pathologies of the LSB, we present one of the largest series published in the English literature, discussing anatomical and surgical considerations for the treatment of this class of diseases.

Keywords: Lateral skull base surgery, pediatric surgery

32.1 Introduction

Pathology that involves the deep parts of the LSB such as the cochlea-vestibular system, facial nerve (FN), internal auditory canal, internal carotid artery, and jugular bulb not only causes functional disturbances that can be devastating in children but also makes extirpation of such tumors a challenging proposition. Considering the early age of the patient, the treating practitioner will always be posed with the dilemma of whether to achieve functional preservation (hearing and FN function) or disease clearance. Fortunately, over the past few decades due to rapid advances in neuroradiology and neuroanesthesia, development of rational surgical approaches and better instrumentation, the objective of LSB surgery has moved from solely being focused on tumor removal to also preservation of cranial nerve functions.[1] Children with LSB pathology have benefitted most from this development because in them, any functional deficit at that age and which remains over a very long period of their life has serious social and psychological consequences.

Pediatric LSB surgery pathology and procedures are relatively rare and there are a very few series dealing with this subject.[2-9] At the Gruppo Otologico we have one of the largest series of pediatric LSB surgery published in English literature. In this chapter we discuss the special considerations in dealing with children with pathologies of the LSB.

LSB surgery in a pediatric population is a challenging proposition because due consideration must be given to hearing and FN preservation in the decision-making process. Treatment challenges become even greater when adopting these procedures to population with longer life expectancies.[2] Most series regarding pathology involving the LSB in the existing literature deal with adult population with very little data regarding the same in children. A review of literature shows that only seven series accounting to up to 156 cases have been presented in the existing peer-reviewed literature.[2,3,5-9] Our series with 65 cases adds substantially to existing literature.

32.1.1 Anatomical Considerations in Pediatric Population

It has been established that most of the growth in the skull base takes place in the first five years of life and continues for at least 10 years after birth.[10,11] Hence adult surgical approaches to the cranial base require modification when implemented in a child.[11] The smaller size and thinness of the bones of the cranial base requires lesser drilling. It is also well known that the mastoid process is absent at birth and is not fully developed until 3 years of age. This renders the FN, which is more superficial and inferior, vulnerable to surgery. The anatomy of the inner ear, though, once formed, changes little in structure or growth throughout life into adulthood. The effect of extensive bony removal and of ossification centers and unfused suture lines may have an unfavorable effect on the growth of the surrounding structures and it is necessary that further studies are focused on this.[1]

32.1.2 Demography

The occurrence of tumor in the skull base expands itself along the entire growing years from birth to the end of adolescence. The age ranges from 1 year to 18 years in our series (▶ Table 32.1), which was also seen in other series.[5,12] Although there is a slight male preponderance in some series, small numbers makes this observation inconclusive.

32.1.3 Clinical Features

There is always a delay in diagnosis of skull base pathology, especially in younger children. This apart, unfortunately, the duration between onset of symptoms and intervention in children is also quite long.[6,9] This is due to multiple factors such as inability of children to express their symptoms adequately, misdiagnosis due to the rarity of pathology of this nature, or reluctance of performing a radical intervention by the treating practitioner because of the tender age of the patients. This is reflected by the fact that prior to surgery at our center, total deafness was

Table 32.1 Patient characteristics and symptoms of the study population

Population characteristics	
Patients	63
Procedures	65
Mean age	13.0 (range 1.5–18)
Males, females	37, 26
Left side, right side	38, 29
Mean symptom duration (range)	25.6 days (range 2–360)
Mean duration of follow-up	42.8 months (range 12–125)
Symptoms	
Hearing loss	29 (44.6%)
Chronic otorrhea	28 (43.1%)
Dizziness/Vertigo	17 (26.2%)
Tinnitus	9 (13.8%)
Facial nerve palsy	7 (10.8%)
Trigeminal palsy	3 (4.6%)
Lower cranial nerve palsy	6 (9.2%)
Headache	4 (6.2%)
Recurrent meningitis	2 (3.1%)
Treatment details	
Patients previously operated elsewhere	21 (32.3%)
Revision surgeries in this series	2 (3.1%)

Table 32.2 Preoperative and postoperative facial nerve and hearing status at the end of 1 year of follow-up (63 patients)

Status	Preoperative; no (%)	Postoperative; no (%)
Facial nerve status		
HB I	52 (80.0%)	44 (67.7%)
HB II	2 (3.1%)	3 (4.6%)
HB III	3 (4.6%)	11 (16.9%)
HB IV	4 (6.2%)	4 (6.2%)
HB V	0 (0%)	0 (0%)
HB VI	4 (6.2%)	3 (4.6%)
Hearing status		
Total deafness	22 (33.8%)	38 (58.5%)
Mean PTA AC	56.3 dB ± 26.4[a]	56.3 dB ± 32.4[b]
Mean PTA BC	33.6 dB ± 16.4[a]	26.7 dB ± 16.0[b]
Mean ABG	22.7 dB ± 16.5[a]	29.5 dB ± 18.0[b]
Speech discrimination score	88.9% ± 13.2[a]	94.6% ± 46.1[b]

Abbreviation: PTA, pure tone audiogram.
[a] Out of the 43 cases with hearing, all had measurable results.
[b] Only 27 cases with hearing preservation procedures included.

seen in 35.4% of cases and a high grade of hearing deterioration in the rest (▶Table 32.2). After a diagnosis, 32.3% of the cases were treated elsewhere by less extensive procedures before they were referred to our center. Fortunately, the FN function fared better with 83.1% of the cases presenting with an HB grade I or II. Lower cranial nerve dysfunction was noted in 9.2% of cases.

The most common complaints are hearing loss, otalgia, headache, pain over the face, facial weakness, upper neck swelling, epistaxis/nasal obstruction, visual disturbances, nausea, and vomiting. The most common clinical findings are ear discharge, mass in the external auditory canal, hearing loss, facial weakness, decreased facial sensation, decreased visual acuity, and hoarseness/swallowing difficulties. Almost all the cranial nerves from the first to the twelfth can be involved in skull base pathology either individually or with others. Acoustic Neuromas and other lesions involving the cerebellopontine angle (CPA) usually involves the acousticofacial bundle (VII, VIII cranial nerves). Lesions involving the jugular foramen like paragangliomas, schwannomas, meningiomas, and chondrosarcomas usually involve the lower cranial nerves (IX, X, XI, XII cranial nerve). Lesions that involve the temporal bone like petrous bone cholesteatomas (PBCs), cholesterol granulomas, chordomas, etc., can involve the trigeminal nerve and the nerves in the cavernous sinus.

32.1.4 Pathology

There is very little data in the modern English literature on pathologies that involve the skull base in children. However, the spectrum of diseases in children is more or less the same as in adults. However, some tumors are reportedly more common in children, like encephaloceles, fibrous dysplasia, esthesioneuroblastomas, astrocytomas, pituitary adenomas, craniopharyngiomas, hemangiomas, giant cell tumors, malignant fibrous histiocytomas, optic nerve gliomas, osteoblastomas, rhabdomyosarcomas, juvenile nasopharyngeal angiofibromas, and Ewing sarcoma.[13] In this chapter we focus on pathologies afflicting the posterior and middle cranial fossa.

The most common tumors arising in children from the posterior cranial fossa and the temporal bone are cholesteatomas, chondrosarcomas, rhabdomyosarcomas, chordomas, vestibular schwannomas (VS), and meningiomas. In our series,[1] nontumoral pathology ($n = 40$) exceeded tumoral pathology ($n = 25$). PBCs were the most common pathology seen in our series, followed by VS. The list of pathologies seen in our series is enlisted in ▶Table 32.3 along with the surgical approaches. Jackson CG et al[2] reported 53.3% of tympanojugular paragangliomas (TJPs) in their series which is contrary to our observation.

Table 32.3 Characteristics of various pathologic conditions and performed surgical approaches[a]

Pathology		No (%)	Surgical approaches
Tumors (n = 25)			
Vestibular schwannoma	Sporadic	5 (7.7%)	TLA (3), TLA (5), TOA (2)
	NF II	5 (7.7%)	
Facial nerve tumors	Schwannoma	4 (6.2%)	TO (1), TO-TPA (1), TC (1), STP (1)
	Neurofibroma	1 (1.5%)	TM-ILA
	Involved by pleomorphic adenoma	1 (1.5%)	STP-TPA
Tympanojugular paraganglioma		3 (4.6%)	ITF- A (1), ITF- A (1), ITF- A + SN graft (1)
Lipoma of cochlear nerve		1 (1.5%)	TLA
Chordoma		1 (1.5%)	ITF- D + OZ + TC
Osteoblastoma		1 (1.5%)	STP
Meningioma meningoteliale		1 (1.5%)	TO-TC
Endolymphatic sac tumor		1 (1.5%)	TLA
Juvenile nasopharyngeal angiofibroma (IIIB)		1 (1.5%)	IFT-D + OZ + SFC
Nontumoral pathology (n = 31)			
Petrous bone cholesteatoma	IL	14 (21.5%)	STP (17), TLA (1), TOA (8)
	SL	5 (7.7%)	
	Massive	7(10.8%)	
Middle ear and mastoid cholesteatoma		1 (1.5%)	STP+CI
Cholesterol granuloma		3 (4.6%)	TM-ILA (3)
Eosinophilic granuloma		1 (1.5%)	TOA
Inflammatory and infectious pathology (n = 4)			
Tuberculosis of temporal bone		1 (1.5%)	TOA
Inflammatory pseudotumor		1 (1.5%)	TOA
Meningoencephalic herniation		1 (1.5%)	STP
Granulation tissue		1 (1.5%)	TM-ILA
Hearing related pathology (n = 5)			
Postmeningitis deafness		1 (1.5%)	TLA+ABI
Bilateral cochlear aplasia		1 (1.5%)	TLA+ABI
Congenital deafness with COM		1 (1.5%)	STP+CI
Mondini deformity, recurrent meningitis		1 (1.5%)	TOA
Traumatic petro-occipital fracture		1 (1.5%)	TOA
Total		**65**	
Gross total disease removal[b]		55 (91.7%)	
Disease-free survival at the end of 3 years		63 (96.9%)	
Duration of surgery (hours) (mean, range)		4.2 (1.5–12)	
Postoperative period (days) (mean, range)		5.5 (4–14)	

Abbreviations: STP, subtotal petrosectomy; TLA, translabyrinthine approach; TOA, transotic approach; TPA, transparotid approach; TM, transmastoid; TC, transcervical; ILA, infralabyrinthine approach; OZ, orbitozygomatic; SFC, subfrontal craniotomy; SN, sural nerve; NF, neurofibromatosis; ABI, auditory brainstem implant; COM, chronic otitis media; CI, cochlear implant; ITF-A, infratemporal fossa approach type A; ITF-D, infratemporal fossa approach type D.
[a] According to modified Sanna classification.[15,16]
[b] Excluding the hearing-related pathology.

32.1.5 Preoperative Workup

All patients must undergo a complete preoperative oto-neurologic evaluation followed by audiometric exam. FN function is graded according to the House-Brackmann (HB) grading system. To precisely evaluate FN function pre- and postoperatively, color photographs of the face are taken in four positions: facial muscles at rest, tight closure of eyes with a grin, raised eyebrows, and pouting lips.[14] At our center, the modified Sanna classification of hearing scores is used for documenting and analyzing audiological data[15,16] wherein audiometric studies include four-frequencies (500, 1,000, 2,000, and 4,000 Hz) pure tone average (PTA) for bone-conduction (BC), air-conduction (AC), and speech discrimination scores (SDS). A high-resolution computed tomography (CT) scan of the temporal bone and magnetic resonance imaging (MRI) are mandatory as a part of the diagnostic battery. Angiography or angio-MRI is indicated in cases where the tumor is in close association with important vasculature.

At our center, PBCs are classified according to the Sanna classification.[17,18] VS are graded according to the Tokyo consensus meeting classification.[16]

32.1.6 Surgical Considerations

The long life span ahead of the patient makes conservative approaches like wait-and-scan and radiotherapy irrelevant in the treatment of majority of benign lesions of the skull base. Petrous apex cholesterol granuloma could be an exception to this as it can be followed up with a wait-and-scan policy. Radiotherapy is ill advised due to the concerns relating to malignant transformation and interference with cranial growth centers that could occur over a long life time.[2] Adult LSB procedures can be safely applied in the pediatric population with minimal comorbidities.[11] Although the surgeon is poised with the dilemma of trying to achieve facial and hearing preservation while dealing with total tumor clearance in an extensive disease, it is important to lean toward total disease clearance. Hearing preservation surgeries, though not used in this series due to the advance nature of pathologies that we encountered, must be however considered wherever feasible. Mastery over LSB surgery can enable complete disease clearance with optimal functional outcomes. In our series, the LSB surgery enabled complete tumor removal in 91.7% of the cases.

32.1.7 Surgical Procedures

A variety of surgical procedures can be employed for extirpation of tumors in the skull base. Although it is desirable to have smaller approaches to minimize surgical sequelae at a tender age, this is not always possible because it is more important to achieve complete disease clearance to avoid recurrent surgeries over a very long follow-up period. Here we will describe the surgical steps of a few important approaches that are routinely used in lateral skull base surgery.

Subtotal Petrosectomy

Subtotal petrosectomy (STP) can be deemed as an interface between middle ear and lateral skull base surgery as it allows drilling out the temporal bone more extensively than in routine middle ear surgery. It has also proven to be of benefit in making hearing CI and active middle ear implantation possible in cases that were previously considered contraindicated. What essentially separates STP from other skull base procedures is that the approach itself is more conservative compared to other lateral skull base procedures. While most of the air cell tracts in the mastoid and middle ear are completely exteriorized in STP, the cortical bony plates over the middle fossa, posterior fossa and the sigmoid, the otic capsule, and the fallopian canal are preserved. They are drilled out only when the disease demands it. On the other hand, other definitive lateral skull base procedures like the translabyrinthine approaches and transotic approaches always involve drilling out the cortical bony plates over the middle and posterior fossa and destruction of the labyrinth, as part of the approach to remove the disease situated in the deeper parts of the temporal bone.

The steps of STP are illustrated step-by-step in ▶ Fig. 32.1 (a–h).

The Eustachian tube is packed with periosteum and the cavity is closed with fat. The skin is closed in layers (▶ Fig. 32.2).

Translabyrinthine Approach

The translabyrinthine approach (TLA) is a lateral approach used for accessing various tumors of the CPA, most commonly VS. There was a developing opinion that while small tumors could be removed through the

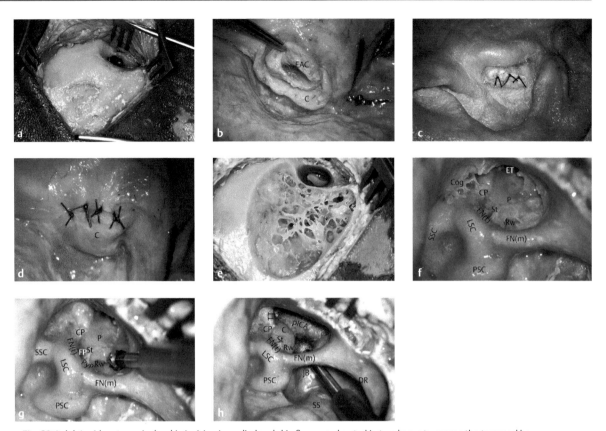

Fig. 32.1 **(a)** A wide retroauricular skin incision is applied and skin flaps are elevated in two layers to expose the temporal bone. **(b)** The external auditory canal (EAC) is cut sharply and the skin is separated from the cartilage (C) layer. **(c)** The skin layer is turned outside and sutured carefully. **(d)** The anterior cartilage (C) is sutured posteriorly to the skin flap to achieve a second layer of closure of the external auditory canal. **(e)** The cortical mastoidectomy is started. **(f)** A canal wall down mastoidectomy is performed. FN (m), mastoid segment of the facial nerve; FN (t), tympanic segment of the facial nerve; LSC, lateral semicircular canal; PSC, posterior semicircular canal; SSC, superior semicircular canal; Rw, round window; St, stapes; CP, cochleariform process; Cog, Cog; P, promontory. **(g)** The hypotympanic bone can be drilled out if necessary. FN (m), mastoid segment of the facial nerve; FN (t), tympanic segment of the facial nerve; LSC, lateral semicircular canal; PSC, posterior semicircular canal; SSC, superior semicircular canal; Rw, round window; St, stapes; FP, foot plate of stapes; CP, cochleariform process; P, promontory. **(h)** The retrofacial cells are drilled out taking care to preserve the bone over the jugular bulb (JB). FN (m), mastoid segment of the facial nerve; FN (t), tympanic segment of the facial nerve; LSC, lateral semicircular canal; PSC, posterior semicircular canal; Rw, round window; St, stapes; CP, cochleariform process; TT, tensor tympani; C, Cochlea; DR, digastric ridge; pICA, petrous internal carotid artery; SS, sigmoid sinus.

TLA, larger lesions were best approached suboccipitally as the TLA failed to provide a large surgical field.[19] To overcome this limitation of the TLA, the proponents of this approach enlarged it by additional bone removal over the middle and posterior fossae and by the addition of the transapical extensions (where bone is drilled out to various degrees around the IAC), thereby obtaining a wider surgical view and a better control over the tumor and surrounding structures. This facilitated removal of even very large tumors with anterior and medial extensions.[20–24]

The steps of the TLA are illustrated step-by-step in ▶Fig. 32.3, ▶Fig. 32.4, ▶Fig. 32.5, ▶Fig. 32.6, ▶Fig. 32.7, ▶Fig. 32.8, ▶Fig. 32.9, ▶Fig. 32.10, ▶Fig. 32.11, ▶Fig. 32.12, ▶Fig. 32.13, ▶Fig. 32.14, ▶Fig. 32.15, ▶Fig. 32.16, ▶Fig. 32.17, ▶Fig. 32.18, and ▶Fig. 32.19. The cavity is obliterated with fat and the skin is closed in layers.

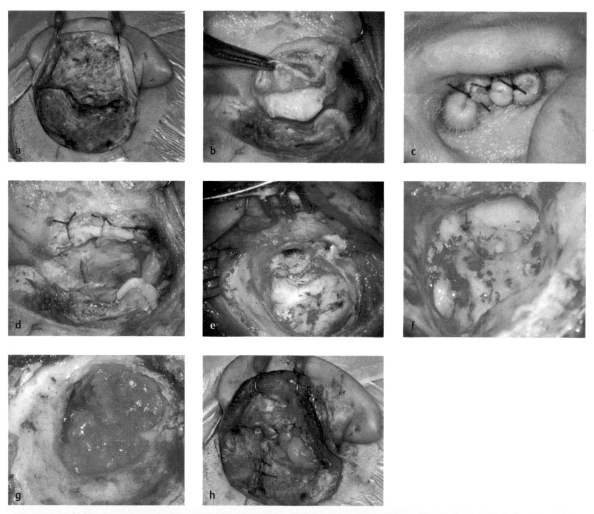

Fig. 32.2 (a–h) The Eustachian tube is packed with periosteum and the cavity is closed with fat. The skin is closed in layers.

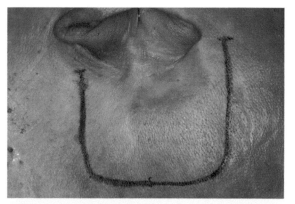

Fig. 32.3 A retroauricular incision is applied, starting from the mastoid tip and ending at the upper border of the helix of the pinna running three finger breadths width behind the pinna and two finger breadths above it.

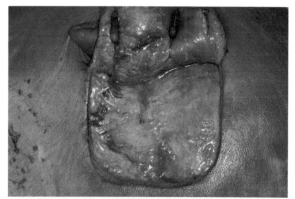

Fig. 32.4 The flaps are elevated between the subcutaneous tissue and the temporoparietal layer.

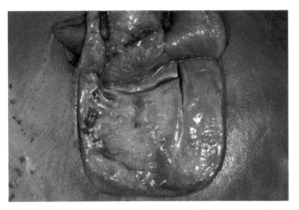

Fig. 32.5 A T-shaped incision is made to the bone to raise the second layer.

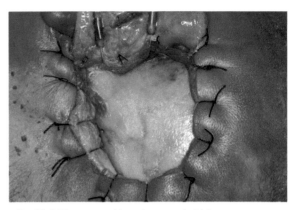

Fig. 32.6 The temporal bone is exposed widely.

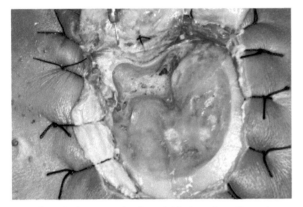

Fig. 32.7 An intact canal wall mastoidectomy is performed with a wide exposure of the middle fossa, sigmoid, and posterior fossa dura.

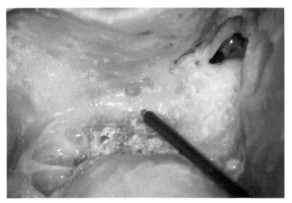

Fig. 32.8 The facial nerve is identified.

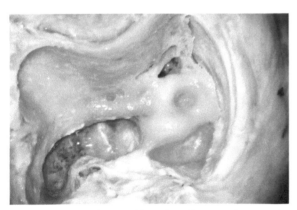

Fig. 32.9 The middle cranial fossa dura, the sigmoid sinus, and the posterior cranial fossa dura (both pre- and postsigmoid dura) are completely decompressed.

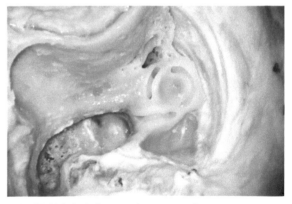

Fig. 32.10 Labyrinthectomy is commenced.

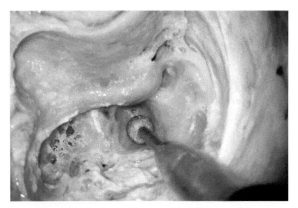

Fig. 32.11 The Jugular bulb is identified and the internal auditory canal is skeletonized.

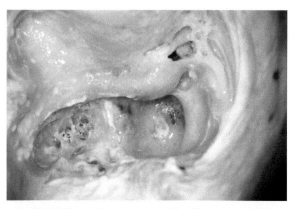

Fig. 32.12 The cochlear aqueduct is identified and opened to let out the cerebrospinal fluid (CSF), thereby reducing the pressure in the posterior cranial fossa.

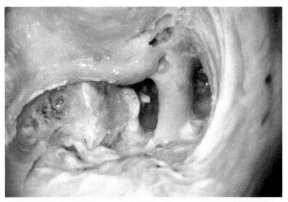

Fig. 32.13 The transapical extension (around the internal auditory canal) is done by drilling between the canal and the jugular bulb and between the canal and the middle fossa dura.

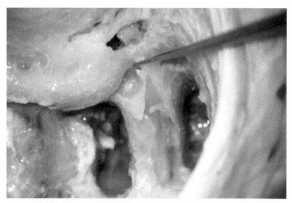

Fig. 32.14 After exposing the dura of the internal auditory canal, the superior ampullary nerve is identified in its canal and is taken down along with the superior vestibular nerve.

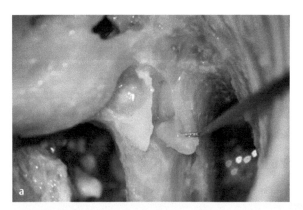

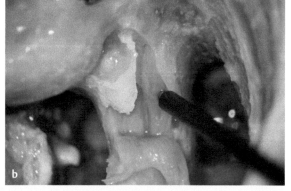

Fig. 32.15 (a, b) The facial nerve is identified just medial to the superior ampullary–superior vestibular nerve complex.

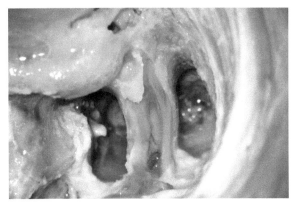

Fig. 32.16 The superior and inferior vestibular nerves are taken down exposing the facial and cochlear nerves.

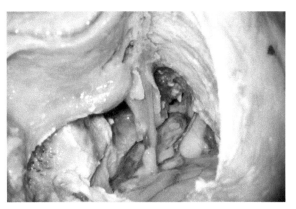

Fig. 32.17 The dura is opened to expose the cerebellopontine angle.

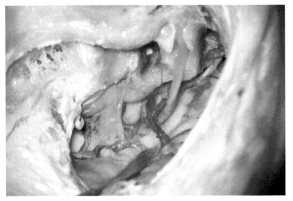

Fig. 32.18 The facial nerve, the lower cranial nerves and the abducens nerves are seen.

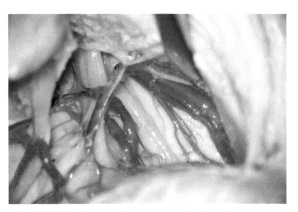

Fig. 32.19 The trigeminal nerve is visualized superiorly.

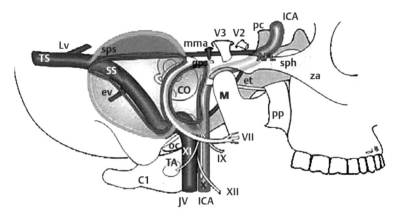

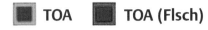

Fig. 32.20 Transotic approach. CO, cochlea; C1, atlas; ev, emissary vein; ICA, internal carotid artery; JV, jugular vein; Lv, vein of Labbe; M, mandible; OC, occipital condyle; pc, clinoid process; PP, pterygoid plate; sph, sphenoid sinus; sps, superior petrosal sinus; TA, transverse process of atlas; TS, transverse sinus; VII, FN; IX, glossopharyngeal nerve; XI, spinal accessory nerve; XII, hypoglossal nerve; V2, maxillary branch of trigeminal nerve; V3, mandibular branch of trigeminal nerve; za, zygomatic arch.

Transotic Approach

This approach is an anterior extension of the translabyrinthine approach at the expense of the cochlea preserving the FN in the fallopian canal. This approach provides better anterior extension compared to the TLA (▶ Fig. 32.20).

327

The steps of transotic approach are illustrated step-by-step in ▸Fig. 32.21, ▸Fig. 32.22, ▸Fig. 32.23, ▸Fig. 32.24, ▸Fig. 32.25, ▸Fig. 32.26, ▸Fig. 32.27, and ▸Fig. 32.28.

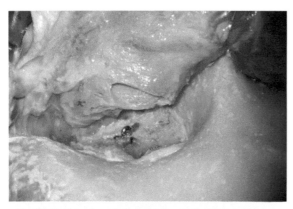

Fig. 32.21 Once the skin flaps are elevated as in a translabyrinthine approach, the external auditory canal is sectioned.

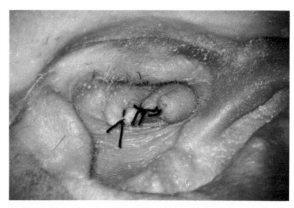

Fig. 32.22 The external canal is sutured in two layers.

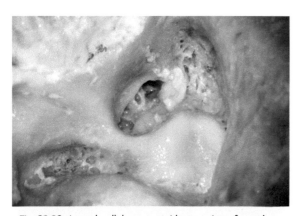

Fig. 32.23 A canal wall down mastoidectomy is performed and the middle ear is eradicated.

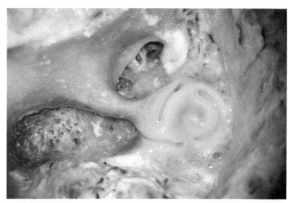

Fig. 32.24 A labyrinthectomy is performed.

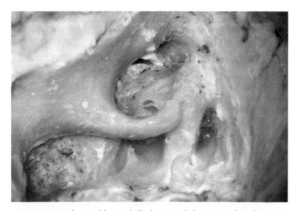

Fig. 32.25 The cochlea is drilled out and the internal auditory canal is skeletonized.

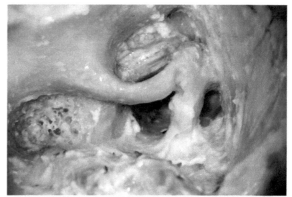

Fig. 32.26 The internal carotid artery is skeletonized. The transapical extensions are performed and drilling is continued till the petrous apex is reached preserving the facial nerve in the fallopian canal.

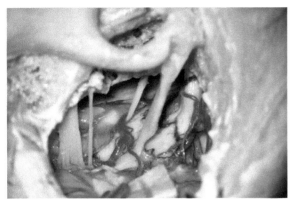

Fig. 32.27 The dura is opened exposing the cerebellopontine angle. The facial nerve, the trigeminal nerve, the abducens, and the lower cranial nerves are identified in the angle.

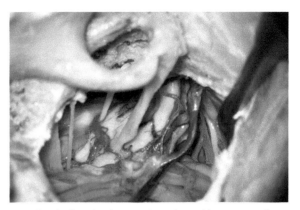

Fig. 32.28 Elevating the tentorium, the trochlear nerve and the Dandy's vein can be identified.

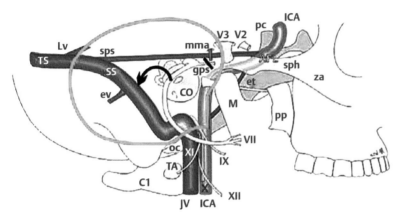

Fig. 32.29 Transcochlear approach. CO, cochlea; C1, atlas; ev, emissary vein; ICA, internal carotid artery; JV, jugular vein; Lv, vein of Labbe; M, mandible; OC, occipital condyle; pc,clinoid process; PP, pterygoid plate; sph, sphenoid sinus; sps, superior petrosal sinus; TA, transverse process of atlas; TS, transverse sinus; VII, FN; IX, glossopharyngeal nerve; XI, spinal accessory nerve; XII, hypoglossal nerve; V2, maxillary branch of trigeminal nerve; V3, mandibular branch of trigeminal nerve; za, zygomatic arch.

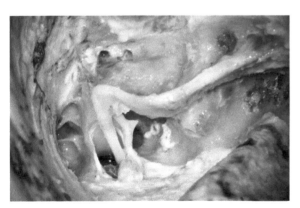

Fig. 32.30 The facial nerve is completely decompressed right up to the cerebellopontine angle.

Transcochlear Approach

The original transcochlear approach described by House and Hitselberger (in 1976) includes identification of the internal auditory canal, posterior re-routing of the FN, and removal of the cochlea and petrous apex with preservation of the middle ear and external auditory canal. The modified transcochlear approach, on the other hand, combines the removal of external auditory canal and middle ear with the posterior re-routing of the FN, thus removing the major impediment to anterior extension of the approach. This allows better control of the vertical and horizontal intrapetrous internal carotid artery and facilitates the total removal of the petrous apex. The extensive anterior bone removal provides an excellent control of the ventral surface of the brainstem without cerebellar and brainstem retraction. It also allows removal of invaded dura and bone and provides excellent control of the intrapetrous internal carotid artery. Modified transcochlear approach type A represents the basic approach. The types B, C, and D are essentially anterior, superior, and inferior extensions, respectively (▶Fig. 32.29).

The steps of transcochlear approach type A are illustrated step-by-step in ▶Fig. 32.30, ▶Fig. 32.31, ▶Fig. 32.32, ▶Fig. 32.33, ▶Fig. 32.34, and ▶Fig. 32.35. The first steps are similar to the transotic approach.

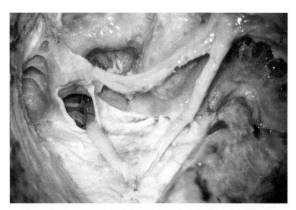

Fig. 32.31 The facial nerve is re-routed posteriorly and the fallopian canal is drilled out completely.

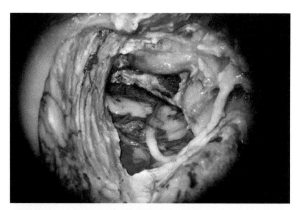

Fig. 32.32 After drilling all the remaining bone up to the clivus, the dura is then opened and the cerebellopontine angle is widely exposed.

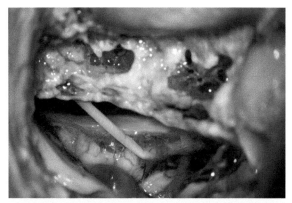

Fig. 32.33 The abducens nerve is seen in the prepontine cistern. The basilar artery is seen medial to the nerve.

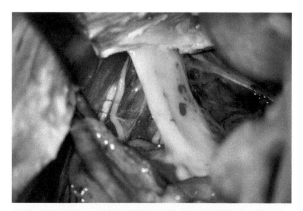

Fig. 32.34 The trigeminal nerve is visualized. The trochlear nerve is identified medial to it by reflecting the tentorium.

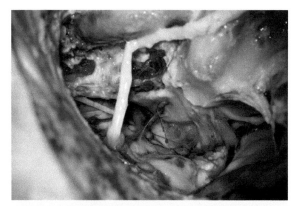

Fig. 32.35 The facial nerve is shown in its original position. The lower cranial nerve is also seen.

Infratemporal Fossa Approach Type A

The ITFA type A has been the mainstay of surgery for TJPs ever since it was described by Fisch and Pillsbury in 1979.[25] The ITFA type A is designed to allow access to the jugular foramen area, the infralabyrinthine and apical compartments of the petrous bone, the vertical segment of the internal carotid artery and the upper jugulocarotid space (▶ Fig. 32.1a). The approach is designed primarily for extensive extradural lesions involving these areas. The key point in this approach is the anterior transposition of the FN to provide optimal control of the targeted areas (▶ Fig. 32.1b). The other structures that prevent lateral access to these areas are shown in ▶ Fig. 32.1c. Besides the FN they include the tympanic bone, the digastric muscle, and the styloid process. These structures are removed to allow an unhindered lateral access. The morbidity associated with the classic ITFA type A includes: conductive hearing loss, temporary or permanent FN dysfunction due to permanent anterior re-routing of the nerve, and temporary masticatory difficulties (▶ Fig. 32.36).

The steps of infratemporal fossa approach are illustrated step-by-step in ▶ Fig. 32.37, ▶ Fig. 32.38, ▶ Fig. 32.39, ▶ Fig. 32.40, ▶ Fig. 32.41, ▶ Fig. 32.42, ▶ Fig. 32.43, ▶ Fig. 32.44, ▶ Fig. 32.45, ▶ Fig. 32.46, ▶ Fig. 32.47, ▶ Fig. 32.48, ▶ Fig. 32.49, ▶ Fig. 32.50, ▶ Fig. 32.51, ▶ Fig. 32.52, ▶ Fig. 32.53, ▶ Fig. 32.54, ▶ Fig. 32.55, ▶ Fig. 32.56, and ▶ Fig. 32.57.

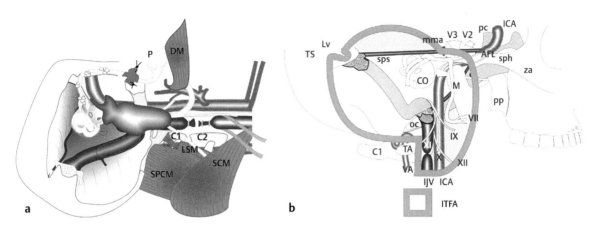

Fig. 32.36 Illustrations for infratemporal fossa approach (ITFA) type A. **(a)** An illustration of surgical view in ITFA. **(b)** An illustration of surgical limit in IT FA. ICA, internal carotid artery; sph, sphenoid sinus; za, zygomatic arch; pc,clinoid process; V2, maxillary branch of trigeminal nerve; V3, mandibular branch of trigeminal nerve; pp, pterygoid plate; M, mandible; CO, cochlea; sps, superior petrosal sinus; Lv, vein of Labbe; TS, transverse sinus; ev, emissary vein; OC, occipital condyle; TA, transverse process of atlas; C1, atlas; C2, axis; VA, vertebral artery; VII, FN; IX, glossopharyngeal nerve; XI, spinal accessory nerve; XII, hypoglossal nerve; IJV, internal jugular vein; TP, transverse process of the atlas; DM, posterior belly of the digastric muscle; SCM, sternocleidomastoid muscle; SP, styloid process; JB, jugular bulb; Ch, cochlea; SPCM, splenius capitis muscle; LSM, levator scapulae muscle; P, parotid gland.

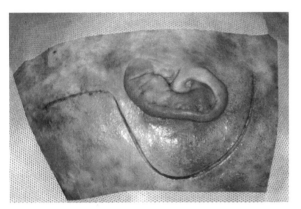

Fig. 32.37 The retroauricular incision is craniotemporocervical.

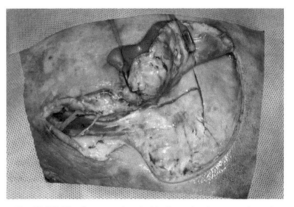

Fig. 32.38 The flaps are elevated in the subcutaneous plane. A T-shaped musculoperiosteal flap is elevated.

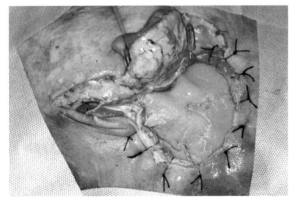

Fig. 32.39 The temporal bone and the neck are exposed.

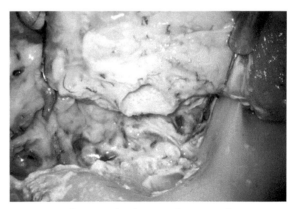

Fig. 32.40 The external auditory canal is sectioned.

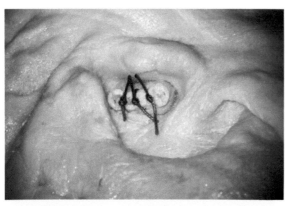

Fig. 32.41 The external auditory canal is closed in two layers.

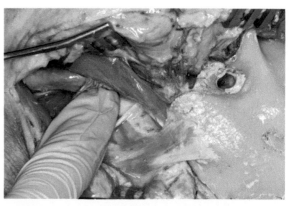

Fig. 32.42 The transverse process of C1 is identified and the internal jugular vein is dissected out just anterior to the process.

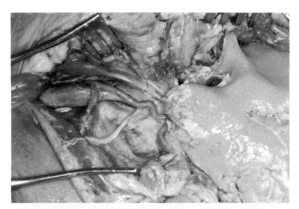

Fig. 32.43 The digastric muscle is excised and transposed, exposing the internal jugular vein, the occipital artery, and the spinal accessory nerve.

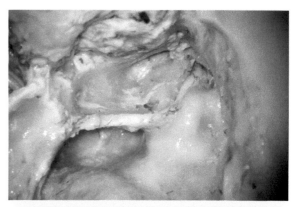

Fig. 32.44 A canal wall down mastoidectomy is performed and the facial nerve is skeletonized along the mastoid and tympanic segments.

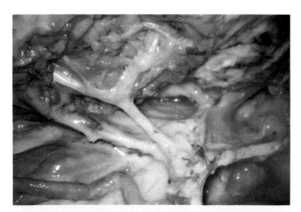

Fig. 32.45 The facial nerve is identified and dissected in the retroparotid and the parotid segments up to the bifurcation.

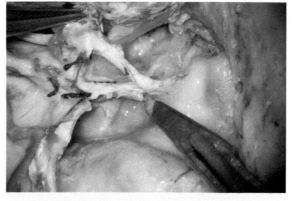

Fig. 32.46 The facial nerve is then dissected sharply and transposed anteriorly.

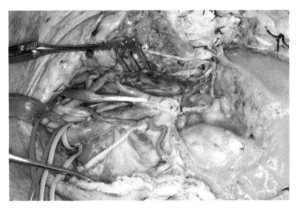

Fig. 32.47 The anteriorly transposed facial nerve provides a complete and unhindered exposure of the area of the jugular bulb.

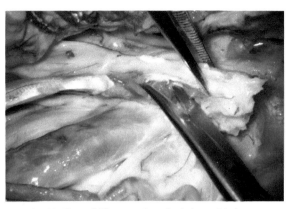

Fig. 32.48 The styloid process is excised along with the muscles attached to it to expose the carotid canal.

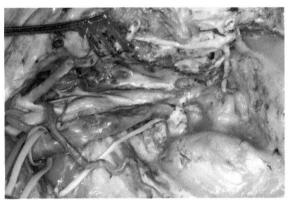

Fig. 32.49 The styloid excision exposes the carotid canal in the parapharyngeal segment up to the petrous segment.

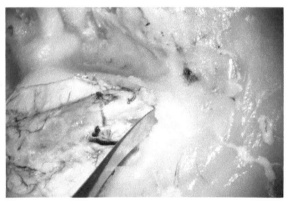

Fig. 32.50 The sigmoid sinus is closed proximally by packing it with Surgicel extraluminally (between the bone and the sinus).

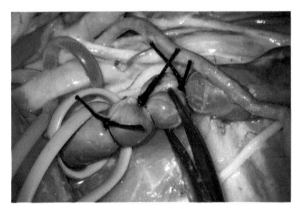

Fig. 32.51 The internal jugular vein is ligated to close the distal segment of the jugulo-sigmoid complex.

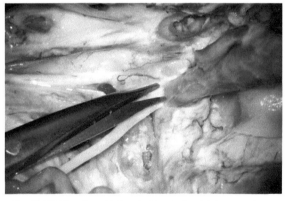

Fig. 32.52 The sigmoid sinus is dissected out right up to the jugular foramen.

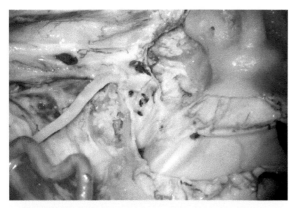

Fig. 32.53 The entire jugulo-sigmoid sinus is resected preserving the medial wall of the jugular bulb. This protects the lower cranial nerves.

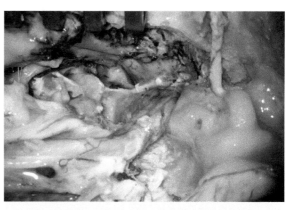

Fig. 32.54 The carotid artery is exposed by drilling out the bone of the carotid canal up to the horizontal portions of the petrous internal carotid artery.

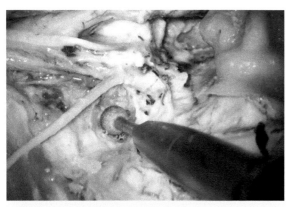

Fig. 32.55 The occipital condyle is drilled out to achieve posteromedial exposure using the transtubercular transcondylar extension.

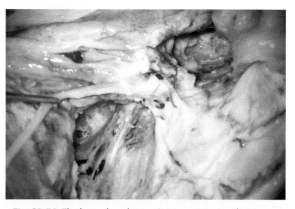

Fig. 32.56 The hypoglossal nerve is seen traversing the occipital condyle.

32.1.8 Functional Preservation

With the advancement of LSB surgery over the past few decades, hearing preservation and FN outcomes have improved tremendously. A review of literature shows that while many series did not analyze hearing results adequately, in the ones that did, hearing preservation rates varied according to the pathology and surgical approach. In case of hearing preservation surgeries for VS, the actual rate of residual hearing after surgery ranged between 20% and 71.4%.[6–8] In our series, we did not perform any hearing preservation surgeries for VS as the tumors were not indicated for such surgeries. However, in all other surgeries, hearing was preserved in 41.5% of the cases. While the mean postoperative AC and ABG worsened, there was improvement in the mean BC and the SDS.

The FN function was well preserved both pre- and postoperatively in most series in literature.

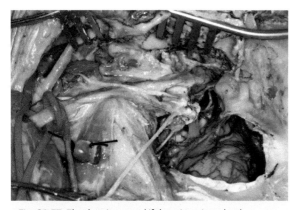

Fig. 32.57 The dura is opened if there is an intradural extension into the posterior cranial fossa converting the approach into a far-lateral approach.

Postoperatively, the review of literature showed that FN HB grade I and II ranged from 79.4% to 100%.[2,6,7,9] In our series, FN HB grade I and II was seen in 72.3%. When the FN tumors were excluded, our FN preservation rates improved to 79.6%.

In the literature, postoperative lower cranial nerve deficits ranged from 4.3% to 40%;[2,6–9] however, the highest deficit was associated with TJPs, which is quite expected considering their close proximity to the nerves.[2] Jackson et al[2] observes that complication rates are higher along with worser incidence of lower cranial nerve preservation in children compared with adults. On the contrary, in our series, we did not have any case with postoperative lower cranial nerve deficits. This could be attributed to the fact that the series by Jackson et al dealt predominantly with paragangliomas unlike ours that had a heterogenous pathology.

32.1.9 Complications

Major postoperative complications in LSB surgery include mortality, cerebrovascular accidents, meningitis, and CSF leaks, and range from 6.9% to 43% in literature. Minor complications include wound breakdown, infection, and abdominal hematoma, and these range between 0.8% and 13.3%. In our series, at the last follow-up, 62 of the 65 patients survived and only one of the 55 cases with gross disease clearance developed a recurrence. The sole case of recurrence was that in a case of supralabyrinthine PBC that developed a recurrence after 5 years and subsequently underwent an STP. Teo et al[3] in their series of predominantly tumoral etiology reported a 2-year tumor-free survival of 81%. In our series, the 3-year disease-free survival that could be calculated in 27 cases was 97.6%.

LSB surgery is a high-risk surgery. However, the quality of life after such surgeries has improved due to developments in subspecialties like phonosurgery, FN reanimation surgeries, and hearing implantology. Also, going by literature, surgery on skull bones did not appear to inflict any long-term morphological sequelae in children.[3]

32.2 Conclusion

LSB surgery in a pediatric population is a surgical challenge. However, results from experienced centers that routinely perform such procedures have yielded good results in terms of disease clearance and functional outcomes. While on one hand, advances in radiology have helped in earlier diagnosis, the silent nature of pathology in the skull base and the inability of children to express themselves must lead the treating practitioner to have a high index of suspicion toward such rare pathologies.

32.3 Highlights

a. Indications
   - Tumors of the lateral skull base.
b. Contraindications
   - Comorbidities which impede general anesthesia.
c. Complications
   - Facial palsy.
   - Hearing loss.
   - Lower cranial nerves palsy.
   - Cerebrospinal fluid leak.
d. Special preoperative considerations
   - Status of the cranial nerves.
   - Hearing status.
   - Involvement of the internal carotid artery.
e. Special intraoperative considerations
   - Depend on the surgical approach.
f. Special postoperative considerations
   - ICU for the first 24 hours.
   - Tight head dressing for the first 8 to 10 days.

References

[1] Grinblat G, Prasad SC, Fulcheri A, Laus M, Russo A, Sanna M. Lateral skull base surgery in a pediatric population: a 25-year experience in a referral skull base center. Int J Pediatr Otorhinolaryngol 2017;94:70–75

[2] Jackson CG, Pappas DG Jr, Manolidis S, et al. Pediatric neurotologic skull base surgery. Laryngoscope 1996;106(10):1205–1209

[3] Teo C, Dornhoffer J, Hanna E, Bower C. Application of skull base techniques to pediatric neurosurgery. Childs Nerv Syst 1999;15(2–3):103–109

[4] Pothula VB, Lesser T, Mallucci C, May P, Foy P. Vestibular schwannomas in children. Otol Neurotol 2001;22(6):903–907

[5] Brockmeyer D, Gruber DP, Haller J, Shelton C, Walker ML. Pediatric skull base surgery. 2. Experience and outcomes in 55 patients. Pediatr Neurosurg 2003;38(1):9–15

[6] Cunningham CD III, Friedman RA, Brackmann DE, Hitselberger WE, Lin HW. Neurotologic skull base surgery in pediatric patients. Otol Neurotol 2005;26(2):231–236

[7] Mazzoni A, Dubey SP, Poletti AM, Colombo G. Sporadic acoustic neuroma in pediatric patients. Int J Pediatr Otorhinolaryngol 2007;71(10):1569–1572

[8] Slattery WH III, Fisher LM, Hitselberger W, Friedman RA, Brackmann DE. Hearing preservation surgery for neurofibromatosis Type 2-related vestibular schwannoma in pediatric patients. J Neurosurg 2007;106(4, Suppl):255–260

[9] Walcott BP, Sivarajan G, Bashinskaya B, Anderson DE, Leonetti JP, Origitano TC. Sporadic unilateral vestibular schwannoma in the pediatric population. Clinical article. J Neurosurg Pediatr 2009;4(2):125–129

[10] Sgouros S, Natarajan K, Hockley AD, Goldin JH, Wake M. Skull base growth in childhood. Pediatr Neurosurg 1999;31(5):259–268

[11] Gruber DP, Brockmeyer D. Pediatric skull base surgery. 1. Embryology and developmental anatomy. Pediatr Neurosurg 2003;38(1):2–8

[12] Hanbali F, Tabrizi P, Lang FF, DeMonte F. Tumors of the skull base in children and adolescents. J Neurosurg 2004;100(2, Suppl Pediatrics):169–178

[13] Tsai EC, Santoreneos S, Rutka JT. Tumors of the skull base in children: review of tumor types and management strategies. Neurosurg Focus 2002;12(5):e1

[14] Sanna M, Khrais T, Mancini F, Russo A, Taibah A. Facial nerve management in middle ear and external auditory canal carcinoma: the facial nerve in the temporal bone and lateral skull base microsurgery. Stuttgart: Georg Thieme Verlag; 2006:270–271

[15] Sanna M, Karmarkar S, Landolfi M. Hearing preservation in vestibular schwannoma surgery: fact or fantasy? J Laryngol Otol 1995;109(5):374–380

[16] Kanzaki J, Tos M, Sanna M, Moffat DA, Monsell EM, Berliner KI. New and modified reporting systems from the consensus meeting on systems for reporting results in vestibular schwannoma. Otol Neurotol 2003;24(4):642–648, discussion 648–649

[17] Pandya Y, Piccirillo E, Mancini F, Sanna M. Management of complex cases of petrous bone cholesteatoma. Ann Otol Rhinol Laryngol 2010;119(8):514–525

[18] Sanna M, Pandya Y, Mancini F, Sequino G, Piccirillo E. Petrous bone cholesteatoma: classification, management and review of the literature. Audiol Neurotol 2011;16(2):124–136

[19] Hardy DG, Macfarlane R, Baguley D, Moffat DA. Surgery for acoustic neurinoma: an analysis of 100 translabyrinthine operations. J Neurosurg 1989;71(6):799–804

[20] Ben Ammar M, Piccirillo E, Topsakal V, Taibah A, Sanna M. Surgical results and technical refinements in translabyrinthine excision of vestibular schwannomas: the Gruppo Otologico experience. Neurosurgery 2012;70(6):1481–1491, discussion 1491

[21] Angeli RD, Piccirillo E, Di Trapani G, Sequino G, Taibah A, Sanna M. Enlarged translabyrinthine approach with transapical extension in the management of giant vestibular schwannomas: personal experience and review of literature. Otol Neurotol 2011;32:125–131

[22] Sanna M, Russo A, Taibah A, Falcioni M, Agarwal M. Enlarged translabyrinthine approach for the management of large and giant acoustic neuromas: a report of 175 consecutive cases. Ann Otol Rhinol Laryngol 2004;113(4):319–328

[23] Falcioni M, Russo A, Mancini F, et al. Enlarged translabyrinthine approach in large acoustic neurinomas. Acta Otorhinolaryngol Ital 2001;21:226–236

[24] Naguib MB, Saleh E, Cokkeser Y, et al. The enlarged translabyrinthine approach for removal of large vestibular schwannomas. J Laryngol Otol 1994;108(7):545–550

[25] Fisch U, Pillsbury HC. Infratemporal fossa approach to lesions in the temporal bone and base of the skull. Arch Otolaryngol 1979;105(2):99–107

33 Surgery of Skull Base Meningoencephalocele

Paolo Castelnuovo, Stefania Gallo, Jacopo Zocchi, Jessica Ruggiero, Davide Locatelli

Summary

Congenital encephaloceles are a rare type of neural tube defect caused by a herniation of the cranial content through areas of arrested bone development in the skull. Nasal encephaloceles in particular are herniations localized to the anterior skull which include frontoethmoidal and basal subtypes. Although there have been no definitive factors implicated in the etiology of these defects, the prevailing theory on their pathogenesis centers around failure of the neuroectoderm to separate from the ectoderm surface during the fourth week post-conception, leading to an area of weakness through which brain and meninges can herniate. The majority of nasal encephaloceles is sporadic, although a small percentage occurs associated with other craniofacial malformations. Given their potential life-threatening complications, which include meningitis and infection of the central nervous system, an early diagnosis is mandatory. Treatment is primarily the surgical resection leading to favorable outcomes in most cases. The endoscopic transnasal approach offers an effective and safe surgical option in selected cases, without major consequences on craniofacial growth.

Keywords: Congenital encephalocele, neurulation, frontoethmoidal encephalocele, basal encephalocele, meningoencephalocele, cranium bifidum, craniofacial malformation, cephalic disorders, pediatric endoscopic transnasal surgery, pediatric skull base reconstruction

33.1 Definition and Historical Notes

Encephaloceles (ECs) are defined as protrusions of the cranial contents beyond the normal confines of the skull through a defect in the cranium and the facial bones.

They account for about 10% to 20% of all craniospinal dysraphisms. The incidence is approximately 1/3,000 to 1/10,000 live births, but the true incidence is likely considerably greater because about 70% of ECs result in loss of pregnancy.[1]

The first documented case was described in the 16th century in a newborn who presented an encephalocele (EC) in the context of a serious clinical picture, today known as Robert syndrome.[2] After that, numerous references can be found in the literature concerning this condition, such as those of Le Dran (1740) who introduced the term *hernia cerebri*, Richter (1813) who described a case of nasal EC, and Spring (1854) who wrote what was probably the first extensive monograph on the subject.[3] Several theories have alternated in order to explain the pathogenesis. In 1827, Saint-Hilaire supposed that an increased intrauterin pressure could cause adhesions between the brain and the germinal membranes, arresting the development of the anterior cranium and allowing herniation of the brain through this opening. Other subsequent speculations pointed to increased organ bulk, ventricular dilatation, rickets, hydrocephalus, and olfactory bulbs residues as putative causes of ECs formation.[4] There have been numerous attempts at classification as well, such as those of Heinecke (1882), Browder (1932), Blumenfeld (1965), until the last more comprehensive classification by Suwanwela and Suwanwela in 1972 which is still used today with minimal rearrangements.[3]

33.2 Classification and Distribution

Encephaloceles have been classified in several subtypes depending on different features.

Related to the onset, ECs may be congenital or acquired. *Congenital* (primary) ECs are the consequence of a defect in the development of the skull during embryogenesis, particularly in the closure of the neural tube. Prevalence is about 0.4–8/10,000 alive infants.[5] *Acquired* (secondary) ECs are usually a consequence of head traumas, even if this is a rare circumstance in children, thanks to the high plasticity of the skull at this age, with an estimated incidence of 0.2%–0.3% of all cerebrospinal fluid (CSF) leaks after trauma in the pediatric population.[6]

Depending on the herniated content and its histology, ECs are divided into *meningocele* (herniation of meninges and CSF), *meningoencephalocele* (herniation of brain tissue and meninges) and *hydromeningoencephalocele* (herniation of a portion of a ventricle, brain tissue, and meninges).[5] Treatment approaches to these entities are functionally identical and a distinction is often not drawn in the clinical literature.

Lastly, ECs are classified based on the location and type of skull defect. They can occur either at the vault and the base of the skull. A commonly accepted system arranges ECs into (1) frontoethmoidal (also known as sincipital), (2) basal, (3) of the cranial vault, and (4) occipital (▶ Table 33.1).

Racial and geographic factors seem to influence the site and the frequency. Indeed, even differences in seasonal patterns or socioeconomic status are supposed to be responsible for the differences in distribution.[7]

About 80% of all ECs occur in the occipital area of the cranial vault.[8] In Southeast Asia, parts of Russia and central Africa, sincipital defects are more common than occipital ones with an incidence of 1/3,500 live births. Contrarily, occipital lesion is the predominant type in the

Table 33.1 Classification of encephaloceles

Frontoethmoidal EC	Nasofrontal
	Nasoethmoidal
	Naso-orbital
Basal EC	Transethmoidal
	Transsphenoidal
	Sphenoethmoidal
	Sphenomaxillary
	Frontosphenoidal/spheno-orbital
EC of the cranial vault	Interfrontal
	Anterior fontanelle
	Interparietal
	Posterior fontanelle
	Temporal
Occipital EC	

Abbreviation: EC, encephalocele.

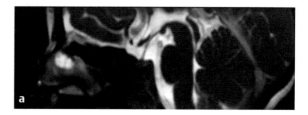

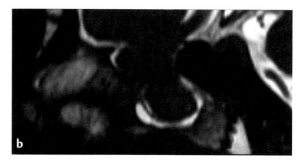

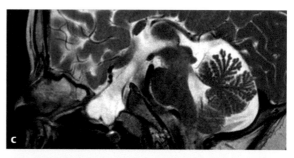

Fig. 33.1 MR sagittal view on the skull midline. **(a)** Sporadic **nasoethmoidal** encephalocele in a 5-month-old baby; the mass was improperly biopsied at another Institute, fact that caused active Cerebrospinal fluid (CSF) rhinorrhea. **(b)** Transethmoidal encephalocele in a 4-month-old baby affected by a complex craniofacial malformation, not identified as a syndrome. The herniation was associated with cleft lip and palate, microphthalmia, hypertelorism, bilateral optic nerve hypoplasia, and severe bilateral deafness. **(c)** Transsphenoidal encephalocele in a 12-year-old child affected by oro-facial-digital syndrome.

white races of North America, Europe, and Australia, representing almost the 85% of all observed ECs.[3,9]

This chapter will focus predominantly on congenital frontoethmoidal and basal ECs, collectively known as nasal encephaloceles, with frontoethmoidal being the most common type of nasal EC encountered, especially in the nasofrontal region.[10,11] Overall, basal defects are rare in all racial groups (2–10% of all reported cases).

These categories, along with their subtypes, are defined based on the specific location of the associated bony defect.

Frontoethmoidal ECs, which are associated with a skull defect at the foramen cecum, are anterior to the cribriform plate and formed by a herniation of the soft tissues of the forehead and nose, and orbit through a defect in the frontal and ethmoid bones. These can be nasofrontal, nasoethmoidal, naso-orbital.[12]

Basal ECs, in contrast, protruding posteriorly to the foramen caecum, present in the nasal cavities as opposed to external masses. Basal ECs include transethmoidal (herniation through the cribriform plate), sphenoethmoidal (herniation at the sphenoethmoid junction), transsphenoidal (herniation through the sphenoid body into the sphenoid sinus or nasopharynx), frontosphenoidal/spheno-orbital (herniation through the superior orbital fissure), sphenomaxillary (herniation through the junction of the sphenoid body and wing into the pterygopalatine fossa)[13] (▶ Fig. 33.1).

A separate mention should be made for the even rarer congenital temporal ECs that arise as a result of any malfunction in the normal bony genesis of the temporal bone. By far, the majority of them manifest in the area of middle ear tegmen and mastoid, where the petrous and squamous aspects of the temporal bone join.[14] Much more uncommon localizations involve the posterior plate of the petrous bone[15] and the petrous apex.[16] More in detail, petrous apex ECs, described either as meningocele or arachnoid cyst, shows connection to Meckel's cave and

may determine secondary erosion of the petrous bone and carotid canal.[17]

Lastly, multiple ECs may coexist complicating the clinical picture.

33.3 Etiology and Embryological Considerations

To date, etiology is still poorly understood but a multifactorial theory, involving genetic and acquired factors during pregnancy, is the most accredited. A number of environmental elements have been reported as being associated with ECs, including maternal malnutrition deficiencies, exposure to various teratogens (such as aflatoxin), advanced paternal age, and long intervals between pregnancies.[18] Other factors have been investigated, such as hyperthermia, viral infection, hypervitaminosis, hypoxia, irradiation, and folic acid insufficiency, but their role is not yet proven.[11]

Some preliminary embryological considerations are necessary in order to better understand developmental anomalies of a complex and not yet fully clarified system.

Summarily, neural development is one of the earliest systems to begin and the last to be completed after birth. The nervous system (NS) develops when the notochord induces its overlying ectoderm to become neuroectoderm and to develop into the neural plate. The neural plate folds along its central axis to form a neural groove lined on each side by a neural fold. The two neural folds fuse together and pinch off to become the neural tube, open initially at each end (rostral and caudal neuropore), both closing before the end of the fourth week (neurulation process). Practically, the original ectoderm divides into three sets of cells: (1) the internally positioned neural tube, which will form the brain and spinal cord, (2) the externally positioned epidermis of the skin (surface ectoderm), and (3) the neural crest (NC) cells in the region that connects the neural tube and epidermis[19] (▶ Fig. 33.2). Before neural folds completely merge to form the neural tube, the rostral population of NC cells migrates to

embryonic pharynx leading to the formation of five pairs of arches, each containing ectoderm, endoderm, and mesenchyme. NC cells of the first two arches contribute to cranial skeletal elements and associated connective tissue.[20] Around the fourth week post-conception, mesenchyme, derived from the paraxial mesoderm and NC, condenses to form the base of the ectomeningeal capsule. This process takes place well after the primordial brain, cranial nerves, eyes, and major intracerebral blood vessels have begun differentiation.[9] The further development of the cranium originates from ossification centers within the mesenchyme of the rudimentary skull, consisting in membranous neurocranium (that will form the flat bones of the skull), cartilaginous neurocranium or chondrocranium (that will form most of the cranial base), and viscerocranium (that will form the facial skeleton), each characterized by a specific ossification mechanism.[21]

Two predominant hypotheses are currently suggested to explain ECs formation.

1. *Neurulation disorder*: Congenital ECs share the common finding of a median skull defect, which corresponds to the site where the neural tube closes along the midline. A disturbance at this level would result in sustained connections between neuroectoderm (brain) and surface ectoderm (epidermal layer of the skin).[22] In addition, Hoving postulated that the

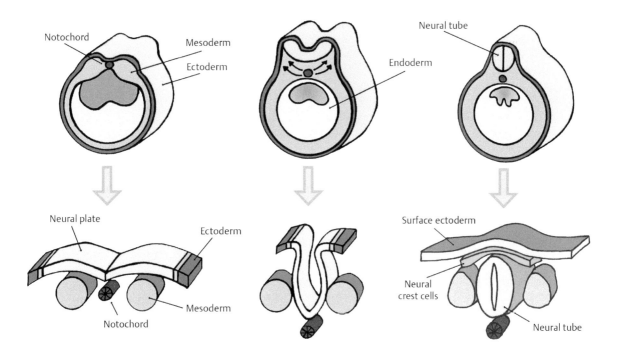

Fig. 33.2 Neurulation and neural crest migration. Notochord forms from mesoderm cell soon after gastrulation is complete. Signals from notochord cause inward folding of the ectoderm at the neural plate. Ends of neural plates fuse and disconnect to form an autonomous neural tube. Near the time of neural tube closure, the neural crest cells go through an epithelial to mesenchymal transition and delaminate from the neural folds or dorsal neural tube and migrate along defined pathways. They will differentiate to form most of the peripheral nervous system as well as cartilages, bones, muscles, and connective tissue.

separation of neural and surface ectoderm occurs focally in the midline through apoptosis mechanisms and not in a zipper-like fashion.[23] Since an imbalanced separation process could happen at any site of the neural tube closure, various kinds of ECs might result.

Recently, several genes, such as SHH (Sonic Hedgehog), have been identified as possible players in the pathogenesis of ECs. SHH, a morphogenetic molecule produced by the notochord, represents an inductive signal for cell growth and differentiation, especially in the brain and spinal cord. During development, a ventrodorsal gradient of SHH directs the neural tube modeling and, by binding to its receptor, it prevents apoptosis.[24]

2. *Post-neurulation disorder*: Since ECs are always covered with skin, mucosa, or at least an epithelial layer, the neural tube must have already closed before EC formation.[22,25] Indeed, Marin-Padilla suggested that a mesodermal insufficiency might be the first event leading to a growth impairment of the chondrocranium and to a delay in the closure of the membranous neurocranium. The subsequent explosive growth of the NS may eventually surpass the accommodative capacity of the neurocranium, and neural tissue may then herniate through the mesenchyme and extracranially.[26]

33.4 Clinical Presentation

Nasal ECs manifest across a broad clinical spectrum, from barely perceptible midface, intranasal or intrapharyngeal masses to severe craniofacial deformity, often evident at birth. However, they may sometimes be asymptomatic.

In detail, most of frontoethmoidal ECs present as skin-covered masses or visible protrusions on the face, over the nose, glabella, or forehead. They show a positive Furstenberg sign, in which compression of bilateral internal jugular veins or Valsalva maneuver leads to enlargement of the protruding mass due to its connection to the subarachnoid space. In other cases, frontoethmoidal ECs present as intranasal, transilluminative, compressible masses near the nasal bridge often associated with hypertelorism.[13]

Basal ECs, on the other hand, are not clinically visible due to their location within the nasal cavities and may present with upper airway obstruction. Other symptoms include snoring, oral breathing, feeding difficulties, and CSF rhinorrhea.[22] As these symptoms may be common in children for other reasons, the definitive diagnosis might be delayed, increasing the risk of dangerous complications. Meningitis or encephalitis develops due to direct communication of the central NS with the external environment, facilitating the entry of pathological microorganisms. The bacteria most commonly associated with such patients are *Streptococcus pneumoniae*, followed by

Staphylococcus aureus and *Neisseria meningitidis*.[3] It is worth to note that recurrent episode of meningitis, even in absence of an active rhinorrhea, has to induce the suspect of a CSF leakage.

Herniation in transsphenoidal ECs may moreover result in endocrine dysfunction or disruption in optic pathways.[22,27] Hypothalamic–pituitary dysfunctions have been observed above all in growth hormone (GH) and antidiuretic hormone (ADH) levels and to a lesser extent in gonadotropins, thyroid stimulating hormone (TSH), and prolactin. Possible causes may be the stretch of pituitary stalk and hypothalamus, with a mechanism similar to the empty sella syndrome, and other unknown congenital conditions.[28]

The majority of nasal ECs is sporadic, although a small percentage occurs associated with other craniofacial malformations (▶Fig. 33.3). About one-third is associated with midline defects such as cleft lip and palate.[5] Additional intracranial anomalies have been reported, mainly observed with frontoethmoidal ECs, with hydrocephalus and corpus callosum agenesis being the most frequent.[10,29]

ECs may also manifest as a part of recognized clinical syndromes, among which the most frequently described are briefly reported here.

• *Septo-optic dysplasia* (or *de Morsier syndrome*) is a rare, congenital, and very heterogeneous syndrome, with a reported incidence of 1 in 10,000 births. The diagnosis can be reached when two or more features of the classical triad of optic nerve hypoplasia, pituitary hormone abnormalities, and midline brain defects (including agenesis of the septum pellucidum and/or corpus callosum) are present.[30,31]

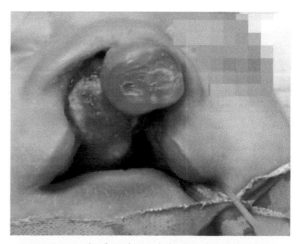

Fig. 33.3 Example of nasal encephalocele associated with a complex craniofacial malformation. This 4-month-old baby presented a complete cleft lip and palate and a deformity of the caudal part of the nose. The nasal cavities were occupied by a voluminous mass that caused distortion of the nasal and skull base anatomy and protruded inside the oral cavity.

- *Morning glory syndrome* is a rare congenital malformation of the optic disc. It is characterized by an enlarged, funnel-shaped optic disc and an elevated pigmented peripapillary tissue annulus, often associated with craniofacial abnormalities, optic nerve atrophy, coloboma, and megalopapilla.[28]
- *Moyamoya disease* is a progressive, steno-occlusive arteriopathy involving the internal carotid artery terminus and its branches that can cause recurrent strokes in children.[32] It is a rare disorder, with an estimated annual incidence of 0.35 to 0.94/100,000 people, often associated with ocular malformations and midline cranial defects.[29,33]

Furthermore, the literature reports cases of nasal ECs associated to other much rarer syndromes, such as craniosynostosis,[5] Dandy–Walker complex,[34] Hunter,[35] Aicardi,[36] Goldenhar[37] syndromes, and lastly with cardiovascular and kidney malformations.[34]

33.5 Diagnosis

A suspect of nasal EC can derive from a detailed clinical evaluation, although a diagnostic confirmation can be reached only through further investigations.

Endonasal endoscopy, either with flexible or rigid-angled scopes, can reveal the presence of an intranasal, usually translucent and pulsating, mass occasionally associated with evident CSF rhinorrhea. *β2-transferrin or β-trace protein dosage* on nasal secretion may represent an additional non-invasive and highly predictive tool to confirm CSF leakage, even in absence of a nasal neoformation. However, limits of this test are that rhinorrhea has to be active and that it is not always so easy to collect nasal fluid samples, especially in pediatric patients.

To better visualize the soft tissue mass, and its contents and boundaries, high-resolution *computed tomography* (CT), or *cone beam CT*, in conjunction with *magnetic resonance* (MR) is recommended in almost all the cases, considering the complementarity of the information provided.[38] Multislice CT scan produces details about the craniofacial skeleton morphology and often allows the identification and the site of a bony defect. Moreover, it functions as operative guide for the surgeon. MR, giving details about soft tissues, is more accurate in enhancing the presence of a brain herniation and a CSF leakage and in excluding other possible coexisting encephalic malformations. In particular T2-weighted, T2-flair, and CISS sequences provide excellent contrast between CSF and other encephalic structures, and they are essential to differentiate between CSF and inflammatory signals in the nose and paranasal sinus cavities; gadolinium sequences allow to rule out tumors. Moreover, and this applies to both the radiological examinations mentioned, the entire skull base (including middle ear roof and mastoid, middle, and posterior cranial fossa) must be checked out in order to detect any multiple skull base defects[6] (▶ Fig. 33.4).

Biopsy is absolutely contraindicated before radiologic evaluations are completed and a diagnostic hypothesis advanced, as it can provoke severe complications, such as CSF leak and ascending infection due to the persisting intracranial communications between the mass and the cranial content.[38] Preoperative intrathecal fluorescein test is rarely necessary.

Histologically, ECs have shown to contain glial cells, cerebral tissue, non-functional neural tissue, choroid plexus, and ependymal cells. Cystic structures with ependymal cells are a distinguishing feature of EC in comparison to gliomas. Glial tissue can be visualized using immunoreactivity for GFAP, S-100 protein, and NSE. Nerve and nasal septum cartilage may also be present.[8]

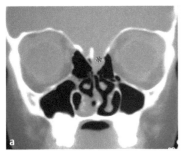
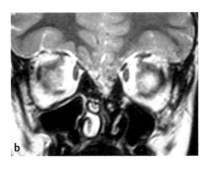
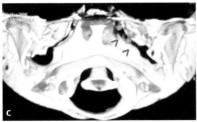
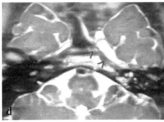

Fig. 33.4 A 9-year-old child, previously operated with a transcranial approach for a left transethmoidal encephalocele (EC), addressed for recurrent episodes of meningitis and persisting CSF rhinorrhea. Radiologic evidence of a persistent/recurrent transethmoidal EC (*red asterisk*) at CT (**a**) and MR (**b**) scans. Simultaneous left petroclival malformation (hypoplasia of petrous bone and diastasis of petroclival suture) conditioning a Cerebrospinal fluid (CSF) leak (*red arrowhead*) at 3D CT reconstruction (**c**) and MR scan (**d**).

Differential diagnosis should include mainly nasal polyps, nasal gliomas, or dermoid cysts.[39] A special mention has to be made for these latter two entities, since they are supposed to share the same pathogenetic mechanism with frontoethmoidal ECs. As discussed above, skull base and facial skeleton development results from a complex interaction of cellular proliferation and regression involving migration of NC cells through ectodermal and mesodermal derived structures. Anteriorly, as the frontal, nasal and ethmoid bones, and nasal capsule fuse together, potential spaces are created that normally regress by birth. Persistence of these spaces including the *fonticulus nasofrontalis* (region between frontal and nasal bones), the *prenasal space* (region between nasal bones and nasal capsule), and the *foramen cecum* (region between frontal and ethmoid bone) may lead to the herniation of intracranial contents or glial tissue, forming either ECs or gliomas. Alternatively, ectodermal and mesodermal tissue may be entrapped in these spaces, leading to the formation of dermoids.[40] From a clinical standpoint, dermoids are the most common midline congenital nasal mass and can present as a non-pulsatile cyst, sinus, or fistula on the external nose (30% of dermoids can communicate with the dura). On the other hand, gliomas represent herniated glial tissue along the skull base and facial skeleton fusion planes but do not have any communication with the CSF. They present clinically as non-pulsatile masses frequently extranasal, but they can be also intranasal or combined (up to 15% of gliomas has attachments to the dura).[41]

33.6 Treatment

Direct surgical repair currently represents the mainstay of nasal ECs treatment. Proper removal and craniofacial reconstruction always require a multi-disciplinary effort involving several specialties, including neurosurgery, otorhinolaryngology, maxillofacial surgery, radiology, and anesthesia.

Treatment options account for several surgical techniques, depending on the location of the defect, including either intracranial or extracranial approaches.[3]

In some cases, only the combination of different approaches appears to be an adequate surgical solution. Indeed, those cases with evident face distortion, resulting from the presence of an EC (such as nasofrontal or naso-orbital types), might require a concomitant correction of the facial deformities, as well as the eventual correction of other associated craniofacial malformations (e.g., cleft lip or palate) (▶ Fig. 33.5).

In many studies, the surgical procedure for frontoethmoidal ECs involves frontal coronal scalp flap incision to gain exposure to the craniofacial skeleton. Any neural or meningeal herniations are cut out and the dura is subsequently closed and repaired.[10,42]

Basal ECs treatment can count on three different approaches, transcranial, endoscopic transnasal, and transpalatal. Conversely, the microscopic transnasal approach in children has been limited by the dimensions of the nares and a sublabial exposure has been favored for pediatric transsphenoidal approaches;[13] nevertheless, thanks to technological improvements, this latter technique also has been progressively abandoned.

Historically, basal ECs have been approached through open techniques (bicoronal incision and frontal craniotomy) and the skull base defect often reconstructed with pericranial flap. However, this approach exposes patients to the risks of blood loss, brain retraction, and injury to the supraorbital/supratrochlear neurovascular complexes. In addition, it potentially causes disruption of growth centers that may result in facial asymmetry.[9]

On the other hand, the transnasal endoscopic approach has been successful in many cases of nasal ECs.[42,43] It gained popularity in time, thanks to its reliability associated to mini-invasiveness, as demonstrated by many studies on the pediatric population.[44,45] Moreover, the degree of limitation for endoscopic techniques seems minimal. Multiple recent quantitative anatomical studies have demonstrated that endoscopic transnasal approaches are minimally restricted in pediatric patients when compared to adults. The nasal aperture in children is almost always sufficient to accommodate pediatric endoscopes and instrumentation.[46] Nevertheless, this technique appears effective when applied to specific subtypes of nasal ECs (basal ECs, nasoethmoidal ECs).

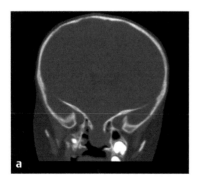
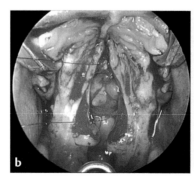

Fig. 33.5 (a, b) Example of combined surgical approach in a 2-year-old toddler affected by de Morsier syndrome. The case was managed with a combined endoscopic transnasal reconstruction of the skull base defect and a contextual transoral correction of the cleft palate.

33.7 Step-by-Step Endoscopic Transnasal Approach

Setting: The surgical procedure is performed under general anesthesia, with controlled arterial blood pressure. Off-label intraoperative intrathecal injection of 5% fluorescein, with a dosage of 0.05–0.1 mL/10 kg, is performed to help identifying the site of the defect (and eventual additional locations in cases of multiple defects) and verifying the watertight seal closure at the end of the procedure.[47] Patient is supine with softly overextended head, slightly turned to the side of the first operator. Rigid 0° and 45° endoscopes with 3 mm diameter (or 4 mm when possible) are used. Tampons soaked with topical anesthetic and, in selected cases, vasoconstrictor drug are inserted in both nostrils using bayonet forceps and kept for 5 to 10 minutes in order to decongest the nasal mucosa. A "four hands" technique is generally practicable[48] (▶ Fig. 33.6).

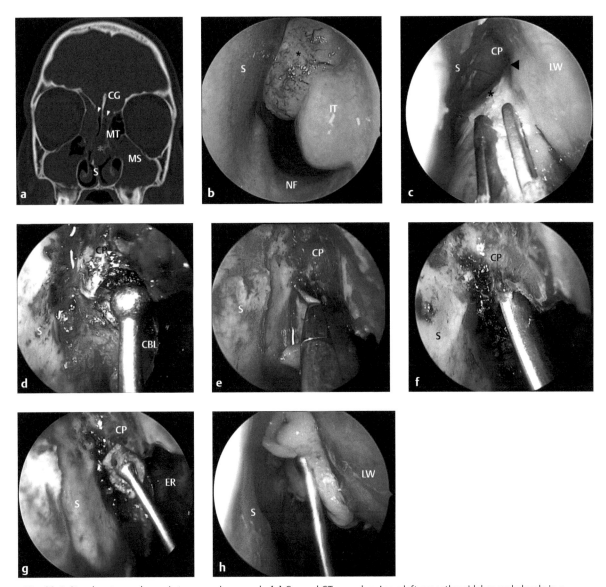

Fig. 33.6 Step-by-step endoscopic transnasal approach. **(a)** Coronal CT scan showing a left nasoethmoidal encephalocele in a 12-year-old child (*red asterisk*). To note the entire incorporation of the middle turbinate inside the encephalic herniation and the asymmetry of anterior skull base (*white arrows*). **(b)** Endoscopic view of the encephalocele occupying the left nasal fossa (*black asterisk*). **(c)** Identification of the origin of herniation (*black asterisk*) and cauterization of the bulging mass. **(d)** Identification of the bony skull base defect which is located, in the presented case, at the level of the insertion of common basal lamella. **(e)** Demucosization of the area nearby the defect. **(f)** Epidural dissection with smooth instrumentation. **(g)** Placement of fascia lata (intracranial layer) and septal cartilage (extradural layer) grafts with gasket-seal technique. **(h)** Placement of an overlay mucoperiosteal graft and stabilization. CG, crista galli; CP, cribriform plate; ER, ethmoidal roof; IT, inferior turbinate; LW, lateral wall; MS, maxillary sinus; MT, middle turbinate; NF, nasal floor; S, septum.

Orientation and space: Before beginning any endoscopic transnasal approach to the skull base, principal landmarks (depending on the approach, maxillary sinus, sphenoid sinus) are identified and exposed, and a good intranasal space is achieved in order to work comfortably.

Exposition: Trying to preserve anatomy and function as much as possible, identification of the EC and its origin, delimitation and exposition of the defect's margins are the first keys for an adequate reconstruction. Depending on its dimension and location, the EC can be cauterized and reduced inside the cranial cavity or resected without any consequence, as it usually contains dysplastic non-functional neural tissue. The only exceptions are represented by cases of transsphenoidal ECs in which the herniated brain might contain the pituitary stalk, the pituitary gland (or some residues), and the hypothalamus. These tissues should always be saved during resection, especially when the endocrine function is preserved. A careful dissection, the intraoperative identification of the ectopic residues of the pituitary gland and a delicate repositioning inside the cranial cavity (with fragment of septal or conchal cartilage) are helpful steps in avoiding postoperative endocrine imbalance.

Margins regularization: Once exposed and well delimited, margins around the defect should be regularized and smoothened and the adjacent mucosa removed in order to receive later on a graft or a flap for reconstruction purposes. This can be done with cutting instruments such as straight and angled Blakesley Thru-Cut forceps and Kerrison rongeur or with diamond burr drills. A delicate epidural dissection is performed, wherever possible, to facilitate the reconstructive step.

Reconstruction: While the above-mentioned principles should be always respected regardless of the kind of defect to face, reconstructive techniques may be selected among a wide spectrum of options, varying from single layer to multilayer plasties, grafts or local vascularized flaps, autologous or heterologous materials. In principle, the ideal material for duraplasty should satisfy a series of criteria: (1) be autologous, to avoid all potential risks of heterogeneous grafts, such as extrusion and infections, (2) be free of biological hazards to avoid communicable diseases, (3) be able to facilitate fibroblastic migration and connective tissue deposition, and (4) exhibit a good cost-effectiveness ratio.[49] In reality, given the rarity and the peculiarity of ECs and the rapid growth rate of the cranial base in pediatric patients, no uniformity of treatment is found in the scientific literature and the surgical choice is more often related to the direct experience of the individual centers that deal with this disease.

Several authors distinguish the repair according to the size of defect, in particular if less or more than 1 cm of diameter; if small, free grafts of fascia (underlay and/or overlay the exposed dura mater), fat, muscle, mucosa, cartilage, bone, or a combination of these materials may be successful, while vascularized tissue is preferable for larger skull base defects or moderate-to-high flow CSF leaks.[21] Furthermore, a local pedicled flap could be located as final layer of reconstruction, in order to obtain a greater stability of the plasty.[38]

In general, the rationale that should drive the choice of the technique is the site and the size of the defect, its relationship with surrounding anatomical structures and the different CSF pressure to which the defect is subjected.

Medication and follow-up: At the end of the reconstructive step, the skull base plasty is stabilized with tabotamp and fibrin glue; expandable packing sponges and silastic sheets (in selected cases) are positioned in the nasal cavities. Bed-rest is mandatory for at least 48 hours, then mobilization is allowed progressively, avoiding all kind of efforts as long as possible. There is no consensus about the indication for lumbar drains, which are suggested mainly in cases of high-flow CSF defects repair.[21] A "second-look" endoscopy[50] may be planned about 3 to 4 weeks after surgery, possibly under sedation (general anesthesia) depending on the patient's age and compliance, in conjunction with an MR. The advantage of this medication includes a detailed inspection of the surgical site and removal of crusting, blood clots, granulation tissue or adhesions, and removal of nasal splints. Serial endoscopic and radiological examinations (MR) are planned at regular intervals (yearly for the first 5 years) until complete craniofacial development is reached.

33.8 Endoscopic Transnasal Surgical Corridors

The knowledge of the exact site of the skull base defect is essential as different localizations can take advantages of different approaches that can be combined accordingly.

- For nasoethmoidal and small transethmoidal ECs, a ***direct paraseptal approach*** to the olfactory cleft is often enough for a good surgical exposure, even preserving the middle turbinate. Whenever needed in order to gain space and orientation, a transethmoidal approach might be taken into account. In this area, the preparation of the receiving site does not include dissection of the dural margin away from the bony border since the dura is extremely fragile, because of the olfactory pores, and any consequent dural tear would mean a useless enlargement of the defect. Reconstruction of defects located around the foramen caecum or defects of the cribriform plate greater than 0.5 cm of diameter are usually repaired in a multilayer fashion (details in the next paragraph), while defects of the cribriform plate smaller than 0.5 cm in diameter are usually repaired with a simple overlay graft (mucoperichondrium or mucoperiostium).[38]
- For transethmoidal and sphenoethmoidal ECs, the surgical steps consider a wider exposure of the ethmoidal roof (***transethmoidal approach***) with resection of the middle turbinate. In these cases, a multilayered

reconstruction is preferable with the underlying principle of re-establishing the tissue barriers. The technique usually involves the application of three layers. The first is made up of fascia (lata or temporal) or dural substitutes placed intracranially and intradurally to serve as a guide for fibroblast migration. In general, this layer should be 30% larger than the dural defect accounting for later shrinkage during healing and prevent recurrences. The second intracranial and extradural layer (underlay) has to be inserted in the previous dissected epidural space and guarantees the plasty with greater stability. Any difficulty encountered when inserting the margins of the fascia in the epidural gap can be overcome by using appropriately shaped fragments of bone or autologous cartilage removed from the nasal cavities or from the ear concha. The third layer, extracranial and intranasal (overlay), facilitates the sealing capacity of the plasty by guiding the repair mechanisms of the nasal mucosa. This layer can be made of fascia or free grafts of septal mucoperichondrium or of septal or turbinal mucoperiostium. It is worth noting that healing and re-epithelialization is much more rapid when mucoperiostium is used as a third layer, rather than fascia, which can sometimes become necrotic even after 1 to 2 months. The "gasket-seal closure" technique is another kind of multilayer reconstruction, used mostly where dural undermining is riskier due to the proximity of neurovascular structures. The planum sphenoidalis represents one of these sites because of the closed proximity to optic nerve and chiasm and superior hypophyseal arteries. This technique allows fixing the graft margins intradurally without risking damage to these neurovascular structures. To accomplish this, the graft is placed on the dural defect and its central portion is pushed inside the defect with the aid of a shaped fragment of septal or conchal cartilage, which is fixed beyond the dural border to seal the closure, while still keeping the margins of the fascia outside the skull base. As with the other closure techniques, it is recommended that no nasal or sinus mucosa be "buried" under any graft or flap to avoid the formation of mucocele.[51]

- For transsphenoidal ECs, a standard bilateral *direct paraseptal sphenoidal approach* is performed, as it is employed to treat sellar lesions. The procedure initially entails partial removal of the vomer (and eventually of the middle turbinate). The septal branch of the sphenopalatine artery is accurately preserved to harvest a nasoseptal flap later on. A wide sphenoidectomy with removal of intersphenoidal septum is performed. In this case a gasket-seal closure combined with a nasoseptal flap can represent a good strategy, considering possible damage of the VI cranial nerves during epidural dissection and a higher intracranial tension at middle and posterior cranial fossa.

- When dealing with sphenomaxillary ECs, exposure is widened through a **trans-ethmoid-pterygoid-sphenoidal approach:** This is a lateral extension of the standard transethmoidal approach. It begins, using a 0° endoscope, with a subtotal uncinectomy, followed by a middle antrostomy extended posteriorly up to the pterygoid process. Then, a complete ethmoidectomy and sphenoidectomy is performed in a standard fashion. After the partial resection of the middle turbinate, sphenopalatine artery is cauterized. The pterygopalatine fossa wall is resected and the posterior wall of the maxillary sinus is partially dissected. Lastly, the base of the pterygoid process is drilled in order to completely expose the lateral recess of the sphenoid sinus. These last steps are performed with the aid of a 45° endoscope, double-angled instruments, and angled drills.[52]

- An infero-lateral extension of this approach is performed when the petroclival or petro-occipital areas have to be reached (**trans-ethmoid-pterygoid-sphenoid-petroclival approach**). In this case by burring the pterygoidal plate and the floor of the sphenoid, following along the Vidian canal, the petroclival region can be approached and, by shifting infero-laterally, the petro-occipital fissure can be reached as well.[53] In both these latter approaches, skull base reconstruction is generally performed through a multilayer technique. However, it is worth noting that in cases of complex petrous bone defects an endoscopic transnasal approach, even wide, might not be sufficient to dominate the defect and a combined external lateral approach is required to achieve a watertight seal reconstruction. The main lateral approaches to be considered are the petro-occipital trans-sigmoid approach, the middle fossa transpetrous approach, the infratemporal fossa approaches (type A, B, C, and D), and the system of modified transcochlear approach.[54]

33.9 Technical Consideration in Pediatric Endoscopic Transnasal Surgery

It is essential to make some clarifications regarding nasal EC's surgery in pediatric age.

33.9.1 Timing of Repair

The exact timing of congenital ECs' repair hasn't been univocally defined yet. In the past, timing depended on a delicate balance between the chance of guaranteeing adequate time for facial development (minimum 3 years old) and the risk of ascending infections or CSF leaks. Nowadays, it is basically dictated by the type of EC and its mode of presentation. In case of life-threatening complications, an early surgery becomes emergent. Besides these conditions, it is probably wiser to postpone surgery until such time that the baby is well enough to tolerate the surgery and blood loss, which is usually around the age of 3 to 4 months.[3] Moreover, given the minimal morbidity of an endoscopic surgical procedure and the low rate of complications reported in the literature, it is recommended that the repair be made as early as possible.[38] In much rarer cases, presenting with hypothalamic and hypophyseal structures' herniation, timing may be dictated by the need to reach an adequate hormonal balance.

33.9.2 Anatomical Aspects

The reduced size of pediatric sinonasal compartments might pose limitations on the ability to approach the skull base endonasally. Until the age of 6 to 7 years old, the nasal aperture is significantly narrower than in adults limiting a surgical approach that requires the passage of many instruments through the piriform aperture.[21] That is why the availability of appropriate surgical instrumentation is unavoidable.[55] Moreover, the endoscopic transnasal approach has long been challenged by the inadequate pneumatization of paranasal sinuses in children since incomplete pneumatization offers smaller working spaces, complicating the endoscopic access through the sinuses to the skull base.[44] This is true specifically for transsphenoidal approaches, related to the variable entity of sphenoid sinus pneumatization. Traditionally, it was accepted that the incomplete sphenoid sinus pneumatization in children under 3 years old would preclude the use of a transsphenoidal approach; however, a study by Tatreau showed that sphenoid sinus dimension doesn't represent an absolute contraindication for expanded endoscopic approaches in pediatric patients, although it requires more drilling during the surgery.[56]

33.9.3 Intraoperative Image Guidance

Intraoperative image guidance systems have been reported as safe and effective tools that facilitate a minimally invasive surgical approach to the skull base in children. Recommendations for their use in pediatric procedures overlap those in adults. Indeed, a particular indication is represented by congenital lesions in which the anatomy and landmarks can be expectedly distorted.[44,57]

33.9.4 Nasoseptal Flap

The nasoseptal flap, pedicled on the posterior septal branches of the sphenopalatine artery, might be used in skull base reconstruction in pediatric patients with high success rate, although poorly described.[21] However, the largest size of nasoseptal flap that can be harvested depends on the dimension and growth level of the nose. A study by Shah, who analyzed craniofacial growth trends in measurements based on CT scans,

showed that the cranial development is rapid in the first few years of life (followed by a leveling off), while skull base continues to increase for at least 10 years after birth. In contrast, the upper midface does not show a dramatic growth early in life, but it accelerates later in time.[58] For this reason, several authors hypothesized that the length of the nasoseptal flap might be insufficient to cover some larger skull base defects in childhood, defining some age limitations for this technique: 6 to 7 years old for a transsellar/transplanum defect and 9 to 10 years old for a transcribriform defect. The flap seems to be insufficient for a clival defect at any pediatric age.[9,21,58] Nevertheless, a few cases in which the flap was successfully used for transsellar/transplanum defects in 4-year-old patients have been described.[21] It is worth noting that nasoseptal flap may be the cause of some local complication such as septal perforation or persistent crusting;[59] thus, it should be reserved for more complex cases, while less invasive grafts remain a reliable technique for simpler defects.

A modification of the nasoseptal flap, pedicled on septal branches of the anterior ethmoidal artery, which has been described for septal perforation repair[60] and covering of posterior wall of frontal sinus during Draf III procedures,[61] might represent an advantageous alternative to reconstruct defects located at the foramen caecum or at the posterior wall of frontal infundibulum (▶ Fig. 33.7).

33.10 Complications and Long-term Outcomes

In general, potential complications after endoscopic transnasal surgery are variable and in part related to the age of the patient, nature of the disease treated (size, type), extent of the surgical intervention, and choice of reconstructive method. Possible complications include those related to sinonasal function, neurovascular injury (hemorrhage, cranial nerve dysfunction), CSF leak, central NS infection (meningitis, cerebritis, abscess), and damage to central NS tissue (endocrinopathy, motor or sensory dysfunction).[13,21] The most thorough discussion on complications associated with endoscopic transnasal surgery has been in a report that encompasses 171 procedures performed in 133 pediatric patients for a variety of anterior skull base pathologies. In the "skull base defect" group (21/133), the rate of complication was much less than in the "skull base tumor" group.[44]

There is an overall good prognosis and a low mortality rate, with 3% surgery-related mortality. Children with nasal ECs have better neurocognitive development compared to those with occipital ECs. Location doesn't represent a significant outcome predictor, but isolated nasal ECs have a better prognosis than those with any other associated defect.[13]

An important consideration in pediatric patients is the potential impact of skull base surgery on

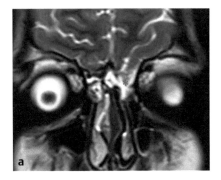
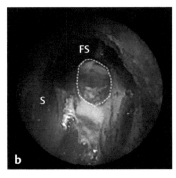
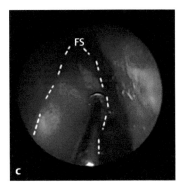
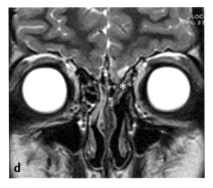

Fig. 33.7 Example of anterior skull base reconstruction with a modified nasoseptal flap pedicled on septal branches of the anterior ethmoidal artery (14-year-old patient). **(a)** T2 MR sequence with evidence of an anterior skull base defect located at the level of left posterior wall of the frontal infundibulum (*red asterisk*). **(b)** Intraoperative view of the defect (*white dashed line*) enhanced by fluorescein. **(c)** Defect repair with an omolateral modified nasoseptal flap (*white dashed line*). **(d)** 4-month MR follow-up which shows a good stability of the reconstruction (*yellow asterisk*). FS, frontal sinus; S, septum.

craniofacial growth. Based on different experiences with open skull base surgery and sinus surgery for inflammatory disease,[62] it seems that endoscopic transnasal surgery can be done safely with little consequences on craniofacial growth, but further longitudinal studies are required to definitively understand the long-term impact.[21,44]

33.11 Highlights

a. Clinical presentation
   - Asymptomatic.
   - Isolated or associated to malformative syndromes.
   - Frontoethmoidal EC: skin-covered masses or visible protrusions, positive Furstenberg sign.
   - Basal EC: snoring, oral breathing, feeding difficulties, CSF rhinorrhea, meningitis or encephalitis.

b. Indications
   - Any diagnosed EC or MEC, confirmed trough a beta-2 transferrin or beta-trace test and/or CT and MRI exam.
   - Early repair.
   - Pure basal and nasoethmoidal EC can benefit from endoscopic transnasal approach.
   - Complex or syndromic cases necessitate of multidisciplinary treatment.
   - Outpatient biopsy is contraindicated.

c. Complications
   - Intranasal or intracranial bleeding.
   - Central NS infection.
   - CSF leak.
   - Endocrinopathy.
   - Motor or sensory nerve dysfunction.
   - Sinonasal synechiae and stenosis.

d. Special preoperative considerations
   - General endotracheal anesthesia.
   - BBB crossing antibiotics.
   - Intrathecal injection of 5% fluorescein in selected cases.

e. Special intraoperative considerations
   - Orientation: exposition of intranasal landmarks.
   - Identification and exposition of EC and skull base defect margins.
   - EC reduction or resection.
   - Margins regularization.
   - Skull base reconstruction through single or multilayer plasty.

f. Special postoperative considerations
   - 48 hours bed rest.
   - "Second look endoscopy" after 2–4 weeks.

References

[1] Sever LE, Sanders M, Monsen R. An epidemiologic study of neural tube defects in Los Angeles County I. Prevalence at birth based on multiple sources of case ascertainment. Teratology 1982;25(3):315–321

[2] Emery JL, Kalhan SC. The pathology of exencephalus. Dev Med Child Neurol Suppl 1970;22(Suppl 22):22–, 51

[3] Singh AK, Upadhyaya DN. Sincipital encephaloceles. J Craniofac Surg 2009;20(Suppl 2):1851–1855

[4] Albright AL, Pollack IF, Adelson PD. Principles and Practice of Pediatric Neurosurgery. Thieme; 2014

[5] Winn HR, Youmans JR. Youmans Neurological Surgery. Saunders; 2004

[6] Locatelli D, Rampa F, Acchiardi I, Bignami M, Pistochini A, Castelnuovo P. Endoscopic endonasal approaches to anterior skull base defects in pediatric patients. Childs Nerv Syst 2006;22(11):1411–1418

[7] Warf BC, Stagno V, Mugamba J. Encephalocele in Uganda: ethnic distinctions in lesion location, endoscopic management of hydrocephalus, and survival in 110 consecutive children. J Neurosurg Pediatr 2011;7(1):88–93

[8] Barnes L. Surgical Pathology of the Head and Neck. M. Dekker, 2001

[9] Gump WC. Endoscopic endonasal repair of congenital defects of the anterior skull base: developmental considerations and surgical outcomes. J Neurol Surg B Skull Base 2015;76(4):291–295

[10] Morina A, Kelmendi F, Morina Q, Dragusha S, Ahmeti F, Morina D. Treatment of anterior encephaloceles over 24 years in Kosova. Med Arh 2011;65(2):122–124

[11] Wang IJ, Lin SL, Tsou KI, et al. Congenital midline nasal mass: cases series and review of the literature. Turk J Pediatr 2010;52(5):520–524

[12] Suwanwela C, Suwanwela N. A morphological classification of sincipital encephalomeningoceles. J Neurosurg 1972;36(2):201–211

[13] Tirumandas M, Sharma A, Gbenimacho I, et al. Nasal encephaloceles: a review of etiology, pathophysiology, clinical presentations, diagnosis, treatment, and complications. Childs Nerv Syst 2013;29(5):739–744

[14] Sdano MT, Pensak ML. Temporal bone encephaloceles. Curr Opin Otolaryngol Head Neck Surg 2005;13(5):287–289

[15] Nadaraja GS, Monfared A, Jackler RK. Spontaneous cerebrospinal fluid leak through the posterior aspect of the petrous bone. J Neurol Surg B Skull Base 2012;73(1):71–75

[16] Jamjoom DZ, Alorainy IA. The association between petrous apex cephalocele and empty sella. Surg Radiol Anat 2015;37(10):1179–1182

[17] Connor SE, Leung R, Natas S. Imaging of the petrous apex: a pictorial review. Br J Radiol 2008;81(965):427–435

[18] Alexiou GA, Sfakianos G, Prodromou N. Diagnosis and management of cephaloceles. J Craniofac Surg 2010;21(5):1581–1582

[19] Gilbert SF, Singer SR, Kozlowski RN. Developmental Biology. Sinauer Associates; 2000

[20] Di leva A, Bruner E, Haider T, et al. Skull base embryology: a multidisciplinary review. Childs Nerv Syst 2014;30(6):991–1000

[21] Rastatter JC, Snyderman CH, Gardner PA, Alden TD, Tyler-Kabara E. Endoscopic endonasal surgery for sinonasal and skull base lesions in the pediatric population. Otolaryngol Clin North Am 2015;48(1):79–99

[22] Hoving EW. Nasal encephaloceles. Childs Nerv Syst 2000;16(10–11):702–706

[23] Broekman ML, Hoving EW, Kho KH, Speleman L, Han KS, Hanlo PW. Nasal encephalocele in a child with Beckwith-Wiedemann syndrome. J Neurosurg Pediatr 2008;1(6):485–487

[24] Bear KA, Solomon BD, Roessler E, et al. Evidence for SHH as a candidate gene for encephalocele. Clin Dysmorphol 2012;21(3):148–151

[25] McLone DG. Neurosurgeons, A.S.O.P., & Neurosurgery, A.A.O.N.S.S.O.P. Pediatric Neurosurgery: Surgery of the Developing Nervous System. Saunders; 2001

[26] Marin-Padilla M, Marin-Padilla TM. Morphogenesis of experimentally induced Arnold-Chiari malformation. J Neurol Sci 1981;50(1):29–55

[27] Policeni BA, Smoker WR. Imaging of the skull base: anatomy and pathology. Radiol Clin North Am 2015;53(1):1–14

[28] Chen CS, David D, Hanieh A. Morning glory syndrome and basal encephalocele. Childs Nerv Syst 2004;20(2):87–90

[29] Bakri SJ, Siker D, Masaryk T, Luciano MG, Traboulsi EI. Ocular malformations, moyamoya disease, and midline cranial defects: a distinct syndrome. Am J Ophthalmol 1999;127(3):356–357

[30] Fadakar K, Dadkhahfar S, Esmaeili A, Keyhanidoust Z. A case of schizencephaly and septo-optic dysplasia presenting with anterior encephalocele. Iran J Child Neurol 2012;6(4):47–50

[31] Periakaruppan A, Pendharkar HS, Gupta AK, Thomas B, Kesavdas C. Septo-optic dysplasia with encephalocele. J Clin Neurosci 2009;16(12):1665–1667

[32] Lee S, Rivkin MJ, Kirton A, deVeber G, Elbers J; International Pediatric Stroke Study. Moyamoya disease in children: results from the International Pediatric Stroke Study. J Child Neurol 2017;32(11):924–929

[33] Teng E, Heller J, Lazareff J, et al. Caution in treating transsphenoidal encephalocele with concomitant moyamoya disease. J Craniofac Surg 2006;17(5):1004–1009

[34] Joy HM, Barker CS, Small JH, Armitage M. Trans-sphenoidal encephalocele in association with Dandy-Walker complex and cardiovascular anomalies. Neuroradiology 2001;43(1):45–48

[35] Manara R, Priante E, Grimaldi M, et al; Italian MPS Neuroimaging Study Group. Closed meningo(encephalo)cele: a new feature in Hunter syndrome. AJNR Am J Neuroradiol 2012;33(5):873–877

[36] Melbourne-Chambers R, Singh Minott I, Mowatt L, Johnson P, Thame M. Aicardi syndrome associated with anterior cephalocele in a female infant. Dev Med Child Neurol 2007;49(6):464–466

[37] Bogusiak K, Puch A, Arkuszewski P. Goldenhar syndrome: current perspectives. World J Pediatr 2017;13(5):405–415

[38] Castelnuovo P, Bignami M, Pistochini A, Battaglia P, Locatelli D, Dallan I. Endoscopic endonasal management of encephaloceles in children: an eight-year experience. Int J Pediatr Otorhinolaryngol 2009;73(8):1132–1136

[39] Steven RA, Rothera MP, Tang V, Bruce IA. An unusual cause of nasal airway obstruction in a neonate: trans-sellar, trans-sphenoidal cephalocele. J Laryngol Otol 2011;125(10):1075–1078

[40] Hedlund G. Congenital frontonasal masses: developmental anatomy, malformations, and MR imaging. Pediatr Radiol 2006;36(7):647–662, quiz 726–727

[41] Saettele M, Alexander A, Markovich B, Morelli J, Lowe LH. Congenital midline nasofrontal masses. Pediatr Radiol 2012;42(9):1119–1125

[42] Baradaran N, Nejat F, Baradaran N, El Khashab M. Cephalocele: report of 55 cases over 8 years. Pediatr Neurosurg 2009;45(6):461–466

[43] Abdel-Aziz M, El-Bosraty H, Qotb M, et al. Nasal encephalocele: endoscopic excision with anesthetic consideration. Int J Pediatr Otorhinolaryngol 2010;74(8):869–873

[44] Chivukula S, Koutourousiou M, Snyderman CH, Fernandez-Miranda JC, Gardner PA, Tyler-Kabara EC. Endoscopic endonasal skull base surgery in the pediatric population. J Neurosurg Pediatr 2013;11(3):227–241

[45] Kassam A, Thomas AJ, Snyderman C, et al. Fully endoscopic expanded endonasal approach treating skull base lesions in pediatric patients. J Neurosurg 2007;106(2, Suppl):75–86

[46] Banu MA, Rathman A, Patel KS, et al. Corridor-based endonasal endoscopic surgery for pediatric skull base pathology with detailed radioanatomic measurements. Neurosurgery 2014;10(Suppl 2):273–293, discussion 293

[47] Wolf G, Greistorfer K, Stammberger H. Endoscopic detection of cerebrospinal fluid fistulas with a fluorescence technique. Report of experiences with over 925 cases Laryngorhinootologie 1997;76(10):588–594

[48] Castelnuovo P, Pistochini A, Locatelli D. Different surgical approaches to the sellar region: focusing on the "two nostrils four hands technique". Rhinology 2006;44(1):2–7

[49] Schick B, Wolf G, Romeike BF, Mestres P, Praetorius M, Plinkert PK. Dural cell culture. A new approach to study duraplasty. Cells Tissues Organs 2003;173(3):129–137

[50] Chang PH, Lee LA, Huang CC, Lai CH, Lee TJ. Functional endoscopic sinus surgery in children using a limited approach. Arch Otolaryngol Head Neck Surg 2004;130(9):1033–1036

[51] Draf W, Carrau RL, Bockmuehl U. Endonasal endoscopic surgery of skull base tumors: an interdisciplinary approach. Thieme; 2015

[52] Castelnuovo P, Dallan I, Pistochini A, Battaglia P, Locatelli D, Bignami M. Endonasal endoscopic repair of Sternberg's canal cerebrospinal fluid leaks. Laryngoscope 2007;117(2):345–349

[53] Castelnuovo P, Dallan I, Bignami M, Pistochini A, Battaglia P, Tschabitscher M. Endoscopic endonasal management of petroclival cerebrospinal fluid leaks: anatomical study and preliminary clinical experience. Minim Invasive Neurosurg 2008;51(6):336–339

[54] Sanna M, De Donato G, Russo A, Taibah AK, Falcioni M, Mancini F. Lateral approaches to the clivus and surrounding areas. Otol Jpn 1999;9(2):116–134

[55] Woodworth BA, Schlosser RJ, Faust RA, Bolger WE. Evolutions in the management of congenital intranasal skull base defects. Arch Otolaryngol Head Neck Surg 2004;130(11):1283–1288

[56] Tatreau JR, Patel MR, Shah RN, et al. Anatomical considerations for endoscopic endonasal skull base surgery in pediatric patients. Laryngoscope 2010;120(9):1730–1737

[57] Benoit MM, Silvera VM, Nichollas R, Jones D, McGill T, Rahbar R. Image guidance systems for minimally invasive sinus and skull base surgery in children. Int J Pediatr Otorhinolaryngol 2009;73(10):1452–1457

[58] Shah RN, Surowitz JB, Patel MR, et al. Endoscopic pedicled nasoseptal flap reconstruction for pediatric skull base defects. Laryngoscope 2009;119(6):1067–1075

[59] Soudry E, Psaltis AJ, Lee KH, Vaezafshar R, Nayak JV, Hwang PH. Complications associated with the pedicled nasoseptal flap for skull base reconstruction. Laryngoscope 2015;125(1):80–85

[60] Castelnuovo P, Ferreli F, Khodaei I, Palma P. Anterior ethmoidal artery septal flap for the management of septal perforation. Arch Facial Plast Surg 2011;13(6):411–414

[61] AlQahtani A, Bignami M, Terranova P, et al. Newly designed double-vascularized nasoseptal flap to prevent restenosis after endoscopic modified Lothrop procedure (Draf III): laboratory investigation. Eur Arch Otorhinolaryngol 2014;271(11):2951–2955

[62] Bothwell MR, Piccirillo JF, Lusk RP, Ridenour BD. Long-term outcome of facial growth after functional endoscopic sinus surgery. Otolaryngol Head Neck Surg 2002;126(6):628–634

34 Brain Stem Implantation

Baishakhi Choudhury, David R. Friedmann, J. Thomas Roland Jr

Summary

Auditory brainstem implants, first intended for auditory rehabilitation in deaf patients with neurofibromatosis-2, have been more recently applied in the pediatric populations who are not candidates for cochlear implantation. Herein we review the history of these devices and surgical techniques in auditory brainstem implantation.

We include a review of recently published literature including outcomes data in this unique population.

Keywords: Auditory brainstem implant, hearing loss, auditory nerve dysfunction, neurofibromatosis type 2

34.1 Introduction

Hearing rehabilitation options are dictated by the nature and etiology of the hearing loss. Patients who do not have a functional auditory nerve connecting the cochlea to the cochlear nucleus in the brainstem cannot benefit from a cochlear implant because they lack a means of sending auditory information centrally. In order to bypass the peripheral auditory system, auditory brainstem implants (ABIs) were developed. This chapter will review ABI technology and potential applications in the pediatric population.

34.1.1 History

The first successful ABI for long-term auditory rehabilitation was performed in 1979 at the House Ear Institute in California.[1,2] The patient was a 51-year-old woman with neurofibromatosis type 2 (NF2) who was undergoing vestibular schwannoma removal in her only hearing ear secondary to tumor growth and development of mild hydrocephalus. She was initially implanted with a platinum electrode pair with 0.5 mm balls separated by 1.5 mm, which was placed within the brainstem in the region that was determined to be the cochlear nucleus. She reported benefit from the implant, with enhanced lip reading and environmental sound awareness, for approximately two months and then unfortunately auditory benefit deteriorated. A new electrode system was designed and constructed and the patient was re-implanted with a new system composed of two 1.7 × 2.0 mm platinum pads mounted on a Dacron mesh, separated by a distance of 3.0 mm. The new design was developed to reduce the problem of electrode migration thought to be the cause of the initial implant failure. Re-implantation was performed in 1981 with the electrode pads positioned on the surface of the cochlear nucleus. Postoperatively, the patient again received similar benefit to the initial implant and per last published report continues to use the implant in her daily life.[2]

Based on further experience with ABI, and documenting safety and potential efficacy, in 2000, the Food and Drug Administration (FDA) approved the use of a multichannel ABI in patients 12 years of age and older who have been diagnosed with NF2. In 2013, the FDA approved an investigational device exemption (IDE) for the use of ABIs in children who are born without an auditory nerve or without a cochlea or who are otherwise not candidates for cochlear implantation. Over 1,000 ABI procedures have been performed worldwide.[3] Results have been mixed, but the ABI continues to offer hope for a population of patients who otherwise do not have access to the auditory world. This can be important from a quality-of-life standpoint, and added safety and security that comes from environmental sound awareness.[4,5] It may also serve as an adjunct to speech reading and enhance total communication approaches. ABI design, placement, and speech processing strategies continue to be a topic of interest in attempt to more consistently maximize results from these devices.

34.1.2 Anatomy

All auditory nerve afferent fibers carry information from the cochlea to the cochlear nucleus (CN) located near the surface of the brainstem.[6] The CN is located at the lateral aspect of the pontomedullary junction, and is divided into a ventral cochlear nucleus (VCN) and a dorsal cochlear nucleus (DCN).[7] The VCN is further subdivided into an anteroventral cochlear nucleus (AVCN) and a posteroventral cochlear nucleus (PVCN).[8] These nuclei are identified next to the lateral recess of the fourth ventricle.[7] There is noticeable variation in the shape of the CN in individuals; however, each CN extends about 8 mm dorsoventrally, 10 mm mediolaterally, and the rostrocaudal extent is less than 3 mm.[9] Each division of the nucleus is composed of different sets of neurons and each cell type encodes specific sound information.[8] The shape of the VCN and its proximity to the surface can be variable in humans.[9] Sound waves of low frequency are relayed to the VCN and sound waves of high frequency are relayed to the DCN.[8,10,11] However, the DCN has another level of complexity as it is also responsible for integrating auditory and multisensory inputs from distinct pathways, and studies have shown neuromodulators are responsible for enhancing inputs from one pathway while inhibiting inputs from another.[12] These excitatory and inhibitory pathways need to be further parsed to determine the optimal stimulation paradigm that an ABI would provide.

A study looking at the morphological and functional maturation of the CN showed that development occurs during mid-gestation and continues up to term.[8] The foramen of Luschka is the pathway to the CN intraoperatively.

The foramen of Luschka projects into the cerebellopontine angle (CPA) at the lateral border of the pontomedullary sulcus.[13] The junction of the glossopharyngeal and vagus nerves with the brainstem is just ventral to the foramen and the junction of the facial and vestibulocochlear nerves with the brainstem is anterior inferior to it. The junction of the accessory and hypoglossal nerves with the brainstem is antero-inferior to the foramen as well. The cerebellar flocculus is directly superior to the foramen. The anterior inferior cerebellar artery (AICA) and the posterior inferior cerebellar artery (PICA) can have close and variable courses with the foramen. The vein of the cerebellomedullary fissure can course between the flocculus and the foramen of Luschka.[14,15]

34.1.3 Auditory Brain Stem Implant Device

Just like a cochlear implant, the components inherent in all ABIs are a microphone, a speech processor, a receiver/stimulator, and an electrode array. The electrode array configuration is the main difference from a cochlear implant since the electrode array is designed to be placed on the surface of the cochlear nucleus. Cochlear Corporation (Sydney, Aus) is the only manufacturer of an ABI with current Food and Drug Administration (FDA) approval in the United States. In 2016, its newest model of the ABI, the Cochlear Nucleus Profile Auditory Brainstem Implant (ABI541) was introduced.[16] It has a paddle that consists of 21 platinum electrodes that is 8.5 × 3.0 mm in area and it's designed to work with the Nucleus 6 sound processor.

MED-EL Corporation (Innsbruck, Au) also manufactures an ABI used elsewhere. The external audio processor is either an OPUS 2 or OPUS 1. The implant itself consists of the receiver/stimulator and an implantable soft silicone matrix with a 12-contact electrode array. The dimensions of the matrix are 5.5 × 3.0 mm. An additional reference electrode is also present to facilitate different stimulation modes.[17]

Oticon medical is the third manufacturer of ABIs. The Digisonic SP ABI brainstem implant is designed with an array of 15 surface electrodes that is positioned on the cochlear nucleus. The Digisonic SP ABI is used with the Saphyr neo collection sound processor.[18]

34.2 Preoperative Evaluation and Anesthesia

ABIs are meant to provide auditory stimulation directly to the cochlear nucleus; therefore, they can be considered in any patient who has an intact cochlear nucleus but does not have functional auditory nerves or in an individual with bilateral cochlear agenesis who cannot undergo cochlear implantation.

Traditionally, the main patients considered for ABIs were NF2 patients who have poor hearing bilaterally and large tumors that do not allow for preservation of the cochlear nerve. In these patients an ABI can be placed at the time of tumor removal from one side. More pediatric non-NF2 patients who are congenitally deaf are now being considered for implantation, such as patients with bilateral cochlear agenesis or absent cochlear nerves on imaging.

There are cases where a cochlea is present and there is a semblance of a cochlear nerve innervating the cochlea on high-resolution MRI. Even in these cases of suspected cochlear nerve deficiency, our current protocol is to perform cochlear implantation on one side as some of these children may receive more auditory benefit than expected with an ABI. The children who do not appear to receive any benefit, or minimal benefit, postcochlear implantation can then be considered for an ABI.

This raises an important clinical consideration relating to where to implant the ABI when other hearing devices are present. Considerations may include the degree of malformation or suspected presence of an adequate cochlear nerve. The side with a more developed lateral recess should be preferred. A more developed lateral recess entails a favorable entrance to the lateral recess or where cerebellar retraction could be minimized. Also the side with more developed neuronal structures should be targeted as this may have implications for the degree of development of other structures inherent to the central auditory pathway.

Among our cohort of pediatric ABI recipients, some continue to use a cochlear implant (CI) contralateral to the ABI while others have their CI device removed at the time of their ABI placement based on the above considerations.

Evaluations must take into account other deficits that the patients have, especially visual and neurocognitive deficits. Evaluation for candidacy should be performed in a multi-disciplinary approach involving pediatric neurotology, neurosurgery, audiology, speech therapy, and neuropsychology. Candidates should be able to undergo postimplant speech and auditory rehabilitation in order to gain the maximum benefit from their implant. Patients and parents of patients undergoing ABI should be counseled with regard to expectations after implantation.

34.3 Surgical Technique

An ABI can be placed using either a translabyrinthine approach or a retrosigmoid approach. In the NF2 population in which tumor removal is being performed simultaneously, a translabyrinthine approach is often preferred. Our protocol in the non-NF2 pediatric population involves a retrosigmoid approach as no tumor removal is involved. General anesthesia without long-term paralytics should be administered to allow for nerve monitoring. As for all skull base surgery, an experienced neuro-anesthesia team and electrophysiologic monitoring team is critical. Pediatric ABI should only be undertaken at centers with prior experience with adult ABI and with pediatric neurosurgery expertise.

Perioperative antibiotics are administered as well as decadron, 0.5 mg/kg up to a max of 10 mg. Mannitol is also given once the craniotomy has begun for brain relaxation. The patient is positioned in the supine position with the head turned to the contralateral side. Continuous electromyograph facial nerve monitor electrodes are applied to the orbicularis oris and oculi on the surgical side and a Prass probe for active stimulation is made available. Subdermal electrodes are also placed for measuring an electrical auditory brainstem response (EABR) once the implant is in place. These electrodes are placed at the vertex of the head, over the seventh cervical vertebrae and the hairline of the occiput. An endotracheal tube with recurrent laryngeal nerve monitoring electrodes is also used for intubation in order to monitor cranial nerve X (▶Fig. 34.1).

The patient is prepped and draped for a standard retrosigmoid incision. If a tumor is present, an appropriate approach is planned with regard to tumor size and location. The abdomen is prepped and draped for abdominal fat graft harvest as well.

The skin is incised down to the level of the temporalis fascia and reflected anteriorly and posteriorly. The incision is then carried through to bone and periosteum is elevated off the bone posteriorly and superiorly to the planned craniotomy site and the lateral sinus. Using a silicone replica of the receiver/stimulator a bony seat is drilled for the device as well as a trough for the electrode lead wire before it enters the dura through the craniotomy site (▶Fig. 34.2). In order to secure the device, a permanent suture is used to close the mouth of the soft tissue pocket in which the receiver-stimulator will reside. The approach to the CPA is performed in the standard fashion and the lower cranial nerves as well as CN VII and VIII (if present) are identified (▶Fig. 34.3). Nerve stimulation can be used to verify cranial nerve positions of VII and X. The foramen of Luschka is found between the roots of CN VII and CN IX, where the choroid plexus is identified. Alternatively, if a remnant of CN VIII is present, this can be followed back to the brainstem where the choroid plexus can then be identified. The choroid can then gently be spread to enlarge the opening into the foramen of Luschka. Often the tinea, a soft tissue arachnoid band is opened to allow access to the foramen. In addition, a vein over the foramen can be dissected away from the opening. To verify correct identification of the lateral recess of the fourth ventricle, a valsalva can be performed and CSF outflow should be noted.

At this point the device can be brought into the field and placed into the well previously made and sutured

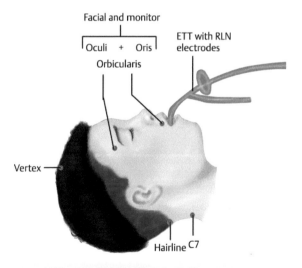

Fig. 34.1 Graphic representation of the electrode positioning for electrophysiologic monitoring intraoperatively. The patient is positioned in the supine position with the head turned to the contralateral side. Continuous electromyograph (EMG) facial nerve monitor electrodes are applied to the orbicularis oris and oculi on the surgical side. Subdermal electrodes are also placed at the vertex of the head, over the seventh cervical vertebrae, and on the hairline of the occiput for measuring an electrical auditory brainstem response (EABR) once the implant is in place. An endotracheal tube with recurrent laryngeal nerve monitoring electrodes is also used for intubation in order to monitor cranial nerve X.

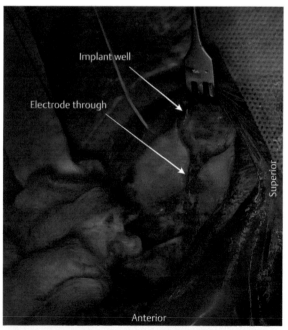

Fig. 34.2 Shows the bony seat that is drilled for the receiver/stimulator as well as a trough for the electrode lead wire before it enters the dura through the craniotomy site. The craniotomy site is anterior and inferior to the well. A silicone replica of the receiver/stimulator can be used as a guide.

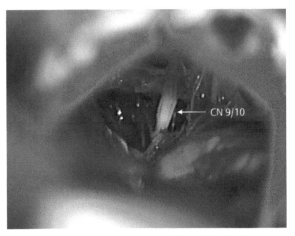

Fig. 34.3 View of the posterior cranial fossa after dural incision and retraction of the cerebellum. The lower cranial nerves are identified.

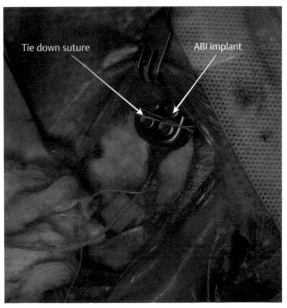

Fig. 34.4 Placement of the device. After the lateral recess of the fourth ventricle has been identified the device can be brought into the field and placed into the well previously made and sutured into place with a permanent suture.

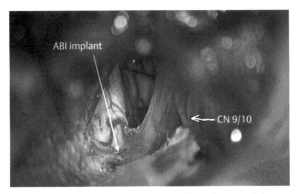

Fig. 34.5 After paddle insertion into the lateral recess of the fourth ventricle. The paddle is inserted with the electrodes facing superiorly and anteriorly.

into place with a permanent suture (▶ Fig. 34.4). Both the suture and the bony seat prevent migration of the receiver/stimulator. The lead wires are placed into the trough and the free ground wire is placed medial to the temporalis muscle periosteum similar to a cochlear implant. We found that proper positioning of the Nucleus 24 Auditory Brainstem Implant required trimming the wings of the mesh on the back of the electrode paddle without damaging the electrodes. We then insert the paddle with the electrodes facing superiorly and anteriorly into the lateral recess of the fourth ventricle (▶ Fig. 34.5). To obtain optimal placement and the least amount of non-auditory stimulation, our audiology colleagues test the electrodes on the device by sending electrical stimulation to bipolar pairs of electrodes and determine whether an (EABR) is evoked or whether non-auditory stimuli patterns are noted such as facial nerve stimulation, myogenic responses, or changes in pulse rate or hemodynamics. The electrode paddle can be shifted if intraoperative EABR implant testing indicates a row or column of electrodes does not evoke any

electrophysiologic responses consistent with auditory stimulation. With this intraoperative feedback, an optimal position of the paddle over the cochlear nucleus is obtained. A paddle-o-gram, which details auditory stimuli and non-auditory stimuli, is made by the audiology team (▶ Fig. 34.6). This assists the team during initial stimulation of the device postoperatively.

A piece of Teflon felt posterior to the electrode paddle can be used to stabilize the paddle in the lateral recess. The matrix of dacron mesh on the electrode paddle provides a scaffold for ingrowth of fibrous tissue that will further stabilize the electrode position.

The electrode lead is brought out through the inferior aspect of the dural flap if a retrosigmoid approach is performed and the dura is closed with 4–0 Neurolon suture with standard technique. The portion of the electrode that spans the dura is wrapped with a piece of muscle to prevent CSF leak from around the electrode insertion through the dura. Tisseal tissue glue is placed over the electrode entry into the dura and over the dural suture line. The bone plate is fixed with miniplates and screws and abdominal fat can be used as needed to pack craniectomy sites and to seal off mastoid air cells. Standard closure of the surgical site is then performed with standard mastoid dressing (▶ Fig. 34.7).

34.4 Postoperative Treatment

Postoperative monitoring and care involves 24-hour monitoring in the pediatric intensive care unit (PICU)

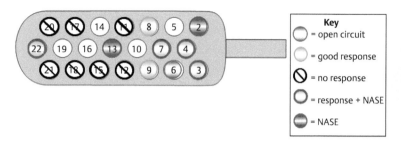

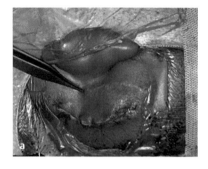 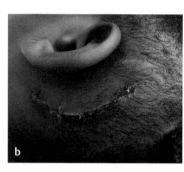

Fig. 34.6 Example of a paddle-o-gram that is obtained from EABR testing intraoperatively. The key is shown in the figure, "good response" indicating a good auditory waveform and "NASE" indicating non-auditory side effect. This key will then be used during the initial stimulation.

Fig. 34.7 Standard closure of the surgical site. **(a)** An intraoperative picture and **(b)** approximately 2 weeks postoperatively.

with frequent neurological checks. Patient is then transferred to the floor on postoperative day 1 and begins to mobilize. Monitoring and mobilization continue on postoperative day 2 and the majority of patients are discharged home on postoperative day 3 once the firm mastoid dressing is removed. Perioperative steroids are routinely administered.

34.4.1 Implant Activation

Implant activation occurs approximately 4 weeks after implantation to allow for healing. The patient is brought back to the operating room for device activation since the manufacturer recommends that patients be connected to vital sign monitors during initial stimulation. Testing is often performed under sedation with dexmedetomidine in pediatrics. Initial testing assesses for EABR responses as well as non-auditory stimulation, such as myogenic responses, facial stimulation, gag reflex/vocal cord stimulation, or bradycardia. The electrophysiologic monitoring setup is similar to that used during operative insertion of the implant except that direct visualization of the vocal cords or soft palate is utilized. Methods of reducing or eliminating non-auditory stimulation if present can be employed, such as changing the reference ground electrode or increasing the stimulus pulse duration. If this initial testing shows no untoward effects, threshold and comfort levels on each electrode are determined and the activation continues on the following day with the patient awake. If the patient is able to report auditory and non-auditory responses, these are recorded for each electrode and stimulation level. If any differences in pitch perception are noted by the patient with different electrode stimulations, these are also recorded. The ability to pitch

rank has implications for speech recognition.[19] If patients report differences in pitch perception, this information is used to program the speech processor. Routine visits for device reprogramming are ideal for the first year after implantation. A typical postimplantation evaluation protocol is initial activation 4 to 6 weeks postimplant, then 1 month, 6 month, and 1 year intervals. Patients should be evaluated annually thereafter.[20]

The programming of young children with ABIs can be more difficult because they are unable to provide verbal feedback with regard to auditory and non-auditory stimuli. An experienced pediatric implant team is needed to determine optimal programming of the implant. Usually EABRs obtained at the time of implant insertion are used as a starting point to establish which electrodes are providing auditory versus non-auditory sensations in a safe and monitored setting. Then careful behavioral testing by trained and experienced audiologists with medical monitoring is needed for safe and optimal stimulation. As with older children and adults, retesting is necessary at least in the initial period as settings can change significantly.

34.4.2 Surgical Complications

The more common postoperative complications are CSF leak, implant migration, and non-auditory stimuli in both adults and children.

CSF leaks may be treated with lumbar drain placement for CSF diversion. Rarely is re-operation for leak repair necessary. CSF leak rates have been reported to be approximately 3.3% to 11%, percentages that are comparable to those from other retrosigmoid and translabyrinthine craniotomies.[21,22]

Implant migration has been improved by dacron backing of the paddle and nonelastic wires. One of 61 patients "lost" more than one electrode over time according to a study by Kuchta et al.[23]

The most common complication reported is non-auditory stimuli, which develops in up to 42% of users.[21,24–26] The most common sensations are dizziness and ipsilateral "tingling." Other sensations described include "jittering" of vision, muscle twitches mainly of CN VII and IX and contralateral "tingling."[20,25,27] Most of this non-auditory stimulation are usually characterized as minimal by the patient and often can be "mapped out" by adjustment of the duration of the stimulus or by selecting a different ground electrode. Removing electrodes with persistent non-auditory side effects from the device map is often required. Reducing the rate of stimulation can also help in some cases.[26] Also, many of these non-auditory sensations often decrease over time, and 9% of patients develop persistent non-auditory sensations.[20,22,27] The incidence of non-auditory stimuli appear to be related to misplacement of the ABI with protrusion from the lateral recess allowing current spread outside of the cochlear nucleus over the surface of the brainstem.[28] Studies have shown that structures within two millimeters of the electrode may be inappropriately stimulated.[28] Non-auditory stimuli more often result from stimulation of the most medial and lateral electrodes.[21,29]

Other more rare complications have been reported to occur such as cerebellar contusion, permanent facial palsy, meningitis, damage of the lower cranial nerves, hydrocephalus, and pseudomeningocele, headache, and tinnitus. Per reports, the complications were significantly less in the nontumor patients than in the NF2 patients.[30]

34.4.3 Outcomes

A multi-institutional study in the United States reported that overall (adults and children) 81% of implants received auditory sensations. Thus far, the ABI appears to provide the most benefit in the form of enhancing lip reading and for providing environmental sound awareness and differentiation. When combined with lip reading, 93% of patients demonstrate improved sentence understanding at 3 to 6 months postimplant. Significant open-set word recognition is rare.[21,29,31] It seems that patients do improve gradually with use of the ABI over time, one study noted improvements in performance seen up to 8 years after implantation.[21,29] Interestingly, patient's subjective evaluation of the ABI is generally higher than would be predicted by objective audiometric data.[32] Preoperative counseling with regard to personal motivation, reasonable expectations, and family support is of particular importance in these candidates. The counseling should stress the following points: (1) some patients do not receive auditory sensations, (2) the ABI does not provide normal sound quality, (3) most ABI patients do not achieve open-set speech recognition, (4) regular follow-ups are required for optimization of the ABI, (5) it will take time and use to develop maximum benefit from the ABI.[22,27,32]

Studies of ABI outcomes seem to show that outcomes of non-NF2 patients implanted with an ABI perform better than those with NF2.[33,34] Given these findings, studies to expand ABI indications to children and infants who are not cochlear implant candidates are being performed. Vittorio Coletti performed the first pediatric ABI surgery for auditory nerve aplasia in 2001.[35] His group reviewed outcomes of ABI implantation in 26 pediatric patients (14 months to 16 years old) with hearing loss caused by a variety of reasons (inner ear malformations/cochlear nerve aplasia, NF2, incomplete cochlear partitioning defects, auditory neuropathy, meningitis-related ossification, and temporal bone fractures with nerve injury) and showed that every child used their implant and achieved environmental sound awareness and language development, including simple words and sentences.[36] Bisyllabic word recognition and comprehension of simple commands was seen in five patients and only one patient achieved open-set word recognition.[36]

The Sennaroglu group in Turkey published a long-term prospective analysis of 64 deaf children implanted with ABIs and followed for up to 12 years. All children in the study showed improvement in auditory perception, with 11% being able to converse on the telephone and 31.3% realizing open-set speech recognition.

Studies out of this group has shown that although ABIs provide some level of auditory benefit in these patients, additional handicaps, such as attention-deficit hyperactivity disorder, seem to limit audiologic progress and should be taken into consideration during preoperative assessment and counseling.

A consensus statement was formed regarding ABI in children and non-NF2 patients after review of 61 pediatric cases in 2009. It was determined that ABI was a viable auditory rehabilitation strategy in two patient categories. The first being prelingual patients with inner ear malformations and cochlear nerve hypoplasia/aplasia. The second was patients deafened postlingually due to meningitis with cochlear ossificans, temporal bone fractures with cochlear nerve avulsion, otosclerosis with gross cochlear destruction, or unmanageable facial nerve stimulation from cochlear implant. The radiologic indications were defined in three groups: well-defined congenital indications, possible congenital indications, and acquired indications. The well-defined group consisted of complete labyrinthine aplasia, cochlear aplasia, cochlear nerve aplasia, and cochlear aperture aplasia. The possible congenital indications are (1) hypoplastic cochleas with cochlear aperture hypoplasia, (2) common cavity and incomplete partition type I cases if the cochlear nerve is not present, (3) common cavity and incomplete partition type I cases if the cochlear nerve is present and if CI fails, (4) if a CI fails in an unbranched cochlear-vestibular nerve, and (5) if the hypo plastic cochlear nerve is less than 50% of the usual size of the cochlear nerve or less than the diameter of the facial nerve. The radiologic acquired indications are deafness due to meningitis with severe ossification of the cochlea, bilateral temporal bone transverse fractures with cochlear nerve avulsion, and cochlear otosclerosis with gross destruction of the cochlea. The group recommended the optimal age to be between 18 and 24 months for prelingually deaf patients, though with an extremely experienced team an ABI could be placed as early as 1 year.

Studies of pediatric ABI implantation in the United States began in 2012, and it is too early to determine open-set speech recognition benefit in these patients. Early outcomes studies are favorable, showing that some patients achieve speech detection thresholds of 25 to 35 dB and all patients develop environmental sound awareness. The Harvard group has reported on early outcomes of four implanted patients, three have demonstrated auditory progression to balling and mimicry with 6 to 12 months of use.[2]

The House group reported on a cohort of five pediatric ABI patients, four of whom showed speech detection thresholds of 30 to 35 dB on their 1-year follow-up. Scores on the IT-MAIS/MAIS ranged from 8 to 31 out of 40, and all the children demonstrated some ability for pattern perception (ability to discriminate between closed-set words that differ by the number of syllables).[1] Our series of children (13) implanted with the ABI reveals that the best performers are those with cochlear nerve deficiency with poor cochlear implant performance on one side and an ABI on the other.

34.5 Conclusion

ABIs provide a safe and effective way to provide some degree of auditory rehabilitation to patients who are not candidates for a cochlear implant or who have failed to benefit from a cochlear implant. However, the degree of auditory rehabilitation can vary significantly and patients should be counseling with regard to realistic expectations and risks of the surgery. A multi-disciplinary approach to these patients is recommended, given the complexity of workup, surgical placement, and postoperative programming and rehabilitation. Multimodal language access should be provided, especially early in the rehabilitation, for all children where ABI placement is being considered.

34.6 Highlights

a. Indications
   - Patients 12 years and older, NF2 diagnosis, studies are being performed with regard to expansion of criteria to include children 1 year and greater with cochlear aplasia or cochlear nerve aplasia or who are otherwise not candidates for cochlear implantation.

b. Contraindications
   - Any patient who has a possibility of benefitting from a cochlear implant, preoperative counseling is very important to set patient expectations, and consideration of comorbidities should be taken into account.

c. Complications
   - Most common are CSF leak, implant migration, and non-auditory stimuli.

d. Special preoperative considerations
   - Careful patient selection with multi-disciplinary evaluation, taking into account comorbidities, patient/parent counseling with regard to expectations.

e. Special intraoperative considerations
   - Experienced neuro-anesthesia team and electrophysiologic monitoring team, correct identification of the foramen of Luschka, testing of the electrodes with EABR to determine most appropriate placement over the cochlear nucleus.

f. Special postoperative considerations
   - Frequent neurological checks in a PICU setting for the first 24 hours, implant activation occurs in the OR approximately 4 weeks postoperatively with monitoring of lower cranial nerves, routine visits for device reprogramming are ideal for at least the first year.

References

[1] Hitselberger WE, House WF, Edgerton BJ, Whitaker S. Cochlear nucleus implants. Otolaryngol Head Neck Surg 1984;92(1):52–54

[2] House WF, Hitselberger WE. Twenty-year report of the first auditory brain stem nucleus implant. Ann Otol Rhinol Laryngol 2001;110(2):103–104

[3] House Research Institute. FDA approves clinical trial of auditory brainstem implant procedure for children in US. Science Daily, 22 January 2013; www.sciencedaily.com/releases/2013/01/130122101334.htm

[4] Lundin K, Stillesjö F, Nyberg G, Rask-Andersen H. Self-reported benefit, sound perception, and quality-of-life in patients with auditory brainstem implants (ABIs). Acta Otolaryngol 2016;136(1):62–67

[5] Fernandes NF, Goffi-Gomez MV, Magalhães AT, Tsuji RK, De Brito RV, Bento RF. Satisfaction and quality of life in users of auditory brainstem implant. CoDAS 2017;29(2):e20160059

[6] Weber PCKS. Anatomy and physiology of hearing. In: Johnson JT RC, ed. Bailey's Head and Neck Surgery Otolaryngology. Vol. 2. Baltimore, MD: Lippincott Williams & Wilkins; 2014:2253–2273

[7] Otto SR, Brackmann DE, Hitselberger WE, Shannon RV, Syms MJ. Auditory brainstem implant. In: Jackler RK, Brackmann DE, eds. Neurotology. 2nd ed. Philadelphia, PA: Mosby; 2005:1323–1330

[8] Mishra S, Roy TS, Wadhwa S. Morphological and morphometrical maturation of ventral cochlear nucleus in human foetus. J Chem Neuroanat 2017

[9] Moore JK. The human auditory brain stem: a comparative view. Hear Res 1987;29(1):1–32

[10] Kandler K, Friauf E. Pre- and postnatal development of efferent connections of the cochlear nucleus in the rat. J Comp Neurol 1993;328(2):161–184

[11] Moore JK, Perazzo LM, Braun A. Time course of axonal myelination in the human brainstem auditory pathway. Hear Res 1995;87(1–2):21–31

[12] Tang ZQ, Trussell LO. Serotonergic modulation of sensory representation in a central multisensory circuit is pathway specific. Cell Reports 2017;20(8):1844–1854

[13] Johal J, Paulk PB, Oakes PC, Oskouian RJ, Loukas M, Tubbs RS. A comprehensive review of the foramina of Luschka: history, anatomy, embryology, and surgery. Childs Nerv Syst 2017;33(9):1459–1462

[14] Sharifi M, Ungier E, Ciszek B, Krajewski P. Microsurgical anatomy of the foramen of Luschka in the cerebellopontine angle, and its vascular supply. Surg Radiol Anat 2009;31(6):431–437

[15] Peris-Celda M, Martinez-Soriano F, Rhoton AL. Rhoton's Atlas of head, neck, and brain: 2D and 3D images. New York, NY: Thieme Medical Publishers, Inc.; 2018

[16] Cochlear Corporation. 2016

[17] Corporation MEDEL. 2017; http://www.medel.com/maestro-components-abi/. Accessed September 2017

[18] Oticon Medical. 2017; https://www.oticonmedical.com/cochlear-implants/solutions/systems/digisonic-sp-abi. Accessed September 2017

[19] Otto S, Staller S. Multichannel auditory brain stem implant: case studies comparing fitting strategies and results. Ann Otol Rhinol Laryngol Suppl 1995;166:36–39

[20] Colletti V, Carner M, Miorelli V, Guida M, Colletti L, Fiorino F. Auditory brainstem implant (ABI): new frontiers in adults and children. Otolaryngol Head Neck Surg 2005;133(1):126–138

[21] Otto SR, Brackmann DE, Hitselberger WE, Shannon RV, Kuchta J. Multichannel auditory brainstem implant: update on performance in 61 patients. J Neurosurg 2002;96(6):1063–1071

[22] Kanowitz SJ, Shapiro WH, Golfinos JG, Cohen NL, Roland JT Jr. Auditory brainstem implantation in patients with neurofibromatosis type 2. Laryngoscope 2004;114(12):2135–2146

[23] Kuchta J. Neuroprosthetic hearing with auditory brainstem implants. Biomed Tech (Berl) 2004;49(4):83–87

[24] Otto SR, Shannon RV, Brackmann DE, Hitselberger WE, Staller S, Menapace C. The multichannel auditory brain stem implant: performance in twenty patients. Otolaryngol Head Neck Surg 1998;118(3 Pt 1):291–303

[25] Otto SR, Brackman DE, Hitselberger WE, Shannon RV. Brainstem electronic implants for bilateral anacusis following surgical removal of cerebello pontine angle lesions. Otolaryngol Clin North Am 2001;34(2):485–499

[26] Colletti V, Carner M, Fiorino F, et al. Hearing restoration with auditory brainstem implant in three children with cochlear nerve aplasia. Otol Neurotol 2002;23(5):682–693

[27] Otto SR, Brackmann DE, Hitselberger W. Auditory brainstem implantation in 12- to 18-year-olds. Arch Otolaryngol Head Neck Surg 2004;130(5):656–659

[28] Shannon RV, Fayad J, Moore J, et al. Auditory brainstem implant: II. Postsurgical issues and performance. Otolaryngol Head Neck Surg 1993;108(6):634–642

[29] Toh EH, Luxford WM. Cochlear and brainstem implantation. Otolaryngol Clin North Am 2002;35(2):325–342

[30] Colletti V, Shannon RV, Carner M, Veronese S, Colletti L. Complications in auditory brainstem implant surgery in adults and children. Otol Neurotol 2010;31(4):558–564

[31] Brackmann DE, Hitselberger WE, Nelson RA, et al. Auditory brainstem implant: I. Issues in surgical implantation. Otolaryngol Head Neck Surg 1993;108(6):624–633

[32] Lenarz M, Matthies C, Lesinski-Schiedat A, et al. Auditory brainstem implant part II: subjective assessment of functional outcome. Otol Neurotol 2002;23(5):694–697

[33] Colletti V, Shannon RV. Open set speech perception with auditory brainstem implant? Laryngoscope 2005;115(11):1974–1978

[34] Colletti V, Shannon R, Carner M, Veronese S, Colletti L. Outcomes in nontumor adults fitted with the auditory brainstem implant: 10 years' experience. Otol Neurotol 2009;30(5):614–618

[35] Colletti L, Shannon RV, Colletti V. The development of auditory perception in children after auditory brainstem implantation. Audiol Neurotol 2014;19(6):386–394

[36] Colletti L, Zoccante L. Nonverbal cognitive abilities and auditory performance in children fitted with auditory brainstem implants: preliminary report. Laryngoscope 2008;118(8):1443–1448

[37] Puram SV, Barber SR, Kozin ED, et al. Outcomes following pediatric auditory brainstem implant surgery: early experiences in a North American Center. Otolaryngol Head Neck Surg 2016; 155(1):133–138

[38] Wilkinson EP, Eisenberg LS, Krieger MD, et al; Los Angeles Pediatric ABI Team. Initial results of a safety and feasibility study of auditory brainstem implantation in congenitally deaf children. Otol Neurotol 2017;38(2):212–220

Suggested Readings

Colletti V, Shannon RV, Carner M, Veronese S, Colletti L. Complications in auditory brainstem implant surgery in adults and children. Otol Neurotol 2010;31(4):558–564

Fernandes NF, Goffi-Gomez MV, Magalhães AT, Tsuji RK, De Brito RV, Bento RF. Satisfaction and quality of life in users of auditory brainstem implant. CoDAS 2017;29(2):e20160059

Lundin K, Stillesjö F, Nyberg G, Rask-Andersen H. Self-reported benefit, sound perception, and quality-of-life in patients with auditory brainstem implants (ABIs). Acta Otolaryngol 2016;136(1):62–67

35 Excision of Fibro-osseous Lesions of the Craniofacial Skeleton

Shahaf Shilo, Dan M. Fliss, Avraham Abergel

Summary

Fibro-osseous lesions of the jaws and craniofacial skeleton are a group of bone and connective tissue proliferative processes, some of which are commonly found in the pediatric population. This chapter focuses on the three main entities of this group: fibrous dysplasia, ossifying fibroma, and osteoma. The chapter reviews the required evaluation, clinical characteristics and management of these lesions with considerations unique to the pediatric population.

Keywords: Fibro-osseous lesions, craniofacial skeleton, pediatric patients, fibrous dysplasia, ossifying fibroma, osteoma

35.1 Introduction

Fibro-osseous lesions of the jaws and craniofacial skeleton occur quite commonly in childhood and adolescence and represent a varied group of bone and connective tissue proliferative processes that result in an aberrant proliferation of a mineralized product and collagen. Fibrous dysplasia, ossifying fibroma, and osteoma are the three classic entities of this group of bony tumors. They are distinguished from each other by different clinical, radiological, and histological characteristics that help arrive at a diagnosis. Although often not readily apparent, accurate diagnosis is imperative, since each entity has different indications for intervention. Surgery is the mainstay of treatment for these lesions once an intervention is indicated, usually due to functional or esthetic impairment caused by the lesion growth. The course of treatment should be planned and individualized based on the manifestations, the type and location of the lesion, the natural history of the disease, and the age of the patient.

35.2 Patient Evaluation

A complete history is an essential part of the preoperative evaluation, and it should include a timeline of lesion growth or any dynamic changes, as well as careful assessment of any symptoms. Some symptoms may not be readily apparent, since most of these lesions tend to grow slowly. The most common clinical presentation for fibro-osseous lesions is facial swelling and asymmetry. Other signs and symptoms include headache, nasal obstruction, visual disturbances, and neurological changes. These lesions are, however, often asymptomatic, and are discovered incidentally when imaging is performed for other reasons.

Physical examination should consist of a complete head-and-neck examination, including a flexible endoscopy, and a careful cranial nerve function assessment. Further evaluation depends on the location of the lesion, and may require a multi-disciplinary assessment. Lesions involving the temporal bone require an audiometric evaluation. A dentist or a maxillofacial surgeon should be part of the treating team when the mandible or maxilla is involved. Lesions involving the orbital bone or the sphenoid bone require a full ophthalmologic evaluation, including best corrected visual acuity, visual field, color vision, and examination of the fundus, all for the early detection of the most subtle changes. Participation of a neurosurgeon in treatment planning and surgery is indicated when the lesion involves the skull base.

For radiographic evaluation, a computerized tomographic (CT) scan is the most appropriate imaging modality for bony lesions. The CT scan may also be used for the intraoperative image-guided navigation system, but it may expose the child to a considerable amount of radiation, especially if repeated periodically. Magnetic resonance imaging (MRI) is useful for avoiding radiation, and also has the benefits of characterizing soft tissue and demonstrating the relation of the lesion to vital structures. Specific features characteristic of each lesion will be discussed separately. Three-dimensional (3D) craniofacial analysis and virtual surgical simulation have been recently integrated into the craniofacial surgery armamentarium, offering the surgeon a more precise surgical and reconstruction planning.[1]

A biopsy may be obtained if the involved site is amenable to biopsy. However, in some cases, obtaining a biopsy may not be possible or necessary. Fibro-osseous lesions consist of a diverse group of conditions with similar histological appearances. Thus, a definitive diagnosis usually cannot be made by histological examination alone, and both clinical and radiological correlations are needed. The surgeon must bear in mind that these lesions may be vascular and tend to bleed, and therefore be prepared for such an eventuality.

35.3 Fibrous Dysplasia

Fibrous dysplasia (FD) is a non-neoplastic bone disease characterized by intramedullary accumulation of fibrous tissue and immature woven bone. It may affect a single bone (monostotic) or multiple bones (polyostotic) throughout the skeleton. Monostotic FD accounts for approximately 80% of cases, of which 10% to 20% occur in the head and neck. Polyostotic FD tends to occur at an earlier age than monostotic FD. It accounts for approximately 20% of cases, and involves the craniofacial bones in about 50% of them, although it can approach 100% in severe cases.[2] When limited to the head and neck and present within several contiguous bones, (e.g., the maxilla, zygoma, frontonasal, and temporal bones) it is termed craniofacial fibrous dysplasia (CFD) and does not constitute a polyostotic disease.[3] Polyostotic FD can be associated with McCune–Albright syndrome, which is also characterized by hyperfunctional endocrinopathies (e.g., precocious puberty, hyperthyroidism, Cushing syndrome, and acromegaly) and cutaneous hyperpigmentation (café au-lait), and usually presents in females.[4,5]

The maxilla and the mandible are the most common sites of FD lesions in the craniofacial bones, followed by the sphenoid, ethmoid, frontal, and temporal bones. Onset is usually during periods of rapid bone growth, typically presenting in teen and adolescent years, although severe forms can arise in infancy. In most cases of CFD, the presenting symptoms are slow-growing painless swelling and craniofacial deformity (▶Fig. 35.1). Other symptoms include facial pain and headache, nasal obstruction and sinusitis, facial numbness, pathological fractures, orbital dystopia, diplopia, proptosis, blindness, epiphora, facial paralysis, loss of hearing, and tinnitus. At the same time, these lesions are often asymptomatic and discovered incidentally when imaging is performed for other reasons. Infrequently, young children and pre-pubertal adolescents may present with an abrupt alteration in the clinical course of the lesion, manifested by rapid growth, cortical bone expansion, and displacement of adjacent structures, resulting in functional deficits. In some patients, this acute change in growth behavior can be associated with secondary pathologies, such as mucoceles, aneurysmal bone cysts, or more rarely with malignant transformation. Malignant transformation, typically into a sarcomatous lesion, is estimated to occur in 0.5% of monostotic FD cases and in 4% of McCune–Albright syndrome cases.[6] Currently, there are no biomarkers to predict the behavior of these lesions, and their histology does not provide reliable prognostic or predictive information.

35.4 Imaging

CT imaging without contrast is the recommended modality for defining the anatomy of individual lesions and for establishing the extent of disease. The most common radiographic characteristic of CFD is a "ground-glass" appearance together with a thin cortex and without distinct borders (▶Fig. 35.2). While different patterns may be observed, with some being mostly sclerotic and some being predominantly cystic or lytic, there is most often a combination of both patterns. This variation of the radiographic appearance of CFD depends on the age of the patient. In pre-pubertal patients, lesions most often appear homogeneous and radiodense. As these patients enter the second decade of life, the lesions progress to a mixed radiodense/radiolucent appearance that stabilizes in adulthood. This natural progression of FD should be differentiated from the development of a secondary disorder (e.g., aneurysmal bone cyst, malignant transformation), which is associated with an abrupt change in the course of development.

MRI may be used for monitoring growth, thus avoiding the exposure of children to ionizing radiation as a result of repeated CT imaging. MRI is also accurate in analyzing the spatial relationship of the lesion with critical neurovascular structures.

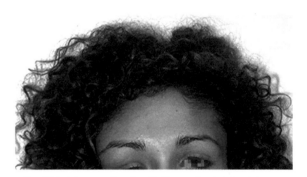

Fig. 35.1 A teenage female with fibrous dysplasia involving the right frontal bone, resulting in craniofacial swelling and deformity.

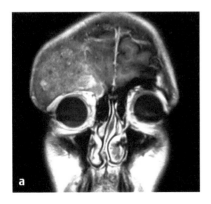
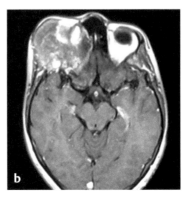

Fig. 35.2 Fibrous dysplasia. Coronal **(a)** and axial **(b)** post-contrast T1-W MRI, respectively, showing right supra-orbital low-intensity mass with characteristic "ground-glass" appearance. Inhomogeneous areas might represent fibrous tissue, cyst formation, or hemorrhage.

Radionuclide bone scintigraphy may be considered at the initial presentation if polyostotic disease is suggested by the clinical course. Increased tissue uptake is nonspecific, and lesions cannot be distinguished from malignancy.

35.5 Management of Fibrous Dysplasia

The clinical and biological behavior and the progression of FD are variable and unpredictable, thereby making the management of this condition difficult with limited published evidence and only few established clinical guidelines. Thus, appropriate treatment for FD is often highly individualized and based on patient-specific presentation. Treatment planning must take into account several factors, including the location of the lesion and its relationship with critical anatomic structures, the lesion's clinical behavior, the nature of symptoms, the assessed potential for reactivation or regrowth, and the patient's age and preferences. Treatment options fall into one of three categories: expectant management, medical treatment, and surgery. Surgery is the mainstay of treatment in FD, with the primary goals of symptom relief, functional restoration or preservation, and esthetic optimization. However, the timing, technique, and, in some instances, indications remain controversial.

It is generally acceptable that small, often incidentally diagnosed lesions that do not seem to progress or cause significant functional or esthetic impairment may be managed with a "watch and wait" approach, which should include periodic clinical and radiographic assessments to evaluate disease progression and obviate potential complications. A more vigilant follow-up by a multidisciplinary team is indicated in asymptomatic patients in whom the lesions involve the orbit, optic canal, skull base, or temporal bone, and it should consist of periodic ophthalmologic, neurologic, or audiometric evaluations, respectively.

No medical treatment is currently available to cure or definitively halt the progression of FD. In recent years, medical therapy with bisphosphonates has been implemented in an attempt to control pain and stabilize the lesions; however, long-term effects are controversial. There has been mixed success in reducing pain and slowing the rate of growth in CFD. Medical management has had a greater role in non-craniofacial FD, in which fractures and chronic pain are more common. Given the increased risk of bisphosphonate-related osteonecrosis, the undetermined efficacy of bisphosphonates in the management of CFD, and the unknown long-term effects of bisphosphonate treatment in children, further studies are necessary before these medications can be recommended.

Radiotherapy must be avoided, since it is ineffective and increases the incidence of malignant transformation 400-fold.[7]

Surgical intervention is advocated once the lesion becomes aggressive or symptomatic, causing functional deficits, such as sinus obstruction, visual disturbances, intracranial complications, and cranial nerve palsies. However, indications and timing for surgical intervention are less clear when the patient presents with a solely esthetic alteration not associated with functional symptoms, especially in children. The surgical treatment of CFD can be broadly categorized into two different approaches. One is the conservative approach, which consists of debulking and contouring of the dysplastic bone tissue and often requires repeat surgery over time. The other is the radical approach, which consists of complete removal of the pathological bone tissue and its reconstruction with an autologous bone graft. In the past, conservative contouring of bone was the preferred treatment for CFD; however, the reported regrowth rates for this approach were up to 25 to 50%.[7,8] Advances in surgical techniques have enabled more radical surgery and immediate reconstruction with good aesthetic and functional outcomes, as well as with significantly lower recurrence rates. Nevertheless, in pediatric patients, each case must be carefully evaluated, and when surgery is indicated, the surgical treatment plan should be as conservative as possible, with the morbidity of the intervention being weighed against its potential benefits.

Only a few treatment algorithms for CFD have been published, and clear and well-established treatment guidelines are still lacking, especially for pediatric patients. In 1990, Chen and Noordhoff[9] divided the craniofacial skeleton into four anatomic zones, and proposed a surgical approach for each zone, based on esthetic, functional, and surgical considerations, thus providing some practical general principles for surgical management of CFD. Zone 1 represents the fronto-orbital, zygomatic, and upper maxillary regions; zone 2 corresponds to the hair-bearing cranium; zone 3 refers to the central cranial base, petrous, mastoid, pterygoid, and sphenoid bones, where major vessels and nerves can be encased by the lesion; and zone 4 comprises the teeth-bearing portions of the skull, the maxilla and mandible. Those authors recommended radical resection and reconstruction for lesions in zone 1, conservative remodeling and bone recontouring for lesions in zones 2 and 4, and surgical treatment only in the presence of symptoms in zone 3. This classification continues to be valid; however, it does not specify special considerations for the management of CFD in children. Additional detailed CFD management guidelines were more recently proposed, based on anatomical sites, clinical behavior, and symptoms, and they also included special considerations for application in the pediatric population.[10–13]

The following are the recommendations for the management and the surgical approach in pediatric CFD, based on the site of involvement. In general, we advocate conservative management in prepubescent patients, and deferral of surgical intervention until after puberty whenever possible. A key principle of our surgical approach in CFD, particularly in children, is to ensure that no greater deformity or functional loss is incurred than that sustained by the lesion itself.

35.5.1 Facial Bones

The most frequent presentation of CFD is a painless facial swelling and asymmetry with no associated functional symptoms. In these cases of a stable non-aggressive lesion that causes facial deformity, the question when to operate arises. Surgical treatment for esthetic indications is usually postponed until after puberty when the patient is skeletally mature and the lesion growth subsides, since interventions at a younger age may require revision surgery sooner. This disadvantage is partially offset by the benefits of early intervention in patients for whom the cosmetic deformity is intolerable. Thus, counseling for patients and their caregivers is imperative, and information regarding the probable regrowth of the lesion requiring further surgery must be provided. The patient and caregivers should also know that there is always some risk of regrowth, even when conservative surgery is performed after puberty, especially in polyostotic disease.[13,14] If surgical intervention is opted for in such cases, conservative surgical remodeling is usually preferred over radical resection with reconstruction, thus enabling esthetical and functional improvements with a less complex surgical intervention and avoiding disruption of craniofacial growth centers.

Surgical intervention in the short term is more clearly indicated for patients with an aggressive and rapidly expanding lesion. Associated symptoms may include new-onset pain or paresthesia, diplopia, proptosis, epiphora, nasal congestion, or malocclusion. Lesions that exhibit aggressive behavior are usually associated with excessive hormonal drive in the setting of underlying endocrinopathy, or, alternatively, with a secondary disorder developing within the primary lesion that includes associated expansile lesions, such as an aneurysmal bone cyst or a mucocele, malignant transformation, or osteomyelitis. The etiology of this change in behavior should be evaluated promptly by a multidisciplinary team and the patient should undergo imaging studies, tissue biopsy, and growth hormone excess assessment prior to surgical intervention. Untreated endocrinopathies should be managed aggressively. In cases of aggressive, rapidly growing lesions, it seems that the best therapeutic option is radical surgical resection with contemporary reconstruction, since it is generally agreed that radical resection is curative with minimal recurrence (▶ Fig. 35.3). Nevertheless, treatment plans for pediatric patients should be individually tailored, and the surgical approach should be determined based on the size and location of the lesion, the anticipated residual defect, and the underlying etiology. Large resections may inflict significant morbidity and disrupt craniofacial growth centers,

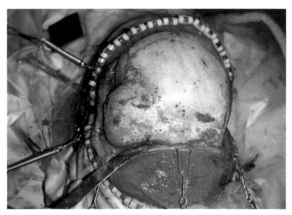

Fig. 35.3 Surgical resection of fibrous dysplasia involving the right frontal bone through an external approach.

resulting in significant functional and cosmetic deficits and facial asymmetry. Furthermore, free flap reconstruction in children, which is often required following large resections of facial bone lesions, is more complicated than in adults, and involves special functional and cosmetic concerns, such as donor-site morbidity, differential craniofacial growth, and the anticipated growth of anastomosed vessels.[15] Thus, despite higher rates of recurrence with contouring procedures, repeated debulking may be associated with less morbidity than a single major surgical procedure. We distinguish between two scenarios. One is when the residual defect is anticipated to be large, in which case conservative debulking and bone remodeling should be considered as the first choice in pediatric patients, thereby delaying the performance of a more aggressive surgical intervention until after puberty. The other is when the lesion and the anticipated residual defect are small, in which case radical resection may be considered, followed by reconstruction using local flaps or bone grafts, such as autogenous rib graft for mandibular reconstruction. These latter cases may require further surgical intervention with free flap reconstruction once skeletal maturity has been reached.

In cases of aggressive behavior due to secondary disorder, the treatment is dictated by the diagnosis. Aneurysmal bone cysts may be managed with curettage of the lesion and contouring of the underlying FD. Malignant transformation, typically into a sarcomatous lesion, requires en bloc resection with adequate oncological margins.

35.5.2 Paranasal Sinuses

Lesions adjacent to the sinuses or involving them can grow and completely obliterate the sinus outflow tract, resulting in nasal congestion, headaches, hyposmia, recurrent or chronic sinusitis, mucocele, or lacrimal obstruction. Surprisingly, the incidence of sinusitis in patients affected by FD is not greater compared with the general population.[10] Treatment options consist of a combination of medical therapy and surgery. Surgery is preferably postponed until the patient is in the late teens if the symptoms are controlled with conservative treatment. However, in symptomatic cases refractory to medical treatment, such as chronic or recurrent infection, surgical intervention is indicated and cannot be delayed.

Over recent decades, traditional and more invasive external approaches, such as craniofacial resection, Caldwell-Luc, and lateral rhinotomy with external ethmoidectomy for sinus lesions, have largely been replaced by minimally invasive transnasal endoscopic approaches that are used in conjunction with image-guided navigational tools. Endoscopic techniques interfere less with the growth of craniofacial skeleton compared to open techniques, which is especially relevant to young patients. Endonasal endoscopic sinus surgery is the preferred approach for lesions involving the sinuses, and its aim is to correct anatomical alterations causing obstruction or associated lesions, such as mucoceles.[16] The extent of resection should be based on the location of the pathological bone and its proximity to important sinus structures, since radical or complete resection may not be necessary or possible. An endoscopic approach may be combined with an external approach, such as in cases when concomitant esthetical corrections are needed.

35.5.3 Optic Canal

There has been significant controversy regarding the management of optic nerve encasement and compression by CFD of the sphenoid bone, particularly in patients whose vision is normal. Traditionally, prophylactic optic nerve decompression was performed whenever an optic nerve encasement was demonstrated radiographically in patients with CFD, even in the absence of visual disturbance. The rate of optic nerve involvement on imaging studies in cases of FD of the sphenoid bone has been reported to be up to 90%.[17] However, several studies have shown that the vast majority of these patients were asymptomatic and had normal ophthalmologic examinations, despite radiological evidence of optic nerve involvement.[17,18] Eventually, in recent years it has been established that surgical optic nerve decompression should be reserved for symptomatic patients.[19] Asymptomatic patients with radiologic evidence of optic nerve encasement should be managed conservatively with repeated ophthalmologic examinations and long-term radiologic follow-up, given that prophylactic decompression unnecessarily puts their optic nerve at risk. Symptomatic patients with abnormal neuro-ophthalmologic examination findings may be considered in two categories: subtle and gradual optic neuropathy, and acute neuropathy with rapid visual changes or vision loss. Excessive growth hormone (GH) levels that typically occur in endocrinopathies have been associated with increased risk for optic neuropathy, and considered to present as a gradual disturbance in vision. Compression or traction on the

optic nerve that accompanies bony expansion of the skull secondary to high GH levels may be the mechanism of gradual vision loss in some patients. Thus, early evaluation and aggressive management of GH excess is essential, with the assumption that control of GH excess may prevent long-term visual impairment.[20] Cases of acute visual change or loss of vision are considered to be associated with a secondary disorder arising within the FD lesion, such as an aneurysmal bone cyst, hemorrhage, or mucocele. Patients presenting acutely with visual disturbance should undergo an immediate CT and MRI of the cranial base and prompt evaluation by a neurosurgeon, otolaryngologist, and neuro-ophthalmologist. Prompt surgical intervention is indicated in both acute and gradual deteriorating vision. Endonasal endoscopic surgery aimed at partial decompression of the optic canal has become widely accepted as the approach of choice. An open or a combined open and endoscopic approach should be considered for cases in which an additional remodeling of the anterior cranial base bone is required.

35.5.4 Temporal Bone

Temporal bone involvement is the least frequently reported type of FD, especially in children (▶Fig. 35.4). Progressive conductive hearing loss is the most common symptom of pediatric temporal bone FD, and is usually secondary to external auditory canal stenosis.[21] Stenosis of the external auditory canal may also result in the formation of an acquired cholesteatoma and further associated complications of the intracranial and intratemporal regions. Other possible complications of temporal bone FD are otitis media or otitis externa, otic capsule invasion

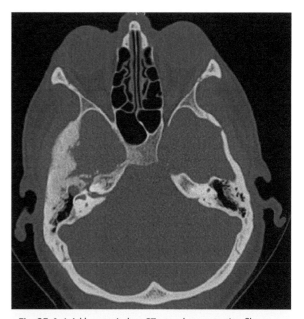

Fig. 35.4 Axial bone-window CT scan demonstrating fibrous dysplasia involving the right temporal bone.

causing a sensorineural hearing loss, vertigo, or tinnitus, intracranial complications (e.g., CSF otorrhea and meningitis) and cranial neuropathy (e.g., facial nerve palsy).[22] Patients with temporal bone involvement should undergo a comprehensive audiologic examination and evaluation of the ear under a microscope, with periodic follow-up assessment. As in most other anatomical regions involved by FD in pediatric patients, observation is the most commonly chosen approach when the disease is limited and progression is slow. Considering the tendency for FD to stabilize after adolescence, surgical intervention in children should be delayed until the patient has progressed beyond puberty. In contrast, surgical intervention is indicated when disease progression is aggressive and FD is accompanied by significant clinical symptoms and complications, including cholesteatoma, progressive stenosis of the external auditory canal causing hearing loss or intractable infection, major cosmetic deformity, neurological symptoms, and cranial neuropathy with radiologic evidence of bony impingement.

The surgical approach should be chosen based on the indication for intervention, and the location, extent, and aggressiveness of the lesion. Canalplasty may be an appropriate surgical option as a first-line treatment for hearing restoration in cases with external auditory canal stenosis, although re-stenosis is common.[23] More radical approaches, such as canal wall down mastoidectomy or subtotal petrosectomy, typically with lower recurrence rates, may be considered in cases of aggressive progression and inadequate response to initial treatment.[24] Tympanoplastic procedures should be attempted if middle ear involvement is present. In case of facial nerve palsy, a high-resolution cranial base or temporal bone CT is indicated, and surgical decompression should be considered.[10,23]

35.6 Ossifying Fibroma

Ossifying fibroma (OF) is a benign fibro-osseous tumor composed of fibrocellular tissue and mineralized material of varying appearances.[25] Conventional OF is the most common subtype, which usually affects female adults in their second to fourth decades of life. It is generally a slow-growing, encapsulated, and well-demarcated expansile tumor, arising in the tooth-bearing areas of the jaws, primarily in the posterior mandible (75%) and the maxilla (25%).[26] Juvenile ossifying fibroma (JOF) is a less common subtype, and unlike conventional OF, it appears at a younger age, is unencapsulated, is more locally aggressive, and potentially has an infiltrative growth pattern.[3] JOF is further classified into two distinct variants, trabecular and psammomatoid. Trabecular JOF is usually seen in children and adolescents with a mean age of 8.5 to 12 years at presentation,[27] and has a predilection mainly for the maxilla (50%) and mandible (44%). Psammomatoid JOF is also mostly seen in children and adolescents; however, the affected individuals tend to be somewhat older than those with the trabecular form. Additionally,

psammomatoid JOF affects a wider patient age range and can appear in older adults as well. The most commonly affected bones are the paranasal sinuses (62%), the anterior skull base and orbits, and, less commonly, the jaws and the cranium.[26] Psammomatoid lesions tend to have a more aggressive biologic behavior.

Presenting signs and symptoms of JOF depend on the location of the tumor and they range from teeth displacement and facial swelling when the jaws are involved, to nasal obstruction and proptosis when the paranasal sinuses are involved. Other signs and symptoms are headaches, epistaxis, and ophthalmologic disturbances, such as diplopia and epiphora. These tumors may also cause serious complications, such as massive mucocele formation, visual loss, and intracranial infections.[28] JOFs are distinguished from other fibro-osseous lesions primarily by their earlier age of onset, their clinical presentation that is characterized by rapid growth, and their potential aggressive behavior that can result in considerable facial disfigurement.

Although multiple recurrences are common for both trabecular and psammomatoid types of JOF, neither tumor type has been reported to undergo malignant transformation.

35.7 Imaging

CT scans of JOFs typically demonstrate well-circumscribed, often multiloculated masses that can have either a radiolucent, ground-glass, or totally radiopaque appearance. These masses often have a rim or "shell" of irregular thickened bone.

35.8 Management of Ossifying Fibroma

The definitive management for OF is surgical resection. For OF lesions restricted to the mandible, treatment is traditionally accomplished with simple curettage or enucleation, due to the favorable results in that particular anatomical location. A "wait and scan" strategy, similar to that recommended for osteomas or FD, has been proposed as an option in select cases of asymptomatic conventional OF that is typically diagnosed in adults and not in children.[29] However, complete surgical resection is the treatment of choice in cases of extra-mandibular OF, and particularly JOF, due to the more aggressive growth behavior and the high recurrence rates, ranging from 30% to 56% after partial or incomplete tumor resection.[27] Total resection is preferably achieved on the first attempt when possible, since a repeat surgery for these lesions is made more difficult by scarring and distortion of anatomic structures and tissue planes. The surgeon's orientation and visualization, as well as the ability to distinguish the tumor from the adjacent normal tissue may be impaired during repeat surgery.

The surgical approach should be dictated by the location of the lesion and the ability to perform complete removal. However, the goal of complete surgical excision should be tempered by the possible risks of attempting complete excision. Traditionally, open approaches have been the mainstay of treatment for these tumors, since they provide wide visibility of the entire mass, thereby allowing complete excision. Various external approaches for sinonasal tumors have been described, such as Caldwell-Luc operation, lateral rhinotomy, and sublabial approach.[30,31] Craniofacial resection has been traditionally performed for extensive disease or when the tumor extends into the cranial cavity.[32] However, JOFs have a predilection for children and can affect even the very young. The pediatric population has special considerations and limitations that must be considered when deciding upon treatment. External approaches are associated with significant morbidity that is less tolerable in children than in adults, and include the risk of disruption of tooth buds and facial growth centers, development of facial asymmetry, and postoperative facial scarring. Open craniofacial resection and frontal craniotomy approaches require retraction of the frontal lobe of the developing child, with the potential for brain injury and resultant encephalomalacia and long-term cognitive changes.

With the advent of endoscopic sinonasal and skull base surgery, the surgical landscape has evolved to now include endoscopic endonasal approaches in the management of JOF. Advancements in endoscopic instrumentation and image-guided navigation, together with refinements of surgical techniques, have enabled complete removal of OFs with good results and acceptable morbidity.[33-35] External approach or a combined endoscopic and external approach may still be required when endoscopic access is limited or contraindicated, such as in cases of frontal or maxillary sinus anterior wall involvement, skull base invasion lateral to the optic nerve, or optic nerve encasement.

Several factors need to be considered when performing endonasal endoscopic excision of JOF. The use of intraoperative image-guided navigation system is imperative. It helps to improve the surgeon's orientation and ability to identify the location of vital structures, thus enabling more reliable preservation of the normal anatomy. This is especially important in children, where the usual anatomic landmarks may be concealed. Furthermore, it helps to distinguish the boundaries of the tumor, and assists in achieving a more complete resection. The resection starts with tumor debulking in order to reduce the tumor mass and to identify anatomical landmarks. The boundary of the tumor is identified with the help of the navigation system, and the outer shell is removed step-by-step. Pathological bone is drilled out with a diamond burr until reaching smooth healthy bone that has a less friable consistency. Maximal resection of JOF is critical for the success of the operation. Possible challenges are posed by the distortion of normal anatomic landmarks by the aggressiveness of

the tumor, the vicinity and adherence of the tumor to vital structures, such as the optic nerve and dura, and the obscuring of the visual field due to bleeding. Intraoperative image-guided navigation system is of vital importance in such circumstances.

Complications of the endoscopic technique include bleeding, injury to the skull base with resultant CSF leak and infection, and injury to orbital structures. JOF can bleed significantly, especially when removed endoscopically by piecemeal resection. Children's smaller blood volume make them less tolerant to intraoperative blood loss, thus blood products should be readily available. Hemostatic techniques include the use of diamond drill bits for bleeding bone removal, infiltration of various hemostatic agents, warm saline irrigation, and packing and compressing the site of hemorrhage. The most effective method to decrease massive bleeding is to resect the tumor as fast as possible to reach the border of the tumor. CSF leaks and orbit injuries usually occur when the tumor infiltrates the skull base or the orbit. A tumor that erodes the anterior cranial fossa and pushes down on the dura should be gently removed from the dura while keeping the dura intact. If CSF leak could not be prevented, a duraplasty using sealing materials such as TachoSil, Duragen, or fascia lata should be performed subsequently. A second layer of mucoperiosteum should be used in cases of a large defect.

Injury to the optic canal, eye, cranial nerves, or internal carotid artery may cause significant morbidity and, in some cases, mortality. Thus, operating in anatomic sites adjacent to these structures should be performed by experienced hands and with the assistance of intraoperative image-guided navigation system, endoscopic Doppler probes, and neuro-monitoring. When necessary, the extent of resection should be compromised in order to preserve these vital structures.

35.9 Osteoma

Osteoma is a benign, slow-growing bone tumor consisting primarily of well-differentiated mature, compact, or cancellous bone. Osteomas are more common in males, and their peak incidence is between the fourth and sixth decades, with an average age at presentation of 50 years. Osteomas are the most common primary bone tumors in the craniofacial skeleton in adults. Nevertheless, osteomas are extremely rare in the pediatric population.[36] They most frequently arise in the fronto-ethmoidal region, but they can also develop in the maxilla, mandible, mastoid sinus, external auditory canal, and cranial vault. These lesions have been identified in 3% of CT scans of the paranasal sinuses.[37,38]

Three main theories have been proposed to explain the mechanism of growth of osteomas. The embryological theory proposes that osteomas develop at the junction between the embryonic cartilaginous ethmoid and the membranous frontal bone. The traumatic theory correlates the development of osteomas with a previous trauma. According to the infective theory, local inflammation may activate adjacent bone osteogenesis.

Osteomas can be associated with Gardner syndrome, an autosomal-dominant disorder characterized by a triad of colon polyps, soft-tissue tumors (including skin cysts and desmoid tumors), and multiple osteomas, typically affecting the jaws. The colon polyps in Gardner syndrome have a high propensity toward malignant transformation; thus, an early gastroenterological evaluation is imperative for these patients and their families. The osteomas themselves have no malignant potential.

Osteomas are usually asymptomatic and discovered incidentally on imaging studies, but they can also cause clinical symptoms, with headache being the most common complaint.[39] Impaired sinus drainage can result in concomitant sinusitis or, more rarely, formation of secondary mucocele. An osteoma may produce an external deformity when it extends beyond the confines of the sinuses. Tumors involving the jaws may cause occlusion disturbances and facial asymmetry, while those involving the orbit can cause epiphora, proptosis, diplopia, and decreased visual acuity. Those extending into the anterior cranial fossa might cause CSF rhinorrhea, meningitis, pneumocephalus, and brain abscess.[40] Temporal bone osteomas may rarely cause conductive hearing loss or ear infections.

35.10 Imaging

Osteomas appear as well-circumscribed masses of heterogeneous consistency on CT, with hyperostotic (high-signal) and spongiotic (lower-signal) components (▶Fig. 35.5). The lower signal components may

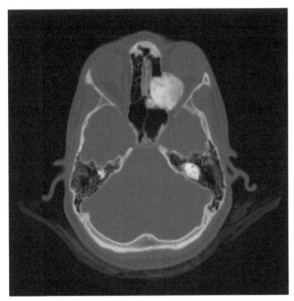

Fig. 35.5 Axial bone-window CT scan demonstrating an osteoma involving the left ethmoid sinus, left sphenoid sinus, and left orbit.

be confused with associated mucoceles. MRI is useful for assessing the extent of the tumor as well as the presence of complications (mucoceles, orbital or intracranial extension). Intravenous contrast shows no enhancement on CT or MRI scans.

35.11 Management of Osteoma

Osteomas are often asymptomatic, and surgical treatment is usually not indicated. In most cases of small, uncomplicated osteomas, a watchful waiting approach with periodic imaging is usually followed. However, a rapidly growing or large osteoma that occupies more than 50% of the frontal sinus may warrant surgical resection. Further indications for operating on asymptomatic osteomas include partial or complete obstruction of the nasofrontal duct, ethmoid sinus involvement, and orbital or intracranial extension.[41-43]

Surgical resection is indicated when the osteoma is symptomatic or associated with complications, including massive headaches with no other explanation, chronic sinusitis due to tumor obstruction, facial deformity, visual symptoms, neurologic symptoms and complications, such as intracranial infection and pneumocephalus.[44]

The choice of surgical technique depends upon the size, location, and extension of tumor, the presence of any complication, and the experience of the surgeon. There are three surgical approaches: external, endoscopic, or combined. External procedures for osteomas in the paranasal sinuses include Lynch procedure, lateral rhinotomy, external ethmoidectomy, bicoronal flap, subcranial approach, and Caldwell-Luc procedure (▶Fig. 35.6). Although external approach allows total tumor resection under direct visual control, it has several disadvantages, especially in children, such as cosmetic deformity, facial growth disruption, higher morbidity, and longer hospital stay. Endoscopic sinus surgery has expended its limits during the last decades, and its indications now include the treatment of paranasal osteomas. As a result, most small- and medium-sized osteomas are now managed endoscopically, and external approaches are mainly indicated in selected cases in which the endoscopic approach is limited. The major advantages of endoscopic approach are better preservation of vital structures, such as the orbit and brain, better cosmetic results, maintenance of the natural endonasal drainage pathways, less bleeding, reduced postoperative morbidity, and shorter hospitalization time. Combined endoscopic and external procedures provide a wide view to the nasofrontal passage, and giant tumors can be excised easily with fewer cosmetic defects compared to the purely external approach.

Endonasal endoscopic resection of a frontal sinus osteoma is feasible when the lesion is medial to a virtual plane through the lamina papyracea and attached at the lower portion of the posterior wall of the frontal sinus.

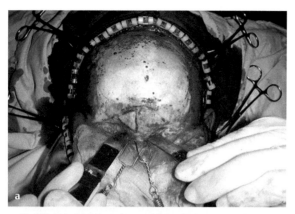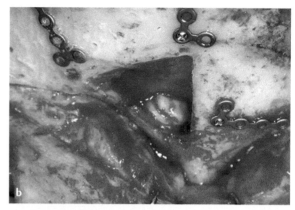

Fig. 35.6 (a, b) External approach for the resection of an osteoma involving the frontal sinus.

Frontal tumors with anterior wall attachment or lateral extent in a well-pneumatized sinus can sometimes be removed using a modified Lothrop procedure. Otherwise, an external or combined external endoscopic approach may be required. Ethmoid sinus osteomas are mostly managed by an endoscopic approach. Tumors involving the cribriform plate or the orbit can also be managed endoscopically by drilling the osteoma gently using a diamond burr. Endoscopic approach is limited by an anterior extension to the nasolacrimal duct and the subcutaneous tissue. In such cases a combined endoscopic external approach is usually required. Maxillary sinus osteomas are usually located on the lateral wall of the sinus. For osteomas located in the floor or the lateral wall of the maxillary sinus, endoscopic approach is difficult and external approach may be necessary. On the other hand, osteomas located in the superior or medial wall of the maxillary sinus can be excised endoscopically. Sphenoid sinus osteomas can usually be safely removed by an endonasal endoscopic approach.

35.12 Acknowledgment

Esther Eshkol, the institutional medical and scientific copyeditor, is thanked for editorial assistance.

35.13 Highlights

a. Special preoperative considerations
  - A multi-disciplinary collaborative team.
  - Neurologic, ophthalmologic, and endocrine function assessment, according to the type and the location of the lesion.
  - Diagnosis is based on the age of onset, clinical manifestations, biological behavior of the lesion, radiographic findings, and histological characteristics.
  - A definitive diagnosis usually cannot be made by histological examination alone since different fibro-osseous lesions has similar histological appearances.
  - 3D simulation for surgical planning.
  - Rapid lesion growth and aggressive biological behavior may be associated with secondary condition such as aneurysmal bone cyst, mucocele, or malignant transformation.
  - Radiotherapy increases the incidence of malignant transformation of fibrous dysplasia.

b. Indications
  - Fibrous dysplasia: Conservative management in prepubescent patients and deferral of surgical intervention until after puberty whenever possible. Immediate surgical intervention is indicated for aggressive behavior, symptoms, and functional deficits.
  - Juvenile ossifying fibroma: Total surgical resection is required.
  - Osteoma: Watchful waiting approach for slow growing asymptomatic lesions. Surgical intervention is indicated for rapidly growing or large lesion, symptomatic lesion, impending functional deficit, and associated complication.

c. Special intraoperative considerations
  - Conservative management in children is advocated whenever possible.
  - The surgical approach is chosen according to the anatomic location of the lesion and the involved craniofacial bones.
  - Surgical treatment of craniofacial fibrous dysplasia is categorized into conservative approach (debulking and contouring of the dysplastic bone tissue) and radical approach (complete removal of the pathological bone tissue with reconstruction).
  - Intraoperative navigation system is used when endoscopic endonasal approach is implemented.
  - Preservation of critical neurological, neurovascular, and endocrine structures' function is of prime importance.
  - Avoiding disruption of craniofacial growth center and tooth buds.

d. Special postoperative considerations
  – Follow-up consisting of clinical examination and periodic imaging.
  – Some lesions such as FD may require repeat surgery.

References

[1] Duek I, Pener-Tessler A, Yanko-Arzi R, et al. Skull base reconstruction in the pediatric patient. J Neurol Surg B Skull Base 2018;79(1):81–90

[2] Lustig LR, Holliday MJ, McCarthy EF, Nager GT. Fibrous dysplasia involving the skull base and temporal bone. Arch Otolaryngol Head Neck Surg 2001;127(10):1239–1247

[3] Hall G. Fibro-osseous lesions of the head and neck. Diagn Histopathol 2017;23(5):200–210

[4] McCune D, Bruch H. Osteodystrophia fibrosa: report of a case in which the condition was combined with precocious puberty, multiple pigmentation of the skin and hyperthyroidism. Am J Dis Child 1937;52:745–748

[5] Albright F, Butler M, Hamptom A, et al. Syndrome characterized by osteitis fibrosa disseminata, areas of pigmentation and endocrine dysfunction with precocious puberty in females. N Engl J Med 1937;216:727–746

[6] Ruggieri P, Sim FH, Bond JR, Unni KK. Malignancies in fibrous dysplasia. Cancer 1994;73(5):1411–1424

[7] Edgerton MT, Persing JA, Jane JA. The surgical treatment of fibrous dysplasia. With emphasis on recent contributions from cranio-maxillo-facial surgery. Ann Surg 1985;202(4):459–479

[8] Park BY, Cheon YW, Kim YO, Pae NS, Lee WJ. Prognosis for craniofacial fibrous dysplasia after incomplete resection: age and serum alkaline phosphatase. Int J Oral Maxillofac Surg 2010;39(3):221–226

[9] Chen YR, Noordhoff MS. Treatment of craniomaxillofacial fibrous dysplasia: how early and how extensive? Plast Reconstr Surg 1990;86(5):835–842, discussion 843–844

[10] Lee JS, FitzGibbon EJ, Chen YR, et al. Clinical guidelines for the management of craniofacial fibrous dysplasia. Orphanet J Rare Dis 2012;7(Suppl 1):S2

[11] Valentini V, Cassoni A, Terenzi V, et al. Our experience in the surgical management of craniofacial fibrous dysplasia: what has changed in the last 10 years? Acta Otorhinolaryngol Ital 2017;37(5):436–443

[12] Fattah A, Khechoyan D, Phillips JH, Forrest CR. Paediatric craniofacial fibrous dysplasia: the Hospital for Sick Children experience and treatment philosophy. J Plast Reconstr Aesthet Surg 2013;66(10):1346–1355

[13] Béquignon E, Cardinne C, Lachiver X, Wagner I, Chabolle F, Baujat B. Craniofacial fibrous dysplasia surgery: a functional approach. Eur Ann Otorhinolaryngol Head Neck Dis 2013;130(4):215–220

[14] Kusano T, Hirabayashi S, Eguchi T, Sugawara Y. Treatment strategies for fibrous dysplasia. J Craniofac Surg 2009;20(3):768–770

[15] Valentini V, Califano L, Cassoni A, et al. Maxillo-mandibular reconstruction in pediatric patients: how to do it? J Craniofac Surg 2018;29(3):761–766

[16] Brodish BN, Morgan CE, Sillers MJ. Endoscopic resection of fibro-osseous lesions of the paranasal sinuses. Am J Rhinol 1999;13(2):111–116

[17] Lee JS, FitzGibbon E, Butman JA, et al. Normal vision despite narrowing of the optic canal in fibrous dysplasia. N Engl J Med 2002;347(21):1670–1676

[18] Cutler CM, Lee JS, Butman JA, et al. Long-term outcome of optic nerve encasement and optic nerve decompression in patients with fibrous dysplasia: risk factors for blindness and safety of observation. Neurosurgery 2006;59(5):1011–1017, discussion 1017–1018

[19] Amit M, Fliss DM, Gil Z. Fibrous dysplasia of the sphenoid and skull base. Otolaryngol Clin North Am 2011;44(4):891–902, vii–viii

[20] Ricalde P, Magliocca KR, Lee JS. Craniofacial fibrous dysplasia. Oral Maxillofac Surg Clin North Am 2012;24(3):427–441

[21] Mierzwiński J, Kosowska J, Tyra J, et al. Different clinical presentation and management of temporal bone fibrous dysplasia in children. World J Surg Oncol 2018;16(1):5

[22] Frisch CD, Carlson ML, Kahue CN, et al. Fibrous dysplasia of the temporal bone: a review of 66 cases. Laryngoscope 2015;125(6):1438–1443

[23] Megerian CA, Sofferman RA, McKenna MJ, Eavey RD, Nadol JB Jr. Fibrous dysplasia of the temporal bone: ten new cases demonstrating the spectrum of otologic sequelae. Am J Otol 1995;16(4):408–419

[24] Kim YH, Song JJ, Choi HG, et al. Role of surgical management in temporal bone fibrous dysplasia. Acta Otolaryngol 2009;129(12):1374–1379

[25] Slootweg PJ, El-Mofty SK. Ossifying fibroma. In: Barnes L, Everson JW, Reichart P, Sidransky D, eds. World Health Organization Classification of Tumours. Pathology and Genetics Head and Neck Tumors. Lyon, France: IARC;2005:319–320

[26] Speight PM, Carlos R. Maxillofacial fibro-osseous lesions. Curr Diagn Pathol 2006;12(1):1–10

[27] El-Mofty S. Psammomatoid and trabecular juvenile ossifying fibroma of the craniofacial skeleton: two distinct clinicopathologic entities. Oral Surg Oral Med Oral Pathol Oral Radiol Endod 2002;93(3):296–304

[28] Manes RP, Ryan MW, Batra PS, Mendelsohn D, Fang YV, Marple BF. Ossifying fibroma of the nose and paranasal sinuses. Int Forum Allergy Rhinol 2013;3(2):161–168

[29] Ledderose GJ, Stelter K, Becker S, Leunig A. Paranasal ossifying fibroma: endoscopic resection or wait and scan? Eur Arch Otorhinolaryngol 2011;268(7):999–1004

[30] Marvel JB, Marsh MA, Catlin FI. Ossifying fibroma of the mid-face and paranasal sinuses: diagnostic and therapeutic considerations. Otolaryngol Head Neck Surg 1991;104(6):803–808

[31] Bhat KV, Naseeruddin K. Sublabial approach to sinonasal juvenile ossifying fibroma. Int J Pediatr Otorhinolaryngol 2002;64(3):239–242

[32] Mehta D, Clifton N, McClelland L, Jones NS. Paediatric fibro-osseous lesions of the nose and paranasal sinuses. Int J Pediatr Otorhinolaryngol 2006;70(2):193–199

[33] Wang H, Sun X, Liu Q, Wang J, Wang D. Endoscopic resection of sinonasal ossifying fibroma: 31 cases report at an institution. Eur Arch Otorhinolaryngol 2014;271(11):2975–2982

[34] Wang M, Zhou B, Cui S, Li Y. Juvenile psammomatoid ossifying fibroma in paranasal sinus and skull base. Acta Otolaryngol 2017;137(7):743–749

[35] Ye P, Huang Q, Zhou B. Endoscopic resection of ossifying fibroma involving paranasal sinuses and the skull base in a series of 15 cases. Acta Otolaryngol 2017;137(7):786–790

[36] Larrea-Oyarbide N, Valmaseda-Castellón E, Berini-Aytés L, Gay-Escoda C. Osteomas of the craniofacial region. Review of 106 cases. J Oral Pathol Med 2008;37(1):38–42

[37] Earwaker J. Paranasal sinus osteomas: a review of 46 cases. Skeletal Radiol 1993;22(6):417–423

[38] Erdogan N, Demir U, Songu M, Ozenler NK, Uluç E, Dirim B. A prospective study of paranasal sinus osteomas in 1,889 cases: changing patterns of localization. Laryngoscope 2009;119(12):2355–2359

[39] Halawi AM, Maley JE, Robinson RA, Swenson C, Graham SM. Craniofacial osteoma: clinical presentation and patterns of growth. Am J Rhinol Allergy 2013;27(2):128–133

[40] Margalit N, Ezer H, Cavel O, Fliss D. Intracranial and orbital complications of bony lesions involving the anterior skull base and paranasal sinuses. Skull Base 2007;17:A173

[41] Georgalas C, Goudakos J, Fokkens WJ. Osteoma of the skull base and sinuses. Otolaryngol Clin North Am 2011;44(4):875–890, vii

[42] Smith ME, Calcaterra TC. Frontal sinus osteoma. Ann Otol Rhinol Laryngol 1989;98(11):896–900

[43] Savić DLJ, Djerić DR. Indications for the surgical treatment of osteomas of the frontal and ethmoid sinuses. Clin Otolaryngol Allied Sci 1990;15(5):397–404

[44] Gil-Carcedo LM, Gil-Carcedo ES, Vallejo LA, de Campos JM, Herrero D. Frontal osteomas: standardising therapeutic indications. J Laryngol Otol 2011;125(10):1020–1027

36 Repair of Pyriform Aperture Stenosis

Robert F. Ward, Marisa Earley

Summary

Congenital nasal pyriform aperture stenosis (CNPAS) is a congenital anomaly that is a rare cause of neonatal nasal obstruction. It is definitively diagnosed by CT scan. If respiratory symptoms are severe, surgical intervention is required. If the symptoms are mild to moderate, watchful waiting can be recommended.

Keywords: Nasal stenosis, respiratory distress, pyriform aperture, central incisor

36.1 Introduction

Congenital nasal pyriform aperture stenosis (CNPAS) is a congenital anomaly that is a rare cause of neonatal obstruction. It was not clinically described in neonates as a cause of congenital nasal obstruction until 1989. More likely causes of neonatal nasal obstruction are choanal atresia, midnasal stenosis, nasal trauma, cysts, skull base defects (i.e., meningoencephalocele and encephalocele), tumors (rhabdomyosarcoma, hemangioma, glioma, lymphangioma, teratoma), nasopharyngeal mass, and nasal hypoplasia. Birth trauma resulting in septal displacement, hematoma or displaced nasal bone fractures can also cause neonatal nasal obstruction and should be differentiated from CNPAS.

The pyriform aperture (PA) is a pear-shaped bony inlet bounded by nasal bone superiorly, nasal process of maxilla laterally, and horizontal process inferiorly. The PA is the narrowest most anterior bony portion of nasal airway. CNPAS most often occurs bilaterally and is typically characterized by bony overgrowth or medial position of the nasal processes of the maxilla. This is thought to occur during the fourth month of fetal development.

Infants are considered obligate nasal breathers until the first few months of life; therefore any narrowing at the PA, which is already the most anterior and narrow portion of the nose, can significantly compromise babies' ability to breathe. Typically oral ventilation appears between 3 and 6 months of age.

CNPAS classically presents with episodic apnea and cyclical cyanosis, sudden total airway obstruction relieved by crying, tachypnea, noisy breathing, and inability to feed. Signs and symptoms often occur immediately after birth. But the degree of narrowing, in combination with any additional comorbidities, dictates severity of presentation, and some patients may present later in infancy.

CNPAS may be an isolated anomaly or may be associated with other midline anomalies such as central incisor (▶ Fig. 36.1) or holoprosencephaly (HPE). HPE is a brain malformation resulting from incomplete cleavage of the prosencephalon into right and left hemispheres. CNPAS may also be associated with craniofacial anomalies in 40% of cases. Other associated comorbidities include shallow sella turcica, craniopharyngeal canal, submucous cleft palate, or hypoplastic maxillary sinuses.

Arlis and Ward identified an association with single maxillary-mega incisor (SMMI) and considered CNPAS to be a developmental field defect along the HPE spectrum or a midfacial dysostosis with associated endocrine and central nervous system abnormalities. HPE usually includes facial dysmorphisms such as ocular hypotelorism, midline cleft lip and/or flat nose, cerebral malformations, learning disabilities, arrhinencephaly, agensis of corpus callosum, hypopituitarism, and a single maxillary central incisor. Chromosomal analysis and magnetic resonance imaging (MRI) to assess hypothalamic–pituitary–thyroid–adrenal axis and brain are indicated when HPE abnormality is suspected. Endocrinology, electrolyte evaluation, and a craniofacial and genetics workup may also be useful.

Diagnosis can be made via clinical exam and computed tomography (CT) findings. Exam will reveal narrow anterior nasal fossae and inability to pass 5 Fr suction catheter or 1.9 mm endoscope. Recommended CT scan should have contiguous thin sections (1–3 mm thick) through midface from palate to orbital roof. CT scan often reveals narrowed anterior nasal inlet and bony overgrowth of maxillary nasal processes. There is some controversy over exact diagnostic measurements, but it is generally accepted that PA width less than 11 mm at the level of the inferior meatus in a term infant is diagnostic of CNPAS. Brown et al reported CNPAS should be diagnosed when maximum transverse diameter of each aperture is </=3 mm in term neonates and in preterm neonates.

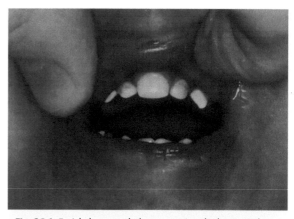

Fig. 36.1 Facial photograph demonstrating the large single central incisor. Sometimes referred to as the megaincisor. (This image is provided courtesy of Dr. Kim Baker.)

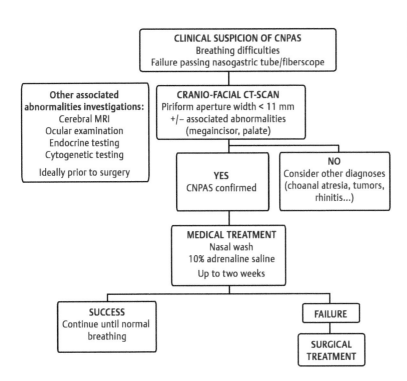

Fig. 36.2 Management algorithm of congenital nasal pyriform aperture stenosis (CNPAS).

Chinwuba et al suggested nasal airway <2 mm is diagnostic. More recently, there has been an increasing diagnostic role for 3D craniofacial CT scan. 3D CT is viewed by some as a better diagnostic tool for CNPAS because it provides more spatial information and preoperative planning information than 2D CT. With 3D CT it is easier to measure distance between the bilateral nasal processes of the maxilla, which can be defined as the interprocess distance (IPD). Lin et al reviewed 40 patients retrospectively and developed a growth curve for the PA. This curve was a cubic curve with two inflection points at 42.9 and 70.9 months and resulted in a formula to estimate growth of IPD. They found no difference in initial IPD between patients who required surgery and those who did not. Further, when IPD fails to progressively increase with age, more aggressive interventions may need to be considered and treatment may progress from observation to conservative management or conservative management to surgical intervention.

Treatment will depend on severity of symptoms. Most authors agree that first-line conservative management should be attempted when possible. This includes use of a McGovern nipple or oral airway with appropriate monitoring in an intensive care unit (ICU) setting. Additional management may include humidification, gentle suctioning, topical steroid and decongestant drops, and gavage feeding if necessary. Some studies suggest that if patients are able to tolerate conservative management, their nasal airway is likely to improve with growth, typically within 6 months of life. The ability to pass a 5 Fr suction catheter is thought to predict success of nonsurgical

management. Ideally, surgery should be delayed when possible until the "rule of 10" is met and the infant is at least 10 lbs, 10 weeks of age, and has a hemoglobin of 10 g. This of course is not always possible. Moreddu et al proposed an algorithm for workup and treatment of CNPAS (▶Fig. 36.2).

Indications for surgery include obstruction refractory to medical therapy, severe degree of obstruction, failure to thrive, and severe obstructive sleep apnea. Contraindications include overall poor prognosis of patient or an unsuitable operative candidate. Since its first clinical description in 1989, surgery has evolved from simple transnasal dilation to sublabial and submucosal approaches. Special instruments typically required are otologic instruments such as small diamond burr drills and a microscope with 300-mm F lens. Other concomitant airway surgeries, neurologic deficits, and other craniofacial anomalies can limit surgical success and prolong hospital course.

36.2 Preoperative Evaluation and Anesthesia

- CT scan with thin cuts (at least 1–3 mm axial sections in a plane parallel to hard palate):
  - This evaluates for dimensions as well as other anomalies (choanal atresia or stenosis, HPE, central maxillary incisor, etc.).
  - If HPE axis abnormalities are noted, endocrine blood work and referral to endocrinologist

to prevent life-threatening complications is recommended.

- If possible, at least 2 weeks of conservative management should be attempted.
- Once CNPAS is diagnosed, other congenital abnormalities involving the pituitary gland, cardiac and urogenital systems should be ruled out.

36.3 Surgical Techniques

36.3.1 Transnasal Approach

This is more often reserved for adults due to poor exposure in infants and increased risk of injury to mucosa and other structures.

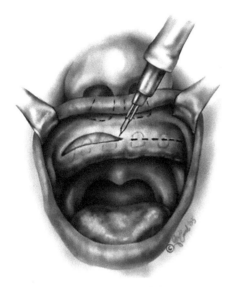

Fig. 36.3 Sublabial incision using electrocautery. (This image is provided courtesy of Dr. Kim Baker.)

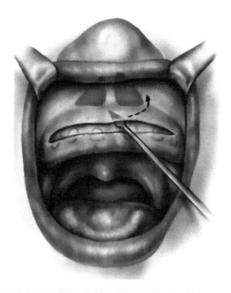

Fig. 36.4 Sublabial approach to the pyriform apertures. Elevation of the soft tissue to expose the boney aperture leaving the nasal mucosa intact. (This image is provided courtesy of Dr. Kim Baker.)

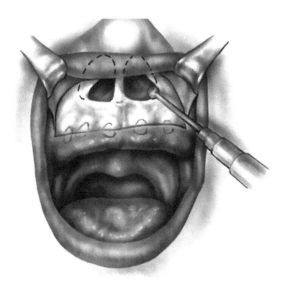

Fig. 36.5 Drilling of the lateral and inferior pyriform aperture. The goal is to stay anterior to the inferior turbinate for the drill out. (This image is provided courtesy of Dr. Kim Baker.)

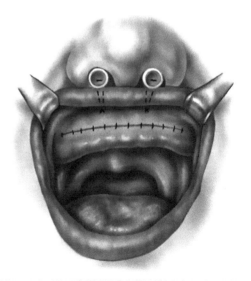

Fig. 36.6 Placement of bilateral nasal stents. (This image is provided courtesy of Dr. Kim Baker.)

36.3.2 Sublabial Approach

Dr. Kim Baker described the following points in her article (▶ Fig. 36.3, ▶ Fig. 36.4, ▶ Fig. 36.5, and ▶ Fig. 36.6):

- Patient should be under general anesthesia with transoral intubation.
- Magnification can be accomplished with 300 mm lens operative microscope or loupe magnification.
- Otologic instruments and microdrill with diamond burr tips of different sizes are utilized.
- Head should be kept in neutral position in donut-shaped headrest with drape to protect eyes.
- Decongest the nose with phenylephrine hydrochloride on pledgets.
- Upper gingival sulcus and PA mucosa are injected with 1% lidocaine with 1:100,000 epinephrine.
- 1.5-cm sublabial incision made in sulcus with needle-tipped cautery; this is extended down to bone.
- Subperiosteal dissection is performed to elevate soft tissue and mucosa exposing anterior nasal spine and floor of each nostril.
- PA should be bilaterally visualized and its bony margin freed up, leaving mucoperiosteum intact along nasal floor.
- 2 mm or other small diamond burr is used to resect bone from inferior and lateral margins of the PA.
- Adequate airway is attained when PA provides passage of 3.5 mm inner diameter endotracheal tube (ETT) stent.
- Keep dissection anterior to head of inferior turbinate to avoid damage to nasolacrimal duct.
- Avoid drilling floor to avoid injury to tooth buds.
- Return soft tissue to original position with releasing mucosal incision in floor of nose.
- Place stent of choice and secure with sutures that originate sublabially in gingival sulcus, pass through the floor of the nose and stent and are tied in the gingival sulcus. Sutures may also be passed through the columella with transverse segment of tubing to prevent compression and pressure necrosis.
  - 3.5 ETT, soft silastic stent or mometasone fuorate nasal stents have been described.
- Stent duration is controversial but is typically 3 to 14 days.
- Close sublabial incision loosely with interrupted absorbable sutures.
- May also use Loupe magnification for drilling (Tate).

36.3.3 Rapid Maxillary Expansion (RME) (Collares et al)

- RME is a common procedure in orthodontics for treatment of transverse maxillary constriction that has the side effect of widening nasal base.

- Collares et al built an acrylic device linked to a mini-expansive screw of 6.5 mm and two lateral surgical orbital plates. The acrylic device was built from patient's dental superior arch mold.
- Device was fixed to palate under general anesthesia, and rapid expansion protocol was used with 0.36 mm expansion per day.
- Active phase was 15 days (stopped based on clinical criteria) and passive phase was 45 days.

36.4 Postoperative Treatment

- Stent should be left in place for up to 2 weeks (some authors say up to 4 weeks):
  - Care must be taken to keep stent clear with frequent saline irrigation, gentle suctioning, and steroid and/or decongestant drops.
- If mometasone fuorate stents are used, they are also secured to septum with 5–0 prolene suture for 2 weeks and will require removal either under anesthesia or secation.
  - These stents are commonly used in sinus surgery and have been described for use after choanal stenosis repair.
  - Mometasone fuorate stents deliver continuous topical steroid to mucosa and some studies suggest it may also impact bony regrowth.
  - This is all off-label usage.
- ICU monitoring is required prior to stent removal as well as immediately after stent removal.
- Feeding difficulty occurs in 90% of infants with congenital nasal obstruction and this is often exacerbated postoperatively.
  - Gavage feeding may be required temporarily.
- Avoid daycare postoperatively or if using conservative management (Lee).

36.5 Highlights

a. Indications
  - Requiring intubation shortly after birth.
  - Inability to extubate or wean from other ventilatory support.
  - Failed at least 2 weeks of conservative management.
  - Severe failure to thrive.
  - Severe OSA.
b. Contraindications
  - Poor prognosis overall.
  - Poor general anesthesia candidate.
  - Soft contraindication: does not meet rule of 10s (10 lbs, Hgb 10, 10 weeks).
c. Complications
  - Injury to nasal mucosa, tooth buds, or nasolacrimal ducts.

- Nasal alar necrosis.
- Retardation of facial growth.
- Restenosis.
- Airway compromise.
- Granulation tissue.
- Blockage of stents.
- Scarring and stenosis.
- May require reoperation or prolonged hospital stay.
d. Special preoperative considerations
   - After the diagnosis is made of pyriform stenosis, it is important to determine whether the patient has an isolated nasal boney obstruction versus a developmental field defect with other CNS abnormalities.
   - If there are any significant CNS problems, these should be addressed prior to any planned surgery.
e. Special postoperative consideration
   - Blockage of stents.
   - Scarring and restenosis.
   - Nasal alar injury.
   - Possible need for revision surgery after stents are removed.

Suggested Readings

Arlis H, Ward RF. Congenital nasal pyriform aperture stenosis: isolated abnormality vs developmental field defect. Arch Otolaryngol Head Neck Surg 1992;118(9):989–991

Baker KA, Pereira KD. Congenital nasal pyriform aperture stenosis. Head Neck Surg 2009;20:178–182

Bharti G, Groves L, Sanger C, Argenta LC. Congenital pyriform aperture stenosis. J Craniofac Surg 2011;22(3):992–994

Brown OE, Myer CM III, Manning SC. Congenital nasal pyriform aperture stenosis. Laryngoscope 1989;99(1):86–91

Collares MVM, Tovo AHS, Duarte DW, Schweiger C, Fraga MM. Novel treatment of neonates with congenital nasal pyriform aperture stenosis. Laryngoscope 2015;125(12):2816–2819

Gonik NJ, Cheng J, Lesser M, Shikowitz MJ, Smith LP. Patient selection in congenital pyriform aperture stenosis repair: 14 year experience and systematic review of literature. Int J Pediatr Otorhinolaryngol 2015;79(2):235–239

Lee JC, Yang CC, Lee KS, Chen YC. The measurement of congenital nasal pyriform aperture stenosis in infant. Int J Pediatr Otorhinolaryngol 2006;70(7):1263–1267

Lee JJ, Bent JP, Ward RF. Congenital nasal pyriform aperture stenosis: non-surgical management and long-term analysis. Int J Pediatr Otorhinolaryngol 2001;60(2):167–171

Lee KS, Yang CC, Huang JK, Chen YC, Chang KC. Congenital pyriform aperture stenosis: surgery and evaluation with three-dimensional computed tomography. Laryngoscope 2002;112(5):918–921

Lin KL, Lee KS, Yang CC, Hsieh LC, Su CH, Sun FJ. The natural course of congenital nasal pyriform aperture stenosis. Laryngoscope 2016;126(10):2399–2402

Moreddu E, Le Treut-Gay C, Triglia JM, Nicollas R. Congenital nasal pyriform aperture stenosis: elaboration of a management algorithm from 25 years of experience. Int J Pediatr Otorhinolaryngol 2016;83:7–11

Shikowitz MJ. Congenital nasal pyriform aperture stenosis: diagnosis and treatment. Int J Pediatr Otorhinolaryngol 2003;67(6):635–639

Smith A, Kull A, Thottam P, Sheyn A. Pyriform aperture stenosis: a novel approach to stenting. Ann Otol Rhinol Laryngol 2017;126(6):451–454

Sultan B, Lefton-Greif MA, Brown DJ, Ishman SL. Congenital nasal pyriform aperture stenosis: feeding evaluation and management. Int J Pediatr Otorhinolaryngol 2009;73(8):1080–1084

Tate JR, Sykes J. Congenital nasal pyriform aperture stenosis. Otolaryngol Clin North Am 2009;42(3):521–525

Visvanathan V, Wynne DM. Congenital nasal pyriform aperture stenosis: a report of 10 cases and literature review. Int J Pediatr Otorhinolaryngol 2012;76(1):28–30

37 Rhinoplasty: Secondary Cleft Nasal Deformity

David Leshem, Sivan Zissman

Summary

Rhinoplasty in patients following cleft deformities is a challenging task requiring an experienced surgeon to restore a normal appearance. Cleft facial deformity may involve the following characteristics: nose deformity, skeletal deformities, dental deformities, and lip deformities.

The ideal timing for rhinoplasty in those patients depends on age, severity of the deformity, understanding of the surgery, and willingness for the surgery.

The open rhinoplasty approach is preferred especially in cleft patients for better exposure, foundation and support reconstruction. We prefer dividing the surgical approach into three stages. First stage: nose foundation. Second stage: structural correction and contouring. Third Stage: aesthetical improvement .The most common complication in cleft rhinoplasty is a residual asymmetry of the nose.

Keywords: Rhinoplasty, secondary cleft deformities, open rhinoplasty, cleft facial deformity

37.1 Introduction

Rhinoplasty in patients following cleft deformities is a challenging task requiring an experienced cleft team to restore a normal appearance. It may be needed due to cleft nose anatomical deformity; growth-related or iatrogenic deformities after primary correction.

Studies have shown that in cleft patients the medial nasal process remains centralized and fails to fuse with the maxillary process. Furthermore, there is discontinuation of the orbicularis oris which affects the aberrant clinical features of the cleft nose.[1-3]

The abnormal insertion of orbicularis oris into the columellar base creates the characteristic view of deformed columella and deviated caudal septum. The insertion of orbicularis into the subalar cartilage results in flattening of the lower lateral cartilage.

Cleft facial deformity may involve the following characteristics:
- Nose deformity: Wide nose, broad and depressed tip, short columella.
- On the cleft side: Wider and retro-displaced nostril, posteriorly and laterally displaced nostril, short medial crus, long lateral crus, deviation of the septum toward the cleft side and inferior turbinate hypertrophy on the non-cleft side.
- Skeletal deformities: Midface retrusion, zygomatic hypoplasia, mandibular pseudo-prognathism, pyriform asymmetry, nasal pyramid deviation.
- Dental deformities: Class III malocclusion, maxillary arch constriction, cleft dental gaps, alveolar fistulae.
- Lip deformities: Short, deficient red or white lip, retracted vermillion, scarred or deviated vermillion.

An example of nasal deformity is shown in ►Fig. 37.1 and ►Fig. 37.2.

37.2 Anatomy of the Nose

The main anatomical structures of the nose are illustrated in ►Fig. 37.3 and ►Fig. 37.4.

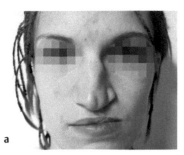 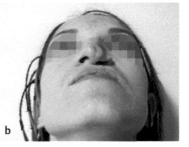 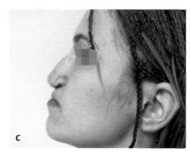

Fig. 37.1 Nasal deformity: preoperative images. **(a)** Frontal view. **(b)** Worm's view. **(c)** Lateral view.

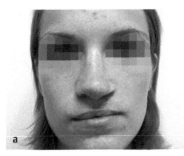 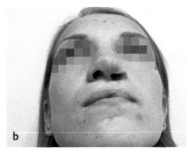 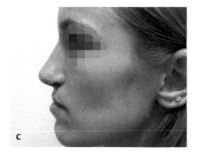

Fig. 37.2 Nasal deformity: postoperative images. **(a)** Frontal view. **(b)** Worm's view. **(c)** Lateral view.

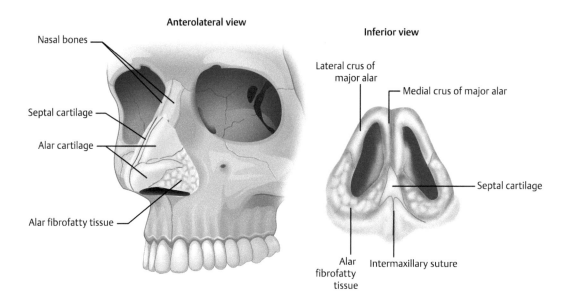

Anterolateral view

Nasal bones

Septal cartilage

Alar cartilage

Alar fibrofatty tissue

Inferior view

Lateral crus of major alar

Medial crus of major alar

Septal cartilage

Alar fibrofatty tissue

Intermaxillary suture

Fig. 37.3 Anatomy of the nose.

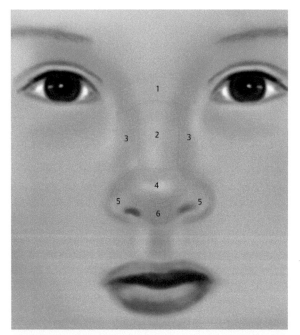

Fig. 37.4 Nasal subunits according to Burget and Menick. **1:** Roof; **2:** Dorsum; **3:** Lateral side wall; **4:** Tip; **5:** Alar lobule; **6:** Columella.

The structural nose component can be divided into three parts:

1. The envelope composed of the outer skin and soft tissue: thinner and mobile skin in the upper two-thirds.
2. Bony and cartilaginous framework.
3. Inner mucosal lining.

Blood supply of the nose is very rich. It is composed of mainly two arteries:

1. Ophthalmic artery: Anterior ethmoidal, dorsal nasal, external nasal arteries—all these arteries supply mainly the proximal part of the nose.
2. Facial artery: Superior labial and angular arteries supply mainly the nasal tip.[4]

37.3 Preoperative Assessment

Preoperative evaluation should include complete history. The surgeon should be familiar with previous operations, and follow standard and systemic nasofacial analysis.[5]

The child's capability of understanding and accepting the surgical procedure and postoperative care is a mandatory condition for proceeding.

There are few basic principles that always guide us during secondary rhinoplasty cases:

- Aesthetics subunits (▶ Fig. 37.4).
- Always look on the whole nose not just on a specific point.
- Previous scars.
- Use cartilage grafts, overdo the support, avoid local flaps for columella, and avoid tissue excision except in alar bases.

37.4 Timing of Surgery

The ideal timing for rhinoplasty in those patients depends on age, severity of the deformity, understanding of the surgery, and willingness for the surgery.

It is usually done around 14 to 16 years old in female patients and 16 to 18 years old in male patients, after facial growth has completed.[6,7]

In rare cases, younger children are operated, such as children with a devastating nose and serious psychosocial difficulties.

37.5 Surgical Approach

The open approach is preferred especially in cleft patients for better exposure, foundation, and support reconstruction. It allows direct visualization of the nasal structures and optimal anatomic reconstruction.

Use of cartilage grafts for structural support is a major part in these patients.

In cleft patients maxillary hypoplasia and alveolar clefts are typically present.

For maxillary hypoplasia correction, Le Fort osteotomies and advancement may be used, prior to definitive rhinoplasty. For bridging the alveolar cleft, bone graft is usually done; it has a role also in supporting the alar base. When the support is inadequate, secondary augmentation using bone, cartilage, or alloplastic implants is a good possibility.

We prefer dividing the surgical approach into three stages:

1. **First stage:** Nose foundation including orthognathic surgical approach for correction of skeletal and dental relationships, fistulae repair, and alveolar bone grafting.
2. **Second stage:** Structural correction and contouring including cleft septorhinoplasty, alloplast / autograft augmentation of zygoma and piriform rim, lower lip reduction, and upper lip augmentation (▶ Fig. 37.5). Skeletal augmentation may be done using materials such as medpor–polyethylene, bone graft, or cartilage.
3. **Third Stage:** Aesthetical improvement including upper lip revision / augmentation, lower lip reduction, and final touch-up nose.

Most of the children during cleft lip repair undergo primary nasal rhinoplasty.

The main goals of primary rhinoplasty are: centralization of the columellar base, symmetrical alar base repositioning in the craniocaudal plane, equalization between the nostrils circumference, release of the attachments of the lower lateral cartilage–accessory cartilage, anteromedial advancement of the cleft-side lateral crus, and creation of the normal overlap of the caudal margin of the upper lateral cartilage.[8]

Various combinations may be used in primary rhinoplasty as indicated by the severity of the primary deformity including presurgical nasoalveolar molding,[9] alar base release, lateral piriform release, inferior turbinate flap, internal nasal valve plication sutures, alar transfixion

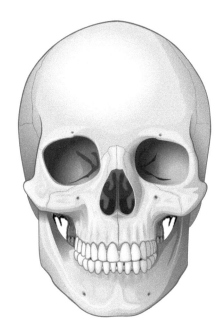

Fig. 37.5 Illustration of skeletal augmentation of zygoma and piriform.

sutures, columellar base–alar base cinch stitch, and postoperative nasal stenting.[8]

37.6 Surgical Technique

Rhinoplasty is done under general anesthesia after incisional marking, local infiltration of the nose with lidocaine 2% epinephrine 1:100,000, and preoperative antibiotic prophylaxis.

Incision: Transcolumellar and infracartilagenous incisions (rim incision) are the most commonly used. After elevation of the skin and mucosa, the nasal structures are exposed and easily visualized.

Septum: The septum is exposed superiorly after detaching the upper lateral cartilages, and a portion of the septum is harvested in subperichondial dissection (submucosal resection) for grafting and tip definition.

Always remember to keep a 1-cm dorsal and caudal strut in order to avoid nasal collapse.

The septum is usually the first option donor site for graft harvesting, others include ear and rib cartilage.

Nasal tip definition is usually done by the combination of suture modification, resection, and cartilage grafts.

Nasal tip suture modification techniques developed by several plastic surgeons[10,11] include: transdomal/interdomal sutures, lateral crural mattress sutures, and columellar septal sutures.

Tip projection and support may be done by various options such as columellar strut, placed in between the medial crura, columellar shield grafts, onlay stacked tip grafts, medial crural strut fold-over graft, cephalic trimming of the lower lateral cartilage, keeping 4 to 6 mm on the caudal region in order to avoid tip collapse, alar batten graft and soft triangle pearls.

The reconstruction options may be used as isolated grafts or combined grafts according to the nasal deformity.

Nasal vestibule: Nasal vestibule asymmetry is a common problem in cleft patients, resulting in nostril stenosis and external nasal valve deformity.

Reconstruction options include: Local tissue rearrangement, excision of redundant tissue followed by placement of a bolster to encourage lateral healing or chondrocutaneous flap.[12,13]

Nasal dorsum: The nasal dorsum is usually deviated toward the cleft side.

In dorsum reconstruction, various manipulations may be done according to the severity of the deformity; excision of excess cartilage, rasping of the bony part and nasofrontal region, and dorsal augmentation using diced cartilage, clavarium, rib, or iliac crest in needed cases.

Osteotomies: Lateral osteotomies (low to high or low to low) are used commonly. Medial osteotomies are used rarely.

Upper lateral cartilages' modification may be done by cartilage trimming and re-approximation, using spreader grafts.

Soft-tissue remodeling includes defatting and alar base excision, usually done bilaterally.

Closure: Sutures for closure—septum 4–0 vicryl, alar rim –5–0 vicryl rapid, intranasal sutures for supra-tip defining suture 5–0 vicryl, transfixation sutures vicryl 3–0, columella 5–0 nylon.

We choose to present an open-approach secondary rhinoplasty in a 17-year-old female who underwent lip-and-cleft palate repair, alveolar bone graft, and le fort 1, in the steps shown in (▶Fig. 37.6).

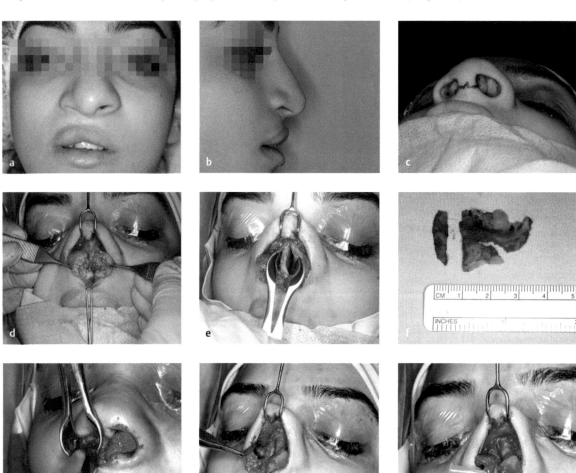

Fig. 37.6 **(a)** Preoperative image frontal view. **(b)** Preoperative image lateral view. **(c)** Transcolumellar incision. **(d)** Exposure of lower lateral cartilage. **(e)** Exposure of the septum. **(f)** Septal graft. **(g)** Lateral osteotomies. **(h)** Marking of cephalic trim of lower lateral cartilage. **(i)** Columellar strut fixation.

(Continued)

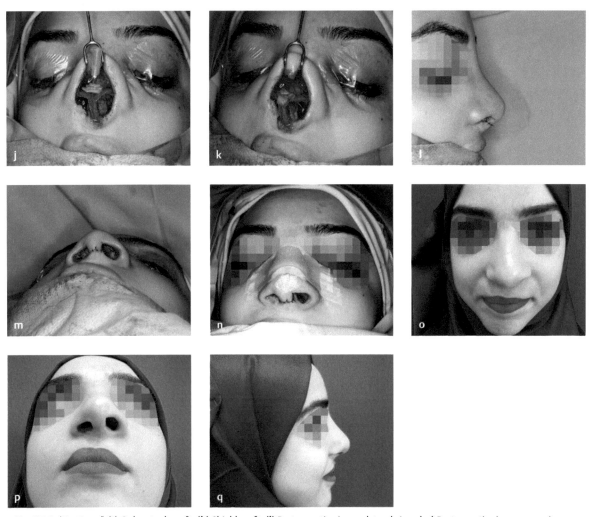

Fig. 37.6 (*Continued*) **(j)** Onlay stack graft. **(k)** Shield graft. **(l)** Postoperative image lateral view. **(m)** Postoperative image worm's view. **(n)** Postoperative dressing. **(o)** Postoperative image following 6 weeks frontal view. **(p)** Postoperative image following 6 weeks worm's view. **(q)** Postoperative image following 6 weeks lateral view.

37.7 Complications

The most common complication in cleft rhinoplasty is a residual asymmetry of the nose. Other complications include nasal obstruction, nasal deviation, unprojected tip, asymmetric and horizontal nostrils, flat ala, short hanging columella, saddle-nose deformity, and patient dissatisfaction.

37.8 Highlights

a. Indications
  – Nose deformity.
b. Contraindications
  – Patient's incapability of understanding and accepting the surgical procedure and postoperative care.
  – Non-cooperative patient.
  – Unrealistic expectations.
c. Complications
  – Residual asymmetry of the nose.
  – Nasal obstruction.
  – Nasal deviation.
  – Unprojected tip.
  – Asymmetric and horizontal nostrils.
  – Fleered ala.
  – Short hanging columella.
  – Saddle-nose deformity.
  – Patient dissatisfaction.
d. Special preoperative considerations
  – Complete history including previous operations.
  – Standard and systemic nasofacial analysis.
  – The child's capability of understanding and accepting the surgical procedure.
e. Special intraoperative considerations
  – Nose foundation.
  – Structural correction and contouring.
  – Aesthetical improvement.
f. Special postoperative considerations
  – Over night hospitalization.
  – Nose cast for 1 week.

References

[1] Rifley W, Thaller SR. The residual cleft lip nasal deformity: an anatomic approach. Clin Plast Surg 1996;23(1):81–92

[2] Johnston MC, Millicovsky G. Normal and abnormal development of the lip and palate. Clin Plast Surg 1985;12(4):521–532

[3] Fisher DM, Sommerlad BC. Cleft lip, cleft palate, and velopharyngeal insufficiency. Plast Reconstr Surg 2011;128(4): 342e–360e

[4] Rohrich RJ, Muzaffar AR, Gunter JP. Nasal tip blood supply: confirming the safety of the transcolumellar incision in rhinoplasty. Plast Reconstr Surg 2000;106(7):1640–1641

[5] Woodard CR, Park SS. Nasal and facial analysis. Clin Plast Surg 2010;37(2):181–189

[6] Kohout MP, Aljaro LM, Farkas LG, Mulliken JB. Photogrammetric comparison of two methods for synchronous repair of bilateral cleft lip and nasal deformity. Plast Reconstr Surg 1998;102(5): 1339–1349

[7] Mulliken JB, Burvin R, Farkas LG. Repair of bilateral complete cleft lip: intraoperative nasolabial anthropometry. Plast Reconstr Surg 2001;107(2):307–314

[8] Fisher DM. Unilateral cleft lip repair: an anatomical subunit approximation technique. Plast Reconstr Surg 2005;116(1):61–71

[9] Grayson BH, Santiago PE, Brecht LE, Cutting CB. Presurgical nasoalveolar molding in infants with cleft lip and palate. Cleft Palate Craniofac J 1999;36(6):486–498

[10] Tebbetts JB. Shaping and positioning the nasal tip without structural disruption: a new, systematic approach. Plast Reconstr Surg 1994;94(1):61–77

[11] Gruber RP, Friedman GD. Suture algorithm for the broad or bulbous nasal tip. Plast Reconstr Surg 2002;110(7):1752–1764, discussion 1765–1768

[12] Sykes JM, Jang YJ. Cleft lip rhinoplasty. Facial Plast Surg Clin North Am 2009;17(1):133–144, vii

[13] Madorsky SJ, Wang TD. Unilateral cleft rhinoplasty: a review. Otolaryngol Clin North Am 1999;32(4):669–682

38 Bilateral Choanal Atresia Repair

Reema Padia, Sanjay R. Parikh

Summary

Common sequelae after bilateral choanal atresia repair are stenosis and granulation tissue formation. A novel endoscopic approach utilizing bilateral nasoseptal flaps allows for vascularized tissue to cover the exposed bone to help reduce this risk.

Keywords: Nasoseptal flap, choanal atresia

38.1 Introduction

Choanal atresia is the most common congenital nasal abnormality that occurs at a frequency of 1 per 8,000 to 10,000 live births and is more common in females.[1,2] Bilateral choanal atresia is suspected in a neonate who has cyanotic spells and respiratory distress with temporary resolution during crying. Inability to pass a 6 French suction catheter and visualization of the atretic plates confirm the diagnosis.[3] Cyanosis and desaturations occur which necessitate early intervention. The obliteration of the choanae by the atretic plates may be bony, membranous, or a combination of the two. The most common presentation is a combination of the two which is confirmed with computed tomography (CT). CT scans can also serve as a guide for endoscopic intervention.[4] Restenosis after repair and development of granulation tissue requiring subsequent interventions are dreaded sequelae. Various mucosal flaps have been described to aid in coverage of the exposed bone that is present after the choanae are opened.[5] A disadvantage of some of these techniques is that the flap is not large enough to withstand manipulation and may fall short in full coverage of the bone. We present our novel endoscopic approach to bilateral choanal atresia repair utilizing nasoseptal flaps as an option to provide well-vascularized, robust tissue around the neo-choanae.

38.2 Surgical Technique

- The patient is intubated under general anesthesia and turned 130 degrees. The endoscopic instruments and towers are set up across from the surgeon. Oxymetazoline-soaked cottonoids are inserted into the nasal passages. Image guidance is not routinely used. 2.7-mm nasal endoscopes are used during the case.
- 1% lidocaine with epinephrine is injected sparingly along the septum and atretic plate mucosa. The sphenopalatine artery is also injected at the base of the middle turbinate (▶ Fig. 38.1).
- Using a sickle knife, a nasoseptal flap is raised from the mid-septum back posteriorly to be pedicled off of the sphenopalatine artery. The flap is elevated posteriorly until the bony plate is visualized and the membranous portion is entered. The same flap is raised on the contralateral side. If a completely bony atresia is encountered, the flap is elevated to the sphenopalatine foramen and a diamond drill is used to penetrate through the atretic plate at the medial and inferior portion (▶ Fig. 38.2).

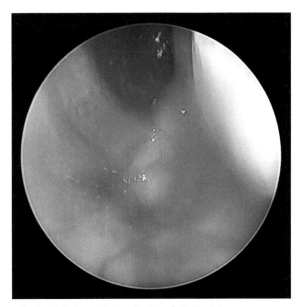

Fig. 38.1 Endoscopic visualization of atretic plate.

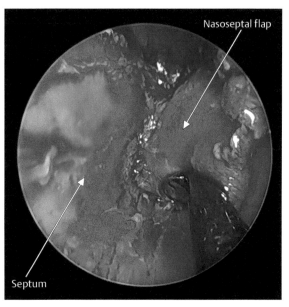

Fig. 38.2 Elevation of nasoseptal flaps.

- The vomer is visualized and the cartilaginous septum is fractured off of the vomer (▶Fig. 38.3). Cutting instruments are used to remove 1 cm of the posterior cartilaginous septum.
- Using a high-speed diamond drill, the vomer is drilled off in order to connect both choanal openings (▶Fig. 38.4).
- Once a large enough choana is created, the left nasoseptal flap is rotated to cover the superior aspect of the nasopharyngeal opening and the right nasoseptal flap is rotated to cover the inferior aspect of the nasopharyngeal opening (▶Fig. 38.5).

- Once the flaps are in the optimal position, a fibrin sealant is applied along the edges of the flap to help prevent collapse (▶Fig. 38.6).
- Stents are not routinely used; however, if there is concern of collapse of the flap or edematous flaps that could create an obstruction, a 2.5 or 3.0 endotracheal tube is fashioned to be placed along one side of the nose through the nasopharynx and is secured to the septum. This is left in place for one week and then removed.

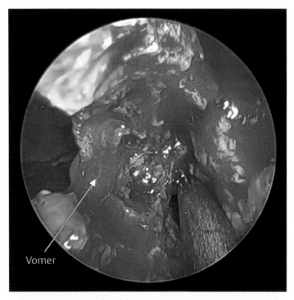

Fig. 38.3 Vomer isolated from posterior cartilaginous septum.

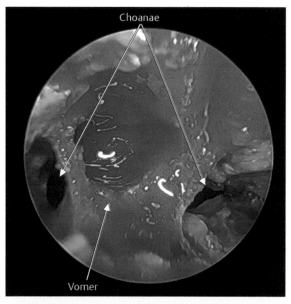

Fig. 38.4 Bilateral choanal openings with residual vomer requiring drill-out.

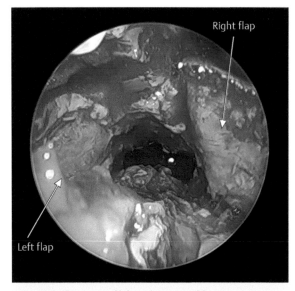

Fig. 38.5 Placement of bilateral nasoseptal flaps.

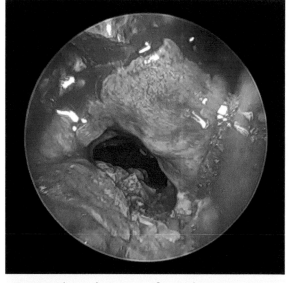

Fig. 38.6 Fibrin sealant to secure flaps in place.

Postoperative care includes saline drops to the bilateral nares twice daily for 3 weeks. Follow-up in clinic is 2 to 3 weeks after surgery when an endoscopic examination is performed. The patient is followed every 3 months for 1 year.

38.3 Discussion

We present our method for bilateral choanal atresia repair. The bilateral nasoseptal flap technique allows for vascularized mucosa to be laid upon the exposed bone. In our experience, the coverage of the bone allows for less crusting that can eventually lead to granulation tissue and stenosis. There is a risk of collapse of the superior flap that can cause obliteration of the nasopharynx; therefore, bedside endoscopic evaluations are indicated if there is clinical concern for worsening nasal obstruction. Should there be evidence of flap collapse, the patient should be taken to the operating room for a more thorough endoscopic evaluation with possible stent placement and/or debridement of the flap. Higher numbers of patients undergoing this technique are needed to determine if healing time and the number of subsequent endoscopic interventions are decreased compared to other techniques.

38.4 Highlights

a. Indications
   - Bony, membranous, or combined choanal atresia.
   - To improve healing after repair to prevent restenosis/granulation tissue.
b. Contraindications
   - Narrow nasal cavities that will not accommodate endoscopic instruments.
c. Complications
   - Collapse of the superior flap causing obstruction.
   - Bleeding.
   - Crusting requiring debridement.
   - Disruption of vascular pedicle of the flaps causing necrosis and infection.
d. Special preoperative considerations
   - Computed tomography with stereotactic image guidance.
   - General endotracheal intubation.
e. Special intraoperative considerations
   - Endoscopic elevation of bilateral nasoseptal flaps with preservation of vascular pedicle.
   - Penetration through atretic plate.
   - Drilling of vomer and removal of posterior septum.
   - Circumferential placement of flaps to cover exposed bone.
   - Fibrin sealant to secure flaps.
f. Special postoperative considerations
   - Intensive care unit monitoring.
   - Saline drops to nares twice daily for 3 weeks.

References

[1] Lee LJ, Canfield MA, Hashmi SS, et al. Association between thyroxine levels at birth and choanal atresia or stenosis among infants in Texas, 2004–2007. Birth Defects Res A Clin Mol Teratol 2012;94(11):951–954

[2] Eladl HM, Khafagy YW. Endoscopic bilateral congenital choanal atresia repair of 112 cases, evolving concept and technical experience. Int J Pediatr Otorhinolaryngol 2016;85:40–45

[3] Benjamin B. Evaluation of choanal atresia. Ann Otol Rhinol Laryngol 1985;94(5 Pt 1):429–432

[4] Ramsden JD, Campisi P, Forte V. Choanal atresia and choanal stenosis. Otolaryngol Clin North Am 2009;42(2):339–352

[5] Nour YA, Foad H. Swinging door flap technique for endoscopic transeptal repair of bilateral choanal atresia. Eur Arch Otorhinolaryngol 2008;265(11):1341–1347

39 Cleft Lip and Palate

Yaniv Ebner

Summary

Clefts of the lip and palate require medical support from birth to adulthood. Attention should be given to multiple concerns such as breathing, feeding, speech, hearing, aesthetic, and orthodontic issues, as well as caregivers' burden, anxiety, and stress. All of these issues can be properly addressed by using a multidisciplinary team.

Clefts can be minor with little affect or can be complete bilateral or with additional craniofacial deformities that might require early and prolonged medical attention.

Clefts of the primary palate have mainly aesthetic, dental, and orthodontic consequences.

Clefts of the secondary palate have mainly feeding, speech, ears, and orthodontic consequences.

Even though for some cleft patients the road is long and sometimes bumpy until completion of medical treatment, proper and dedicated treatment should bring the great majority of patients to normal aesthetic and function.

Keywords: Cleft palate, cleft lip, craniofacial deformities

39.1 Introduction

Clefts of the lip and palate result from incomplete closure process of the palate and lip components between weeks 7 and 10 of pregnancy. The palate is divided according to embryological origins to primary palate (originating from the nasofrontal process) that includes the prolabium (premaxilla and median upper lip) and the secondary palate (originating from the maxillary shelves) that includes the palate posterior to the foramen incisivum, both hard and soft. During embryonic development the primary palate starts to fuse with the maxillary shelves from the foramen incisivum forward. Secondary palate is created by midline fusion of the bilateral maxillary shelves from the foramen incisivum backward. If fusion process of the primary and/or secondary palates is interrupted, complete or incomplete clefts occur.

Clefts of the primary palate (include lip) have mainly cosmetic, dental, and orthodontic concerns. Cleft of the secondary palate have mainly speech, feeding, swallowing, ears, and sometimes orthodontic concerns.

Treatment of cleft patient starts at birth and usually continues to late adolescence. The patients and caregivers are guided and supported through this prolong process by a dedicated multidisciplinary team. The team includes medical and paramedical members: experts in otolaryngology, maxillofacial surgery, plastic surgery, orthodontic, pediatric dentistry, genetics, speech and language pathology, occupational therapy, pediatric dietitian, audiology, nurse, social worker, and patients and team coordinator.

Primary and secondary clefts require different surgeries and medical care. General timeline for potential surgeries and medical care:

- 1 week of age: Presurgical orthodontic—Nasoalveolar molding (NAM) adjust and fixation (primary palate).
- 10 to 12 weeks: Cleft lip repair (primary palate).
- 10 to 12 months: Cleft palate repair and myringotomy tubes placement (secondary with/without primary palate).
- 2 to 6 years: Second set of myringotomy tubes in about 50% of secondary cleft palate patients.
- 4 years: Pharyngeal flap (in case of velopharyngeal insufficiency) (secondary palate).
- 7 to 8 years: Orthodontics (primary and/or secondary palate).
- 9 to 10 years: Alveolar ridge bone graft (primary palate).
- 17 years: Rhinoplasty for cleft lip nasal deformity (CLND) (primary palate).
- Early adulthood: Orthognathic surgery—bimaxillary advancement (mainly secondary palate).

39.2 Unilateral Cleft Lip Repair

39.2.1 Introduction

Cleft lip comprises a range of deformities:
- Microform: Slight depression in the vermilion or the column of the philtrum.
- Incomplete cleft lip: A cleft of the lip tissue—vermilion and skin, but not including the floor of the nose.
- Complete cleft lip: A cleft of the whole lip and anterior nasal floor. The cleft includes all layers of the lip—skin, muscle, and mucosa.

Closure addresses three main issues: lip cosmesis, orbicularis oris muscle continuity and function, and nasal deformity (cleft lip nasal deformity—CLND).

The cleft gap is closed by advancing and rotating adjacent tissues.

39.2.2 Preoperative Evaluation and Anesthesia

Soon after birth and prior to surgery, presurgical orthopedics is applied. Nasoalveolar molding (NAM) device is customized to the patient in order to improve nostril symmetry, as well as premaxilla and maxillary shelf position.

Repair usually takes place at 3 to 4 months of age. The patient should be evaluated by the pediatric anesthesiologist to ensure that the infant gained enough weight and is generally healthy in order to make the anesthesia and surgery at optimal safety, taking into consideration that the surgery is elective and mainly cosmetic.

39.2.3 Surgical Technique

Surgery is done under general inhalational anesthesia with an oral endotracheal RAE tube secured to the mandible but without distorting the lower lip. A shoulder roll is placed under the supine patient for a Rose position. The surgeon is positioned in front of the head of the bed, either sitting or standing.

Markings

The upper lip landmarks are carefully marked with an extra-fine marker and calipers.

The Millard rotation-advancement technique is widely used and is depicted in ▶ Fig. 39.1:
- Point 1: Non-cleft side (NCS) commissure.
- Point 2: NCS Cupid's bow peak.
- Point 3: Cupid's bow nadir (midline).
- Point 4: Cleft-side (CS) Cupid's bow medial peak.
  - Distance 2 to 3 equals 3 to 4.
- Point 5: CS base of columella.
- Point 6: NCS base of columella.
- Point 7: CS alar base.
- Point 8: CS Cupid's bow lateral peak.
- Point 9: CS commissure.
  - Distance 1 to 2 equals 8 to 9.
- Point 10: Base of rotation flap should not cross midline of columella.
  - Length of curved line 4 to 10 equals 7 to 8.

At points 4 and 8 the white roll usually attenuates and the vermilion is starting to narrow superiorly.

After marking the landmarks and the curved 4 to 10 rotation flap line on the NCS, lidocaine–adrenaline mixture is injected to the lip slowly in order not to get the tissue too swollen and distorted, and is rubbed in. This should reduce bleeding allowing clear and accurate incisions.

Incisions

Incisions are done as described in ▶ Fig. 39.2:
- From point 4 vertically in the vermilion up to red line of wet mucosa.
- From point 4 along the vermilion border up to its insertion to the columella at point 5.
- From point 4 along the curved line up to point 10; a small back cut can be made if necessary.
- From point 8 vertically in the vermilion.
- From point 8 along the vermilion border up to its insertion to the ala nasi at point 7.
- Short horizontal incision from point 7 laterally and curving around the ala nasi base to create advancement flap (marked green). Length of incision as required for tension free release of CS lip.

The vermilion mucosa is peeled posteriorly. Later excessive mucosa can be discarded ▶ Fig. 39.3.

The distorted edges of the orbicularis oris muscle are exposed and then its insertion to the columellar base and ala nasi base should be released ▶ Fig. 39.4. By holding the edge with a forceps or a hook and pooling it to its appropriate place, it is easy to appreciate if the muscle was released enough from the base of the nose. A good bulk

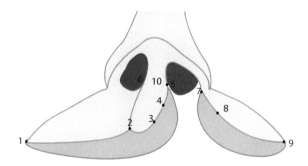

Fig. 39.1 Lip markings for modified Millard repair.

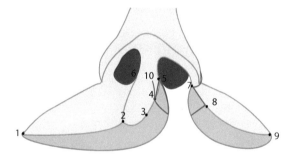

Fig. 39.2 Lip incisions.

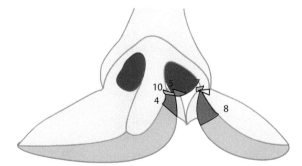

Fig. 39.3 Flap raised.

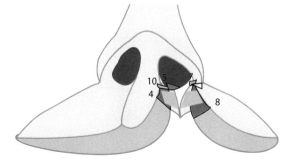

Fig. 39.4 Muscle released.

of muscle should easily fill the vermilion without being tethered to the nasal base. Excessive or hypotrophic edges of the muscle can be cut and discarded to get fresh and bulky muscle edges. Free edges can be created by undermining the muscle from the mucosa. Small horizontal incisions can be done in order to create muscle digits that will be later used for interdigitation suturing. In order to reduce bleeding from the labial arteries, pinching the lip lateral to the incision could be done.

The skin C-flap is raised (marked purple).

At this point the landmarks are approximated to make sure that they are readily juxtaposed without tension and with good symmetry:

- Orbicularis oris muscle edges.
- Points 4 and 8.
- Corner of C-flap and 7.
- Superior corner of advancement flap and point 10.

Sutures

Suturing starts at the posterior wet vermilion mucosa (▶Fig. 39.5), then muscle edges (▶Fig. 39.6), then lip skin, and finally nasal sill which is created by the C-flap (▶Fig. 39.7). Mucosa can be sutured by dissolvable suture, such as *vicryl*, muscle by long-term dissolving sutures, and skin by either 7–0 nondissolving monofilament sutures that should be later removed, or by 6–0 rapidly dissolving sutures.

Good tensionless eversion of the philtrum column skin edges would promise the best esthetic result.

39.2.4 Postoperative Care

Before the patient emerges from anesthesia, arm restraints are placed in order to prevent the infant from touching the surgical wound. Feeding is continued by syringe with attached soft rubber tube for 2 weeks. Breastfeeding can be continued after surgery, but it should be taken into consideration that some suckling infants would be uncomfortable with suckling during the few days after surgery and might not want to go back to breastfeeding after the postoperative recovery period.

If nondissolving sutures were used, the patient is brought back to the operating room or sedation suite after 1 week to remove the skin sutures under general anesthesia or sedation.

Prevention from the scar being exposed to sun is recommended and silicon gel (such as Kelo-cote or Mederma) can be recommended as well.

Antibiotic treatment is not routinely prescribed.

39.3 Bilateral Cleft Lip Repair

39.3.1 Introduction

Bilateral cleft lip deformity is characterized by extrusion of the premaxilla, symmetric deformed nostrils, and short columella. Degree of anterior deviation

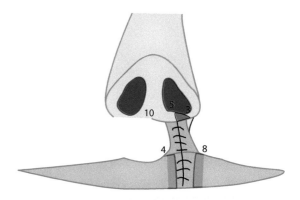

Fig. 39.5 Suturing of posterior wet vermilion mucosa.

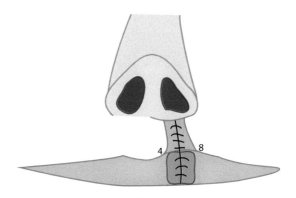

Fig. 39.6 Suturing of orbicularis oris muscle edges.

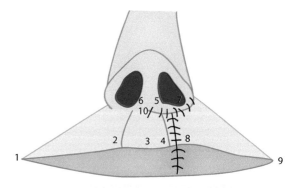

Fig. 39.7 Suturing of lip vermilion and skin. Nasal sill is created by the C-flap.

of the premaxilla significantly influences the perceived deformity and ease of repair. Suckling might be affected. Cleft lip is bilateral in about 25% of cases and more common in males.

39.3.2 Preoperative Evaluation and Anesthesia

Soon after birth and prior to surgery, presurgical orthopedics is applied. Nasoalveolar molding (NAM) device is customized to the patient in order to improve nostril shape, as well as premaxilla and maxillary shelf position.

Repair usually takes place at 3 to 4 months of age. The patient should be evaluated by the pediatric anesthesiologist to ensure that the infant gained enough weight and is generally healthy in order to make the anesthesia and surgery at optimal safety, taking into consideration that the surgery is elective and mainly cosmetic.

39.3.3 Surgical Technique

Surgery is done under general inhalational anesthesia with an oral endotracheal RAE tube secured to the mandible but without distorting the lower lip. A shoulder roll is placed under the supine patient for a Rose position. The surgeon is positioned in front of the head of the bed, either sitting or standing.

Markings

The upper lip landmarks are carefully marked with an extra-fine marker and calipers (▶ Fig. 39.8).

Prolabium

- Point 1: Midpoint of the vermilion-cutaneous junction.
- Point 2: On the vermilion-cutaneous junction, 2 to 2.5 mm lateral to point 1 to the right.
- Point 3: On the vermilion-cutaneous junction, 2 to 2.5 mm lateral to point 1 to the left.
  - The distance from 1 to 2 is equal to 1 to 3 (for a symmetric cupid bow).
- Point 4: Right prolabium columella junction.
- Point 5: Left prolabium columella junction.
  - The distance from 2 to 4 is equal to 3 to 5 (for symmetric philtral columns).

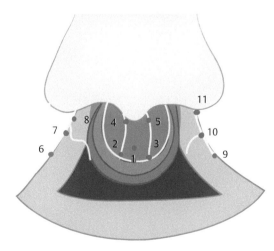

Fig. 39.8 Markings for bilateral cleft lip repair.

Lateral Lip Segments

- Point 6: Right vermilion-cutaneous junction where the white roll starts to attenuate and the vermilion starts to narrow superiorly.
- Point 7: On the vermilion-cutaneous junction, 2 to 2.5 mm superior to point 6.
- Point 8: Junction of vermilion-cutaneous border and right nostril.
- Point 9: Left vermilion-cutaneous junction where the white roll starts to attenuate and the vermilion starts to narrow superiorly.
- Point 10: On the vermilion-cutaneous junction, 2 to 2.5 mm superior to point 9.
- Point 11: Junction of vermilion-cutaneous border and left nostril.
- The distances 6 to 7 and 9 to 10 are equal to the length of 1 to 2 and 1 to 3.
- The distances 6 to 8 and 9 to 11 are equal to the length of 2 to 4 and 3 to 5.

After marking the landmarks, lidocaine–adrenaline mixture is injected to the lip and base of prolabium slowly in order not to get the tissue too swollen and distorted, and is rubbed in. This should reduce bleeding allowing clear and accurate incisions.

Incisions

Incisions are done as described in ▶ Fig. 39.9.
- Central prolabium superiorly based flap:
  - From point 1 to 2.
  - Point 1 to 3.
  - Point 2 to 4.
  - Point 3 to 5.
- Forked superiorly based flaps (used as tissue bank for columella and nasal sill reconstruction; might be later discarded if found unnecessary):
  - Point 2 lateral-superiorly along the vermilion-cutaneous border up to the nostril.
  - Point 3 lateral-superiorly along the vermilion-cutaneous border up to the nostril.
- The three cutaneous flaps are undermined.
- Lateral lip:
  - 6 to 8 full thickness.
  - From 7 vertical full-thickness incision through the vermilion. Vermilion segment 7 to 8 is discarded.
  - From 8 laterally along the alar crease. The length is modified as needed for adequate advancement.
  - 9 to 11 full thickness.
  - From 10 vertical full-thickness incision through the vermilion. Vermilion segment 10 to 11 is discarded.
  - From 8 laterally along the alar crease. The length is modified as needed for adequate advancement.

Incisions of the gingivobuccal sulcus ("elastic flaps") are made for adequate advancement medially. Remnant muscular insertion to nostril is dissected and soft tissue can be gently dissected from the maxilla for adequate relaxation.

Sutures

Suturing starts at the posterior wet vermilion mucosa, beginning at the superior aspect and continuing inferiorly (▶ Fig. 39.9).

Then orbicularis oris muscle edges are advanced medially anterior to the prolabium and sutured with a 4–0 dissolving braided suture (▶ Fig. 39.10).

Skin and vermilion is closed with attention to the continuity of the vermilion border. Skin is closed with either 7–0 nondissolving monofilament suture or 6–0 rapid dissolving suture.

Vermilion is closed with 5–0 dissolving suture (▶ Fig. 39.11).

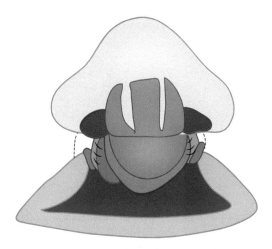

Fig. 39.9 Incisions and suturing of posterior wet vermilion mucosa for bilateral cleft lip repair.

39.3.4 Postoperative Care

Before the patient emerges from anesthesia, arm restraints are placed in order to prevent the infant from touching the surgical wound. Feeding is continued by syringe with attached soft rubber tube for 2 weeks. Breastfeeding can be continued after surgery, but it should be taken into consideration that some suckling infants would be uncomfortable with suckling during the few days after surgery and might not want to go back to breastfeeding after the postoperative recovery period.

If nondissolving sutures were used, the patient is brought back to the operating room or sedation suite after 1 week to remove the skin sutures under general anesthesia or sedation.

Prevention from the scar being exposed to sun is recommended and silicon gel (such as Kelo-cote or Mederma) can be recommended as well.

Antibiotic treatment is not routinely prescribed.

39.4 Highlights of Cleft Lip Repair

a. Indications
   – Unilateral or bilateral cleft lip.
b. Contraindications
   – General medical condition not safe for general anesthesia.
c. Complications
   – Wound infection.
   – Hematoma.
   – Dehiscence.
   – Whistle deformity.
   – Hypertrophic scar.

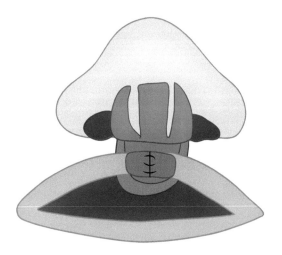

Fig. 39.10 Sutures of orbicularis oris muscle edges.

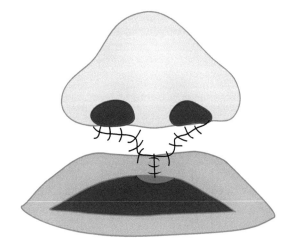

Fig. 39.11 Skin and vermilion sutures.

- Other not satisfying aesthetic results.
- Pain preventing from sufficient oral intake.

d. Special preoperative considerations
- General endotracheal anesthesia with RAE tube.
- Supine rose position.

e. Special intraoperative considerations
- Accurate skin marking.
- Skin and mucosal incisions.
- Flaps elevation.
- Orbicularis oris muscle insertion detachment.
- Mucosal sutures.
- Muscle sutures.
- Skin sutures.

f. Special postoperative considerations
- An overnight hospitalization.
- Suckling can be continued but might be less comfortable for the infant.
- Feeding can be done by a syringe or a special bottle with straw, preferably on the not operated side.

39.5 Cleft Palate Repair

39.5.1 Introduction

Cleft palate breaches the natural partition of the oral cavity from the nasal cavity and also split the soft palate that results in disorientated insertion of the split levator veli palatini muscle. Hence, symptoms include suckling difficulties, nasal regurgitation, speech disturbance, including resonance and articulation problems. Due to the dysfunction of the levator veli palatini muscle in the routine opening of the Eustachian tubes during swallowing, the normal pressure equalization of the middle ear (tympanic cavity) is compromised and this results in effusion build-up and conductive hearing loss. During the first year of life, the main concern is proper feeding. Normal suckling process involves the production of negative pressure in the infant's oral cavity by bringing the tongue to a full contact with the palate and then retracting the tongue from the palate—recreating oral space—which results in vacuum and movement of milk from the nipple to the infant's mouth. This process is affected by the cleft palate deformity and special feeding solution should be suggested. Most of the cleft palate infants are managed by feeding with a special bottle and nipple that actively pushes the milk into the infant's mouth (e.g., Haberman, Mid-Johnson). Feeding is done in a sitting position to reduce nasal regurgitation.

At about one year of age the infant is neurologically capable of speech development. To provide normal speech development, cleft palate repair and myringotomy tubes placement is scheduled to about 10 to 12 months of age. Three main concepts should be in mind: suturing cleft edges without tension, reorienting and attaching the levator veli palatini muscle, and lengthening posteriorly the soft palate as much as possible. The pediatric

otolaryngology surgeon has an added advantage of assessing and relating to the pharyngeal airway. Approximating the soft palate edges medially changes the pharyngeal airway anatomy and might reposition tonsils medially in an obstructing way or narrowing the nasopharyngeal passage in case of adenoid hypertrophy. Rarely, the otolaryngology surgeon might consider reducing the superior part of the adenoid or doing a partial tonsillotomy in order to prevent postoperative obstructive sleep apnea.

39.5.2 Preoperative Evaluation and Anesthesia

Prior to surgery the patient is assessed for cleft extension and width in order to plan a suitable surgery. Ears and hearing are assessed for making decision regarding myringotomy tube placement. Mandible size and tongue location are assessed to rule out glossoptosis and potential difficult airway for orotracheal intubation or postoperative airway obstruction.

General anesthesia is usually by volatile gas through an RAE tube placed in the midline and secured to the chin. The endotracheal tube will be stabilized also by the grooved tongue depressor during the surgery. Local anesthesia with a mixture of lidocaine and adrenaline is also used, reducing pain in addition to the systemic analgesia agent.

39.5.3 Surgical Technique

The patient is laid in Rose position—supine with cervical extension by a shoulder roll.

The surgeon is standing or seated at the head of the operating table. Head light and magnifying loups enhance visibility. Dingman mouth gag is inserted, sliding the mouth retractor groove over the RAE tube, mouth opened and the mouth gag is stabilized over a Mio table, held in position using the Draffin bipod stand, or supported by rolled towels.

Palate is injected with lidocaine–adrenaline mixture. Waiting several minutes would improve hemostasis and reduce local swelling.

Three main techniques are described below:
- Pushback technique for clefts of the secondary palate.
- Two-flap technique for clefts of the primary and secondary palates.
- Furlow double-opposing Z-plasty for narrow clefts of the soft palate or submucous cleft palate.

Pushback Palatoplasty

Incisions

Incisions are made in the oral mucosa along the medial edges of the cleft along the maxillary shelves (▶ Fig. 39.12). The incisions are made not on the exact border of the

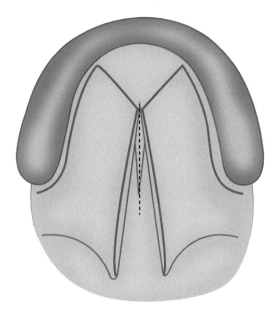

Fig. 39.12 Incisions for pushback palatoplasty.

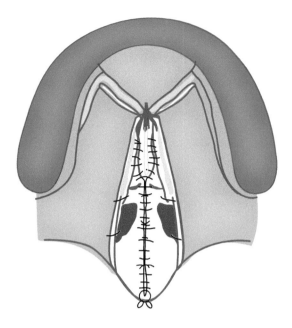

Fig. 39.13 Sutures of nasal mucosal flaps.

oral and nasal mucosa but few millimeters into the oral mucosa in order to lengthen the tender and immobile nasal mucosa on expense of the oral mucosal flap that is more robust and more easily mobilized. Then incisions are made medial to the alveolar ridge in a beveled angle, when the bevel is more lateral as it goes deeper. This technique allows sliding the oral mucosal flap medially with minimal exposure of the palatal bone, which should enhance healing as well as prevent excessive scarring that might result later in constricted maxilla. Finally an incision is made diagonally along the maxilla–premaxilla suture, connecting the other incisions of each maxillary shelf.

Oral mucosal flaps are raised from the maxillary shelf bone in a subperiosteal plane. When reaching posteriorly, caution is taken not to harm the neurovascular bundle while isolating it to improve flap mobility.

When reaching the soft palate, dissection continues along the same plane between the oral mucosa and the muscular bundle of the levator veli palatini which is attached at each side to the hard palate. Next, the muscle is separated from the bluish nasal mucosa which is much more gentle and thin than the oral mucosa so tears should be avoided. When the levator veli palatini insertion to the hard palate is properly exposed, the muscle is detached from the posterior edge of the hard palate. If the insertion continues anteriorly along the medial edge of the maxillary shelf, the muscle is detached from there as well. By grabbing the anterior edge of the muscle with a forceps, it is possible to evaluate its mobility. Dissection is continued from any tethering attachment to the hard palate, oral or nasal mucosa. The muscle is pulled posteromedially. If further release is required, the hamulus process is exposed with an incision and it is either

fractured or the tensor veli palatini tendon is released from the hamulus process.

Same is done on the contralateral side.

In case of bilateral cleft the septum is "floating" between the maxillary shelves, median incision is made along the inferior edge of the bony nasal septum which is seen through the cleft, and vomer mucoperiosteal flaps are raised bilaterally anteriorly up to the premaxilla.

In case of unilateral cleft the septum is attached on the "non-cleft" side (NCS) to the maxillary shelf so at this side a vomer mucoperiosteal flap is raised unilaterally.

Sutures

Suturing starts at the nasal mucosa flaps which are sutured together with a 4-0 dissolving braided suture (►Fig. 39.13). Knots should preferably be placed on the nasal cavity side. Posterior to the septum the nasal mucosal flaps are sutured one to the other. In case of bilateral cleft, when reaching the septum the nasal flap on each side is sutured to the vomer flaps. In case of unilateral cleft, nasal flap on the cleft side is sutured to the vomer flap previously raised from the NCS.

The two edges of the levator veli palatini muscle are sutured one to the other with a 3-0 dissolving braided suture (►Fig. 39.14). The muscle should be pushed as much posteriorly as possible and as tense as possible. About three vertical mattress sutures are usually required.

Next, the oral mucosal flaps are sutured with a 4-0 dissolving braided suture starting at the uvula and

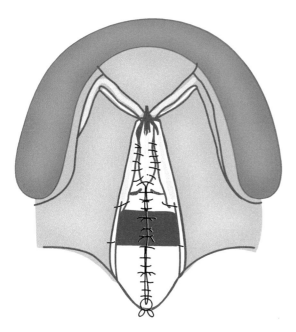

Fig. 39.14 Sutures of levator veli palatini muscle edges.

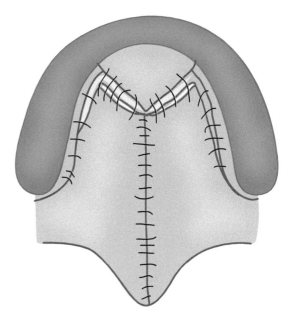

Fig. 39.15 Sutures of oral mucosal flaps.

Two-Flap Palatoplasty

Incisions

This technique is similar to pushback palatoplasty regarding the secondary cleft repair.

Incisions are modified on the primary palate and extend along the cleft up to the alveolar ridge (▶Fig. 39.16).

Incisions are made in the oral mucosa along the medial edges of the cleft along the maxillary shelves of the secondary palate and extend continuously along the primary palate cleft all the way to the posterior border of the alveolar ridge. The incisions are made not on the exact border of the oral and nasal mucosa but few millimeters inferior to this border in order to lengthen the tender and immobile nasal mucosa on expense of the oral mucosal flap that is more robust and more easily mobilized. Then incisions are made medial to the alveolar ridge in a beveled angle, when the bevel is more lateral as it goes deeper. This technique allows sliding the oral mucosal flap medially with minimal exposure of the palatal bone, which should enhance healing as well as prevent excessive scarring that might result later in constricted maxilla.

Oral mucosal flaps are raised from the maxillary shelf bone in a subperiosteal plane. When reaching posteriorly, caution is taken not to harm the neurovascular bundle while isolating it to improve flap mobility (▶Fig. 39.17).

When reaching the soft palate, dissection continues along the same plane between the oral mucosa and the muscular bundle of the levator veli palatini which is attached at each side to the hard palate. Next, the muscle

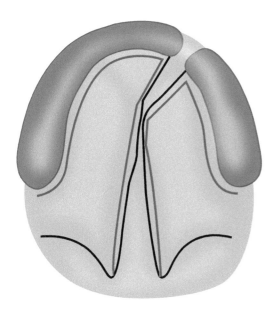

Fig. 39.16 Incisions for two-flap palatoplasty.

advancing anteriorly (▶Fig. 39.15). Vertical mattress sutures would ensure proper eversion of the edges. The suture line should be tension-free. This creates a V to Y repair.

The lateral and anterior incisions are sutured loosely to avoid adding tension to the median suture line or to pull the palate anteriorly. Microfibrillar collagen can be tacked to those incisions to prevent oozing.

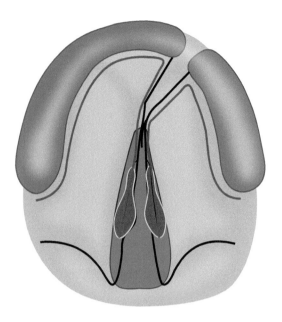

Fig. 39.17 Flaps elevated.

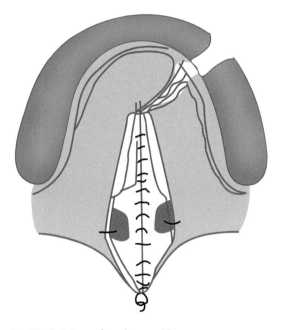

Fig. 39.18 Sutures of nasal mucosal flaps.

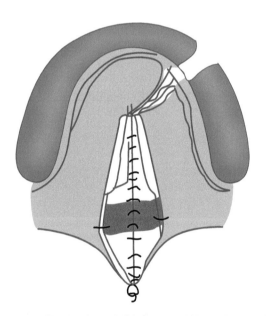

Fig. 39.19 Sutures of levator veli palatini muscle edges.

is separated from the bluish nasal mucosa which is much more gentle and thin than the oral mucosa so tears should be avoided. When the levator veli palatini insertion to the hard palate is properly exposed, the muscle is detached from the posterior edge of the hard palate. If the insertion continues anteriorly along the medial edge of the maxillary shelf, the muscle is detached from there as well. By grabbing the anterior edge of the muscle with

a forceps, it is possible to evaluate its mobility. Dissection is continued from any tethering attachment to the hard palate, oral or nasal mucosa. The muscle is pulled posteromedially. If further release is required, the hamulus is exposed with an incision and it is either fractured or the tensor veli palatini tendon is released from the hamulus.

Same is done on the contralateral side.

In case of bilateral cleft the septum is "floating" between the maxillary shelves, median incision is made along the inferior edge of the bony nasal septum which is seen through the cleft, and vomer mucoperiosteal flaps are raised bilaterally anteriorly up to the premaxilla.

In case of unilateral cleft the septum is attached on the "non-cleft" side (NCS) to the maxillary shelf so at this side a vomer mucoperiosteal flap is raised unilaterally.

Sutures

Suturing starts at the nasal mucosa flaps which are sutured together with a 4–0 dissolving braided suture (▶Fig. 39.18). Knots should preferably be placed on the nasal cavity side. The most anterior side of the cleft is the most hard to reach zone, so suturing starts there and continues posteriorly. In case of bilateral cleft, when reaching the septum the nasal flap on each side is sutured to the vomer flaps. In case of unilateral cleft, nasal flap on the cleft side is sutured to the vomer flap previously raised from the NCS. Posterior to the septum the nasal mucosal flaps are sutured one to the other.

The two edges of the levator veli palatini muscle are sutured one to the other with a 3–0 dissolving braided suture (▶Fig. 39.19). The muscle should be pushed as

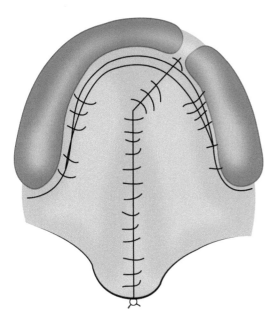

Fig. 39.20 Sutures of oral mucosal flaps.

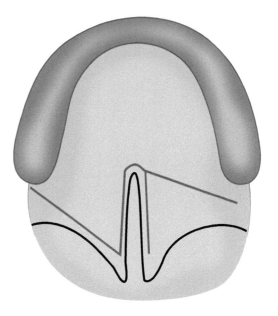

Fig. 39.21 Incisions for double-opposing Z-palatoplasty.

The lateral-anterior relaxation incisions are sutured loosely to avoid adding tension to the median suture line or to pull the palate anteriorly. Microfibrillar collagen can be tacked to those incisions to prevent oozing.

Double-Opposing Z-Palatoplasty

Incisions

On the left side a diagonal incision is made with the tip anteriorly (▶ Fig. 39.21). In case of submucosal cleft a midline incision is made, i.e., oral mucosa only. In case of an overt cleft of the soft palate, incisions are made in the oral mucosa of the median edge of the cleft, several millimeters away (anatomically inferolateral) of the oral-nasal border.

A posteriorly based triangular musculomucosal flap containing the oral mucosa attached to the levator veli palatini muscle is raised from the bluish nasal mucosa (▶ Fig. 39.22).

On the right side, a diagonal incision is made in the oral mucosa only, with the tip posteriorly, and an anteriorly based triangular oral mucosal flap that includes the submucosal layer of minor salivary glands is raised from the muscle, leaving the muscle attached to the nasal mucosa.

On the left side a diagonal incision is made in the nasal mucosa with the tip posteriorly to create an anteriorly based triangular nasal mucosal flap.

On the right side a diagonal incision is made in the nasal mucosa with the tip anteriorly to create a posteriorly based triangular musculomucosal flap containing the nasal mucosa attached to the levator veli palatini muscle.

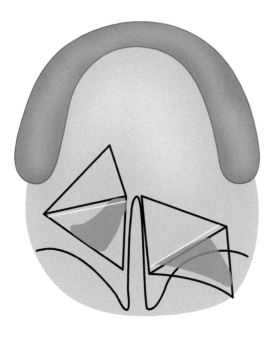

Fig. 39.22 Oral mucosal flaps elevated.

much posteriorly as possible and as tense as possible. About three vertical mattress sutures are usually required.

Next, the oral mucosal flaps are sutured with a 4–0 dissolving braided suture starting at the uvula and advancing anteriorly all the way to the alveolar ridge (▶ Fig. 39.20). Vertical mattress sutures would ensure proper eversion of the edges. The suture line should be tension-free.

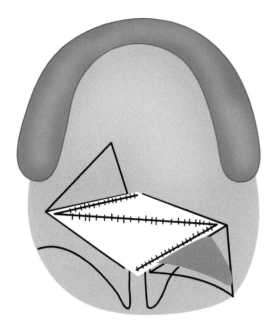

Fig. 39.23 Sutures of nasal mucosal flaps.

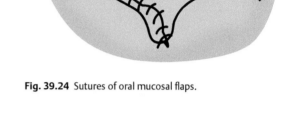

Fig. 39.24 Sutures of oral mucosal flaps.

Sutures

The left nasal mucosal flap tip is sutured to the right lateral corner and the anterior edge of the flap is sutured to the nasal mucosa of the soft palate (▶Fig. 39.23).

The right musculomucosal flap tip is sutured to the left lateral corner and the posterior edge of the flap's nasal mucosa is sutured to the nasal mucosa of the soft palate.

The nasal mucosa of the anterior edge of the musculomucosal flap is sutured to the posterior edge of the nasal mucosal flap.

The left musculomucosal flap tip is sutured to the right lateral corner and the posterior edge of the flap's oral mucosa is sutured to the oral mucosa of the soft palate (▶Fig. 39.24).

The right oral mucosal flap tip is sutured to the left lateral corner and the anterior edge of the flap is sutured to the oral mucosa of the soft palate.

The oral mucosa of the anterior edge of the musculomucosal flap is sutured to the posterior edge of the oral mucosal flap.

39.5.4 Postoperative Care

Before the patient emerges from anesthesia, arm restraints are placed in order to prevent the infant from touching the surgical wound. Feeding is started several hours after surgery with liquids only using a cup for 3 weeks. Pacifier and bottle should not be used during this period. When sufficient oral intake and adequate oral pain control is achieved, the patient can be discharged. Follow-up visit is scheduled to about 3 weeks postoperative.

39.6 Highlights of Cleft Palate Repair

a. Indications
   - Unilateral or bilateral cleft lip.
b. Contraindications
   - General medical condition not safe for general anesthesia.
c. Complications
   - Bleeding.
   - Edema.
   - Dehiscence.
   - Pain preventing from sufficient oral intake.
   - Wound infection.
d. Special preoperative considerations
   - General endotracheal anesthesia with RAE tube.
   - Supine rose position.
e. Special intraoperative considerations
   - Mucosal incisions.
   - Nasal and oral mucosa flaps elevation with preservation of palatine neurovasclar bundle.
   - Nasal mucosa flaps midline sutures.
   - Levator veli palatini muscle insertion detachment, reorientation and reattachment.
   - Oral mucosa flaps midline sutures.
   - Uvuloplasty.
f. Special postoperative considerations
   - An overnight hospitalization.
   - Analgesics (IV, suppository or oral).
   - Elbows restrains.
   - Liquid diet for 2 weeks by a syringe or a soft spoon.

40 Mandibular Distraction Osteogenesis

Craig Senders, Mary Roz Timbang, Mohammad Abraham Kazemizadeh Gol

Summary

Micrognathia is the main feature of Pierre Robin sequence. When the micrognathia is severe, the neonate typically has severe upper airway obstruction. Traditionally, these patients would require a tracheotomy and gastrostomy tube. Over the past two decades distraction osteogenesis of the mandible has proven a replacement for a tracheostomy. This chapter describes the surgical technique.

Keywords: Micrognathia, Pierre Robin sequence, distraction osteogenesis, surgical technique

40.1 Micrognathia and Pierre Robin Sequence

In the simplest terms, micrognathia is defined as a small mandible. When present at birth, etiologies fall into two main categories—from an inherent growth defect or from physical restriction of mandibular growth in utero. Micrognathia is a main feature of Pierre Robin sequence, which is a chain of developmental malformations, one contributing to the next. Pierre Robin sequence begins with micrognathia, which results in backward displacement of the tongue, causing respiratory insufficiency and feeding difficulties. The tongue's abnormal position may prevent appropriate closure of the palate, causing a cleft palate.[1] Although Pierre Robin officially named the Sequence in 1923, it had been described by many others prior. Lannnelongue and Menard first described infants with Pierre Robin features in 1891, and Fiarbarn first included cleft palate in 1911.[1,2] Pierre Robin sequence can be isolated or be part of a named congenital syndrome such as Goldenhar, Treacher-Collins, or Stickler syndrome.[3]

Severity of airway obstruction in Pierre Robin sequence correlates with size and retrusion of the mandible. Since upper airway obstruction hinders swallowing, many of these patients also have feeding difficulties. Often, they require placement of a gastronomy tube for sufficient nutrition. Surgical treatment is considered when conservative measures fail to improve obstruction. Surgical options include glossopexy, subperiosteal floor of mouth release, tracheostomy, or mandibular distraction osteogenesis. Success rates for the first two procedures are inconsistent. Until reversed, glossopexy worsens swallowing issues because it restricts tongue mobility. While tracheostomy is the gold standard for treatment of severe airway obstruction, it carries significant long-term morbidity, mortality risk, and overall cost.[4,5] Mandibular distraction osteogenesis is gaining popularity as the primary treatment for airway obstruction due to micrognathia.

40.2 Mandibular Distraction Osteogenesis

Mandibular distraction osteogenesis is a surgical technique that involves mandibular osteotomies, placement of mandibular hardware for distraction, and subsequent lengthening of the mandible by gradual separation of the segments. The Law of Tension-Stress Effect governs the principle behind mandibular distraction. Constant but gradual tension and stress on segments of healing bone promote tissue growth and regeneration, while mechanical load and blood supply influence its shape.[6]

After proof of concept in animal models, McCarthy introduced mandibular osteotomy followed by distraction in humans as a treatment option for micrognathia in 1992.[7,8] Since then, it has gained popularity as a primary surgical option for patients with micrognathia, particularly bilateral mandibular distraction osteogenesis for pediatric patients with Pierre Robin sequence.

Over the past two decades, several advances in the mandibular distraction have been made, including options for either internal or external distractors, development of multidirectional distractors, improved surgical tools allowing for more precise and controlled osteotomies, development of 3D imaging and planning technology, and better data on long-term results.[9] Recent follow-up data has confirmed long-term benefit for patients with craniofacial abnormalities with an acceptable rate of complications. These studies have also provided more information regarding preoperative patient characteristics that may confer better surgical outcomes.[9-12]

40.3 Preoperative Evaluation and Management

Preoperative evaluation of patients with micrognathia is multifaceted. At our institution, members of a multidisciplinary cleft and craniofacial team work together when evaluating and managing these patients to provide high-quality treatment in all aspects of their care. Consideration of eligibility for surgery is based on probable success of treatment. We deem mandibular distraction osteogenesis completely successful in children with severe airway obstruction when it prevents tracheostomy placement or results in decannulation. Improvement in associated feeding difficulties is often a corollary. Studies have shown different results, mostly depending on patient age and comorbidities. Therefore, the evaluation of neonates will be different than older children.

A number of studies have shown improved outcomes in younger patients, particularly those younger than 3 months.[10] In neonates, distraction is often considered if a micrognathic child has persistent airway obstruction despite conservative treatment. Preliminary airway management includes the following: lateral or prone positioning, nasopharyngeal airway placement, high flow oxygen, noninvasive positive pressure ventilation, and intubation if necessary. Additional management with antireflux medication can be considered. Often additional abnormalities can contribute to the respiratory compromise. One study found ~20% of patients with micrognathia, cleft palate, and glossoptosis had an associated syndrome.[3] Therefore, it is imperative one considers additional syndromes and comorbidities.

Multiple studies have shown poorer outcomes in patients with additional syndromes and comorbidities compared to patients with isolated Pierre Robin sequence. Patients with Pierre Robin sequence as part of a syndrome such as Stickler or Goldenhar consistently had decreased rates of decannulation and increased need for placement of tracheostomy after mandibular distraction osteogenesis. Similar results were found for children with associated neurologic, cardiac, and pulmonary disease. These patients also had increased rates of complications. Thus, performing mandibular distraction osteogenesis on these patients is less straightforward and requires careful consideration of risk-to-benefit ratio. Evaluating for additional sites of airway obstruction with flexible laryngoscopy under sleep conditions is ideal. The jaw thrust maneuver can show potential benefit of mandibular distraction osteogenesis. Unfortunately, this is not possible for many candidates as they are already intubated or their obstruction is so severe that they would not tolerate the procedure.

Prior to making a final decision on treatment, the team should monitor pulse oximetry, and the frequency and degree of oxygen desaturations should be documented. Obtaining an accurate sleep study in a neonate can be challenging and treatment decisions can often be made without a formal sleep study in this age group.[13] If obstructive symptoms are mild or moderate, a sleep study is reasonable to determine additional causes of desaturation such as central sleep apnea. Monitoring capillary carbon dioxide levels can also help determine efficacy of preliminary interventions or help confirm the need to proceed with a more invasive treatment. Typically, persistent carbon dioxide levels greater than 50 milliequivalent units per liter of blood necessitate additional intervention. However, in the setting of cardiac or pulmonary disease a higher carbon dioxide threshold can be accepted.

As aforementioned, there exist other surgical options to consider. A tongue lip adhesion surgery suspends the obstructing base of tongue by suturing the tongue to the anterior lower lip. Tongue lip adhesion is a relatively simple procedure with low surgical risk, but there is controversy as to which patients benefit from it and its negative effects on speech and swallow. Furthermore, critics of the technique contend the benefit of tongue lip adhesion is also achievable with a nasopharyngeal airway. At UC Davis, nasopharyngeal airways are rarely offered in the outpatient setting.

Although feeding difficulty is not a direct reason to proceed with mandibular distraction osteogenesis, neonates will not feed effectively or gain weight appropriately if they are struggling with upper airway obstruction. Evaluation in conjunction with feeding and swallowing specialists, monitoring for oxygenation desaturations while feeding, and monitoring for coughing, sputtering, or startling with feeding can be clues that the airway is not sufficient and is limiting feeding.

In older children, the decision for proceeding with mandibular distraction osteogenesis is often based on a combination of the degree of micrognathia (usually at least 10 mm of maxillary overjet) and severity of the sleep study (severe obstruction sleep apnea with apnea-hypopnea index greater than 10, or frequent oxygen desaturations less than 90%). It is not uncommon for a child to have a tracheotomy placed earlier in life because of upper airway obstruction and to subsequently undergo mandibular distraction osteogenesis to allow for safe repair of a cleft palate or in an attempt to improve the airway sufficiently to allow for decannulation.

There is also the question of whether to use an internal or external distraction device (image/table). External devices have pins that extrude from the mandible to the skin. The main advantages of the newer internal devices are the lack of a large cumbersome external device and scar formation from the pins.[14] However, internal devices require removal of the device in the operating room. Not only is the second incision larger as the device has increased in size with distractions, the fascial planes are distorted after healing from the initial surgery (image). Theoretically, this would increase risk of injury to the marginal mandibular nerve. Additionally, the internal device only has a unidirectional vector of movement and thus placement of screws has very little room for error. Because of this, 3D computerized planning is typically used with the internal device. A copy of the patient's computerized topography scan with 3-dimensional re-formatting is sent to a company that makes a model of the mandible. The surgeon collaborates with an engineer at the company to determine vector of distractions, osteotomy, and pin sites. The model is created along with distraction guides, all of which are then needed to perform the surgery. This usually takes 3 weeks. Therefore, at our institution, we only offer internal distraction to patients who do not need immediate results. For example, if we are trying to avoid tracheostomy in an infant, then external devices are placed. For children who require distraction for safe palate repair or for mild/moderate airway obstruction, there is time to plan for internal distraction. ▶ Table 40.1 shows internal vs. external device.

Table 40.1 Internal vs. external device

	Internal device	External device
Model	Internal distraction device.	External distraction device.
Placement and removal	• Need preoperative model (increased cost) for exact vectors • Difficult exposure • Need second surgery for removal • Periosteal envelope disrupted twice (for placement and removal)	• No need for preoperative model • Better exposure • No need for second surgery, can remove in office • Periosteal envelope only disrupted once
Distraction	• Precise vector of distraction, determine preoperatively • Limitations in adjustments	• Vectors may be adjusted during distraction • Multidirectional adjustment possible
Other risks	• Increased risk for tooth injury • Fewer scars	• Decreased risk of injuring teeth as vector and pin site are separate • Multiple scars from incision and pin sites

40.4 Surgical Technique

The following is the surgical technique employed by the senior author (CS):

- Room preparation
  - Equipment
    - Distractor, pins, screws.
    - Cutting guides if using internal device with official 3-dimensional planning.
    - Saw:
      - i. Ultrasonic bone saw.
      - ii. Reciprocating saw.
    - Straight Osteotomies: 3 to 6 mm.
    - Malleable retractors.
    - Soft-tissue instruments:
      - i. 15 blade:
      - ii. Needle tip Bovie.
      - iii. Dissectors and pickups.
      - iv. Wide double prong retraction needles.
    - Sterile pencil.
    - Nerve hook.
    - Periosteal elevator (Molt #9, freer, Cottle).
    - Drill.

- Discuss airway with anesthesia
  - Nasotracheal vs. orotracheal intubation:
    - i. Nasotracheal intubation allows for better monitoring of occlusion and mandibular symmetry during the distraction phase.
  - Turn bed 180 degrees.
  - Perioperative antibiotics within 30 minutes of the incision.
  - No ongoing neuromuscular paralysis during the case.
  - Determine postoperative airway plan. At our institution, if used for airway obstruction, we leave the patient intubated until appropriate amount of distraction performed (see postoperative section).
- Positioning, prepping, and draping
  - Place a shoulder roll.
  - Iodine based prep.
  - Drape to include the following in the field:
    - Upper and lower lips with a clear adhesive over the mouth.
    - Ear lobule.
    - Mastoid process and cervical skin back to the anterior edge of trapezius.
    - Inferiorly to the clavicles.

- The anesthesia circuit can be passed through a sterile circuit bag over the surgical field allowing for easy visualization of the circuit and turning the head from side to side.
- Incision planning
  - Submandibular incision
    - 2 cm below the inferior boarder of the mandible to stay below the marginal mandibular branch of the facial nerve for neonates, 2 finger breadths for older children and adults.
    - 2 to 3 cm long in a skin crease if present.
    - Extend about 5 mm posterior to the mandibular angle.
  - Inject local anesthetic and vasoconstrictive agent (0.25% bupivacaine with 1:200,000 epinephrine using appropriate dosing).
  - It is helpful to mark out both incisions at the same time for symmetry.
- Surgical approach to the mandible
  - Sharply make a skin incision and carry the incision through the subcutaneous fat down to the level of the platysma.
  - Either sharply or using electrocautery divide the platysma the entire length of the skin incision.
  - Identify submandibular gland. The marginal mandibular nerve will run in the fascia overlying the submandibular gland. Often the facial vein and artery need to be divided to reflect the fascia off the submandibular gland. Staying deep to the vessels will protect the nerve. It is imperative to not inadvertently transition to a more superficial plane in order to keep the nerve safe.
  - Maintaining a plane under the submandibular fascia, the pterygomasseteric sling is identified.
  - Bovie or bipolar cautery is used to divide the pterygomasseteric sling on the inferior boarder. Dividing along the inferior boarder as opposed to the lateral mandibular boarder adds additional protection to the marginal mandibular nerve. A 2 cm opening is usually sufficient, since the opening can often be safely stretched with retractors while preforming the subperiosteal dissection.
  - Elevate in a subperiosteal plane to expose the outer mandibular angle, inner mandibular angle, sigmoid notch, subcondylar mandible, posterior ½ to 1/3 of the mandibular body, and medial surface of the mandible. The periosteum needs to be circumferentially elevated off the mandible along the planned osteotomy site. For external distractors, a minimum of 1.5 cm of exposed bone should be visible on either side of the osteotomy. Wider exposure is required if cutting templates or an internal distractor will be used. For internal distractors, enough elevation should be done to allow for the entire footplate to sit directly on mandibular bone.
  - Close attention to the medial surface of the mandible often will reveal the location where the inferior alveolar nerve enters the mandible just lateral to the lingula.
- Design the osteotomy and mark it with a pencil. Confirm there is adequate subperiosteal dissection. Osteotomies can be angulated, reversed L-shaped, or vertically oriented. Preoperative imaging can be used to create cutting guides or to help determine the ideal locations for the osteotomies. The senior author prefers an angulated, cortical osteotomy from the inner angle to just anterior to the outer angle in neonates and children. When the mandible is larger, a through-and-through reversed osteotomy gives best results. Distraction works best when the osteotomy creates a large surface area for healing. The ramus is relatively thin in neonates and young children.
  - An angulated osteotomy (▶ Fig. 40.1) extends from the inner mandibular angle. The osteotomy can overlap with the posterior tooth bud, by design the majority of the bud should remain in the anterior segment. With distraction, the buds should move with the anterior segment. It allows for multidirectional distraction. The final part of the osteotomy is completed by fracturing the bone to prevent injury to the inferior alveolar nerve (see Step 7). A criticism of this osteotomy is that after distraction is complete, the mandibular angle is not well defined.
  - A reversed L-shaped osteotomy (▶ Fig. 40.2) is through and through, and it starts with its horizontal segment above the lingual nerve and extends posteriorly. Then it turns inferiorly for its vertical segment after the lingua nerve and tooth buds are passed. The degree of angulation at the turn can be as much as 90 degrees, but in younger patients a less acute turn is used (i.e., 30 degrees) to help maintain better posterior bone stock. L-shaped

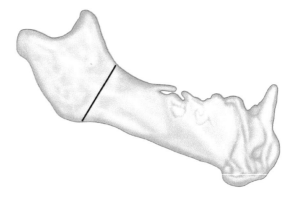

Fig. 40.1 Angulated osteotomy.

osteotomies are more technically demanding and difficult in neonates.

– The senior author does not perform vertical osteotomies.

• Distractor placement: The distractors need to be positioned before the osteotomies are completed in order to optimally control their orientation.

– External distractors

◦ Pin placement

i. Pin site choice is important (▶Fig. 40.3). The pins should be at least 0.5 mm from the osteotomy site. Ideally, they are placed in thick bone just posterior to the inferior alveolar nerve and at the inferior borders of the mandible. With distraction, the pins will migrate with the direction of the vector of distraction. The posterior pins will migrate posteriorly and the anterior pins anteriorly. However, since the inferior border of the mandible is solid thick bone, it is unlikely that they will erode through the bone during migration. The posterior pins should be placed just posterior to the course of V3 in the subcondylar buttress about 8 mm from the posterior border of the mandible. If preoperative imaging is available, the course of the inferior alveolar nerve can be approximated to help determine pin site placement that will not violate the nerve intraoperatively or via pin migration during distraction.

ii. Place posterior pins first. The ideal orientation for the pins is perpendicular to the midsagittal plane. This orientation can be difficult to accurately identify and therefore we find it more reliable to place the pins perpendicular to the plane of the ascending ramus. Placing the pins perpendicular to the body will create an angulated vector and cause binding and tension on the pins (▶Fig. 40.4).

iii. A small hemostat is bluntly passed from internally and a small skin incision is made. The path is stretched by opening the hemostat. The hemostat tines are placed into the hole of the trocar which guides the trocar through the soft tissue.

iv. Using the trocar to maintain correct orientation, a drill is used to make a shallow cortical opening. Without the cortical opening, the self-drilling pins often create small microfractures.

v. A self-drilling pin is then placed bi-cortically through the trocar, taking care to maintain perpendicular orientation in both the superior–inferior and anterior–posterior planes. It is helpful to have a second observer confirm correct orientation. A malleable can be placed medial to the mandible during pin placement for protection and for tactile feedback. The posterior pins are threaded for 10 mm, while the anterior pins need to be threaded about 15 mm.

◦ The multidirectional distractor is adjusted, and then positioned on the pins in the intended orientation and position. Make sure the distractor driver is positioned along the distraction arm in a way that allows for sufficient subsequent distraction (i.e., the distractor driver can inadvertently be positioned at the completion end of the arm leaving no additional room for distraction).

◦ Place the distractor on the pins in the intended final position and mark the pins with a surgical site marker.

◦ Remove the distractor and complete the osteotomies (see below for details on completing osteotomies).

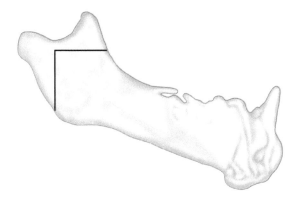

Fig. 40.2 Reverse L osteotomy.

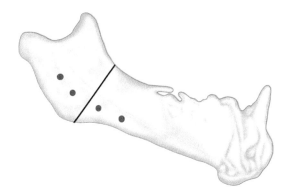

Fig. 40.3 External distractor pin placement.

– Internal distractors
  o Determine the desired distraction vector—usually, parallel to or in a plane slightly inferior to the plane of the inferior border of the mandible is chosen.
  o During 3D computer planning:
    i. Determine the intended orientation of the distraction arm. Anteriorly positioned distractor arms will leave a more visible anterior scar but are further away from the facial nerve. Posteriorly positioned distraction arms are preferred unless the vector and osteotomy would irritate the auricle.
    ii. Determine screw location and length. Ideally, four screws locations on each plate are available in case one location is not useable intraoperatively.
    iii. The distractor footplates are customized by the surgeon. The inferior set of screw holes is typically removed. Using the 3D model, the footplates are pre-bent to exactly fit the mandible.

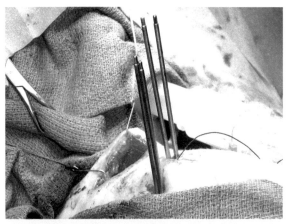

Fig. 40.4 External pins are all parallel.

  o Confirm there is adequate mandibular periosteal dissection for the distractor footplate
  o The guide is placed over the mandible and two screw locations are marked by a monocortical drill hole.
• Preform the osteotomies. Preoperatively osteotomy guides can be created to help avoid the inferior alveolar nerve, tooth buds, and allow for precise internal distractor positioning.
  – Make the cortical osteotomy with the ultrasonic bone or reciprocating saw:
    o At the superior and inferior border of the mandible, it is through both cortices.
    o Over the tooth buds and the inferior alveolar nerve, it is monocortical on both the lateral and medial surface. Because of exposure, the entire medial cortical osteotomy is often not feasible (▶ Fig. 40.5 and ▶ Fig. 40.6).
  – A straight osteotome is wedged into the osteotomy site and gently twisted to break the cancellous bone. Care should be taken to not fracture cortical bone while twisting the osteotome. If it appears that adjacent cortical bone is beginning to fracture, one should confirm the cortical osteotomies are complete. Often there is additional cortical bone along the superior and/or inferior border of the mandible that needs to be cut. This final portion of the cortical osteotomy can be finished with the piezo-electric saw or sharply with the osteotome.
  – The mandible should be freely mobile at the osteotomy site. **It is important to verify a complete fracture, as a greenstick fracture will not distract.**
  – A right angle nerve hook can be used to confirm integrity of the inferior alveolar nerve.
  – Occasionally, there are tooth buds visible in the osteotomy line. If upon widening the osteotomy

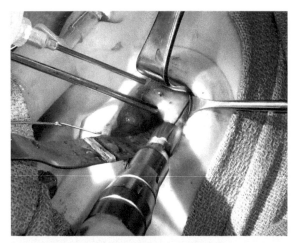

Fig. 40.5 Monocortical osteotomy, lateral surface.

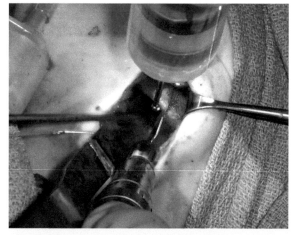

Fig. 40.6 Monocortical osteotomy, medial surface.

they stay in the ramus segment, they can be pushed anteriorly into the body to keep them in a more anatomic location after distraction.

- Place the distractor
  - External distractor
    - ○ The distractor is placed at the marked lines on the pins.
    - ○ Activate the distractor and confirm there is uniform distraction along the osteotomy.
    - ○ Close the osteotomy gap back down to 1 mm.
  - Internal distractor
    - ○ Place the distractor across the osteotomy by loosely placing the previously marked screws. Typically, a 3 to 7 mm hex head screws are used depending on the proximity of tooth buds or the inferior alveolar nerve.
    - ○ Ideally the foot plates are secured with three screws per plate.
    - ○ Activate the distractor and confirm there is uniform distraction along the osteotomy. Uneven distraction suggests a greenstick fracture.
    - ○ Close the osteotomy gap back down to 1 mm.
    - ○ Place a multidirectional elbow and distraction arm. The distraction arm can exit through the incision, but we prefer a separate stab site. Ideally the arm is positioned to allow for the elbow to be completely under soft tissues, so after distraction is completed and the distraction arm is removed, no additional hardware is exposed.
    - ○ Adjust the distractor pin to ensure non-reversing ratcheting.
- Close the incisions in multiple layers
  - The pterygomasseteric sling does not necessarily need to be closed.
  - Close the platysmal layer.
  - Close the skin with deep dermal sutures and a subcuticular suture followed by skin glue.
  - A drain is not usually needed for external distractors. If needed for internal distractors, a quarter inch Penrose drain is preferred.
- Dressing
  - Antibiotic ointment and gauze is placed around the pin sites or distractor arm followed by xeroform gauze for external distractors (▶Fig. 40.7).

40.5 Postoperative Care and Distraction Monitoring

Postoperative care varies depending on the patient's age and severity of preoperative respiratory distress. For all patients, the skin around the pins is protected with Xeroform gauze and bacitracin ointment. We do not administer prophylactic postoperative antibiotics. If there are signs of superficial infection at pin sites such as skin erythema or drainage, Bactrim or Keflex is started.

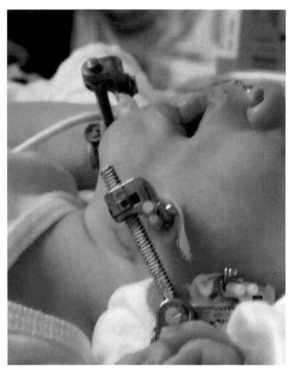

Fig. 40.7 Early results 13 days postoperatively.

In neonates, distraction can begin immediately. Distraction is usually done at 8 or 12 hour intervals with a total of between 1 and 2 millimeters of lengthening a day. If a neonate required intubation before surgery, we distract at least 8 mm before attempting extubation. Steroids are given on a case-by-case basis depending on the anticipated degree of airway edema. Typically, a 24 course of dexamethasone dosed at 0.25 to 0.5 mg/kg q8hrs is used. If a feeding tube is in place, feeding can begin when bowel sounds are heard. After extubation, feeding can begin immediately. Pain is typically controlled with ibuprofen and Tylenol, but occasionally narcotics are given for breakthrough pain. ▶Table 40.2 shows postoperative distraction rates.

Older children typically present with severe OSA with or without a tracheotomy tube already in place. If the patient is intubated for surgery, the surgeon and anesthesiologist make the joint decision at the conclusion of surgery regarding whether to extubate in the operating room. If minimal airway edema is expected and it is not late in the evening these patients can be extubated in the operating room. However, if there are airway concerns it is not uncommon to leave a patient intubated at least overnight while treating with a course of peri-extubation steroids. Distraction is typically not started in older children until postoperative day 3 to 7 to allow for the bone to transition to the regenerative phase (neonates do not need this transitional waiting period).

Wound care and distraction instructions are taught to the patient's caregivers. After the patient meets

Table 40.2 Postoperative distraction rates

Age	Latency (days)	Rate (millimeters/day)
Neonate to 3 months	0	2
3 months–2 years	0	1.5
2–6 years	3–5	1.5
Greater than 6 years	5–7	1.0

nutritional, respiratory, and pain control criteria, they can be discharged home to complete the remainder of the desired distraction.

If external distractors are placed, the distraction vectors can be adjusted mid-course to correct any developing cross bite or open bite. The distraction vectors oftentimes cross to some degree; therefore, periodically adjusting the transverse hinges on a multidirectional external distractor every few days can minimize this binding and help relieve unnecessary strain on the pins. The longer the distraction distance, the greater the binding.

Ideally distraction proceeds to the point of slight over correction because the distracted mandibular bone grows slower than the remainder of child's facial bones and recurrence of the micrognathia can develop. Distracting until the alveoli lineup end to end or even to the point of 2 to 3 mm underjet is a typical goal. Oftentimes the amount of distractor arm lengthening does not correlate in a 1:1 ratio with the overjet correction because of variations in the planes of the distractor and the mandible, and pin and screw migration. For example, one might need to distract 15 mm to correct a 12 mm overjet.

With external distractors, the pins should be monitored at least every few days during the distraction process to make sure they are not loosening. If they start to loosen distraction should be stopped—in our experience, this has not significantly affected outcome. Once the mandible is close to the desired position, or if the mandible is overcorrected, the distractor arms can be adjusted a few mm in either direction to correct asymmetries if needed.

In some cases, both mandibular height and lengthening are needed. In this scenario, ideally the vertical distraction is completed first to prevent binding of the teeth while distracting.

For external distractors, after the mandible has reached the desired position either a consolidation bar is placed to maintain the distracted position or the distractor device is simply left on without making additional adjustments. For internal distractors the distract arms are removed, which ideally allows for soft tissue to cover all the hardware. Consolidation usually takes 6 to 8 weeks. The external hardware can be removed in clinic. Internal hardware is removed by reopening the previous incision in the operating room. Occasionally, there is bony overgrowth over the parts of the internal hardware that requires a drill to remove.

40.6 Complications

Mandibular distraction osteogenesis is a complex and demanding surgery that requires comprehensive training and experience in order to minimize complications. However, even the most experienced centers experience a variety of complications. A 2015 systemic review of mandibular distraction osteogenesis performed for congenital abnormalities estimated that some degree of complication is present in about 34% of cases. However, most of these are minor and manageable, or temporary. Complications most commonly cited include dental injury (ex. Tooth loss, dentigerous cyst), nerve injury (ex. facial nerve paralysis, inferior alveolar nerve paresthesias), poor aesthetic outcome (ex. hypertrophic scar), open-bite deformity, and need for repeat surgery.[9,15]

It has been our experience that inferior alveolar nerve paresthesia is not often clinically noticeable (i.e., drooling, incidental lip biting, or subjective descriptions of a difference in sensation between the two sides). Marginal mandibular nerve weakness is seen, but usually resolves with time. Occasionally the weakness begins part way through the distraction. In this scenario, a judgment call must be made regarding whether or not to proceed with additional distraction. Although TMJ ankylosis has been described in the literature, it is not frequently seen in our distracted patients. Potentially this can be avoided by trying to distract in a more anterior direction rather than a vertical direction. The surgical scars are often noticeable for the first year or two, but with massage and routine wound care they usually heal nicely and are not disfiguring several years out. Damage to the molars is frequently seen in early distraction (i.e., before 6 months of age). Pin loosening is also more frequently seen in early distraction. Waiting until the child is older (at least 12 months old) can minimize risk to the molars and allow for more robust bone stalk to place the pins or screws into, but can require tracheotomy placement in the meantime.

40.7 Conclusion

Bilateral mandibular distraction osteogenesis is surgically challenging but excellent results are achievable. It is a relatively safe and effective means of treating airway obstruction and feeding difficulty in patients, especially infants with Pierre Robin sequence. Traditionally, tracheostomy has been performed for the most severe or refractory cases of upper airway obstruction. However, given significant morbidity, cost, and caregiver burden associated with long-term tracheostomy, mandibular distraction osteogenesis is becoming increasingly used as the primary treatment for severe airway obstruction caused by micrognathia.

40.8 Highlights

a. Micrognathia
   - Pierre Robin sequence.
   - Airway obstruction.
b. Mandibular distraction osteogenesis
   - History of distraction osteogenesis.
   - Mandibular distraction osteogenesis.
c. Preoperative evaluation
   - Neonates.
   - Outcomes.
   - Preop tests.
   - Tongue lip adhesion.
   - Internal vs. external distraction.
d. Surgical technique
   - Equipment.
   - Incision.
   - Exposure.
   - Osteotomy designs.
   - Distractor placement.
e. Postoperative care
   - Distraction rates and latency.
   - Wound care.
   - Goal for final incisor position.
f. Complications
   - Tooth loss.
   - Inferior alveolar nerve injury.
   - Facial nerve injury, mandibular branch.

References

[1] Robin P. Glossoptosis due to atresia and hypotrophy of the mandible. Am J Dis Child 1934;48(3):541–547
[2] Forrest H, Graham AG. The Pierre Robin syndrome. Scott Med J 1963;8:16–24
[3] Bütow KW, Morkel JA, Naidoo S, Zwahlen RA. Pierre Robin sequence: subdivision, data, theories, and treatment. Part 2: syndromic and nonsyndromic Pierre Robin sequence. Ann Maxillofac Surg 2016;6(1):35–37
[4] Hartnick CJ, Bissell C, Parsons SK. The impact of pediatric tracheotomy on parental caregiver burden and health status. Arch Otolaryngol Head Neck Surg 2003;129(10):1065–1069
[5] Gianoli GJ, Miller RH, Guarisco JL. Tracheotomy in the first year of life. Ann Otol Rhinol Laryngol 1990;99(11):896–901
[6] Natu SS, Ali I, Alam S, Giri KY, Agarwal A, Kulkarni VA. The biology of distraction osteogenesis for correction of mandibular and craniomaxillofacial defects: a review. Dent Res J (Isfahan) 2014;11(1):16–26
[7] Karp NS, Thorne CH, McCarthy JG, Sissons HA. Bone lengthening in the craniofacial skeleton. Ann Plast Surg 1990;24(3):231–237
[8] McCarthy JG, Schreiber J, Karp N, Thorne CH, Grayson BH. Lengthening the human mandible by gradual distraction. Plast Reconstr Surg 1992;89(1):1–8, discussion 9–10
[9] Verlinden CR, van de Vijfeijken SE, Jansma EP, Becking AG, Swennen GR. Complications of mandibular distraction osteogenesis for congenital deformities: a systematic review of the literature and proposal of a new classification for complications. Int J Oral Maxillofac Surg 2015;44(1):37–43
[10] Scott AR, Tibesar RJ, Lander TA, Sampson DE, Sidman JD. Mandibular distraction osteogenesis in infants younger than 3 months. Arch Facial Plast Surg 2011;13(3):173–179
[11] Tibesar RJ, Scott AR, McNamara C, Sampson D, Lander TA, Sidman JD. Distraction osteogenesis of the mandible for airway obstruction in children: long-term results. Otolaryngol Head Neck Surg 2010;143(1):90–96
[12] Lam DJ, Tabangin ME, Shikary TA, et al. Outcomes of mandibular distraction osteogenesis in the treatment of severe micrognathia. JAMA Otolaryngol Head Neck Surg 2014;140(4):338–345
[13] Scott AR, Tibesar RJ, Sidman JD. Pierre Robin sequence: evaluation, management, indications for surgery, and pitfalls. Otolaryngol Clin North Am 2012;45(3):695–710, ix
[14] Hong P, Bezuhly M. Mandibular distraction osteogenesis in the micrognathic neonate: a review for neonatologists and pediatricians. Pediatr Neonatol 2013;54(3):153–160
[15] Ow AT, Cheung LK. Meta-analysis of mandibular distraction osteogenesis: clinical applications and functional outcomes. Plast Reconstr Surg 2008;121(3):54e–69e

Suggested Readings

Runyan CM, Uribe-Rivera A, Karlea A, et al. Cost analysis of mandibular distraction versus tracheostomy in neonates with Pierre Robin sequence. Otolaryngol Head Neck Surg 2014;151(5):811–818 10.1177/0194599814542759
Saman M, Abramowitz JM, Buchbinder D. Mandibular osteotomies and distraction osteogenesis: evolution and current advances. JAMA Facial Plast Surg 2013;15(3):167–173– [Peer Reviewed Journal]

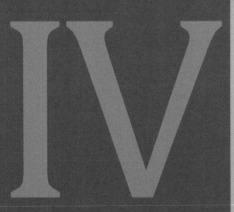

41 Surgery for Velopharyngeal Insufficiency

Gadi Fishman

Summary

There is not one single surgical technique to correct velo-pharyngeal insufficiency. The surgical approach typically depends on the pattern of the vellopharyngeal closure, its location and size, as well as on the surgeon's surgical experience. The goal is to achieve the best possible outcome without causing upper airway obstruction and sleep apnea.

Keywords: Velopharyngeal insufficiency, pharyngeal flap, sphincter pharyngoplasty, Furlow palatoplasty

41.1 Introduction

Attaining optimal outcomes and low long-term morbidity in surgical intervention for velopharyngeal insufficiency (VPI), requires the surgeon's ability to tailor the surgical correction to the specific defect of the child. Various surgical procedures are performed depending on the pathology contributing to VPI. As the pattern of VPI closure impact the surgical type of correction that is planned, recognition of basic closure patterns of the velo-pharynx is essential.[1]

41.2 Patterns of Velopharyngeal Closure

- Coronal closure is the most common closure pattern, and is present in 55% of patients with normal velar function. The major contribution to closure is from the soft palate as it contacts a broad area of the posterior pharyngeal wall. Little medial motion of the lateral pharyngeal walls occurs. A coronal closure pattern is often present with an enlarged adenoid pad.
- Circular closure is present in approximately 20% of individuals with normal closure. It involves contributions from both the soft palate and the lateral pharyngeal walls. This results in a closure that resembles a circle getting smaller.
- Circular closure with the Passavant ridge occurs in 15% to 20% of the population. It is a circular pattern that involves anterior motion of the posterior pharyngeal wall (known as Passavant ridge).
- Sagittal closure is the least common pattern, and is present in 10% to 15% of people. Here, palatal elevation is minimal. The main contribution is from medial motion of the lateral pharyngeal walls. This is the pattern seen most commonly in patients with persistent velopharyngeal dysfunction (VPD) after repair of a cleft palate. See ▶ Fig. 41.1.

41.3 Velopharyngeal Assessment

The assessment of velopharyngeal function is best performed in the setting of a multispecialty team evaluation composed of a speech-language pathologist (SLP), otolaryngologist, prosthodontist, and plastic surgeon. Multiple modalities should be utilized to perform a complete evaluation of the patient. After a thorough review of the patient's history, the standard workup involves perceptual speech evaluation, followed by video nasoendoscopy (VNE) and multiview speech videofluoroscopy (SVF).[3,4]

There is considerable variation in the utilization of imaging studies to guide treatment of VPD. Different institutions will preferentially utilize VNE or SVF or other novel imaging modalities; other institutions use both studies for comprehensive evaluation. Lipira et al[5] evaluated the relative benefits of videofluoroscopy versus nasoendoscopy and concluded that both studies were best used in tandem to optimally evaluate patients with VPD.

41.4 Surgical Treatment Options

Patients with a history of previously repaired cleft palate and anatomic findings of VPD are frequently candidates for surgical intervention. Once the decision for surgery has been established, a choice must be made as to which intervention would best fit the needs of the patient. The two most commonly discussed procedures for correction of VPD remain the posterior pharyngeal flap and the sphincter pharyngoplasty. Both procedures aim to decrease the size of the residual velopharyngeal port.

More recently, procedures designed to improve palatal closure have gained increasing popularity. The Furlow palatoplasty and palatal re-repair are two techniques performed to either lengthen the palate or otherwise tighten the levator sling. Some authors have also reported a success with posterior pharyngeal wall augmentation procedures.

Surgical procedures should be tailored to the patient's specific anatomy, as visualized on VNE and SVF studies. Based upon these studies, a pattern of closure can be determined as well as the size of the defect.

Pharyngeal flaps are designed to bring tissue into the central portion of the velopharynx. Therefore, they are best utilized to correct central gaps (sagittal or circular patterns of closure) where good lateral pharyngeal wall motion is visualized on VNE or SVF in the AP dimension.[6] Sphincter pharyngoplasty, on the other hand, brings in tissue laterally toward the center and appears most useful for lateral defects (coronal and bowtie patterns), especially when lateral wall motion is poor. Furlow

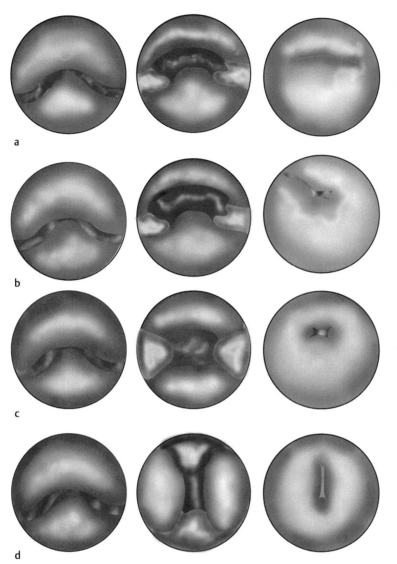

Fig. 41.1 The velopharyngeal valve as seen on nasopharyngoscopy at rest and during partial and complete closure. The posterior pharyngeal wall and adenoid tissue are at the top of the circle and the soft palate is at the bottom. **(a)** Coronal pattern, **(b)** circular pattern, **(c)** circular pattern with Passavant ridge, and **(d)** sagittal pattern.[2]

palatoplasty has shown success primarily in smaller central gaps, especially in circumstances where evidence exists of diastasis of the levator muscle sling (i.e., midline notch on VNE). Posterior pharyngeal augmentation procedures are similarly utilized for very small residual defects. Little consensus exists in regards to the treatment of large "black hole" deformities, which tend to have the poorest results when reconstruction is attempted. Some have noted success with sphincter pharyngoplasty alone[7] or with wide, nearly obstructing pharyngeal flaps. Others have suggested that results are best when palatal lengthening procedures such as Furlow palatoplasty are performed in conjunction with a sphincter pharyngoplasty.[8]

Despite the theories and preferences for reconstruction that have been noted above, little evidence exists suggesting whether pharyngeal flap or sphincter pharyngoplasty is superior to the other. Rather, both procedures appear to have equivalent efficacy when performed by experienced surgeons.[9,10]

41.5 Surgical Procedures

41.5.1 Superiorly Based Pharyngeal Flap

Indications

Central gaps (sagittal or circular patterns of closure) with good lateral pharyngeal wall motion.

Preparation and Anesthetic Considerations

- Adenotonsillar hyperplasia may require adenotonsillectomy before flapplacement to prevent postoperative obstructive apnea. A 4- to 6-week interval for healing should elapse between procedures.
- General endotracheal anesthesia.

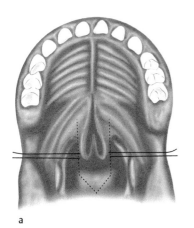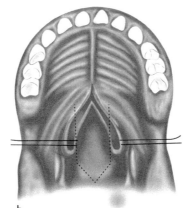

a   b

Fig. 41.2 (a, b) Splitting the soft palate and placing traction sutures.

- There is a high prevalence of velo-cardio-facial syndrome (chromosomal microdeletion 22q11.2) in VPI patients. Phenotypic expression includes VPI, submucous cleft palate, learning disabilities, cardiac anomalies, retrognathia, malar flattening, pharyngeal hypotonia, slender hands and fingers, small stature, and medialized carotid arteries.[11] Cardiac status should be investigated.
- Antibiotic prophylaxis is often necessary to prevent subacute bacterial endocarditis.
- The patient is positioned on a shoulder roll to maintain hyperextension of the neck.

Procedure

- A mouth gag is inserted, and the patient is placed into suspension.
- The posterior pharyngeal wall is visualized and palpated to identify any significant vessels in the operative field. The internal carotid arteries may be medialized in velo-cardio-facial syndrome patients. These vessels will be deep to the prevertebral fascia and not interfere with the operation, but increased care in raising the flap is necessary.
- Proposed posterior pharyngeal wall incision lines as well as the soft palate are infiltrated with 1% lidocaine with 1:100,000 units of epinephrine to affect vasoconstriction and ease the raising of the flap.
- Nasal stents are placed transnasally into the hypopharynx to size the lateral ports. Smaller endotracheal tubes, 3.5, are used for children, and 4.0 endotracheal tubes are used for adolescents.
- A midline vertical incision is made to split the soft palate from the edge of the uvula to a point close to the junction of the hard palate. This is an important step in order to expose the posterior nasopharyngeal wall and enable measuring the length of the flap and raising it high enough for optimal closure of the velopharynx. Traction sutures placed on the free edge of the soft palate can improve visualization (▶Fig. 41.2).

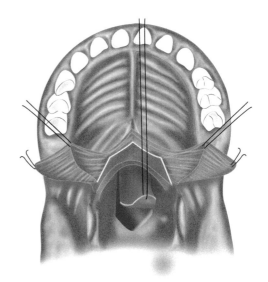

Fig. 41.3 Elevation of superiorly based pharyngeal flap.

- The standard flap width should not be larger than the distance between the nasal stents.
- The length of the flap can be checked by measuring the distance from the posterior pharyngeal wall to the free margin of the soft palate, and then measuring down from the level of velopharyngeal closure.
- The superiorly based pharyngeal flap is elevated by incising down to the prevertebral fascia. This fascial layer is white in color, and the plane will be essentially avascular.
- Flap elevation needs to be high into the nasopharynx, to the natural level of velopharyngeal closure. Failure to raise the flap high enough will result in an inferior tethering of the free edge of the soft palate, further compromising velopharyngeal function. This will also cause the flap to be located in a position precluding its participation in velopharyngeal closure (▶Fig. 41.3).

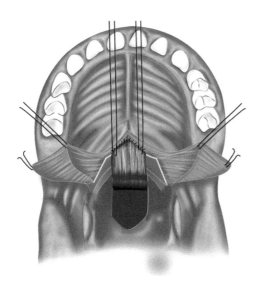

Fig. 41.4 Suturing the oral mucosa and muscle of the flap to the anterior nasopharyngeal mucosa of the soft palate.

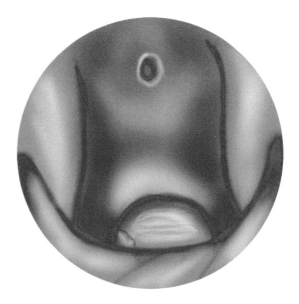

Fig. 41.6 High location of the pharyngeal flap in the nasopharynx.

Fig. 41.5 (a, b) Suturing the donor site.

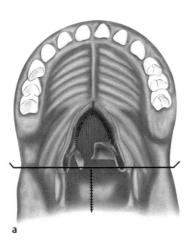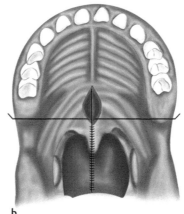

a   b

- 4–0 Vicryl sutures are used to sew the oral mucosa and muscle of the flap to the anterior nasopharyngeal mucosa of the soft palate (▶Fig. 41.4).
- The donor site is closed with 3–0 Vicryl suture (▶Fig. 41.5).
- Overzealous closure of the donor site superiorly can lead to nasopharyngeal stenosis.
- A mirror is used to evaluate the lateral ports.
- At the conclusion of the procedure, the pharyngeal flap should not be visible in the oropharynx; it must be high in the nasopharynx (▶Fig. 41.6).
- The palate is closed in three layers. Meticulous technique is necessary to minimize fistula formation.
- The nasal stents are positioned with their distal end in the mid-oropharynx, and are then secured with tape to the nose.

Postoperative Care

The patient is admitted for postoperative observation.
- Perioperative oral antibiotics are prescribed for 1 week.
- The nasal stents are irrigated with normal saline and suctioned as necessary.
- The nasal stents are removed the following morning if no airway obstruction occurred overnight.
- The patient is observed in the hospital without the nasal stents for an additional night.
- Patients return for a postoperative check at 3 weeks.
- Speech therapy begins 1 month postoperatively.
- A repeat office evaluation for objective resonance testing occurs at 3 months. Repeat nasopharyngoscopy is performed if continued hypernasality or nasal emission is detected.

Complications

- Obstructive sleep apnea (OSA): Adenotonsillar hyperplasia must be addressed prior to performing a pharyngeal flap to prevent OSA. Snoring is expected, but obstructive events must be treated. Continuous positive airway pressure (CPAP) can alleviate the problem until postoperative edema subsides.
- Stenosis or too small lateral ports may cause prolonged airway obstruction. Revision surgery and sometimes cutting and separating the flap is necessary.
- Narrowing of the flap may cause inadequate obturation of the velopharyngeal defect. In some patients, the secondary intention healing of the raw surface of the flap causes the flap to narrow. If a wide flap is determined to be necessary preoperatively, an additional step of lining the flap with mucosal flaps, based on the free margin of the soft palate, minimizes the raw surface of the flap left to granulate, and can more predictably maintain the width of the flap (▶ Fig. 41.3).

41.5.2 Sphincter Pharyngoplasty

Indications

Central gaps (coronal pattern of closure) with poor or absent lateral pharyngeal wall motion.

Preparation and Anesthetic Considerations

- General endotracheal anesthesia.

- Cardiac evaluation should be performed since there is a high prevalence of VCF syndrome in these patients.
- Antibiotic prophylaxis is often necessary to prevent subacute bacterial endocarditis.
- The patient is positioned on a shoulder roll to maintain hyperextension of the neck.

Procedure

- A mouth gag is inserted, and the patient is placed into suspension. The posterior pharyngeal wall is visualized and palpated to identify any significant vessels in the operative field.
- Catheters are placed transnasally and brought out through the mouth to symmetrically retract the soft palate.
- Proposed incision lines are infiltrated with 1% lidocaine with 1:100,000 units epinephrine to affect vasoconstriction. The incisions entail rectangular flaps encompassing each posterior tonsillar pillar. A horizontal incision is made connecting the medial limbs of the incisions at the level of velopharyngeal closure (▶ Fig. 41.7).
- The soft palate may be split in the midline to facilitate visualization within the nasopharynx.
- The mucosa is incised to the prevertebral fascia on the medial incisions. The palatopharyngeus muscle is incorporated into the flap. Lateral dissection is limited in the area of the tonsil (▶ Fig. 41.8).

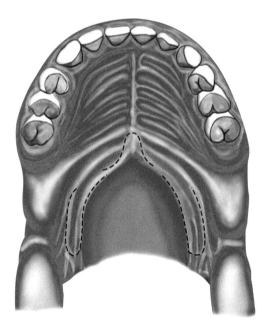

Fig. 41.7 Incision lines for sphincter pharyngoplasty.

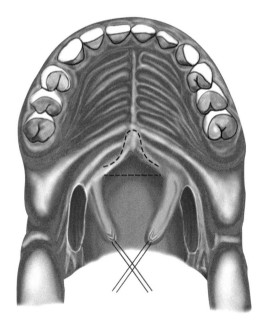

Fig. 41.8 Incorporating the palatopharyngeus muscle into the flap.

- After making the transverse incision at the level of velopharyngeal closure, the surrounding tissue is elevated superiorly to create a bed within which the flaps may be inset. Inferior dissection is avoided to prevent insetting the flaps below the level of velopharyngeal closure.
- The base of each flap is undermined superiorly and laterally to effectively narrow the lateral velopharyngeal walls when the flaps are rotated medially.
- The inferior edge of each flap is medially rotated and sewn to the lateral limit of the recipient horizontal incision of the opposite side. One flap will reside above the other (▶Fig. 41.9).
- The donor sites are closed with interrupted 3–0 Vicryl sutures.
- If the palate was divided for improved exposure, it is closed in three layers. Meticulous technique is necessary to minimize fistula formation.

Postoperative Care

- Perioperative oral antibiotics are prescribed for 1 week.
- Postoperative neck pain is expected as the prevertebral fascia has been irritated.
- Patients return for a postoperative check at 3 weeks.
- Speech therapy begins 1 month postoperatively.
- A repeat office evaluation for objective resonance testing occurs at 3 months. Repeat nasopharyngoscopy is performed if continued hypernasality or nasal emission is detected.

Complications

- Nasopharyngeal stenosis may occur and cause airway obstruction.
- VPI may persist if the sphincteroplasty is not positioned at the level of velopharyngeal closure or if inadequate narrowing of the lateral nasopharynx was achieved.

41.5.3 Posterior Pharyngeal Wall Augmentation

Biocompatible or homologous tissues are used to augment the posterior pharyngeal wall and to bring this structure closer to the velum during maximal closure of the velum, thereby aiding in speech and preventing escape of air and sound energy. Since Passavant described an unsuccessful attempt to do so utilizing adjacent soft tissues in 1879,[12] many products have been tried in an attempt to optimize speech function. This has included petroleum jelly, paraffin, cartilage, fat and/or fascia, silastic, Teflon, and Proplast.[13-23]

Indications

- Small gaps (less than 4 mm) along the posterior pharyngeal wall.
- Touch closure of the velopharyngeal mechanism that cannot withstand increased intraoral pressure.

Preparation and Anesthetic Considerations

- General endotracheal anesthesia is required.
- Cardiac evaluation should be performed since there is a high prevalence of VCF syndrome in these patients.
- Antibiotic prophylaxis is often necessary to prevent subacute bacterial endocarditis.
- Medical grade Teflon carries the risk of infection, granuloma formation, inferior displacement over time,[24] or theoretically, embolization.[25]
- Commercially available collagen products are available from manufacturers, but little experience exists concerning their use in the posterior pharyngeal wall.
- Homologous fat may be injected and can be harvested from the abdomen or buttock. The amount of absorption and tissue viability vary, and the need for repeat procedures should be discussed with patients and families.
- The patient is positioned on a shoulder roll to maintain hyperextension of the neck.

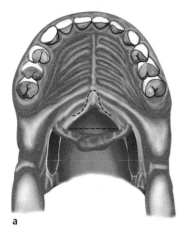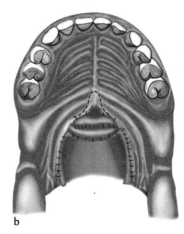

a b

Fig. 41.9 (a, b) Rotation and suturing of sphincter flaps.

Procedure

- A mouth gag is inserted, and the patient is placed into suspension.
- The posterior pharyngeal wall is visualized and palpated to identify any significant vessels in the operative field. The internal carotid arteries may be medialized in velo-cardio-facial syndrome patients.
- Catheters are placed transnasally and brought out through the mouth to retract the soft palate symmetrically.
- A Bruening syringe is loaded with Teflon or fat; a spinal needle is used to inject collagen. The needle is inserted into the exact site of deficiency and introduced to the level of the prevertebral fascia. The fascia offers increased resistance compared to the overlying mucosa and muscle. A single-needle puncture per injection site is important to minimize the amount of material escaping during the injection.
- A metal tongue blade is pushed against the posterior pharyngeal wall immediately inferior to the injection site. This creates a broad barrier to displacement of the injected material in an inferior direction.
- The augmentation material is slowly injected onto the prevertebral fascia. Generally, 1 to 2 cc of material are injected at each site. Over correction is necessary.
- After the material has been deposited, the needle should not be removed for an additional 1 minute to allow the pressure in the tissues to disperse, thus minimizing the amount of material expelled through the injection puncture site.
- Additional sites are injected as required. Central defects will require two injections, one on either side of the median raphe that prevents the material from crossing the midline.

Postoperative Care

- Perioperative oral antibiotics are prescribed for 1 week.
- Postoperative neck pain is expected because the prevertebral fascia has been irritated.
- Patients return for a postoperative check at 3 weeks.
- Speech therapy begins 1 month postoperatively.
- A repeat office evaluation for objective resonance testing occurs at 3 months. Repeat nasopharyngoscopy is performed if continued hypernasality or nasal emission is detected.

Complications

- VPI may persist if the injection is not positioned at the level of velopharyngeal closure.
- VPI may re-develop if resorption of the injected material re-opens an area for nasal escape.

41.5.4 Furlow Palatoplasty

The Furlow double-opposing Z-plasty repair of the palate was originally proposed as a surgical technique for primary cleft palate repair.[26] It offers both considerable palatal lengthening and correction of the abnormal anterior direction and insertion of the levator veli palatini muscles by repositioning the fibers into a transverse orientation. It is thought that lengthening the palate may allow it to more effectively span and occlude the velopharyngeal gap during speech production.

In general, the Furlow technique is preferred in palates that are kinetic, with evidence of anterior orientation of the levator muscle fibers. It offers a lower risk of obstructive sleep apnea than either the pharyngeal flap or sphincter pharyngoplasty, and has a low rate of oronasal fistulas.

Indications

- Small gaps (less than 1 cm) with good palatal movement.

Preparation and Anesthetic Considerations

- General endotracheal anesthesia.
- Cardiac evaluation should be performed since there is a high prevalence of VCF syndrome in these patients.
- Antibiotic prophylaxis is often necessary to prevent subacute bacterial endocarditis.
- The patient is positioned on a shoulder roll to maintain hyperextension of the neck.

Procedure

- A mouth gag is inserted, and the patient is placed into suspension.
- The palate is visualized and palpated to identify the hamuli prior to the injection of local anesthetic.
- The soft palate is then divided at the midline (▶ Fig. 41.10a), typically along a previous scar from initial cleft repair, up to the region of the hard/soft palate junction.
- Oral Z-plasty incisions are then designed from the hamuli, with the posteriorly-based musculomucosal flap drawn to the posterior edge of the hard palate and the anteriorly-based mucosal flap extending posteriorly toward the divided uvula (▶ Fig. 41.10b).
- The levator muscle is then carefully released from the posterior edge of the hard palate and separated from the nasal mucosa. During this process, the tensor veli palatine attachments are automatically divided and separated from the levator.
- After myomucosal flap elevation, the nasal mucosal flap is then elevated on the ipsilateral side. This limb

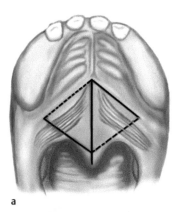 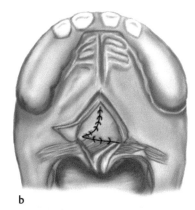 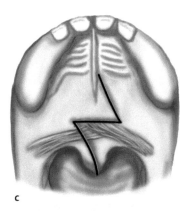

a   b   c

Fig. 41.10 Furlow palatoplasty stages: **(a)** midline division of the soft palate, **(b)** oral and nasal Z-plasty incisions, **(c)** transposition and suturing of oral and nasal Z-plasty flaps.

is incised from the base of the uvula to the lateral edge of the exposed levator (▶Fig. 41.10b).

- Attention is turned to the opposite side, where an oral mucosal flap is elevated from the base of the uvula to the hamulus, using care to avoid any elevation of muscle. Following this, the final nasal myomucosal flap is developed. The muscle is carefully released from the hard palate and the nasal mucosa is divided, taking care to leave a small cuff of mucosa along the hard palate edge to suture to during closure. Once the dissection has been completed, the nasal Z-plasty flaps are transposed and sutured. The oral flaps are similarly transposed (▶Fig. 41.10c). In the process, the levator musculature is mobilized from an oblique orientation to a transverse dimension, with significant overlap of the muscle occurring on the oral and nasal layers.

Postoperative Care

- Perioperative oral antibiotics are prescribed for 1 week.
- Patients return for a postoperative check at 3 weeks.
- Speech therapy begins 1 month postoperatively.
- A repeat office evaluation for objective resonance testing occurs at 3 months. Repeat nasopharyngoscopy is performed if continued hypernasality or nasal emission is detected.

Complications

- Oro-nasal fistula.
- VPI persistence.

41.6 Highlights

a. Indications
   - Chronic nasal regurgitation of food and/or liquids which are refractory to conservative treatment accompanied by VPI findings on nasoendoscopy.

   - Significant speech disturbance accompanied by hypernasality and VPI findings on nasoendoscopy.
b. Contraindications
   - Neurological and other general severe comorbidities.
c. Complications
   - Obstructive sleep apnea.
   - Narrowing of the flap may cause inadequate obturation of the velopharyngeal defect.
   - Oro-nasal fistula.
   - VPI persistence.
d. Special preoperative considerations
   - General endotracheal anesthesia.
   - Adenotonsillar hyperplasia may require adenotonsillectomy before flap placement to prevent postoperative obstructive apnea. A 4- to 6-week interval for healing should elapse between procedures.
   - There is a high prevalence of velo-cardio-facial syndrome (chromosomal microdeletion 22q11.2) in VPI patients. Cardiac status should be investigated.
   - Antibiotic prophylaxis is often necessary to prevent subacute bacterial endocarditis.
e. Special intraoperative considerations
   - The patient is positioned on a shoulder roll to maintain hyperextension of the neck.
   - The posterior pharyngeal wall is visualized and palpated to identify any significant vessels.
   - Nasal stents are placed transnasally into the hypopharynx to size the lateral ports.
f. Special postoperative considerations
   - The patient is admitted for postoperative observation.
   - Perioperative oral antibiotics are prescribed for 1 week.
   - The nasal stents are irrigated with normal saline and suctioned as necessary.
   - The nasal stents are removed the following morning if no airway obstruction occurred overnight.

- The patient is observed in the hospital without the nasal stents for an additional night.
- Patients return for a postoperative check at 3 weeks.
- Speech therapy begins 1 month postoperatively.
- A repeat office evaluation for objective resonance testing occurs at 3 months.
- Repeat nasopharyngoscopy is performed if continued hypernasality or nasal emission is detected.

References

[1] Bluestone CD, Simons J. Bluestone and Stool's pediatric otolaryngology. 5th ed. Volume 2: 1968

[2] Witzel MA, Posnick JC. Patterns and location of velopharyngeal valving problems: atypical findings on video nasopharyngoscopy. Cleft Palate J 1989;26(1):63–67

[3] Havstam C, Lohmander A, Persson C, Dotevall H, Lith A, Lilja J. Evaluation of VPI-assessment with videofluoroscopy and nasoendoscopy. Br J Plast Surg 2005;58(7):922–931

[4] Sommerlad BC. Evaluation of VPI-assessment with videofluoroscopy and nasoendoscopy. Br J Plast Surg 2005;58(7):932–933

[5] Lipira AB, Grames LM, Molter D, Govier D, Kane AA, Woo AS. Videofluoroscopic and nasendoscopic correlates of speech in velopharyngeal dysfunction. Cleft Palate Craniofac J 2011; 48(5):550–560

[6] Argamaso RV, Shprintzen RJ, Strauch B, et al. The role of lateral pharyngeal wall movement in pharyngeal flap surgery. Plast Reconstr Surg 1980;66(2):214–219

[7] Marsh JL. The evaluation and management of velopharyngeal dysfunction. Clin Plast Surg 2004;31(2):261–269

[8] Gosain AK, Arneja JS. Management of the black hole in velopharyngeal incompetence: combined use of a Furlow palatoplasty and sphincter pharyngoplasty. Plast Reconstr Surg 2007; 119(5):1538–1545

[9] Ysunza A, Pamplona C, Ramírez E, Molina F, Mendoza M, Silva A. Velopharyngeal surgery: a prospective randomized study of pharyngeal flaps and sphincter pharyngoplasties. Plast Reconstr Surg 2002;110(6):1401–1407

[10] Abyholm F, D'Antonio L, Davidson Ward SL, et al; VPI Surgical Group. Pharyngeal flap and sphincterplasty for velopharyngeal insufficiency have equal outcome at 1 year postoperatively: results of a randomized trial. Cleft Palate Craniofac J 2005;42(5):501–511

[11] Shprintzen RJ, Goldberg RB, Lewin ML, et al. A new syndrome involving cleft palate, cardiac anomalies, typical facies, and learning disabilities: velo-cardio-facial syndrome. Cleft Palate J 1978;15(1):56–62

[12] Passavant G. Über die Verbesserung der Sprache nach der Uranoplastik. Deutch Geselschaft Chirurgie. 1879;23:771–780

[13] Gersuny R. Über eine subcutane Prosthese. Zeitschrift fur Heilkunde. 1900;21:199–204

[14] Eckstein H. Hartparaffininjecktionen in der hintere Rachenwand bei angeborenen und etwarbenen Gaumendefekten. Deutsch med. Wochenschrift. 1922;1:1186–1187

[15] Hollweg E, Perthes G. Tübingen: Pietzcker. Beitrag zur Behandlung von Gaumenspalten; 1912

[16] Bentley FH, Watkins I. Speech after repair of cleft palate. Lancet 1947;2(6485):862–865

[17] Denny AD, Marks SM, Oliff-Carneol S. Correction of velopharyngeal insufficiency by pharyngeal augmentation using autologous cartilage: a preliminary report. Cleft Palate Craniofac J 1993;30(1):46–54

[18] Von Gaza WV. Transplanting of free fatty tissue in the retropharyngeal area in cases of cleft palate. Paper presented at German Surgical Society, April 9, 1926; Berlin, Germany

[19] Halle H. Gaumennaht und gaumenplastik. Ztschr Hals, Nasen-U. Ohrenheilk. 1925;12:377–389

[20] Blocksma R. Correction of velopharyngeal insufficiency by Silastic pharyngeal implant. Plast Reconstr Surg 1963;31:268–274

[21] Blocksma R, Braley S. The silicones in plastic surgery. Plast Reconstr Surg 1965;35:366–370

[22] Lewy R, Cole R, Wepman J. Teflon injection in the correction of velopharyngeal insufficiency. Ann Otol Rhinol Laryngol 1965;74(3):874–879

[23] Wolford LM, Oelschlaeger M, Deal R. Proplast as a pharyngeal wall implant to correct velopharyngeal insufficiency Cleft Palate J 1989;262:119–126

[24] Smith JK, McCabe BF. Teflon injection in the nasopharynx to improve velopharyngeal closure. Ann Otol Rhinol Laryngol 1977;86 (4 Pt 1):559–563

[25] Borgatti R, Tettamanti A, Piccinelli P. Brain injury in a healthy child one year after periureteral injection of Teflon. Pediatrics 1996;98(2 Pt 1):290–291

[26] Furlow LT Jr. Cleft palate repair by double opposing Z-plasty. Plast Reconstr Surg 1986;78(6):724–738

42 Pediatric Tracheostomy

Blake Smith, Paul Krakovitz

Summary

Pediatric tracheostomy persists as a necessary armament of the airway surgeon despite evolving indications over the past several decades. The primary indications for tracheostomy include airway obstruction, pulmonary toilet, and prolonged need for assisted ventilation. Knowledge of relevant variants between pediatric and adult laryngotracheal anatomy is essential. Multiple techniques for tracheostomy exist, each aimed toward minimization of complication. In patients with anticipated long-term need for tracheostomy or low likelihood of decannulation, a formalized stoma or starplasty tracheostomy should be considered. Early complications of tracheostomy include tube obstruction, air leak, hemorrhage, accidental decannulation, and infection. Late complications include granulomata, tube obstruction, accidental decannulation, tracheal erosion, and airway stenosis or collapse. Tracheostomy-related mortality in pediatric patients occurs at a reported rate of approximately 3%, most commonly from accidental decannulation. The risk of complication from accidental decannulation can be minimized by formalization of the tracheostoma. Successful home care of a child with a tracheostomy depends on careful education of the caregivers prior to discharge on tracheostomy management. In addition, the availability of necessary medical supplies and skilled caregivers is essential. Following tracheostomy, continued airway surveillance in a multi-disciplinary setting facilitates optimal care with regard to daily management, long-term strategic planning for decannulation, and the patient's global health needs. Ten to 30% of patients in whom decannulation is achieved will have persistence of a tracheocutaneous fistula which may require surgical repair.

Keywords: Pediatric tracheostomy, starplasty, starplasty tracheostomy, decannulation, accidental decannulation, tracheocutaneous fistula

42.1 Introduction

When considering pediatric tracheostomy, one must mind the mantra that children are not just small adults. Children undergoing tracheostomy have a higher rate of morbidity than their adult counterparts, and differences in anatomy, pathophysiology, and perioperative management complicate surgical decision-making. Effective interdisciplinary and parental communications are essential to patient well-being. In a field with ever-improving medicine, evolving indications, and growing patients, a thoughtful and individualized approach to airway management is essential.

42.2 Indications

The primary indications for pediatric tracheostomy are airway obstruction, pulmonary toilet, and prolonged need for assisted ventilation. The etiology of airway obstruction can be congenital, acquired, or infectious in nature. With the widespread implementation of vaccination for *Haemophilus infuenzae* and *Corynebacterium diphtheriae* and greater facility with endotracheal intubation, there has been a significant decrease in the number of tracheostomies performed for upper airway infections including epiglottitis, laryngotracheobronchitis, and diphtheria over the last 50 years.[1-3]

Alternatively, increased survival of neonates and children with complex medical needs has led to a commiserate uptrend in the need for tracheostomy in the setting of chronic medical conditions and long-term ventilatory requirement.[1-3] Children with neurologic or neuromuscular disorders suffering from hypotonia or inability to manage secretions may require long-term tracheostomy for pulmonary toilet if not obstruction. Similarly, cardiopulmonary disorders including bronchopulmonary dysplasia, respiratory distress syndrome (RDS), and cardiomyopathy may necessitate prolonged ventilator support for which tracheostomy would be indicated.

Currently, established guidelines do not exist regarding the timing of tracheostomy in the intubated pediatric patient. While the pliability of the pediatric airway accommodates longer intubation than an adult, close attention to endotracheal tube selection, cuff pressure, and positioning is required to prevent complications including laryngeal edema, granulation, mucosal ischemia, ulceration, and airway stenosis. The authors recommend evaluation for tracheostomy candidacy following 2 weeks of intubation or more than two unsuccessful attempts at extubation; however, more prolonged intubation, particularly in the neonatal population, may be necessary.

42.3 Surgical Technique

42.3.1 Anatomy

The cartilages of the pediatric laryngotracheal complex are smaller and more pliable than those of their adult counterparts. Their compressibility makes palpation more difficult and increases risk of injury to adjacent structures in comparison to adults. Furthermore, the pediatric larynx is positioned more superiorly in the neck and is often shielded by the hyoid cartilage. The cricoid cartilage is the most prominent structure on palpation and the narrowest point of the airway lumen. It should be noted that due to the small caliber of the pediatric airway, mucosal edema alone can cause significant obstruction; trauma to the airway mucosa should be minimized during all airway procedures.

42.3.2 Traditional Tracheostomy

The patient is positioned on the bed with a roll beneath the shoulders to facilitate extension of the neck, thus bringing the laryngotracheal complex more anterosuperior. In patients with cervical spinal instability or immobility, use of a neutral position may be necessary. A vertical or horizontal incision is marked between the sternal notch and the cricoid cartilage and infiltrated with 1:100,000 epinephrine (▶ Fig. 42.1).

Following skin incision, the subcutaneous tissues are divided with monopolar cautery and the anterior jugular veins are retracted laterally or ligated if needed. Dissection is carried onto the strap muscles, which are divided vertically in the midline raphe and also retracted laterally.

The cricoid cartilage and thyroid isthmus are then identified. The isthmus may be retracted superiorly in some patients, facilitating exposure of the trachea, or dissection may be carried out in the pretracheal plane to elevate the isthmus and divide it with monopolar cautery or suture ligation.

Meticulous hemostasis should be obtained prior to entering the airway, and FiO_2 should be reduced to a maximum of 30% in the event electrocautery is needed after incision of the airway. Monopolar cautery is contraindicated in the event that FiO_2 cannot be reduced below 30%.

Non-absorbable 3.0 stay sutures are then placed on either side of the planned midline vertical incision through two tracheal cartilages. Tracheal rings 2 and 3 or 3 and 4 may be used depending on exposure. These are labeled "left" and "right" accordingly. A vertical incision is then made in the midline anterior tracheal wall (▶ Fig. 42.2).

During incision, one should avoid rupture of the endotracheal tube balloon. Deflating the balloon prior to incision or advancement of the endotracheal tube past the fourth tracheal ring is the commonly used technique to avoid rupture. The endotracheal tube is then partially withdrawn under direct visualization via the newly created tracheotomy until it is superior to the incision. The tracheostomy tube is inserted, the ventilatory circuit is connected, and the return of end tidal CO_2 is confirmed. The endotracheal tube may then be completely withdrawn from the oral cavity.

The tracheostomy tube is secured using four-point fixation with non-absorbable sutures. The stay sutures are taped to the chest. The skin of the neck is then circumferentially dressed, the authors favor Allevyn or Duoderm, to prevent pressure injury and either a foam or a ribbon collar is placed around the neck, further securing the tracheostomy tube.

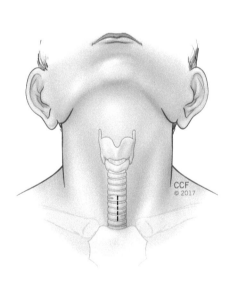

Fig. 42.1 A vertical incision marked between the cricoid cartilage and sternal notch. (Reproduced with permission, Cleveland Clinic Center for Medical Art & Photography © 2017. All Rights Reserved.)

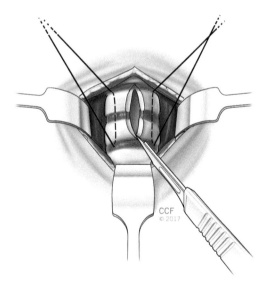

Fig. 42.2 Non-absorbable 3.0 stay sutures are then placed on either side of the planned midline vertical incision through two tracheal cartilages, and a vertical incision is then made in the midline anterior tracheal wall. (Reproduced with permission, Cleveland Clinic Center for Medical Art & Photography © 2017. All Rights Reserved.)

42.3.3 Bjork Flap

In older children with adequate tracheal width to accommodate an inferiorly based tracheal flap, the above technique may be modified. As an alternative to vertical tracheal incision, a horizontal incision may be made between rings 2 and 3 or 3 and 4. Using curved Mayo scissors, an inferiorly based flap is created with the cartilaginous ring below the tracheal incision. An absorbable suture is then thrown around the tracheal ring incorporated in the flap and through the inferior midline dermis and secured. This flap aims at safe replacement of a displaced cannula.[4] While commonly used in adult tracheostomy, few direct comparisons of tracheostomy techniques exist, and there is insufficient evidence to consider it standard of care in adult tracheostomy.[5]

42.3.4 Starplasty Tracheostomy

Starplasty tracheostomy, originally described by Koltai, is based on the geometry of three-dimensional Z-plasty. A cruciate or x-shaped skin incision is marked halfway between the sternal notch and cricoid cartilage and infiltrated with 1% lidocaine with 1:100,000 epinephrine (▶Fig. 42.3). Skin is incised and the resulting triangular skin flaps are undermined with scissors (▶Fig. 42.4). The subcutaneous fat overlying the strap musculature is excised (▶Fig. 42.5) and the strap muscles are vertically divided in the midline raphe and retracted. The thyroid isthmus, if encountered, is divided.

The pretracheal connective tissues are then dissected bluntly from the trachea and incision is made in the anterior tracheal wall vertically through four tracheal rings. A horizontal incision is then created in the middle of the vertical incision (two tracheal rings above and two below) forming a plus "+" shape (▶Fig. 42.6). The triangular skin flaps and triangular tracheal flaps

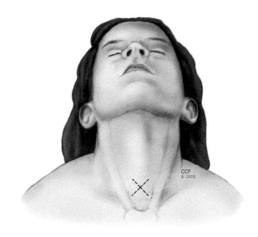

Fig. 42.3 A cruciate or x-shaped skin incision is marked halfway between the sternal notch and cricoid cartilage. (Reproduced with permission, Cleveland Clinic Center for Medical Art & Photography © 2017. All Rights Reserved.)

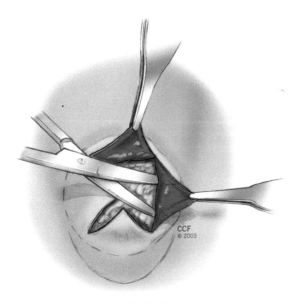

Fig. 42.4 Following skin the resulting triangular skin flaps are undermined with scissors. (Reproduced with permission, Cleveland Clinic Center for Medical Art & Photography © 2017. All Rights Reserved.)

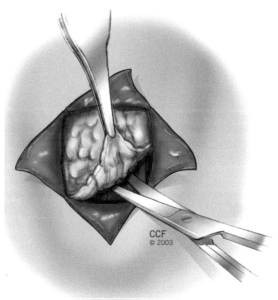

Fig. 42.5 The subcutaneous fat overlying the strap muscles is excised. (Reproduced with permission, Cleveland Clinic Center for Medical Art & Photography © 2017. All Rights Reserved.)

are then circumferentially interdigitated with mattressed 5.0 vicryl suture approximating first the tip of the upper tracheal flap to the trough of the upper skin flap (▸Fig. 42.7a), followed by the trough of the adjacent tracheal flap to the tip of the adjacent skin flap (▸Fig. 42.7b). The remaining flaps are then approximated in a similar manner until the entire stoma is formalized (▸Fig. 42.7c).

The authors favor starplasty tracheostomy in patients with an anticipated long-term need for cannulation or low likelihood of decannulation. This technique has been shown to reduce the rate of major complications including pneumothorax and more importantly death from accidental decannulation. However, this technique

results almost universally in tracheocutaneous fistula, should the patient no longer require tracheostomy.[6–8]

In the setting of a formalized stoma, some patients may be candidates for long-term tube-free tracheostomy. This technique was developed by Eliachar for adult patients with obstructive sleep apnea.[9] There are anecdotal uses of tube-free tracheostomy in children, but it remains far from standard of care. Starplasty tracheostomy with its high rate of permanent tracheocutaneous fistula has been used by the authors for tube-free tracheostomy in selected patients.

42.4 Intraoperative Complications

Intraoperative complications consist primarily of injury to adjacent structures and hemorrhage. Landmarks of the laryngotracheal complex must be carefully identified and frequently palpated throughout a midline dissection to avoid inadvertent injuries. High tracheostomy can result in airway stenosis.[10] Injuries to the laryngeal cartilages, recurrent laryngeal nerve, and esophagus have been reported.[3,11] Overdissection of the fascial planes or inadvertent injury of the pleural apex can result in pneumothorax. Avoidance of a potentially high-riding innominate artery and excellent hemostatic technique is essential. These complications can be generally avoided by meticulous surgical technique.

42.5 Postoperative Complications

Reported complications for pediatric tracheostomy range from 15 to 66%.[1,3,12–14] Complications can be generally divided into early complications, those occurring within 1 week of surgery, and late complications. Common early

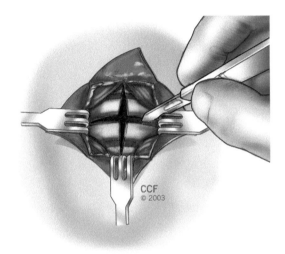

Fig. 42.6 A horizontal incision is then created in the middle of the vertical incision (two tracheal rings above and two below) forming a plus "+" shape. (Reproduced with permission, Cleveland Clinic Center for Medical Art & Photography © 2017. All Rights Reserved.)

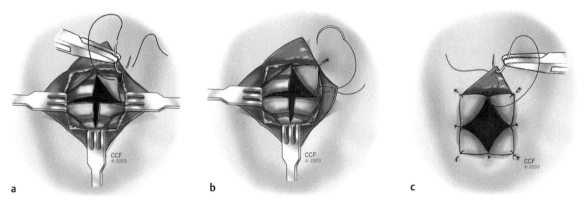

a   b   c

Fig. 42.7 The triangular skin flaps and triangular tracheal flaps are then circumferentially interdigitated with mattressed 5.0 vicryl suture approximating first the tip of the upper tracheal flap to the trough of the upper skin flap **(a)**, followed by the trough of the adjacent tracheal flap to the tip of the adjacent skin flap **(b)**. The remaining flaps are then approximated in a similar manner until the entire stoma is formalized **(c)**. (Reproduced with permission, Cleveland Clinic Center for Medical Art & Photography © 2017. All Rights Reserved.)

complications include tube obstruction, air leak, hemorrhage, accidental decannulation, and infection. Late complications include granulomata, tube obstruction, accidental decannulation, tracheal erosion, and airway stenosis or collapse. Wetmore et al reviewed the experience at The Children's Hospital of Pennsylvania and found that early complications occurred in 19% of patients and late complications in 57%.[12] Crysdale et al found an overall complication rate of 44%.[13]

42.6 Early Complications

42.6.1 Tube Obstruction

Tube obstruction is the most commonly reported early complication, but can occur at any time. Meticulous attention to suctioning, humidification, and saline lavage prevents the vast majority of mucous plugging and crusting; however, constant supervision is necessary and two caregivers must be facile with care and management of the tracheostomy in the event of an obstruction.

42.6.2 Air Leak

Pneumothorax, pneumomediastinum, and subcutaneous emphysema are inherent risks in the tracheostomy procedure which creates confluence between the facial planes of the neck and the airway. Dissection of air can occur into the surrounding soft tissues, mediastinum, and even into the pleural space. These are relatively common early complications when taken as a group, which occur in approximately 3 to 9% of cases.[3,13] Prevention of air leak involves minimizing dissection particularly in the pre and para-tracheal planes, atraumatic insertion of the cannula, and avoidance of excessive positive pressure ventilation. A routine chest X-ray should be obtained postoperatively.

42.6.3 Hemorrhage

Hemorrhage from the tracheostomy site in the immediate postoperative period is most often the result of inadequate intraoperative hemostasis or anticoagulation. In these instances, bleeding that is not self-limited may respond to packing with a hemostatic agent or a purse-string suture; however, significant or persistent bleeding would necessitate return to operating room for control.

After the immediate postoperative period, more common causes of bleeding include granulomata, tracheitis, and suction trauma. These can typically be managed conservatively. Granulomas easily accessible through the tracheostoma often respond to silver nitrate cautery or topical steroid creams. Suction trauma can be prevented by carefully measuring the length of the tracheostomy tube and appropriately restricting the depth of suction passage. Any bleeding from the tracheostomy

site warrants flexible endoscopy for further evaluation to exclude more sinister etiology such as a sentinel bleed from tracheoinnominate erosion.

42.6.4 Accidental Decannulation

Accidental decannulation particularly in the immediate postoperative period can have devastating results and is a significant contributor to tracheostomy-related mortality. Four-point fixation with suture, tracheostomy ties, and stay sutures or more formalized somatization forms the first line of defense against accidental decannulation and risk of subsequent replacement into a false passage that could preclude ventilation and potentially cause pneumomediastinum. Having a second tracheostomy tube of the same or smaller caliber and an obturator at the bedside is an absolutely necessary precaution. Variables that can influence successful replacement include depth of the surgical wound, adequacy of illumination, and caregiver experience.[6] Flexible endoscopy to ensure appropriate positioning after replacement is advisable.

As the stoma matures, risk from decannulation decreases. However, maintaining a secure neck tie and constant supervision remains essential to patient safety. Caregivers should have a replacement plan in the event of accidental decannulation after discharge from the hospital. Regardless of the setting, the tracheostomy tube should always be replaced in a calm, controlled manner under direct visualization.

42.6.5 Infection

Local infection requiring antibiotic therapy as a result of tracheostomy is uncommon and antibiotic prophylaxis is not generally recommended. However, direct communication of the airway with the external environment and presence of a foreign body can predispose to local inflammation and result in bacterial superinfection. Pneumonia, tracheitis, and peristomal cellulitis are reported complications,[2,12] but can be prevented by careful attention to routine tracheostomy care and treated with topical or systemic antibiotics.

42.7 Late Complications

42.7.1 Granulomata

Granulomas are the most common late complication of pediatric tracheostomy. Wetmore et al and Crysdale et al reported granulomas in over 50% of patients in their series.[2,13] Granulomas of the suprastoma, stoma, and trachea are typically the result of friction and chronic inflammation. They can often be managed conservatively by avoiding suction trauma, repositioning of the tracheostomy tube, or applying topical antibiotics and steroids. Granulation tissue easily accessible through the stoma may respond to silver nitrate cautery in the office setting or topical steroid cream; however, obstructing granulomas or those that fail conservative management are best removed endoscopically in the operating room.

42.7.2 Airway Stenosis or Collapse

Airway stenosis can occur at the level of the subglottis or trachea. High tracheostomy can result in stenosis of the subglottis[13] and over-resection of tracheal cartilage may contribute to airway collapse. However, chronic low-grade inflammation also creates an environment prone to stenosis and softening of the cartilages regardless of technique.[6] In addition, prolonged intubation or acid reflux may also cause inflammation.[3] Patients with subglottic stenosis often benefit from steroid injection and balloon dilatation; however, more distal stenoses may require tracheal resection or reconstruction with autologous cartilage grafting to achieve adequate patency.

42.7.3 Peristomal and Tracheal Erosion

An inappropriately sized or positioned tracheostomy tube places the surrounding soft tissues at risk for erosion. The peristomal skin may develop pressure ulceration at any point of prolonged contact with the tube. Meticulous attention to the peristomal soft tissue must be emphasized as part of routine tracheostomy care. The authors advocate a circumferential skin dressing in the immediate postoperative period. After the first tracheostomy change, close monitoring ensues, and any sign of early skin breakdown should prompt immediate intervention. A variety of absorbent protective dressings can be used in the event of early tissue injury, or the tracheostomy tube may need to be replaced or modified to alleviate pressure. In the setting of severe tissue erosion, wet to dry dressings should be used to encourage healing by secondary intention.

Distal malposition of the tracheostomy tip or overinflation of the balloon can result in erosion of the posterior tracheal wall. Erosion of the posterior tracheal wall into anterior esophageal wall, while rare, may lead to formation of a tracheoesophageal fistula. Patients with irradiated tissues, cervical spine abnormalities, or indwelling esophageal tubing are at increased risk.

Anterior tracheal wall erosion occurs by the same mechanism but with more devastating complication. Proximity of the innominate artery to the anterior tracheal wall can result in life-threatening hemorrhage, should erosion progress into the vessel. Sentinel bleeding may herald massive hemorrhage. Any bleeding from the tracheostomy should prompt flexible endoscopy and evaluation of the anterior tracheal wall for evidence of erosion. Concern for tracheoinnominate fistula may prompt computed tomography-arteriogram for evaluation.[3] However, massive hemorrhage should be managed immediately by tamponade, with digital pressure and distal placement of a cuffed endotracheal tube followed by emergent surgical repair in coordination with thoracic surgery. Mortality is high.

42.8 Mortality Rate

All-cause mortality in pediatric patients with tracheostomy has approximated 20% (ranging from 13 to 25%).[1,3,6,15] However, a large percentage of these deaths are attributable to primary or comorbid disease. Tracheostomy-related mortality, most commonly from accidental decannulation, accounts for generally <3% of deaths (0.5–3.6%).[1,6] However, the risk of mortality with tracheostomy tubes approximates 1–2% annually.

42.9 Home Care

Adequate preparedness for home care of a child with tracheostomy depends largely on caregiver education prior to discharge. Two caregivers must be instructed on routine management of the tracheostomy and detection of airway-related complications. Caregivers should demonstrate necessary skills for suctioning, cleaning, and tube replacement prior to leaving the hospital. A dislodgement plan should be in place as well as coordination for adequate supervision of the child. In addition, instruction on basic cardiopulmonary resuscitation may prove invaluable in the event of an arrest. Depending on familial circumstances and patient comorbidities, skilled nursing, home health, or use of a rehabilitation or nursing facility may be indicated.

Appropriate disposition to home requires arrangement of home medical supplies. A suction machine and supply of suction catheters must be available to the family by the time of discharge to enable routine care and prevent obstruction. Caregivers should be equipped with a spare tracheostomy tube and obturator in the event one is necessary for urgent exchange, replacement, or use during routine cleaning. Sterile saline for tracheal lavage, Velcro tracheostomy ties, and any other sponges or dressings used while inpatient should also be arranged.

The health of the lower respiratory mucosa and secretions depends on humidification of inspired air through the tracheostomy. This can be achieved by use of a heat and moisture exchange (HME) device or "nose" for the tracheostomy tube. Alternatively, humidification of room air or supplemental oxygen may also be used. In the setting of tenacious secretions or crusting, nebulized therapies such as isotonic or hypertonic saline is a helpful adjunct.

42.10 Surveillance

Following tracheostomy, continued airway surveillance in a multi-disciplinary setting facilitates optimal care in regard to daily management and long-term strategic planning for decannulation or other needs. An ideal multi-disciplinary team consists of pediatric otolaryngologists, pulmonologists, gastroenterologists, speech therapists, respiratory therapists, and nutritionists. Multi-disciplinary clinics reduce travel time for patients and encourage interdisciplinary management addressing patients' global health.

We recommend patients be seen within 1 month of discharge for their initial visit and then followed at increasing intervals depending on their level of complication. If doing well, patients should be evaluated at least biannually for surveillance. This facilitates any necessary changes in the tracheostomy tube size as the child grows and enables close monitoring for late complications. We recommend evaluation for suprastomal granulomas annually either with a sedated exam or with office-based retroflexed tracheostomy to evaluate the subglottis.

42.11 Decannulation

When and if a patwient's underlying need for tracheostomy has resolved, candidacy for decannulation may be considered. Crysdale et al reported an overall decannulation rate of 41% and Gupta et al reported decannulation rates as high as 28% in patients with underlying neurologic diagnoses.[8,13] Criteria and technique for decannulation vary widely. We recommend an observation period of 3 to 6 months during which the patient does well without apparent necessity of the tracheostomy before consideration of decannulation. Decannulation should be preceded by endoscopy. In cooperative patients, adequate endoscopy may be obtained in office. However, formal airway evaluation in the operating room may be needed for sufficient examination and allows for any necessary endoscopic intervention to be made simultaneously.

Most pediatric patients undergoing decannulation should be admitted for 24 to 48 hours of observation with continuous pulse oximetry. Some practitioners opt for downsizing or capping. The site is dressed with steri strips, gauze, and tape, which may be changed or reinforced as needed.

42.12 Tracheocutaneous Fistula

Persistent tracheocutaneous fistula persisting 6 months after decannulation warrants surgical repair. Tracheocutaneous fistula occurs frequently following traditional tracheostomy, with a reported incidence ranging from 10 to 30% and is more common in the setting of a formalized stoma.[1,6,8] Various techniques for surgical repair exist, but all invariably involve excision of excess skin with obliteration of the fistula tract. Regardless of technique it is critical to have an egress for air escape following the surgical repair to reduce the risk of pneumo-mediastinum.

42.12.1 Technique—Repair of Tracheocutaneous Fistula

An elliptical incision is marked around the fistula site and infiltrated with 1% lidocaine with 1:100,000 epinephrine. Incision is made through the skin and subcutaneous tissues and the tract identified (▶ Fig. 42.8a). Dissection of the tract is carried down to the airway without violation of the tract itself (▶ Fig. 42.8b). The fistula tract may then be imbricated on itself using Connell stitch if sufficient tissue exists (▶ Fig. 42.8c) or may be oversewn primarily (▶ Fig. 42.8d). Strap muscles are reapproximated. The deep dermal layer is then reapproximated and the skin closed primarily. A Penrose or rubber band drain is placed to allow passive egress of any air leak and may be removed the following day (▶ Fig. 42.8e).

42.13 Highlights

a. Indications
   - Airway obstruction.
   - Pulmonary toilet.
   - Prolonged need for assisted ventilation.
b. Contraindications
   - Bleeding disorder (relative).
   - Hemodynamic instability.
c. Complications
   - Tube obstruction.
   - Air leak.
   - Hemorrhage.
   - Accidental decannulation.
   - Infection.
   - Tracheal or peristomal erosion.
   - Tracheoinnominate fistula.
   - Granulomata.
   - Airway stenosis.
d. Special preoperative considerations
   - General endotracheal anesthesia.
   - No antibiotic prophylaxis necessary.
e. Special intraoperative considerations
   - Placement of shoulder roll to facilitate neck extension.
   - Protect the endotracheal tube balloon on airway incision.
   - Tracheotomy: vertical incision through two tracheal rings, Bjork flap, or starplasty technique.

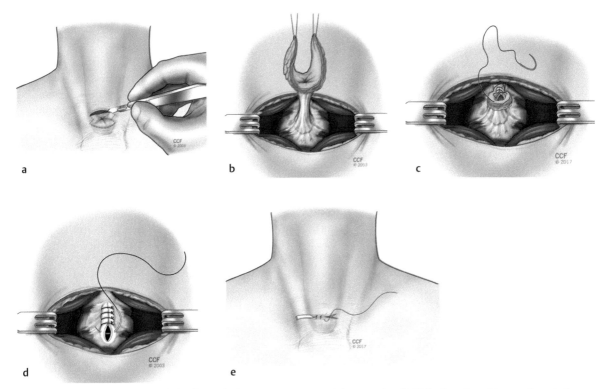

Fig. 42.8 Incision is made through the skin and subcutaneous tissues and the tract identified **(a)**. Dissection of the tract is carried down to the airway without violation of the tract itself **(b)**. The fistula tract may then be imbricated on itself using Connell stitch if sufficient tissue exists **(c)** or may be oversewn primarily **(d)**. Following approximation of the strap muscles, a Penrose or rubber band drain is placed to allow passive egress of any air leak and may be removed the following day **(e)**. (Reproduced with permission, Cleveland Clinic Center for Medical Art & Photography © 2017. All Rights Reserved.)

  – Withdrawal of endotracheal and placement of tracheostomy tube.
  – Confirmation of end tidal CO_2.
f. Special postoperative considerations
  – Four-point fixation with suture, tracheostomy ties, and stay sutures until stoma maturation.
  – Immediate availability of secondary tracheostomy tube of the same or smaller caliber and an obturator at the bedside in the event of decannulation.

References

[1] Carron JD, Derkay CS, Strope GL, Nosonchuk JE, Darrow DH. Pediatric tracheotomies: changing indications and outcomes. Laryngoscope 2000;110(7):1099–1104
[2] Wetmore RF, Handler SD, Potsic WP. Pediatric tracheostomy: experience during the past decade. Ann Otol Rhinol Laryngol 1982;91(6 Pt 1):628–632
[3] Watters KF. Tracheostomy in infants and children. Respir Care 2017;62(6):799–825
[4] Bjork VO. Partial resection of the only remaining lung with the aid of respirator treatment. J Thorac Cardiovasc Surg 1960;39:179–188
[5] Au JK, Heineman TE, Schmalbach CE, St John MA. Should adult surgical tracheostomies include a Bjork flap? Laryngoscope 2017;127(3):535–536
[6] Koltai PJ. Starplasty: a new technique of pediatric tracheotomy. Arch Otolaryngol Head Neck Surg 1998;124(10):1105–1111
[7] Solares CA, Krakovitz P, Hirose K, Koltai PJ. Starplasty: revisiting a pediatric tracheostomy technique. Otolaryngol Head Neck Surg 2004;131(5):717–722
[8] Gupta A, Stokken J, Krakovitz P, Malhotra P, Anne S. Tracheostomy in neurologically compromised paediatric patients: role of starplasty. J Laryngol Otol 2015;129(10):1009–1012
[9] Eliachar I. Unaided speech in long-term tube-free tracheostomy. Laryngoscope 2000;110(5 Pt 1):749–760
[10] Jackson C. High tracheostomy and other errors: the chief causes of chronic laryngeal stenosis. Surg Gynec Obster 1921
[11] Kremer B, Botos-Kremer AI, Eckel HE, Schlöndorff G. Indications, complications, and surgical techniques for pediatric tracheostomies: an update. J Pediatr Surg 2002;37(11):1556–1562
[12] Wetmore RF, Marsh RR, Thompson ME, Tom LW. Pediatric tracheostomy: a changing procedure? Ann Otol Rhinol Laryngol 1999;108(7 Pt 1):695–699
[13] Crysdale WS, Feldman RI, Naito K. Tracheotomies: a 10-year experience in 319 children. Ann Otol Rhinol Laryngol 1988;97(5 Pt 1):439–443
[14] Mahida JB, Asti L, Boss EF, et al. Tracheostomy placement in children younger than 2 years: 30-day outcomes using the National Surgical Quality Improvement Program Pediatric. JAMA Otolaryngol Head Neck Surg 2016;142(3):241–246
[15] McPherson ML, Shekerdemian L, Goldsworthy M, et al. A decade of pediatric tracheostomies: indications, outcomes, and long-term prognosis. Pediatr Pulmonol 2017;52(7):946–953

43 Tracheocutaneous Fistula Repair

Christine Fordham, Anna H. Messner

Summary

Tracheocutaneous fistula (TCF) repair is indicated in pediatric patients who have a persistent TCF 3 to 6 months following tracheostomy decannulation. The surgical repair can be primary, with a four-layer closure, including the tracheal wall, strap muscles, subcutaneous tissue, and skin, or it can be secondary, with excision of the TCF tract and delayed closure by secondary intention. The secondary type of repair is often advocated in an effort to decrease the risk of postoperative pneumothorax/pneumomediastinum, but no statistically significant difference is seen when primary repair and secondary repair are compared.

Keywords: Fistula, repair, tracheostomy, primary, secondary, subcutaneous emphysema, pneumothorax, pneumomediastinum

43.1 Introduction

TCF (▶Fig. 43.1) is the result of a non-healing epithelized tracheostomy stoma after decannulation. In recent years the indications for tracheostomy have changed in the pediatric population. There has been a decrease in the rate of tracheostomy for infections, and an increase in tracheostomy for children with congenital anomalies. Currently, common reasons for placement of a tracheostomy in pediatric patients include upper airway obstruction related to craniofacial dysmorphism, vocal fold paralysis, neurologic impairment, and subglottic stenosis. Another sizable group of children require prolonged mechanical ventilation due to cardiac or pulmonary illnesses, and a tracheostomy is placed to assist with ventilation. The result is an increased number of younger children requiring tracheostomy for a longer period of time.[1-3] If pediatric patients meet criteria for decannulation, the rate of developing a TCF after tracheostomy removal is reported from 13.1 to 37.8%.[1-3] The rate of TCF increases if the tracheostomy is performed in children younger than 6 months of age or if the tracheostomy is in place for a longer duration of time.[1-4] Carron et al showed a 70% TCF rate in children that had a tracheostomy cannulation for greater than 2 years and 8.1% TCF rate if the tracheostomy was in place less than 2 years.[4]

In addition to young age at tracheostomy creation and duration of cannulation, it is also thought that the type of tracheostomy procedure affects the incidence of TCF after decannulation. Procedures that are concerning for increased TCF are stoma maturation with sutures to the trachea, Bjork cartilage flap, and starplasty. Colmen et al found that stoma maturation did not have an impact on the incidence of TCF formation.[5] Conversely, Sautter et al reported 28 patients who underwent decannulation after starplasty tracheostomy with stoma maturation and 25/28 patients had a persistent TCF.[6] Clearly, there are differences in the reported outcomes after decannulation in the literature for patients who underwent stoma maturation. In patients with likely resolution of the underlying disease requiring tracheostomy, stoma maturation techniques including starplasty, should be used cautiously secondarily to the increased risk of TCF.

TCF should be repaired in pediatric patients with a non-healing fistula that is no longer needed. The persistent fistula has several potentially negative sequela including: (1) recurrent aspiration with subsequent respiratory infections, (2) skin irritation secondary to exposure to tracheal mucus, (3) ineffective cough, (4) difficulty in phonation, (5) inability to be submerged in water, and (6) cosmetic and social acceptance concerns. Repair generally should not be performed prior to 3 to 6 months after decannulation because many TCFs will heal spontaneously during this time period.

43.2 Preoperative Evaluation for TCF repair

After a period of several months following decannulation, and before surgical repair of the TCF, the patient should be evaluated for upper airway obstruction. Potential sources of upper airway obstruction include tonsil/adenoid hypertrophy, vocal fold paralysis, laryngomalacia, subglottic stenosis, subglottic cysts/hemangiomas, and suprastomal collapse of the trachea. Premature closure of a TCF that the patient is dependent on for ventilation could lead to acute airway obstruction and an urgent need for recannulation or endotracheal intubation.

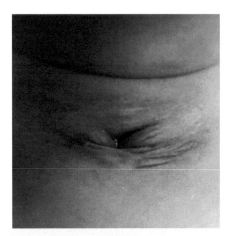

Fig. 43.1 Tracheocutaneous fistula.

A diagnostic microdirect laryngoscopy with bronchoscopy should be performed prior to TCF repair. The endoscopic evaluation can be performed during the same procedure as the repair of the TCF to spare the patient a separate anesthesia. In addition, an overnight sleep apnea study or sleep endoscopy with occlusion of the fistula is indicated preoperatively if there are concerns on history for obstructive sleep apnea. Gallagher and Hartnick[7] recommend against closure in patients with persistent cough and patients with anatomic obstruction or severe trismus that would make reintubation difficult.

43.3 Tracheocutaneous Fistula Repair

Several methods of TCF repair have been described. The methods can be divided into two primary groups: primary and secondary closure. Primary closure is typically a four-layer closure including the tracheal wall, strap muscles, subcutaneous tissue, and skin. Secondary repair is performed by excising the skin of the TCF tract, then allowing the fistula to close spontaneously during the postoperative period.

43.3.1 Secondary Closure—Description of Procedure

The patient is taken to the operating room and microdirect laryngoscopy and bronchoscopy, with or without sleep endoscopy, is performed. Assuming there is no evidence of airway obstruction that would preclude repair of the TCF the patient is nasally or orally intubated with a cuffed tracheostomy tube. The endotracheal tube balloon is placed inferior to the TCF. A rolled towel is positioned behind the patient's shoulders to better expose the neck. An elliptical incision is created around the

TCF incorporating any associated scar tissue. To improve hemostasis and anesthesia, the planned incision is injected with 1% lidocaine with 1:100,000 epinephrine. A scalpel is used to incise the tissue to the level of the subcutaneous tissue (▶Fig. 43.2). Due to the risk of airway fire, the use of cautery is minimized and avoided if possible. With circumferential blunt dissection, the tract is exposed as it approaches the anterior tracheal wall (▶Fig. 43.3). The tract is then truncated at the level of the anterior tracheal wall (▶Fig. 43.4). The tracheal defect is evaluated for persistent epithelial tissue and any additional identified skin removed. Hemostasis is obtained and the wound covered. The patient is awakened and extubated. He/she is admitted to the hospital, typically the intensive care unit, overnight for monitoring with continuous pulse oximetry.

43.3.2 Primary Closure

The initial surgery is the same as the secondary closure technique. After truncating the tract at the anterior

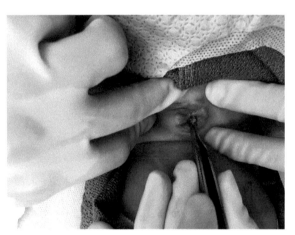

Fig. 43.2 Dissection of the tracheocutaneous fistula (TCF) tract.

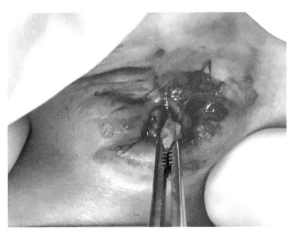

Fig. 43.3 Dissection of the tracheocutaneous fistula (TCF) tract to the level of the anterior tracheal wall.

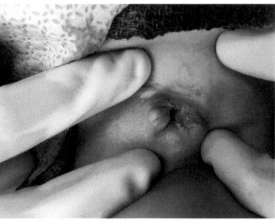

Fig. 43.4 Neck wound after truncating of the tracheocutaneous fistula (TCF) at the anterior tracheal wall.

tracheal wall the trachea is evaluated. The endotracheal tube is then slowly withdrawn to position the balloon immediately superior to the TCF. The tracheal defect is closed with 3–0 or 4–0 polyglactin 910 (Vicryl®). The wound is irrigated and the airway pressure increased to 30 cm of water by anesthesia personnel to evaluate for an air leak. Once no air leak is present, the strap muscles are closed in the midline. The subcutaneous tissue is then loosely approximated and the skin closed with absorbable suture. The placement of a drain is often advocated due to the theoretical benefit of preventing subcutaneous air and/ or pneumothorax, but has been shown to be ineffective in preventing postoperative air-related complications.[7,8] After primary closure, all patients are admitted to the intensive care unit overnight for monitoring.

43.4 Complications of Tracheocutaneous Fistula Repair

Complications of tracheocutaneous fistula repair are rare but potentially fatal. Major complications include subcutaneous emphysema, hemorrhage, pneumomediatinum/pneumothorax, need for urgent intubation or recannulation, and repeated surgical intervention. Minor complications include persistent TCF, unfavorable scar, wound infection, granuloma, oxygen dependence, and wound dehiscence. Due to the high risk nature of potential major complications, the appropriate surgical technique to minimize complications is often debated.

Traditionally, primary closure was advocated due to a reported low complication rate, increased TCF closure rate, improved scar, and decreased need for wound care. Several studies have shown the effectiveness of primary closure.[3,6,8,9] Concern arose for increased risk of pneumomediastinum/pneumothorax associated with primary closure; thus, some authors have advocated for secondary TCF closure.[10] Recently, however, several reviews have shown no significant difference in the primary and secondary closure methods with regard to TCF closure rates and major complications.[8–12] Specifically, no difference was seen in subcutaneous emphysema and urgent airway problems.[7] Notably, secondary closure has been associated with decreased operating room time and shorter hospital stay.[6] Due to the severity of complications observed in primary closure, secondary closure is advocated at major institutions despite the similar risk profile of the two techniques.[10]

43.5 Highlights

a. Indications
  – Persistent tracheocutaneous fistula (TCF) after tracheostomy decannulation.

b. Contraindications
  – Concern that the patient is requiring the TCF for adequate ventilation.
  – Severe trismus or other anatomic obstruction that would make oral intubation difficult.

c. Complications
  – Postoperative subcutaneous air, pneumothorax, pneumomediastinum.
  – Need for urgent intubation or recannulation.
  – Oxygen dependence.
  – Wound infection.
  – Wound dehiscence.
  – Unfavorable scar.
  – Persistent/recurrent TCF.

d. Special preoperative considerations
  – Evaluate the child for sources of upper airway obstruction (e.g., tonsil/adenoid hypertrophy, vocal fold paralysis, laryngomalacia, etc.).
  – Consider sleep endoscopy and/or polysomnogram with stoma occluded.

e. Special intraoperative considerations
  – Microdirect laryngoscopy/bronchoscopy prior to TCF closure.
  – Position the endotracheal tube balloon inferior to the TCF.
  – Minimize/avoid the use of cautery to avoid an airway fire.
  – Consult with the anesthesiologist to ensure the lowest oxygen settings possible (to minimize fire risk).
  – If primary closure is performed obtain an airtight closure of the trachea.

f. Special postoperative considerations.
  – Overnight hospitalization in a monitored unit.
  – Closely observe for subcutaneous emphysema.

References

[1] Mahadevan M, Barber C, Salkeld L, Douglas G, Mills N. Pediatric tracheotomy: 17 year review. Int J Pediatr Otorhinolaryngol 2007;71(12):1829–1835

[2] Al-Samri M, Mitchell I, Drummond DS, Bjornson C. Tracheostomy in children: a population-based experience over 17 years. Pediatr Pulmonol 2010;45(5):487–493

[3] Carron JD, Derkay CS, Strope GL, Nosonchuk JE, Darrow DH. Pediatric tracheotomies: changing indications and outcomes. Laryngoscope 2000;110(7):1099–1104

[4] Tasca RA, Clarke RW. Tracheocutaneous fistula following paediatric tracheostomy: a 14-year experience at Alder Hey Children's Hospital. Int J Pediatr Otorhinolaryngol 2010;74(6):711–712

[5] Colman KL, Mandell DL, Simons JP. Impact of stoma maturation on pediatric tracheostomy-related complications. Arch Otolaryngol Head Neck Surg 2010;136(5):471–474

[6] Sautter NB, Krakovitz PR, Solares CA, Koltai PJ. Closure of persistent tracheocutaneous fistula following "starplasty" tracheostomy in children. Int J Pediatr Otorhinolaryngol 2006;70(1):99–105

[7] Lewis S, Arjomandi H, Rosenfeld R. Systematic review of surgery for persistent pediatric tracheocutaneous fistula. Laryngoscope 2017;127(1):241–246

[8] Geyer M, Kubba H, Hartley B. Experiences of tracheocutaneous fistula closure in children: how we do it. Clin Otolaryngol 2008;33(4):367–369

[9] Gallagher TQ, Hartnick CJ. Tracheocutaneous fistula closure. Adv Otorhinolaryngol 2012;73:76–79

[10] Osborn AJ, de Alarcón A, Hart CK, Cotton RT, Rutter MJ. Tracheocutaneous fistula closure in the pediatric population: should secondary closure be the standard of care? Otolaryngol Head Neck Surg 2013;149(5):766–771

[11] Wine TM, Simons JP, Mehta DK. Comparison of 2 techniques of tracheocutaneous fistula closure: analysis of outcomes and health care use. JAMA Otolaryngol Head Neck Surg 2014;140(3): 237–242

[12] Cheng J, Setabutr D. Tracheocutaneous fistula closure in children. Int J Pediatr Otorhinolaryngol 2016;89:107–111

44 Pediatric Bronchoscopy

Annabelle Tay Sok Yan, Christine Barron, Tulio A. Valdez

Summary

Rigid bronchoscopy provides an excellent visualization of the airway. With the advancement in medical technology, the indications and uses continue to expand. This has resulted in a shift in paradigm in airway surgeries. The development of flexible bronchoscopy has come in timely to resolve some of the limitations with rigid bronchoscopy such as its ability to be used in children with unstable spine and its ability to be passed to the distal airway. However, each instrument has its own limitations and together they can be complementary.

Keywords: Rigid bronchoscopy, flexible bronchoscopy, difficulty airway, endoscopic, foreign body, airway stenosis

44.1 Introduction

The father of modern bronchoscopy is considered to be Gustav Killian, who in 1897 developed a direct ocular mechanism for extracting foreign bodies from a patient's airway.[1] Chevalier Jackson is often considered the father of endoscopy and was central to the development of safe and effective techniques of bronchoscopy and esophagoscopy. Since then, numerous physician scientists have expanded the capabilities of this technology.[2] In 1966, Shigeto Ikeda revolutionized the field with the development of the flexible fiberoptic bronchoscope, paving the way for imaging and video bronchoscopy.[3] This was followed in the early 1980s by the development of transbronchial needle aspiration and the use of lasers to coagulate endobronchial lesions.[4] Today, bronchoscopy has become an integral part of numerous subspecialties for the diagnosis and treatment of airway pathologies.

For many decades, rigid endoscopy has been the main tool used in the evaluation of airway disease. However, in recent years, with the introduction of flexible fiberoptic endoscopy, the role of rigid endoscopy has become much more clearly defined and the two types of endoscopy have proven complementary. Traditionally, rigid bronchoscopy has been used in the evaluation of airway disease, operative airway procedures, and removal of foreign body. Recent technologic advances and the development of specialized endoscopic tools have resulted in a new era of endoscopic airway surgery. This chapter will discuss the equipment and techniques used in rigid and flexible bronchoscopy in the evaluation and management of pediatric airway conditions.

Table 44.1 Airway cart contents

Laryngoscopes

- Benjamin
- Parsons
- Lindholm
- Miller

Micrognathia, anterior larynx

- Anterior commissure laryngoscopes

Bronchoscopes

- Sizes 2.5–5
- Pharyngeal suctions
- Laryngeal suctions
- Tracheal suctions

Hopkin rods

Light box

Light cables

Microlaryngeal instruments

Foreign body forceps

Tooth guards

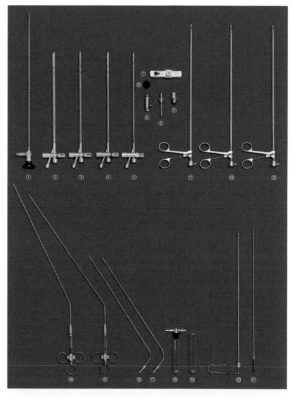

Fig. 44.1 Basic pediatrics bronchoscopy set, with Hopkins rod, light prism, bridge with window, suctions, and foreign body forceps. (Reproduced with permission of Karl storz SE and Co KG, Tuttlingen, Germany.)

44.2 Instruments

A list of commonly used laryngoscopes and broncho-scopes recommended for the pediatric endoscopic air-way cart is presented in ▶Table 44.1 and ▶Fig. 44.1 and ▶Fig. 44.2.

44.2.1 Laryngoscopes

The Parsons, Benjamin, Lindholm, Phillips, or Miller blades are the most common laryngoscopes used in pedi-atric laryngoscopy. Most pediatric airway cases can be managed with the aforementioned laryngoscopes. How-ever, in certain patients with difficult exposure, such as patients with micrognathia or Pierre Robin sequence, the slotted anterior commissure scope or the anterior commissure C-Mac D blade scope may be useful. The McIntosh blades are not commonly used by otolaryngolo-gist as the curved blades make passing a telescope or rigid bronchoscope more difficult.

The Parsons and Lindholm are suspension laryngo-scopes. The Parsons is a slotted scope and is preferred by some surgeons who enjoy the additional room for a sec-ond instrument (▶Fig. 44.3). When a suspension laryn-goscope is employed, the larynx can be examined with a microscope or a rigid telescope, such as the Hopkins rod telescopes. A microscope with 400 mm lens is recom-mended when two hands are needed for manipulation

and surgical intervention. For routine examination, a Hopkins rod telescope connected to a camera and video monitor system gives superior image and improved abil-ity to inspect the subglottis and the distal trachea.

44.2.2 Bronchoscopes

Rigid bronchoscopes come in a variety of diameters and lengths. A list of the common sizes and accesso-ries is presented in ▶Table 44.2. Regardless of the type of scopes used, it is important to remember the outer diameter of the scope is larger than the listed size of the scope. For example, a size 3.5 bronchoscope has an inner diameter (ID) of 5.0 mm and outer diameter (OD) of 5.7 mm (▶Fig. 44.4). The shorter length 18.5 cm scope should be used for small neonates and prema-ture infants, and the 30 cm should be used for an older child. A common and easy to remember cut-off is the age of 6 months. An appropriately sized bronchoscope is crucial to ensure safe passage and minimal trauma to the airway.

When performing a diagnostic rigid bronchoscopy in the operating room, it is important to have various sizes of bronchoscopes available. Specifically, a bronchoscope

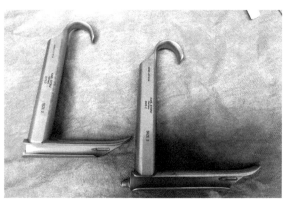

Fig. 44.3 Parsons laryngoscopes with a lateral insufflation channel for anesthetic gas and oxygen supply. Parsons laryngoscopes are slotted on one side facilitating instruments introduction.

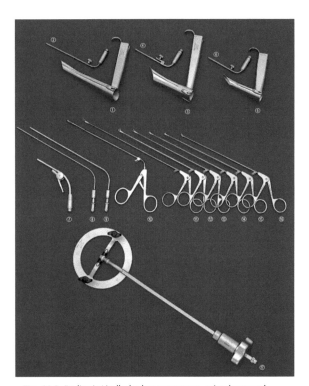

Fig. 44.2 Pediatric Lindholm laryngoscopes, microlaryngeal instruments, light clip, and suspension system. (Reproduced with permission of Karl storz SE and Co. KG, Tuttlingen, Germany.)

Table 44.2 Bronchoscope sizes

Age bronchoscopes sizes outer diameter (mm)

Premature 2.5 (4.0)

Full-term newborn 3.0 (5.0)

6 months–1 year 3.0–3.5 (5.0)

1 year–2 years 3.5 (5.7)

2 years–3 years 3.5–4.0 (5.7–6.7)

3 years–5 years 4.0 (6.7)

10 years 5.0 (7.8)

14 years 5.0 (7.8)

appropriate for patient's age as well as two sizes down should be readily available.

44.2.3 Ancillary Tools

A list of ancillary tools such as suction devices, light cords, anti-fog solutions, topical lidocaine sprays, tooth guards, saline-soaked gauze sponges, endotracheal tubes (ETT), and microsurgical instruments should be present. Depending on the patient's diagnosis, microde-briders, airway balloons, optical forceps, and laser setup may be necessary.

44.2.4 Imaging System

The high-definition camera and video system provide for a magnified view of the airway, allowing everyone in

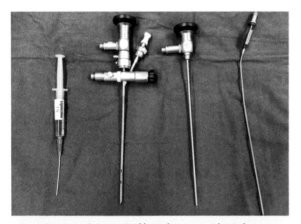

Fig. 44.4 A size 3.5 mm rigid bronchoscope with a 0 degree 2.9 mm Hopkins telescope, lidocaine, and tracheal straight suction.

the operating room to visualize the airway and remain cognizant of where the surgeon is working (▶Fig. 44.5). High-quality images captured during the procedures are especially valuable for patients with complex airway issues who make repeated trips to the operating room. Photographs can be shown to patient family members to enhance their understanding of the child's problem and the management plans. Video recording is ideal to document dynamic processes such as tracheomalacia or bronchomalacia. There are a variety of imaging systems on the market. Fundamentally, it is important to ensure the system purchased can be integrated with the system utilized in the operating room. Ease of use and access to technical support are important points to consider.

44.3 Technique

For diagnostic evaluation of the airway, a ventilating bronchoscope is used less frequently than a Hopkins rod Telescope. The advantages of using the bare telescope are that it minimizes the chance for trauma to the airway because of its small diameter and allows for better visualization with its 360-degree field of vision. The greatest disadvantage is that the patient cannot be ventilated using this technique.

44.3.1 Types of Anesthesia

Communication with anesthesiologist is important and the key to a successful airway procedure. In many cases, the patient's airway may be unstable or abnormal, and a discussion with the anesthesiologist prior to induction ensures awareness of the contingency plans should the need arise. In general, rigid bronchoscopy is conducted in the operating room under general anesthesia, whereas flexible bronchoscopy may be performed under general

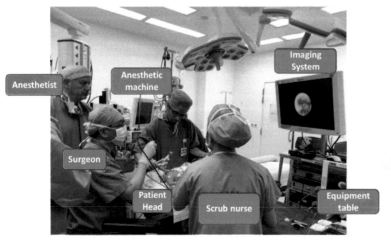

Fig. 44.5 Operating room setup during microdirect laryngoscopy and bronchoscopy.

anesthesia or conscious sedation in bronchoscopy suite or intensive care unit.[5-7]

Intravenous induction is preferred in older children, though inhalational induction may be necessary in infants. A rapid onset inhalational agent such as Sevoflurane is commonly used. Once the rigid bronchoscope is in place, it is appropriate to switch to intravenous anesthesia in order to prevent contamination as the anesthetic circuit is not closed. Remifentanil and Propofol are preferred because of its quicker recovery, reduced nausea and vomiting, and decreased postoperative delirium. In addition, corticosteroids may be given at induction to reduce the edema generated from manipulation.[5]

Topical Lidocaine spray (5 mg/kg) can be applied to the larynx. In pediatric patients, nebulized fentanyl (2 mg/kg) in combination with the lignocaine (4 mg/kg) has been shown to improve hemodynamic stability and reduce the cough reflex in children undergoing foreign body removal.[5] After induction, the anesthetic level can be maintained with total intravenous anesthesia (TIVA) using Propofol and Remifentanil. This technique is well tolerated even in children with preoperative respiratory impairment.

Spontaneous ventilation is often preferred for patients since it maintains the respiratory drive avoiding unnecessary emergencies in cases with a difficult airway or in the presence of a foreign body.[5]

Supplemental oxygen can be provided during the procedure either through the side port of the laryngoscope or via an endotracheal tube placed in the nose or in the oral cavity. Most units now use spontaneous respiration, but practice varies between centers. Ventilation strategies include spontaneous ventilation, closed-circuit positive pressure ventilation, high-frequency jet ventilation, and use of a venturi jet. Complications can occur specific to anesthesia such as cough, laryngospasm, and airway fires.[6,7] To prevent airway fires during airway procedures, it is important to maintain an FIO_2 below 35% and to communicate with anesthesia when a laser or cautery is going to be used.

44.4 Surgical Technique

Once the child is adequately anesthetized, he or she is positioned with the head at the top of the bed, slightly extended and the neck slightly flexed ("sniffing position"). A mouth guard is placed if the child has teeth and if not, a wet-gauze may be placed to protect the gum. The laryngoscope is held in the left hand and the right hand is used to pry open the mouth. The tongue is swept to the left side and the tip of the blade is placed into the vallecula (▶Fig. 44.6). If a rigid ventilating

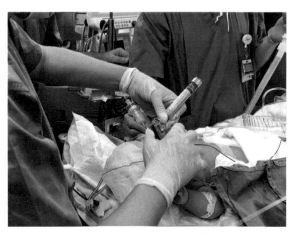

Fig. 44.6 Laryngoscopy in a neonate using standard laryngoscopy technique.

bronchoscope is used, the bronchoscope should be rotated 90 degree at the level of the vocal folds to avoid traumatizing the vocal folds as it is passed into the subglottis.

It is important to perform a systematic examination. The examination begins in the oral cavity and progresses through the rest of the airway. The supraglottis, glottis, subglottis, trachea, right and left main stem bronchus should be evaluated, and findings recorded during the endoscopy (▶Fig. 44.7). To examine the right main stem bronchus, the patient's head is rotated to the left and the opposite rotation is performed to examine the left main stem bronchus.

A caveat is that during rigid laryngoscopy, the blade of the laryngoscope can affect the anatomy of the supraglottis and may affect the appearance of the larynx. Dynamic evaluation of the airway and assessment of the vocal fold movements are better assessed in the office using a flexible laryngoscope in an awake patient.

44.5 Indications

Rigid bronchoscopy can be performed for diagnostic and therapeutic purposes.

Endoscopy allows for a careful evaluation of the airway for underlying pathology and structural abnormalities. Congenital stridor is the most frequent indication for bronchoscopy in infancy, of which the most common etiologies include laryngomalacia and vocal cord paralysis.[8,9] For other conditions such as subglottic stenosis (▶Fig. 44.8), subglottic hemangioma (▶Fig. 44.9), cystic lesions, inflammation, scarring, or laryngeal stenosis, laryngeal webs (▶Fig. 44.10), rigid endoscopy, and passage of an endotracheal tube

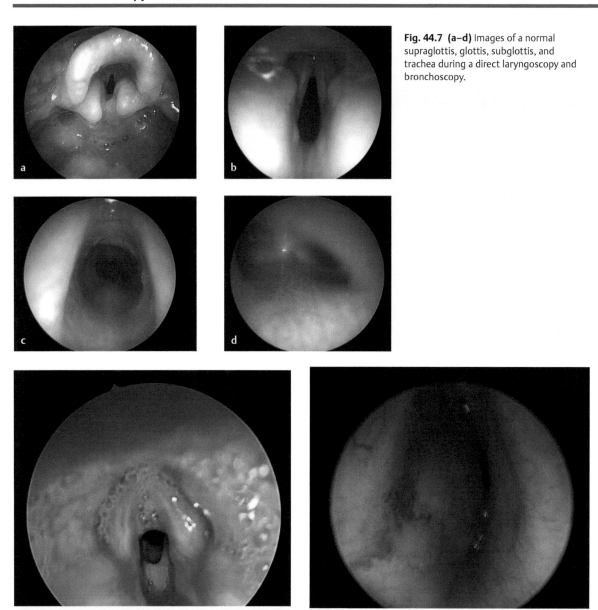

Fig. 44.7 (a–d) Images of a normal supraglottis, glottis, subglottis, and trachea during a direct laryngoscopy and bronchoscopy.

Fig. 44.8 Subglottic stenosis.

Fig. 44.9 Subglottic hemangioma.

Fig. 44.10 Congenital laryngeal web.

can quantify the size of the airway and degree of stenosis. It is important to avoid causing swelling in areas. A right-angle probe can be used to palpate for laryngeal cleft (▶Fig. 44.11), which may not be obvious on flexible endoscopy. Failure to extubate is an indication for bronchoscopy, and in such situations, the airway should be assessed for iatrogenic subglottic stenosis, subglottic cyst (▶Fig. 44.12), and posterior glottic stenosis. In children with recurrent pulmonary infections, rigid laryngoscopy and palpation as well as bronchoscopy are performed to exclude the presence of laryngeal clefts or tracheoesophageal fistulas (▶Fig. 44.13). Finally, rigid bronchoscopy can be used to diagnose tracheomalacia often in conjunction with flexible bronchoscopy. In cases of a suspected vascular or mass compressing the airway, a CT angiography or MRI is often recommended.[10,11]

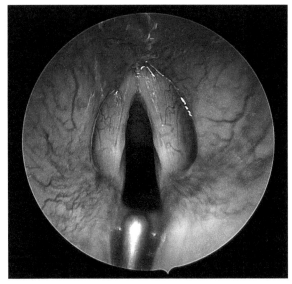

Fig. 44.11 Palpating for laryngeal cleft using a right angle probe.

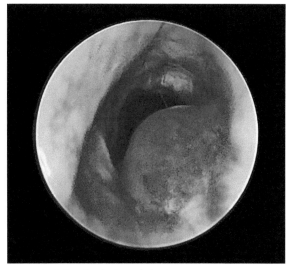

Fig. 44.12 Post-intubation subglottic cyst.

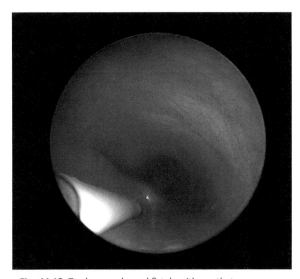

Fig. 44.13 Tracheoesophageal fistula with a catheter cannulating the fistula tract.

In addition to serving as a useful diagnostic tool, rigid endoscopy also provides the surgeon with the opportunity to perform treatment at the same setting. One of the most common uses is the removal of a foreign body using a bronchoscope with optical forceps.[1,12] The rigid bronchoscope with optical forceps may also be used to take biopsies or remove granulation tissues following an open airway surgery. A list of different types of optical forceps is presented in ▶ Fig. 44.14.

The development of the airway dilatation balloon (▶ Fig. 44.15) and microdebrider had also revolutionized the endoscopic opportunities in pediatric airway management. The airway balloon may be used to augment a postsurgical airway patency, dilate a freshly acquired subglottic stenosis, or place an endoscopic posterior graft. The microdebrider and KTP laser has enabled endoscopic removal of papilloma with much precision, hence achieving a better postoperative outcome.

44.6 Limitations

44.6.1 Disadvantages

The primary limitation of rigid endoscopy is the inability to reach the distal airways, precluding its examination. It can also be more traumatic when compared with flexible endoscopy. Rigid bronchoscopy must be done under general anesthesia, so it is not an option for children with absolute contraindications to general anesthesia. In addition, children with cervical spine abnormalities or instability may not be suitable candidates for rigid endoscopy due to their inability to mobilize the neck necessary for the procedure. In such situations, the flexible endoscopy is a useful alternative.[8]

44.6.2 Complications

The overall complication rate for rigid endoscopy is 2% to 3%. These include hemorrhage, perforation, cardiac arrhythmias, and respiratory complications (▶ Table 44.3).

44.7 Flexible Endoscopy

44.7.1 Introduction

The flexible bronchoscope was introduced by Dr. Shigeto Ikeda in 1966.[4] In contrast to rigid bronchoscopy, flexible bronchoscopy allows visualization of the dynamic movement of the airway with minimal distortion from instrumentation. It can be passed into the smaller airways and allows visualization of the distal airways. In the past, flexible bronchoscopy can be done only in the endoscopy

Special Features:
- Newly designed forceps enable removing of foreign bodies under precise optical control not previously possible
- Small size of forceps allows them to be introduced through pediatric bronchoscopes as of size 3.5 and larger in lengths ranging from 18.5 up to 30 cm

- Foreign bodies can be removed quickly and with utmost safety
- Better assessment of the depth of cut when taking biopsies

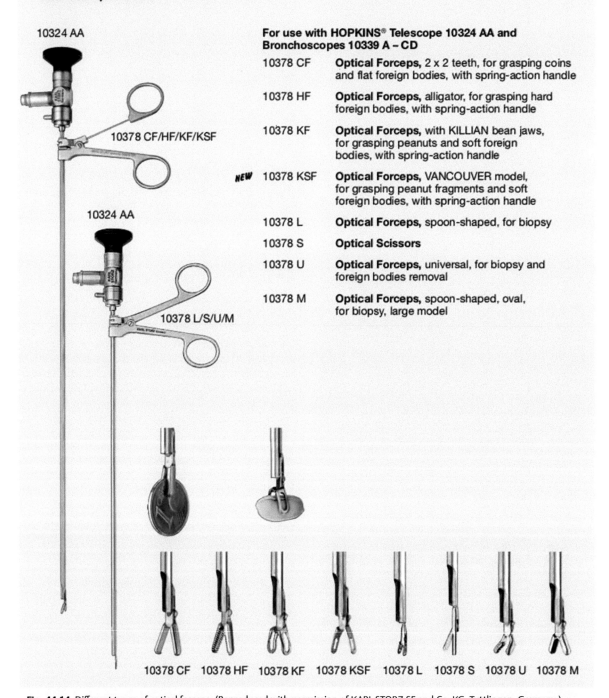

10324 AA

10378 CF/HF/KF/KSF

10324 AA

10378 L/S/U/M

For use with HOPKINS® Telescope 10324 AA and Bronchoscopes 10339 A – CD

10378 CF	**Optical Forceps,** 2 x 2 teeth, for grasping coins and flat foreign bodies, with spring-action handle
10378 HF	**Optical Forceps,** alligator, for grasping hard foreign bodies, with spring-action handle
10378 KF	**Optical Forceps,** with KILLIAN bean jaws, for grasping peanuts and soft foreign bodies, with spring-action handle
NEW 10378 KSF	**Optical Forceps,** VANCOUVER model, for grasping peanut fragments and soft foreign bodies, with spring-action handle
10378 L	**Optical Forceps,** spoon-shaped, for biopsy
10378 S	**Optical Scissors**
10378 U	**Optical Forceps,** universal, for biopsy and foreign bodies removal
10378 M	**Optical Forceps,** spoon-shaped, oval, for biopsy, large model

10378 CF   10378 HF   10378 KF   10378 KSF   10378 L   10378 S   10378 U   10378 M

Fig. 44.14 Different types of optical forceps. (Reproduced with permission of KARL STORZ SE and Co. KG, Tuttlingen, Germany.)

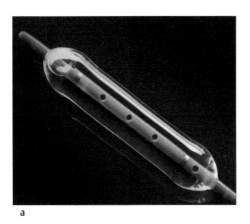

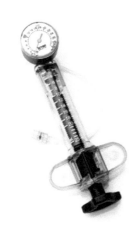

Fig. 44.15 (a, b) Aeris Airway Balloon. (Reproduced with permission of Bryan Medical.)

Table 44.3 Complications of rigid bronchoscopy

Trauma to teeth
Trauma to lips
Trauma to base of tongue
Trauma to epiglottis
Trauma to tracheobronchial tree
Pneumomediastinum

suites. However, with increasing experience with its use, flexible bronchoscopy is now commonly performed in intensive care units, emergency departments, and in the office setting.[8-10]

44.7.2 Instrument

The flexible bronchoscopes come in different sizes. The smaller ones such as a 2.5 mm diameter scope can be used in the neonates and premature infants. It can be threaded through small endotracheal tubes (ETT) such as a size 3 ETT or tracheostomy tube. The limitations include poor illumination and image quality and the lack of a suction port. The larger flexible bronchoscope has the advantage of having better image quality, illumination, a suction port, and the ability to deliver topical anesthesia to the lower airway, allowing it to be used for bronchoalveolar lavage. The same channel also allows biopsy forceps to be passed for endobronchial biopsies.

44.7.3 Indications

The ability to thread an endotracheal tube over a flexible bronchoscope allows it to be used in intubating patients with difficult airways such as patients with Hunter disease or with other craniofacial abnormalities. Other indications include evaluation of a child with persistent stridor, wheezing, recurrent pneumonia, atelectasis, chronic cough, and hemoptysis and in suspected airway anomalies.

It is also commonly done as part of the triple endoscopy in children with aerodigestive pathology since it provides better ability to image the distal airways and does not distort the airway by stenting it as rigid bronchoscopy does.

44.7.4 Technique

Most of the flexible bronchoscopy can be done under sedation. The technique varies depending on the patient and physician preference. The bronchoscope can be introduced through the nose, mouth, or through a laryngeal mask. It can also be readily performed through an endotracheal tube or tracheostomy tube.

44.7.5 Complications

Flexible bronchoscopy is a safe procedure with less than 2% major complications. Desaturations, laryngospasm, bronchospasm, epistaxis, coughing, and postbronchoalveolar lavage fever. Severe complications such as pneumothorax or bronchial hemorrhage rarely occur and are usually associated with biopsy procedures.

44.8 Highlights

- When performing a diagnostic rigid bronchoscopy in the operating room, it is important to have various sizes of bronchoscopes available. Specifically, a bronchoscope appropriate for patient's age as well as two sizes down should be readily available.
- Patients with difficult exposure, such as patients with micrognathia or Pierre Robin, the anterior-commissure scope or the C-Mac® D blade scope may be useful.
- Communication with anesthesiologist is important and the key to a successful airway procedure. In many cases, the patient's airway may be unstable or abnormal, and a discussion with the anesthesiologist prior to induction ensures awareness of the contingency plans, should the need arise.

- It is important to perform a systematic examination. The examination begins in the oral cavity and progresses through the rest of the airway. The supraglottis, glottis, subglottis, trachea, right and left main stem bronchus should be evaluated and findings recorded during the endoscopy.
- Flexible endoscopy is a useful alternative for children with cervical spine abnormalities or instability who may not be suitable candidates for rigid endoscopy due to their inability to mobilize the neck necessary for the procedure.

References

[1] Tang LF, Xu YC, Wang YS, et al. Airway foreign body removal by flexible bronchoscopy: experience with 1027 children during 2000–2008. World J Pediatr 2009;5(3):191–195

[2] Boyd AD. Chevalier Jackson: the father of American bronchoesophagoscopy. Ann Thorac Surg 1994;57(2):502–505

[3] Antony P, Deshmukh H. Bronchoscopic findings of flexible bronchoscopy: a one-year retrospective study in a tertiary care hospital. Int J Res Med Sci 2018;6(2):591–596

[4] Panchabhai TS, Mehta AC. Historical perspectives of bronchoscopy: connecting the dots. Ann Am Thorac Soc 2015;12(5):631–641

[5] José RJ, Shaefi S, Navani N. Anesthesia for bronchoscopy. Curr Opin Anaesthesiol 2014;27(4):453–457

[6] Chai J, Wu XY, Han N, Wang LY, Chen WM. A retrospective study of anesthesia during rigid bronchoscopy for airway foreign body removal in children: propofol and sevoflurane with spontaneous ventilation. Paediatr Anaesth 2014;24(10):1031–1036

[7] Bakan M, Topuz U, Umutoglu T, et al. Remifentanil-based total intravenous anesthesia for pediatric rigid bronchoscopy: comparison of adjuvant propofol and ketamine. Clinics (São Paulo) 2014;69(6):372–377

[8] Cohen S, Pine H, Drake A. Use of rigid and flexible bronchoscopy among pediatric otolaryngologists. Arch Otolaryngol Head Neck Surg 2001;127(5):505–509

[9] Nicolai T. The role of rigid and flexible bronchoscopy in children. Paediatr Respir Rev 2011;12(3):190–195

[10] Cakir E, Ersu RH, Uyan ZS, et al. Flexible bronchoscopy as a valuable tool in the evaluation of persistent wheezing in children. Int J Pediatr Otorhinolaryngol 2009;73(12):1666–1668

[11] Singh V, Singhal KK. The tools of the trade: uses of flexible bronchoscopy. Indian J Pediatr 2015;82(10):932–937

[12] Grego MG, Meji AL, Roge P. Bronchoscopic techniques for removal of foreign bodies in children's airways. Pediatr Pulmonol 2012;62:59–62

45 Surgery of Laryngomalacia

Yoram Stern, Moshe Hain

Summary

Laryngomalacia is a common cause of neonate stridor and is usually managed conservatively. Severe cases with an indication for surgery are best managed by a multidisciplinary team. Supraglottoplasty is the mainstay surgery of choice and should be tailored to the specific sites of the obstruction dynamics. Surgery has good overall outcomes with a low complication rate. Care must be taken to select the appropriate patients for surgery, taking into account the risk factors for failure and complications.

Keywords: Laryngomalacia, supraglottoplasty, gastroesophageal reflux disease, synchronous airway lesions, pulmonary hypertension

45.1 Introduction

Laryngomalacia is the most common cause of neonatal stridor, comprising up to 75% of all causes of congenital stridor.[1-4] Inspiratory collapse of supraglottic structures causes narrowing of the airway lumen resulting in inspiratory stridor. Due to its typically benign natural history of gradual improvement and eventual resolution by age 2 years old, laryngomalacia is most often managed conservatively. In approximately 10% to 15% of cases surgery is indicated because of dyspnea, failure to thrive (FTT), feeding difficulties, and other significant morbidity.[5-9]

45.2 Pathophysiology

The pathophysiology of laryngomalacia has not been completely elucidated. Hypotheses proposed to explain the seemingly weak supraglottic structures address issues of deficient cartilage maturation, weak muscle tone, and effects of laryngopharyngeal reflux (LPR). Although these processes may play a role, the more accepted current understanding suggests that altered laryngeal tone and sensorimotor integrative functions are the underlying cause. Laryngomalacia patients were found in clinical testing to have increased laryngopharyngeal sensory thresholds and submucosal nerve hypertrophy on histology, strengthening the neurological explanation.[10,11] These changes are thought to cause altered vagally mediated resting laryngeal tone. LPR is thought to play a role in this process.[12-15]

45.3 Presentation

Although stridor caused by laryngomalacia may be present at birth, the typical clinical course begins with normal breathing at birth and inspiratory stridor appearing by age 2 to 3 weeks. In some cases stridor may appear as late as several months of age. The severity of the stridor and airway obstruction may then increase gradually, plateauing by age 4 to 6 months. Most cases thereafter gradually improve until complete resolution by age 2 years. The stridor is described as an inspiratory high-pitched fluttering sound usually worse in the supine position with improvement when placed face down (this maneuver is used clinically to help characterize the stridor).

There are also other subtypes of laryngomalacia presenting differently such as late-onset laryngomalacia,[16-18] exercise-induced laryngomalacia,[19,20] and laryngomalacia presenting as obstructive sleep apnea.[21-24] These cases are managed differently but when surgery is indicated the same surgical principles as in infant laryngomalacia are applied.[17,25-27]

45.4 Symptoms

Activities increasing respiratory demands such as crying, feeding, agitation, and physical activity worsen the stridor. Airway obstruction with overt dyspnea is the hallmark of severe laryngomalacia and a clear indication for surgery. The work of breathing in moderate-to-severe cases often causes FTT, making severity more apparent. In the more severe cases apneic events and cyanosis may be present. Even in milder cases, patients may suffer from an array of feeding difficulties which may include dysphagia, choking episodes, and regurgitation that may also lead to FTT.

Comorbid conditions often associated with laryngomalacia include gastroesophageal reflux disease (GERD)/LPR, obstructive sleep apnea, neurologic or neuromuscular disease.[28-30]

These comorbidities may directly affect the management of laryngomalacia.

Pectus excavatum, cor-pulmonale, and pulmonary hypertension may develop in severe longstanding cases, secondary to chronic obstruction and must be evaluated preoperatively in order to avoid operative and postoperative complications.

Incidence of synchronous airway lesions (SALs) ranges from 12% to 50% and therefore thorough examination of the entire airway is mandatory.[31-34]

Many classifications and categorizations have been proposed for laryngomalacia.[35-38] The purpose of classification is to create a common language to describe and assess severity, assist with the management decision-making process, and in cases operated on to help apply appropriate pathology-specific tailored surgery. The classifications refer to both static and dynamic findings on endoscopy. Both of these elements are necessary towards understanding each child's specific pathology and thus enabling correct surgical treatment. We find most useful the classification of Monnier who divides laryngomalacia into three types which associate with three different supraglottoplasty elements.

Type I: Inward collapse of aryepiglottic folds on inspiration.

Type II: Curled tubular epiglottis with shortened aryepiglottic folds, which collapses circumferentially on inspiration.

Type III: Overhanging epiglottis that collapses posteriorly, obstructing the laryngeal inlet on inspiration.

Diagnosis is usually confirmed by awake, office flexible laryngoscopy. Although this usually provides an accurate assessment, "sleep endoscopy" consisting of flexible fiberoptic laryngoscopy under general anesthesia with spontaneous breathing may be superior in providing the most accurate view of the true dynamic pathology.[39,40]

Less common laryngomalacia may appear at later age, present as cause or partial cause of OSA, and may be better recognized using sleep endoscopy.[16,17,21,22]

45.5 Indications for Surgery

Clinical assessment of laryngomalacia severity is best when viewed as a spectrum. The severity of laryngomalacia must be assessed firstly and most importantly based on its clinical effect on breathing, feeding, development, and growth and any other systemic parameter attributable to laryngomalacia. Flexible endoscopy is not only crucial for confirming diagnosis but also is an important adjunct to grade severity. One must correlate the clinical with endoscopic severity and when a discrepancy is seen, seek other pathology.

Indications for supraglottoplasty are severe stridor with respiratory compromise, feeding difficulties, FTT (when other causes are ruled out), and obstructive sleep apnea. Severe respiratory distress with suprasternal retractions, hypoxemia, or hypercapnia requires urgent surgery. The management of the laryngomalacia patient should be done by an aerodigestive team which may include a pediatrician, pediatric pulmonologist, pediatric gastroenterologist, pediatric intensivist, pediatric dietician/nutritionist, speech pathologist, social worker in addition to other professionals depending on comorbidities. Decision-making should be performed jointly after assessment and discussion with the team. Parents must be involved in the process and counseled. They must be provided with all pertinent information regarding their child's health status, treatment options, complications, and realistic expectations. When the decision to perform surgery has been made, they must sign on informed consent.

45.6 Preoperative Evaluation and Anesthesia

When the decision to perform surgery has been made, the patient undergoes a thorough anesthesiologist evaluation. As with all pediatric airway procedure, precise, fine-tuned teamwork with all professionals in the operating suite is of utmost importance and a prerequisite for proceeding with the surgery. Pediatric airway surgery proposes a unique challenge to the anesthesiologist who must at times have the patient without a definitive airway, must "share" the airway with the otolaryngology surgeon, and good surgeon-anesthesiologist team-work cannot be over stressed.

The preferred surgical procedure is endoscopic supraglottoplasty, which is the focus of this chapter. When contraindicated the other surgical option is tracheotomy, which is described elsewhere.

45.7 Supraglottoplasty

Endoscopic supraglottoplasty is performed via suspension laryngoscopy under general anesthesia using spontaneous breathing. The anesthesiologist may use any of a large variety of methods to ventilate as needed, including bag ambo, intermittent LMA (laryngeal mask), intermittent intubation, jet ventilation. It is not in the scope of this chapter to fully describe anesthetic technique for pediatric airway surgery.

45.8 Airway Safety

If the appropriate setting for performing safe airway surgery is lacking, transferring the patient to an appropriate center should be considered including intubation or tracheotomy to secure the airway for transport.

45.9 Stages of Surgery

Setup for standard airway surgery: Setup should include preparation of endotracheal tube (ETT) in place over a narrow (2.7–2.9 mm) rigid endoscope, should urgent intubation be required during the procedure.

Tooth guard in place: Use an intubation blade laryngoscope to gain direct vision of the larynx.

Application of topical lidocain 2% at a volume of 0.2 mL/kg to supraglottis and glottis.

Preceding suspension laryngoscopy, perform preliminary rigid endoscopic examination with 4 mm 0 degree optics with blade laryngoscope to assess laryngeal structures, rule out any unexpected anomaly,[41] observe degree of obstruction in order to allow anesthesiologist a view of the airway.

Perform suspension laryngoscopy with a supraglottoscope (Benjamin-Lindholm laryngoscope or Parson laryngoscope) to achieve optimal exposure of the entire pharyngolarynx allowing surgical access to all supraglottic structures. The laryngoscope must be carefully positioned with the anterior blade in the vallecula, so as not to distort the epiglottic position or form. In order to achieve optimal exposure of the entire surgical field one may at times need to adjust degree of neck extension, at times removing extension totally. One may also apply pressure to the anterior neck at the cricoid level (similar to Selik maneuver) to help bring anterior laryngeal structures into direct view. This maneuver may be sustained during surgery by applying tape across the neck securing this position.

Once optimal exposure has been obtained, the airway should be examined by rigid endoscopy including the subglottis and trachea to rule out additional airway lesions.[31,42]

Bring the operating microscope with 400 mm lens into place. We find the work with the CO_2 laser most accurate with minimal collateral damage for supraglottoplasty. This surgery has also been described using cold metal instruments, microdebrider, and coblation, and the surgeon must choose the tool he is most comfortable with and the tool that in his hands brings the best results.[43,44]

As mentioned the surgery is best performed under general anesthesia with spontaneous breathing without an ETT. Due to the small size of the larynx when an ETT is in place the structures may be distorted and access to precise areas of resection difficult and therefore it is not recommended. Ideally, spontaneous breathing can be maintained with oxygen applied through side piece of suspension laryngoscope and/or via nasal airway. Another technique is to operate in an apneic state using intermittent intubation to re-oxygenate the patient. In this technique careful intubation is required with a small ETT (at least 0.5 of size less than the estimated ETT size for this patient).

When working with CO_2 laser, all necessary safety precautions must be taken, including covering the patient's exposed areas with wet drapes or gauze, using safety goggles, etc.

Use of the CO_2 laser may begin after reduction of O_2 supply when anesthesiologist confirms FIO_2 drops below 40% to prevent potentially disastrous airway fire, and give OK to proceed.

CO_2 laser settings: Superpulse mode. Continuous or 10 Hz repetitious rate. Power should be set at 1.5–2.5. An additional suction should be placed through laryngoscope to evacuate smoke from laser use.

The tools used to manipulate the mucosa to be resected to bring in line with the laser include microlaryngoscopic triangular lt/rt graspers, micro-Hartman (alligator) forceps, laser-protected suction tube, as needed.

45.10 Type of Supraglottoplasty[45–47]

45.10.1 Type 1

Surgery should be tailored according to specific dynamic pathology. In type 1 laryngomalacia the redundant mucosa of arytenoid and aryepiglottic fold is removed (▸Fig. 45.1). The reduction of mucosa along with the stiffening effect of postoperative scaring combine to resolve the dynamic obstruction.

Use the triangular microforceps to gently grasp the redundant arytenoid mucosa laterally, make incision with laser medially and posteriorly, adjusting retraction medially while incising laterally. Extreme caution must be taken to spare sufficient healthy mucosa medially near the intra-arytenoid area to avoid the severe complication of citarical supraglottic stenosis. The excision of mucosa is

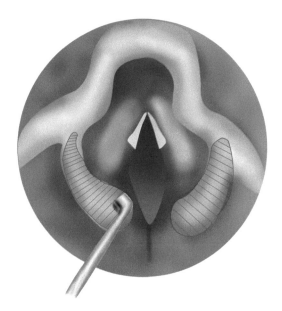

Fig. 45.1 Type 1 laryngomalacia. Resection of redundant mucosa. Must be careful to spare adequate intra-arytenoid mucosa as to prevent citarical scarring.

extended until the superior/anterior border of dissection which is the lateral base of epiglottis. The surgeon should take into account the specific anatomy of each case and may choose to excise more or less mucosa depending on the amount of mucosal redundancy. In some cases the area of excision may be limited to the corniculate area of the arytenoids, sparing incision of the aryepiglottic fold if deemed not significant in the laryngomalacia dynamics.

Care should be taken to never incise the pharyngoepiglottic fold, which can increase risk of aspiration. In addition to removing the excess mucosa, one may vaporize the cuneiform cartilage causing additional favorable scarring to approximate the edges of healthy mucosa. If bleeding should occur, hemostasis is obtained using small pledgets soaked in diluted adrenalin (1:10,000: use ampule of 1 mg/1 mL adrenalin and dilute 1 mL adrenaline into 9 mL of NaCl).

45.10.2 Type 2

In type 2 laryngomalacia (▶Fig. 45.2) the curled tubular epiglottis narrows the supraglottic inlet so the goal of surgery is to widen the inlet circumferentially by trimming the mucosa not only of the aryepiglottic folds but also of the epiglottic lateral edges.

The first stage of the procedure for type 2 laryngomalacia is identical to type 1.

The dissection and removal of mucosa of the aryepiglottic folds is carried upward from the free lateral borders of the epiglottis sparing the apical rim of the epiglottis. Only a thin rim of mucosa should be removed, with being careful not to include epiglottic cartilage in the dissection. Once again care should be taken not to incise the pharyngoepiglottic fold.

45.10.3 Type 3

In type 3 laryngomalacia (▶Fig. 45.3) there is dynamic posterior collapse of the epiglottis toward the posterior glottis and posterior pharyngeal wall. This collapse causes the dynamic inspiratory obstruction.

Depending on the static and dynamic elements of the particular laryngomalacia, the surgery is planned. The addition of type 3 is epiglottopexy.[48,49]

Suspension laryngoscopy is performed carefully to obtain adequate exposure of the epiglottis, vallecula, and posterior third of base of tongue. This part of the surgery may be performed with a transnasal ETT in place, but the ETT must be protected from the laser with wet gauzes. The settings of laser are changed to a weaker power in order to enhance coagulation necrosis and reduce bleeding.

Laser settings:
- CW mode, 3 to 5 W power.
- Slightly defocused laser beam.

Using the defocused laser beam, mucosal denudation of the vallecula is performed, including the base of lingual surface of epiglottis and most posterior base of tongue. The goal is to achieve a raw surface on both sides of the vallecula, the lingual and epiglottic surfaces to cause anterior traction and stiffening of the epiglottis with scarring of denuded area. In addition, it is recommended to add two 4–0 vicryl sutures through the lingual surface of epiglottis (▶Fig. 45.4) and the base of tongue to firmly approximate the epiglottis to the base of tongue. An endoscopic needle holder is used. Placing these sutures may be challenging but the added effect is worthwhile.

The final position of the epiglottis should be an upright one without posterior prolapse on breathing. One must

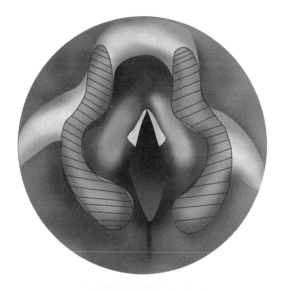

Fig. 45.2 Type 2 laryngomalacia. Extended resection of mucosa to include lateral surface of epiglottis and aryepiglottic folds.

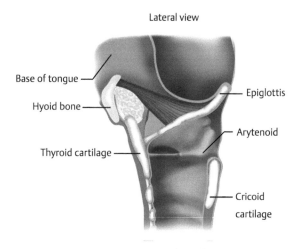

Lateral view

Base of tongue

Hyoid bone

Thyroid cartilage

Epiglottis

Arytenoid

Cricoid cartilage

Fig. 45.3 Type 3 laryngomalacia. Posterior collapse of the epiglottis toward the posterior glottis and posterior pharyngeal wall causing obstruction.

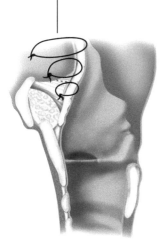

Suturing epiglottis to base of tongue

Fig. 45.4 Type 3 laryngomalacia. Perform epiglottopexy by first removing base of tongue-vallecular mucosa creating a "raw" surface. Follow by suturing epiglottis anteriorly to the base of tongue.

avoid being overly aggressive with the sutures to avoid anterior prolapse of the epiglottis in order to avoid the potential complication of postoperative aspirations.

45.11 Postoperative Treatment

When surgery has been completed the patient should be extubated with spontaneous breathing and transferred to the Pediatric Intensive Care Unit (PICU) for overnight monitoring.[50,51] In cases with comorbidities or SALs, there may be need for ventilation support with intubation and a longer PICU stay, as indicated. Corticosteroids should be initiated during surgery and continued for a few days following surgery. Antibiotics are not routinely prescribed perioperatively with the exception of cases of type 3 laryngomalacia where epiglottopexy is performed and the risk of infection is greater. Most laryngomalacia patients that require surgery have already begun anti-LPR treatment (proton pump inhibitors or H_2 antagonists) prior to surgery and should be continued until complete healing postop and resolution of symptoms. Those who were not previously treated should begin treatment perioperatively and continue through follow-up until resolution of symptoms.

45.12 Complications

Complications after supraglottoplasty are relatively rare at about 8% but meticulous care must be taken at all stages of the surgical care to keep this rate as low as possible.[29] Most complications are related to the surgical site such as aberrant scarring with band or web

formation, granulation tissue formation, bleeding, and infection. The severe complication of supraglottic stenosis has been reported at 4% and a few factors have been implicated. Excessive reduction of mucosa in the intra-arytenoid area without leaving sufficient tissue untouched is the main cause. In cases where granulation tissue forms in this area, early meticulous removal may help to prevent the excessive scarring. As discussed earlier anti-reflux treatment is mandatory in all supraglottoplasty cases and failing to treat adequately may also play a role in pathologic healing. Perioperative systemic steroids are indicated for this same reason. Unilateral supraglottoplasty has been proposed to reduce this complication rate but has not been proven to do so.[52,53] When managing an evolving complication of stenosis, removal of scar bands, dilation, and local steroid injection may be helpful. Unfortunately, supraglottic stenosis may be very difficult to treat due to the lack of rigid structures to work with and difficulty in grafting healthy tissue to expand this area. Sometimes aggressive attempts to prevent or manage the stenosis result in worsening stenosis and a decision to perform tracheostomy to allow the scarring to finalize and leave restorative surgery for a later date is legitimate and in some cases superior.

Patients with comorbidities especially neuromuscular disorders, genetic disorders, or cardiac disease are at a much higher risk for complications.[28-30] This risk must be preoperatively evaluated by the multidisciplinary team and performing a tracheostomy should be considered.[54-57] Other complications encountered are aspiration, pneumonia, and bronchiolitis. A transient dysphagia with or without aspiration has been reported in a significant number of supraglottoplasty patients but is usually self-resolved and does not require treatment.[58] Mortality is rare and is usually in complex patients with significant comorbidities.

45.13 Surgical Results

Success rates for supraglottoplasty are high and resolution of inspiratory stridor, dyspnea, and feeding difficulties should be expected.[30,59,60] The improvement in feeding and weight gain may take the longest, at times several months and anti-reflux medication should be continued through to full resolution of symptoms.[61,62] When choosing between being less or more aggressive in surgery, we recommend being on the more conservative side. When the results of surgery are not sufficient, revision surgery may be safely done without raising the risks of major complications. There are reports of 3% to 12% needing revision surgery after supraglottoplasty with rates of up to 50% for those having unilateral surgery initially.[57] The rates of complete failure requiring tracheostomy are 1% to 3% and as mentioned earlier these are usually cases with comorbidities.[63]

45.14 Highlights

a. Indications
   - Absolute:
     ○ Respiratory compromise (may include).
     ○ Pulmonary hypertension.
     ○ Cor-pulmonale.
     ○ Pectus excavatum.
     ○ Hypoxia.
     ○ Apnea.
     ○ Cyanosis.
   - Relative:
     ○ Aspiration.
     ○ Feeding difficulty failed medical intervention.
     ○ Weight loss with feeding difficulty.
     ○ Failure to thrive.
     ○ Severe obstructive sleep apnea.
b. Relative contraindications.
   - Significant comorbidity.
   - Neuromuscular disorder.
   - Cardiac anomaly.
   - Genetic disorder.
   - Synchronous airway lesion (SAL).
c. Complications.
   - Local surgical site.
   - Bleeding.
   - Aberrant scarring.
   - Granulation tissue formation.
   - Infection.
   - Supraglottic stenosis.
   - Airway related.
   - Pneumonia.
   - Acute/persistent aspiration.
   - Airway fire.
   - Failure to extubate.
   - Mortality.

References

[1] Zoumalan R, Maddalozzo J, Holinger LD. Etiology of stridor in infants. Ann Otol Rhinol Laryngol 2007;116(5):329–334
[2] Reardon TJ. Congenital laryngeal stridor. Am J Med Sci 1907; 134:242–252
[3] Holinger LD. Etiology of stridor in the neonate, infant and child. Ann Otol Rhinol Laryngol 1980;89(5 Pt 1):397–400
[4] Landry AM, Thompson DM. Laryngomalacia: disease presentation, spectrum, and management. Int J Pediatr 2012;2012:753526
[5] Holinger LD, Konior RJ. Surgical management of severe laryngomalacia. Laryngoscope 1989;99(2):136–142
[6] Roger G, Denoyelle F, Triglia JM, Garabedian EN. Severe laryngomalacia: surgical indications and results in 115 patients. Laryngoscope 1995;105(10):1111–1117
[7] Sichel JY, Dangoor E, Eliashar R, Halperin D. Management of congenital laryngeal malformations. Am J Otolaryngol 2000;21(1): 22–30
[8] Solomons NB, Prescott CA. Laryngomalacia: a review and the surgical management for severe cases. Int J Pediatr Otorhinolaryngol 1987;13(1):31–39
[9] McSwiney PF, Cavanagh NP, Languth P. Outcome in congenital stridor (laryngomalacia). Arch Dis Child 1977;52(3):215–218
[10] Thompson DM. Abnormal sensorimotor integrative function of the larynx in congenital laryngomalacia: a new theory of etiology. Laryngoscope 2007;117(6 Pt 2, Suppl 114):1–33
[11] Munson PD, Saad AG, El-Jamal SM, Dai Y, Bower CM, Richter GT. Submucosal nerve hypertrophy in congenital laryngomalacia. Laryngoscope 2011;121(3):627–629
[12] Giannoni C, Sulek M, Friedman EM, Duncan NO III. Gastroesophageal reflux association with laryngomalacia: a prospective study. Int J Pediatr Otorhinolaryngol 1998;43(1):11–20
[13] Bibi H, Khvolis E, Shoseyov D, et al. The prevalence of gastroesophageal reflux in children with tracheomalacia and laryngomalacia. Chest 2001;119(2):409–413
[14] Hartl TT, Chadha NK. A systematic review of laryngomalacia and acid reflux. Otolaryngol Head Neck Surg 2012;147(4):619–626
[15] Hadfield PJ, Albert DM, Bailey CM, Lindley K, Pierro A. The effect of aryepiglottoplasty for laryngomalacia on gastro-oesophageal reflux. Int J Pediatr Otorhinolaryngol 2003;67(1):11–14
[16] Richter GT, Rutter MJ, deAlarcon A, Orvidas LJ, Thompson DM. Late-onset laryngomalacia: a variant of disease. Arch Otolaryngol Head Neck Surg 2008;134(1):75–80
[17] Gessler EM, Simko EJ, Greinwald JH Jr. Adult laryngomalacia: an uncommon clinical entity. Am J Otolaryngol 2002;23(6):386–389
[18] Revell SM, Clark WD. Late-onset laryngomalacia: a cause of pediatric obstructive sleep apnea. Int J Pediatr Otorhinolaryngol 2011;75(2):231–238
[19] Smith RJ, Bauman NM, Bent JP, Kramer M, Smits WL, Ahrens RC. Exercise-induced laryngomalacia. Ann Otol Rhinol Laryngol 1995;104(7):537–541
[20] Mandell DL, Arjmand EM. Laryngomalacia induced by exercise in a pediatric patient. Int J Pediatr Otorhinolaryngol 2003;67(9):999–1003
[21] Smith JL II, Sweeney DM, Smallman B, Mortelliti A. State-dependent laryngomalacia in sleeping children. Ann Otol Rhinol Laryngol 2005;114(2):111–114
[22] Zafereo ME, Taylor RJ, Pereira KD. Supraglottoplasty for laryngomalacia with obstructive sleep apnea. Laryngoscope 2008; 118(10):1873–1877
[23] Goldberg S, Shatz A, Picard E, et al. Endoscopic findings in children with obstructive sleep apnea: effects of age and hypotonia. Pediatr Pulmonol 2005;40(3):205–210
[24] Chan DK, Truong MT, Koltai PJ. Supraglottoplasty for occult laryngomalacia to improve obstructive sleep apnea syndrome. Arch Otolaryngol Head Neck Surg 2012;138(1):50–54
[25] Mandell DL, Arjmand EM. Laryngomalacia induced by exercise in a pediatric patient. Int J Pediatr Otorhinolaryngol 2003;67 (9):999–1003
[26] Golz A, Goldenberg D, Westerman ST, et al. Laser partial epiglottidectomy as a treatment for obstructive sleep apnea and laryngomalacia. Ann Otol Rhinol Laryngol 2000;109(12 Pt 1):1140–1145
[27] Valera FC, Tamashiro E, de Araújo MM, Sander HH, Küpper DS. Evaluation of the efficacy of supraglottoplasty in obstructive sleep apnea syndrome associated with severe laryngomalacia. Arch Otolaryngol Head Neck Surg 2006;132(5):489–493
[28] Day KE, Discolo CM, Meier JD, Wolf BJ, Halstead LA, White DR. Risk factors for supraglottoplasty failure. Otolaryngol Head Neck Surg 2012;146(2):298–301
[29] Denoyelle F, Mondain M, Gresillon N, Roger G, Chaudre F, Garabedian EN. Failures and complications of supraglottoplasty in children. Arch Otolaryngol Head Neck Surg 2003;129(10):1077–1080, discussion 1080
[30] Thompson DM. Laryngomalacia: factors that influence disease severity and outcomes of management. Curr Opin Otolaryngol Head Neck Surg 2010;18(6):564–570
[31] Dickson JM, Richter GT, Meinzen-Derr J, Rutter MJ, Thompson DM. Secondary airway lesions in infants with laryngomalacia. Ann Otol Rhinol Laryngol 2009;118(1):37–43
[32] Krashin E, Ben-Ari J, Springer C, Derowe A, Avital A, Sivan Y. Synchronous airway lesions in laryngomalacia. Int J Pediatr Otorhinolaryngol 2008;72(4):501–507
[33] Schroeder JW Jr, Bhandarkar ND, Holinger LD. Synchronous airway lesions and outcomes in infants with severe laryngomalacia

requiring supraglottoplasty. Arch Otolaryngol Head Neck Surg 2009;135(7):647–651

[34] Rifai HA, Benoit M, El-Hakim H. Secondary airway lesions in laryngomalacia: a different perspective. Otolaryngol Head Neck Surg 2011;144(2):268–273

[35] Shah UK, Wetmore RF. Laryngomalacia: a proposed classification form. Int J Pediatr Otorhinolaryngol 1998;46(1–2):21–26

[36] Kay DJ, Goldsmith AJ. Laryngomalacia: a classification system and surgical treatment strategy. Ear Nose Throat J 2006;85(5):328–331, 336

[37] Erickson B, Cooper T, El-Hakim H. Factors associated with the morphological type of laryngomalacia and prognostic value for surgical outcomes. JAMA Otolaryngol Head Neck Surg 2014;140(10):927–933

[38] van der Heijden M, Dikkers FG, Halmos GB. The groningen laryngomalacia classification system: based on systematic review and dynamic airway changes. Pediatr Pulmonol 2015; 50(12):1368–1373

[39] Lima TM, Gonçalves DU, Gonçalves LV, Reis PA, Lana AB, Guimarães FF. Flexible nasolaryngoscopy accuracy in laryngomalacia diagnosis. Rev Bras Otorrinolaringol (Engl Ed) 2008;74(1):29–32

[40] Sivan Y, Ben-Ari J, Soferman R, DeRowe A. Diagnosis of laryngomalacia by fiberoptic endoscopy: awake compared with anesthesia-aided technique. Chest 2006;130(5):1412–1418

[41] Yuen HW, Tan HK, Balakrishnan A. Synchronous airway lesions and associated anomalies in children with laryngomalacia evaluated with rigid endoscopy. Int J Pediatr Otorhinolaryngol 2006;70 (10):1779–1784

[42] Mancuso RF, Choi SS, Zalzal GH, Grundfast KM. Laryngomalacia: the search for the second lesion. Arch Otolaryngol Head Neck Surg 1996;122(3):302–306

[43] Groblewski JC, Shah RK, Zalzal GH. Microdebrider-assisted supraglottoplasty for laryngomalacia. Ann Otol Rhinol Laryngol 2009;118(8):592–597

[44] Zalzal GH, Collins WO. Microdebrider-assisted supraglottoplasty. Int J Pediatr Otorhinolaryngol 2005;69(3):305–309

[45] Richter GT, Thompson DM. The surgical management of laryngomalacia. Otolaryngol Clin North Am 2008;41(5):837–864, vii

[46] Monnier P, ed. Pediatric Airway Surgery. Berlin, Heidelberg: Springer-Verlag; 2011: 99–106

[47] Potsic WP, Cotton RT, Handler SD, Zur KB, eds. Surgical Pediatric Otolaryngology. 2nd ed. New York, NY: Thieme Medical Publishers Inc.; 2016

[48] Whymark AD, Clement WA, Kubba H, Geddes NK. Laser epiglottopexy for laryngomalacia: 10 years' experience in the west of Scotland. Arch Otolaryngol Head Neck Surg 2006;132(9):978–982

[49] Zalzal GH, Anon JB, Cotton RT. Epiglottoplasty for the treatment of laryngomalacia. Ann Otol Rhinol Laryngol 1987;96(1 Pt 1):72–76

[50] Fordham MT, Potter SM, White DR. Postoperative management following supraglottoplasty for severe laryngomalacia. Laryngoscope 2013;123(12):3206–3210

[51] Albergotti WG, Sturm JJ, Stapleton AS, Simons JP, Mehta DK, Chi DH. Predictors of intensive care unit stay after pediatric supraglottoplasty. JAMA Otolaryngol Head Neck Surg 2015;141(8):704–709

[52] Kelly SM, Gray SD. Unilateral endoscopic supraglottoplasty for severe laryngomalacia. Arch Otolaryngol Head Neck Surg 1995;121(12):1351–1354

[53] Reddy DK, Matt BH. Unilateral vs. bilateral supraglottoplasty for severe laryngomalacia in children. Arch Otolaryngol Head Neck Surg 2001;127(6):694–699

[54] Preciado D, Zalzal G. A systematic review of supraglottoplasty outcomes. Arch Otolaryngol Head Neck Surg 2012;138(8):718–721

[55] Durvasula VS, Lawson BR, Bower CM, Richter GT. Supraglottoplasty outcomes in neurologically affected and syndromic children. JAMA Otolaryngol Head Neck Surg 2014;140(8):704–711

[56] Escher A, Probst R, Gysin C. Management of laryngomalacia in children with congenital syndrome: the role of supraglottoplasty. J Pediatr Surg 2015;50(4):519–523

[57] Hoff SR, Schroeder JW Jr, Rastatter JC, Holinger LD. Supraglottoplasty outcomes in relation to age and comorbid conditions. Int J Pediatr Otorhinolaryngol 2010;74(3):245–249

[58] Chun RH, Wittkopf M, Sulman C, Arvedson J. Transient swallowing dysfunction in typically developing children following supraglottoplasty for laryngomalacia. Int J Pediatr Otorhinolaryngol 2014;78(11):1883–1885

[59] Lee KS, Chen BN, Yang CC, Chen YC. CO_2 laser supraglottoplasty for severe laryngomalacia: a study of symptomatic improvement. Int J Pediatr Otorhinolaryngol 2007;71(6):889–895

[60] Richter GT, Wootten CT, Rutter MJ, Thompson DM. Impact of supraglottoplasty on aspiration in severe laryngomalacia. Ann Otol Rhinol Laryngol 2009;118(4):259–266

[61] Eustaquio M, Lee EN, Digoy GP. Feeding outcomes in infants after supraglottoplasty. Otolaryngol Head Neck Surg 2011; 145(5):818–822

[62] Suskind DL, Thompson DM, Gulati M, Huddleston P, Liu DC, Baroody FM. Improved infant swallowing after gastroesophageal reflux disease treatment: a function of improved laryngeal sensation? Laryngoscope 2006;116(8):1397–1403

[63] Douglas CM, Shafi A, Higgins G, et al. Risk factors for failure of supraglottoplasty. Int J Pediatr Otorhinolaryngol 2014;78(9):1485–1488

46 Unilateral and Bilateral Vocal Fold Paralysis

Carol Nhan, Jean-Paul Marie, Karen B. Zur

Summary

This chapter will describe the evaluation, management, and surgical procedures used by the senior authors for the management of unilateral vocal fold immobility (Section 46.1) and bilateral vocal fold immobility (Section 46.2), highlighting non-selective and selective laryngeal nerve reinnervations, respectively.

Keywords: Reinnervation, selective, non-selective, unilateral vocal fold immobility, bilateral vocal fold immobility

46.1 Part 1 Unilateral Vocal Fold Paralysis

Carol Nhan, Karen B. Zur

46.1.1 Introduction

Unilateral vocal fold paralysis (UVFP) presents with dysphonia (weak, breathy or hoarse voice, stridor in infants) and sometimes aspiration. The primary surgical options are injection medialization and recurrent laryngeal nerve reinnervation (RLN). Due to chance of recovery and concern for a child's developing laryngeal structures, the authors do not advocate for laryngeal framework procedures or arytenoid adduction, which carry risks of scarring or disruption of the laryngeal mechanism as well as prosthesis migration, airway obstruction and granulation formation.

46.1.2 Preoperative Evaluation

- If there is no clear etiology to explain the vocal fold immobility (history of thoracic or neck surgery, cardiopulmonary disease, etc.), an MRI or CT scan from the brainstem to the carina should be obtained to determine whether there is a lesion along the vagus or RLN.
- The symptoms and their severity will determine the treatment indicated.
  The clinical significance of the vocal fold paralysis is measured by:
  - The severity of the voice disorder as assessed by several acoustic and quality-of-life parameters including:
    - Pediatric voice handicap index (pVHI).
    - Maximal phonation time (MPT).
    - Grade-Roughness-Breathiness-Aesthenia-Strain evaluation (GBRAS) or Consensus Auditory-Perceptual Evaluation of Voice (CAPE-V).
  - Aspiration on fiberoptic endoscopic evaluation of swallowing (FEES) or videofluoroscopic swallowing study (VFSS).
  - History of pneumonia.

- Laryngoscopy or stroboscopy. Note the configuration of the vocal folds and arytenoids on laryngoscopy (example: injection medialization laryngoplasty is not as effective for a large posterior glottic gap).
- In patients with comorbidities or a history of prematurity, other factors such as breath support may be contributory. It is important to set realistic expectations regarding therapy and surgical outcomes in these patients.
- Formal swallowing assessment by a speech language pathologist (SLP).
- Medical clearance for anesthesia.
- Microlaryngoscopy and bronchoscopy with palpation of the cricoarytenoid joint to distinguish vocal fold paralysis/palsy from vocal fold fixation and to ensure there is no defect relating to intubation injury.
- Laryngeal electromyography (LEMG) to confirm chronic denervation of the affected vocal fold.

46.1.3 Surgical Options

When conservative management (voice therapy or thickening of feeds for those who aspirate) fails, surgical options are considered.

46.1.4 Injection Medialization Laryngoplasty

Introduction

Injection medialization is a temporary measure to improve glottic insufficiency and thus treat dysphonia or aspiration in vocal fold immobility. It is a good option even when there is a possibility for recovery of vocal fold function.

Preoperative Evaluation and Anesthesia

- See section 46.1.2 preoperative evaluation.
- Discussion regarding injection as a temporary treatment, and consideration of possible materials and their duration of effectiveness (short-term 2–3 months vs. long-term 1–2 years). Disclosure that injection material use in children is "off-label" use of an FDA-approved (United States Food and Drug Administration) procedure in adults.
- Injection medialization may be of limited effectiveness when the problem is caused by a large posterior glottic gap.
- Short-term injection with gel-type material often provides better voice outcomes and better plumping of

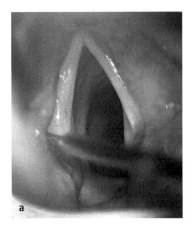
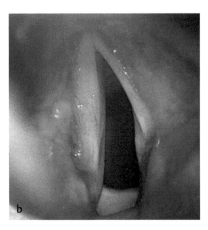

Fig. 46.1 (a) Insertion of transoral needle for an injection laryngoplasty. (b) Mild plumping noted after the injection is complete. Mild posterior subglottic stenosis is noted as well in this patient.

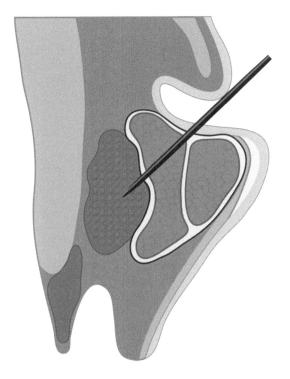

Fig. 46.2 Schematic representation of the placement of an injection material immediately lateral to the vocal fold, allowing medial displacement and plumping of the vocal fold to reduce a glottic gap. (Reproduced from Potsic, Cotton, Handler, and Zur. *Surgical Pediatric Otolaryngology*. 2nd ed. ©2016, Thieme Publishers, New York. Illustration by Susan Shapiro Brenman/Birck Cox/Eo Trueblood.)

- Suspension microlaryngoscopy or suspension with visualization of a telescope rod is used. Palpation to rule out cricoarytenoid fixation and other lesions causing immobility is performed.
- The injection material is prepared and the needle primed. Some materials come pre-packaged with a long transoral needle. Otherwise, bruning syringe or a 25-gauge butterfly needle with cut flanges and grasped with a cupped or alligator forceps may be used.
- Injection is performed anterior and lateral to the involved vocal process (▶ Fig. 46.1a). This is best done by using the side of the needle to slightly lateralize the false vocal fold on the affected side, aiming to inject lateral to the thyroarytenoid muscle (▶ Fig. 46.2). Make sure that the needle is not too deep that the material extrudes intraluminally on the undersurface of the vocal fold or too superficial such that it goes into the lamina propria causing a poor voice outcome by disrupting the mucosal wave. With gentle continuous pressure on the syringe plunger, plumping of the vocal fold and reduction of the glottis gap is achieved (▶ Fig. 46.1b and ▶ Video 46.1).

Postoperative Treatment

- No postoperative restrictions are necessary.
- The family should be advised that the voice may be strained in the first 2 weeks.

46.1.5 Highlights

a. Indications
  - Dysphonia or aspiration secondary to vocal fold immobility or paralysis with glottic insufficiency.
b. Contraindications
  - Medical contraindication to general anesthesia.
c. Complications
  - Inadequate or no improvement in dysphonia/dysphagia; foreign body reaction with certain injection materials; low risk of over-injection and airway compromise in infants.

the vocal fold in children compared to the longer-term more viscous injectates.
- Spontaneous ventilation without endotracheal tube by anesthesia is recommended. Insufflation via an endotracheal tube placed in the hypopharynx may be helpful.

Surgical Technique

- Vocal fold mobility is assessed before deepening anesthesia.

d. Special intraoperative considerations
   – Spontaneous ventilation with insufflation, deepened plane to anesthesia to prevent laryngospasm. While unlikely to impact laryngeal EMG (electromyography) recordings, the author does not routinely use 2% lidocaine topical spray for patients undergoing an EMG.

46.1.6 Unilateral Ansa Cervicalis to Recurrent Laryngeal Nerve Reinnervation

Introduction

Unilateral recurrent laryngeal nerve reinnervation allows for improving posterior glottic closure at the inter-arytenoid level and maintaining increased tone of the paralyzed vocal fold to improve voice and to manage aspiration. Most commonly, one of the ansa cervicalis nerve roots is used to anastomose and innervate the affected recurrent laryngeal nerve. Since this procedure requires transection of the recurrent laryngeal nerve (RLN), it is imperative that irreversible damage to the nerve is

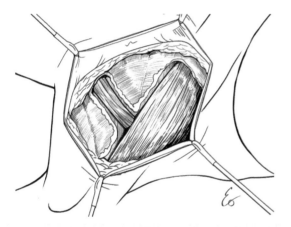

Fig. 46.3 Surgical exposure of the anterior border of the sternocleidomastoid (SCM) muscle and the omohyoid muscle. (Reproduced from Potsic, Cotton, Handler, and Zur. *Surgical Pediatric Otolaryngology.* 2nd ed. ©2016, Thieme Publishers, New York. Illustration by Susan Shapiro Brenman/Birck Cox/Eo Trueblood.)

ascertained before proceeding. This is confirmed with an intraoperative laryngeal EMG (electromyography). Often, patients have already undergone an injection medialization laryngoplasty to confirm its effectiveness before deciding to undergo a more definitive surgery such as a unilateral recurrent laryngeal nerve reinnervation.

Preoperative Evaluation and Anesthesia

- See above section 46.1.2 preoperative evaluation.
- A laryngeal electromyography (LEMG) is obtained intraoperatively to confirm paralysis.
- This procedure is generally performed in conjunction with a temporary vocal fold injection medializaton to allow for immediate improvement while reinnervation takes effect.
- No paralysis to allow nerve stimulation.

Surgical Technique

- A shoulder roll is placed and the head turned to the opposite side. Standard prepping and draping is performed.
- Mark the point along the sternocleidomastoid (SCM) where the omohyoid muscle crosses the carotid sheath. This is the midpoint of your curvilinear incision (approx. 3 cm). Subplastysmal flaps are elevated.
- The anterior border of the SCM is dissected to allow posterior retraction and the omohyoid muscle is dissected where it crosses under the SCM and is retracted medially and inferiorly (▶Fig. 46.3).
- The ansa cervicalis can be found overlying the internal jugular vein (IJV). Its inferior loop and its branches (to omohyoid, sternohyoid, and sternothyroid) are located (▶Fig. 46.4a, b and ▶Video 46.2). A nerve stimulator may be used to confirm the integrity of the ansa cervicalis donor nerve roots.
- Next, the RLN is identified in the tracheoesophageal groove by elevating the straps from the thyroid gland (from a lateral approach), and dissecting caudal to the inferior pole of the ipsilateral thyroid lobe (▶Fig. 46.5 and ▶Video 46.3). In cases where the nerve is not easily found, you may need to identify it at its insertion into larynx by the cricothyroid joint after reflecting the superior thyroid pole inferiorly

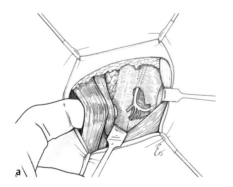
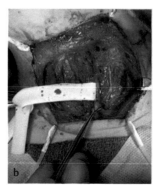

Fig. 46.4 (a) Schematic representation of the ansa cervicalis branches and the tunnel created by dissection of the strap muscles. (Reproduced from Potsic, Cotton, Handler, and Zur. Surgical Pediatric Otolaryngology. 2nd ed. ©2016, Thieme Publishers, New York. Illustration by Susan Shapiro Brenman/Birck Cox/Eo Trueblood.) **(b)** Surgical exposure of the ansa cervicalis branches, and retraction of the strap muscles using a penrose drain.

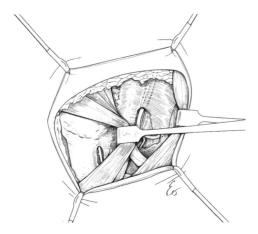

Fig. 46.5 Schematic representation of the exposure of the recurrent laryngeal nerve after retraction of the strap muscles off of the inferior thyroid gland. (Reproduced from Potsic, Cotton, Handler, and Zur. *Surgical Pediatric Otolaryngology*. 2nd ed. ©2016, Thieme Publishers, New York. Illustration by Susan Shapiro Brenman/Birck Cox/Eo Trueblood.)

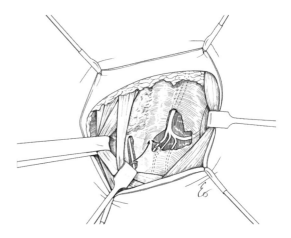

Fig. 46.6 Schematic representation of the arc of rotation of the cut donor ansa cervicalis branch and the cut recurrent laryngeal nerve. (Reproduced from Potsic, Cotton, Handler, and Zur. *Surgical Pediatric Otolaryngology*. 2nd ed. ©2016, Thieme Publishers, New York. Illustration by Susan Shapiro Brenman/Birck Cox/Eo Trueblood.)

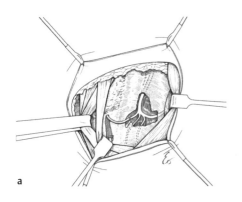

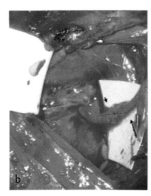

Fig. 46.7 (a) Schematic representation of the anastomosis of the recurrent laryngeal nerve and ansa cervicalis. (Reproduced from Potsic, Cotton, Handler, and Zur. *Surgical Pediatric Otolaryngology*. 2nd ed. ©2016, Thieme Publishers, New York. Illustration by Susan Shapiro Brenman/ Birck Cox/Eo Trueblood.) **(b)** Surgical depiction of the anastomosis. *Arrow end* shows the recurrent laryngeal nerve, the *arrow* shows the ansa cervicalis branch.

and medially and performing retrograde dissection to achieve a nerve segment that is 1 to 2 cm to ensure tension-free anastomosis. Care should be taken to avoid injury to the parathyroid glands.

- A tunnel is created under the strap muscles to allow anastomosis between the ansa cervicalis and RLN (▶Fig. 46.6 and ▶Video 46.4). A ¼-inch penrose may be used to retract the straps medially so that the anastomosis can be performed with good exposure of both nerves.
- A sterile-draped microscope and microinstruments are used to perform the anastomosis (▶Fig. 46.7 a, b and ▶Video 46.5).
- Determine which ansa cervicalis branch has the best caliber match to the RLN, verifying that it can be mobilized to create a tension-free anastomosis. Transect it distally.
- Transect the RLN with a 1- to 2-cm stump to allow rotation toward the lateral neck.
- The author tags both nerves with a micro-ligature clip so that the nerve does not retract, making it difficult to find. Once ready for the actual microneurography, the ligature is cut and the nerve edge freshened.

- Use a BV 100–4, 9–0 monofilament nylon suture to approximate the epineuria of the proximal ansa cervicalis nerve end to the distal RLN nerve end. Depending on the nerve caliber, one suture or two sutures placed at two points approximately 180 degrees apart can be used. Tissue glue may be placed around the anastomosis.
- Remove the penrose drain retractor and lay the strap muscles back over the anastomosis.
- The straps, platysma and skin are closed. No drain is needed.

Postoperative Treatment

- Patients are discharged on the day of surgery with no significant limitations.
- The child is allowed to resume the diet that they were cleared to have preoperatively. That is, if a child was on a thickened liquid diet due to aspiration, then she should continue that diet until cleared postoperatively for an un-restricted diet. If the diet was not restricted, then it can be resumed postoperatively with no re-evaluation by the swallowing specialist.

- The voice will likely be strained for 1 to 2 weeks due to the injection. Then, the family should expect the voice to worsen once the temporary injection resorbs in about 2 to 3 months. Improvement in voice from the reinnervation will start to show 3 to 6 months postoperatively and should gradually improve over the next 18 to 20 months.

46.1.7 Highlights

a. Indications
  - Persistent dysphonia or aspiration secondary to *confirmed* vocal fold paralysis with glottic insufficiency unresponsive to medical management.
b. Contraindications
  - Medical contraindication to general anesthesia, extensive postsurgical neck scarring with inability to identify the RLN stump; vocal fold scarring.
c. Complications
  - Inadequate or lack of improvement in dysphonia/dysphagia; wound infection.
d. Special preoperative considerations
  - Workup for etiology if unclear; confirm UVFP with LEMG; consider injection medialization for immediate symptomatic improvement.
e. Special intraoperative considerations
  - No paralysis to be given to patient.
f. Special postoperative considerations
  - It can take 3 to 20 months to hear full voice benefit.

Suggested Readings

Alghonaim Y, Roskies M, Kost K, Young J. Evaluating the timing of injection laryngoplasty for vocal fold paralysis in an attempt to avoid future type 1 thyroplasty. J Otolaryngol Head Neck Surg 2013;42:24

Arviso LC, Johns MM III, Mathison CC, Klein AM. Long-term outcomes of injection laryngoplasty in patients with potentially recoverable vocal fold paralysis. Laryngoscope2010;120(11):2237–2240

Butskiy O, Mistry B, Chadha NK. Surgical interventions for pediatric unilateral vocal cord paralysis: A systematic review. JAMA Otolaryngol Head Neck Surg 2015;141(7):654–660

Cates DJ, Venkatesan NN, Strong B, Kuhn MA, Belafsky PC. Effect of vocal fold medialization on dysphagia in patients with unilateral vocal fold immobility. Otolaryngol Head Neck Surg 2016;155(3):454–457

Farhood Z, Reusser NM, Bender RW, Thekdi AA, Albright JT, Edmonds JL. Pediatric recurrent laryngeal nerve reinnervation: A case series and analysis of post-operative outcomes. Int J Pediatr Otorhinolaryngol 2015;79(8):1320–1323

Li M, Chen S, Wang W, et al. Effect of duration of denervation on outcomes of ansa-recurrent laryngeal nerve reinnervation. Laryngoscope 2014;124(8):1900–1905

Lisi C, Hawkshaw MJ, Sataloff RT. Viscosity of materials for laryngeal injection: A review of current knowledge and clinical implications. J Voice 2013;27(1):119–123

Miaśkiewicz B, Szkiełkowska A, Piłka A, Skarżyński H. Assessment of acoustic characteristics of voice in patients after injection laryngoplasty with hyaluronan. Otolaryngol Pol 2016;70(1):15–23

Paniello RC, Edgar JD, Kallogjeri D, Piccirillo JF. Medialization versus reinnervation for unilateral vocal fold paralysis: A multicenter randomized clinical trial. Laryngoscope 2011;121(10):2172–2179

Setlur J, Hartnick CJ. Management of unilateral true vocal cord paralysis in children. Curr Opin Otolaryngol Head Neck Surg 2012;20(6):497–501

Smith ME, Houtz DR. Outcomes of laryngeal reinnervation for unilateral vocal fold paralysis in children: Associations with age and time since injury. Ann Otol Rhinol Laryngol 2016;125(5):433–438

Smith ME, Roy N, Houtz D. Laryngeal reinnervation for paralytic dysphonia in children younger than 10 years. Arch Otolaryngol Head Neck Surg 2012;138(12):1161–1166

Smith ME. Pediatric ansa cervicalis to recurrent laryngeal nerve anastomosis. Adv Otorhinolaryngol 2012;73:80–85

Stephenson KA, Cavalli L, Lambert A, et al. Paediatric injection medialisation laryngoplasty: Recent Great Ormond Street Hospital experience. Int J Pediatr Otorhinolaryngol 2017;100:86–90

Zur KB, Carroll LM. Recurrent laryngeal nerve reinnervation in children: Acoustic and endoscopic characteristics pre-intervention and post-intervention. A comparison of treatment options. Laryngoscope 2015;125(Suppl 11):S1–S15

Zur KB, Cotton S, Kelchner L, Baker S, Weinrich B, Lee L. Pediatric Voice Handicap Index (pVHI): A new tool for evaluating pediatric dysphonia. Int J Pediatr Otorhinolaryngol 2007;71(1):77–82

Zur KB. Recurrent laryngeal nerve reinnervation for unilateral vocal fold immobility in children. Laryngoscope 2012;122(Suppl 4):S82–S83

46.2 Part 2 Bilateral Vocal Fold Paralysis

Carol Nhan, Karen B. Zur, Jean-Paul Marie

Most cases of pediatric Bilateral vocal fold paralysis (BVFP) present at birth. Due to chance of recovery and desire to avoid disruption of a growing laryngeal framework, management strategies in pediatrics are unique. For these reasons, the authors do not advocate for procedures that could permanently affect vocal function such as cordotomy or cordectomy, arytenoidectomy, vocal fold lateralization and type II thyroplasty.

When there is no obvious iatrogenic etiology, an MRI brain is needed to rule out an Arnold–Chiari malformation. Imaging from base of skull to mediastinum will rule out lesions along the vagus and recurrent laryngeal nerves.

In cases of respiratory distress, a tracheostomy is sometimes necessary; however there are numerous other options. In infants, a cricoid split and stenting (see Chapter 47 that refers to endoscopic cricoid split and stenting with endotracheal tube) may provide sufficient augmentation of the airway. Open or endoscopic laryngotracheal reconstruction (see Chapter 49) with placement of a posterior cartilaginous graft is an excellent method of augmenting the posterior airway in patients with bilateral vocal fold immobility. Placing a small enough posterior graft (usually no more than 2 mm width is needed in a child) can help prevent significant voicing issues and possible aspiration in these children.

Botox injection into laryngeal adductor muscles has been described in a few case series. Its premise is that weakening synkinetic innervation to the thyroarytenoid and lateral cricoarytenoid would allow better unopposed abduction by the posterior cricoarytenoid muscles. Currently this appears to provide marginal airway improvement.

Laryngeal pacing is a procedure undergoing clinical trials that uses an external pacemaker implanted into the chest wall to stimulate the posterior cricoarytenoid muscle. Trials employing unilateral pacing in patients with BVFP show promising ventilation outcomes without sacrifice to voice.

46.2.1 Bilateral Selective Recurrent Laryngeal Nerve Reinnervation

Introduction

This procedure is an exciting concept for reinnervating the nerves that are either paralyzed or exhibiting synkinetic motion abnormalities. Bilateral selective recurrent (BSR) allows physiologic abduction of the vocal folds with breathing. It uses a root of the phrenic nerve to innervate the posterior cricoarytenoid (PCA) muscles and stimulate abduction with each breath. The diaphragm is unique, in that it is the only inspiratory muscle that functions during involuntary breathing including sleep. A nerve graft is needed to connect a root of the phrenic nerve to the PCA by implantation of the nerve graft into the muscle (neurotization). The interposition nerve graft used is the greater auricular nerve since it has a bifurcation which allows just one single phrenic nerve root to reinnervate both the right and left PCA muscles. To augment vocalization and interfere with laryngeal synkinesis, anastomosis of the RLNs to the thyrohyoid branch of the hypoglossal nerve is also performed bilaterally. This is a lengthy and intricate surgery that will likely continue to gain momentum in the years to come.

Preoperative Evaluation and Anesthesia

- If the etiology is unclear, obtain MRI imaging of the brain down to mediastinum.
- Pulmonary reserve should be ascertained by a pulmonary function test (PFT) since a branch of the phrenic nerve will be used.
- A laryngeal electromyography (LEMG) is obtained intraoperatively to confirm paralysis before proceeding. Residual synkinetic innervation does not preclude BSR.
- Antibiotic prophylaxis is provided intraoperatively.
- No paralysis is given during surgery to allow nerve stimulation.

Surgical Technique

- Position with a shoulder roll for neck extension, midline. Prepare and drape widely up to the preauricular/cheek region and down below the clavicles.
- Perform a tracheostomy if patient doesn't already have one.
- A curvilinear incision at the level of the cricoid cartilage or slightly higher is made, staying a good distance from the tracheostomy site. Subplatysmal flaps are raised to the level of the hyoid and to the clavicles.
- The right sternocleidomastoid muscle (SCM) is dissected and the omohyoid muscle located and sectioned. The phrenic nerve is located deep to the posterior belly of the omohyoid muscle, overlying the anterior scalene muscles posterolateral to the carotid artery and jugular vein.
- Retrograde dissection of the right phrenic nerve is performed to find the nerve roots. The uppermost root is used to allow adequate remaining innervation to the diaphragm. Nerve stimulation of the roots is helpful to confirm the chosen root as well as ensure good contraction of the diaphragm with stimulation of the remaining roots. Once identified, place a thread around the chosen phrenic nerve root (▶ Fig. 46.8).
- Next, the right thyrohyoid branch off the hypoglossal nerve is identified at its insertion into the posterolateral aspect of the thyrohyoid muscle, 1 to 2 cm from the hyoid bone (▶ Fig. 46.9a, b). This nerve is very tiny and confirmed by nerve stimulation. Retrograde dissection is performed and a thread is gently and loosely placed around it.

- The right recurrent laryngeal nerve (RLN) is identified. In cases where there is scarring from previous surgery, identification at its insertion into larynx with retrograde dissection is performed. This is facilitated by rotation of the larynx with a hook on the posterior border of the thyroid alar cartilage, palpation of the cricothyroid joint as a landmark, and splitting the cricopharyngeal muscle to find the RLN deep to the inferior horn of the thyroid cartilage. Retrograde dissection of the recurrent laryngeal nerve is performed. Care should be taken to avoid injury to the parathyroid glands.
- The posterior cricoarytenoid (PCA) muscle is exposed posteriorly.
- A retrocricoid tunnel is made between the esophagus and the cricoid cartilage and a thread is placed through the tunnel.
- On the left side, the nerve to the thyrohyoid nerve and the RLN are dissected as above.
- Next, either the right or left greater auricular nerve is harvested all the way up to the parotid to encompass the bifurcation of the nerve. Ideally, a 7- to 8-cm graft is harvested.

- The greater auricular nerve interposition graft is placed retrocricoid. Starting in the left neck, the single end of the graft is placed on the thread that was left retrocricoid and gentle traction is used to pull it through the retrocricoid tunnel to the right.
- One arm of the "Y"-shaped interposition nerve graft is implanted into the vertical fibers of the left PCA muscle using a 9–0 monofilament nylon suture and tissue glue.
- The left RLN is transected, leaving enough length to anastomose its distal end to the proximal end of the left nerve to thyrohyoid (if the length is insufficient, an interposition free nerve graft will be needed). The nerve anastomosis is performed with 1 to 2 stitches through the epineurium using a 9–0 (BV100–4) monofilament nylon suture, and tissue glue may be placed around the anastomosis.
- Now the same anastomoses are performed on the right: the other arm of the "Y"-shaped interposition nerve graft is implanted into the vertical fibers of the right PCA, and the distal end of the transected right RLN is anastomosed to the proximal end of the nerve to thyrohyoid (with interposition graft as needed).
- On the right, a tunnel is created below the jugular vein or carotid artery.
- The chosen phrenic nerve root is transected and anastomosis of its proximal end is made with the single end of the greater auricular transposition nerve graft.
- The platysma and skin are closed. No drain is needed. ▸ Fig. 46.10 shows the overview of the anastomoses.

Postoperative Treatment

- Patients are admitted for approximately 1 week postoperatively with decannulation at approximately postoperative day 5 (there is immediate improvement of the laryngeal airway due to relaxation associated with section of the RLNs).
- It takes 6 to 9 months for nerve function due to the long interposition graft and time required to regenerate along its length.
- Normally, patients do not have dysphagia and swallowing assessment is not required unless clinical symptoms present.

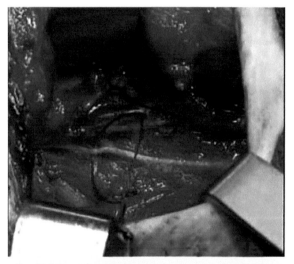

Fig. 46.8 Loop placed around the chosen upper phrenic nerve root.

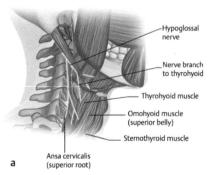

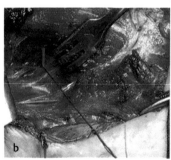

Fig. 46.9 (a) Schematic representation of the thyrohyoid nerve branch. (b) The right thyrohyoid branch off the hypoglossal nerve is identified at its insertion into the posterolateral aspect of the thyrohyoid muscle, 1 to 2 cm from the hyoid bone.

Hypoglossal nerve

Nerve branch to thyrohyoid

Thyrohyoid muscle

Omohyoid muscle (superior belly)

Sternothyroid muscle

Ansa cervicalis (superior root)

a

b

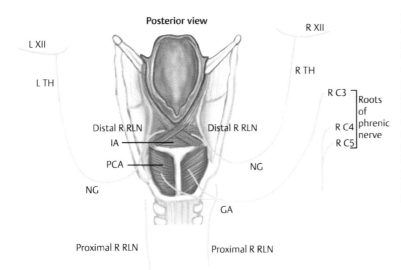

Posterior view

Fig. 46.10 Diagrammatic illustration of bilateral selective laryngeal nerve reinnervation. C3-5 cervical nerve roots of the phrenic nerve; XII, hypoglossal nerve; GA, greater auricular nerve interposition graft; IA, interarytenoid muscle (in this diagram representing the insertions of the RLN into the intrinsic laryngeal muscles except the cricothyroid); NG, cable nerve graft (used if insufficient length to anastomose TH to distal RLN, often a branch of the ansa cervicalis is used); PCA, posterior cricoarytenoid muscle; RLN, recurrent laryngeal nerve; TH, thyrohyoid nerve branch.

46.2.2 Highlights

a. Indications
   - *Confirmed* BVFP of irreversible cause with airway compromise otherwise requiring a tracheostomy.
b. Contraindications
   - Medical contraindication to general anesthesia; extensive postsurgical neck scarring causing inability to identify RLN stumps; poor pulmonary reserve/function.
c. Complications
   - Inadequate or lack of airway improvement; dysphagia; wound infection.
d. Special preoperative considerations
   - Workup for etiology if unclear; confirm BVFP with LEMG; confirm good pulmonary reserve.
e. Special intraoperative considerations
   - No paralysis given during the surgery.
f. Special postoperative considerations
   - Reinnervation effect takes 4+ months.

Suggested Readings

Ekbom DC, Garrett CG, Yung KC, et al. Botulinum toxin injections for new onset bilateral vocal fold motion impairment in adults. Laryngoscope 2010;120(4):758–763

Engin O, Ipekci F, Yildirim M, et al. Phrenic-recurrent nerve anastomosis in animal models with unilateral cutting of the recurrent nerve. Indian J Surg 2010;72(5):362–366

Li M, Chen S, Zheng H, et al. Reinnervation of bilateral posterior cricoarytenoid muscles using the left phrenic nerve in patients with bilateral vocal fold paralysis. PLoS One 2013;8(10):e77233

Li Y, Garrett G, Zealear D. Current treatment options for bilateral vocal fold paralysis: A state-of-the-art review. Clin Exp Otorhinolaryngol 2017;10(3):203–212

Marie JP. Reinnervation: New frontiers. In: Diagnosis and Treatment of Voice Disorders. 4th ed. By John S. Rubin, Robert T. Sataloff, Gwen S. Korovin. Plural Publishing Inc., 2014

Marie JP, Lacoume Y, Laquerrière A, et al. Diaphragmatic effects of selective resection of the upper phrenic nerve root in dogs. Respir Physiol Neurobiol 2006;154(3):419–430

Marina MB, Marie JP, Birchall MA. Laryngeal reinnervation for bilateral vocal fold paralysis. Curr Opin Otolaryngol Head Neck Surg 2011;19(6):434–438

Mueller AH. Laryngeal pacing for bilateral vocal fold immobility. Curr Opin Otolaryngol Head Neck Surg 2011;19(6):439–443

Mueller AH, Hagen R, Pototschnig C, et al. Laryngeal pacing for bilateral vocal fold paralysis: voice and respiratory aspects. Laryngoscope 2017;127(8):1838–1844

Ongkasuwan J, Courey M. The role of botulinum toxin in the management of airway compromise due to bilateral vocal fold paralysis. Curr Opin Otolaryngol Head Neck Surg 2011;19(6):444–448

Smith ME, Park AH, Muntz HR, Gray SD. Airway augmentation and maintenance through laryngeal chemodenervation in children with impaired vocal fold mobility. Arch Otolaryngol Head Neck Surg 2007;133(6):610–612

47 Endoscopic Airway Surgery

K. A. Stephenson, M. E. Wyatt

Summary

Advances in instrumentation and anesthetic techniques have expanded the boundaries of endoscopic airway surgery. Specialized microinstruments, the dilating balloon, laser, and powered microdebrider are key tools. Primary endoscopic surgery has several advantages over an open approach including potential for improved vocal outcomes and avoidance of the morbidity of an external incision. The need for tracheostomy, intensive care, and hospital stay may also be reduced.

This chapter focuses upon the concepts, considerations, and equipment relating to endoscopic, 'minimally invasive, and endoluminal airway surgery. Careful patient selection and preoperative planning is essential. Significant disorders of the laryngotracheal framework are more likely to be successfully treated by open surgery while endoluminal concerns may be better suited to an endoscopic approach. The role of endoscopic surgery as an adjunct to open airway surgery is well acknowledged. As with open surgery, the individual surgeon's experience and the resources of the institution in which care is delivered are crucial considerations along with the personal circumstances of the patient and family.

Keywords: Airway lasers, airway anesthesia, balloon dilatation, endoscopy, cricoid split, graft, infant, child, endoscopes, microdebrider, Coblation

47.1 Introduction

47.1.1 History and Evolution

While endoscopic airway surgery is very much a current "hot topic" and exciting area of pediatric ENT, it has a long history. Endoluminal techniques have been used to dilate and treat laryngotracheal stenosis since the 19th century. Inspired and innovative approaches were devised to tackle the effects of infections–namely diphtheria – and trauma. In the 1920s and 1930s the advancement of electrically heated esophageal bougies and the placement of upper airway stents were explored. The concept of scar tissue incision by a "laryngeal dilating knife" followed in the 1950s. The pace of development of airway surgery in the 20th century was driven by two main factors: the intensive care and increased survival of premature infants accompanied by advancements in technique. The survival of premature infants was associated with the need for prolonged endotracheal intubation of a vulnerable airway, which could result in significant acquired laryngotracheal stenosis, principally of the glottis and subglottis.

Endoluminal "minimally invasive" techniques logically evolved alongside open laryngotracheal surgery. From the 1970s onwards, procedures to correct laryngotracheal stenosis developed and progressed rapidly. These open laryngotracheal framework expansion surgeries and the related use of stents were frequently associated with the development of endoluminal granulation tissue and stenosis at anastomotic sites; these pathologies are naturally accessible endoscopically. Outcomes of open surgery can be improved by the use of subsequent endoscopic procedures, which allow for visualization of areas of concern and intervention if necessary.

In order for endoscopic airway surgery to be feasible, the surgeon needs to be able to assess the pathology to be operated upon and then maintain this exposure in order to perform surgery. The operating microscope has been the traditional workhorse for surgery of the supraglottis and glottis and enables both depth perception and two-handed working. The advent of the rigid endoscope, the Hopkins rod, revolutionized the direct visualization of the subglottis and trachea. Harold Hopkins patented his lens system in 1959 however it wasn't until the later 1960s that the manufacturing and distribution of these revolutionary instruments began. The excellent image and bright illumination, coupled with a wide field of view, proved to be a new and exciting addition to the operating microscope. For the purposes of this chapter, the term "endoscopic" will be used broadly to cover all endoluminal surgery, regardless of whether the microscope or rigid endoscope is used.

In the past 20 to 30 years, both the use and scope of endoscopic airway surgery have increased significantly, facilitated by better anesthetic techniques, tailored instruments and "endoscopic" medications such as steroids and Mitomycin C. The 1980s saw a major interventional advance: endoscopic balloon dilatation. Previous dilatation methods included the advancement of bougies (e.g., esophageal or urethral dilators) or the rigid bronchoscope. Dilatation in this fashion relies upon the conversion of longitudinal to radial force and has the disadvantages of mucosal trauma and shearing forces. Mucosal and submucosal injury can then lead to further fibrosis and increase the likelihood of restenosis. The amount of radial pressure that can be applied is also limited and difficult to gauge.

47.1.2 Relationship of Endoscopic to Open Airway Surgery

Historically, tracheostomy has been the workhorse of airway surgery providing a means of bypassing obstruction to allow direct access for ventilation of the lungs. Pediatric ENT surgeons have concentrated both their open and endoscopic efforts either to enable decannulation or to avoid such intervention in the first place. Improvements in technology broadened the capabilities of endoscopic approaches. Coupled with the Hopkins rod endoscope and the binocular operating microscope, the tools to treat disease have become more varied. Examples include the carbon dioxide laser, which can now be delivered via a flexible fiber allowing improved access while the thulium laser has the advantage of improved hemostasis. The Coblation wand and microdebrider have delivery systems for endoscopic use and the introduction of the non-compliant airway balloon has been invaluable. Cold steel instruments such as Blitzer and lancet knives have been designed for use in the pediatric airway.

The potential advantages of an endoscopic procedure include a shorter operating time, a decreased length of intensive care, and an overall hospital stay. The morbidity of an external neck incision is also avoided. The significant effect on voice from the disruption to the laryngeal framework that occurs with open surgery, particularly the classic full laryngofissure, is well recognized; endoscopic approaches have the obvious benefit of avoiding this. The need to improve vocal outcomes seen with open surgery is acknowledged as an ongoing goal in pediatric ENT.

Another favorable aspect of the endoscopic approach is that it is possible to assess the effects of surgery on a more frequent basis and then to treat further if required. Current understanding of scar development and wound healing indicates that early and frequent intervention enhances the likelihood of a successful outcome. Direct application of adjuvant therapy (e.g., injectable or topical steroid) is also possible.

The combination of endoscopic and open approaches (combined approach or "hybrid" surgery) is a definite step forward. A more accurate midline division of a congenital laryngeal web is achieved endoscopically, while placement of an anterior cartilage graft to treat the associated subglottic stenosis requires the open approach. A further prime example is the use of the endoscope in the airway while the posterior cricoid is being divided in an open surgery; this again improves the quality of the procedure.

If the main concern to be corrected is intraluminal, this is likely to be amenable to endoscopic surgery. As a rule, if the laryngotracheal framework ("exoskeleton") is not intact, primary endoscopic surgery alone is unlikely to be successful, and this situation may be best treated by open surgery. Endoscopic cricoid splits and posterior cricoid grafting are however challenging this general principle. Endoscopic surgery as an adjunct to open surgery, for example balloon dilatation or the removal of granulations a few weeks after an open reconstruction, is well recognized as improving long-term outcomes.

This chapter is directed toward the concepts involved in endoscopic airway surgery, but it is important to balance these alongside existing and developing open techniques. Each approach has its merits and the outcome achieved for an individual patient may be best reached by either or from a combination of both. The individual surgeon's experience and that of the institution in which care is delivered are crucial considerations along with the personal circumstances of the patient and their family.

47.2 Preoperative Evaluation and Anesthesia

47.2.1 History and Examination

Once a diagnosis of upper airway pathology requiring intervention has been made, the aim of a detailed history is twofold; first, the suitability of the pathology to endoscopic surgery must be judged, and second, the patient's general eligibility for endoscopic surgery needs to be assessed.

The Pathology

Mature and congenital laryngotracheal stenoses, particularly of higher grades, are unlikely to be improved by endoscopic surgery alone. Congenital cartilaginous stenoses such as a congenital subglottic stenosis will not be improved by dilatation alone as it will not impact upon the abnormally thickened cartilage and may risk rupture.

A detailed history of previous endoscopic and open airway surgery is vital. In cases of laryngotracheal stenosis that have been treated by balloon dilatation and no degree of improvement seen, consideration of an alternative technique is suggested. Experience shows that further endoscopic dilatation is not prudent if correction of a stenosis has not been adequate after three serial dilatations, separated by a number of weeks.

It is imperative to check for secondary airway lesions such as malacia or vocal fold immobility. In combination with comorbidities, these may influence both the choice and timing of an approach and the likelihood of treatment success.

The Patient

Whether primary endoscopic, combined endoscopic and open surgery, or endoscopic surgery as an adjunct to open surgery is being considered, careful patient selection is essential. The patient's neck movement, mouth opening and dentition are all-important access considerations. In order for endoscopic airway surgery to be possible, a "line-of-sight" access is required from the lips to the operative field (▶ Fig. 47.1). Micrognathia, retrognathia, and a significant overjet (an anterior–posterior overlap of the maxillary central incisors over the mandibular central incisors) are all likely to increase the difficulty of access.

If the child has a tracheostomy this will facilitate administration of oxygen and anesthetic gases. The

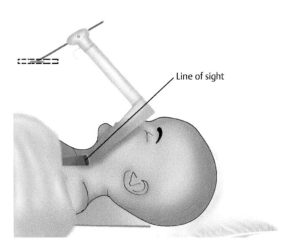

Fig. 47.1 Line of sight required for endoscopic airway surgery.

tracheostoma is also an additional potential port of access to the upper airway for the endoscope and for instruments.

As with open airway surgery, laryngopharyngeal reflux should be identified and treated. This may require medical treatment (e.g., proton pump inhibitor therapy) or in severe cases, surgical management with a gastric fundoplication. Similarly, the presence of infection within the airway should also be preoperatively identified. An infected airway is often apparent on inspection. Microbiological cultures using swabs or aspirates are recommended to enable effective treatment prior to surgery. In patients with long-term tracheostomies, airway colonization and infection is often a concern. Many experienced surgeons advise proactive investigation of infection and prophylactic antibacterial treatment prior to any airway surgery.

Deferral of surgery is advisable in cases where there is an "active larynx". This may be evidenced by generalized edema and erythema; a cobblestoned appearance of the mucosa of the epiglottic base and eversion of the laryngeal ventricles are also suggestive signs. Work in such an inflamed and reactive airway is likely to be technically more difficult in terms of visualization and surgical intervention. It also risks poorer mucosal healing with its concomitant worries of restenosis and granulation formation. An "active larynx" is known to be a risk factor for surgical failure and warrants investigation and treatment of infection, gastro-esophageal reflux disease (GERD), and eosinophilic esophagitis. In some cases, this "angry state" is idiopathic; deferral of surgical intervention and a waiting period of several months are recommended. Experts have suggested trials of a variety of anti-inflammatory medications such as steroids and antibiotics such as azithromycin.

The pulmonary, nutritive, and cardiac states of the patient should be optimized as far as possible. The age of the child may also be an important consideration, with implications for surgical access, technical feasibility, and

postoperative care. Preoperative evaluation and documentation of the patient's ability to swallow and voice is also crucial. This may not only influence surgical planning but also enable comparison of pre- and postoperative function. The monitoring and recording of these factors is an important consideration in outcome reporting, facilitating the pooling and comparison of research data.

A multi-disciplinary "airway forum" is an ideal discussion opportunity for difficult surgical cases and may aid in planning. Potential complications should be identified and postoperative care preparations made. Intensive care facilities may be required; the patient may require close airway monitoring, tracheostomy care, or remain intubated for a number of days following surgery. The surgical plan including perioperative care must be discussed in detail with the family and child, if applicable. The importance of both effective communication and the management of expectations cannot be emphasized strongly enough. This is often aided by the use of clinical photographs and diagrams.

47.2.2 Investigations

In addition to pulmonary, cardiac, and nutritive assessments of the patient, several targeted investigations may also be of use when preparing for potential endoscopic airway surgery.

Flexible Endoscopic Evaluation

Flexible laryngoscopy is particularly useful to assess dynamic abnormalities such as vocal cord immobility and laryngomalacia. This may be performed without sedation in the infant or in the older cooperative child, or under anesthesia. Per-oral passage of an endoscope may be performed in the edentulous neonate using a finger between the gums to protect the instrument. It is essential to note the basic but important point that a good laryngeal or tracheal view gained at flexible endoscopic evaluation does not translate to adequate access with the rigid endoscope and/or transoral instrumentation.

Cross-Sectional Imaging

Use of CT and MRI of the neck and chest in the preoperative preparation of the child for airway surgery varies widely from center to center. These scans may aid in the evaluation of airway lesions although they are not usually sufficiently sensitive to fully characterize a lesion or stenotic segment. Helical or multidetector CT with multiplanar and 3D reconstruction offers increasingly better definition of fixed tracheal lesions, and can provide "virtual bronchoscopy". Dynamic changes—primary and secondary tracheobronchomalacia—are not well evaluated by cross-sectional imaging. The degree, maturity, and mucosal quality of a stenosis can be more accurately assessed at endoscopy.

47.2.3 Anesthesia

Endoscopic airway surgery is a prime example of "shared airway working", which requires close cooperation and understanding between the surgeon and anesthetist. Safe, efficient, and successful surgery is facilitated by a long-term working relationship with a skilled pediatric anesthetist with a special interest in ENT.

We recommend that the anesthetist is either able to view the screen displaying the endoscopic image, or is able to view a second screen. Depth of anesthesia can be gauged not only by the presence and effort of respiration but also by the degree of vocal cord movement when the larynx is in view. Periods of airway occlusion, for example by balloon dilatation, can also be monitored. This real-time visual feedback complements the close verbal communication between surgeon and anesthetist.

Careful timing of endoscopic airway surgery involves optimization of respiratory fitness and airway irritability. Steady anesthetic conditions with good oxygenation, minimal airway secretions, and lack of mucosal inflammation are the goals. Elective surgery should be deferred in the presence of a current upper or lower respiratory tract infection. Airway irritability, predisposing to coughing, and laryngospasm may persist for a number of weeks following such an illness.

A variety of anesthetic techniques exist for endoscopic airway surgery and vary from center to center. It is probably more important that a theater team work together effectively than that one particular technique is followed. Intubation may be used at the start of the procedure in some centers; however, most units would now use spontaneous respiration throughout rather than neuromuscular blockade and paralysis. Spontaneous respiration has much to recommend itself as a technique; it maintains muscle tone, promotes gas exchange, and is essential to detect dynamic conditions.

Induction of Anesthesia

Some units will use an anticholinergic premedication such as atropine or glycopyrrhonium bromide to facilitate a dry surgical field and improve the efficacy of topical anesthesia; this may impact upon the heart rate. Perioperative steroids are a good precaution, particularly in cases of significant stenosis or when there is likely inflammation and edema. Intravenous induction is preferable for older children though gaseous induction is best in infants, younger children, those with poor venous access, and those with a precarious airway. Topical local anesthetic spray (typically lidocaine) should be applied to the vocal cords when the anesthetic level is sufficiently deep for this to be tolerated. This amount needs to be carefully measured as the preparations used in adults can easily result in overdosage.

Minimum patient monitoring includes temperature, electrocardiogram (ECG), non-invasive blood pressure, and peripheral oxygen saturation (SpO_2). Accurate monitoring of end-tidal carbon dioxide is not possible in the absence of endotracheal intubation.

Maintenance of Anesthesia

Two principal anesthetic techniques are used for general anesthesia with spontaneous respiration—maintenance with a volatile agent (e.g., sevofluorane) or total intravenous anesthesia (TIVA) with an infusion such as propofol and remifentanil.

A volatile agent and oxygen mix can maintain a level of anesthesia that allows examination and endoscopic intervention in a child who is breathing spontaneously. Sevoflurane is nonirritant to the airway and has the advantages of rapid onset and no pungency, allowing immediate delivery of high concentrations. This advantage of rapid induction may be offset by a variable effect during periods of relative hypoventilation or airway obstruction.

Airway Tube Technique

An endotracheal tube may be used as a nasopharyngeal airway or "prong' to provide oxygen and volatile anesthetic agents. This should be carefully positioned above the supraglottis (▶ Fig. 47.2). Should transnasal passage not be possible, an oropharyngeal tube may be used, placed at the corner of the mouth. A significant advantage of this non-intubation technique is that the endoscopist has a view of an airway that has not been altered by the passage of an endotracheal tube. An alternative technique is to intubate the child and withdraw the tube for periods of endoscopic work (apneic anesthesia with intermittent ventilation); this method is not routinely used in our institutions.

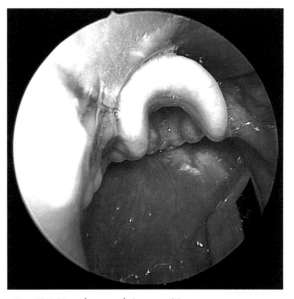

Fig. 47.2 Nasopharyngeal airway position.

Jet ventilation can allow the patient to be paralyzed, preventing coughing. In a pediatric setting it is broadly associated with barotrauma and carbon dioxide retention concerns. This practice is not widespread and use varies significantly from region to region; it is not used in our centers.

47.3 Surgical Techniques

47.3.1 Preparation and Positioning

Great care and time should be taken in the positioning of the child for endoscopic airway surgery. Positioning may significantly improve or hinder access and differs from case to case, depending on the individual anatomy and the region of the upper airway to be focused upon. Hyperextension of the neck—especially for prolonged periods of time—must be avoided, particularly in children with skeletal concerns or trisomy 21. The head must be well supported at all times. A "sniffing the morning air" position often enables good access in the older child while a more neutral position often suits the infant. The degree of soft padding required under the shoulders and/or head of the child depends on the relative size of the occiput. Sandbags or pads can be placed either side of the head to support it in a midline position, if required. A malleable "U"-shaped cushion that conforms when suction is applied is ideal for tailored positioning (▶Fig. 47.3). If suspension laryngoscopy is employed, a Mayo table or custom-made platform supports the laryngostat clear of the chest (▶Fig. 47.4).

An elastic tape secured across the larynx may improve visualization of the anterior commissure and avoid the need for an assistant to exert pressure on this area. It also provides constant pressure and avoids unwanted movement during surgery. Care should also be taken that the child's body is squarely supine on the operating table and not rotated.

47.3.2 Endoscopic Airway Evaluation

Laryngeal examination and access for endoscopic surgery is usually begun by gently inserting a laryngoscope with integrated illumination, taking care to protect the teeth and lips and to keep the tongue in the midline to provide a well-centered view. As in adults, it is important to check the overall appearance of the pharynx and supraglottis during introduction of the laryngoscope. If an endotracheal tube is present, it can be followed to the tip of the epiglottis. The epiglottis should be gently lifted forwards making certain that it does not curl up in front of the laryngoscope, preventing a complete view of the anterior commissure.

Laryngeal examination without an endotracheal tube in place provides a superior view, and by using a probe to move the arytenoids independently, the mobility of the cricoarytenoid joints can be assessed. If an interarytenoid scar is present, the arytenoids will not move independently. A posterior laryngeal cleft is assessed by passing a probing instrument between the arytenoids, comparing the lower limit of the interarytenoid groove with that of the posterior commissure, and palpating the underlying cricoid cartilage. Finally, great care should be taken when passing through the vocal cords using a rigid endoscope to inspect the subglottis, trachea, and main bronchi.

The time available for the examination will depend on the airway, the respiratory reserve, and anesthetic technique. In a child breathing spontaneously with a normal airway and normal lung function, anesthesia can be maintained solely by the use of inhalational or intravenous agents and a nasopharyngeal airway. In some cases the time may be very limited and it is essential to be prepared to move ahead with other techniques such as ventilating bronchoscopy or intubation. If there is significant laryngotracheal stenosis, use of an ultra-fine rigid endoscope is likely to cause less trauma than a bronchoscope.

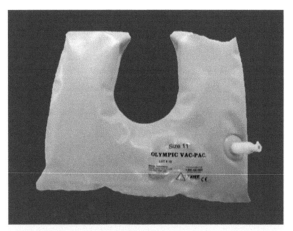

Fig. 47.3 Example of surgical positioning system—Olympic Vac-Pac, Natus GmbH, Planegg, Germany.

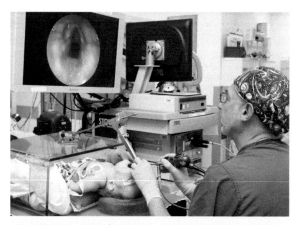

Fig. 47.4 Suspension laryngoscopy: positioning and endoscopic visualization of the larynx using a Hopkins rod rigid endoscope (This image is provided courtesy of Mr. David Albert).

47.3.3 Endoscopic Airway Surgery

General Principles

Endoscopic airway surgery is a highly technical procedure. The whole team (surgeon, anesthetist, and theatre nurses) need to work together closely. A high-definition camera coupled either to the rigid endoscope or the operating microscope with a high-definition screen is both essential for this technically demanding surgery and is also invaluable in training and team working. The anesthetist and theatre team can view the live image and may be able to anticipate interventions required.

It is important to prepare and check all equipment prior to the procedure and prepare for all eventualities. The range of Hopkins rod rigid endoscopes should include all lengths and diameters that could be needed. A 0° endoscope is most commonly used and is technically easiest to work alongside using a straight instrument. An angled 30° or 45° telescope has certain advantages; it may better assess the supraglottic larynx and provide useful visualization around and beneath a pathology, or into the laryngeal ventricle, for example.

The Hopkins rod rigid endoscope coupled to a camera head is typically held in the non-dominant hand. An instrument (e.g., probe, needle-holder, forceps, or scissors) is then used in the dominant hand. This approach restricts the surgeon to one-handed surgery, which may be technically challenging. It is also possible for the endoscope to be held by an assistant, allowing the surgeon to use instrumentation in both hands. Access and instrumental crowding may restrict this method. In comparison, use of the operating microscope enables two-handed surgery. If a microscope is used, a 400-mm lens allows the use of standard laryngeal instruments; however, a closer focal length of 300 to 350 mm may be better suited to surgery in children.

Application of topical epinephrine (1:10,000 concentration) is a key technique in endoscopic airway surgery. A neuropatty (a small flat absorbent pad on a thread) can be soaked and used as a vehicle to deliver epinephrine to the surgical site (▶Fig. 47.5). This reduces mucosa l edema and promotes hemostasis by vasoconstriction. It may also help to clean and better visualize the surgical field and remove charring associated with laser use. Epinephrine may also be used in the distal airway and introduced through a small flexible catheter. Use of epinephrine, even topically, should be communicated to the anesthetist.

Surgical simulation of endoscopic airway work using either animal or artificial models has potential both for training surgeons and for development of new techniques. This is becoming increasingly widespread in the teaching and assessment of otorhinolaryngologists and is likely to become more widely employed as simulation quality and availability improves.

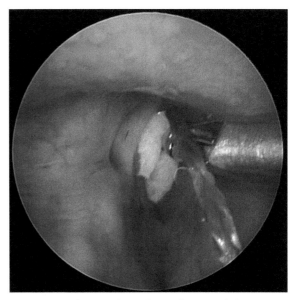

Fig. 47.5 Application of topical epinephrine to subglottic inflammation using a small neuropatty prior to endoscopic surgery.

Equipment

Laryngoscopes

Several pediatric laryngoscopes are available and can be tailored to the anatomical upper airway site to be exposed and the individual anatomy of the child. The placement of the tip of the laryngoscope can be varied according to laryngoscope type and surgical exposure needed. Careful adjustment of the laryngoscope to achieve optimal exposure is time very well spent prior to commencement of any endoscopic surgery. Small alterations in laryngoscope depth in the vallecula may result in significant improvements or deteriorations in epiglottic position. In cases with difficult transoral laryngeal access—often those with craniofacial abnormalities and a significant overjet or retrognathia—a right-sided paraglossal approach may be useful. It is often necessary in difficult cases to trial several sizes and shapes of laryngoscopes in order to achieve the best possible access, along with adjustments in patient positioning.

Parsons laryngoscopes are specifically designed for the pediatric airway with a broad, flat upper blade, a wide proximal opening, and a side opening to accommodate instrumentation. Gas delivery through a side port and suspension laryngoscopy is possible. They are ideal for diagnostic work and can be used for endoscopic surgery, with the side opening facilitating instrumental access. Other specialized pediatric laryngoscopes include the Lindholm-Benjamin, Kleinsasser, and Holinger-Benjamin laryngoscopes. The Lindholm-Benjamin laryngoscope is particularly suited to suspension laryngoscopy and lends itself to endoscopic airway surgery, offering a wide view of the larynx and good working space. ▶Fig. 47.6 shows examples of pediatric laryngoscopes.

Microinstruments

A variety of microlaryngeal instruments is essential for successful endoscopic airway surgery. Choice of instrument is very much tailored to the task. The Bouchayer set describes a collection of many of these tools. Recommended microinstruments include:

- Endoscopic needle holder (e.g., Lichtenberger, Kleinsasser).
- Vocal fold retractor forceps ("laryngeal spreader").
- Endoscopic knot pusher.
- Alligator forceps.
- Cupped forceps.
- Heart-shaped forceps.
- Endoscopic scissors: straight, angled, and curved.
- Probes.
- Elevators.
- Fine rigid suction.
- Endoscopic knives (e.g., lancet knife, sickle knife, Beaver blade, Blitzer knife).

"Laryngeal spreaders" are a vital microinstrument for endoscopic airway surgery and warrant special mention (▶Fig. 47.7). They may be placed either with the instrument handle toward the floor of the operating room or may be inverted and suspended from the laryngostat when the patient is in a suspension laryngoscopy position. Different sizes and shapes of laryngeal spreader are available. This instrument can be carefully placed to retract either the false vocal cords or the true cords and is often crucial for good exposure of the glottis and subglottis, for example for an endoscopic laryngeal cleft repair or a posterior cricoid split.

Sutures with a small needle and with long thread length are best suited to endoscopic suturing. Matching of the length and curvature of the needle to the endoscopic suturing task is likely to improve what is a technically demanding task.

Laser

Historically the workhorse laser used in endoscopic airway surgery has been the carbon dioxide (CO_2) laser, coupled to the operating microscope by a micromanipulator. It has a depth of penetration of 0.9 mm and its thermal effect can be limited by careful choice of settings; low power, small spot size, and use in short and interrupted pulses ("ultra-pulse" mode) are all advantageous. Specific advantages of the CO_2 laser include its hemostatic action on small vessels, its delivery from the microscope, and that it does not crowd the operative field. Precise microsurgical action can be achieved. Drawbacks include the need for direct line of sight (when used with a micromanipulator), cost and setup considerations, and crucially, the associated risk of airway fire and burns.

Carbon dioxide laser use is well established in a wide range of endoscopic airway procedures, such as supraglottoplasty, arytenoidectomy, and cordotomy, radial incision of a stenosis, and the debulking and/or excision of upper airway tumors. As with any technique, maximum preservation of mucosa is essential as large defects will heal principally by secondary intention and thus be prone to fibrosis and contracture.

Laser safety is of highest importance and a full description is beyond the scope of this chapter. We aim to highlight the central considerations. In brief, the operating room personnel must have specific training for its use and the operating room must be appropriately prepared and designed for laser use—signage, "black-out" of doors and windows, eye protection, and smoke evacuation equipment are some of the many important preparations. Other precautions include the protection of the

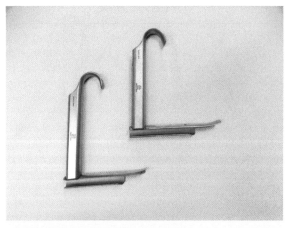

Fig. 47.6 Parsons laryngoscopes.

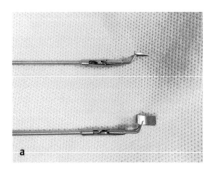

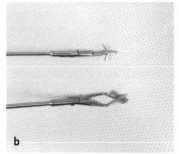

Fig. 47.7 (a, b) Vocal fold retractor ("Laryngeal spreader") forceps: lateral and superior views.

patient's eyes, face, and chest with moist swabs or towels. Checking of both the laser machine and the beam alignment is mandatory. A further essential component of laser safety is the action plan in the event of airway fire. This includes immediate extubation (if applicable), saline application into the airway, and the removal of supplementary oxygen.

There are numerous anesthetic considerations for laser use. The oxygen content in the anesthetic gas delivered should be decreased as far as possible. If an endotracheal tube or tracheostomy tube is in place, this should be as "laser-safe" as possible. If there is danger of laser "overshoot," which could strike either normal distal mucosa or an endotracheal tube, moistened neuropatties can be placed in this area as a protective barrier.

Use of the micromanipulator-coupled CO_2 laser beyond the subglottis has been described; however, its potential for distal application is very limited. A flexible delivery system for the CO_2 laser has been developed and enabled bronchoscopic use. A number of other lasers can also be used by flexible delivery systems and used for application in the lower airway, for example in the distal trachea and bronchi. This flexible fiber can either be directed through the bronchoscope or directed by a handheld instrument to a target point at close range. These include the potassium-titanyl-phosphate (KTP) laser and the Nd:YAG (neodymium-doped yttrium aluminum garnet) laser, which have particular hemostatic advantages and are useful for vascular lesions. Another laser with desirable properties and increasing use in the pediatric airway is the thulium laser; it is reported to have more controllable effects, can be fiber-delivered, and has good ablative properties with a small margin of coagulation.

Powered Microdebrider

Use of the microdebrider has significantly expanded endoscopic surgical capabilities and in many situations offers an alternative to laser use. The integrated suction, coupled with endoscopic or microscopic control, enables precise visualization and work. Contamination of the upper airway by blood and debulked material is also reduced. With careful application, mucosal trauma is minimized when compared to a "cold steel" instrumental technique. Through choice of working length, tip angulation, and "ferocity" (skimming or cutting type) of the debriding blade, the microdebrider can be tailored to the endoluminal task. Having evolved from initial ENT use in sinus surgery, several microdebriders for laryngeal and tracheal work have been developed.

The microdebrider is typically introduced transorally. Trans-stomal use in patients with an existing tracheostomy has also been described; this is particularly advantageous in the removal of a suprastomal granuloma. It is ideal for the debulking of recurrent respiratory papillomatosis and has become part of the standard of care for this disease. Advantages over the carbon dioxide laser in

treatment of recurrent respiratory papillomatosis have been found to include reductions in procedure time and postoperative pain alongside good disease clearance.

Other expanding applications of the microdebrider include use in select cases of subglottic hemangioma, suprastomal collapse, granulation tissue, cysts, and other endoluminal tumors. A skimming-type blade is particularly suitable to fine work on a soft pathology, such as a papilloma, while a more aggressive cutting blade lends itself to debulking of mature granulomata and stenotic tissue.

Coblation

Like the powered microdebrider, the Coblation wand is directly applied to tissues under endoscopic vision. Deriving its name from "controlled ablation," this relatively new medical technology achieves the removal of tissue at a relatively low temperature and with some hemostasis. A thin plasma layer of 100 to 200 μm thickness is generated at the working tip of the instrument by the application of electrical energy to normal saline, supplied by an integrated delivery system. The handpieces ("wands") are available in varying sizes and the action is foot pedal–controlled with ablation and coagulation modes. Coagulation is achieved by electrocautery between fine metal bars at the working tip. Integrated suction retrieves the saline and is a useful adjunct. Coblation also avoids the risk of airway fire associated with laser use.

Robotics

Transoral robotic surgery (TORS) use is gradually expanding in the head-and-neck surgical field. In select centers TORS application to pediatric airway surgery has been explored, given the appealing potential advantages of tremor-free, controlled and delicate working in difficult to reach areas. Attempted robotic-assisted surgeries include endoscopic laryngeal cleft repair, posterior cricoid split, arytenoidectomy, and cordotomy. Successful management of upper airway benign tumors, lymphatic malformations, and saccular cysts has also been described. Limited transoral access in the child has been found to be a key factor and in the few reported cases to-date, a fair proportion needed to be abandoned due to these constraints. Robotic technology will however progress; smaller and more sophisticated equipment is likely to lead to increasing interest and applications in airway surgery.

Examples of Endoscopic Airway Surgery

Uncapping of Subglottic Cysts

Subglottic cysts are a frequent cause of postextubation upper airway obstruction in the neonate, particularly in cases of prolonged intubation related to prematurity. It is thought that the process of mucosal damage from

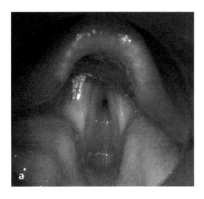
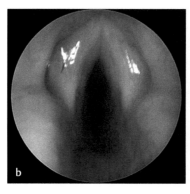

Fig. 47.8 (a, b) Uncapping of subglottic cysts: pre- and postoperative views.

intubation and subsequent healing leads to obstruction of the ducts of the mucous glands, alongside the potential development of subglottic stenosis. These cysts may be multiple and occlude the airway, requiring emergency surgery. Following an endoscopic diagnostic assessment, topical epinephrine is applied to the area. Microinstruments such as cupped forceps and microscissors are then used to uncap the cysts, taking care to avoid tearing of the mucosa toward the true vocal cords (▶Fig. 47.8). Use of the powered microdebrider has been described for subglottic cyst surgery; however, it is typically necessary for a working edge to be created by a microinstrument before the microdebrider can be engaged. Repeat applications of topical epinephrine are used during and following the debulking to reduce bleeding and improve visualization. Vocal cord spreaders can be used to improve visualization of the subglottis, if needed. It is important to assess whether the cysts are associated with a subglottic stenosis; balloon dilatation and serial endoscopies may be indicated.

Balloon Dilatation

Several types of balloon have been used for endoscopic airway dilatation. Balloon angioplasty catheters were initially applied and have been followed by airway-specific balloons. A noncompliant balloon is recommended to achieve effective and safe airway dilatation; this expands to a fixed diameter and then varies radial pressure at this set size. In comparison, a compliant balloon will continue to expand with increasing pressure and may therefore be associated with over-stretching of the airway and a greater risk of rupture. The size and length of the balloon is matched to the purpose; a variety of balloon lengths (e.g., 2/4 cm) and diameters (e.g., 4–10 mm) are available for pediatric use.

Careful balloon sizing is crucially important. Undersizing will lead to a suboptimal effect while over-sizing risks undesirable soft-tissue damage and airway rupture—principally within the closed cricoid ring—as demonstrated in animal models. Similarly, complete tracheal and bronchial rings are associated with significant danger of rupture. In the initial years of endoscopic balloon dilatation use, choice of balloon size has been

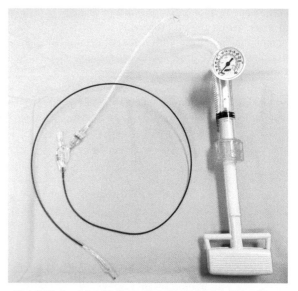

Fig. 47.9 Example of balloon dilatation apparatus (Powerflex Pro PTA [percutaneous transluminal angioplasty] catheter, Cordis, Cardinal Health Inc. Dublin, Ohio, USA).

based on individual experience, reflective of the normal airway size expected for the age of the child, the diameter of the airway and stenosis as gauged by endotracheal tube size and the stenosis site. Evidence is building in this area; an example of a balloon size guideline based on a large number of clinical cases uses the outer diameter of an age-appropriate endotracheal tube plus 1 mm for the larynx or subglottis and plus 2 mm for the trachea (Great Ormond Street Hospital 2017).

Titration and optimization of the pressure applied by the balloon is a second variable. The balloon must be inflated with water and not air, with care that air has been expelled from the inflation circuit. A compatible balloon inflation device with integrated pressure gauge is required (▶Fig. 47.9). A size-specific pressure guide in atmospheres typically accompanies the balloon, given that balloons may have varying properties according to size and degree of compliance.

Test inflation of the balloon prior to use is not necessary and unfurls the balloon from its manufactured low-profile, streamlined shape that facilitates passage through a tight stenosis. The balloon is advanced to the area of stenosis under direct endoscopic visualization and placed evenly across the narrowed airway segment. As the balloon has very narrow connecting tubing, it is easy to observe the balloon with the endoscope for the entire duration of the procedure. Stabilization of the balloon may be necessary as it can be prone to "watermelon seeding" (slippage out of the stenotic segment either proximally or distally when inflated). ▶ Fig. 47.10 shows placement of a balloon into an immature subglottic stenosis. The recently developed Aeris balloon (Tracoe medical GmbH, Germany) aims to avoid this slippage by "gripping" the stenosis; two "hubs" appear at either end of the balloon upon inflation and aim to lock the balloon in place across the stricture. A series of multiple dilatations may be of use within the same surgical episode (e.g., two to three times), with endoscopic monitoring of the result after each intervention.

The dilatation time is a further area of uncertainty. As balloon dilatation results in complete upper airway obstruction, the duration of use is typically limited and dictated by desaturation. Pre-oxygenation is recommended to combat this. Dilatation times of 30 to 120 seconds are typically reported.

Endoscopic radial incision of a stenosis prior to balloon dilatation can increase efficacy. This was published in the 1980s and continues to be cited as a useful technique. Several radial incisions are made in a circumferential stenosis, with maximum preservation of the mucosal bridges between these incisions (▶ Fig. 47.11). These are typically three ("Mercedes Benz emblem type") or four incisions in a concentric stenosis. Given the concern of thermal injury and subsequent increased fibrosis, "cold steel" incision may be preferable to laser incision, if technically feasible.

Endoscopic balloon dilatation is particularly useful for the primary treatment of immature, acquired laryngotracheal stenoses and is a common adjunctive procedure following open airway surgery. To achieve effective dilatation in the anterior glottis, for example, after division of an anterior web, a further useful tip is to place a small dilating balloon anterior to an endotracheal tube.

Endoscopic Cricoid Splits and Grafts

Anterior and posterior cricoid splits were first performed by open surgery. With increased endoscopic surgical capabilities and confidence came the realization by pioneers of pediatric airway surgery that these procedures could be performed endoscopically. These techniques are providing an alternative to open laryngotracheal surgery in a proportion of cases and also have advantages over ablative procedures to increase the laryngeal airway such as cordotomy and arytenoidectomy.

An endoscopic cricoid split can be either anterior, posterior, or both, and is guided by the pathology. For example, a posterior glottic stenosis may be best treated by a posterior cricoid split and grafting while combined anterior and posterior splits have been found to achieve airway expansion in some infants with bilateral vocal cord palsies. A particular benefit of the anterior cricoid split is its ability to enable extubation and avoid tracheostomy in select cases of the intubated neonate (▶ Fig. 47.12).

Endoscopic cricoid splits require adequate access in suspension laryngoscopy. The mucosa is prepared by topical vasoconstriction. Local anesthetic with epinephrine injection of the mucosa over the cricoid plate has also been suggested as helpful in reducing mucosal bleeding. Vocal cord spreaders provide essential exposure.

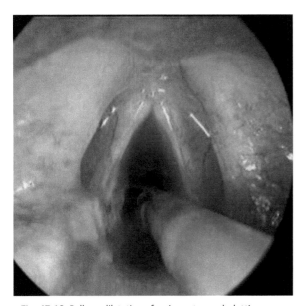

Fig. 47.10 Balloon dilatation of an immature subglottic stenosis.

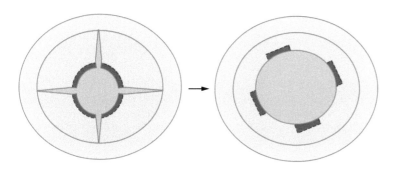

Fig. 47.11 Radial incision of a stenosis prior to balloon dilatation ("Shapshay's endoscopic technique").

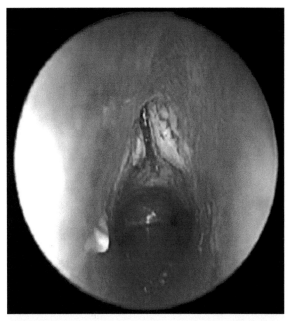

Fig. 47.12 Completed endoscopic anterior cricoid split.

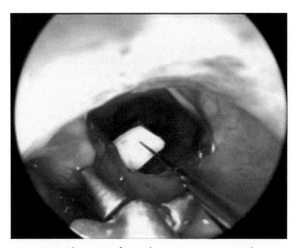

Fig. 47.14 Placement of an endoscopic posterior cricoid rib graft.

Gentle pre-split balloon dilatation is advocated by some surgeons with the aim of compressing mucosal edema. A number of instruments can be used to divide the cricoid cartilage including CO_2 laser, endoscopic knives, and scissors. Gentle external pressure on the neck angulates the anterior cricoid plate more vertically and facilitates its division. Use of a cold steel technique enables tactile feedback to determine when the split is complete. Post-split balloon dilatation then aims to expand the opened cricoid ring. In cases where both an anterior and posterior splits are to be performed, it is sensible to perform the posterior split first so that bleeding from the anterior split does not obscure the operative field posteriorly.

Endoscopic placement of a costal cartilage graft into the posterior cricoid gives greater framework

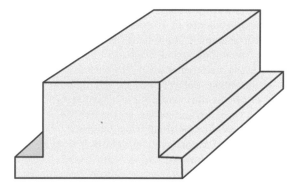

Fig. 47.13 Posterior cricoid rib graft shape.

expansion. The rib graft is fashioned into a "keystone" or "T" shape in order to sit as securely as possible within the posterior cricoid gap (▶Fig. 47.13, ▶Fig. 47.14). Placement of this graft is technically challenging and may require some force. The graft width needs to be carefully balanced so that it is wide enough to achieve sufficient expansion and to be held tightly in place by the cricoid cartilage, but not overly broad so as to risk significant deterioration in voice and swallowing function. Balloon inflation anterior to the graft has been proposed as a useful tip to "click" the graft into place. This has been described as a two-stage procedure and as a tracheostomy-avoiding single-stage surgery, where the patient remains intubated for several days postoperatively.

In cases of open surgery, which are often dictated by the need for significant framework expansion and anterior grafting, the cricoid split and laryngofissure position can still be marked endoscopically; this may better protect the anterior commissure and achieve a more accurate midline split.

Other common pediatric airway surgeries that employ endoscopic techniques are covered in detail in this section: bronchoscopy, aryepiglottoplasty, surgery for vocal cord paralysis, surgery for papillomatosis, and laryngeal cleft repair.

Adjuncts
Mitomycin C

This is an antibiotic derived from a strain of actinomyces that is metabolized into an alkylating compound. It impedes fibroblast proliferation by inhibition of DNA and protein synthesis and is used as chemotherapy for several malignancies, including urological and ophthalmological tumors. It can be used as a topical agent in the pediatric airway with the hope that the quality of mucosal healing is improved and the risk of restenosis thus reduced. The degree of efficacy of Mitomycin C continues to be a topic of clinical debate. Its use is widespread but may vary significantly from center to center. Given the complexity of factors that influence clinical outcomes with patients with upper airway disease, it is difficult for high-quality supporting evidence to be generated. Despite multiple animal and human studies, uncertainties include the dosage, the duration, and frequency of application, and whether the area treated should be cleansed with saline post-application. Delayed wound healing and development of a bulky fibrin layer in the area of application are reported concerns, and may be particularly significant in the obstruction-prone small pediatric airway. The long-term effects of Mitomycin C have also been cited as a potential worry; however, in over 20 years of use a single case of carcinoma of the larynx has been documented in an adult patient who had previously received topical Mitomycin C. No systemic toxicity has been reported in relation to topical upper airway use.

Steroids

Corticosteroids have multiple complex and wide-ranging anti-inflammatory effects. The desirable properties of glucocorticoids, such as dexamethasone and prednisolone, include inhibition of collagen synthesis and reduction of fibroblast activity. Intralesional injection using a long-acting steroid (e.g., triamcinolone) may be employed during or following endoscopic airway surgery with the aim of improving outcome through a reduction in subsequent fibrosis. Steroid can be applied topically as either a liquid or ointment while systemic steroids should be used in short courses to avoid significant side effects that include adrenal suppression, growth retardation, and Cushingoid features. As with Mitomycin C, it is difficult to discern the exact efficacy of this adjuvant treatment without adequately powered randomized controlled trials.

Stents

Success in airway surgery for laryngotracheal stenosis depends upon the stability of the postoperative airway. Stents may be employed in the hope of supporting the new shape and/or preventing the recurrence of scarring. Stents are associated with a number of inherent drawbacks, including granulation tissue and biofilm formation, stent migration, and the need for a secure airway. Any period of stenting should be limited as far as possible. An endotracheal tube can function as a short-term stent and has a greater role in single-stage airway surgery where laryngotracheal framework support is required. Stenting, other than by intubation, is far less frequently associated with primary endoscopic airway surgery.

Numerous types of airway stent have been used and continue to evolve. The anatomical region, the nature of the surgery, stent cost, and availability alongside surgeon preference dictate stent choice. Segments of endotracheal tube, which may be oversewn at either end, can be employed. Silastic or silicone sheet can be a useful material and is particularly useful in the avoidance of re-webbing at the anterior commissure. Preformed keels, laryngeal molds, and solid stents are also options. Naturally, solid upper airway stents necessitate a covering tracheostomy while hollow stents should be used with extreme caution if a tracheostomy is not in place. Stent migration or occlusion risks disastrous consequences.

47.4 Postoperative Treatment

To successfully undertake endoscopic procedures in the pediatric airway it is vital to have the appropriate care setting. It is well recognized that there can be postoperative issues with airway swelling and bleeding; identification of these problems and early intervention is essential.

A high-care (HDU) setting is recommended with the support of an intensive care unit (ICU) ideal. The administration of steroid such as dexamethasone at a weight-appropriate dose and nebulized epinephrine can smooth the immediate postoperative recovery. Overnight stay is typically advisable but highly dependent on the nature of the case.

Early endoscopic review following endoscopic surgery is linked to successful outcomes. Repeat visualization under general anesthetic with further intervention such as balloon dilatation within a few weeks of the initial procedure should be considered. The general consensus is that if a favorable outcome has not been achieved by three surgeries then an alternative open technique should be considered.

47.5 Highlights

a. Indications
   - Endoluminal pathologies such as laryngeal clefts, masses and stenoses are frequently suited to endoscopic airway surgery.
   - Endoscopic surgery can assist an open surgical procedure.
   - Potential advantages include avoidance of external incisions, decreased length of intensive care, and overall hospitalization.
   - Voice outcomes may be improved if a laryngofissure is avoided.
b. Contraindications
   - Poor access can prevent endoscopic surgery.
   - Significant disorders of the laryngotracheal framework are likely to be more successfully treated by open surgery.
   - Higher-grade mature stenoses are unlikely to be significantly improved by endoscopic surgery alone.
c. Complications
   - Surgery in the inflamed larynx is linked to poorer healing outcomes.
   - Special considerations relate to laser safety.

- Intraoperative complications may include bleeding, airway deterioration, pneumothorax (rib graft harvest), and airway rupture (balloon dilatation).
- Postoperative complications are procedure-specific.
- Serial procedures may be necessary.

d. Special preoperative considerations
- Pulmonary, nutritive, and cardiovascular optimization is recommended prior to surgery.
- Preoperative flexible and rigid endoscopic evaluation facilitates planning.
- Antibiotics and antireflux treatment may be advisable.
- Voice and swallowing assessments should be undertaken.

e. Special intraoperative considerations
- Close working with the anesthetic and theatre team is required.
- A range of pediatric laryngoscopes and microinstruments should be available.
- Endoscopic and microscopic visualization options should be considered.
- Techniques such as balloon dilatation have been significant advances.
- Vocal cord retractors are a useful tool.

f. Special postoperative considerations
- Appropriate care settings may vary from a general ward to high or intensive care.
- Short-term steroid administration can reduce postoperative airway edema.
- Early postoperative endoscopic review is often helpful.

Suggested Readings

Cotton RT, Seid AB. Management of the extubation problem in the premature child. Anterior cricoid split as an alternative to tracheotomy. Ann Otol Rhinol Laryngol 1980;89(6 Pt 1):508–511

Dahl JP, Purcell PL, Parikh SR, Inglis AF Jr. Endoscopic posterior cricoid split with costal cartilage graft: A fifteen-year experience. Laryngoscope 2017;127(1):252–257

De S, Bailey CM. Trends in paediatric airway surgery: a move towards endoscopic techniques. J Laryngol Otol 2010;124(4):355–360

Monnier P, ed. Pediatric Airway Surgery. Management of Laryngotracheal Stenosis in Infants and Children. Berlin, Heidelberg: Springer-Verlag; 2011

Quesnel AM, Lee GS, Nuss RC, Volk MS, Jones DT, Rahbar R. Minimally invasive endoscopic management of subglottic stenosis in children: success and failure. Int J Pediatr Otorhinolaryngol 2011;75(5): 652–656

Rutter MJ, Cohen AP, de Alarcon A. Endoscopic airway management in children. Curr Opin Otolaryngol Head Neck Surg 2008;16(6):525–529

Rees CJ, Tridico TI, Kirse DJ. Expanding applications for the microdebrider in pediatric endoscopic airway surgery. Otolaryngol Head Neck Surg 2005;133(4):509–513

Sharma SD, Gupta SL, Wyatt M, Albert D, Hartley B. Safe balloon sizing for endoscopic dilatation of subglottic stenosis in children. J Laryngol Otol 2017;131(3):268–272

Wentzel JL, Ahmad SM, Discolo CM, Gillespie MB, Dobbie AM, White DR. Balloon laryngoplasty for pediatric laryngeal stenosis: case series and systematic review. Laryngoscope 2014;124(7):1707–1712

48 Surgical Approach to Juvenile Onset Recurrent Respiratory Papillomatosis

Seth M. Pransky, Jeffrey D. Bernstein

Summary

Juvenile onset recurrent respiratory papillomatosis (JORRP) is caused by human papillomavirus (HPV) types 6 and 11. Transmission is believed to occur vertically from mother to newborn at birth with slow and progressive growth of the papilloma leading to hoarseness and airway obstruction. At present there is no proven medical therapy to "cure" this infectious disease, and the mainstay of treatment is surgical debulking and use of a variety of adjuvant treatments. The goals of treatment stress conservative resection avoiding injury to critical laryngeal structures, achieving a safe and patent airway, preserving voice quality and avoiding the need for a tracheotomy, while prolonging the intersurgical interval. Multiple modalities are available for surgical resection of JORRP with no single option proving to be superior. Indeed, multiple modalities are often combined at any single procedure to optimize the debulking while ensuring no injury to the larynx. It is critical to be fully prepared for an airway emergency and to have all equipment available prior to starting the case. Since surgical resection is not curative, a variety of "adjuvant" treatments have been used in an effort to achieve durable remission or reduce disease burden. Cidofovir and Bevacizumab (Avastin) are the two most widely used intralesional injection "adjuvant" therapies. In the past it was felt appropriate to wait for "severe" disease to be present, requiring repetitive intervention for airway management prior to introducing "adjuvant" therapy. However, the senior author has advocated for early introduction of adjuvant medical therapy to help reduce the number of procedures, and reduce the likelihood of iatrogenic injury to laryngeal structures and potentially achieve durable remission. Communication and coordination with anesthesia for these procedures is critical to successfully managing the airway, as the "shared airway" concept is overtly at play in these patients. Medical personnel should be familiar with HPV as a sexually transmitted disease and understand that the future management of this disease is prevention through vaccination prior to exposure to the virus.

Keywords: Recurrent respiratory papillomatosis, human papillomavirus (HPV), cidofovir, avastin, vaccination

48.1 Introduction

48.1.1 General

Juvenile onset recurrent respiratory papillomatosis (JORRP) is the most common benign neoplasm of the aerodigestive tract. These lesions are caused by human papillomavirus (HPV) in a process marked by slow, progressive growth leading to voice changes with persistent hoarseness and, if not managed, airway obstruction. Though infectious in etiology, no proven predictive curative medical therapies have arisen to date, with surgical debulking for airway and voice preservation being the mainstay of treatment. Disease presentation varies greatly in both extent and location; lesions may be sessile or pedunculated, located in multiple locations within the airway, and focal, multifocal, or diffuse. A key characteristic of JORRP is its persistence in the basal epithelium, resulting in recurrence of the lesions or expression in previously normal-appearing tissue. The natural history is that of persistent and recurrent disease that usually requires multiple surgeries, which often can lead to both physical impairment and psychological trauma.

Although there are many surgical modalities available to treat JORPP, given the variability of involvement of laryngeal structures, no single option is best to debulk the diseased areas. Being knowledgeable about and having available a combination of tools and techniques ensure the optimal management of each unique presentation of disease. Unfortunately, surgical resection of papilloma does not lead to "cure." The average number of surgeries to remission lies near 20, and it is not uncommon for patients to have 70 to 100 or more lifetime surgeries for this condition.[1] To achieve optimal outcome, the discerning surgeon must account for the nature of the disease, assess the needs and goals of the individual patient, and guide the approach appropriately. This translates into removing disease while avoiding iatrogenic damage to the airway. True remission is likely brought about by as yet unidentified immunologic factors (▶ Fig. 48.1, ▶ Fig. 48.2, and ▶ Fig. 48.3).

48.1.2 Pathophysiology

JORRP is caused by HPV types 6 and 11. The infection is widely considered to be transmitted vertically from mother to newborn during childbirth through an infected cervix/vagina. However, delivery by C-section is not fully protective and, although far less common, C-section births can develop JORRP. Respiratory papilloma initially presents as exophytic cauliflower-like growths primarily at and around the vocal folds, but can involve both the supraglottic and subglottic/tracheal airway. Common sites of disease include: the upper and lower ventricle margins, undersurface of the vocal cord, laryngeal surface of the epiglottis, carina, bronchial spurs, nasal limen vestibule, and the nasopharyngeal surface of the soft palate.[2]

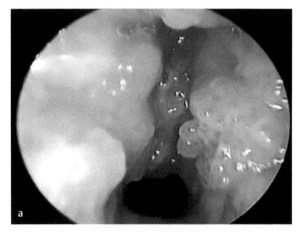
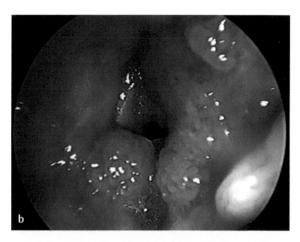

Fig. 48.1 (a, b) Diffuse papillomatosis.

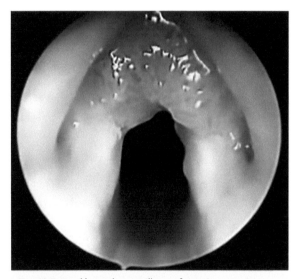

Fig. 48.2 Focal horseshoe papilloma of anterior commissure region.

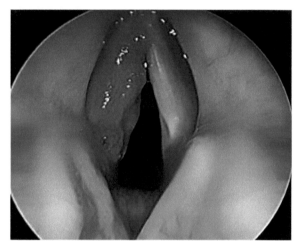

Fig. 48.3 Sessile papilloma along left true vocal cord.

48.1.3 Epidemiology

Incidence of RPP in the United States has traditionally been estimated at 4.3 per 100,000 in children and 1.8 per 100,000 in adults. However, with the introduction and wide implementation of HPV vaccination, these numbers are believed to be decreasing.[3]

48.1.4 Presentation

Initial presentation in the child occurs on average at 3 years of age, with 75% of patients diagnosed by age 5.[4] The most common presenting symptom is varying severity of progressive dysphonia, or in severe cases, progressive inspiratory or biphasic stridor. Misdiagnosis is common, as presentation may be mistaken for asthma, recurrent croup, or bronchitis. Definitive diagnosis is often delayed for up to one year from initial symptomatology.

48.1.5 Clinical Assessment

In the child with hoarseness, stridor, or airway symptoms, it is critical to distinguish JORRP from other causes of these symptoms. A comprehensive history will address the nature and timing of symptoms, history of prior airway trauma or intubation, congenital anomalies or prematurity, significant comorbidities such as gastroesophageal reflux or history of "recurrent croup", and associated symptoms. Maternal history of condyloma acuminatum or abnormal Pap testing should be elicited.

Unless acute respiratory distress is present, flexible nasolaryngoscopy with video recording should be done to identify areas of involvement and extent of disease. These images can be reviewed with the parents and shared with anesthesia prior to surgery.

Patients presenting with acute respiratory distress should be stabilized in an emergency department and taken directly to the operating room for management.

48.1.6 Patient Discussion

Once the diagnosis is confirmed histologically, the surgeon should meet with the family to discuss the natural history of JORRP along with expectations and goals of treatment, including the anticipated need for repetitive surgical debulking. Adjuvant therapies can be discussed and a schedule of planned interventions created. The impact of this chronic disease, including the potential affect on voice and the emotional and psychological burden to the patient and family should be addressed. Therefore, expectations ought to be properly framed for the patient: treatment may not be curative, repeat operations are expected, and papilloma may be left behind initially and serially removed in an effort to minimize scarring and long-term mucosal changes.

48.2 OR Preparation

The removal of laryngeal papilloma can be both challenging and stressful for all operating room personnel. Even experienced endoscopists will encounter cases that require the ability to manage an unexpectedly compromised airway.

Prior to the patient entering the OR, it is the responsibility of the surgeon to select and inspect the appropriate instrumentation, brief all involved operative personnel as to the status of the airway, and establish a well-developed plan with anesthesia with contingencies for "the unexpected."

Specifically, the surgeon and anesthesiologist must partner and discuss how best to share the airway. The goals of anesthesia include providing alveolar ventilation and anesthesia through a potentially compromised airway, while the goals of the otolaryngologist are to obtain an unobstructed view of the airway to permit removal of disease and avoid injury to non-involved tissue. To achieve these goals, the anesthesiologist should be shown a picture or drawing of the involved portion of the airway and review the degree of airway compromise. This permits a thorough discussion regarding an agreed-upon approach to the anesthetic technique (spontaneous ventilation vs. other techniques). The use of paralytic agents, such as succinylcholine, should be discussed as loss of muscle tone in a markedly obstructed larynx could result in the inability to ventilate the patient and precipitate an airway crisis. Fire risks for laser and management of FiO_2 during the procedure should also be reviewed. Ideally both the anesthesiologist and otolaryngologist should be comfortable with difficult airway management and spontaneous ventilation technique to best share and manage the airway.

48.3 OR Setup

The OR setup may vary from OR to OR but requires having all possibly needed instruments set up and available.

Table 48.1 Basic instrument needs for RRP endoscopic surgery

Instruments
Telescopes: 0° and 30°
Bronchoscopes of appropriate size
Laryngeal spreader
Ventilating laryngoscopes: Parsons; Benjamin-Lindholm
Cup forceps: straight, angled and up biting; small and large sizes
Various sized laryngeal suctions
Cotton pledget (radiographic markers)
Topical adrenaline or oxymetazoline for hemostasis
Monitor and picture/video capability
Additional supplies for laser therapy
Water basin filled with saline
Cloth wrapping for patient facial protection
Eye protection for OR personnel

The basic tools needed for RRP endoscopy are listed in ▶Table 48.1. The video monitors should be placed such that the surgeon, the scrub nurse, and anesthesiologist can see the airway during the procedure. The setup should have the O_2 saturation monitor near the surgeon and loud enough for the surgeon to hear.

48.3.1 Tools for Removal of Papilloma

Due to the variability of disease severity and location, there is no single universal modality for papilloma removal. Rather than taking a one-size-fits-all approach, individualized therapy means choosing the best combination of tools and techniques to meet the stated goals of conservative treatment. Bulky and sessile disease will be best managed with different tools. See ▶Table 48.2 for summary of advantages and disadvantages of each tool.

Microdebrider: Ideal for addressing bulky exophytic disease rapidly and efficiently. Sessile lesions and papilloma located within the ventricles or at the anterior commissure may be difficult to remove effectively and safely with the microdebrider. There are two sizes of rotating blades (2.9 and 3.5) and two types of blades available (skimmer and cutting). Most often the 2.9 skimmer blade will be used at a setting of 500 to 800 RPM. There is a learning curve when first utilizing the microdebrider to ensure no damage to normal tissue. Bleeding that occurs is best controlled with topical adrenaline or oxymetazoline on cotton pledgets (▶Fig. 48.4).

CO_2 laser: CO_2 laser ablates tissue via thermal destruction.[5] These lasers have been used for >40 years and are familiar to most laryngeal surgeons. Although still available to be coupled to a microscope with a micromanipulator, visualization with this approach is limited to line-of-sight only. Many prefer the use of a flexible

Table 48.2 Advantages and limitations of tools for papilloma removal

	Microdebrider	CO₂ laser	KTP laser	Coblation	Cup forceps
Hemastatis	No	Yes	Yes	Yes	No
Precision	Limited	Yes	Yes	Limited	Yes
Bulky disease	Yes	Only if used as "knife" to separate from underlying tissue	Only if used as "knife" to separate from underlying tissue	Yes	+/-
Sessile lesions	No	Yes	Yes	No	Yes
Maneuverability	Limited	Yes (with flexible fiber)	Yes	Limited	Yes
Biopsy	No	Yes (when used as cutting knife)	Yes (when used as cutting knife)	No	Ideal
Possible thermal damage	No	Yes	Yes	Limited	No
Additional personnel required	No	Yes	Yes	No	No
Fire hazard	No	Yes	Yes	No	No

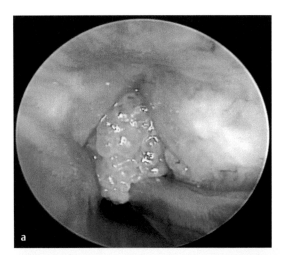
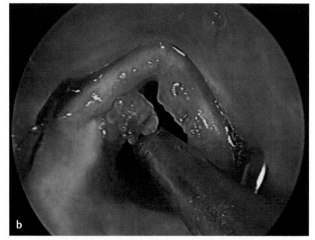

Fig. 48.4 (a, b) Microdebrider for bulky papilloma.

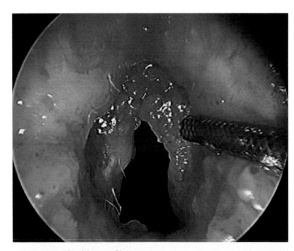

Fig. 48.5 Flexible CO₂ fiber.

fiber placed through an appropriate hand piece or suction. Working with telescopes, the flexible fiber permits access to difficult to visualize areas and is excellent for removal of sessile lesions. It is manually focused 1 to 2 mm above the papilloma and permits precision ablation of the lesions. Using the laser on bulky disease may be time consuming and the heat generated and depth of laser penetration (100–300 μm) may cause thermal injury. However, the laser can be used as a surgical knife to separate the papillomatous lesion from the underlying tissue if a clean tissue plane is available. It is best to reduce the wattage and use in pulsed delivery mode to reduce injury to deeper tissue planes (▶ Fig. 48.5).

532 nm Potassium-titanyl-phosphate (KTP) laser: An angiolytic laser which penetrates epithelium to photocoagulate microvasculature. The 532-nm wavelength targets oxyhemoglobin, disrupting blood supply while achieving hemostasis and sparing surrounding tissue.[6] The 400 to 600 μm depth of penetration is ideal for blood vessel ablation. The KTP laser settings include power, pulse width (ms), and pulse frequency. Classic settings are 30 to 35 W/15 ms/2 Hz. The KTP is available with 0.4- and 0.6-mm-sized fibers. As hemoglobin absorbs this laser wavelength, it is best used when there is no bleeding present. Bulky lesions can be difficult to manage with the KTP, yet the various benefits include the ability to manage sensitive areas such as the anterior commissure and true vocal cord, access of difficult-to-reach regions such as the ventricles or infraglottis, and its precision for small lesions and tissue-sparing properties (▶ Fig. 48.6).

Laser safety: Due to risk of catastrophic fire, the use of laser technology requires additional intraoperative personnel, equipment, and patient precautions. The Association of Surgical Technologists' Standards of Practice for Laser Safety includes the following measures:

A well-trained laser safety officer, eye protection for both OR personnel and patient, personal protective equipment, and a nonflammable teeth protector.

To prevent accidental injury to the eyes and face, the patient's head should be wrapped in a moistened towel. Combustible material must not be present in the airway when a laser is used, including an endotracheal tube (ETT) or cotton pledgets. If the patient cannot be managed with spontaneous ventilation, an appropriate laser-resistant wrapped ETT must be used. Prior to the surgeon initiating use of the laser, the anesthesiologist should reduce the inhaled fraction of inspired oxygen (FiO_2) to

the minimum amount tolerated by the patient to maintain safe hemoglobin oxygen saturation. A syringe filled with saline and a basin filled with sterile water should be immediately available for operative personnel to rapidly extinguish an airway fire.[7,8]

Laryngeal cold ablation (Coblation): A novel method using localized radio frequency energy transduction to denature viral proteins and destroy papilloma without compromising hemostasis.[9] Best used at a power level of 7 to 9 with a slow drip of saline to ensure an appropriate environment for the coblation plasma field. To ablate papilloma, place the tip of the wand over the lesions at a 90° angle where possible to minimize surrounding thermal damage. Coblation wands come in pediatric and adult sizes with one or three electrodes, respectively. Classically the smaller pediatric wand is used in JORRP patients. Depending on the location of the papilloma, one may see tissue quivering when the energy is applied (▶ Fig. 48.7, ▶ Fig. 48.8, and ▶ Fig. 48.9).

Cup forceps: The primary surgical mode prior to advent of the laser, cup forceps are used to take biopsies for histopathologic assessment and HPV typing, remove larger bulky exophytic lesions, or to remove small irregular tissue that remains after using other modalities. Straight,

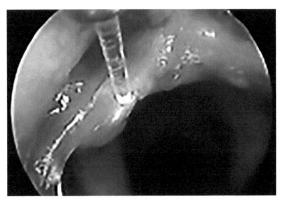

Fig. 48.6 400 µm KTP fiber.

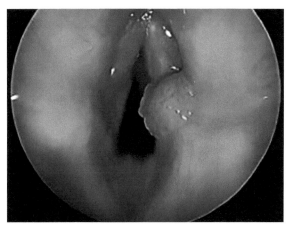

Fig. 48.7 Focal bulky papilloma.

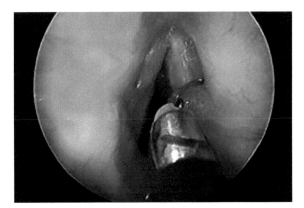

Fig. 48.8 Pediatric coblation wand.

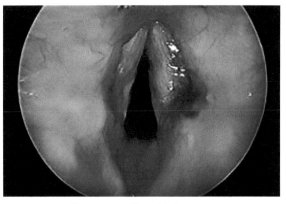

Fig. 48.9 Papilloma removed by coblation.

up-biting and left or right-angled cup forceps are available. The cup grasps the lesion and gently separates the abnormal tissue from the underlying epithelium. If the papilloma does not detach easily with gentle force, release grip and reposition to prevent underlying tissue damage. Bleeding can occur and, as with a microdebrider, is controlled with topical hemostatic agents on cotton pledgets (▶ Fig. 48.10).

48.4 Intraoperative Approach

48.4.1 General Treatment Principles

The surgical approach to JORRP removal centers on employing a conservative technique to establish an airway and improve phonation by removing obstructive papilloma while avoiding injury to noninvolved tissue and taking great care to avoid generating web formation at the anterior commissure. The primary goals of care are to reduce tumor burden, create a safe and patent airway, decrease the chance for distal spread of disease, increase the interval between procedures, and preserve vocal

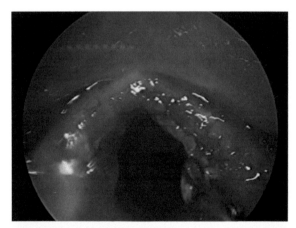

Fig. 48.10 Cup forceps removal.

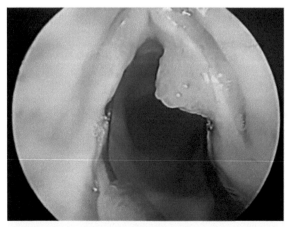

Fig. 48.12 Use of laryngeal spreader.

integrity and quality of life for the patient. To reduce iatrogenic damage to the larynx, leave papilloma where opposing tissue approximates and return for planned interval debulking. Importantly, it is best to avoid a tracheostomy if at all possible, as this generates tracheal mucosal injury, which permits further spread of disease into the tracheal airway, especially at the tracheostomy site.

48.4.2 General Technique "Pearls"

There should be no extraneous noise (such as music playing) during the procedure so that the surgeon may listen to the tone of the O_2 sat monitor and anticipate a drop in oxygen saturation level. A monitor (▶ Fig. 48.11) should be available for both the surgeon and anesthesiologist as oftentimes one will see that the vocal cords begin to quiver prior to the O_2 saturation level overtly dropping and is an indication that the anesthesia is "too light." During the procedure, care should be taken not to continuously suction the airway, as this will remove the inhaled anesthetic gas. It is quite helpful when using the telescopes, laryngeal instruments, and suction for the scrub nurse to support the cables to prevent tension and pull on the cables. All operating room personnel should be focused on the monitor to ensure complete involvement in the procedure and to anticipate any difficulties that might arise.

The procedure is begun with the patient anesthetized with inhaled sevoflurane. Then, an IV is started. Local

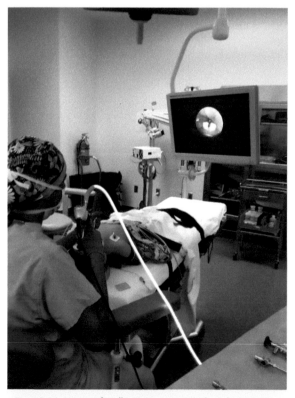

Fig. 48.11 Monitor for all in OR to see. Anesthesiologist is to left with O_2 sat monitor by left ear of surgeon.

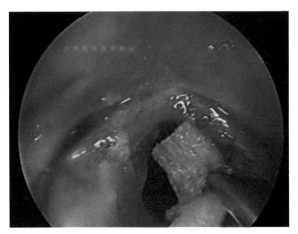

Fig. 48.13 Use of adrenaline pledget to clean laryngeal tissue after ablation.

anesthesia is applied to the larynx via topical 4% lidocaine (40 mg/mL dosed at a maximum of 4–5 mg/kg). Ideally, anesthesia is maintained by intravenous propofol along with inhaled sevoflurane and spontaneous ventilation throughout. A complete airway assessment is done with either telescopes or bronchoscopes to the subsegmental bronchi. Once completed, an appropriately sized suspension laryngoscope is placed and a complete laryngeal assessment is repeated using both the 0° and 30° telescopes. Throughout the procedure, high-quality images and video of the larynx and any distal lesions should be obtained. The decision is then made as to what instrumentation is best for managing the papilloma for the patient. To improve exposure and to reduce chance of injury to normal laryngeal tissue, a laryngeal spreader is essential (▶Fig. 48.12). Intermittently during the case, use a cotton pledget with epinephrine or oxymetazoline to control bleeding, dry the field, and wipe away excess char, blood, and debrided tissue (▶Fig. 48.13).

At the initial procedure, and intermittently during the ongoing management of the patient, a biopsy should be done prior to debulking and sent for histopathology and HPV typing, if available. Staging is determined using the Staging and Assessment Scale for RRP[10] (see ▶Fig. 48.14). Use of steroids: Steroids are routinely used intraoperatively to reduce postoperative nausea and vomiting and in airway cases for control of airway edema. This is controversial in JORRP, as immunosuppression in the setting of a known viral infection could potentially increase the rate of disease recurrence.[11]

48.4.3 Adjuvant Therapy

Although surgery is the primary modality used to control JORRP, at least 20% of patients have refractory disease requiring additional therapeutic intervention.[12,13] Current adjuvant therapies involve disruption of viral replication, disruption of angiogenesis, and immunomodulation.

Surgical adjuvant therapy involves intralesional injection into the papilloma. There are multiple nonsurgical adjuvants that have been used with limited success and more recent use of intravenous bevacizumab for very severe extensive airway disease.

48.4.4 Note on Adjuvant Treatment

Historically, adjuvant therapy has been reserved for only the most "aggressive and severe" disease, typically interpreted as more than four to six surgeries per year or disease spread beyond the larynx.[14] However, in light of modern therapeutic options and our enhanced understanding of the natural history of JORRP, this principle begs revision. By its nature, most forms of recurrent respiratory papillomatosis may be considered "severe and aggressive." Repeated surgery inflicts physical, emotional, and financial hardship upon the patient and their family, often requiring a "long road" of surgical procedures. To achieve the best long-term outcomes, perhaps it is time to rethink the principles of treatment and initiate adjuvant therapy early in the course of the disease.

48.4.5 Technique of Intralesional Injection

Injection of adjuvant medications into laryngeal tissue is classically done following debulking of the lesions. Using an appropriately sized minimally beveled laryngeal needle (Zeitels' vocal fold infusion needle, Storz Kleinsasser injection needle, …) the adjuvant is injected into the submucosa where the lesion was located, raising a small bleb. While taking great care not to overinject or obstruct the airway, injections are continued circumferentially around the larynx where overt papilloma has been removed. Tracheal lesions are managed in a similar fashion with removal followed by injection (▶Fig. 48.15, ▶Fig. 48.16).

48.4.6 Cidofovir

Intralesional injection of Cidofovir is the most commonly used adjuvant therapy for JORRP. An analogue of cytosine, Cidofovir blocks proliferation of DNA viruses by inhibiting viral DNA polymerase within rapidly dividing cells. Though FDA approved for treatment of CMV retinitis in HIV patients, off-label use in RRP has been routinely used (with knowledge and consent from the family). One may see a dramatic initial response to treatment, with marked reduction in severity and extent of papilloma recurrence. In 40% to 45% of cases, patients achieve lasting remission (>5 year disease-free) although multiple injections are routinely needed.[15] Approximately five injections of 1 to 2 mL at 5 to 7.5 mg/mL are planned at 2 to 4 week intervals and modified depending on disease response. Although durable remission is desired,

STAGING ASSESSMENT FOR RECURRENT LARYNGEAL PAPILLOMATOSIS

PATIENT INITIALS:____   DATE OF SURGERY:____   SURGEON:____
PATIENT ID #:____   INSTITUTION:____

1. How long since the last papilloma surgery? ____days, ____weeks, ____months, ____years,
   ____don't know, ____1st surgery
2. Counting today's surgery, how many papilloma surgeries in the past 12 months? ____
3. Describe the patient's voice today: ____aphonic, ____abnormal, ____normal, ____other
4. Describe the patient's stridor today: ____absent, ____present with activity, ____present at rest,
   ____don't know
5. Describe the urgency of today's intervention: ____scheduled, ____urgent, ____emergent

FOR EACH SITE, SCORE AS: 0 = none, 1 = suface lesion, 2 = raised lesion, 3 = bulky lesion

LARYNX
>   **Epiglottis**
>>   Lingual surface_____ Laryngeal surface_____
>   Aryepiglottic folds: Right____ Left____
>   False vocal cords: Right____ Left____
>   True vocal cords: Right____ Left____
>   Arytenoids: Right____ Left____
>   Anterior commisure_____ Posterior commisure_____
>   Subglottis _____

TRACHEA:
>   Upper one-third_____
>   Middle one-third_____
>   Lower one-third_____
>   Bronchi: Right_____ Left _____
>   Tracheotomy stoma_____

OTHER:
>   Nose _____
>   Palate _____
>   Pharynx _____
>   Esophagus_____
>   Lungs _____
>   Other _____

TOTAL SCORE ALL SITES:_____

Fig. 48.14 (a, b) Staging assessment for recurrent laryngeal papillomatosis. (Provided courtesy of Derkay et al. 1998.)[10]

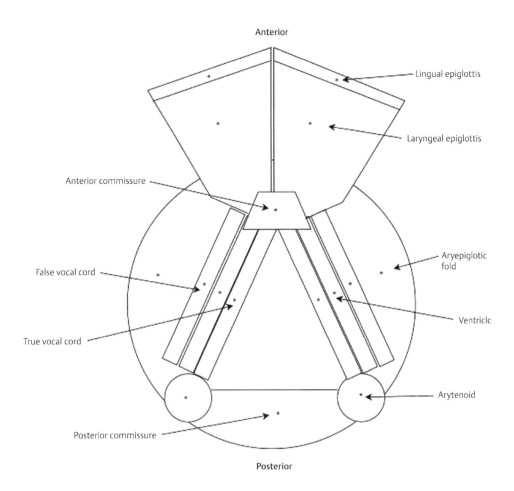

Anterior

Lingual epiglottis

Laryngeal epiglottis

Anterior commissure

Aryepiglotic fold

False vocal cord

Ventriclc

True vocal cord

Arytenoid

Posterior commissure

Posterior

Fig. 48.14 (*continued*)

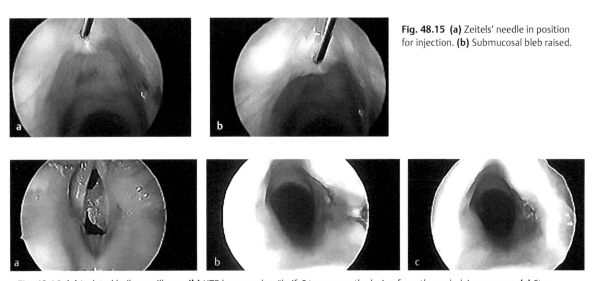

Fig. 48.15 **(a)** Zeitels' needle in position for injection. **(b)** Submucosal bleb raised.

Fig. 48.16 **(a)** Isolated bulky papilloma. **(b)** KTP laser used as "knife" to remove the lesion from the underlying mucosa. **(c)** Storz laryngeal needle raising a submucosal bleb where papilloma is removed.

Cidofovir should be considered to control extent of disease, increase intersurgical interval, and decrease the amount of intervention in total.

48.4.7 Safety Concerns

It has been hypothesized that incorporation of Cidofovir into cellular DNA may disrupt genomic integrity of the host cell, increasing risk of carcinogenesis. While malignant transformation is a concern with Cidofovir use, recent reviews have demonstrated that risk of dysplastic transformation and development of malignancy is greater with naturally progressive disease than with Cidofovir adjuvant therapy.[16–18] Without treatment, adult-onset RRP has a known 2% to 4% risk of malignant degeneration, most commonly in extensive tracheal and pulmonary disease.[18] There have been no documented cases of malignant degeneration in pediatric patients treated with Cidofovir. Concerns have been raised regarding Cidofovir-induced scarring of the larynx, but it is not clear if this scarring is due to the multiple surgical interventions or Cidofovir itself.

Choosing when to initiate Cidofovir requires consideration of extent of disease, regrowth rate, impact on the patient, and the philosophy of the attending surgeon. In 2013, a consensus statement was published that reviewed the many questions associated with Cidofovir use including dosage, interval of treatment, number of injections, precautions, and consent[19] (see ▶Table 48.3). However, control of disease and the many psychosocial aspects of JORRP must be weighed heavily against potential side effects. In light of these issues, the senior author has evolved his practice in recent years to initiate adjuvant therapy much earlier in the course of disease than noted in the consensus statement.

Bevacizumab (Avastin): Like Cidofovir, intralesional injection with bevacizumab has been shown to effectively impact the growth of JORRP. Bevacizumab is a human monoclonal antibody that binds VEGF, thus inhibiting vascular endothelial growth in tissue. It is FDA approved for use in various cancers, including colorectal, renal, lung, and certain brain malignancies. Like other neoplastic processes, RRP growth is dependent upon vascular supply, inhibition of which has been hypothesized to reduce the rate of proliferation of the papillomatous disease.[20,21]

For focal disease, bevacizumab is delivered via intralesional injection after debulking. The current approach and injection technique is similar to the protocol for Cidofovir, employing a series of approximately five injections of 1 to 2 mL at 25 mg/mL, given at 4 to 6 week intervals. Bevacizumab has been shown to reduce disease severity and prolong the intersurgical interval, with the rare case report of complete resolution of disease.[22] Of note, there have been no reported side effects of intralesional bevacizumab to date, making it an effective and potentially safe option for managing severe disease without expectation for remission.

For extensive tracheal or distal bronchiolar disease, a nonsurgical, systemic adjuvant therapy should be considered. Reports of intravenous bevacizumab for treatment of RRP have shown promising results, including significantly prolonged intersurgical interval, reduced disease bulk and extent, improved quality of life, and rare complete resolution of disease.[23,24,25] IV bevacizumab is administered by our Hematology-Oncology colleagues at 3 week intervals with variable duration of treatment from 5 to 21 months. Surveillance endoscopy and disease removal is intermittently done during the course of treatment and varies depending on response to therapy. Unlike intralesional injection, however, IV bevacizumab is not without concern for side effects. Though generally well tolerated, patients receiving therapy have reported fatigue, hypertension, and proteinuria.[25] Blood pressure and urine output should be monitored at regular intervals in patients undergoing a course of therapy.

Other nonsurgical adjuvant treatments include pegylated interferon, artemisinin, and Indole-3-Carbinol. Each has been shown to have limited, intermittently reproducible effects on disease burden without evidence of cure.[26,27] Though they are not currently accepted as first-line adjuvant therapy, further research may be warranted.

HPV vaccination has been tried as a therapeutic modality in patients with RRP. By its nature, the viral-like protein of

Table 48.3 Consensus statement for Cidofovir use[19]

Indications	6+ surgeries/year, intersurgical interval decreasing, or presence of extralaryngeal spread in a pediatric patient
Method	Intralesional local injection following debridement
Dosing	20–40 mg in <4 mL for adults; <20 mg in <2 mL for pediatric patients (<3 mg/kg); 2.5–7.5 mg/ml
Scheduling	5 injections per protocol; 2–6 week scheduled interval
Biopsy	At first procedure in all patients, every procedure in adults
Routine blood work	Not recommended if dosing is below 3 mg/kg
Special consent	Required to address dysplasia/malignancy issues, possible renal toxicity, and "off label" use of the drug
Follow-up	Long-term follow-up of all patients receiving Cidofovir is critical

the vaccine will not generate an immune response against active disease. However, some anecdotal case reports suggest some effect. In a systemic review of studies of adolescent and adult patients with active HPV disease (of any form) who received the HPV vaccine, 9 out of 12 studies suggested that vaccine treatment decreased burden of disease, decreased disease recurrence, and increased the intersurgical interval.[28] As the safety parameters of the vaccine are so well established, vaccination earlier than the approved initiation at age 9 likely has minimal drawback.

48.4.8 The Future of JORRP Management

The future of JORRP eradication lies in vaccination. Vaccination programs have proven to reduce the incidence of JORRP. In 2007, Australia implemented the first nation-wide vaccination program, which was a resounding success. Over a 10-year period, nearly 80% of the school-age population received the vaccine, and the incidence of JORRP decreased significantly from 0.16 per 100,000 to 0.022 per 100,000 ($p < 0.001$). Of the 15 reported cases who did develop JORRP, all were of unvaccinated mothers, suggesting that greater vaccination uptake may further reduce incidence of RRP.[3] Similar studies are ongoing in the United States and Canada. At present HPV vaccine adherence has been estimated at only 60% in the United States, 20% to 30% less than other adolescent vaccines. Despite less than ideal rates of vaccination in the United States, in the 10 years since introduction of HPV quadrivalent vaccine, there has been a greater-than-expected reduction in HPV-related disease.[29] The current 9-valent vaccine is approved for both males and females age 9 to 45 given in three separate injections for patients older than 15 and two injections for those less than 15.

Moving beyond the 9-valent vaccine, new DNA vaccines are being developed that induce a robust immune response and prevent or treat active HPV disease. The current research uses a calreticulin-linked HPV-11 E6E7 vaccine to generate a significant CD8+ T cell response in HPV-infected mice.[30]

Research into checkpoint inhibitors is being actively pursued as a treatment modality for HPV disease. In accordance with the antigen-tolerance theory of HPV proliferation, active and aggressive papilloma has been shown to overexpress PD-L1 and PD-1 proteins that join to negatively regulate the immune system response and permit disease proliferation. These same proteins are targeted by numerous drugs used in cancer therapy, including the PD-1 inhibitor Pembrolizumab that blocks interaction of PD-1 and PD-L1/L2. Trials for their efficacy in RRP are ongoing and may offer a new avenue for management.[31]

The future of JORRP management is also extending into the realm of personalized medicine. One groundbreaking study harvested tissue from laryngeal and distal bronchial papillomata in a single patient with severe, advanced, and extensive RRP. Using these samples, authors grew clones of both healthy and diseased cell lines in vitro. With these "conditionally reprogrammed cells," authors were able to identify the unique genomes of these papillomata as well as screen and test the efficacy of various drugs for treatment.[32] Papilloma cell growth is currently being investigated by the senior author as well as in several institutions around the United States.[33]

48.5 Highlights

a. Indications
   - Identification of papillomatosis in children with stridor or hoarseness.
   - Assess the entire airway for papilloma.
   - Maintain airway patency.
   - Reduce risk for spread to other parts of the airway.
   - Preserve vocal quality.
   - Prevent need for tracheostomy.
b. Contraindications
   - None.
c. Complications
   - Airway edema/obstruction/bleeding.
   - Structural damage to the larynx.
   - Intraoperative fire.
   - Chronic dysphonia.
   - Distal spread of papilloma.
   - Malignant degeneration.
d. Special preoperative considerations
   - Discussion with anesthesia regarding:
      ○ Technique of anesthesia, ability to perform spontaneous ventilation.
      ○ Risks of use of paralyzing agents.
      ○ Fire hazard and management.
      ○ Review of current status of the airway.
      ○ Review of prior anesthetic episodes.
   - Discussion with operating room personnel regarding equipment needed:
      ○ Suspension apparatus, 0/30 degree telescopes, laryngeal spreader.
      ○ Laryngeal needles for injection.
      ○ Adjuvant therapy ordered and prepared.
      ○ Microdebrider, laser, coblation availability.
      ○ Video monitor(s) for anesthesiologist and OR personnel to watch the procedure and anticipate needs or next portion of the procedure.
   - Discussion/preparation for emergent airway compromise/fire.
e. Special intraoperative considerations
   - Reduce extraneous noise and distractions (no radio...).
   - Topical 4% lidocaine spray for the larynx/airway.
   - O_2 sat monitor loud enough for surgeon to hear.
   - Laser safety precautions for patient and operating room personnel.

- Appropriate high-filtration masks for all OR personnel.
- Handling of biopsy specimens.
- Video monitor and picture taking and recording prepared.

f. Special postoperative considerations
- Airway status.

References

[1] Larson DA, Derkay CS. Epidemiology of recurrent respiratory papillomatosis. APMIS 2010;118(6–7):450–454

[2] Kashima HK, Shah F, Lyles A, et al. A comparison of risk factors in juvenile-onset and adult-onset recurrent respiratory papillomatosis. Laryngoscope 1992;102(1):9–13

[3] Novakovic D, Cheng ATL, Zurynski Y, et al. A prospective study of the incidence of juvenile-onset recurrent respiratory papillomatosis after implementation of a National HPV Vaccination Program. J Infect Dis 2018;217(2):208–212

[4] Cohn AM, Kos JT II, Taber LH, Adam E. Recurring laryngeal papillopa. Am J Otolaryngol 1981;2(2):129–132

[5] Strong MS, Jako GJ, Polanyi T, Wallace RA. Laser surgery in the aerodigestive tract. Am J Surg 1973;126(4):529–533

[6] Burns JA, Zeitels SM, Akst LM, Broadhurst MS, Hillman RE, Anderson R. 532 nm pulsed potassium-titanyl-phosphate laser treatment of laryngeal papillomatosis under general anesthesia. Laryngoscope 2007;117(8):1500–1504

[7] Lee GS, Irace A, Rahbar R. The efficacy and safety of the flexible fiber CO2 laser delivery system in the endoscopic management of pediatric airway problems: Our long term experience. Int J Pediatr Otorhinolaryngol 2017;97:218–222

[8] Association of Surgical Technologists' Guidelines for Best Practices in Laser Safety. Association of Surgical Technologists April 12, 2019

[9] Carney AS, Evans AS, Mirza S, Psaltis A. Radiofrequency coblation for treatment of advanced laryngotracheal recurrent respiratory papillomatosis. J Laryngol Otol 2010;124(5):510–514

[10] Derkay CS, Malis DJ, Zalzal G, Wiatrak BJ, Kashima HK, Coltrera MD. A staging system for assessing severity of disease and response to therapy in recurrent respiratory papillomatosis. Laryngoscope 1998;108(6):935–937

[11] Derkay CS. Recurrent respiratory papillomatosis. Laryngoscope 2001;111(1):57–69

[12] Schraff S, Derkay CS, Burke B, Lawson L. American Society of Pediatric Otolaryngology members' experience with recurrent respiratory papillomatosis and the use of adjuvant therapy. Arch Otolaryngol Head Neck Surg 2004;130(9):1039–1042

[13] Katsenos S, Becker HD. Recurrent respiratory papillomatosis: a rare chronic disease, difficult to treat, with potential to lung cancer transformation: apropos of two cases and a brief literature review. Case Rep Oncol 2011;4(1):162–171

[14] Derkay CS, Darrow DH. Recurrent respiratory papillomatosis. Ann Otol Rhinol Laryngol 2006;115(1):1–11

[15] Pransky SM, Magit AE, Kearns DB, Kang DR, Duncan NO. Intralesional cidofovir for recurrent respiratory papillomatosis in children. Arch Otolaryngol Head Neck Surg 1999;125(10):1143–1148

[16] Lindsay F, Bloom D, Pransky S, Stabley R, Shick P. Histologic review of cidofovir-treated recurrent respiratory papillomatosis. Ann Otol Rhinol Laryngol 2008;117(2):113–117

[17] Broekema FI, Dikkers FG. Side-effects of cidofovir in the treatment of recurrent respiratory papillomatosis. Eur Arch Otorhinolaryngol 2008;265(8):871–879

[18] Karatayli-Ozgursoy S, Bishop JA, Hillel A, Akst L, Best SR. Risk factors for dysplasia in recurrent respiratory papillomatosis in an adult and pediatric population. Ann Otol Rhinol Laryngol 2016;125(3):235–241

[19] Derkay CS, Volsky PG, Rosen CA, et al. Current use of intralesional cidofovir for recurrent respiratory papillomatosis. Laryngoscope 2013;123(3):705–712

[20] Zeitels SM, Barbu AM, Landau-Zemer T, et al. Local injection of bevacizumab (Avastin) and angiolytic KTP laser treatment of recurrent respiratory papillomatosis of the vocal folds: a prospective study. Ann Otol Rhinol Laryngol 2011;120(10):627–634

[21] Best SR, Friedman AD, Landau-Zemer T, et al. Safety and dosing of bevacizumab (avastin) for the treatment of recurrent respiratory papillomatosis. Ann Otol Rhinol Laryngol 2012;121(9):587–593

[22] Sidell DR, Nassar M, Cotton RT, Zeitels SM, de Alarcon A. High-dose sublesional bevacizumab (avastin) for pediatric recurrent respiratory papillomatosis. Ann Otol Rhinol Laryngol 2014;123(3):214–221

[23] Mohr M, Schliemann C, Biermann C, et al. Rapid response to systemic bevacizumab therapy in recurrent respiratory papillomatosis. Oncol Lett 2014;8(5):1912–1918

[24] Zur KB, Fox E. Bevacizumab chemotherapy for management of pulmonary and laryngotracheal papillomatosis in a child. Laryngoscope 2017;127(7):1538–1542

[25] Best SR, Mohr M, Zur KB. Systemic bevacizumab for recurrent respiratory papillomatosis: a national survey. Laryngoscope 2017;127(10):2225–2229

[26] Ivancic R, Iqbal H, deSilva B, Pan Q, Matrka L. Current and future management of recurrent respiratory papillomatosis. Laryngoscope Investig Otolaryngol 2018;3(1):22–34

[27] Rosen CA, Bryson PC. Indole-3-carbinol for recurrent respiratory papillomatosis: long-term results. J Voice 2004;18(2):248–253

[28] Dion GR, Teng S, Boyd LR, et al. Adjuvant human papillomavirus vaccination for secondary prevention: a systematic review. JAMA Otolaryngol Head Neck Surg 2017;143(6):614–622

[29] Markowitz LE, Gee J, Chesson H, Stokley S. Ten years of human papillomavirus vaccination in the United States. Acad Pediatr 2018;18(2S):S3–S10

[30] Ahn J, Peng S, Hung CF, Roden RBS, Wu TC, Best SR. Immunologic responses to a novel DNA vaccine targeting human papillomavirus-11 E6E7. Laryngoscope 2017;127(12):2713–2720

[31] Ahn J, Bishop JA, Roden RBS, Allen CT, Best SRA. The PD-1 and PD-L1 pathway in recurrent respiratory papillomatosis. Laryngoscope 2018;128(1):E27–E32

[32] Yuan H, Myers S, Wang J, et al. Use of reprogrammed cells to identify therapy for respiratory papillomatosis. N Engl J Med 2012;367(13):1220–1227

[33] Attra J, Hsieh LE, Luo L, et al. Development of human-derived cell culture lines for recurrent respiratory papillomatosis. Otolaryngol Head Neck Surg 2018;159(4):638–642

49 Laryngotracheal Reconstruction

Diego Preciado, George Zalzal

Summary

This chapter will review the preoperative, intraoperative, and postoperative considerations for successfully carrying out laryngotracheal reconstruction. Key points of consideration to ensure success while avoiding potential pitfalls will be highlighted.

Keywords: Larynx, cartilage, stents

49.1 Introduction

The management of laryngotracheal stenosis in children is often challenging and best managed at a tertiary institution with expertise in pediatric airway disorders, requiring a high level of integration of multiple medical services, led by an otolaryngologist. In general, multidisciplinary expertise in anesthesia, surgery, pulmonology, intensive care management, and pediatric hospitalist medicine is requisite to adequately manage these patients. Furthermore, expertise in nursing and speech therapy is essential for education, counseling tracheotomy care instruction, and home care integration. Although there has been an emerging trend toward the endoscopic management of these pathologies with airway balloons, open airway reconstruction remains the definitive tool for the long-term repair of pediatric laryngotracheal stenosis. In the long term, severe stenosis in particular appears to do better with open approaches. This chapter will focus primarily on open surgical approaches for laryngotracheal stenosis, focusing specifically on laryngotracheal reconstruction (LTR), which is not a single technique but a collection of multiple approaches depending on the nature of the stenosis (Video 49.1).

49.2 Definition and Classification

The incidence of laryngotracheal stenosis in neonates remains around 0.1% to 1% with a majority caused by long-term intubation. In some cases, the child may be born with congenital laryngeal stenosis—due to thickening of the cricoid ring or lack of recanalization of the airway during development. These instances of congenital stenosis are more frequent as part of some syndromes such as Down syndrome. The grading scale most universally employed to categorize subglottic stenosis (SGS), based on endotracheal tube size, was proposed by Myer and Cotton in 1994. They described Grade 1 SGS as 0% to 50% narrowing, Grade 2 SGS as 50% to 75% narrowing, Grade 3 SGS as 75% to 99% narrowing, and Grade 4 SGS as no-identifiable lumen as shown in ▶ Fig. 49.1. This grading scheme is important in comparative outcomes assessment, for planning surgical approach, and for objectively classifying disease severity. In 2009 Moniere introduced a modification of the Myer Cotton Scale, whereby each level of stenosis is further subclassified (a) for isolated stenosis, (b) for presence of medical comorbidities, (c) for glottic involvement, and (d) for both comorbidities and glottic involvement. This modified scale can add objectivity and lend important information when one counsels families regarding expected outcomes, or inform surgical decisions such as electing between a single- and a double-stage approach.

49.3 Evaluation, Preoperative, and Anesthesia Considerations

The evaluation of children with suspicion of laryngotracheal stenosis should include a careful history and physical assessment. Preoperative radiographic imaging plays a limited role in the diagnosis of laryngotracheal stenosis except to help characterize and determine the length of a stenotic airway segment. Undoubtedly, the gold standard in the preoperative airway evaluation for SGS characterization is rigid direct microlaryngoscopy and bronchoscopy (DLB) under general anesthesia. The preferred anesthetic management method for this evaluation is with children under spontaneous ventilation anesthesia with oxygen insufflation using a combination of inhalational agents and propofol or dexmedetomidine. This approach allows for a dynamic assessment of the laryngotracheobronchial tree while manipulating the airway without needing intubation or ventilation through a rigid bronchoscope. The surgeon is able to simply utilize

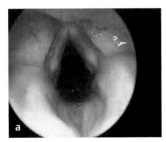 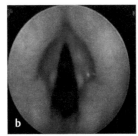 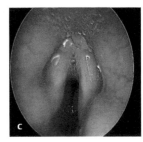 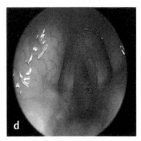

Fig. 49.1 Subglottic stenosis grading scale. (a–d) Left to right: Grade 1 (0–50%), Grade 2 (51–75%), Grade 3 (76–99%), and Grade 4 (100%) stenosis.

narrow rigid fiberoptic "naked" telescopes for diagnostic purposes, minimizing airway trauma associated with the larger diameter ventilating bronchoscope. Usage of the ventilating bronchoscope is then reserved for cases where therapeutic or interventional maneuvers have to be performed in the trachea and mainstem bronchi. After DLB is performed, in order to objectively determine the severity of the stenosis, the lumen of the stenotic airway is typically sized with endotracheal tubes (ETTs). Direct microlaryngoscopy and bronchoscopy is supplemented in select patients by flexible nasopharyngolaryngoscopy, both done under sleep and awake. Sleep flexible endoscopy can help assess the tongue base level of the airway along with the nasopharyngeal and hypopharyngeal levels of the airway without laryngeal manipulation/suspension. Flexible nasopharyngolaryngoscopy is important in nonintubated patients where one should carefully assess the nasopharynx, oropharynx, and particularly the vocal cord level. Abnormalities of glottic mobility due to neurologic problems, scarring of the glottis, or involvement of the cricoarytenoid joints complicate surgical therapy. Flexible laryngobronchoscopy under anesthesia is also best accomplished without intubation, under spontaneous ventilation with oxygen insufflation through the side port of the flexible scope, most efficiently using a combination of dexmedetomidine and Propofol. This is particularly useful in patients with severe micrognathia to assess the degree of possible obstruction at the tongue base. Awake flexible laryngoscopy is important to rule out vocal cord immobility. Most infants with acquired SGS will have had a history of neonatal intubation. For neonates presenting with inflammatory SGS and multiple failures to extubate, close cooperation needs to occur among the neonatology and otolaryngology teams. Close attention should be paid to the patient's medical condition, with emphasis on cardiopulmonary status, ventilation status, oxygen requirements, and the details of previous extubation failures. Possible concomitant presence of gastroesophageal reflux (GERD) should be investigated and treated, as many have reported a correlation between the presence of GERD and SGS and that GERD may affect surgical healing after LTR. Patients with dysphagia, or severe laryngeal and hypopharyngeal inflammation should be considered for eosinophilic esophagitis, as this emerging disorder has also recently been shown to be associated with SGS and influence negative healing and outcomes after LTR.

For patients with laryngotracheal stenosis without an existing tracheotomy tube, further and definitive reconstructive management is based upon the clinical picture and the severity of the stenotic segment. Presence of chronic pulmonary disease, often represented by baseline oxygen requirement in the setting of bronchopulmonary dysplasia and poor pulmonary functional reserve, is a contraindication for single-stage LTR, necessitating placement of a tracheotomy prior to or during the LTR. This is because reconstructive laryngotracheal surgery requires lung function adequate enough to withstand not only the surgery but also the postoperative course in ICU and subsequent extubation. Indeed, those children with significant pulmonary disease should undergo consultation by a pediatric pulmonologist. In general, it is inadvisable to perform LTR in children with anything more than a mild nighttime oxygen requirement; in selected cases, continued oxygen administration may be possible by nasal prongs after decannulation.

49.3.1 Timing of Reconstruction

The ideal timing of LTR surgery remains somewhat ill-defined. Although some have demonstrated that children younger than 24 months have higher rates of reconstruction failure despite lesser degrees of stenotic pathology when compared to older children, other series have suggested that although younger children have a higher rate of re-intubation after single-stage procedures, age alone may not be a stand-alone predictor for reconstructive failure (defined as failure to decannulate or avoid tracheotomy). In children with existing tracheotomies, any LTR timing decisions must consider the fact that severe SGS managed with tracheotomy, where formal LTR is deferred, is potentially life-threatening as yearly tracheotomy-specific mortality in children due to tracheotomy tube obstruction is purportedly in the 1% to 3.4% range. Associated tracheotomy tube morbidity also includes the need for comprehensive nursing care and monitoring, delayed speech and language development, feeding difficulties, and infection. Therefore, now many authors propose that reconstruction as early as possible is recommended so as to avoid tracheotomy-related complications.

49.4 Surgical Management

49.4.1 Role for Endoscopic Treatment

In general, endoscopic treatment is limited to acquired (and not congenital) airway stenoses. Classically, endoscopic treatment has taken the form of laser ablation of narrowing lesions, but is only useful for nonmature, noncircumferential, short soft lesions that comprise mild Grade 1 or 2 stenoses. Recent case series have also described the usage of balloon dilating catheters as potential tools that may successfully treat some patients with SGS, even if severe, but larger confirmatory studies are necessary to validate this approach. Comparative, retrospective studies have concluded that for severe SGS (grade 3 and 4), endoscopic balloon dilation has limited application compared with LTR in terms of achieving a long-term adequate airway lumen, and in some cases failed balloon dilation is perhaps even detrimental, increasing the risk

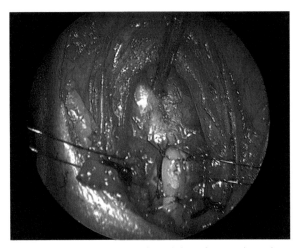

Fig. 49.2 Thyroid ala graft. A thyroid ala graft sutured into the anterior airway split. The suction device depicts the thyroid cartilage notch.

of unplanned urgent interventions compared with LTR.[1] In any circumstance, dilation may certainly help temporize obstructive symptoms. Multiple, serial repeated dilations may eventually weaken the airway lateral walls, effectively making the pathology worse.

49.5 Open Surgical Techniques

49.5.1 Anterior Cricoid Split

The anterior cricoid split (ACS) procedure was introduced by Cotton and Seid in 1980 as an alternative approach to tracheotomy in the failing to extubate premature neonate with healthy lungs but laryngeal obstruction due to edema and early stenosis. In order to qualify for this procedure, the only reason for extubation failure must be laryngeal obstruction, and neonate should have grown to 1.5 kg, required no assisted ventilatory support for 10 days, have no supplemental oxygen need greater than an FiO2 of 35%, and have no evidence of congestive heart failure. The procedure consists of making an anterior vertical split through the first tracheal ring, cricoid cartilage, and lower thyroid cartilage followed by nasotracheal intubation for 10 to 14 days in the NICU. If criteria are strictly and carefully followed, case series have demonstrated ACS to be successful in avoiding tracheotomy in neonates. During ACS, placement of a small piece of thyroid ala cartilage into the vertical split (▶ Fig. 49.2) has also been described and may improve the success of the surgery.

49.5.2 LTR with Cartilage Grafting

LTR with interposition of cartilage graft was introduced by Fearon and Cotton in 1972 as a means to expand an otherwise narrowed subglottic airway segment. The principle of the procedure is to distract the cricoid cartilage either anteriorly and/or posteriorly by placing cartilaginous grafts over a luminal, appropriately sized stent. This procedure can be performed in either a single-stage (without a tracheotomy tube in place) or in a double-stage approach (where a tracheotomy tube is left in place postoperatively).

If carefully selected, the reported overall success rates of LTR in preventing tracheotomy or decannulation ranges from 81% to 100%. In general, the more severe the stenosis, the lower the likelihood of successful outcomes with LTR expansion techniques. For grade 3 and 4 stenoses, success rates are reportedly in the 75% to 85% range. Indeed, in these severe cases, when an adequate distance (at least >3 mm) exists between the lower margin of the vocal cords and the stenotic segment of the airway a consideration should be given to partial airway resection techniques, such as cricotracheal resection (CTR), as these reportedly have higher success rates than LTR for severe grade 3 and 4 stenoses, in the 90% to 95% range.[2,3] However, as opposed to CTR, when LTR procedures fail, there are more options for revision surgery—where LTR with re-grafting can be performed multiple times, resection techniques such as CTR can only be performed once.

Cartilage is the most frequently employed graft material to expand the laryngotracheal lumen during LTR procedures. While the use of thyroid alar and auricular cartilage grafts has been proposed, costal cartilage grafts remain the workhorse for LTR.[4] This is due to their availability, access, well-matched thickness, and generally robust rigidity requisite for reconstructing the laryngotracheal framework. Thyroid alar cartilage may be used for isolated anterior grafting, as a spacer graft during anterior cricoid splits in neonates or in select grade II or III stenosis, but its thin profile renders it difficult to carve/mold with flanges and inadequate for support of the posterior cricoid lamina. Hyoid bone has also been used with variable success in adult patients; however, its thinness limits expansive potential, bone is also difficult to carve to specification, and ossification may limit integration and neo-epithelialization along with significant resorption.

49.5.3 Anterior Grafts

Isolated graft expansion of the anterior cricoid is typically employed when there is mild stenosis of the subglottic airway, or when the scar limits the anterior aspects of the cricoid ring, which is the case in a minority of cases only. In some instances of congenital glottic and subglottic stenosis, such as partial laryngeal atresia with failure of airway recanalization during embryonic development, the thickened cartilage is often mostly located anteriorly and anterior grafting may suffice as reconstructive approach.

The surgical approach for anterior LTR proceeds as follows. After performance of DLB to confirm the position/extent of stenosis, and to rule out any active laryngeal inflammation (which would prohibit proceeding with the open reconstruction) a transverse/horizontal incision is made over the level of the cricoid, usually about 2 to 3 cm in length. In cases where a tracheotomy tube is in place, and a double-stage approach is planned, then this incision is placed 1 to 2 cm above the tracheostoma, so as to not violate the stoma. This allows for ongoing routine tracheotomy tube changes and care in the postop period, prevents the need for placing a new tracheotomy, and avoids potential complications associated with fresh tracheotomy wounds such as false tracts and accidental decannulation. On the other hand, in cases where an existing tracheotomy tube is in place preoperatively, but a single-stage approach is planned, then the tracheostoma is incorporated into the initial LTR incision, in preparation to remove the stoma during the reconstruction. After the skin incision, superior and inferior subplatysmal flaps are elevated, strap muscles and thyroid isthmus divided in the midline, and retracted laterally until the upper tracheal rings, cricoid, and thyroid cartilages can be plainly visualized. Next, the anterior cricoid incision is made with a beaver blade, extending through the extent of the scarred airway superiorly, most often to immediately below the anterior commissure. Inferiorly, the incision extends to the superior aspect of the tracheal stoma in a single-stage technique, or just through the scarred segment if keeping a tracheotomy. As in anterior cricoid split, prolene stay sutures are placed lateral to this incision and gently secured with hemostats. In some cases, such as congenital laryngeal atresia with concomitant SGS, a formal complete laryngofissure through the stenotic anterior commissure may need to be performed. Importantly, superior and inferior extension of the incision proceeds under direct visualization, employing a right-angle forceps to visualize the lumen, ensure that the anterior commissure is not violated, and assess extent of scarring. The intraoperative use of a direct laryngeal endoscope by an assistant to guide the split may be helpful as well. After splitting the airway, and confirming the entire vertical length of the scarred airway segment has been split, the stenosis is examined carefully. It is critical to determine the vertical length of the stenosis, the rigidity of the tracheal side walls, the status of the posterior cricoid luminal surface, and the absence of concomitant airway mucosal lesions such as cysts. A helpful method is to gently slide an appropriately sized endotracheal tube (ETT) in a retrograde fashion so as to confirm adequate release of the scar—with a loosely fitting ETT. At this point, the graft is harvested.

The costal cartilage graft is harvested (▶ Fig. 49.3) by making a 2- to 3-cm skin incision in the right inframammary crease. In cases where there is a ventriculoperitoneal shunt in place (almost universally on the right side) traversing the right chest wall, one may have to harvest the costal graft on the left side. After the skin incision, subcutaneous fat and intercostal muscles are divided over the surface of the fifth or sixth rib, exposing the anterior surface of the rib from the osseocartilagenous junction laterally to the sternal attachment medially. At this point, the perichondrium over the superior surface of the rib is incised along the length of the rib, and a subperichondrial plane is established over the superior margin of the rib and extended over the posterior surface of the rib. This subperichondrial tunnel protects the pleural membrane. The same exact subperichondrial tunnel is then established on the inferior margin of the rib and extended over the posterior surface of the rib, connecting to the previously established tunnel that had been started from the superior aspect. Care is taken to ensure the anterior perichondrium is left in place, fully attached to the rib. Next, a Doyen-type rib retractor/elevator is inserted into the tunnel and the rib is transected at the osseocartilaginous junction. The rib is lifted off of the inner perichondrium and chest cavity from lateral to medial, detaching the intercostal muscles as one dissects medially and finally completely detached from the sternum. The remaining wound/bed is flooded with saline, and positive intrathoracic pressure is applied to demonstrate no leak of air through the pleura, confirming no injury to the pleura has occurred. The intercostal muscles are then reapproximated with absorbable suture, and the skin is closed in layers over a passive drain placed at the edge of the wound.

The graft is carved to fit the anterior incision (▶ Fig. 49.4) with flanges at each end to avoid prolapse into the airway with the perichondrium facing the lumen. The inset is carved in a typical "boat" or "tear-drop" fashion, with a

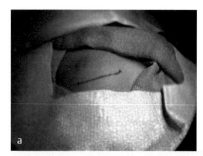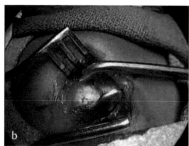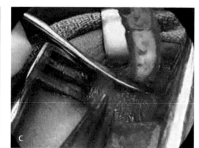

Fig. 49.3 Rib graft harvest. **(a–c)** Incision in right infra-mmary crease; exposure of the fifth rib from osseocartilaginous junction to sternal insertion; harvest of rib from lateral to medial in a posterior subperichondrial plane.

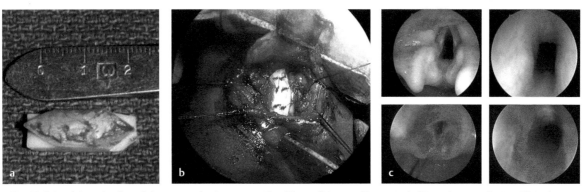

Fig. 49.4 (a–c) Anterior rib graft laryngotracheal reconstruction. The graft is carved into a typical boat shape, and sutured into the anterior airway split. Right panel shows airway lumen healing over time.

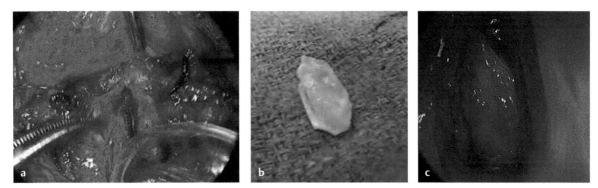

Fig. 49.5 (a–c) Posterior graft laryngotracheal reconstruction. The posterior cricoid lamina is split without the need for a complete laryngofissure through the anterior commissure. The carved posterior graft has small flanges. Right panel shows the graft "snapped" into position without sutures.

typical insert depth of 2 to 3 mm. After carving the graft, it is sutured in place distracting the airway split. Typically, mattress sutures are used for this step. Some surgeons prefer absorbable suture material such as vicryl, while others employ permanent suture material such as prolene. For single-stage surgery, the graft is sutured over an appropriately sized ETT which has been placed in the airway nasotracheally. For double-stage surgery, the graft is sutured over a suprastomal stent in cases where a posterior graft is being placed (▶ Fig. 49.5). After completing the graft placement and suturing, the thyroid gland isthmus is repaired, the strap muscles are sutured closed over the midline, the platysma is reapproximated, and the wound is closed in layers. A dependent drain is also left in place to allow for egress of any air from the peritracheal space. For single-stage procedures, patients are kept nasotracheally intubated in the pediatric intensive care unit (PICU) for a period of 5 to 6 days. In this postoperative period, it is critical to avoid paralysis, while maintaining an appropriate level of sedation commensurate to avoiding excessive thrashing of the patient on or pulling on the ETT. Patients older than 3 years of age, and certainly most teenagers and adults, can often be managed mostly awake while intubated in the PICU with minimal sedation and anxiolysis on board. The recent advent of dexmedetomidine usage as a primary sedative agent in the PICU after single-stage LTR has reduced the incidence of withdrawal and sedation-related complications in these patients.

49.5.4 Posterior Grafts

In most cases of severe SGS requiring open expansion, especially in cases of concomitant posterior glottic stenosis, the posterior cricoid level of the airway needs to be grafted[4,5] to achieve an adequate airway lumen (▶ Fig. 49.5). Indeed a majority of cases of neonatal acquired stenosis will include a posterior glottic/subglottic component to the scar. This is due to the fact that the pressure and ulceration exerted by the ETT leading to stenosis in neonates and infants is most often posterior. Surgical approach for placement of the posterior expansion grafts proceeds in the same fashion for anterior LTR. After completing the anterior vertical airway split and partial laryngofissure, the posterior larynx is infiltrated with 1% lidocaine with 1:100,000 epinephrine. The posterior larynx, posterior glottis, subglottic scar, and full length of posterior lamina of the cricoid are divided down to the level of the hypopharyngeal mucosa. If the interarytenoid area is fibrosed, incision may be carried superiorly to divide the scarred muscular fibers.

Inferiorly, the incision may extend about 1 cm into membranous tracheoesophageal septum. Critically, in order to obtain adequate exposure of the posterior cricoid, it is NOT necessary to perform a complete laryngofissure through the anterior commissure.

Posterior cartilage grafts are carved with small flanges on the nonperichondrial side with the perichondrium inset to be facing luminally. The flanges for posterior graft are small, and meant to be wedged behind the posterior cricoid lamina as the posterior graft is inserted snugly into the distracted cricoid segments. The recoil effect of the posterior cricoid cartilage ring grips the graft in place, preventing its prolapse into the airway. Using this approach, it is feasible to "snap" the posterior graft in place, without having to place sutures. A disadvantage of having to suture the posterior graft into place has to do with surgical exposure, in most cases necessitating a complete laryngofissure through the anterior commissure. Even when sutured, posterior grafts require support in the form of a stent, typically for 10 to 14 days postoperatively. The stent used in single-stage reconstruction is an ETT placed nasotracheally, and a suprastomal stent sutured transluminally for double-stage procedures.

49.5.5 Use of Stents

Laryngeal stents are primarily used adjunctively during LTR. For single-stage procedures, the nasotracheal ETT is used as the primary form of stenting, for 7 to 14 days. For double-stage surgery, a stent is sutured across the airway with a large prolene suture above the stoma, but the stent is not attached to the trach tube. Although an ideal suprastomal stent does not exist, the very useful stents that have been around for over 40 years remain the most popular today. These are primarily the Aboulker-type stents and the soft silicone Montgomery T-tube (▸Fig. 49.6). For the latter, one of the limbs of the T-tube is cut and used

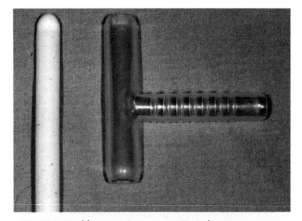

Fig. 49.6 Double-stage airway stents. Typical stents employed in double-stage laryngotracheal reconstruction (LTR), including an Aboulker-type stent on the left and a Montgomery T-tube on the right.

as the stent above the trach. Ideally, stents used after LTR should be rigid enough to keep the reconstructed area and grafts stable in position, permit vocalization, allow for oral intake of food without aspiration, be easy to examine and remove, minimize granulation tissue formation, and be compatible with tracheotomy tube cares and changes. In double-stage cases, the use of suprastomal stent types sutured postoperatively in position at the reconstruction site with some distance between it and the tracheal stoma (i.e., a "short" suprastomal stent) is associated with the formation of granulation tissue and potential stenosis at its distal end in the suprastomal location. For this reason, stenting duration is limited to 3 to 4 weeks.

In cases when the reconstructed tracheal walls are flaccid, or where then there is poor graft stability, or if the anatomy is highly distorted due to previous multiple failed reconstruction attempts, longer stenting periods than 4 weeks may be warranted. To prevent the suprastomal, distal stent granulation tissue formation associated with the "short" suprastomal stents, and allow for longer periods of stenting, a modification in the use of the Aboulker-type stent, where a tracheotomy tube is inserted through a fenestration in a long Aboulker stent encompassing the stomal region and securely wired in position, has been described (i.e., a "long" Aboulker stent). The stenting duration with this "long stent" type could be extended to greater than 2 months. However, due to the inability to change the tracheotomy tube postoperatively and to anecdotal instances of stent fracture, the use of this fenestrated, tracheotomy wired, "long" Aboulker stent has fallen out of favor. Traditionally in adults the most commonly used long-term laryngotracheal stent has been the full Montgomery T-tube. It has also been demonstrated to be an effective, reliable stent in children[6] allowing for long-term stenting (>2 months). T-tubes provide for stable, long-term laryngeal stenting with the possibility of vocalization. They can be readily removed and changed. However, they also have several disadvantages. Due to the potential for mucous plug obstruction associated with smaller T-tubes, they can only be used in children older than 4 years of age and require meticulous postoperative and home care. Failure to maintain plugging of the T-tube's anterior limb invariably results in mucous obstruction. Given that in children there is rarely enough distance between the reconstructed segment of the airway and the free margin of the vocal folds, in order to prevent glottic and supraglottic granulation tissue formation, the T-tube's superior limb has to be positioned above the false vocal cords, leading to a higher potential for significant aspiration. Finally, if the T-tube has to be modified intraoperatively to attain an appropriate superior or inferior limb length, the resulting cut, "nonmachined," edges of the T-tube can result in a significantly higher rate of airway granulation tissue formation.

Large outcome studies demonstrate success (defined by avoidance of tracheotomy need) of single-stage LTP surgery in over 80% of children.[7] The only factor associated with surgical failure was found to be the presence of tracheomalacia. Management of the child in the postoperative period while intubated in the PICU is often difficult and continually evolving. Reports suggest that older children (>3 years old) tolerate the intubation period better and often require minimal sedation or ventilatory assistance (▶Fig. 49.7).

In double-stage procedures, a tracheotomy tube is either placed or left in place after the surgery. As a stent, a sutured indwelling suprastomal stent is left in place postoperatively while the grafts heal (▶Fig. 49.8). Usually the stents are left in place for a period of 2 to 4 weeks with the top of the stent sitting at the level of the arytenoid domes (▶Fig. 49.9). Double-stage approaches are necessary when the child has a need for prolonged stenting, more complex airway lesions, concomitant airway pathology (such as tracheomalacia, impaired vocal cord

mobility, or tongue base obstruction), or in revision surgical cases.

49.5.6 Cricotracheal Resection

Resection of a narrowed laryngotracheal airway segment was first introduced in adults by Conley in 1953 and later popularized in children by Monnier in the 1990s.[2] Multiple reports have since demonstrated that this procedure is more likely to achieve decannulation or avoid a tracheotomy tube in children with severe grade 3 or grade 4 stenosis,[3,8–10] where success rates of greater than 90% have been reported. The concept of this procedure is to resect the narrowed subglottic airway, including the anterolateral cricoid cartilage ring, sparing the posterior cricoid cartilaginous plate, maintaining functional cricoarytenoid joints. As with LTR procedures, CTR can be done in a single- or double-stage fashion. Added postoperative considerations include the usage of chin-to-chest sutures for 7 to 10 days postoperatively to prevent neck extension and anastomotic dehiscence.

49.5.7 Decannulation

For double-stage procedure, the decannulation process begins once DLB indicates an adequate airway including adequate vocal cord movement. The first step is typically a reduction in size of the tracheotomy tube in a controlled environment with usage of a speaking valve, followed by plugging of the tracheotomy tube in a monitored setting. The tube is plugged initially while the patient is awake. The tracheotomy tube remains plugged as long as the

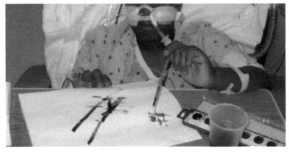

Fig. 49.7 Single-stage anterior graft with intubation. Postoperative day 4, 12-year-old child nasotracheally intubated, able to tolerate the intubation awake in the intensive care unit.

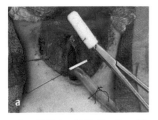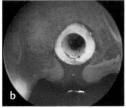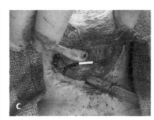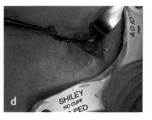

Fig. 49.8 (a–d) Optimal position of stent. Picture demonstrates where the top of the stent should sit in the airway during double-stage surgery.

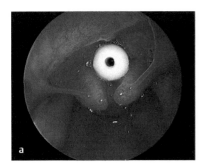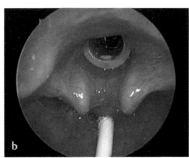

Fig. 49.9 (a, b) Placement of suprastomal stent. Picture demonstrates from left to right how the stent is sutured in place. A large prolene stitch is placed transtracheally securing the stent in place. A small plastic angiocatheter tube helps keep the knot toward the right edge of the trachea. A long knot is tied, protruding on the right edge of the skin incision. The knot is cut at the time of transoral, endoscopic stent removal 2 to 4 weeks after placement.

child shows no clinical evidence of respiratory distress or oxygen desaturation. If the child tolerates plugging while awake then nighttime plugging of the tracheotomy tube is appropriate in a monitored setting including pulse oximetry. Decannulation itself is carried out in a monitored setting (for at least 49 hours) to evaluate for any significant oxygen desaturations.

If a child fails plugging at some point during this process, several possibilities should be considered including supraglottic collapse, inadequate vocal cord movement, residual laryngeal stenosis, suprastomal collapse, and tracheobronchomalacia. If there is any question about the adequacy of the airway or the ability of the child to clear secretions, then plugging the tracheotomy tube for a period of 3 months is advisable during which time the child should be able to tolerate an upper respiratory infection without unplugging. Following decannulation, the child should be evaluated endoscopically for intratracheal granulation tissue.

49.5.8 Postoperative Considerations

The postoperative considerations of patients undergoing laryngotracheal reconstructive procedures depend on the nature of the surgery. For those patients undergoing single-stage procedures, the usage of sedation protocols for PICU management is likely to be helpful in minimizing complications. Children who require high doses of sedation, paralytic agents, and controlled, assisted ventilation are at higher risk of pneumonia, narcotic withdrawal, and need for reintubation. These morbidities are especially salient in the young neonates and infants less than 3 years of age. Older children are less likely to require high levels of ventilatory and anesthetic support.

For double-stage patients, meticulous care of the tracheotomy tube is mandatory. This is especially the case considering the presence of a suprastomal stent above the tracheotomy tube a fact which further confers the child completely tracheotomy tube dependent for an airway. In this setting, accidental decannulation or tracheotomy mucous plugging are potentially lethal events without the appropriate level of nursing and monitoring. Given that children with suprastomal stents, and certainly those with Montgomery T-tubes, are likely to aspirate to a varying degree, a small risk of pneumonia also exists. Careful cooperation with a speech-and-language pathologist to gauge the child's ability to swallow or aspiration

risk is critical in postoperative double-stage patients with indwelling stents. It is not unusual for systemic antibiotics to be needed during the period of stenting. Importantly, after stent removal, the airway will typically display a fair amount of irritation and granulation as a reaction to the stent. Systemic steroids prescribed after stent removal will help alleviate and dissipate this inflammatory reaction. It is critical to surveil the healing graft site 7 to 10 days after stent removal to assess for clearance of the granulation and for adequacy of the reconstructed airway lumen (▶Fig. 49.10).

Long-term, the grafts should epithelialize by 3 months and fully integrate into the airway framework by 6 months (▶Fig. 49.11).

Potential long-term laryngeal complications from grafting and expansion LTR techniques include anterior commissure incongruence (in cases where a complete laryngofissure was required, or if the scarring included the anterior glottis), re-stenosis of the subglottis (fairly unusual, as the reconstructed airway is expected to grow over time), and arytenoid prolapse. The latter is a fairly common long-term sequela of posterior grafting with a reported incidence of 1% to 3%. In some cases the prolapsed arytenoid will cause symptoms of obstruction, especially during exertion and physical activity. Partial CO_2 laser removal of the prolapsed segment of the arytenoid may be required to relieve the symptoms (▶Fig. 49.12).

49.6 Highlights

a. Indications
   - Moderate-to-severe SGS failing to respond to endoscopic techniques such as balloon dilation.
   - Severe posterior glottic stenosis.
   - Bilateral vocal cord paralysis.
b. Contraindications
   - Active airway inflammation.
   - MRSA tracheitis.
   - Untreated reflux or eosinophilic esophagitis.
   - Chronic cardiopulmonary disease (for single-stage procedures).
c. Complications
   - Arytenoid prolapse.
   - Graft prolapse into the airway lumen.
   - Poststent removal airway granulation.
   - Pneumothorax (from rib graft harvest).
   - Graft infection.

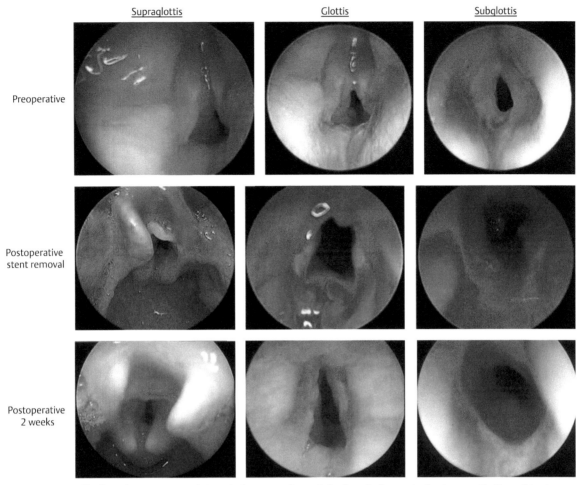

	Supraglottis	Glottis	Subglottis
Preoperative			
Postoperative stent removal			
Postoperative 2 weeks			

Fig. 49.10 Typical healing after stent removal. A marked amount of granulation is typically seen in the airway at the time of stent removal in double-stage cases (*middle row*). It is important to surveil and examine the airway endoscopically 7 to 14 days after stent removal to ensure the inflammation and granulation tissue has cleared (*bottom row*).

d. Special preoperative considerations
   - Examine for other potential airway obstructive levels.
   - Ensure cardiopulmonary maturity and adequacy.
   - Perform preoperative DLB.
e. Special intraoperative considerations
   - Avoid laryngofissure through the anterior commissure if possible.
   - In cases of planned double-stage surgery with an existing tracheotomy, do not violate the mature stoma so as to allow for safe tracheotomy changes in the postoperative period.
   - Assess the split airway segment for lateral wall rigidity, posterior cricoid scarring, and length of the stenosis to inform amount of cartilage needed for grafting.
f. Special postoperative considerations
   - In single-stage surgery, avoid paralysis and consider the use of dexmedetomidine as a primary sedative agent in the intubation period.
   - Keep suprastomal stents for only up to 4 weeks so as to minimize granulation tissue formation, surveil the airway 7 to 10 days after stent removal.
   - Minimize steroid usage perioperatively, but prescribe airway dose steroids at the time of extubation or stent removal.

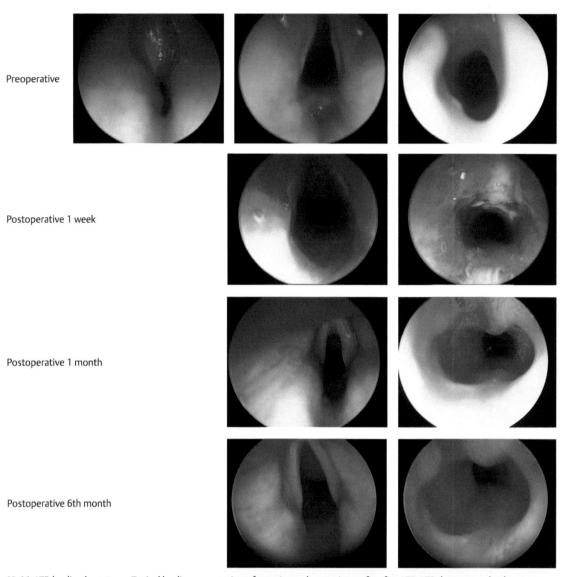

Preoperative

Postoperative 1 week

Postoperative 1 month

Postoperative 6th month

Fig. 49.11 LTR healing long-term. Typical healing progression of anterior and posterior grafts after LTR. LTR, laryngotracheal reconstruction.

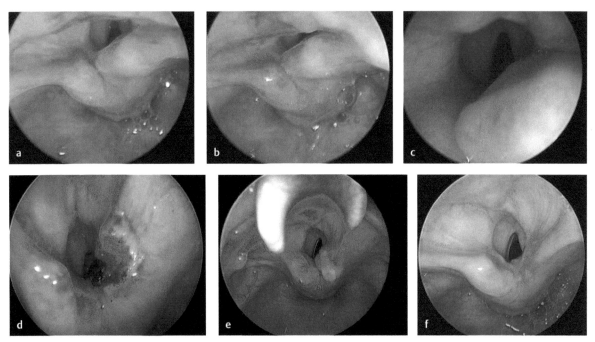

Fig. 49.12 (a–f) Arytenoid prolapse after LTR. Typical arytenoid prolapse into the airway lumen. This is potential long-term complication after posterior graft placement. The bottom row depicts treatment and healing (from left to right) of this complication with CO$_2$ laser partial arytenoidectomy. LTR, laryngotracheal reconstruction.

References

[1] Maresh A, Preciado DA, O'Connell AP, Zalzal GH. A comparative analysis of open surgery vs endoscopic balloon dilation for pediatric subglottic stenosis. JAMA Otolaryngol Head Neck Surg 2014;140(10):901–905

[2] Monnier P, Savary M, Chapuis G. Partial cricoid resection with primary tracheal anastomosis for subglottic stenosis in infants and children. Laryngoscope 1993;103(11 Pt 1):1273–1283

[3] Rutter MJ, Hartley BE, Cotton RT. Cricotracheal resection in children. Arch Otolaryngol Head Neck Surg 2001;127(3):289–292

[4] Zalzal GH. Rib cartilage grafts for the treatment of posterior glottic and subglottic stenosis in children. Ann Otol Rhinol Laryngol 1988;97(5 Pt 1):506–511

[5] Rutter MJ, Cotton RT. The use of posterior cricoid grafting in managing isolated posterior glottic stenosis in children. Arch Otolaryngol Head Neck Surg 2004;130(6):737–739

[6] Stern Y, Willging JP, Cotton RT. Use of Montgomery T-tube in laryngotracheal reconstruction in children: is it safe? Ann Otol Rhinol Laryngol 1998;107(12):1006–1009

[7] Gustafson LM, Hartley BE, Liu JH, et al. Single-stage laryngotracheal reconstruction in children: a review of 200 cases. Otolaryngol Head Neck Surg 2000;123(4):430–434

[8] White DR, Cotton RT, Bean JA, Rutter MJ. Pediatric cricotracheal resection: surgical outcomes and risk factor analysis. Arch Otolaryngol Head Neck Surg 2005;131(10):896–899

[9] Hartley BE, Rutter MJ, Cotton RT. Cricotracheal resection as a primary procedure for laryngotracheal stenosis in children. Int J Pediatr Otorhinolaryngol 2000;54(2–3):133–136

[10] Bailey M, Hoeve H, Monnier P. Paediatric laryngotracheal stenosis: a consensus paper from three European centres. Eur Arch Otorhinolaryngol 2003;260(3):118–123

50 Partial Cricotracheal Resection

Ian N. Jacobs

Summary

The mainstay for repair of severe laryngotracheal stenosis is either laryngotracheal reconstruction (LTR) with cartilage expansion using autologous cartilage or partial cricotracheal resection (CTR) where the scarred segment is excised and the trachea is brought up to replace the resected portion of the cricoid leaving a normal intact posterior cricoid plate. Both procedures are useful in specific clinical situations. The workup, indications, relative contraindications, as well as step-by-step surgical approach is reviewed.

Keywords: Partial cricotracheal resection (pCTR), laryngotracheal reconstruction (LTR)

50.1 Indications

- Severe grades of stenosis, including Grades III and IV (complete stenosis), involving the larynx and upper trachea.
- Normal glottic function and ability to phonate and protect the airway.
- Competent larynx and swallow.
- Some degree (at least 5 mm) of separation from the glottis.
- Resectable portion—less than 50% of trachea.
- Better pulmonary function for older children being considered for single stage (SS).

50.2 Relative Contraindications

- Mild grades of subglottic stenosis (Cotton Grades I and II).
- Infants.
- Poor glottic function or glottic scarring.
- Active gastroesophageal reflux disease (GERD) or eosinophilic esophagitis (EE).
- Active inflammatory airway.
- Multiple previous surgeries making mobilization difficult.
- Previous tracheoesophageal fistula (TEF) or laryngeal cleft repair.
- Bilateral vocal cord (VC) paralysis or fixation.
- At least five to seven normal tracheal rings.
- Poor pulmonary or cardiac function.
- Supraglottic stenosis.
- Extensive length of disease where resection would not be possible (greater than 50% of the trachea).
- Severe cervicospine neck problems or scarring limiting mobilization.

50.3 Comparison to LTR Best Handles

- Less severe grades of stenosis.
- Glottic stenosis/restriction which is so common.
- Bilateral VC paralysis.
- Tracheotomy-related problems, such as severe suprastomal prolapse.[1,2]

50.4 Grades of Stenosis III, IV

50.4.1 Diagnostic Evaluation

- **Outpatient clinical evaluation:** The evaluation starts with the multidisciplinary aerodigestive clinic where the patient is screened by phone call triage and care is coordinated ahead of time. Previous studies, as well as the parent's goal, are reviewed (i.e., "The goal is to get the tracheotomy out"). The patient is then seen by otolaryngology, gastroenterology, pulmonary, speech, nutrition, and a nurse practitioner. Awake flexible laryngoscopy is performed to examine the nasopharynx, pharynx, and larynx, and the results are recorded. The exam is performed to detect enlarged adenoids, tonsils, tongue base collapse, and pooling of secretions. The larynx is examined awake to determine vocal fold mobility and supraglottic stenosis.
- **Swallow evaluation:** First clinical evaluation in the aerodigestive clinic by a speech and swallow therapist (SLP). He/she will take a feeding history and may observe the child swallowing, looking for signs such as aspiration and congestion. Functional endoscopic evaluation of swallowing (FEES) or modified barium swallow is then performed to detect gross or silent aspiration.
- **GERD workup:** The gastroenterologist will take an extensive history and physical examination. He/she may order a number of diagnostic studies including upper gastrointestinal tract radiography (upper GI), esophagogastroduodenoscopy (EGD), and/or impedance. During triple scope, EE and uncontrolled GERD are ruled out.
- **Triple endoscopy:** Pulmonary laryngoscopy, bronchoscopy, and EGD. The otolaryngologist will place the patient into suspension and perform a detailed examination of the pharynx, larynx, and trachea. First, tongue base collapse, enlarged lingual, and/or pharyngeal tonsils are ruled out or in. Then the supraglottis is examined dynamically during the flexible laryngoscopy under general anesthesia (sleep endoscopy)

for epiglottic prolapse or supraglottic stenosis. During rigid microlaryngoscopy, the larynx is suspended and the vocal folds are evaluated for normal mobility versus fixation or paralysis. The arytenoids may be palpated for fixation or prolapse. The stenosis is then examined with a thin telescope. In severe Grade III stenosis, a 2.7-mm Hopkins rod telescope may be placed. If possible, the approximate distance from the end of the stenosis to the tracheotomy site is determined. Evidence of normal distal tracheal rings is examined. Also the trachea and bronchi are examined for tracheobronchomalacia. Appropriate surveillance cultures of the distal right middle lobe bronchus are taken during the pulmonary lavage for preoperative antibiotic planning. EGD is performed with multilevel biopsies and then an impedance probe is placed.[3–5]

50.4.2 General Surgical Approach

- Single stage (SS) vs. double stage (DS).
- Microlaryngoscopy and bronchoscopy (MLB).
- Surgical procedure (Standard pCTR).[6]

1. The patient undergoes an initial MLB. The stenosis and surgical plan are reviewed with the team. The airway is also checked for infection and distal secretions. The airway is then secured with either an oral endotracheal tube that fits the stenosis or a cuffed flexible anode tube in the stoma, if an in-dwelling trach is present. The patient is given IV antibiotics consisting of appropriate anti-pseudomonas and anaerobic coverage, such as IV ceftazadime and clindamycin. The patient is placed in a hyper-extended position and an esophageal bougie is placed (▶Fig. 50.1).

2. After prepping and draping a standard wide-field apron, the incision is made and a superior and inferior subplatysmal flap is elevated and sutured in place. The laryngotracheal complex is then dissected free. Under endoscopic control, a midline cricoid incision is made in case a decision is made to convert to LTR. The final decision is made intraoperatively (▶Fig. 50.2). CTR would be necessary if the cricoid block was not expandable with rib grafts.

3. The airway is inspected and, if it appears that the segment would do better with resection, lateral cuts are made removing the anterior of the cricoid leaving the lateral buttress (▶Fig. 50.3). This depends on whether the airway can be best expanded or it must be resected.

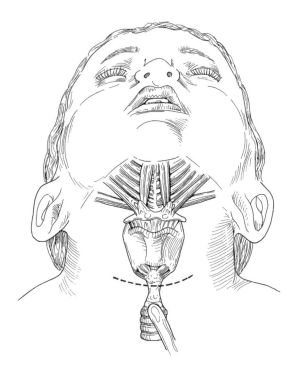

Fig. 50.1 Partial cricotracheal resection is performed under general anesthesia administered through a reinforced endotracheal tube in the tracheostomy site. (Reproduced from Potsic, Cotton, Handler, and Zur, Surgical Pediatric Otolaryngology, 2nd edition, ©2016, Thieme Publishers, New York. Illustration by Susan Shapiro Brenman/Birck Cox/Eo Trueblood.)

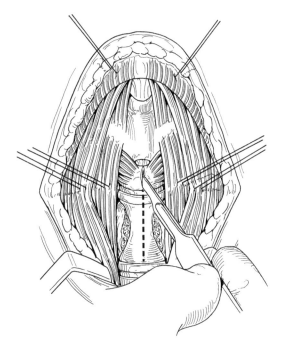

Fig. 50.2 A vertical incision is made through the cricoid and stenotic segment extending to the normal trachea below. (Reproduced from Potsic, Cotton, Handler, and Zur, Surgical Pediatric Otolaryngology, 2nd edition, ©2016, Thieme Publishers, New York. Illustration by Susan Shapiro Brenman/ Birck Cox/Eo Trueblood.)

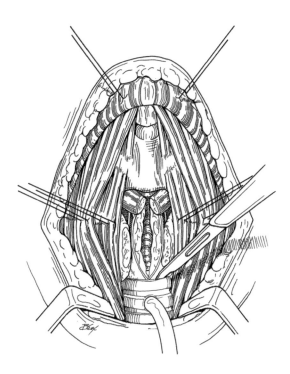

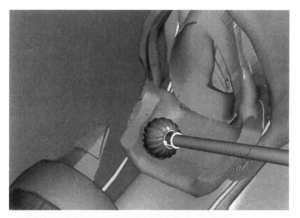

Fig. 50.4 Oblique view of the subglottis after resection of the stenotic cricotracheal segment. The uppermost posterior section of the mucosa is made just below the cricoarytenoid joints. A diamond burr is used to widen the denuded cricoid plate, and a triangular wedge of cartilage is kept attached anteriorly to the tracheal ring used for the anastomosis. (Reproduced with permission of W.B./SAUNDERS CO. Monnier P, Lang F, Savary M. Cricotracheal resection for adult and pediatric subglottic stenosis: Similarities and differences. *Operative Techniques in Otolaryngology Head Neck Surgery*.)

Fig. 50.3 The trachea is transected below the stenosis with a knife, preserving the integrity of the esophagus. (Reproduced from Potsic, Cotton, Handler, and Zur, Surgical Pediatric Otolaryngology, 2nd edition, ©2016, Thieme Publishers, New York. Illustration by Susan Shapiro Brenman/Birck Cox/Eo Trueblood.)

4. The lateral shelves are shaved down and the posterior cricoid is drilled flat as well. All firm scar tissue is simply removed with the drill. The airway is sculpted and the cricoid is taken down to a thin plate. This prepares the posterior cricoid plate for acceptance of the trachea (▶ Fig. 50.4).

5. If necessary, a suprahyoid release is performed to relieve tension on the suture line (▶ Fig. 50.5). The distal trachea is mobilized as well and a hilar release may be performed if necessary.

6. The common party space is entered and the esophagus is separated from the trachea going down to the mediastinum (▶ Fig. 50.6).

7. The trachea is brought up to replace the cricoid and two traction sutures are placed on both lateral tracheal rings (▶ Fig. 50.7).

8. The posterior tracheal mucosa is sutured to the superior cricoid with 4–5 interrupted vicryl sutures, which are first placed and then tied. The suture is placed through the trachealis mucosal flap and anchored to the posterior cricoid cartilage (▶ Fig. 50.8).

9. The ventilating tube is taken out when the sutures are tied and then replaced.

10. A decision is made whether to do the procedure single stage over an endotracheal tube or double stage over a Montgomery T-tube.

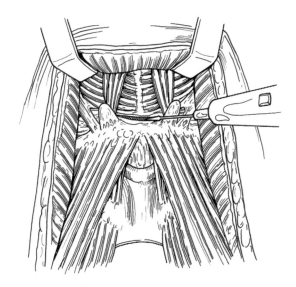

Fig. 50.5 The larynx is then released from its suprahyoid attachments. A transverse incision is made just above the hyoid bone using electrocautery, releasing the geniohyoid and hyoglossal muscles from the hyoid bone. (Reproduced from Potsic, Cotton, Handler, and Zur, Surgical Pediatric Otolaryngology, 2nd edition, ©2016, Thieme Publishers, New York. Illustration by Susan Shapiro Brenman/Birck Cox/Eo Trueblood.)

11. Next the lateral tracheal suture is placed through the lateral cricoid shelve taken care to avoid the recurrent laryngeal nerve (RLN). These are placed and then tied to pull up the tracheal segment (▶ Fig. 50.9).

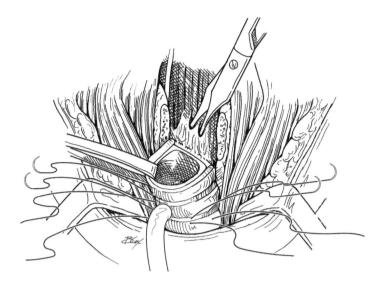

Fig. 50.6 The inferior portion of the trachea is released by careful dissection of soft tissue of the party wall to facilitate the anastomosis. (Reproduced from Potsic, Cotton, Handler, and Zur, Surgical Pediatric Otolaryngology, 2nd edition, ©2016, Thieme Publishers, New York. Illustration by Susan Shapiro Brenman/Birck Cox/Eo Trueblood.)

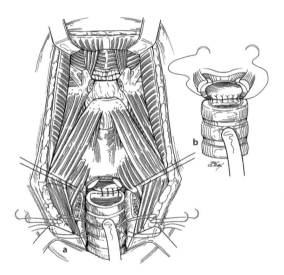

Fig. 50.7 (a, b) A running continuous suture technique using a double-armed 4–0 PDS suture is used to complete the anastomosis from posterodistally to anteroproximally. (Reproduced from Potsic, Cotton, Handler, and Zur, Surgical Pediatric Otolaryngology, 2nd edition, ©2016, Thieme Publishers, New York. Illustration by Susan Shapiro Brenman/Birck Cox/Eo Trueblood.)

12. The anterior lateral sutures are placed in vertical mattress fashion. They are placed and tied at the end (▶Fig. 50.10).
13. Fibrin glue on the suture line.
14. The polydioxanone suture (PDS) suture is used to reduce internal tension. This is done by suturing the lateral trachea to the thyroid cartilage with two 2.0 PDS sutures (▶Fig. 50.11).
15. Repeat scope and nasotracheal intubation with an age-appropriate tube.

16. External chin to chest (Grillo suture) or neck immobilization collar (▶Fig. 50.12).
17. The child is kept intubated with the neck in a flexed or neutral position for 7 to 10 days and then rescoped and extubated if single stage.

50.4.3 Major Pearls of the Surgery

- Avoidance of the RLN: stay right on the cartilage of the laryngotracheal complex and avoid going lateral; RLN should be avoided. Also take care with the lateral sutures, stay medial and somewhat anterior to the space where the RLN goes in.
- Don't burn a bridge until you decide to CTR. Important to start with vertical midline split in the cricoid until you decide that CTR is most optimal and doable.
- Tension release: Imperative to have a tension-free anastomosis. Ample mobilization can be obtained by the laryngeal release. Further maneuvers on the trachea can get more mobilization, but be careful of tracheal blood supply.
- Posterior plate can be shaved down to "sculpt" the airway, making sure all scar tissue is reduced.
- Airway approach: Single stage is best for most uncomplicated cases where the patient is not a high risk for re-stenosis.

50.5 Single Stage verses Double Stage

Most cases can be done in single-stage fashion as long as the stenosis is simple and not multilevel, where an extended CTR would be performed. Also the medical and pulmonary status would need to be optimal. In these cases, the anastomosis is closed around an

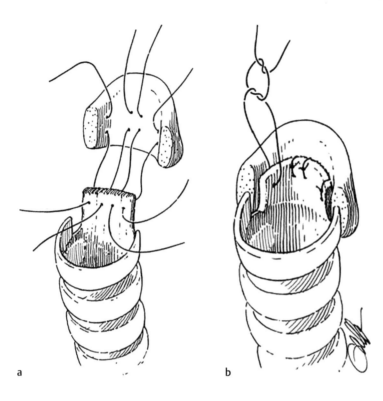

Fig. 50.8 (a, b) Anterior views of posterior anastomosis suture placement. (Reproduced with permission of Boseley ME, Hartnick CJ. Pediatric partial cricotracheal resection: A new technique for the posterior cricoid anastomosis. *Otolaryngology Head Neck Surgery* 2006; 135:320.)

a

b

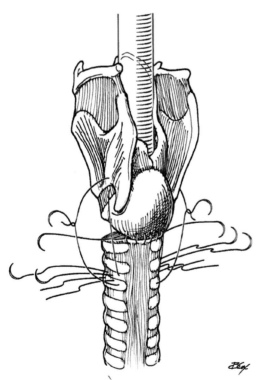

Fig. 50.9 The anastomosis is completed by running the 3–0 PDS suture anteriorly through the lower thyroid cartilage and lateral cricoid cartilage to connect to the tracheal rings. (Reproduced from Potsic, Cotton, Handler, and Zur, Surgical Pediatric Otolaryngology, 2nd edition, ©2016, Thieme Publishers, New York. Illustration by Susan Shapiro Brenman/ Birck Cox/Eo Trueblood.)

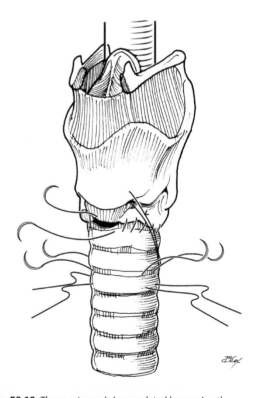

Fig. 50.10 The anastomosis is completed by running the 3–0 PDS suture anteriorly through the lower thyroid cartilage and lateral cricoid cartilage to connect to the tracheal rings. (Reproduced from Potsic, Cotton, Handler, and Zur, Surgical Pediatric Otolaryngology, 2nd edition, ©2016, Thieme Publishers, New York. Illustration by Susan Shapiro Brenman/ Birck Cox/Eo Trueblood.)

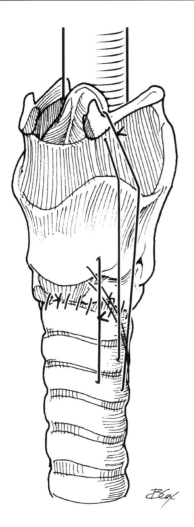

Fig. 50.11 The tension-releasing sutures placed above are now tied. Additional tension-releasing sutures are placed bilaterally in the posterolateral trachea using 3–0 PS that is passed through the posterolateral aspect of the thyroid cartilage. (Reproduced from Potsic, Cotton, Handler, and Zur, Surgical Pediatric Otolaryngology, 2nd edition, ©2016, Thieme Publishers, New York. Illustration by Susan Shapiro Brenman/Birck Cox/Eo Trueblood.)

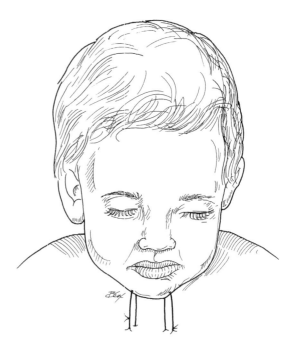

Fig. 50.12 Two sutures are placed from the skin of the chin to the skin of the chest with 0-Prolene to prevent extension of the neck. If the anastomosis is not under undue tension, a cervical collar is a good alternative. (Reproduced from Potsic, Cotton, Handler, and Zur, Surgical Pediatric Otolaryngology, 2nd edition, ©2016, Thieme Publishers, New York. Illustration by Susan Shapiro Brenman/Birck Cox/Eo Trueblood.)

50.7 Combined LTR and CTR

In situations where there is both glottic and subglottic stenosis, a CTR can be combined with an LTR with posterior grafting (combined LTR/pCTR). This will require extended periods of stenting typically with a Montgomery T-tube.

50.8 Postoperative Care

It's imperative to keep the patient's neck in a neutral or flexion position at all times. The "Grillo" suture from the chest to the chin prevents hyperextension, flexion, or brace. This may be discontinued in approximately in 7 to 10 days (▶Fig. 50.13).

The intubated older child or teen may be kept awake with a humid cuff on the nasotracheal tube. The T-tube requires frequent suctioning and irrigations.

IV antibiotics are continued for 72 hours until drains are removed. In cases of methicillin-resistant *Staphylococcus aureus* (MRSA), appropriate coverage is necessary, such as vancomycin, for that period. Repeat MLB is performed at 7 days right before extubation or later for children who are stented for longer periods of time with a Montgomery T-Tube.

age-appropriate endotracheal tube and the patient is kept intubated for 5 to 7 days. In more complex cases, the procedure can be double-staged over a Montgomery T-tube. It is imperative not to use a size smaller than a 7 as they may plug frequently.

50.6 Extended CTR

The limits of resection can be extended to include and treat stenosis involving the glottis and supraglottis and distal trachea. The extended procedures may involve longer periods of stenting and are less often amenable to single-stage approaches.

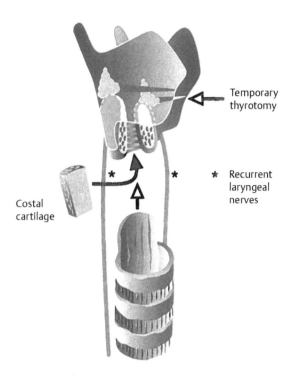

Fig. 50.13 Cricotracheal resection (CTR) with posterior costal cartilage graft (according to Rethi) for the cure of combined subglottic and posterior glottic stenoses. CTR is performed according to the conventional technique. A pedicled flap of membranous trachea is obtained by removing two more rings of the tracheal stump distally. A posterior midline incision of the cricoid plate is made through a temporary thyrotomy, and a costal cartilage graft is interposed between the two parts of the posterior cricoid (*black arrow*). The trachea is advanced upward (*open arrow*), and its membranous portion is sutured to the mucosa of the posterior commissure of the larynx. The lateral and anterior anastomosis is completed as in conventional CTR. A full mucosal lining of the subglottis is obtained in this way. A laryngeal stent is used for 3 to 4 weeks if the tracheostoma site remains in place. Stenting with a nasotracheal tube for 1 week proved sufficient in the two cases treated thus far without tracheotomy. (Reproduced with permission of W.B./SAUNDERS CO. Monnier P, Lang F, Savary M. Cricotracheal resection for adult and pediatric subglottic stenosis: Similarities and differences. *Operative Techniques in Otolaryngology Head Neck Surgery*.)

50.9 Results

The published results and outcomes for standard partial CTR used to treat Grades III and IV pure subglottic stenosis are quite good. The success rate is generally listed as over 90% for all grades of stenosis percentage.[2,3] Revision and extended CTR does not do quite as well. Generally, the operation outperforms LTR for the severe grades of stenosis. However, CTR is a more complicated surgery than LTR, and therefore a steep learning curve is found. A surgeon's first CTR should be straightforward one.

When something goes wrong it can really go wrong rapidly. Complications are listed below.[4,5]

50.10 Complications

Frequent complications (temporary) include:
- Temporary dysphagia or aspiration.
- Atelectasis.
- Neuromuscular weakness.
- Pneumonia or respiratory issues.
- Wound infection.
- Airway edema.
- Suture line granulation.

Severe complications (less common) include:
- Postop stridor.
- Voice change.
- Glottic edema—conus elasticus from close resection to glottis or very young patients—less than 2 years.
- Chronic aspiration.
- Anastomotic dehiscence.
- Re-stenosis.
- Late arytenoid prolapse.
- Wound infection.
- Spinal cord injuries from positioning.

Postoperative edema can be managed with steroids and watchful waiting when not severe. Occasionally, balloon dilation may be needed to press out glottic or conus elasticus edema. This may need to be repeated more than once. Chronic aspiration may be treated with temporary nasogastric (NGT) feeds and the use of thickeners with thin liquids. Anaptotic dehiscence will require emergency reoperation to repair the dehiscent region and cover it with vascularized muscle grafts. Re-stenosis may need repeated balloon dilations with steroid injections. Occasionally, it may require revision surgery with augmentation cartilage grafts. Wound infections will need to be drained, cultured, and treated with IV antibiotics. Spinal cord injuries are best avoided in the first place by avoiding extreme hyperextension on the operating table and severe flexion.[5]

50.11 Conclusion

In summary, partial CTR is a great operation for severe grades of subglottic stenosis and often outperforms laryngotracheal reconstruction with cartilage grafts. The operation is more technically difficult and requires a high level of expertise, being more detailed than LTR, but when done well, may be better than LTR. Meticulous patient selection and postoperative care are essential to an optimal outcome. Overall, extended approaches may manage multilevel stenosis as well, although it is best performed in a double-stage rather than single-stage fashion.

50.12 Highlights

a. Indications
   - Severe grades of subglottic stenosis—grades III and IV.
   - Normal competent glottis and ability to phonate and protect the airway.
   - Competent swallow.
   - Some degree of separation (at least 5 mm) of the stenosis from the glottis.
   - Resected portion less 50 % of the trachea.
   - Good cardiopulmonary function for single-stage.

b. Contraindications
   - Bilateral vocal cord paralysis.
   - Mild grades of stenosis—grade I and II.
   - Active inflamed airway.
   - Previous tracheal esophageal fistula (TEF).
   - Previous multiple surgeries making mobilization difficult.
   - Poor glottic function or scarring.
   - Active inflamed larynx or uncontrolled GERD.
   - Supraglottic stenosis.
   - Extensive length of tracheal resection.
   - Severe cervical spine problems limiting extension or neck mobilization.
   - Infants.

c. Complications
   - Postoperative stridor.
   - Late arytenoid prolapse.
   - Restenosis.
   - Voice change.
   - Wound infection.
   - Anastomotic dehiscence.
   - Recurrent laryngeal nerve paralysis.

d. Special preoperative considerations
   - Preoperative triple scope with ENT, GI and pulmonary, impedance probe and biopsies.
   - Cultures to determine antibiotic coverage.
   - Antibiotics and short acting relaxants.

e. Special intraoperative considerations
   - Head extension and placement of esophageal bougie.
   - Establish airway with cuffed ventilation tube in tracheostome site.
   - Dissection of the cricoid first and midline incision to explore stenosis opening.
   - Resection anterior arch of cricoid and include scarred upper tracheal rings.
   - Laryngeal release maneuvers to free up tension.
   - Mobilization of the larynx and trachea.
   - Separation of the esophagus from the trachea.
   - Dissection on the trachea and no need to dissect RLN's or monitor RLN.
   - Resection of the stenotic segment.
   - Remove esophageal bougie and reduce head extension.
   - Crico-tracheal anastomosis with lateral sutures tension releasing sutures posterior and then anterior suturing with ventilating tube taken in and out.
   - Head flexion with possible Grillo suture.
   - Nasotracheal intubation.
   - Staged repair with T-tube for extended CTR.

f. Special postoperative considerations
   - Maintain head flexion for 7 days.
   - Rescope and extubate when healed.

References

[1] Gallagher TQ, Hartnick CJ. Cricotracheal resection and thryotracheal anastomosis. Adv Otorhinolaryngol 2012;73:42–49

[2] Jaquet Y, Lang F, Pilloud R, Savary M, Monnier P. Partial cricotracheal resection for pediatric subglottic stenosis: long-term outcome in 57 patients. J Thorac Cardiovasc Surg 2005;130(3):726–732

[3] Bajaj Y, Cochrane LA, Jephson CG, et al. Laryngotracheal reconstruction and cricotracheal resection in children: recent experience at Great Ormond Street Hospital. Int J Pediatr Otorhinolaryngol 2012;76(4):507–511

[4] Hartley BE, Cotton RT. Paediatric airway stenosis: laryngotracheal reconstruction or cricotracheal resection? Clin Otolaryngol Allied Sci 2000;25(5):342–349

[5] George M, Ikonomidis C, Jaquet Y, Monnier P. Partial cricotracheal resection in children: potential pitfalls and avoidance of complications. Otolaryngol Head Neck Surg 2009;141(2):225–231

[6] Potsic WP, Cotton RT, Handler SD, Zur KB, eds. Surgical pediatric otolaryngology. 2nd ed. New York, NY: Thieme; 2016:385–395

51 Harvesting Costal Cartilage for Laryngotracheal Reconstruction

Anat Wengier, Ari DeRowe

Summary

Laryngotracheal reconstruction (LTR) includes a variety of techniques for expanding the laryngotracheal complex and stabilizing the resultant airway, in cases of laryngotracheal stenosis.

Cartilage interposition grafting for treatment of subglottic stenosis was pioneered in 1972, and has since become the work horse for LTR.

The chapter will describe surgical technique for costal cartilage graft harvest and discuss the postoperative care and possible complications of the procedure.

Keywords: Laryngotracheal stenosis, costal cartilage, laryngotracheal reconstruction

51.1 Introduction

Pediatric laryngotracheal stenosis involves a wide variety of pathologies caused by scar tissue formation in most cases but can also be a result of congenital anomalies.[1-3]

Various techniques for surgical management exist and will be discussed in other chapters.

Laryngotracheal reconstruction (LTR) is a procedure in which the thyroid, cricoid, and tracheal cartilages are split and the framework is expanded with various combinations of cartilage grafts and stents.

LTR has evolved to include a variety of techniques for expanding the laryngotracheal complex and stabilizing the resultant airway.

Different materials have been used in LTR over the years including short- and long-term stents, silastic sheaths, and auricular, thyroid, or costal cartilage grafts.[4]

Cartilage interposition grafting for treatment of subglottic stenosis was pioneered by Fearon and Cotton in 1972,[5] and has since become the work horse for LTR.[6-9]

In this section, we wish to describe the surgical technique for costal cartilage graft harvest and discuss the postoperative care and possible complications of the procedure.

51.2 Indications and Contraindications

Costal cartilage grafting is indicated in patients with subglottic or tracheal stenosis who are planned for laryngotracheoplasty or LTR.[10,11] Contraindications include recent pulmonary infection and restrictive lung disease. Special consideration should be taken in children with prior cardiothoracic surgery as pleural adhesions may exist with resulting pleural tears during surgery.

51.3 Surgical Technique

To accurately describe surgical procedure it is imperative to include both stenotic site and donor site.

First, direct laryngoscopy and bronchoscopy under general anesthesia is performed, while maintaining spontaneous ventilation (▶Fig. 51.1). After determining the location, degree, and length of stenosis, the patient is ventilated either through an existing tracheostomy tube or via an endotracheal tube.

The patient is then prepped and draped for the procedure at two separate sites.

Incisions are marked; horizontal neck incision in skin crease and costal cartilage donor site incision over the forth rib just lateral to the synchondrosis (▶Fig. 51.2).

Surgical sites are injected with 1% lidocaine with 1:100,000 epinephrine.

The neck incision is made at the level of an existing tracheostomy tube or just below the cricoid. Subplatysmal flaps are elevated to expose the thyroid cartilage superiorly and the thyroid inferiorly. The trachea is exposed by dividing strap muscles at the midline raphe and 2–0 silk sutures are placed through strap musculature to facilitate exposure (▶Fig. 51.3).

A thyroid isthmectomy is performed and the gland is separated from the trachea.

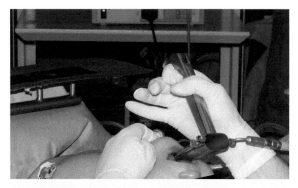

Fig. 51.1 Direct laryngoscopy setup.

The trachea is entered using a #15 or #11 blade and stenotic segment is incised precisely in the midline (▶Fig. 51.4), while a direct laryngoscopy is performed to re-evaluate the airway and location and adequacy of the vertical tracheolaryngeal incision. Adrenalin-soaked pledgets are placed along mucosal edges for hemostasis.

Next the length of cartilage graft necessary to repair stenosis is measured. At this point graft position and architecture is planned, determining whether anterior graft will suffice or posterior graft may also be needed.

The neck surgical site is covered and costal cartilage graft is harvested.

Right costal cartilages are preferred due to cardiac location. A 3- to 4-cm incision is made at the level of the fourth to fifth rib (▶Fig. 51.5); the incision continues through skin, subcutaneous tissue, and fascial layers to the level of external oblique muscles. Costal cartilage is exposed while carefully preserving outer perichondrium (▶Fig. 51.6). The bony-cartilaginous junctions are identified to evaluate graft potential length. A rectangular segment of cartilage exceeding the size of the measured stenosis is carefully separated with a periosteal elevator from the posterior wall of the rib, taking care not to penetrate the inner perichondrium and injure

the pleura. In order to free the costal cartilage, a curved rib dissector is used (▶Fig. 51.7). The rib cartilage is incised at the bony-cartilaginous junction and then dissected toward the sternum where another incision is performed after measuring and attaining adequate length (▶Fig. 51.8).

The cartilage segment is then harvested and the donor site is evaluated for pleural competency by placing saline

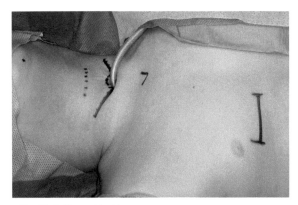

Fig. 51.2 Planned incisions.

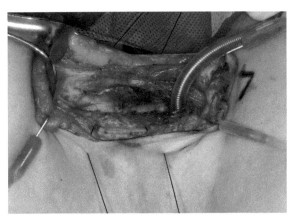

Fig. 51.3 Anterior tracheal wall exposure.

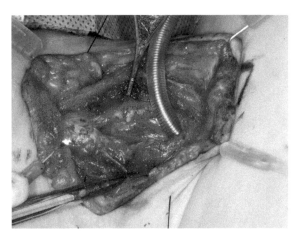

Fig. 51.4 Midline incision of anterior tracheal wall.

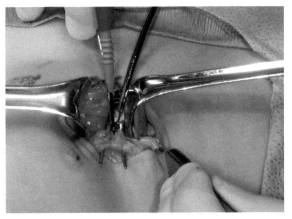

Fig. 51.5 Chest incision in inframammary line.

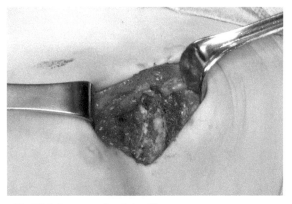

Fig. 51.6 Exposure of costal cartilage.

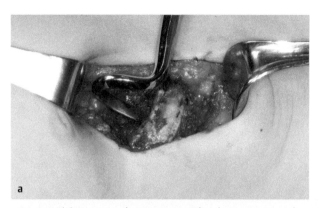
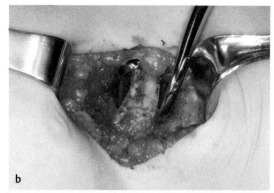

Fig. 51.7 (a) Preserving the posterior perichondrium—superior release. **(b)** Inferior and posterior release.

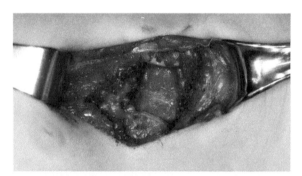

Fig. 51.8 Graft segment incised, pleura preserved.

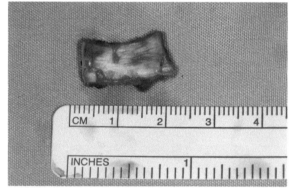

Fig. 51.9 Costal cartilage harvested graft.

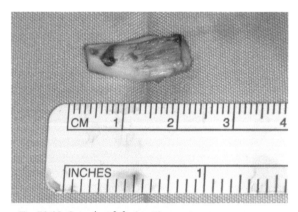

Fig. 51.10 Carved graft for insetting.

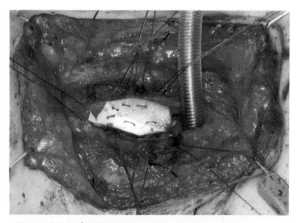

Fig. 51.11 Graft insetting.

in the surgical wound and applying 40-cm positive-pressure ventilation while looking for bubbles.

Following meticulous hemostasis, the wound is closed in a layered fashion. No drain is needed.

The costal cartilage graft is then designed to fit the airway defect, usually carved in an elongated boat-shape and the edges are graded to avoid graft dislodgement (▶ Fig. 51.9 and ▶ Fig. 51.10).

Prior to graft placement the cartilage is placed in Cefazolin solution.

The graft is positioned in the anterior airway defect with perichondrium lining the airway. 4–0 PDS mattress sutures are first placed in graft circumference and then secured individually once the graft is in place (▶ Fig. 51.11). The ties should be performed on the tracheal/laryngeal cartilage and not on the graft. Usually the external surface of the graft will project above adjacent trachea.

If tracheotomy is present, tracheotomy site may be incised and fistula closed in layered fashion for one-stage repair followed by a leak test to verify adequacy of seal with an endotracheal tube left as stent for approximately 1 week.[1,2] If a two-stage repair is performed, either a T-tube is inserted in place of the tracheostomy tube or a stent is sutured at the level of the graft, to be later removed.

Surgical wound is closed in a layered fashion, with a Penrose catheter left as drain deep to the strap muscles.

51.4 Donor Site Postoperative Care

Chest X-ray is obtained in the recovery room or intensive care unit to ensure there is no pneumothorax.

Donor site is examined for signs of infection daily.

Consideration should be given regarding postoperative pain management.

51.5 Donor Site Complications

Surgical complications of costal cartilage harvest are rare and include minor and major complications. While the list of minor complications include postoperative pleuritic pain, seroma formation, surgical site infection, pleural tear, chest wall deformity, and keloid formation; pneumothorax is the one major donor site complication of this procedure.[1,3,1,4]

To avoid pneumothorax formation, a leak test is performed as mentioned above. If pleural injury is detected, a small caliber catheter is inserted through the pleural tear into the chest cavity with its free end placed in saline solution. The pleura is then sutured around the catheter, while the anesthesiologist performs positive pressure ventilation until the air bubbling in the saline container disappears once air from the chest cavity is completely drained. The catheter is removed as the suture is tied.

If the pleural repair fails and pneumothorax evolves, a chest tube is inserted and left until resolved.

51.6 Highlights

- Bony-cartilaginous junction should be identified to maximize graft length.
- Great care should be taken during dissection to avoid pleural tear.
- When identified, pleural tears should be repaired to avoid pneumothorax formation.
- Graft design should include grading of graft edges to avoid dislodgement.
- Pain should be managed diligently in the postoperative period.

References

[1] Cotton RT, Myer CM III, O'Connor DM. Innovations in pediatric laryngotracheal reconstruction. J Pediatr Surg 1992;27(2):196–200

[2] Cotton RT, Myer CM III, O'Connor DM, Smith ME. Pediatric laryngotracheal reconstruction with cartilage grafts and endotracheal tube stenting: the single-stage approach. Laryngoscope 1995;105(8 Pt 1):818–821

[3] Hartley BE, Cotton RT. Paediatric airway stenosis: laryngotracheal reconstruction or cricotracheal resection? Clin Otolaryngol Allied Sci 2000;25(5):342–349. Review

[4] Javia LR, Zur KB. Laryngotracheal reconstruction with resorbable microplate buttressing. Laryngoscope 2012;122(4):920–924

[5] Fearon B, Cotton R. Surgical correction of subglottic stenosis of the larynx. Preliminary report of an experimental surgical technique. Ann Otol Rhinol Laryngol 1972;81(4):508–513

[6] Schmidt RJ, Shah G, Sobin L, Reilly JS. Laryngotracheal reconstruction in infants and children: are single-stage anterior and posterior grafts a reliable intervention at all pediatric hospitals? Int J Pediatr Otorhinolaryngol 2011;75(12):1585–1588

[7] Bailey M, Hoeve H, Monnier P. Paediatric laryngotracheal stenosis: a consensus paper from three European centres. Eur Arch Otorhinolaryngol 2003;260(3):118–123

[8] Gustafson LM, Hartley BE, Liu JH, et al. Single-stage laryngotracheal reconstruction in children: a review of 200 cases. Otolaryngol Head Neck Surg 2000;123(4):430–434. Review

[9] Lewis S, Earley M, Rosenfeld R, Silverman J. Systematic review for surgical treatment of adult and adolescent laryngotracheal stenosis. Laryngoscope 2017;127(1):191–198

[10] Hartley BE, Gustafson LM, Liu JH, Hartnick CJ, Cotton RT. Duration of stenting in single-stage laryngotracheal reconstruction with anterior costal cartilage grafts. Ann Otol Rhinol Laryngol 2001 May;110(5 Pt 1):413–416

[11] Gallagher TQ, Hartnick CJ. Costal cartilage harvest. Adv Otorhinolaryngol 2012;73:39–41

[12] Wee JH, Park MH, Oh S, Jin HR. Complications associated with autologous rib cartilage use in rhinoplasty: a meta-analysis. JAMA Facial Plast Surg 2015;17(1):49–55

[13] Varadharajan K, Sethukumar P, Anwar M, Patel K. Complications associated with the use of autologous costal cartilage in rhinoplasty: a systematic review. Aesthet Surg J 2015;35(6):644–652

[14] Yang HC, Cho H-H, Jo SY, Jang CH, Cho YB. Donor-site morbidity following minimally invasive costal cartilage harvest technique. Clin Exp Otorhinolaryngol 2015;8(1):13–19

52 Laryngotracheal Cleft Repair

Nikolaus E. Wolter, Reza Rahbar

Summary

Laryngotracheal cleft (LC) represent a spectrum of anomalous connections of the trachea and esophagus extending from laryngeal inlet. In general, the degree of symptoms varies with length of the LC. Diagnosis requires a high index of suspicion. Shallow clefts maybe treated with conservative or medical management but longer clefts will require surgical repair. Surgery can be done endoscopically or open and depends on the cleft size and the experience of the surgeon. In all cases, management requires a multidisciplinary approach.

Keywords: Laryngeal cleft, laryngotracheal cleft, laryngotracheoesophageal cleft

52.1 Introduction

LC represents a spectrum of anomalous connections of the trachea and esophagus extending from laryngeal inlet. In general, the degree of symptoms varies with the length of the LC. LCs are typically classified based on their length in relation to surrounding structures (▶Table 52.1). The most commonly employed classification was described by Benjamin and Inglis[1] and is outlined in detail below (▶Fig. 52.1). However, each LC must be viewed in the context of the child's overall health as a shallow LC will impact an otherwise healthy child differently than a child with concomitant cardiac disease.[2,3] The most common sequelae include recurrent aspirations, pneumonia, and bronchiectasis. Children often undergo multiple investigations prior to diagnosis and are often hospitalized with infection. Type 1

and even some type 2 LCs may go unnoticed for prolonged periods, and diagnosis is often quite delayed. It is critical for physicians to be cognizant of LCs when considering children with recurrent aspiration or else they are likely to be missed.[2] Deeper LCs are often more symptomatic. Type 3 or type 4 LC will often present within days after birth; however, patients presenting later in life have been described.[2]

LCs are rare with estimates ranging from 1:10,000 to 1:20,000 live births.[8] However, considering the subtle presentation of many type 1 and type 2 LCs, the true incidence is not known. Among children undergoing direct laryngoscopy for recurrent respiratory symptoms, the incidence ranges from 0.2% to 7.6%.[2,9] It is believed that there is a slight male predominance for LCs, but no genetic inheritance patterns have been confirmed.[2]

52.2 Embryology of Laryngotracheal Clefts

The etiology of LC is controversial, as the understanding of how the tracheoesophageal septum forms remains incomplete.[10,11] Traditionally, it was felt that the aerodigestive tracts became separated by the outgrowth and fusion of lateral ridges from the sidewalls of the primitive foregut.[10,11] It was believed that incomplete fusion of these ridges led to the formation of LC. Subsequent embryological studies have not found evidence of these ridges and this theory has fallen from favour.[6,11] More recent studies have suggested that at approximately 28 days gestation a

Table 52.1 Classification systems for laryngeal tracheal clefts

Benjamin and Inglis (1989)[1]	Monnier (2010)[4]	Pettersson (1955)[5]	Armitage (1984)[6]	Evans (1985)[7]
Type 1—Supraglottic interarytenoid cleft extending down to the level of the vocal cords	Type 1—Supraglottic interarytenoid cleft extending down to the level of the vocal cords	Type 1—Partial cricoid cleft involving the interarytenoid muscles and cricoid lamina	Type 1a—Absence of the interarytenoid muscle Type 1b—Absence of the interarytenoid muscle and partial cleft of the cricoid cartilage	Type 1—Interarytenoid and supraglottic cleft
Type 2—Partial cricoid cleft extending beyond the level of the vocal cords	Type 2—Partial cricoid cleft extending beyond the level of the vocal cords		Type 1c—Absence of the interarytenoid muscle and cricoid cartilage is incomplete posteriorly	Type 2—Cleft penetrates below vocal cords through cricoid into cervical tracheal
Type 3—Cleft extends down into the cervical trachea	Type 3a—Total cricoid cleft Type 3b—Cleft extending into the extrathoracic trachea	Type 2—Cleft extends into the cervical trachea involving some tracheal rings	Type 2—Cleft extends into the cervical trachea involving some tracheal rings	
Type 4—Cleft extends down into the thoracic trachea	Type 4a—Cleft extends to the carina Type 4b—Cleft extends into one main-stem bronchus	Type 3—Total cleft extends to carina involving all tracheal rings	Type 3—Total cleft extends to carina involving all tracheal rings	Type 3—Total cleft extending to the thoracic trachea

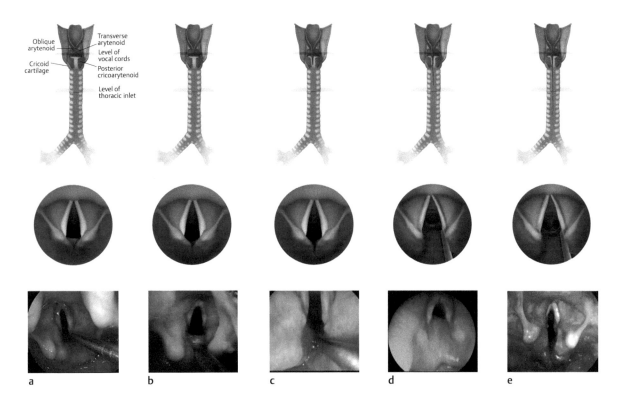

Fig. 52.1 The Benjamin–Inglis Classification. Top row: Posterior view; Middle row: Superior view; Bottom row: Endoscopic view. **(a)** A normal larynx. **(b)** Type 1 Laryngotracheal cleft (LC) extend to the level of the vocal cords. **(c)** Type 2 LC extends below the vocal cords into the cricoid cartilage. **(d)** Type 3 extends through the cricoid cartilage to the cervical trachea/esophagus. **(e)** Type 4 LC extends to the level of the thoracic trachea/esophagus. Note the esophageal mucosa herniating through the type 4 cleft that can make diagnosis difficult. (Figure adapted from Johnston et al 2014.)

series of folds develop on the ventral wall of the endodermic foregut just distal to the fourth pharyngeal pouches.[12] This results in the formation of the respiratory diverticulum which continues to descend ventrocaudally through the mesenchyme of the surrounding foregut. The intervening mesenchyme between the trachea and esophagus becomes the septum and maintains a constant height via rapid proliferation of the caudal fold. If growth in this area cannot match the descent of the respiratory diverticulum, this can result in a range of tracheoesophageal anomalies including LCs.[10] This process may explain the significant rate (12%) of concomitant LC and tracheoesophageal fistula.[8] For type 1 and 2 LCs, the defects likely represent impairments in the structural components of the larynx itself which are derived from the neural crest cells of the fourth and sixth pharyngeal arches.[12] The mesenchyme here proliferates rapidly and forms arytenoid swellings which grow upwards toward the tongue and for a brief period become completely occluded. Recanalization of the larynx appears to be complete by the tenth week. The epithelial lining of the larynx develops from the endoderm at the cranial end of the laryngeal tube. The cricoid develops from two lateral cartilage centers which fuse ventrally and then dorsally approximately one week later. The development of the interarytenoid muscle depends

to some extent on this process and cannot occur in the absence of cartilaginous fusion. Incomplete formation of the interarytenoid muscle without absence of the interarytenoid mucosa would form a deep LC. The incomplete formation of both the interarytenoid muscle and mucosa results in a type 1 LC. The addition of incomplete formation of the posterior cricoid cartilage results in a type 2 LC.

52.3 Presentation

Presenting signs and symptoms of an LC are most often respiratory in nature. Chronic cough is common, especially during feeding. The degree of associated respiratory distress typically depends on the depth of the LC; however, in a child with significant comorbidities, cough can be associated with frank cyanosis.

Roughly 90% of patients with type 1 to 3 LCs have respiratory symptoms including aspiration, recurrent pneumonia, stridor, and cyanosis.[13] Specifically, type 1 and 2 LCs are associated with respiratory symptoms such as wheezing and cough in 50% to 60% of children.[14] Admission to hospital is reported in 15% of children with type 1 LCs and 25% of those with type 2 LCs.[14] Smaller LCs usually do not have significant symptoms until at least several months of age and diagnosis commonly established between 2 and 5 years of age. Significant delay in diagnosis can occur if LC is not included on the differential diagnosis of patients with recurrent respiratory symptoms and may not be picked up until later in life. Type 3 and 4 LCs usually present within the first few days of life are invariably associated with greater respiratory symptoms including recurrent pneumonia and often excessive mucus.[2]

Over half (58–68%) of patients with LCs have an associated congenital defect.[9,14,15] These defects can be conceptually grouped as other anatomic malformations or coincident pathology. Gastrointestinal anomalies are the most commonly associated anatomic malformations and can include esophageal atresia, microgastia, tracheoesophageal fistula, imperforate anus, and intestinal malformation. Genitourinary defects are less common and included: hypospadias and kidney malformations. Cardiac abnormalities such as aortic coarctation, transposition of the great vessels, patent ductus arteriosus, and septal defects have also been described. Particular attention must be made to vocal cord function in children who have undergone repair of these conditions as unilateral vocal focal paralysis may occur in as many as 30% of these patients.[16]

One of the most common coincident pathologies seen with LCs is laryngomalacia which was found in up to 90% of patients with type 1 LC in one study.[17] Over half of those patients had tracheobronchomalacia and gastroesophageal reflux disease (GERD). The abnormal configuration of the posterior larynx and possibly tracheal can result in redundant arytenoid, posterior laryngeal, and esophageal mucosa, which results in prolapse during inspiration and associated airway narrowing. Given the greater chance of aspiration of gastric contents in the setting of LC, the coincidence of clinically significant GERD is likely quite high. "Cobble stoning" of the airway mucosa and aspirated saliva is often seen on endoscopy; however, pH probe proven disease is usually not established.

Although genetic causes of LCs have not been identified and most cases are sporadic, a number of syndromic associations that include LCs have been identified (▶Table 52.2). Opitz G/BBB syndrome (hypertelorism, hypospadias, cleft lip, and palate), Pallister–Hall syndrome (hypothalamic/pituitary abnormalities,

poly- and syndactyly, imperforate anus, cardiac, pulmonary, renal abnormalities), VACTERL syndrome (vertebral anomalies, anal atresia, cardiac anomalies, renal anomalies, limb anomalies), and CHARGE syndrome (coloboma, heart anomalies, choanal atresia, growth and mental retardation, genitourinary anomalies, and ear anomalies) have all been described.

52.4 Preoperative Evaluation and Management

It is critical to maintain a broad differential diagnosis for patients with recurrent respiratory issues and may include laryngomalacia, GERD, neuromuscular swallowing disorders, and reactive airway disease, all of which are more common than LCs. However, unless a high index of suspicion is maintained, diagnosis may be delayed. Most diagnostic practices include a comprehensive history and physical examination paying close attention to the characteristics of the breathing around feeding, chest X-ray, swallowing assessment, and flexible fiberoptic laryngoscopy. Although these are important in understanding the global picture of aerodigestive health in these patients, the cornerstone of diagnosis of LC is direct laryngoscopy with palpation of the interarytenoid area.

52.4.1 Investigations

The majority of children who present with the above respiratory symptoms are usually accompanied by a chest X-ray. Recurrent, chronic aspiration will be identified as pneumonia or peribronchial cuffing. It is important to note that 25% of children with type 1 LCs and 13% of type 2 LCs will have a normal chest X-ray.

A feeding assessment via videofluoroscopic swallowing study (VFSS) is a critical part of the evaluation of LC patients. In this study, the speech/swallowing pathologist will administer varying consistencies of food containing radiolabelled tracers that can be identified under fluoroscopy. Anteroposterior and lateral views are obtained to study oral, pharyngeal, esophageal, and gastric phases of swallowing. However, as it represents a single picture

Table 52.2 Syndromes with possible laryngeal tracheal clefts

Syndrome	Inheritance	Genetic changes	Frequency	Description
Opitz G/BBB syndrome	AD X-linked	22q11.2 deletion MID1 mutation	1:10,000– 1:50,000	Hypertelorism, hypospadias, cleft lip and palate
Pallister–Hall syndrome	AD	GLI3 mutation	Unknown	Hypothalamic-pituitary abnormalities, poly-syndactyly, bifid epiglottis, imperforate anus, cardiac, pulmonary, renal abnormalities
VACTERL	Sporadic	Multifactorial	1:10,000– 1:40,000	Vertebral anomalies, anal atresia, cardiac anomalies, tracheoesophageal fistula, ear anomalies, renal anomalies, limb anomalies
CHARGE	AD	CHD7 (~50%)	1:8,500–1:10,000	Coloboma, heart anomalies, choanal atresia, growth and mental retardation, genital anomalies, ear anomalies

Abbreviation: AD, autosomal dominant.

in time, it may be normal in children who aspirate intermittently. VFSS can also be used to identify patients who have a discoordinated swallow, which is commonly found in children with other neurodevelopmental delays. This can be helpful when counseling patient who will under surgical intervention, as continued work with the speech/swallowing pathology team may be needed postoperatively.[18] In an otherwise healthy child, a positive swallow study for aspiration has a strong correlation with an anatomic abnormality. Overall, over 75% of patients with a type 1 and type 2 LC will display aspiration on VFSS.[2] Children with LC will often require multiple VFSS studies and the cumulative radiation dose must be kept in mind when ordering these tests.[2,19]

Flexible fiberoptic laryngoscopy is critical for obtaining a dynamic view of the larynx. In particular, it is essential for determining vocal cord function which can lead to decreased laryngeal sensation and aspiration. It can also be done while a speech/swallow pathologist administers dyed food in the form of a flexible endoscopic evaluation of swallow (FEES). In this way, pooling or penetration/aspiration of swallowed food can be observed directly.

The gold standard of LC diagnosis is operative endoscopy via direct laryngoscopy and palpation of the interarytenoid area. As many of the presenting symptoms overlap across a number of clinical entities, patients undergo "triple endoscopy" by otolaryngology (direct laryngoscopy), pulmonology (flexible bronchoscopy), and gastroenterology (flexible esophagogastroduodenoscopy) under the same general anesthetic. At our institution, direct laryngoscopy is often performed with spontaneous ventilation to achieve a dynamic view of the airway. A Parson's laryngoscope and 0° degree 4 mm telescope (Karl Storz Co., Tuttlingen, Germany) is used to visualize the larynx. After direct laryngoscopy, telescopic tracheobronchoscopy is usually done to assess for edema, cobble stoning, rigid or malacic stenosis, blunting of tracheal rings, and tracheoesophageal fistula. A blunt-tipped laryngeal probe is then used to palpate the depth of the interarytenoid groove. Palpation must be done gently to avoid excessive pressure that would distort or deepen the interarytenoid mucosa. During this process the presence of and extent of the LC can be determined. The extent of the LC can be classified in a number of ways (▶Table 52.1), the most common being the Benjamin–Inglis classification (▶Fig. 52.1a–e).[1] Type 1 LCs involve an interarytenoid defect to the level of the true vocal folds. Differentiation of a type 1 LC from a deep groove can be challenging. It is helpful to keep the patient's symptoms in mind while making this assessment. Type 2 LCs extend beyond the true vocal cords into the posterior cricoid. Type 3 LCs extend completely through the posterior cricoid into the cervical trachea. Finally, type 4 LCs involve an extension into the thoracic trachea. Monnier has further subclassified type 3 and type 4 LCs based on their extent.[4] Type 3a LCs penetrate completely through the cricoid and type 3b LCs go through the cricoid into the extrathoracic trachea.

Type 4a LCs extend into the thoracic trachea up to the carina; however, type 4b LCs extend beyond the carina into the mainstem bronchus. Paradoxically, although long, type 3 and type 4 LCs can be challenging to diagnose because redundant mucosa herniation through the LC obscures the surgeon's view (▶Fig. 52.1e).

52.4.2 Preoperative Medical Management

Medical management is critical for these children, not only to optimize patients for surgical intervention, but also to maintain optimal respiration, prevent the pulmonary complications of recurrent pneumonia, and ensure adequate nutrition.[20,21]

Medical management is primarily aimed at type 1 and select type 2 LCs and includes feeding therapy involving thickening of liquid and food consistency. A trial of medical management in type 1 LCs may help obviate the need for surgical management in some patients.[9,14,17] At our institution, we usually allow for at least 6 months of feeding and medical therapy before re-evaluation of swallowing competence via VFSS.[14] This period of time also allows for patient growth and development of swallowing function. If pulmonary aspiration and/or infection persist, the patient is scheduled for endoscopic repair. Medical management also includes treating comorbid conditions that may contribute to swallowing dysfunction. For example, treatment with proton pump inhibitor for treatment of GERD, treatment of reactive airway disease, and treatment of food allergies can reduce aerodigestive edema and irritation and may improve swallow function.

52.4.3 Anesthetic Considerations

Airway surgery typically demands an experienced anesthetic team familiar with the requirements and nuances of the procedures. For endoscopic repair of type 1, 2, and select type 3 LCs the anesthetic requirements are immobility, analgesia, lack of airway reflexes such as cough and wheeze, ventilation and oxygenation, and a full view of the laryngeal inlet.[20] At our institution we prefer a "tubeless" anesthesia with the patient maintaining spontaneous respiration throughout the procedure. Oxygen is delivered via constant flow throughout the procedure via a side port. Alternatively, jet ventilation can be employed as well and should be in the room in case of emergency if using spontaneous respiration.[20] Intermittent intubation by the surgeon can also be performed, but it is cumbersome and may prolong the duration of the procedure. Unconsciousness is induced by inhalational agents (e.g., nitrous oxide or sevoflurane) by mask while maintaining spontaneous respiration. After induction, total intravenous anesthesia (TIVA) using remifentanil or propofol is optimal. Throughout the procedure, ventilation must be monitored visually by chest rise and auscultation.

For open repairs, airway management depends to some extent on the size of the LC and experience of the institution. For type 3 and select type 4 LCs, intubation over a flexible bronchoscope or rigid telescope can be performed to allow direct visualization and precise placement of the endotracheal tube. At the time of laryngofissure and tracheal division, a new endotracheal tube can be inserted into the distal airway and secured in place.[22,23] Some surgical and anesthetic teams will use extracorporeal membrane oxygenation or cardiopulmonary bypass particularly for type 4 LCs.[2] This allows an unobstructed view of the trachea but also avoids trauma and pressure on the suture line.

52.5 Surgical Technique

Surgical management should be considered for type 1 LCs that fail a trial of medical management. Type 2 to 4 LCs will almost inevitably require surgical intervention because aspiration is common. Endoscopic repair should be considered for type 1, 2, and select type 3 LCs. Three factors are important to consider when determining if a type 3 LC can be repaired endoscopically. The first is the ability to maintain anesthesia with spontaneous ventilation as is necessary for endoscopic repair.[24] Prior to considering an endoscopic approach, a conversation with the anesthesiologist is necessary to determine if this approach is possible from a cardiopulmonary perspective. The anesthetic team must be comfortable with maintaining the patient with this anesthetic technique for 1.5 to 2 hours. The second factor is the ability to achieve adequate posterior glottic exposure. The depth of the LC must be visualized and made accessible for suture placement while the patient is in suspension.[24] After a diagnosis of type 3 LC is made on preoperative endoscopic exam, it is advisable

to determine if adequate exposure is possible by inserting a Lindholm laryngoscope (Karl Storz Co., Tuttlingen, Germany) at that time and delicately manipulating the LC. Finally, conditions with more severe LC can be associated with more severe coincident anatomic abnormalities, and surgical management may include additional procedures such as tracheotomy or gastrostomy tube, or even repair of esophageal atresia, or micrognathia.

52.5.1 Endoscopic Repair

The appropriate microlaryngeal instrumentation is required to facilitate endoscopic repair. Our microlaryngeal set contains 10 instruments: three Kleinhauser needle holders (Karl Storz Endoscopy-America, Inc., El Segundo, CA) for suture manipulation (▶Fig. 52.2a), knot pusher (Karl Storz Endoscopy-America, Inc.) (▶Fig. 52.2b), alligator forceps (small and large) (▶Fig. 52.2b), two scissors (straight and curved) (▶Fig. 52.2c), Jako probe (Pilling Surgical Instruments, Teleflex Medical, Durham, NC) for LC palpation (▶Fig. 52.2d), and a Lindholm vocal cord retractor (Karl Storz Endoscopy-America, Inc.) to splay the LC open if excessive mucosa is present (▶Fig. 52.2d). A range of laryngeal suctions (Karl Storz Endoscopy-America, Inc.) should also be available.

Topical 4% lidocaine is applied to the larynx for local anesthesia. A Lindholm suspension laryngoscope is seated in the valleculae (▶Fig. 52.3). Direct communication with an experienced anesthetist facilitates obtaining the proper anesthetic level. Positioning of the laryngoscope is critical for success and must be done keeping three factors in mind: (1) airway—a direct line is best for instilling oxygen into the airway particularly for jet ventilation; (2) beam—the surgeon must be able to visualize the extent of the LC particularly if CO_2 laser is to be used

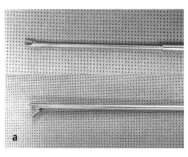
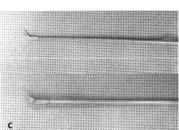
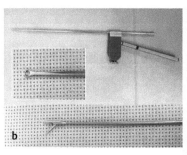
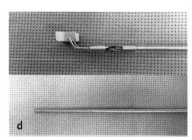

Fig. 52.2 Instrumentation set up for endoscopic laryngeal cleft repair. **(a)** Kleinhauser needle holders: straight (above), right and left (below). **(b)** Knot pusher (above), large and small (not shown) alligator forceps (below). **(c)** Curved (above) and straight (below) scissors. **(d)** Vocal cord retractor (above) and Jako probe (below).

for preparing the mucosal edges; (3) closure—the laryngoscope must be positioned such that there is sufficient space posteriorly to place sutures.

Visualization can either be achieved using a microscope or 4-mm 0-degree Hopkins telescope. To prepare the edges of the LC for closure, a CO_2 micromanipulator laser set to 3 to 5 W in pulse mode with 10 to 30 ms pulses is used to denude mucosa on both sides of the LC (▶Fig. 52.4a).[3] A CO_2 laser with flexible fiber delivery, e.g., an OmniGuide laser (OmniGuide surgical, Lexington, USA) set to 6 to 8 W, 100-ms single pulse can also be used. Extreme care must be taken to ensure complete eradication of mucosa down to the apex of the LC. The charred tissue can be removed using a 1/8 inch

oxymetazoline-soaked pledget. Closure can be done using either a one-layer[2,3,14] or two-layer[15,25] closure technique. We employ a one-layer closure using a deep absorbable 3-0 or 4-0 vicryl on a short half curve P1 or P3 needle suture (Ethicon Inc., Johnson & Johnson Co, Somerville, New Jersey) (▶Fig. 52.4b–e). A deep, one-layer closure provides adequate strength without compromising the laryngeal lumen diameter significantly. For type 1 and 2 LCs two to three sutures are usually sufficient. Simple interrupted sutures are used passing the needle from posterior to anterior, and then anterior to posterior. Occasionally, a figure-of-eight–type suture is used if there is difficulty placing an interrupted suture. This involves passing the needle from posterior to anterior on both sides of the LC. Knots are tied on the pharyngeal surface of the larynx using the knot pusher, with an assistant securing the free end of the suture string (▶Fig. 52.5). While placing the sutures, care must

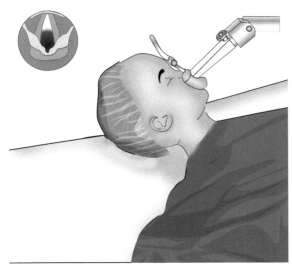

Fig. 52.3 Suspension laryngoscopy and position is critical for endoscopy repairs of Laryngotracheal cleft (LC). Three conditions must be met: (1) a direct line is best for instilling oxygen into the airway particularly for jet ventilation; (2) the surgeon must be able to visualize the extent of the LC particularly if CO_2 laser is to be used for preparing the mucosal edges "(inset: laryngoscopic view)"; (3) the laryngoscope must be positioned such that there is sufficient space posteriorly to place sutures.

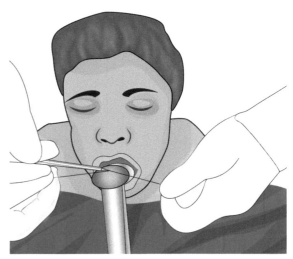

Fig. 52.5 Knot tying. The surgical assistant (gray glove) grasps one end of the suture as the surgeon guides the knot down toward the surgical site with the knot pusher (▶Fig. 52.2b). The surgeon must direct the surgical assistant to increase and decrease the tension as the knot is adjusted towards the site.

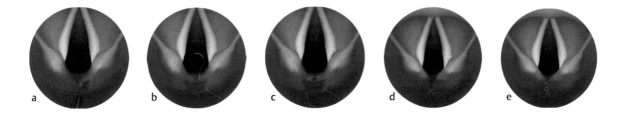

Fig. 52.4 Endoscopic CO_2 laser repair of a Type 1 Laryngotracheal cleft (LC). **(a)** Laser-denuded cleft mucosa. **(b)** First suture on one side. **(c)** First suture through both sides. **(d)** Inferior suture tied with inferior edges of cleft approximated. **(e)** Superior suture tied with superior part of cleft approximated. (Figure adapted from Johnston et al 2014.)

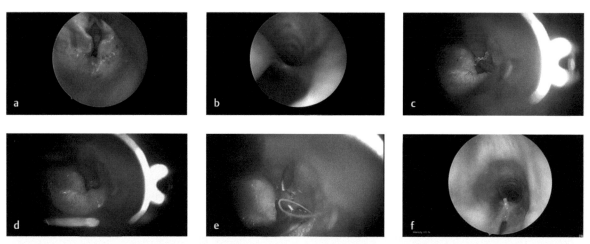

Fig. 52.6 Staged endoscopic repair of a type 3 Laryngotracheal cleft (LC). **(a)** Endoscopic view of the type 3 LC. **(b)** Endoscopic view of the apex of the type 3 LC within the cervical trachea. **(c)** The OmniGuide laser is used to denude the mucosa of the apex. **(d)** The extent of the laser-denuded mucosa for stage 1. **(e)** The suture is placed through the second side in a figure-of-eight fashion (first side not shown). **(f)** Endoscopic view at the end of the first stage of repair.

be taken to avoid inadvertently injuring the epiglottis, which will cause bleeding and obscure visualization. Once the repair is complete the 4-mm 0-degree Hopkins telescope is used to re-examine the trachea for any blood or secretions that need to be suctioned out.

For type 3 LCs that are appropriate for endoscopic repair, suspension microlaryngoscopy with the administration of general anesthesia can be performed with spontaneous ventilation using the anesthesia technique described above. Similarly, the larynx is visualized with a Lindholm laryngoscope (▶Fig. 52.6a). The microscope is preferable in this case as a two-handed technique is required so that one hand may distract the tissues while the other hand applies the laser (▶Fig. 52.6b). Alternatively, a vocal fold retractor or a curved fine microlaryngeal alligator forceps can be used to spread the mucosa during ablation with the laser (▶Fig. 52.6c). A small, malleable retractor can be placed into the esophagus to prevent inadvertent laser damage to the lining of the esophagus. An OmniGuide Surgical CO_2 laser set at 6 W at 3 to 4 ms in pulse mode is used to denude the mucosal lining beginning at the apex of the LC and extending cranially (▶Fig. 52.6b, c). Given the length, the OmniGuide is particularly useful for in this case. Cotton pledgets soaked with oxymetazoline are applied to the area for hemostasis and to remove char. Again, it is important to remove the mucosa completely at the apex of the LC to prevent development of a fistula at the distal end of the repair. Absorbable interrupted sutures (4–0, 5–0, and/or 6–0 vicryl on P1 or P3 needles (Ethicon Inc.) are used to re-approximate the mucosal edges (▶Fig. 52.6d). The first suture is the most important and placed at the most caudal extent of the LC. We generally place three to four sutures in a distal-to-proximal fashion (▶Fig. 52.6e, f). Depending on the depth and access offered, these repairs can be done as a single procedure or as a planned staged repair.[24] A staged approach may also lead to less

postoperative edema and avoid subsequent airway compromise.[24] In the single-stage approach with a long suture line, tracheostomy or G-tube insertion must be considered to avoid pressure from an endotracheal tube or NG tube, respectively, in the postoperative period.

52.5.2 Open Repair

The goal of surgical therapy for type 3 and 4 LCs is to recreate separate, functional tracheal and esophageal lumens. This dual repair results in two suture lines and with that a greater chance for anastomotic leak compared with a single suture line. Anterior approaches with cervical and/or thoracic incisions are employed for the best exposure, but lateral approaches to the pharynx and cervical and thoracic trachea have been described.[7] Type 4 clefts have been approached through the neck.[22,26] Alternatively, in long LCs the cervical and thoracic portions can also be approached separately by a right cervical approach and right posterolateral thoracotomy, respectively.[27,28] Anterior approaches via laryngofissure have the advantage of lower risk to the recurrent laryngeal nerves, but may have increased risk for postoperative tracheomalacia. Various tissues have been used as interposition grafts to allow for a more robust tension-free closure, including pericardium, sternocleidomastoid muscle flaps, pleura, strap muscle, jejunum, clavicular periosteum, and tibial periosteum, to name a few.[22,23,27-31] Techniques for LC closure include a two-layer or three-layer closure with either symmetric or asymmetric flaps with or without complete separation of the tracheal and esophageal lumens.[26] Asymmetric flaps have the advantage of avoiding overlapping suture lines. Even in open approaches, exposure to the distal apex can be challenging. Therefore, thorough diagnostic operative endoscopy must be done at the outset with an aim to determine the subsequent surgical approach and if general or cardiothoracic surgery team involvement will be required.

At our institution, tibial periosteum is most commonly used. Patients are initially intubated by orotracheal or nasotracheal intubation taking care to position the endotracheal tube distal to the LC. For harvest of the periosteal patch, a vertical incision is made along the anteromedial face of the tibia on the medial surface of the leg. The subcutaneous tissue is then dissected away from the tibia keeping the periosteum intact. A rectangular piece of tibial periosteum, approximately 3 × 1 cm is sharply dissected and then released using a freer elevator. The skin is closed in layers using a 3–0 vicryl for the subcutaneous layer and a 4–0 monocryl in a running subcuticular fashion. If there is insufficient length to the tibial periosteum, sternal or clavicular periosteum can often be easily accessed through a cervical approach.[22,26]

A horizontal incision is made in a skin crease at the level of the cricoid, and the laryngeal frame work is exposed from the thyroid notch to the trachea (▶Fig. 52.7a, b). An anterior laryngofissure extending from the thyroid cartilage, through cricoid, and down to the first two to three tracheal rings is made depending on the length of LC (▶Fig. 52.7c). An endotracheal tube is then inserted directly in the trachea and the anesthesia circuit is connected, allowing exposure to the posterior part of the larynx and trachea. The two mucosal borders of the LC are secured with traction sutures and the folds of excess mucosa are scored with monopolar cautery. The mucosal margins are dissected in two planes: a posterior plane of pharyngoesophageal mucosa and an anterior plane of laryngotracheal mucosa. This allows interposition of one

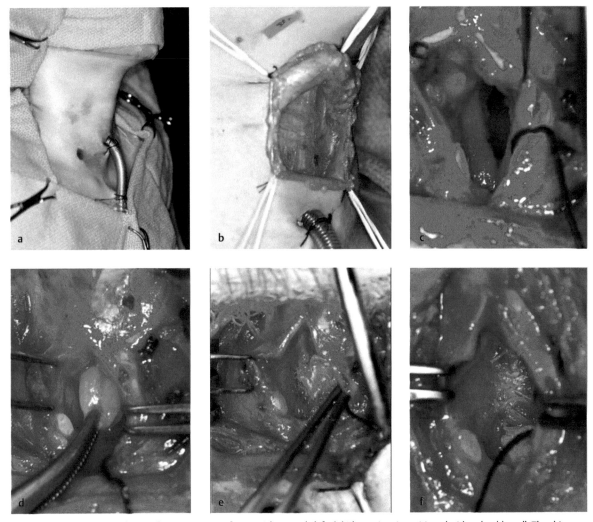

Fig. 52.7 Intraoperative photos of an open repair of a type 3 laryngeal cleft. **(a)** The patient is positioned with a shoulder roll. The chin is at top edge of photo and endotracheal tube sewn into tracheotomy incision at the bottom edge of the photo. **(b)** Exposure of strap muscles in a midline approach. **(c)** Cleft seen in middle of photo deep to divide anterior tracheal wall with retraction sutures in place. **(d)** Retractors hold open anterior tracheal wall and forceps grasp tibial periosteum to be used for repair of cleft. **(e)** Retractors hold open the anterior tracheal wall with the tibial periosteum tacked down in deep portion of photo. **(f)** Retractors hold open the anterior tracheal wall with repaired cleft and tied sutures in deep portion of photo.

of the graft materials outlined above to prevent juxtaposition of the two suture lines (▶ Fig. 52.7d). The posterior part is closed with a 5–0 polydioxanone suture (PDS) (Ethicon Inc.) in an interrupted fashion. The tibial periosteum is interposed as the middle layer of the closure, stretched, and fixed laterally by four interrupted sutures at each corner (▶ Fig. 52.7e). The laryngeal mucosa is then sutured so that it covers the tibial periosteum using an interrupted 5–0 PDS suture burying the knots (▶ Fig. 52.7f). The patient is then reintubated transorally or transnasally. The larynx and trachea are closed with a 4–0 vicryl suture over the endotracheal tube, which is left in place for one week. Immediately after the surgical procedure, laryngoscopy is performed in order to confirm the upper level of the closure of the LC. In both endoscopic and open approaches, the repaired laryngeal introitus must be examined to ensure that it has not been overly narrowed. In instances where it has become too narrow, releasing incisions can be made into the aryepiglottic folds.

52.6 Postoperative Treatment

Following endoscopic repair, spontaneous respiration is maintained and the patient is awakened from anesthetic without intubation. They are then admitted to the intensive care unit for the first 24 hours for close airway observations, then transferred to the floor for an additional 24 hours. Intravenous antibiotics (ampicillin/sulbactam) are administered for 48 hours and then continued orally for the length of the patients stay in hospital. Three doses of intravenous steroid (dexamethasone 0.5 mg/kg) are given. Antireflux medication has been recommended but is not used at our center. The patient's preoperative feeding regime is restarted once the patient is fully awake. Flexible laryngoscopy is performed in the clinic in 1 to 2 weeks to inspect the repair site. VFSS is performed in 2 to 3 months or at the discretion of the speech/swallowing pathology team. It is important to counsel the family that often feeding issues may continue for a short time postoperatively, despite successful surgical repair of the LC, due to neuromuscular discoordination of the swallowing reflex.[2,18]

Following open repairs of type III or IV LCs, care consists of a variable period of endotracheal intubation (either transnasal or transoral). The endotracheal tube effectively functions as a stent during the initial healing process. Some authors prefer a tracheotomy tube. If ECMO has been used, patients can remain free from intubation for approximately 7 days. Enteral feeding with a nasogastric/nasoduodenal tube or preexisting gastric/duodenal/jejunal tube is maintained for several weeks to avoid anastomotic breakdown due to exposure to gastric refluxate. Coincident gastric abnormalities can significantly alter gastric emptying and can result in continued aspiration from refractory esophageal reflux, along with pressure and inflammation at the anastomotic sites, which may, among other things, contribute to the lower success of closure in type 3 and 4 LCs. Although it is not a common practice at our institution, we would not hesitate to perform tracheotomy and/or gastrostomy in type 3 and 4 LC patients as prolonged treatment courses should be expected and these interventions offer life sustaining airway and nutritional support. Diet advancement is conservative, yet complicated due to frequent gastric abnormalities, feeding diversion, and medical complexities.

Success rates for endoscopic repair of type 1 and 2 LCs exceed 90% but are predicated on continued work with the speech/swallowing pathology team. Reported complications are rare in the literature. The most feared complication is dehiscence of the repair but this can typically be addressed via the same endoscopic approach. For type 3 and 4 LCs common complications include tracheoesophageal fistula, which has been improved with the use of interposition grafts. These fistulas can result in recurrent aspiration, chronic lung disease, and the need for multiple revision procedures. Tracheotomy dependence is common, largely due to significant tracheomalacia (preexisting or iatrogenic) or occasionally chronic lung disease, as well. Other complications of surgical repair include recurrent laryngeal nerve injury, granulation tissue formation, esophageal stricture, and continued aspiration. Mortality rates for type 3 and 4 LCs can reach 50% to 75% in the literature due to coincident congenital anomalies and the complex operative and perioperative care of these children.

52.7 Highlights

a. Indications for surgical intervention
   – Failure of medical management for type 1 LC (e.g., recurrent issues: pneumonia, respiratory distress).
   – Failure to maintain age-appropriate weight.
   – Type 2, 3, or 4 LC.
b. Contraindications to endoscopic repair
   – Inadequate endoscopic exposure.
   – Inability to achieve adequate anesthetic conditions due to medical or anatomical factors.
   – Some type 3 and all type 4 laryngeal cleft.
c. Complications
   – Endoscopic repair:
     ○ Dehiscence of repair.
     ○ Damage to lips or teeth.
     ○ Postoperative atelectasis or pneumonia.
   – Open repair:
     ○ Dehiscence of repair.
     ○ Recurrence laryngeal nerve injury (lateral approach).
     ○ Scar.
d. Special preoperative considerations
   – During diagnostic endoscopy, the interarytenoid area must be palpated but care must be taken to not distort the mucosa and create the appearance of a cleft.

– During diagnostic endoscopy, access must be considered. Can the cleft be accessed endoscopically? Can it be accessed transcervically? Or does it require a sternotomy or thoracotomy?
– After diagnosis of a type 3 cleft, it is helpful to re-examine the cleft with a Lindholm laryngoscope inconsideration for a possible endoscopic approach.
– Maximize pulmonary function and reduce gastric reflux as much as possible in the preoperative period.

e. Special intraoperative considerations for endoscopic repair
– Anesthetic considerations: immobility, analgesia, lack of airway reflexes such as cough and wheeze, ventilation and oxygenation, and a full view of the laryngeal inlet.[20]
– Positioning considerations: Positioning of the laryngoscope is critical for success:
   ○ Airway—A direct line is best for instilling oxygen into the airway particularly for jet ventilation.
   ○ Beam—The surgeon must be able to visualize the extent of the LC particularly if CO_2 laser is to be used for preparing the mucosal edges.
   ○ Closure—The laryngoscope must be positioned such that there is sufficient space posteriorly to place sutures.
– Laser safety considerations:
   ○ Patient.
   ○ Completely cover patients face with water-soaked towels to prevent off-target laser strikes.
   ○ Eye shields.
   ○ Laser-safe tube if tubeless anesthetic is not possible.
   ○ Use smallest tube possible and fill balloon with saline.
– Surgeon/anesthetist:
   ○ Laser safety training.
   ○ Cognizance of anesthetic gas mixture.
   ○ O_2, N_2O, and volatile anesthetic agents are all combustible agents.
   ○ Total intravenous anesthetic with a mixture of 25% O_2 and 75% N_2 is a safe option.
   ○ Establish fire risk and plan of action with OR team.
– Operating room:
   ○ Warning signs on entry ways.
   ○ Eye protection for all OR personnel.
   ○ Laser safety trained nurse.
   ○ Basin of saline on field.
– Tight closure of the cleft apex is critical and is predicated on good access.
– Avoid "over-closure" of the laryngeal introitus—releasing incisions in the aryepiglottic folds may be necessary.

– Repeat telescopic examination of the trachea must be done at the end of the procedure to ensure that no blood or crusts have been aspirated during the procedure.

f. Special intraoperative considerations for open repair
– Use of robust interposition graft.
– Keep low threshold for tracheostomy or gastrostomy tube insertion.
– Recurrent laryngeal nerve—in lateral approaches, great care must be taken to identify and preserve the nerve.

g. Special postoperative considerations
– Postoperative monitoring:
   ○ Endoscopic repair—ICU monitoring for the first 24 hours then transferred to the floor for an additional 24 hours.
   ○ Open repair—Typically remain intubated for 3 to 5 days in ICU.
– Postoperative medications:
   ○ Intravenous antibiotics (ampicillin/sulbactam) administered for the length of stay and oral antibiotics are continued at home for 2 weeks.
   ○ Three doses of intravenous steroid (dexamethasone 0.5 mg/kg).
– Postoperative feeding:
   ○ Preoperative feeding regime is restarted once the patient is fully awake and diet is advanced conservatively with the speech/swallowing pathology team.
– Postoperative follow-up:
   ○ Flexible laryngoscopy is performed at 1 to 2 week to inspect the repair site.
   ○ MBS is performed in 2 to 3 months or at the discretion of the speech/swallowing pathology team.

References

[1] Benjamin B, Inglis A. Minor congenital laryngeal clefts: diagnosis and classification. Ann Otol Rhinol Laryngol 1989;98(6):417–420
[2] Johnston DR, Watters K, Ferrari LR, Rahbar R. Laryngeal cleft: evaluation and management. Int J Pediatr Otorhinolaryngol 2014;78(6):905–911
[3] Watters K, Ferrari L, Rahbar R. Minimally invasive approach to laryngeal cleft. Laryngoscope 2013;123(1):264–268
[4] Monnier P. Pediatric Airway Surgery (Monnier P, ed.). Berlin, Heidelberg: Springer Science & Business Media; 2010
[5] Pettersson G. Inhibited separation of larynx and the upper part of trachea from oesophagus in a newborn: report of a case successfully operated upon. Acta Chir Scand 1955;110(3):250–254
[6] Armitage EN. Laryngotracheo-oesophageal cleft. A report of three cases. Anaesthesia 1984;39(7):706–713
[7] Evans JN. Management of the cleft larynx and tracheoesophageal clefts. Ann Otol Rhinol Laryngol 1985;94(6 Pt 1):627–630
[8] Fraga JC, Adil EA, Kacprowicz A, et al. The association between laryngeal cleft and tracheoesophageal fistula: myth or reality? Laryngoscope 2015;125(2):469–474
[9] Parsons DS, Stivers FE, Giovanetto DR, Phillips SE, Type I. Type I posterior laryngeal clefts. Laryngoscope 1998;108(3):403–410
[10] Merei JM, Hutson JM. Embryogenesis of tracheo esophageal anomalies: a review. Pediatr Surg Int 2002;18(5–6):319–326

[11] Metzger R, Wachowiak R, Kluth D. Embryology of the early foregut. Semin Pediatr Surg 2011;20(3):136–144

[12] Moore KL, Persaud TVN, Torchia MG. The Developing Human. Elsevier Health Sciences; 2015; 10th edition, Philadephia, PA

[13] Rahbar R, Rouillon I, Roger G, et al. The presentation and management of laryngeal cleft: a 10-year experience. Arch Otolaryngol Head Neck Surg 2006;132(12):1335–1341

[14] Rahbar R, Chen JL, Rosen RL, et al. Endoscopic repair of laryngeal cleft type I and type II: when and why? Laryngoscope 2009;119(9):1797–1802

[15] Evans KL, Courteney-Harris R, Bailey CM, Evans JNG, Parsons DS. Management of posterior laryngeal and laryngotracheoesophageal clefts. Arch Otolaryngol Head Neck Surg 1995;121(12):1380–1385

[16] Strychowsky JE, Rukholm G, Gupta MK, Reid D. Unilateral vocal fold paralysis after congenital cardiothoracic surgery: a meta-analysis. Pediatrics 2014;133(6):e1708–e1723

[17] van der Doef HP, Yntema JB, van den Hoogen FJ, Marres HA. Clinical aspects of type 1 posterior laryngeal clefts: literature review and a report of 31 patients. Laryngoscope 2007;117(5):859–863

[18] Osborn AJ, de Alarcon A, Tabangin ME, Miller CK, Cotton RT, Rutter MJ. Swallowing function after laryngeal cleft repair: more than just fixing the cleft. Laryngoscope 2014;124(8):1965–1969

[19] Hersh C, Wentland C, Sally S, et al. Radiation exposure from videofluoroscopic swallow studies in children with a type 1 laryngeal cleft and pharyngeal dysphagia: a retrospective review. Int J Pediatr Otorhinolaryngol 2016;89:92–96

[20] Ferrari LR, Zurakowski D, Solari J, Rahbar R. Laryngeal cleft repair: the anesthetic perspective. Paediatr Anaesth 2013;23(4):334–341

[21] Leboulanger N, Garabédian E-N. Laryngo-tracheo-oesophageal clefts. Orphanet J Rare Dis 2011;6(1):81

[22] Propst EJ. Repair of short type IV laryngotracheoesophageal cleft using long, tapered, engaging graft without need for tracheotomy. Laryngoscope 2016;126(4):1006–1008

[23] Garabedian E-N, Ducroz V, Roger G, Denoyelle F. Posterior laryngeal clefts: preliminary report of a new surgical procedure using tibial periosteum as an interposition graft. Laryngoscope 1998;108(6):899–902

[24] Adil E, Al Shemari H, Rahbar R. Endoscopic surgical repair of type 3 laryngeal clefts. JAMA Otolaryngol Head Neck Surg 2014;140(11):1051–1055

[25] Garabedian E-N, Pezzettigotta S, Leboulanger N, et al. Endoscopic surgical treatment of laryngotracheal clefts: indications and limitations. Arch Otolaryngol Head Neck Surg 2010;136(1):70–74

[26] Propst EJ, Ida JB, Rutter MJ. Repair of long type IV posterior laryngeal cleft through a cervical approach using cricotracheal separation. Laryngoscope 2013;123(3):801–804

[27] Kawaguchi AL, Donahoe PK, Ryan DP. Management and long-term follow-up of patients with types III and IV laryngotracheoesophageal clefts. J Pediatr Surg 2005;40(1):158–164, discussion 164–165

[28] Ryan DP, Muehrcke DD, Doody DP, Kim SH, Donahoe PK. Laryngotracheoesophageal cleft (type IV): management and repair of lesions beyond the carina. J Pediatr Surg 1991;26(8):962–969, discussion 969–970

[29] Simpson BB, Ryan DP, Donahoe PK, Schnitzer JJ, Kim SH, Doody DP. Type IV laryngotracheoesophageal clefts: surgical management for long-term survival. J Pediatr Surg 1996;31(8):1128–1133

[30] Geller K, Kim Y, Koempel J, Anderson KD. Surgical management of type III and IV laryngotracheoesophageal clefts: the three-layered approach. Int J Pediatr Otorhinolaryngol 2010;74(6):652–657

[31] Hashizume K, Kanamori Y, Sugiyama M, Ito M, Kamii Y. Successful repair of the esophagus in type-IV laryngo-tracheo-esophageal cleft using interposed jejunum. Pediatr Surg Int 2003;19(3):211–213

53 Slide Tracheoplasty

Michael Rutter, Claudia Schweiger

Summary

Slide tracheoplasty is a surgical technique originally designed by Goldstraw in the 1980s to repair congenital tracheal stenosis caused by complete tracheal rings. It is a versatile operation with expanding indications in the setting of congenital tracheal stenosis, tracheoesophageal fistulas, or acquired tracheal injury. It consists of overlapping stenotic segments of the trachea, shortening it but doubling the diameter of the narrowed area, and can be performed through a sternotomy or through the neck. Slide tracheoplasty is a safe and reliable technique, with a high success rate. Its morbidity and mortality are related to the underlying health status of the child.

Keywords: Slide tracheoplasty, trachea, stenosis, complete tracheal rings

53.1 Introduction

Slide tracheoplasty was originally described by Tsang et al[1] and popularized by both Grillo et al[2] and by our team at Cincinnati Children's Hospital.[3] This operation overlaps stenotic segments of the trachea, shortening it but doubling its diameter (▶ Fig. 53.1). Slide tracheoplasty is currently the operation of choice for tracheal stenosis attributed to complete tracheal rings (CTRs), but its indications has been broadening and recent publications show that it can be used for the treatment of acquired tracheal stenosis, absent tracheal rings, sleeve trachea, and tracheoesophageal fistulas (TEFs).[4]

This technique has a number of advantages relative to other methods. These advantages include immediate tracheal reconstruction with rigid, vascularized tissue with a normal mucosa; ability to extubate patients early in many cases; less postoperative granulation tissue

formation; less risk of dehiscence; and growth potential of the reconstructed trachea.[2] In addition, it is a versatile technique: one can perform a short-segment slide, an oblique slide, or even an inverse slide if circumstances dictate. The slide can also extend into the membranous trachea or into the carina if required. The whole length of the trachea may be slid, even past the carina.

At Cincinnati Children's, we have been performing slide tracheoplasty under cardiopulmonary bypass since 2001, mainly for patients with distal tracheal stenosis and those who require concomitant cardiovascular repair. Cervical slide tracheoplasty has also been performed since 2003. This procedure is an adaptation of the standard slide procedure and can be used for cervical tracheal stenosis, tracheal "A frame" deformities, and multilevel laryngotracheal stenosis.

Our experience has demonstrated that the slide tracheoplasty can be performed with very low mortality despite the complexity of the patient population. In our 2011 cohort study with 80 patients who underwent slide tracheoplasty on bypass, 48 patients (60%) had associated cardiac or great vessels anomalies, and only 5 (6.2%) required a revisional open surgery. Twenty-three percent of our population required endoscopic airway re-intervention within 12 months of the initial procedure, which involved balloon dilation, endoscopic resection of granulation tissue, or temporary stent placement. Four deaths (5%) were reported.[5] This mortality rate was much lower than the previously reported mortality rate of up to 24% in some series.[6,7] More recently, we published our series with 130 patients, which included 76 (58%) patients with associated cardiac or vascular anomaly and 18 (13.8%) with pulmonary malformations. The stenosis rate was again very low (6.9%), with a mortality rate of 6.1%.[8]

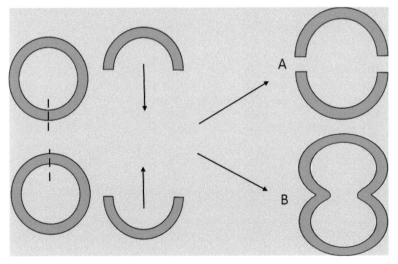

Fig. 53.1 Overlapping of the stenotic segments of the trachea, increasing the diameter and the airflow. A: Typical postoperative airway. B: "Figure 8" airway.

A series of 101 children who underwent a slide procedure at Great Ormond Street Hospital was published in 2014. Seventy-two of their patients (71.3%) had associated cardiovascular anomalies. Thirty-three children (33%) had residual stenosis at 3 months, and 8 (8%) had residual stenosis at 9 months after the surgery. Stenting was required in 21.8%, mainly in patients with preoperative bronchomalacia. The mortality rate was 11.8%, and bronchomalacia and the need of preoperative extracorporeal membrane oxygenation (ECMO) were associated with this outcome.[9]

In our cohort published in 2012 about cervical slide tracheoplasties, we described 29 patients who underwent this procedure. Operation-specific success rate was 79% (23 of 29 patients), including all 10 patients with long-segment acquired tracheal stenosis. Lower operative success occurred in patients with concomitant subglottic stenosis, posterior glottic stenosis, and multilevel airway lesions. Four patients (14%) experienced complications: one patient had a minor wound infection; one had a dehiscence that was managed with a revision tracheoplasty; one had an innominate artery injury that was successfully treated intraoperatively without sequelae; and one had a symptomatic "figure 8" deformity that required revision therapy.[10]

53.2 Preoperative Evaluation and Anesthesia

Optimal management of children with tracheal stenosis requires comprehensive evaluation prior to repair. The temptation is to proceed straight to definitive repair should the child deteriorate. However, if the airway permits intubation with a 2.0 endotracheal tube or bigger, this should be performed via nasotracheal route in order to temporarily stabilize the child. When this approach is not possible, an endotracheal tube sized to accommodate the cricoid cartilage, but placed shallow and proximal to the complete rings, can still permit positive pressure ventilation. It is rare that the first two tracheal rings are affected in children with CTR, and therefore most children can be intubated proximal to the complete rings. If ventilation remains difficult, ECMO is advisable but should not be taken lightly. Clearly, tracheotomy is rarely helpful as the smallest CTRs tend to be more distal, and the smallest available commercial tracheotomy tube is 3.6 mm in outer diameter. In an airway compromised enough to consider tracheotomy, the stenotic segment is typically 2.0 to 2.5 mm in diameter, and therefore not amenable to tracheotomy placement. More importantly, tracheotomy may further compromise the options of subsequent operative repair.

Preoperative bronchoscopy is universally relied on for the diagnosis and definition of airway anatomy. Both flexible and rigid instrumentation can be used to determine the type of lesion, localization, extension, and severity. However, this evaluation must be the most careful as possible, not to cause edema of the airway and to turn a stable airway into an emergency.

Contrast chest computed tomography scans with three-dimensional reconstruction and echocardiography should be performed in all cases to aid in defining airway and great vessels anatomy and also to define cardiac malformations.

All patients with a tracheotomy (typically older children with acquired cervical tracheal stenosis) should undergo methicillin-resistant *Staphylococcus aureus* (MRSA) screening and treatment before the surgery. MRSA infection in open airway procedures can be a devastating complication, resulting in dehiscence, and weakening of the cartilaginous structure of the laryngotracheal complex.

Regarding the anesthetic technique, although current methods, including jet ventilation, may allow for repair of distal and long-segment tracheal stenosis, these can often be obtrusive and cumbersome for the surgeon. Cardiopulmonary bypass is a safe alternative that allows partial deflation of the heart and lungs so that exposure of the complete trachea is optimized. Conversion of ECMO to cardiopulmonary bypass is also recommended for the procedure for this same reason. Successful surgical management thus depends upon close collaboration of the airway surgeon and the cardiovascular surgeon. For the cervical slide tracheoplasty, endotracheal intubation should be used.

53.3 Surgical Techniques

53.3.1 Intrathoracic Slide Tracheoplasty

▶ Fig. 53.2 illustrates the surgery technique. Typically, a sternotomy allows for exposure of the trachea, placement of atrial and aortic cannulas (if cardiopulmonary bypass is required) (▶ Fig. 53.3a), and repair of any coexisting cardiovascular anomalies. The trachea is exposed by dissecting between the ascending aorta and the superior vena cava. In the process, removal of the right paratracheal lymph nodes facilitates tracheal exposure. The carina is identified deep to the right pulmonary artery and the anterior trachea is exposed from the carina to the upper aspect of the CTRs.

Intraoperative bronchoscopy is then performed to define the upper and lower limits of the CTR segment. A 30-gauge needle is placed through the anterior tracheal wall as it is visualized by a 2.8-mm flexible bronchoscope to define the proximal and distal CTRs. At this point, with the patient stabilized on cardiopulmonary bypass, a more comprehensive evaluation of the distal airway can also be performed if desired.

The length of the stenosis is then measured and the trachea is transected at the midpoint of the segment of

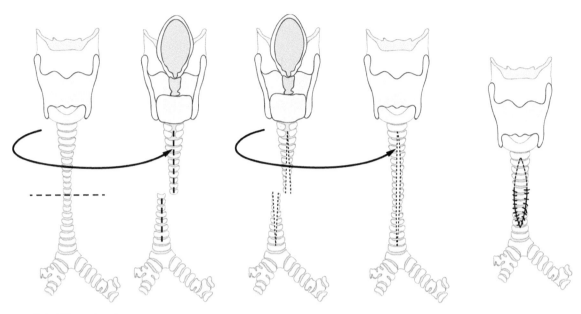

Fig. 53.2 Slide tracheoplasty.

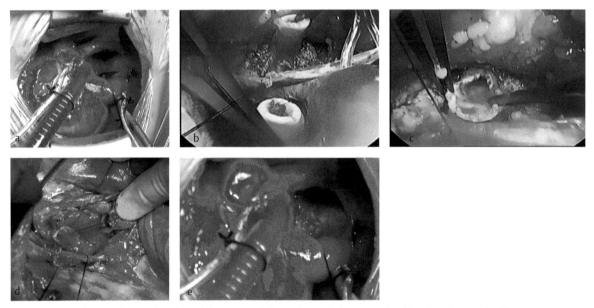

Fig. 53.3 Intrathoracic slide tracheoplasty. **(a)** Exposure of the trachea and placement of atrial and aortic cannulas (if cardiopulmonary bypass is required). **(b)** Transection of the trachea at the midpoint of the segment of complete rings/tracheal stenosis. **(c)** Vertical anterior incision of the proximal tracheal segment. **(d)** Double-armed 5.0 or 6–0 PDS sutures. **(e)** Intrathoracic slide tracheoplasty: completed anastomosis.

complete rings (▶Fig. 53.3b). Each end of the transected trachea is then mobilized. The lateral vascular attachments to the trachea are preserved in this process. The anterior wall of the proximal tracheal segment is incised vertically (▶Fig. 53.3c). The posterior wall of the distal segment is cut vertically toward the carina. Cartilage is then trimmed from the corners of the proximal and distal segments, and the segments then slid over each other.

Depending upon the length of the stenotic segment, this requires additional tracheal mobilization from both superior and inferior attachments. The carina is displaced superiorly by temporary stay sutures.

The anastomosis is commenced from distal posterior (carinal) in a running fashion using appropriate-sized double-armed polydioxanone sutures (5.0 or 6–0 PDS in infants) (▶Fig. 53.3d). Four to six throws of the suture are

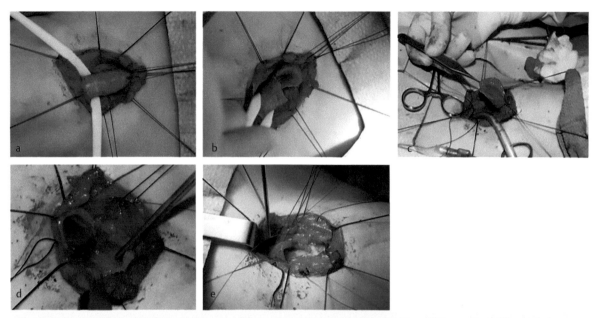

Fig. 53.4 Cervical slide tracheoplasty. **(a)** Exposure of the trachea via horizontal cervical incision. **(b)** Transection of the cervical trachea at the midpoint of the stenotic segment. **(c)** Vertical anterior incision of the proximal tracheal segment. **(d)** Double-armed 5.0 or 6–0 PDS sutures. **(e)** Intubation prior to the closure of the anterior wall.

generally placed at the carina and tightened with a nerve hook. The anastomosis is then continued up the left and right sides of the trachea, with the sutures placed through cartilage and mucosa, therefore being exposed intraluminally. An effort is made to evert the lateral sides of the anastomosis to prevent internal bunching of the anastomotic lines (a "figure 8" trachea). Before the anastomotic suture lines rejoin in the midline at the proximal anterior aspect of the repair, the trachea is suctioned clear and the patient is intubated with an age-appropriate endotracheal tube, and the tip of the tube positioned under direct visualization. The anastomosis is completed (▶Fig. 53.3e) with a single proximal knot being thrown, leak tested (to 35-cm water pressure), and marked with Ligaclips applied to the proximal and distal ends of the anastomosis (to help identify the extent of the anastomosis on postoperative radiographs). Fibrin glue is then applied to the anastomosis. The patient is then removed from bypass, the chest closed, and the patient is transferred to the intensive care unit. At completion of the procedure, the airway is re-evaluated with a flexible bronchoscope to ensure that the repair is adequate and that blood and secretions are suctioned.

Even with near full-length tracheal reconstruction, it is unusual to need a suprahyoid release or chin-to-chest sutures. Extension of the slide into a bronchus or cricoid cartilage has been performed successfully at our institution and may assist with repairing these concomitant stenoses. In children with an associated pig bronchus, a modified slide can also be performed, with the rings being split slightly oblique to the midline, so as not to compromise the orifice to the bronchus. The proximal

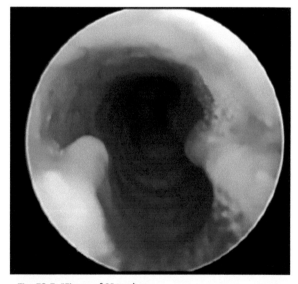

Fig. 53.5 "Figure of 8" trachea.

extent of the slide should extend at least 2 rings into normal trachea beyond the pig bronchus.

53.3.2 Cervical Slide Tracheoplasty

This technique is very similar to the intrathoracic slide tracheoplasty described above (▶Fig. 53.4a–e). In older children with a more proximal stenosis, the risk of developing a "figure 8" trachea (▶Fig. 53.5) is higher, and a temporary silicone stent may be placed for a week or more if required. In long segment acquired cervical stenosis, part of the stenosis may be resected, and the remaining may be slid. If scarred trachea is slid into normal trachea, the outcome will be acceptable. If scarred trachea is slid into scarred trachea, the result is less predictable.

53.3.3 Slide Tracheoplasty for Tracheoesophageal Fistula

Slide tracheoplasty can also be used for the repair of tracheoesophageal fistulas (TEFs), mainly complex cases and previously repaired fistulas. Modifications have been made to the standard technique to address the TEF. Microscopic direct laryngoscopy, bronchoscopy, and esophagoscopy are initially performed to verify the location of the fistula. An esophageal bougie is placed. The technique varies depending upon the surgical approach. Patients undergoing a cervical incision will be intubated orally, or in the case of an existing tracheostomy, through the stoma site. Patients requiring a sternal incision and cardiopulmonary bypass will be intubated orally with the stoma sutured shut. In these patients, cardiopulmonary

bypass is established prior to the beginning of tracheal work. In both approaches, the anterior wall of the trachea is freed from surrounding tissue as distal as possible. For patients with a cervical approach, mobilization often continues into the mediastinum and to the carina. In all patients, care is taken to preserve lateral tracheal attachments to maintain the blood supply and avoid damage to the recurrent laryngeal nerves. Retraction sutures using 2–0 Prolene are placed through the distal tracheal rings to retract the trachea. Flexible bronchoscopy through the endotracheal tube or rigid bronchoscopy can be repeated to confirm the location of the fistula. A needle is placed through the anterior tracheal in the corresponding location of the fistula. The trachea is then divided both superior and inferior to the fistula tract, leaving a small portion of trachea attached to the tract (▶Fig. 53.6a). The trachealis of the superior and inferior tracheal segments is then separated from the esophagus and mobilized. The trachea that remains attached to the fistula is then freed of it and mucosa and the cartilage portion is removed (▶Fig. 53.6b). The edges of the esophageal side of the fistula are freshened in preparation of closure. The tracheal mucosa is then inverted and folded into the

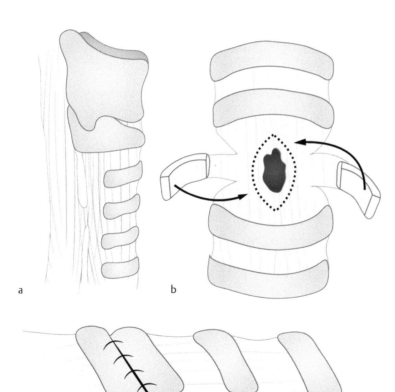

Fig. 53.6 Slide tracheoplasty for TEF: **(a)** The trachea is divided superior and inferior to the fistula site. A small portion of the trachea remains attached at the fistula and is used to reinforce the fistula repair. **(b)** The tracheal mucosa is removed from the cartilaginous rings and folded into the denuded fistula to reinforce the closure. In some instances the cartilage can also be used to reinforce the closure site. **(c)** The sternal periosteum is placed between the tracheal and esophageal closure to reinforce the repair. Tracheal closure occurs through an oblique running anastomosis. The trachea mucosa that had been removed from the tracheal cartilage has been folded into the esophageal side of the fistula and incorporated into the repair. TEF, tracheoesophageal fistula.

a

b

Graft

c

esophageal portion of the fistula. Closure is performed with a series of interrupted vicryl sutures. In cases of large fistulas, the cartilage can be kept in continuity with the mucosa and used in the closure for added support. Periosteum is harvested from the sternum and placed on top of the esophageal closure (▶ Fig. 53.6c).

Approximately 1 cm of the posterior wall of the inferior tracheal segment and the anterior wall of the superior segment are then divided vertically. The corners of the two segments are removed in order to achieve better approximation during closure. A running PDS is then used to close the anastomosis beginning with the posterior aspect of the trachea. The resulting, oblique anastomosis is longer than a corresponding end-to-end anastomosis, thereby distributing the tension across a longer area. Once all sutures are placed, fibrin glue is then applied across the tracheal closure. If occurring through a cervical incision, the previously placed Prolene retraction sutures can be placed around the hyoid as internal Grillo sutures. When performed through a sternotomy, the retraction sutures can be removed as the hyoid is not exposed.

53.4 Postoperative Treatment

Complications that occur after slide tracheoplasty most commonly reflect the underlying health status of the child. These infants may be critically ill prior to tracheal repair, and often remain critically ill following tracheal repair. The tracheal repair may also cause problems, including granulation tissue along suture lines and restenosis or collapse at the anastomosis site. Temporary or permanent injury to the recurrently laryngeal nerve is also possible. Failure of extubation usually results from one of these issues. A worrisome complication is dehiscence of the anastomosis. However, this is extremely uncommon, because of the long oblique suture line. Granulation tissue is usually amenable to serial bronchoscopic management. Stenosis or collapse at the anastomosis site may require either periodic dilation of the trachea or placement of a tracheotomy tube, with the tip of the tracheotomy tube bypassing the area of concern. However the primary predictors for poor outcomes were revision surgery, unilateral pulmonary agenesis, and bronchial stenosis.

Following open tracheal repair, the aim is to extubate the child at the conclusion of the procedure, or within 24 to 48 hours. While the patient is intubated in the pediatric intensive care unit, the child's head is maintained in forward flexion on a pillow, and it is advisable to maintain peak ventilation pressures below 30 cm of water pressure so as not to damage the anastomosis. Ideally, chest drains are left in place until after the extubation. In the setting of an extremely unstable preoperative ventilated child, postoperative ECMO may be required. The aim is to establish endotracheal ventilation and remove the child from ECMO as soon as possible.[5]

Follow-up endoscopy to examine the repair is routinely performed 1 and 2 weeks after the operation. Gentle balloon dilation is sometimes useful during the recovery phase if the figure-8 tracheal deformity at the repair is significant. This intervention helps prevent left and right lateral suture lines from coming into contact and adhering. Children without cardiopulmonary anomalies are typically discharged from the hospital 2 to 3 weeks postoperatively.

A good tracheal outcome at 3 months probably predicts an excellent long-term tracheal outcome. However, as these children have often concomitant cardiopulmonary pathologies, an excellent tracheal outcome does not guarantee an excellent overall outcome.

53.5 Highlights

a. Indications
   - Congenital tracheal stenosis/complete tracheal rings.
   - Absent tracheal rings.
   - Sleeve trachea.
   - Acquired tracheal stenosis.
   - Tracheoesophageal fistula.
   - A-frame deformities (most common post-tracheostomy).
b. Contraindications
   - Inadequate cartilage structure to the trachea.
   - Recent tracheal resection is a relative contraindication.
c. Complications
   - Granulation tissue formation.
   - Restenosis.
   - Dehiscence.
   - "Figure 8" trachea.
   - Recurrent laryngeal nerve injury.
d. Special preoperative considerations
   - Careful bronchoscopy for evaluation of the airway anatomy (better to "inadequately" assess than to compromise the airway).
   - Evaluation of cardiac and great vessels anatomy with chest CT with three-dimensional reconstruction should always be performed prior to surgery.
   - Screening for MRSA should be performed in children with tracheostomy.
   - Stabilize the child with severe symptoms with intubation (above rings preferentially) or ECMO. If there are ventilation problems, pull the tube back, do not advance it.
   - In the intubated child with distal tracheal stenosis, a longer inhalation and exhalation time (I time and E time) is recommended, and higher peak pressure may be tolerated. Mucus plugging is a concern, and maximal humidity is therefore recommended.

e. Special intraoperative considerations
   - If there are severe ventilation problems prior to initiating cardiopulmonary bypass, 1 mL of 1:10,000 epinephrine down the endotracheal tube is helpful. A longer I time and E time is also useful.
f. Special postoperative considerations
   - Extubate early.
   - If early extubation cannot be achieved, prevention of mucus plugging with saline down the endotracheal tube is critical.
   - A follow-up bronchoscopy should be performed 1 week postslide.
   - A good tracheal outcome at 3 months probably predicts an excellent long-term tracheal outcome. However, an excellent tracheal outcome does not guarantee an excellent overall outcome.

References

[1] Tsang V, Murday A, Gillbe C, Goldstraw P. Slide tracheoplasty for congenital funnel-shaped tracheal stenosis. Ann Thorac Surg 1989;48(5):632–635

[2] Grillo HC, Wright CD, Vlahakes GJ, MacGillivray TE. Management of congenital tracheal stenosis by means of slide tracheoplasty or resection and reconstruction, with long-term follow-up of growth after slide tracheoplasty. J Thorac Cardiovasc Surg 2002;123(1):145–152

[3] Rutter MJ, Cotton RT, Azizkhan RG, Manning PB. Slide tracheoplasty for the management of complete tracheal rings. J Pediatr Surg 2003;38(6):928–934

[4] Provenzano MJ, Rutter MJ, von Allmen D, et al. Slide tracheoplasty for the treatment of tracheoesophageal fistulas. J Pediatr Surg 2014;49(6):910–914

[5] Manning PB, Rutter MJ, Lisec A, Gupta R, Marino BS. One slide fits all: the versatility of slide tracheoplasty with cardiopulmonary bypass support for airway reconstruction in children. J Thorac Cardiovasc Surg 2011;141(1):155–161

[6] Chiu PP, Kim PC. Prognostic factors in the surgical treatment of congenital tracheal stenosis: a multicenter analysis of the literature. J Pediatr Surg 2006;41(1):221–225

[7] Kocyildirim E, Kanani M, Roebuck D, et al. Long-segment tracheal stenosis: slide tracheoplasty and a multidisciplinary approach improve outcomes and reduce costs. J Thorac Cardiovasc Surg 2004;128(6):876–882

[8] DeMarcantonio MA, Hart CK, Yang CJ, et al. Slide tracheoplasty outcomes in children with congenital pulmonary malformations. Laryngoscope 2017;127(6):1283–1287

[9] Butler CR, Speggiorin S, Rijnberg FM, et al. Outcomes of slide tracheoplasty in 101 children: a 17-year single-center experience. J Thorac Cardiovasc Surg 2014;147(6):1783–1789

[10] de Alarcon A, Rutter MJ. Cervical slide tracheoplasty. Arch Otolaryngol Head Neck Surg 2012;138(9):812–816

Section V

Pediatric Trauma

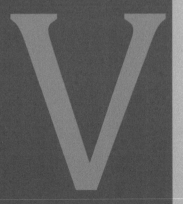

54 Facial Trauma in Pediatric Patient

Amir Laviv, Amir Shuster, Vadim Reiser

Summary

Pediatric craniofacial skeleton fractures can be challenging to manage. The patterns of trauma and the possible long-term growth disturbances, makes the clinical considerations and treatment approach unique. This chapter describes the common facial fractures in the growing child, and the recommended treatment.

Keywords: Pediatric facial trauma, maxillofacial fractures, craniofacial fractures

54.1 Introduction

Facial injuries in children are relatively rare compared with adults.[1,2] This relatively low incidence is related to anatomic reasons on one hand, such as facial bone flexibility, the lack of paranasal sinuses pneumatization, and the protection of the buccal fat pad in infants, and environmental reasons on the other hand, such as parents' close supervision, and "child friendly environment." Later in childhood, when involvement at school and playground rises, children become more vulnerable to facial trauma, and therefore the incidence of facial trauma increases.[3,4]

During the past few decades, there have been considerable advances in the diagnosis and treatment of craniofacial injuries. Diagnosis improved by using new imaging techniques, with computer tomography (CT) availability, which provides better understanding of fracture complexity using three-dimensional reconstruction.[5,6] The introduction of rigid internal fixation has changed the treatment outcomes, allowing reduction and fixation of bone fractures, without the need for long period of maxillomandibular fixation (MMF).

The management of pediatric maxillofacial fractures is complex. In a growing patient, soft tissue and periosteal injury, both because of the trauma itself, as well as for fracture exposure and fixation reasons, may cause scarring and possible growth disturbances. Moreover, fracture mobilization, reduction, and fixation (with hardware) may also alter future growth of the facial skeleton.[2,7,8,9]

The presence of tooth buds inside the jaws reduces the available bone for fracture fixation. The relatively small, sometimes mobile deciduous teeth do not retain wires as good as permanent dentition due to its shape (with minimal undercut area needed for the wire retention). Children's comprehension of their situation may be also problematic, and MMF (with the mouth wired shut) is not tolerated well in the pediatric population.[10]

However, malocclusion problems can be compensated by growth of the patient, and fractures tend to heal much quicker in children. Longitudinal follow-up is mandatory in this population, in order to identify, treat, and avoid any possible complications or growth disturbances.

In the past, and to some degree today, the management of pediatric maxillofacial trauma was relatively more conservative, with nonsurgical management preferred sometimes to prevent disruption in growth and development of the growing child. However today, with the increasing use of rigid fixation techniques, displaced fractures can be reduced accurately and fixated with rigid fixation (screws and plates), avoiding the usage of MMF.[10]

This chapter describes common fracture types in pediatric maxillofacial trauma, and their treatment, as recommended by the authors. Dentoalveolar fractures and dental trauma are not discussed in this chapter. It is beyond the scope of this chapter to describe all fracture subtypes and all possible treatment plans. The reader should bear in mind that each patient is unique, and the treatment plan should be tailored to a specific case.

54.2 Growth and Development

In early life, facial development is closely linked to the functional demands of the growing child.

The cranial vault (neurocranium) develops through intramembranous bone ossification, and grows rapidly in the first year of life as the brain tissues expand. Head circumference reaches about 86% by the first year of life, and 90% of its adult size by the age of 3 to 5 years. Growth of the cranial vault reaches a plateau by the age of 5 to 7 years. The cranium width further develops until the age of 14 years in girls and 15 years in boys.[5,6,9,11]

The skull base is the junction between the cranial vault and the facial skeleton. It is formed mainly by endochondral ossification. It includes the structures of the brain, orbits, and olfactory system and expands in the synchondrosis areas of the frontal, sphenoid, ethmoid, and occipital bones. Once ossified, the inner and outer surfaces of each bone extend their growth and remodel through appositional growth.[7,12,13]

The orbit consists of both cranio-orbital and nasomaxillary complexes. Most of the growth occurs at the sutures between these bones. As in the growth of the neurocranium, so do the orbits rapidly grow through the first year of life and reaches its adult volume by the age of 5 to 7 years. Intercanthal width is about 93% of its adult size by the age of 5 years, and is fully mature by 8 years of age in girls and 11 years of age in boys.[7,13]

Zygomatic bones' growth is more gradual compared to the cranium. The bizygomatic width reaches 83% of its mature size by the age of 5 years, and its final maturation is at 13 years in girls and 15 years in boys.

The maxillary growth is by intramembranous ossification, with forward and downward suture growth and surface remodeling. Its final maturation is at 13 years in girls and 15 years in boys.

The mandible is unique by having different areas of bone growth. The temporomandibular joint (TMJ) is formed by endochondral ossification, whereas the other parts of the mandible are formed by remodeling and apposition of bone. At the end of the first year, symphysial cartilage is replaced by bone. During the coming years, appositional growth occurs on the posterior border of the ramus and on the alveolar ridge, while resorption occurs along the anterior border of the ramus. Condyles grow upward and backward to maintain contact with the skull base.

Mandibular width is reached by the age of 1 year; however, its height is not complete until the teenage years. Mandibular depth (anterior posterior position) is 85% complete at the age of 5 years. Its mature dimensions are not final until 14 to 16 years in girls and 16 to 18 years in boys.

As the child is growing, the cranium-to-face ratio becomes less prominent.[10–12] The cranium-to-face ratio is about 8:1 in infancy and becomes around 2.5:1 in adulthood (▶ Fig. 54.1).

This is the main reason for higher incidence of cranial trauma in early childhood, and increasing incidence of midface and mandibular fractures with decreasing cranial trauma as the child grows up. Other well-accepted reasons for the low incidence of fractures in the early childhood are the retrusive position of the midface, the gradual pneumatization of the paranasal sinuses, and the elasticity of the child's facial bones.

The theory of functional matrix growth (Moss 1960) has gained general acceptance. It proposes that "origin, growth and maintenance of skeletal units are always secondary, compensatory and mechanically obligatory responses to prior events and processes occurring in related non-skeletal tissues, organs and functional spaces." Facial bones grow in response to the expansion of the cranium and development of the facial masticatory and oropharyngeal apparatus. Therefore, scar tissue, traumatically or surgically induced, can restrict further skeletal growth in the growing child. Surgical attention should be addressed to avoid scar formation and allowing normal function, in order to maintain functional growing tissue.

54.3 Epidemiology

Facial trauma comprises up to 11% of pediatric emergency department visits, and about 4% of pediatric trauma admissions.[13] Out of all maxillofacial fracture patients, children younger than 17 years old comprise about 14% of patients. However, most of the emergency department visits are related to soft tissue or dentoalveolar injury.

The proportion of patients with facial fractures increases substantially with age, with the peak in the age group of 6 to 12 years. Fractures in children younger than 5 years are rare with rate of up to 1.4%.[9] The risk to sustain facial fracture in a child increases by 14% with every year of age.

The etiology of trauma changes with age, but the most common causes are sport injuries and falls. The various etiologies depend on the age groups examined. Young children sustain injuries from low-velocity forces like falls, while older children are more exposed to high-velocity forces like road traffic accidents and sports injuries.[8,9,12,14–15]

Male gender also increases the likelihood of maxillofacial trauma. Boys are twice more injured than girls (2:1 ratio). This is related to more participation in sports events, and a tendency in attending dangerous activities.[7,16,17]

Fracture sites change with different age groups. Nasal fractures and dentoalveolar fractures are the most common facial fractures in children, but are not reported as frequently as expected, because most of these fractures can be treated on an outpatient basis, and therefore these fractures are under-reported in the hospital and admission statistics. Mandibular fractures are the most

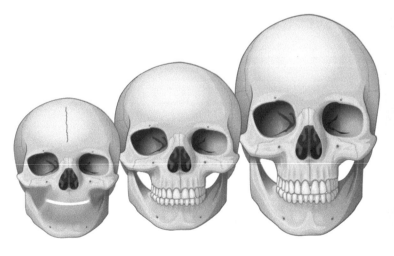

Fig. 54.1 Left to right: Infant, mixed dentition, and adult human skulls illustrate the decreasing cranium-to-face ratio as the infant grows up.

common facial fractures reported in hospitalized children. Their incidence increases with age. Zygomatic complex fractures and orbital fractures are the next prevalent fracture type, whereas midface and Le Fort fractures (at all levels) are uncommon, and can occur in children of 13 to 15 years of age. Orbital roof fractures and cranial vault fractures occur in young children, with undeveloped frontal sinus, usually before the age of 7 years, because of the relatively prominent frontal bone.[16,18,19]

54.4 Preoperative Evaluation

As in every trauma patient, life-threatening injuries should be addressed first, before treatment of the facial injury. Advanced trauma life support algorithm should be used. The small size of the face relative to the cranium usually indicates that whenever facial trauma occurs, it is probably caused by high-energy impact. It has been found that up to 57% of children younger than 5 years of age with facial fractures have concomitant intracranial injury, whereas concomitant cervical spine injury is less likely (0.9–2.3%).[2,9,18,20]

Airway maintenance, bleeding control, and early resuscitation in children are very important due to the higher metabolic rate, oxygen demand (with less oxygen reservation), and lower blood volume and stroke volume. Intubation is preferred in all cases of airway compromise. Cricothyroidotomy is contraindicated in children less than 12 years of age, because of the risk of subglottic stenosis. Hypothermia in resuscitation of trauma in children is common, so elevation of room temperature, warmed normal saline for intravenous use, and warming devices are recommended. As for IV access which may be difficult in children, intraosseous access can be a good alternative. Blood transfusion and fluid resuscitation should be considered for possible volume loss. Maintenance fluids in babies are usually one-quarter normal saline with dextrose, and one-half normal saline for older children and teenagers. Urine output should be around 1 to 2 mL/kg/h.[7,12,14]

Assessment of craniofacial injury begins with history and physical examination. However, sometimes an adult may not have witnessed the trauma, and obtaining history from a child can be very difficult. Moreover, physical examination may be compromised because of poor cooperation, especially shortly after experiencing a traumatic injury.

A comprehensive thorough facial physical examination is mandatory. The examination should start from the scalp and proceed in a systematic fashion to the lower face and neck. Special focus should be addressed to facial lacerations, orbital exam, sensory disturbances, bone stability and step-offs, and occlusion of the teeth. Orbital examination should include pupils' reactivity, visual acuity, extraocular muscle function, possible diplopia, and

assessment of exophthalmos and hypoglobus. In case of questionable extraocular muscle restriction, forced-duction test should be considered; however, the exam cannot be performed when the child is awake, so consider doing it when the child is under sedation for imaging purposes or before definitive treatment. Children with orbital injury may also experience pain with eye movement, nausea, vomiting, and bradycardia. Bony step-offs of the orbits should be palpated, in addition to malar bone prominence evaluation and zygomatic arch continuity, in order to assess for zygomatico-maxillary fractures. Paresthesia of cranial nerve V distributions can suggest for possible fracture, with V1 (ophthalmic) suggestive for possible frontal fracture, V2 (maxillary) for orbital floor and zygomatico-maxillary fracture, and V3 (mandibular) for mandibular body or angle fracture. Intraoral examination should evaluate the dentition and occlusion, possible fractured teeth or alveolar bone fractures with malocclusion and inability to close the teeth, different than premorbid occlusion. Any hemorrhage should alert for possible adjacent fracture, such as sublingual hematoma as a sign for mandibular fracture, and palatal hematoma for maxillary or palatal fracture.

Plain radiographs are no longer the selected imaging modality, as the CT scan has become the standard of care in pediatric population.[21] The plain films are unreliable in pediatric trauma because of the undeveloped sinuses, incompletely ossified areas, potential green stick fractures, possible soft tissue entrapment, and the developing teeth buds. The CT scan is quick, provides good resolution, and the radiation dose decreases as technology improves. Sometimes, especially in young children, sedation or general anesthesia is essential for the CT scan.

This chapter will discuss different fracture types in the pediatric population and the recommended treatment. It is beyond the scope of this chapter to discuss multiple fractures treatment or panfacial trauma in children.

54.5 Fractures Sites and Surgical Treatment (by Fracture Site)

54.5.1 Frontal Bone, Frontal Sinus, and Superior Orbital Fractures

In the years of infancy, there is rapid expansion of the cranial vault and skull base. As this process proceed, the non-pneumatized frontal sinus (before the age of 6 years), and the relative prominent frontal bone and superior orbital rim, orbital roof fractures are more common in children younger than 10 years of age (▶ Fig. 54.2). These fractures are cranial fractures, and as such, neurosurgical and ophthalmologic evaluation is mandatory. It can also involve the globe and lead to muscle entrapment, exophthalmos, and in severe cases even to direct globe injury.[22–24]

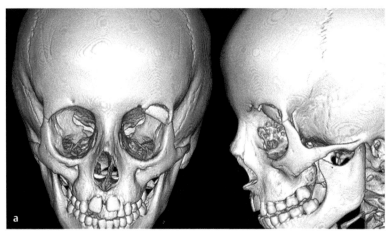

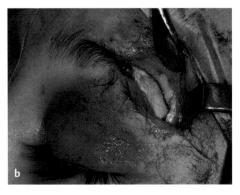
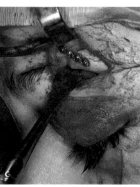

Fig. 54.2 Seven-year-old patient involved in bicycle accident, sustained left supraorbital frontal fracture, displaced into the orbital area with upper gaze diplopia. **(a)** 3D CT scans showing the fracture displaced into the superior orbit. **(b)** Fracture exposed through existing upper eyebrow laceration. **(c)** Fracture reduced and fixated with miniplate.

In general, indications for frontal and orbital roof fracture reduction include possible ocular involvement, and a fracture displaced more than full-thickness width of the bone involved. Ocular muscle entrapment can result in increased ocular pressure, diplopia, exophthalmos, and in severe cases even in superior orbital fissure syndrome. Fracture displaced more than full-thickness width can result in future esthetic concerns. Surgery should be coordinated with neurosurgeons to evaluate possible dural tear, CSF leak, or brain injury. The patient should have long-term neurosurgical follow-up because of the possibility of future brain herniation to the site of dural tears (and sometimes may need cranioplasty).

As the child grows up and the frontal sinus develops (after the age of 6 years), frontal sinus fractures are more common. Treatment indications and approach are the same as in adults. For posterior table fractures, if there are dural tears (with possible CSF leak), it should be treated by cranialization. It is important to seal the anterior cranial fossa to minimize the risk for postoperative meningitis. For displaced anterior table fractures, simple reduction and stabilization can be performed. This can be performed through an existing incision, or through a coronal flap. Minimally displaced anterior table fractures that will probably have no aesthetic

concern can be treated with observation only. Significant disruption of the nasofrontal duct will mandate intervention. Sinus obliteration is generally avoided in children. With the new endoscopic technologies, preservation of the sinus is preferred, with regular follow-up visits and imaging as needed, in order to assure proper sinus function.

Step by Step: Superior Orbital Roof Fracture

- Evaluation—Is there an indication for fracture reduction: fracture displacement more than full-thickness width, ocular involvement, increased ocular pressure, or neurosurgical brain involvement?
- Surgical approach—If laceration exists in the area of the fracture, try using it (extend as needed). If the fracture is on the mid-to-lateral side of the rim, use supraorbital eyebrow or upper eyelid approach. If neurosurgical intervention is also needed or fracture cannot be approached through the above incisions, coronal flap should be considered.
- Fracture reduction and fixation.
- Wound closure.
- Follow-up (including neurosurgery follow-up).

54.5.2 Naso-Orbito-Ethmoid Fractures

Naso-orbito-ethmoid (NOE) fractures in children are relatively rare. Ophthalmologic consultation to rule out globe injury, and assessment of the nasolacrimal aperture is mandatory. NOE fractures can cause medial canthal tendon disruption (with a fractured bone segment), which can cause telecanthus.

Treatment is similar as in adult patients. It should not be delayed after healing has been established, because late fixation or revision of these fractures can be very difficult, with suboptimal results compared to immediate treatment.[25] If the fractured nasal pyramid feels stable, or the fracture is minimally displaced, closed reduction and close follow-up should be considered. For a displaced fracture, with medial canthal tendon disruption, "open reduction internal fixation" (ORIF) should be considered (▶Fig. 54.3). The approach to the NOE area should be through an existing laceration (if present), or through coronal approach. The main treatment goals are restoration of medial canthal attachment and nasal projection. In cases of open reduction internal fixation, fracture sites should be approached, reduced, and fixated. Transnasal wiring of the medial canthal tendon with or without external bolsters to splint the underlying bony fragments may be necessary for restoration of the medial canthal attachment. The fixation should be held in place for 4 to 6 weeks. Unsupported nasal bone fracture may need strut bone graft (e.g., calvaria, rib graft). As for the nasolacrimal aperture, stenting is usually not necessary during immediate repair in children (not for all cases); however, long-term follow-up is mandatory.

Step by Step: Naso-Orbito-Ethmoidal Fractures

- Evaluation—Is there ocular or neurosurgical brain involvement? Is the fracture displaced?
- Surgical approach for "open reduction internal fixation"—If laceration exists in the area of the fracture, try using it (extend as needed). If no evident laceration, use coronal flap for exposure.

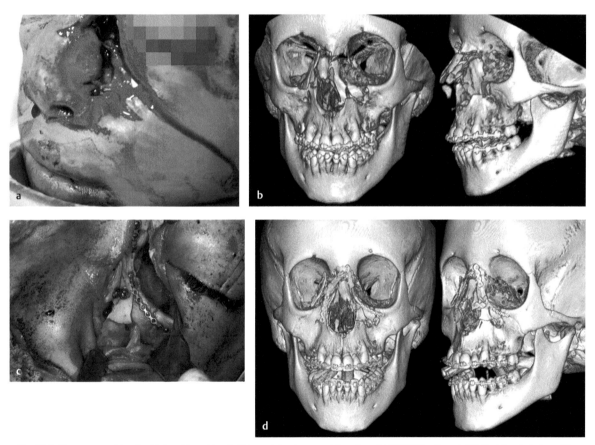

Fig. 54.3 Eleven-year-old patient injured by rubber bullet, sustained naso-orbito-ethmoidal (NOE) fracture. **(a)** Patient in admission with large lateral nasal soft tissue laceration, comminuted nasal and frontal process of the maxilla. **(b)** 3D CT reconstructions with bilateral NOE fractures, clinically—the medial canthus was attached to the large ethmoidal segment. **(c)** Intraoperative picture with reduction and fixation of the fractures through the existing laceration. **(d)** 3D CT reconstructions postop with adequate fracture reduction.

- Fracture reduction and fixation—If unstable nasal fracture after reduction, use bone strut in order to support the nose.
- Fracture reduction and fixation—Pay attention to the medial canthal tendon: if it is attached to a large bony segment, reduction and fixation of the bony segment will be adequate. If the canthal tendon is free or attached to a small piece of bone, reduce the large bony segments, and after wound closure, use a bolster (not always necessary) on the soft tissue of the nose bilaterally, and fixate it with a through-and-through wire from the left side of the nose to the right side of the nose.
- Wound closure.
- Follow-up (including ophthalmology follow-up, postop X-rays).

Highlights

Possible complications

- Traumatic telecanthus, nasal collapse, nasolacrimal obstruction.
- In order to avoid possible complications, fractures should be reduced correctly, making sure for correct intercanthal distance and proper nasal projection. Late fixation can be much more difficult. When nasolacrimal obstruction occurs, dacryocystorhinostomy should be considered.
- Encephalocele, globe protrusion.
- If detected during surgery, fixation of bone perforation or bone protrusion should be addressed.

54.5.3 Orbital Floor and Blowout Fractures

Orbital fractures are common in children. After the age of 5 years, most orbital fractures involve the floor of the orbit, and most of these fractures are located medial to the infraorbital nerve.[15,22,26–27] For all the patients with orbital fractures, ophthalmologic evaluation is mandatory to rule out any damage to the globe, ocular muscles, or optic nerve. Many children may have nausea and vomiting after orbital fractures due to vagal response to pain associated with extraocular muscle traction (oculocardiac reflex). This entity comprises triad of bradycardia, nausea and syncope.[27,28] Another possible unique feature in children is the "trapdoor" fracture, when muscle is entrapped through an orbital green stick fracture, caused by the elasticity of the orbital floor or medial wall. This may cause "white eyed orbital fracture" in children, which comprises diplopia and restriction in either vertical gaze (in orbital floor fracture) or lateral gaze (in medial wall fracture), with no evidence of soft tissue trauma (and no signs of subconjunctival hemorrhage).[9,28]

Surgical approach to the orbit is similar as in adult patients. Existing lacerations should be used whenever possible in order to avoid new incisions. The subciliary approach is common; however, the transconjunctival approach (with or without lateral canthotomy) is favored for esthetic reasons (and in pure blowout fractures). Coronal incision is favored whenever approach to the medial, lateral, and superior orbit is necessary.

Small orbital fractures in children should be managed conservatively and nonoperatively in the case of minimal displacement, good mobility of the globe, and no ophthalmologic indications.

In fractures involving the optic canal with possible visual compromise, canal decompression should be considered with or without corticosteroids administration to reduce the swelling and pressure.

Patients demonstrating oculocardiac reflex require emergent repair. Trapdoor fracture or white eyed blowout fracture, should be operated within 24 to 48 hours (▶ Fig. 54.4).

Delay in intervention may cause ischemic necrosis and muscle shortening within a few days, which may lead to permanent diplopia.[12,22,26–27] Release of the entrapped tissue is the main goal of the operation. Endoscopic approach through the maxillary sinus may be efficient to visualize the reduction of small trapped tissue reduction, and inaccessible areas, such as the posterior orbital floor.

Large orbital floor defect usually does not cause muscle and soft tissue entrapment, but may cause orbital diplopia and enophthalmos, and the main reason for treatment is to prevent these complications. The fractures can be explored after edema subsides (up to 1 week). The fracture should be reduced and reconstructed. Reconstruction can be performed using alloplastic implant or autologous graft. Children younger than 7 years, who may continue their orbital growth, should be treated with autologous bone graft, such as calvarial split bone graft. After the age of 7 years, when the orbit is adult size, open reduction can be performed without concern for growth disturbances. Different reconstruction materials can be used for floor reconstruction including autogenous bone graft, alloplastic titanium mesh, or porous polyethylene with the advantage of the latter two with no donor site involvement and morbidity. Today, the surgeon can also use preform, printed titanium mesh for a specific patient using the 3D reconstruction of the CT scan.

Step by Step: Orbital Floor and Blowout Fracture

- Evaluation—Ophthalmology consult.
- Evaluation—If oculocardiac reflex, emergent repair.
- Evaluation—If "white eyed orbital fracture" or "trap-door fracture," surgical intervention within 24 to 48 hours.
- Evaluation—For small fracture without diplopia, follow-up only.
- Evaluation—For large orbital floor fractures, surgical intervention within 5 to 7 days.
- Surgical approach—If laceration exists in the area of the fracture, try using it (extend as needed).

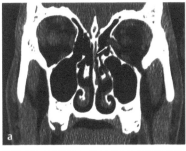
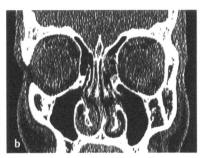
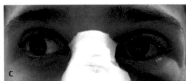
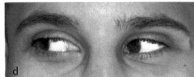

Fig. 54.4 Seventeen-year-old patient post–head collision during football play, sustaining medial wall orbital blowout fracture (and nasal fracture), with diplopia on lateral and medial gaze on presentation. Transconjunctival approach performed within 4 hours from presentation, with exploration and reduction of the fracture, without plate fixation. **(a)** Preoperative CT scan coronal view, demonstrating the left medial wall orbital blowout fracture, with the medial rectus entrapped in the fractured bone (*white arrow*). **(b)** Postoperative CT scan demonstrating good reduction of the fractured area, with intact medial rectus. **(c)** Immediate postoperative clinical picture with slight remnant of medial gaze limitation. **(d)** Three months postoperative without eye movement limitation. (These images are provided courtesy of Dr. Zachary S. Peacock.)

Otherwise use subciliary or transconjunctival approach. Using minimal endoscope through maxillary sinus can facilitate direct vision of the orbital floor to assess the quality of reduction.

- Fracture reduction and fixation—If floor reconstruction needed for patients younger than 7 years, autologous bone graft is recommended. For patients older than 7 years, autograft or alloplast can be used.
- Wound closure.

Highlights

Possible complications

- Exophthalmos, persistent diplopia (due to soft tissue entrapment), scar cicatrization of herniated content, ocular injury.
- To avoid complications, perform surgery in the recommended timeframe. Make sure the exploration is sufficient to elevate the entrapped/dropped soft tissue back to the orbit, and place adequate support for the fractured bone area. Late fixation can be very hard to achieve. Forced-duction test is recommended before the surgery and immediately after the surgery (in the operating room) to check for free eye movements. Ocular injury is more probable in the initial trauma. However, globe injury should be avoided during surgery, especially during dissection of the orbital walls, and when releasing orbital content from fracture site.

54.5.4 Nasal Fractures

Nasal fractures are the most common facial bone fracture in the pediatric population. The incidence of nasal fractures is underreported, because most of the patients are treated on an outpatient basis, and therefore, the fracture is not documented as a hospital admission for facial fracture.[12]

Most nasal fractures can be diagnosed on physical examination. The clinical findings suggestive of nasal fracture include overlying skin laceration, nasal crepitus and bone mobility, swelling, epistaxis, septal hematoma, and intranasal laceration. Palpation of the nasal bone area can miss underlying fracture because of absence of crepitus in children, and lack of cooperation. Septal hematoma, if present, requires early drainage in order to avoid septal necrosis, and subsequent saddle nose. After hematoma evacuation, compressive bolster should be used to eliminate dead space and blood accumulation, and provide perichondrial healing.

The nasal septum is an important growth center. Untreated injury may cause lack of nasal projection, and may lead to growth disturbances. Full growth of the nose is achieved by the age of 16 to 18 years in girls, and 18 to 20 years in boys.

Treatment of choice for nasal bone fractures is early closed reduction. This can be performed under sedation and local anesthesia, once the swelling resolves, or under general anesthesia. The purpose of treatment is to realign the nasal bones, and straighten the nasal septum.

Step by Step: Nasal Fracture

- Evaluation—Inspection and palpation. Look for overlying skin laceration, swelling, epistaxis, septal hematoma, and intranasal laceration. Use a speculum for intranasal examination.
- In case of septal hematoma, early drainage is mandatory, with compressive bolster in place.
- In case of displaced nasal fracture, closed reduction is recommended after swelling resolves (usually 5 to 7 days). Nasal bone alignment, and straightening the nasal septum.
- Use intranasal packing and a splint to cover the nose.

Highlights

Possible complications
- Nasal deformity, septal deviation, nasal airway obstruction, and growth disturbances (because of naso-ethmoidal or septovomerine sutures involvement).
- Secondary rhinoplasty may be required. Functional rhinoplasty can be performed as soon as needed, whereas esthetic rhinoplasty should be delayed until growth completion.

54.5.5 Midface and Zygomaticomaxillary Complex Fractures

The small paranasal sinuses, unerupted teeth, and the prominent forehead relative to the midface, all make zygomaticomaxillary fractures in children uncommon, but increase in adolescence. If present, it is usually the result of high-velocity trauma. Isolated zygomatic fractures can occur more frequently (up to 40% of pediatric midface injury) than isolated maxillary fractures (up to 20% of pediatric midface injury), and Le Fort fractures are very rare.[12]

Zygomatic fractures may appear with different clinical signs such as transconjunctival hemorrhage, edema, ecchymosis, exophthalmos, palpable step-offs in the orbital rim, paresthesia in maxillary division of the trigeminal nerve, diplopia with inferior rectus or inferior oblique entrapment. Zygomatic arch fracture can result in mouth opening limitation by being a hard stop, interfering with the coronoid process of the mandible moving forward during mouth opening.

For all zygomatic fractures, ophthalmologic consult should be performed to rule out any globe injury.

Approach to access midface fractures are similar to those in adults, and include the superior eyelid or supratarsal incision, the subciliary or transconjunctival incision, and the transoral vestibular incision. For zygomatic arch fractures, Gillies approach (closed reduction through a hairline incision) is effective. Severely comminuted fractures may benefit from a coronal incision.[12]

Periosteal stripping in young children should be avoided in order to avoid possible growth restriction by scar tissue formation. It is debatable, but some authors even recommend removing titanium plates and screws at 3 to 4 months after open surgery in order to avoid future growing problems.

Indications for treatment include possible future esthetic concerns (cheek asymmetry) and orbital functional problems. Treatment should be initiated within 5 to 7 days, before fracture consolidation, and after the swelling resolves.

Fractures with significant displacement in the buttresses area require open reduction and internal fixation. However, in patients in the age of 6 to 12 years, care should be taken with screw placement in order to avoid possible damage to the developing dentition.

Minimally displaced fractures should be treated conservatively.

Zygomatic arch fracture can be reduced with closed reduction using the Gillies approach in the first few days after the trauma, or through intraoral incision (Keene approach). Usually, the zygomatic arch fractures are stable after reduction, and plating is unnecessary.

For displaced zygomatic fractures, open reduction is recommended, through incisions as described above (▶ Fig. 54.5). After reduction of the fractures, microplates and miniplates with screws are used to fixate at least one fracture site. Usually, one plate is adequate fixation in children.

Le fort fractures in children younger than 6 years rarely require surgical intervention. If needed, MMF or suspension on the zygomatic arches or superior piriform rim can be used. For Le Fort fractures with mobile maxilla, "open reduction internal fixation" is needed. In few different long-term follow-up studies of pediatric Le Fort fractures treated with rigid fixation, it appeared that midface fractures without tissue loss and with adequate reduction did not result in long-term midface growth impairment.

Step by Step: Zygomatic and Maxillary Fractures

- Evaluation—Ophthalmology consult as needed.
- Isolated zygomatic arch fracture—Closed reduction using Gillies approach or transoral approach in the first few days after the trauma. Usually, no plating necessary.
- Zygomatic fracture—Minimally displaced, no ocular injury, follow-up.
- Zygomatic fracture—Displaced fracture with possible future esthetic consequences, "open reduction internal fixation." Usually one plate is sufficient.
- Le Fort fracture—Before 6 years of age, usually follow-up only with soft diet (case selection, not always follow-up only). If fixation is needed, suspension is required on zygomatic arch or piriform rim. Mobile fracture in adolescent, "open reduction internal fixation." Try to avoid screw fixation in the area of tooth bud formation.
- Wound closure.

54.5.6 Mandibular Fractures

Mandibular fractures are the most commonly reported facial fractures in children, with increasing incidence with age.[12,13] Fractures of the mandible can appear on the different parts: symphysis and parasymphysis area (anterior area between the mental foramina bilaterally), body of the mandible (between the mental foramen and the area of the second molar tooth on each side), angle (distal to the second molar tooth and back to the ascending ramus of the mandible), ascending ramus, coronoid process (the most anterior superior part on the ascending

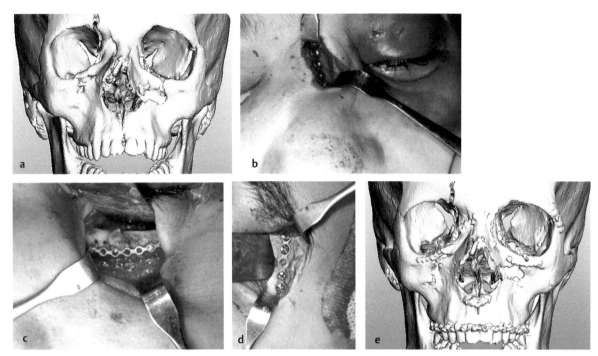

Fig. 54.5 Fourteen-year-old patient after motor vehicle accident as a pedestrian hit by a track. **(a)** 3D reconstruction CT scan showing the facial fractures: right frontal fracture, bilateral zygomatic fractures, left maxillary fracture, and midpalatal fracture. **(b–d)** Intraoperative pictures, reduction and fixation of maxillary fracture through existing laceration, infraorbital rim fracture through subciliary incision, frontozygomatic fracture through supraorbital eyebrow incision, respectively. **(e)** Postoperative 3D reconstruction CT scan. (These images are provide courtesy of Dr. Eran Regev.)

part of the mandible), and condylar process (the articulation of the mandible with the glenoid fossa). The different areas of the jaw can be affected, with mandibular condylar fractures being the most common, followed by (in decreasing order) fractures of the symphysis (and parasymphysis), angle, and body. Compared to adults, symphysis and parasymphysis fractures occur more often in children than adults, while body fractures in children are uncommon. Fractures of the coronoid process and ascending ramus in children are very rare.[9,29,30]

Clinical signs of mandibular fractures may include malocclusion, limited mouth opening, dental or mandibular segment mobility, paresthesia in the inferior alveolar nerve distribution, swelling, and sublingual or buccal hematoma.[12]

In the past, mandibular fracture confirmation was based on plain X-rays which included panorex, posterior anterior (PA), Townes view, occlusal, and lateral oblique X-rays. However, intracapsular condylar fracture, as well as green stick fractures and small minimally displaced fractures could be misdiagnosed in plain radiographs. Nowadays, and for the past few decades, CT scan has become the imaging modality for facial fractures. The axial, coronal, sagittal, and 3D reconstructions make it an efficient accurate tool, showing details of the fracture site, shape, amount of displacement, and anatomic structure proximity.

Treatment of mandibular fractures may be challenging, and the surgeon should take into consideration the bony growth potential, and future dental development, as the mandible is the last facial bone to reach skeletal maturity.

In contrast to adults, many pediatric mandibular fractures can be treated with conservative measures. In general, nondisplaced fracture, with no malocclusion, can be treated with liquid soft diet, physical activity avoidance, and close observation.[9]

Alveolar Process Fractures

Alveolar process fracture can be identified by mobility of bone segments with the teeth in the segment, and will result in premature contact of the teeth with the opposing jaw in that area. It can be treated with open or closed reduction and immobilization by acrylic splints and arch bars for 4 to 6 weeks. If relatively more rigid fixation is needed, the surgeon can use acrylated arch bar, which is an arch bar in place, reinforced with acrylic resin. Prior panorex or periapical X-ray is advised, in order to identify possible teeth affected in the fracture—either intact teeth, fractured teeth, or developing teeth involved in the fracture site.

Mandibular Condylar Fractures

The condyle is the most common mandibular fracture in children, occurring bilaterally in about 20% of the cases. However, fracture location can change with age. Children have relatively thick and short condylar neck, and therefore condylar fracture in patient younger than 6 years of age is more likely to be intracapsular, whereas older adolescents are more likely to sustain condylar neck fractures.[7,16]

Fall on the chin is a red alert for possible condylar fracture because of impact transfer from the chin area to the articulation of the mandible (the condylar head) with the base of the skull (temporal fossa). Condylar fractures are characterized by shortening of the affected side, causing ipsilateral deviation on mouth opening, premature contact on the ipsilateral (shortened affected) side, with open bite on the contralateral side. Bilateral condylar fractures may cause bilateral shortening of the ramus, causing an anterior open bite by the pull of the infrahyoid muscles.

Occasionally, despite condylar fracture, a child can maintain symmetry and occlusion of the mandible, and can be treated conservatively with soft diet and close observation. The main significant parameter for treatment of condylar fracture is to maintain functional soft tissue envelope in order to assure growth potential continuity.

The main treatment for condylar fractures is closed reduction with MMF followed by physical therapy, and close follow-up. Intracapsular and high subcondylar fractures (with malocclusion) should be treated with 1 to 2 weeks of tight MMF converted to functional elastics for occlusal guidance—alternating with physical therapy. This treatment allows early mobility of the joint to avoid joint ankylosis while maintaining the correct occlusion with the elastics occlusal guidance. Close follow-up should continue with regular intervals until completion of mandibular growth, to find out possible asymmetry development during growth. Low subcondylar fractures (with malocclusion) should be treated by MMF for 3 to 4 weeks, followed by physical therapy and close follow-up. Open reduction of condylar fracture should be considered rarely, when occlusion cannot be reestablished due to condylar segment position, when the segment is displaced into the middle cranial fossa, or when a foreign body is present.

The condyle in children is a primary growth center, and therefore growth disturbances after condylar fractures are a major concern. It has been documented that condylar fractures during active vertical growth of the mandible may require future orthognathic surgery. Up to 10% of adult patients with dentofacial deformity had evidence of condylar fracture in the past.

Mandibular Fractures other than the Condylar Fracture (▶ Fig. 54.6)

Displaced fractures should be treated by reduction and immobilization. In general, closed reduction is recommended for younger patients because the tooth buds within the mandible may be damaged by plates and screws fixation. After closed reduction, stability of the fracture site should be maintained for 3 to 4 weeks, and can be achieved by traditional arch bars, or acrylic splint fixed either to the teeth or with circummandibular wires (especially in cases when primary dentition cannot tolerate dental wiring). Manufacturing of acrylic splint is time consuming, and mandate for three general anesthesia appointments in children: the first for dental impressions (model fabrication), the second for placement and fixation of the splint, and the third for splint removal.

In general, "open reduction internal fixation" (ORIF) is applied to displaced fractures that cannot be properly reduced and stabilized with closed reduction technique. If the patient has reached skeletal and dental maturity, ORIF can be performed similarly to an adult patient.

ORIF can be performed in the symphysis area after eruption of permanent incisors (around 6 years), parasymphysis ORIF can be performed after eruption of permanent canines (around 9 years), and body and angle ORIF can be performed after eruption of posterior dentition (around 12 years). When the patient is more than 12 years old, the fracture should be treated as adult with MMF if the occlusion is stable, and MMF with or without ORIF for malocclusion, displaced fractures. Third molars should be evaluated for possible damage or involvement in angle fractures. In case of ORIF in children, usually a single miniplate in the inferior border can be sufficient for stabilization, with monocortical screws to avoid damage to tooth buds. Additional arch bar in the superior border (dentition) will prevent rotation of the fractured segment.

Hardware removal is controversial, and there is no evidence-based research for possible growth restriction when hardware is kept in place.[10,29,31,32]

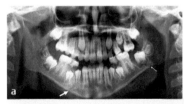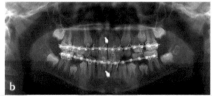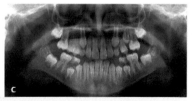

Fig. 54.6 Ten-year-old patient after violence attack. (a) Preoperative panorex with right parasymphysis fracture (*wide white arrow*), and left mandible angle fracture involving the erupting second molar tooth (*narrow white arrow*). (b) Postoperative panorex after MMF application (with arch bars, and two IMF screws), with good and stable occlusion. The right parasymphysis area seems to be well reduced, the left angle fracture is reduced, but not ideal. There was not enough space below the second molar in order to perform ORIF with plate and screws fixation, and if ORIF was performed, the tooth would have probably been extracted during the procedure. (c) Six weeks postoperative panorex, after MMF removal. Fracture of the right parasymphysis area has recovered uneventfully and there is no sign of the fracture. The left angle fracture area—callus with continuity of the lower border of the jaw can be detected. IMF, Intermaxillary fixation; MMF, maxillomandibular fixation; ORIF, open reduction internal fixation.

Step by Step: Mandibular Fractures

- Evaluation: Look for clinical signs for mandibular fracture: malocclusion, limited mouth opening, dental or mandibular segment mobility, paresthesia in the inferior alveolar nerve distribution, swelling, and sublingual or buccal hematoma.
- Define fractured area:
- *Dentoalveolar fracture*—Reduction and immobilization. X-ray advised to rule out teeth pathology in the fractured segment. Immobilization by acrylic splint/arch bar/acrylated arch bar for 4 to 6 weeks.
- *Condylar fracture*—Stable occlusion—soft diet, physical therapy after 2 to 3 weeks, close follow-up.
- *Condylar fracture*—Malocclusion:
  - *Intracapsular fracture or high subcondylar fracture*: MMF for 1 to 2 weeks, converted to functional elastics for occlusal guidance alternating with physical therapy.
  - *Low subcondylar fracture*: MMF for 3 to 4 weeks, followed by physical therapy.
  - *Open reduction of condylar fracture*: When occlusion cannot be reestablished because of the condylar segment position, when the segment is displaced into the middle cranial fossa, or when a foreign body is present.
- *Mandibular fracture other than condylar fracture—stable occlusion:*
  - *Nondisplaced fracture*: Until the age of 12 years, soft diet +/– MMF. After 12 years, MMF +/– ORIF.
- *Mandibular fracture other than condylar fracture—malocclusion:*
  - *Displaced fracture*: Closed reduction and MMF versus ORIF monocortical plate on the inferior border +/– arch bar on superior border. Avoid ORIF in the symphysis area before 6 years of age, parasymphysis area before 9 years of age, body of mandible before 12 years of age.
- Patient should remain in close follow-up.

Highlights

Possible Complications

- Growth disturbances, TMJ ankylosis.
- Growth disturbances are reported in 15% of TMJ fractures, especially in intracapsular fractures of children below 2.5 years. As a result, there may appear mandibular asymmetry by under or over growth of the affected side. TMJ ankylosis is reported in up to 7% of the condylar fractures. Therefore, early mobilization in children is important. It may appear with prolonged MMF, and in very young patients (below 5 years of age), due to lack of cooperation, especially in physical therapy. When it appears, ankylosis release is recommended. Bone graft to restore vertical dimension should be considered (e.g., rib graft, fibula).

Long-term Follow-up

- Long-term follow-up after pediatric maxillofacial trauma is recommended until skeletal maturity. Even patient with nondisplaced or minimally displaced fracture treated conservatively may develop facial skeleton growth problems. Such problems should be addressed as early as possible, because it can become much of a problem later in growth, and early fixation should be considered.

54.5.7 Resorbable Plates

Currently, the use of resorbable plates in pediatric maxillofacial surgery is in debate. The plates have been first introduced in cranial vault remodeling in neurosurgery, and created interest for application in pediatric maxillofacial surgery. The plates and screws are made of polymers of polylactic and polyglycolic acids, and many articles have reported on the successful use of plates in pediatric maxillofacial surgery. However, the plates and screws are weaker than titanium. The plates are bulkier, have little shape-memory which makes overbending almost impossible. The screws require tapping and handling which is more technique sensitive.

As discussed in this chapter, the use of plates and screws is limited in pediatric maxillofacial fractures, and there is not enough significant data for the advantage or disadvantage of using resorbable plates versus titanium plates, and no significant data indicating maxillofacial growth restrictions using titanium plates.[10,12,29,32,34]

Complications

Apart from site-specific possible complications (see highlights above), other complications may appear.

Early complications, such as malunion and infection, are rare in children compared to adults, because of faster bone healing and compensatory potential with growth and teeth eruption. Possible injury to the developing tooth buds is unique to the pediatric population and can be caused by screws secured to the bone for "open reduction internal fixation." Malocclusion is attributed to short fixation period in alveolar fractures, and can also be seen due to growth disturbances postcondylar fracture. As teeth erupt, the malocclusion can be fixed sometimes spontaneously. Great care should be addressed during MMF or reduction of the fractures, and the goal is to get the closest occlusion (bite) as possible to the premorbid bite.

Nerve injury is sometimes seen on injury presentation. However, surgery can also result in nerve injury, because of different reasons such as fracture exposure, screws of plating, etc. Great care should be taken on exploration and fixation.[10]

Frequent postoperative follow-up is recommended in order to find the complications as early as possible, and to treat them as soon as possible, in order to avoid future growth disturbances.

References

[1] Gassner R, Tuli T, Hächl O, Rudisch A, Ulmer H. Cranio-maxillofacial trauma: a 10 year review of 9,543 cases with 21,067 injuries. J Craniomaxillofac Surg 2003;31(1):51–61

[2] Gassner R, Tuli T, Hächl O, Moreira R, Ulmer H. Craniomaxillofacial trauma in children: a review of 3,385 cases with 6,060 injuries in 10 years. J Oral Maxillofac Surg 2004;62(4):399–407

[3] Grunwaldt L, Smith DM, Zuckerbraun NS, et al. Pediatric facial fractures: demographics, injury patterns, and associated injuries in 772 consecutive patients. Plast Reconstr Surg 2011;128(6):1263–1271

[4] Vyas RM, Dickinson BP, Wasson KL, Roostaeian J, Bradley JP. Pediatric facial fractures: current national incidence, distribution, and health care resource use. J Craniofac Surg 2008;19(2):339–349, discussion 350

[5] Waitzman AA, Posnick JC, Armstrong DC, Pron GE. Craniofacial skeletal measurements based on computed tomography: Part I. Accuracy and reproducibility. Cleft Palate Craniofac J 1992;29(2):112–117

[6] Waitzman AA, Posnick JC, Armstrong DC, Pron GE. Craniofacial skeletal measurements based on computed tomography: Part II. Normal values and growth trends. Cleft Palate Craniofac J 1992;29(2):118–128

[7] Miloro M, Ghali GE, Larsen P, Waite P. Peterson's Principles of Oral and Maxillofacial Surgery. 3rd ed. PMPH USA, Ltd. 2012

[8] Tanaka N, Uchide N, Suzuki K, et al. Maxillofacial fractures in children. J Craniomaxillofac Surg 1993;21(7):289–293

[9] Zimmermann CE, Troulis MJ, Kaban LB. Pediatric facial fractures: recent advances in prevention, diagnosis and management. Int J Oral Maxillofac Surg 2005;34(8):823–833

[10] Kellman RM, Tatum SA. Pediatric craniomaxillofacial trauma. Facial Plast Surg Clin North Am 2014;22(4):559–572

[11] Costello BJ, Rivera RD, Shand J, Mooney M. Growth and development considerations for craniomaxillofacial surgery. Oral Maxillofac Surg Clin North Am 2012;24(3):377–396

[12] Kaban LB, Troulis MJ. Pediatric Oral and Maxillofacial Surgery. Philadelphia, PA: W.B. Saunders; 1990

[13] Imahara SD, Hopper RA, Wang J, Rivara FP, Klein MB. Patterns and outcomes of pediatric facial fractures in the United States: a survey of the National Trauma Data Bank. J Am Coll Surg 2008;207(5):710–716

[14] Morris C, Kushner GM, Tiwana PS. Facial skeletal trauma in the growing patient. Oral Maxillofac Surg Clin North Am 2012;24(3):351–364

[15] Burm JS, Chung CH, Oh SJ. Pure orbital blowout fracture: new concepts and importance of medial orbital blowout fracture. Plast Reconstr Surg 1999;103(7):1839–1849

[16] Boffano P, Roccia F, Zavattero E, et al. European Maxillofacial Trauma (EURMAT) in children: a multicenter and prospective study. Oral Surg Oral Med Oral Pathol Oral Radiol 2015; 119(5):499–504

[17] Thorén H, Iizuka T, Hallikainen D, Nurminen M, Lindqvist C. An epidemiological study of patterns of condylar fractures in children. Br J Oral Maxillofac Surg 1997;35(5):306–311

[18] Posnick JC. Management of facial fractures in children and adolescents. Ann Plast Surg 1994;33(4):442–457

[19] Posnick JC. Craniomaxillofacial fractures in children. Oral Maxillofac Clin North Am 1994;1:169

[20] Thorén H, Schaller B, Suominen AL, Lindqvist C. Occurrence and severity of concomitant injuries in other areas than the face in children with mandibular and midfacial fractures. J Oral Maxillofac Surg 2012;70(1):92–96

[21] Braun TL, Xue AS, Maricevich RS. Differences in the management of pediatric facial trauma. Semin Plast Surg 2017;31(2):118–122

[22] Koltai PJ, Amjad I, Meyer D, Feustel PJ. Orbital fractures in children. Arch Otolaryngol Head Neck Surg 1995;121(12):1375–1379

[23] Messinger A, Radkowski MA, Greenwald MJ, Pensler JM. Orbital roof fractures in the pediatric population. Plast Reconstr Surg 1989;84(2):213–216, discussion 217–218

[24] Wright DL, Hoffman HT, Hoyt DB. Frontal sinus fractures in the pediatric population. Laryngoscope 1992;102(11):1215–1219

[25] Liau JY, Woodlief J, van Aalst JA. Pediatric nasoorbitoethmoid fractures. J Craniofac Surg 2011;22(5):1834–1838

[26] Grant JH III, Patrinely JR, Weiss AH, Kierney PC, Gruss JS. Trapdoor fracture of the orbit in a pediatric population. Plast Reconstr Surg 2002;109(2):482–489, discussion 490–495

[27] Hatton MP, Watkins LM, Rubin PA. Orbital fractures in children. Ophthal Plast Reconstr Surg 2001;17(3):174–179

[28] Bansagi ZC, Meyer DR. Internal orbital fractures in the pediatric age group: characterization and management. Ophthalmology 2000;107(5):829–836

[29] Goth S, Sawatari Y, Peleg M. Management of pediatric mandible fractures. J Craniofac Surg 2012;23(1):47–56

[30] Oji C. Fractures of the facial skeleton in children: a survey of patients under the age of 11 years. J Craniomaxillofac Surg 1998;26(5):322–325

[31] Bayram B, Yilmaz AC, Ersoz E, Uckan S. Does the titanium plate fixation of symphyseal fracture affect mandibular growth? J Craniofac Surg 2012;23(6):e601–e603

[32] Fernandez H, Osorio J, Russi MT, Quintero MA, Castro-Núñez J. Effects of internal rigid fixation on mandibular development in growing rabbits with mandibular fractures. J Oral Maxillofac Surg 2012;70(10):2368–2374

[33] Siy RW, Brown RH, Koshy JC, Stal S, Hollier LH Jr. General management considerations in pediatric facial fractures. J Craniofac Surg 2011;22(4):1190–1195

[34] Yerit KC, Hainich S, Enislidis G, et al. Biodegradable fixation of mandibular fractures in children: stability and early results. Oral Surg Oral Med Oral Pathol Oral Radiol Endod 2005;100(1): 17–24

Suggested Readings

Ellis E III, Zide MF. Surgical Approaches to the Facial Skeleton. Philadelphia, PA: Williams & Wilkins; 1995

Horswell BB, Jaskolka MS. Pediatric head injuries. Oral Maxillofac Surg Clin North Am 2012;24(3):337–350

55 The Management of Temporal Bone Fractures

Gil Lahav, Ophir Handzel

Summary

Traumatic insults to the temporal bone (TB) in the pediatric population are not rare. TB trauma can result in life-threatening complications and severe functional loss. Correct and timely diagnosis and treatment may help reduce the risks and impact associated with these injuries. The focus of this chapter is to present the diagnostic and therapeutic approaches to TB trauma for the otolaryngologist, and to cite typical issues that need to be addressed for comprehensive patient assessment and treatment.

Keywords: Temporal bone trauma, facial nerve palsy, CSF leak, pediatric patients

55.1 Introduction

55.1.1 Epidemiology

Temporal bone fractures in the pediatric population differ from those of adults in etiology and consequences.

The frequency of skull base fractures varies from 5% to 14% in children with head injuries, with a high prevalence of the temporal bone (as high as 62%), followed by the occipital, sphenoidal, and sphenoethmoidal complex and orbital portion of frontal bone. [1]

Most traumatic injuries are blunt, and the common mechanisms are motor vehicle accidents, followed by falls, and bicycle and other recreational vehicle-related injuries. Frequency varies among the different age groups, with falls being a more frequent cause in young children (<5 years of age) and collision accidents in the older ages.[2,3]

It is important to note that abuse is a common cause of traumatic brain injury and skull fractures in all age groups, especially in younger children where it accounts ~14% of cases.[4,5]

55.1.2 Pathophysiology

Apart from the common head contusion–related injuries, there are specific aspects of temporal bone trauma which are related to the different structures that reside in or are adjacent to the temporal bone. These include the inner ear structures, the dura and CSF-containing spaces, blood vessels, nerves, middle ear structures, and the Eustachian tube.

The anatomical properties of children's skulls differ from those of adults, thereby resulting in different skull base and temporal bone fractures characteristics. These differences vary with age, being most significant in infants, whose skull sutures are still open. The pediatric skull is more deformable, which enhances its energy absorption ability. An exception being the petrous part of the temporal bone, which is the most compact bone in the skeleton, and already well-developed in the newborn. This makes the forces that play a role in head trauma different specifically relative to the temporal bone.[6] The dissimilarity between adult and pediatric trauma mechanism is demonstrated by the lower incidence of facial nerve (FN) injury, and the higher rate of conductive hearing loss (CHL) in children compared to adults.[7]

55.1.3 Classification

Historically, temporal bone fractures have been categorized as longitudinal or transverse, relative to the axis of the petrous ridge of the temporal bone.[8] Longitudinal fracture lines classically run through the mastoid bone cortex and air cells, squamous part of the temporal bone and the external canal wall (typically postero-superior), with frequent involvement of the tympanic membrane. The fracture line of transverse fractures typically runs through the petrous bone (and commonly the otic capsule), and may also involve the foramen magnum posteriorly, the jugular foramen and the foramen lacerum anteriorly. A third type of fracture is the oblique or mixed, which according to some studies is actually the most frequent.[9] To improve the clinical relevance, the classification scheme has been modified according to the otic capsule involvement: otic capsule violating (OCV) vs. otic capsule sparing (OCS) fractures. According to several studies, the new classification method can better predict the risk for sensorineural hearing loss (SNHL), FN involvement, as well as cerebrospinal fluid (CSF) leak (all of which are more prevalent in OCV fractures).[8,10] These, however, do not separate adult from pediatric patients. In a study by Dunklebarger et al comparing the two systems, the OCS/OCV system had a better predictive value regarding SNHL, but neither system predicted CHL and FN involvement well.[11] This study showed 90:10 percent proportion of OCS/OCV fractures and 75:25 percent proportion of longitudinal/transverse fractures. Another study by Wexler et al found that neither system was a better predictor of FN injury, SNHL or CHL.[12]

55.2 Diagnostic Approach

55.2.1 Initial Evaluation

- Since temporal bone fracture is usually only part of a more complicated trauma, the primary concern should always focus on other more pressing life-threatening issues. The clinician must act according to the ATLS scheme, before approaching the specific temporal bone injury.

A temporal bone fracture could potentially pose a life danger if a main blood vessel is involved, namely the carotid artery or sigmoid sinus, but this is quite rare. Recording facial nerve function as early as possible is imperative. Particularly in unconscious patients or ones that are about to be sedated and/or intubated. An effort to establish facial nerve function will facilitate appropriate management of the paralyzed nerve. The window for this very early assessment typically closes before the otolaryngologist is involved, and should be included in the initial assessment by the trauma team.

- Traumatic brain injury (TBI): Relating to head trauma, once the patient's airway, breathing, and circulation status are stable, a neurological assessment should be performed. A detailed description of the neurologic examination is beyond the scope of this chapter; however, the main points are mentioned.

The Glasgow Coma Scale (GCS) is widely used to assess consciousness level. It has been adapted for children, and is easy to use for a general evaluation of the patient's current neurological state: a score of 3 to 7 is severe, 8 to 12 is moderate, and 13 to 15 is mild. Other symptoms and signs to observe are confusion, somnolence, or irritability, as well as vomiting and pallor. With relation to temporal bone fractures, loss of consciousness and other intracranial injuries are present in about 60% of cases.[13] The wide spectrum of brain injury and neurological signs ranges from subtle focal deficits to signs of brain herniation. Either way, when TBI is suspected, further investigations and management are warranted. A key point, even in mild head trauma cases, where initial evaluation does not lead to the diagnosis of TBI, is repeating the neurologic examination several times during the first few hours, since the appearance of new neurological signs may indicate complications such as progressive brain edema or secondary intracranial hemorrhage or thrombosis.[6]

55.2.2 Temporal Bone Fracture

Once the initial evaluation and stabilization are completed (principally by other members of the trauma team), it is time for the otolaryngologist to focus on the evaluation of the injured temporal bone. The diagnosis can be suspected on the basis of history and physical findings, although in some cases an imaging-based diagnosis may already be made at the time of the evaluation. The possibility of bilateral temporal fractures mandates the evaluation of both sides.

A detailed evaluation of each subsite is required, and will be further discussed, but at the initial "survey" two key-points require immediate attention: establishing the functional status of the facial nerve, and the presence of CSF leak. The management of the immediately completely paralyzed FN may require surgical intervention more frequently than the delayed paralyzed nerve. Other possible injuries require less urgent diagnosis and treatment.

Evaluation starts with a history if the patient is alert and cooperative. The patient (and/or parents) should be questioned about otalgia, ear fullness, loss of hearing, dizziness or vertigo, mechanism of trauma, past otologic history, and the presence of prior facial nerve dysfunction.

Next, a full ENT examination is performed, with a focus on neurotologic relevant pathologies:

- External ear: The auricle should be inspected for lacerations. Postauricularly, ecchymosis which signifies base of skull fracture (Battle sign) may be seen. Next, the ear canal is examined. As mentioned, it is important to diagnose the presence of CSF otorrhea as early as possible, so one should look for the presence of a clear discharge.

Canal laceration and/or bony fragments may be present with or without stenosis of the canal (which will require further intervention). Foreign bodies may be detected in the external auditory canal (EAC).

- Tympanic membrane (TM) and middle ear: The TM is often involved in temporal bone trauma, with a perforation more frequently encountered in longitudinal fractures. This will normally present with signs of fresh blood or clots in the canal. When the TM is not perforated, the pathognomonic hemotympanum is seen in about 80% of cases of temporal bone fractures.[7] Other middle ear involvement, including ossicular chain damage, will be difficult to diagnose with otoscopy at the time of initial evaluation.

Damage to middle ear structures is the most common reason for hearing loss. In most series, a CHL is the more common type (>50% of documented HL), followed by sensorineural hearing loss (SNHL) and mixed hearing loss (MHL).[3,7,12] In most instances, CHL is mild and resolves spontaneously. When the presentation is more severe, an ossicular disruption is the most probable pathology (▶Fig. 55.1), and complete improvement is less likely.[14,15]

- Inner ear: Otic capsule violation may include both the vestibular and cochlear components of the inner ear.

Vestibular bedside assessment in head trauma patient should take into account the possibility of concurrent central vestibular system involvement. Also, when

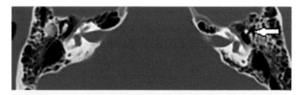

Fig. 55.1 A 37-year-old male sustained blunt trauma to the left side of the head falling off a bicycle at a low speed. He noticed an immediate hearing loss. Otoscopy was normal. Audiometry revealed a 45-dB conductive hearing loss. Imaging depicts a separation of the incus body from the malleus head. No temporal bone fracture was present. Transcanal ossiculoplasty was successful in closing most of the air-bone gap (axial bone window temporal bones CT scan).

examining the patient, head movements should be performed with caution, accounting for possibility of spinal injury. The bedside assessment includes the routine tests: evaluation of nystagmus, fistula test, Dix-Hallpike test, head thrust test, and post–head-shaking nystagmus. The most useful components to record in the initial evaluation are the characteristics of spontaneous nystagmus and head impulse test in the plane of the horizontal canal. Pathologic findings are expected in cases of acute vestibular paralysis, even without a fracture. The most common vestibular pathologies following temporal bone trauma are BPPV and vestibular hypofunction.

Hearing loss is present as a symptom in up to 33% to 80% of cases.[7,14] A bedside evaluation with the tuning fork test's results may vary in different situation: unilateral vs. bilateral fractures, and type of hearing loss: conductive, mixed, or sensorineural (SN), but it is important to perform and document it at least for follow-up purposes.

An audiometry must be performed when possible. It is not urgent, since the patient's cooperation is needed and hearing rehabilitation (surgical or conservative) will usually be done at a later stage. SNHL, second to CHL in incidence, may present on a wide scale, with temporary, mild, high tone loss to irreversible deafness. In general the more severe the hearing loss is on presentation, the higher the risk of some sort of sequelae.

- CSF leak: CSF leak is not rare in temporal bone fractures in children (~20% of cases).[15] The natural history of quick spontaneous resolution probably contributes to its under-diagnosis.[15] A high index of suspicion is required.

Principally, a CSF leak resulting from temporal bone fracture can present as either otorrhea or rhinorrhea. In the latter, where the CSF drains through the Eustachian tube to the nasal cavity, the bedside diagnosis is more challenging because of a wider differential diagnosis of clear nasal discharge (rhinitis, which is very common in children, tears, etc.).

On examination one should look for clear discharge in the external canal. Irrigation of the canal should therefore be avoided. If the discharge is bloody and not clear, the long known halo or sign may a useful bedside tool. A small amount of discharge is placed on a white gauze pad. Blood will concentrate in the middle and a clearer halo will appear. However, the specificity of the ring sign is not ideal (it depends on the CSF concentration, and may be positive for fluids other than CSF), and usually more definitive tests are used.[16,17] Rhinoscopy and endoscopic nasal examination aid in determining the nature and source of nasal discharge, with direct visualization of the Eustachian tube orifices.

Collecting and testing the fluid for the presence of beta-2-transferrin is considered the gold standard laboratory test for diagnosis because of its high sensitivity and specificity. The presence of the protein in the discharge makes the diagnosis of a CSF leak certain. However, a negative test does not rule out a leak, as sampling and other technical errors may result in a falsely negative test. Former tests such as the fluid glucose levels have been abandoned since their accuracy is very low.

Once the diagnosis of CSF leak has been established, imaging studies are performed to locate its source. These are especially important when planning surgical intervention, when conservative management fails. The different modalities, namely CT and MRI scans including the use of intrathecal injections will be discussed in the management section.

- Facial nerve injury: Facial nerve paralysis is one of the most devastating sequelae of temporal bone fractures, especially in the pediatric population. In most series, the incidence of FN paralysis is lower in children compared to adults, although the reported incidence varies greatly from 3% to 25%).[7,9,12,14,18]

The facial nerve is the motor nerve with the longest intraosseous course in human body. As the Fallopian canal leaves no space for expansion of an edematous nerve, complete dysfunction of the nerve may result from injuries that do not significantly disrupt its continuation. The two most important factors influencing treatment of the injured FN are the timing of the onset of injury and its extent. An immediate complete paralysis may represent a complete transection (▶Fig. 55.2). Delayed paralysis or paresis represents other injury mechanisms such as edema or hematoma. The determination of presence and/or timing of nerve injury can be impossible if the patient is unconscious when examined, although if some degree of consciousness exists, a facial movement can be elicited by a painful stimulation. Although it was originally developed for other purposes, the House-Brackman grading system is the most commonly used and best known. An important part of this is the degree of eye closure, which, if incomplete, may require protective eye measures.

Further investigations include imaging studies and electrophysiologic tests—electroneurography (ENOG) and electromyography (EMG). The combination of both helps the decision making regarding surgical intervention.

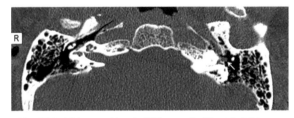

Fig. 55.2 A 24-year-old male fell from a significant height. He suffered multiorgan and life-threatening injuries and loss of consciousness. Two weeks after his injury, facial nerve function could be evaluated and revealed complete peripheral paralysis on the left. The left facial nerve is severed at the proximal tympanic segment (*arrow*). Spontaneous recovery is impossible (axial bone window temporal bones CT scan).

55.2.3 Management

Generally, the need for early interventions in temporal bone fractures is rare, especially in children. Surgery is indicated early in some cases of penetrating trauma, bleeding, large defects (with displaced fractures), brain herniation, or blocking CSF leaks complicated with meningitis.[19] In most cases, however, the indication will be a failure of conservative management. The preoperative assessment and decision making depends greatly on hearing status and imaging findings.

55.3 CSF Leak

The rate of traumatic CSF leaks resulting in meningitis is 10%. Most cases present immediately (within 48 hours of the trauma), but some may present later, if a clot, brain tissue, or scar tissue which initially sealed a dural tear dissolve or move.[19] The majority of cases (95–100%) resolve with conservative management: bed rest, head elevation (to ~25 degrees), and avoidance of maneuvers that might increase intracranial pressure: straining, nose blowing, sneezing, and coughing.[7,15] This is expected within a week.

The use of prophylactic antibiotic treatment during the period of conservative management of the leak is controversial. In the pediatric-specific case series, there was no advantage to prophylactic antibiotic treatment, although some patients were treated with antibiotics for other reasons. Brodie et al in a series of 820 cases (not specifically pediatric) reported a 23% increased risk for meningitis in patients whose CSF leak persisted for more than a week, or in patients who had a concurrent infection. They concluded that the use of antibiotics should be considered.[20] A meta-analysis of data from several studies discussing the use of prophylactic antibiotics for post-traumatic CSF fistula showed that antibiotic treatment contributed to a significant reduction of the incidence of meningitis from 10% to 2.5%. The authors of this chapter refrain from the use of prophylactic antibiotic.

When the leak does not cease within a week, the use of a lumbar drainage should be considered, with intermittent drainage preferred over continuous drainage due to lower complication rate.[19] The success rate of CSF drainage is high, and the leak is expected to resolve within another week to ten days.

In the uncommon case of persistent CSF leak despite conservative management it must be surgically sealed. The choice of approach for repair is dependent on the location of the source of the leak and the hearing status.

The source of a leak is localized with imaging. The most useful modality is high-resolution CT (HRCT) of the temporal bone. However, very small defects may not be apparent on the HRCT and often multiple defects are present, making it difficult to decide which of the defects is the likely source of the leak. In these circumstances, additional imaging modalities can be useful. CT cisternogram (CTC) is performed before and after intrathecal administration of nonionic myelographic iodinated contrast. The goal is to visualize the contrast-enhanced CSF leak egressing the dural space to the neighboring air-containing spaces. CTC, which was once a major diagnostic tool in the setting of CSF leaks lost its popularity. Its disadvantages: high radiation dose, low sensitivity in cases of an intermittent leak, need for lumbar puncture and its complications, potential side effects of intrathecal contrast use, and a difficulty of distinguishing between bone and contrast. CTC has been replaced by MR cisternogram (MRC) in some cases, although it is not approved in all countries in the pediatric population. Diluted gadolinium is injected intrathecally. Heavily T2-weighted images are acquired, depicting a bright trail of CSF communicating the subarachnoid space and the extracranial space, with or without an accompanying meningoencephalocele. This information is combined with the osseous details gathered by HRCT.

Similarly to CTC, MRC is contributory only when the leak is active. But differently to CTC, in cases of intermittent of low-output leaks, it is possible to suspend the scan for up to 24 hours after the intrathecal injection, thus increasing the sensitivity. Also, the differentiation between bone and contrast is better, and there is no exposure to ionizing radiation.[21]

CSF leak can be stopped by sealing either the source of the leak or TB air spaces' communication with the respiratory system or to the breached skin. The choice of approach depends on the site of the leak or leaks, and the hearing status. If the source of the leak is identified, closure of the defect is considered. The interface of dura and adjacent air spaces must be identified and sealed. When hearing preservation is a goal, tegmental defects can be approached through the middle fossa approach. The wide exposure from the Meckel's cave via the petrous ridge to the posterior border of the TB is useful in verifying the location and sealing most leaks originating in the roof of the TB.

When the fracture involves the otic capsule, hearing and vestibular function is completely and irreversibly lost, and the translabyrinthine (TL) approach can be ideal. Through the TL approach almost all sources of leaks can be approached: both the dura of the middle and the posterior fossa, jugular bulb, carotid canal, and the Eustachian tube and its neighboring air cells are all readily accessible. Labyrinthectomy does not eliminate the possibility of hearing rehabilitation with a cochlear implant.

Subtotal petrosectomy (SP) with blind sac closure of the meatus of the EAC segregates the CSF-filled spaces from potential source of infection. A thorough removal of as much air-cells as possible from the mastoid and epitympanum is performed. The closure of the EAC meatus must be water-tight. It can be supported by rotating a musculo-periosteal flap from the mastoid cortex to support the closed lateral EAC. The orifice of the Eustachian tube is plugged with a combination of muscle and fascia. Wedging the incus into the tissue plug can support it. If peritubal air cells, as seen on HRCT scans, extend along the ET, the bony opening of the ET can be widened to allow for deeper plugging of the ET lumen. The surgical cavity is packed with subcutaneous abdominal fat. In both TL and subtotal approaches CSF is likely to be present in the surgical field and water-tight skin suturing is mandatory. SP is very effective in controlling CSF leaks, and is commonly used in other skull base procedures.

The leak is dealt with even if the source isn't specifically identified. The main disadvantage is the associated CHL, which is especially critical in pediatric patients. Hearing is rehabilitated with one of the variety of bone-conducting hearing aids (implantable or not) available. Hearing rehabilitation can be staged, especially if the chosen device requires breaching the integrity of the scalp (i.e., BAHA connect, Cochlear Bone Anchored Solutions AB, Mölnlycke Sweden).

When the source of the leak can be completely accessed through the mastoid, a mastoidectomy with hearing preservation can be considered. A complete mastoidectomy is performed and the source of the leak in the dura isolated. In order to seal the leak effectively, it must be free of surrounding bone. The dural tear is covered with fascia and suitable glue. The mastoidectomy cavity is tightly packed with abdominal fat and pedicled muscle flap (i.e., temporalis). Particular attention is paid to sealing air cells in the facial recess, perifacial nerve, antrum, and attic regions.

When the source is in the posterior cranial fossa, mostly in transverse fractures TL, mastoidectomy, or SP approach is best suited depending on the hearing status. An intracranial repair through a posterior cranial fossa approach is an additional option if hearing is to be preserved,[19] although it is rarely utilized. A combined intracranial and transmastoid approach has been suggested.

55.4 Facial Nerve

55.4.1 Choice of Management

As mentioned earlier, facial nerve (FN) injury is not very common, especially one which necessitates surgical intervention. The FN can be severed or distracted and in these cases, without surgical re-establishment of its continuity, the prognosis will be poor. These injuries will present with immediate and complete paralysis. Most FN injuries will be delayed and/or partial paresis, both of which are likely to resolve with observation and conservative management. In these cases, treatment with systemic corticosteroids is recommended. Hence, even in cases of a temporal bone fracture complicated by facial nerve involvement, surgery is usually not necessary. Of note is the fact that surgery for decompressing a paralyzed facial nerve can add an additional insult to the nerve that often may be under-appreciated at the time of surgery.

The data in literature does not provide high-level evidence regarding the specific management of pediatric cases. Therefore, the description below follows the general approach which does not differ between pediatric and adult patients.

Furthermore, there are still controversies with regards to the correct management in adults (where much more data is available), including the role of surgery.[22]

The conventional management scheme in most centers suggests that some patients could benefit from a nerve exploration. The accepted indications for surgery are:

- Immediate complete paralysis (caused by a transected or severely crushed nerve), with >95% degeneration.
- Delayed complete paralysis (caused by progressive edema of hematoma), with electrophysiological test analysis suggesting a poor prognosis. However, there is a trend toward conservative management for delayed paralysis even if complete.

The electrophysiological tests that are used are electroneurography (ENOG) and electromyography (EMG). These are indicated only when complete paralysis is present. The utilization of these tests originates from the experience gained in the management of Bell palsy,[23] but data to support their use in temporal bone trauma also exists.[24] Serial ENOG testing is performed from the fourth or fifth day to two weeks post-trauma.

If these show a deterioration of 95% or more of lost nerve fibers on the injured side as compared to the contralateral normal side, the prognosis is considered poor, indicating surgery. If the ENOG shows less than 95% degeneration, or when this level of degeneration takes longer than 14 days to develop, the prognosis is better, and surgery is not indicated.

EMG starts being informative only 2 to 3 weeks post-trauma. When signs of denervation (fibrillations) are observed, surgery is also indicated.

A patient with a severed or distracted nerve has poor prognosis and is the one most likely to benefit from intervention. Functional testing cannot differentiate these lesions from impingements and similar lesions associated with more favorable outcomes.

Electric-based functional testing can be difficult or impossible to administer in a child. They may cause significant discomfort, limiting the child's ability to cooperate, (i.e., in efforts to maximally contract a given facial region), making results difficult to interpret. Most commonly, decision will be made without these tests performed.

In cases of immediate paralysis, the location of nerve injury is expected to be seen on HRCT. The area of the first genu (geniculate ganglion), or second genu are most commonly involved, especially in longitudinal fractures,[25,26] with the former in 66% and the latter in 20% of cases. The tympanic and mastoid segments were involved in 8% and 6%, respectively. More than one segment may be involved. In transverse fractures, the IAC, meatal, or labyrinthine segment may be involved.

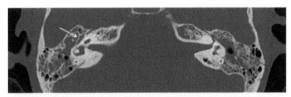

Fig. 55.3 A 17-year-old male sustained multiorgan trauma in a motorcycle accident. Upon presentation both facial nerves were completely paralyzed. CT scan verified the anatomical continuation of the Fallopian canal (*arrow*). Surgery was deferred. A year following the injury the patient had close to normal facial nerve function on the right side and grade 2 House Brackmann function on the left with synkinesis (axial bone window temporal bones CT scan).

Although imaging is the best accepted test for pointing to the site of injury, the role of HRCT in identifying patient with lesions associated with poor prognosis (and hence good candidates for surgery) has not been established. That being said, we believe HRCT does have an important role in the decision to intervene.

A 24-year-old patient suffered blunt trauma after falling from a height of fifth floor. He had a complete facial nerve palsy, probably immediate. HRCT depicts a clearly severed nerve in the proximal tympanic segment (▶Fig. 55.2). The nerve function never recovered. In contrast a 17-year-old male was injured in an accident operating a motorcycle. He was wearing a full face helmet and suffered from bilateral complete facial nerve paralysis. Functional nerve testing showed complete denervation on the left and a minor residual function of the temporal branch on the right. HRCT depicted fracture line on both TB but the integrity of the fallopian canal was not breached (▶Fig. 55.3). He recovered completely on the right and to a grade 2 by House Brackmann on the left.

55.4.2 Surgical Technique

Optimal timing for surgery remains debatable. Evidence favoring early intervention conflicts with the possibility of spontaneous recovery and the time required for its appearance (>6 months).

The approach for exploration depends on hearing status: in anacoustic ears, a TL approach allows exposure and handling of the whole temporal nerve including intracranial segments if needed. A middle-cranial fossa allows relative convenient approach to the geniculate ganglion, labyrinthine segment, and meatal foramen, if hearing is to be preserved. Exploration of the nerve is performed with isolation of the involved segment. After removal of bone fragments, granulations, and scar tissue, the extent of damage is assessed: if the nerve isn't cut, or more than 50% of its area is intact, decompression by opening of the nerve sheath is performed. When more than 50% of the damaged segment is involved, the injured segment is resected, and mobilization should be performed in order to achieve tension-free neurorrhaphy.

A nerve graft needs to be used in some cases, when tension-free single anastomosis cannot be achieved. The greater auricular or sural nerves are both possible donor sites. The usual neurorrhaphy technique is perineural suturing, but success of facial nerve neurorrhaphy has also been reported in cases of vestibular schwannoma surgery using a stitchless fibrin glue technique[27].

In cases with persistent paralysis after surgery or when denervation already occurred, other facial reanimation solutions should be offered. These include interpositional nerve grafting, nerve transfers, muscle transfers, free tissue flaps, and static slings, weights, and tissue rearrangement.[28]

55.5 Hearing Loss

- Conductive hearing loss: CHL is the most common type of hearing loss in children with temporal bone fracture. This makes sense in view of the fact that hemotympanum is the most common clinical sign. In the majority of patients (72%) the loss of hearing resolves spontaneously.[7] Initially, observation and local treatment of the external ear canal are required, in order to allow good conditions for hearing assessment. Once CHL or MHL are persistent, middle ear exploration and ossiculoplasty can be offered, taking into account the child's age, the size of air-bone gap, and the patient and parent's preference of rehabilitation. Tympanoplasty is indicated if a traumatic perforation does not heal properly spontaneously.

On exploration, the most common ossicular pathology is incudostapedial joint dislocation, but incudal dislocation or fracture of the stapes suprastructure has also been described,[14,29] and separation of the incus from the malleus is seen as well (▶Fig. 55.1). Incus interposition or a prosthesis are both accepted for reconstruction. Prosthetic ossicular replacement requires cartilage support of the tympanic membrane interface.

- Sensorineural hearing loss: SNHL is mostly a mild, temporary, high tone loss, although moderate and even severe cases have been reported to improve over a period of months. Generally, OCV and transverse fractures tend to present with a more severe SNHL and worse chances (~33%) of recovery.[14,15,30] When SNHL presents without a fracture, the mechanism is cochlear concussion, the result is usually mild, and prognosis is better.[14,31]

In cases of unilateral profound hearing loss, resulting in single-sided deafness, a variety of interventions for rehabilitation exist: contralateral routing of signal (CROS) hearing aids, bone conduction implants, and cochlear implant are all possible solutions. With bilateral temporal bone fracture and bilateral deafness, cochlear implantation is clearly indicated. However, special consideration regarding posttemporal bone fracture cochlear implant is required. Histologically, OCV fractures result in severe loss of hair cells, ganglion cells, and other supporting cells in the inner ear. Labyrinthitis ossificans may also occur, especially in cases complicated by infection.[32] In such cases, the basal turn of the scala tympany may be ossified, necessitating its drilling to facilitate insertion.[32,33] Preoperative CT and MRI aid in assessing cochlear patency prior to implantation. Although these cases may be more complex, including the possibility of facial nerve stimulation due to altered petrous bone anatomy, the success and usage rates are satisfactory.[33]

A potentially treatable post-traumatic hearing loss is the perilymphatic fistula, presenting with fluctuating or deteriorating hearing loss accompanied by vertigo. Such a diagnosis requires a high index of suspicion, and when suspected or evident, a closure of the fistula is indicated and may solve the problem.[34]

Another interesting entity with post-traumatic hearing loss is SNHL in the ear contralateral to the trauma-inflicted side.[35] This may result from cochlear concussion. In some cases the mechanism is *sympathetic hearing loss*, which is caused by an autoimmune response to inner ear antigens that have been exposed to the immune system following trauma. It has been reported to happen in 1% to 10%, responsive to corticosteroid therapy, but in some cases progressive up to deafness. This entity emphasizes the need for long-term follow-up of patients post-trauma.

55.6 External Ear Injury

The pinna and the external ear canal—cartilaginous and osseous can all be involved in temporal bone fractures. Potential long-term sequelae are esthetic pinna deformities, canal stenosis, and fistula between the external canal and mastoid air cells. The pinna is usually treated with primary suturing and debridement. Canal stenosis can be dealt with immediately by removal of detached cartilage, skin and bone fragments, alignment of canal skin, and packing. Care should be taken in cases of posterior canal wall involvement not to damage the facial nerve, especially in younger patients in whom the nerve can be more superficial. Posterior wall defects reconstruction with cartilage helps preventing a canal-mastoid fistula. Major posterior wall damage may necessitate canal wall down (CWD) mastoidectomy.

Anterior bony canal involvement can pose a significant therapeutic challenge. Reduction of bony fragments is compromised by the mandibular condyle movements. A CWD mastoidectomy may be indicated as a means to prevent stenosis or collapse.

A delayed intervention is also possible with meatoplasty or canaloplasty, with the different approaches according to the specific case and surgeon's preference.[36]

55.7 Other Complications

Some rare, mostly late complications are worth mentioning. These may present at a very late stage, even years after trauma, usually in more severe cases. This is specifically important in the pediatric population, and underscores the role of long-term follow-up.

Cholesteatoma may develop in the external ear, middle ear, attic, or mastoid. It may be secondary acquired when skin is entrapped in the middle ear cleft through a traumatic perforation which later heals. It can also be a result of Eustachian tube insufficiency secondary to its involvement in the fracture. Canal cholesteatoma may develop if the canal skin is mal-aligned or layered when the involved canal heals unfavorably.

Late CSF leak with or without meningocele or meningoencephalocele presents as otorrhea, rhinorrhea, or meningitis. Meningitis may also present latently without evidence of CSF leak. This is due to spread of infection from the middle ear to the inner ear and IAC post-OCV fractures. The healing of the petrous bone leaves fibrous, unossified fracture lines that become pathways to spread of infection.[37]

55.8 Highlights

a. General considerations
   – TB trauma in children is not rare, and can result in life-threatening complications and severe functional loss.
   – The main serious outcomes of temporal bone trauma are cerebrospinal fluid (CSF) and meningitis, facial nerve (FN) injury, and hearing and vestibular loss.
   – Most cases resolve with conservative management.
b. Clinical approach
   – The initial approach to the patient adheres to the advanced trauma life support procedures.
   – In the early assessment of TB trauma, it is most important to determine the presence of CSF leak and FN injury.
   – The timing (immediate vs. delayed) and extent of FN injury are the most important factors to determine.
c. Indications for surgical intervention
   – CSF leak not resolving with conservative management.
   – Facial nerve paralysis:
     ○ Immediate complete paralysis (caused by a transected or severely crushed nerve).
     ○ Delayed complete paralysis (relative indication).
     ○ Imaging supports an unfavorable outcome (i.e., severed nerve).
   – Nonresolving CHL.
   – External canal stenosis and injury.
d. Special preoperative considerations
   – Hearing status may influence the choice of surgical approach for controlling CSF leak or facial nerve repair.

- Imaging studies are utilized to locate the source of CSF leak.
- Electrophysiologic tests may not be possible to perform in children, although they are considered good predictors of prognosis and important decision-making tools.

e. Special intraoperative considerations
- Commonly, SP with blind sac closure of the external ear meatus and Eustachian tube orifice plugging can be a superior option to direct closure of a CSF leak.
- Facial nerve neurorrhaphy is performed when more than 50% of the damaged segment is involved.
- In selected severe cases of external ear canal injury, a CWD mastoidectomy may be indicated as a means to prevent stenosis or collapse.

f. Special postoperative considerations
- Prolonged follow-up is needed in some cases in order to rule out the development of late complications such as cholesteatoma and meningocele or meningoencephalocele.

References

[1] Perheentupa U, Kinnunen I, Grénman R, Aitasalo K, Mäkitie AA. Management and outcome of pediatric skull base fractures. Int J Pediatr Otorhinolaryngol 2010;74(11):1245–1250

[2] Temporal bone fractures | SpringerLink. Available at: https://link-springer-com.kaplan-ez.medlcp.tau.ac.il/article/10.1007/s10140-008-0777-3. Accessed May 29, 2017

[3] Waissbluth S, Ywakim R, Al Qassabi B, et al. Pediatric temporal bone fractures: a case series. Int J Pediatr Otorhinolaryngol 2016;84:106–109

[4] Leventhal JM, Martin KD, Asnes AG. Fractures and traumatic brain injuries: abuse versus accidents in a US database of hospitalized children. Pediatrics 2010;126(1):e104–e115

[5] Marx J, Hockberger R, Walls R. Rosen's Emergency Medicine: Concepts and Clinical Practice. Elsevier/Saunders, 2014; Philadelphia, USA

[6] Pinto PS, Poretti A, Meoded A, Tekes A, Huisman TAGM. The unique features of traumatic brain injury in children: review of the characteristics of the pediatric skull and brain, mechanisms of trauma, patterns of injury, complications and their imaging findings—part 1. J Neuroimaging 2012;22(2):e1–e17

[7] Lee D, Honrado C, Har-El G, Goldsmith A. Pediatric temporal bone fractures. Laryngoscope 1998;108(6):816–821

[8] Dahiya R, Keller JD, Litofsky NS, Bankey PE, Bonassar LJ, Megerian CA. Temporal bone fractures: otic capsule sparing versus otic capsule violating clinical and radiographic considerations. J Trauma 1999;47(6):1079–1083

[9] Williams WT, Ghorayeb BY, Yeakley JW. Pediatric temporal bone fractures. Laryngoscope 1992;102(6):600–603

[10] Little SC, Kesser BW. Radiographic classification of temporal bone fractures: clinical predictability using a new system. Arch Otolaryngol Head Neck Surg 2006;132(12):1300–1304

[11] Dunklebarger J, Branstetter B IV, Lincoln A, et al. Pediatric temporal bone fractures: current trends and comparison of classification schemes. Laryngoscope 2014;124(3):781–784

[12] Wexler S, Poletto E, Chennupati SK. Pediatric temporal bone fractures: a 10-year experience. Pediatr Emerg Care 2016

[13] Lee J, Nadol JB Jr, Eddington DK. Factors associated with incomplete insertion of electrodes in cochlear implant surgery: a histopathologic study. Audiol Neurotol 2011;16(2):69–81

[14] McGuirt WF Jr, Stool SE. Temporal bone fractures in children: a review with emphasis on long-term sequelae. Clin Pediatr (Phila) 1992;31(1):12–18

[15] McGuirt WF Jr, Stool SE. Cerebrospinal fluid fistula: the identification and management in pediatric temporal bone fractures. Laryngoscope 1995;105(4 Pt 1):359–364

[16] Sunder R, Tyler K. Basal skull fracture and the halo sign. CMAJ 2013;185(5):416

[17] Dula DJ, Fales W. The 'ring sign': is it a reliable indicator for cerebral spinal fluid? Ann Emerg Med 1993;22(4):718–720

[18] Glarner H, Meuli M, Hof E, et al. Management of petrous bone fractures in children: analysis of 127 cases. J Trauma 1994;36(2):198–201

[19] Youmans and Winn Neurological Surgery. 4-Volume Set. 7th Ed. Available at: https://www.elsevier.com/books/youmans-and-winn-neurological-surgery-4-volume-set/winn/978-0-323-28782-1. Accessed July 25, 2017

[20] Brodie HA, Thompson TC. Management of complications from 820 temporal bone fractures. Am J Otol 1997;18(2):188–197

[21] Reddy M, Baugnon K. Imaging of cerebrospinal fluid rhinorrhea and otorrhea. Radiol Clin North Am 2017;55(1):167–187

[22] Nash JJ, Friedland DR, Boorsma KJ, Rhee JS. Management and outcomes of facial paralysis from intratemporal blunt trauma: a systematic review. Laryngoscope 2010;120(7):1397–1404

[23] Gantz BJ, Rubinstein JT, Gidley P, Woodworth GG. Surgical management of Bell's palsy. Laryngoscope 1999;109(8):1177–1188

[24] Nosan DK, Benecke JE Jr, Murr AH. Current perspective on temporal bone trauma. Otolaryngol Head Neck Surg 1997;117(1):67–71

[25] Darrouzet V, Duclos JY, Liguoro D, Truilhe Y, De Bonfils C, Bebear JP. Management of facial paralysis resulting from temporal bone fractures: our experience in 115 cases. Otolaryngol Head Neck Surg 2001;125(1):77–84

[26] Coker NJ, Kendall KA, Jenkins HA, Alford BR. Traumatic intratemporal facial nerve injury: management rationale for preservation of function. Otolaryngol Head Neck Surg 1987;97(3):262–269

[27] Ramos DS, Bonnard D, Franco-Vidal V, Liguoro D, Darrouzet V. Stitchless fibrin glue-aided facial nerve grafting after cerebellopontine angle schwannoma removal: technique and results in 15 cases. Otol Neurotol 2015;36(3):498–502

[28] Gordin E, Lee TS, Ducic Y, Arnaoutakis D. Facial nerve trauma: evaluation and considerations in management. Craniomaxillofac Trauma Reconstr 2015;8(1):1–13

[29] Cannon CR, Jahrsdoerfer RA. Temporal bone fractures: review of 90 cases. Arch Otolaryngol 1983;109(5):285–288

[30] Schell A, Kitsko D. Audiometric outcomes in pediatric temporal bone trauma. Otolaryngol Head Neck Surg 2016;154(1):175–180

31 Vartiainen E, Karjalainen S, Kärjä J. Auditory disorders following head injury in children. Acta Otolaryngol 1985;99(5–6):529–536

[32] Morgan WE, Coker NJ, Jenkins HA. Histopathology of temporal bone fractures: implications for cochlear implantation. Laryngoscope 1994;104(4):426–432

[33] Camilleri AE, Toner JG, Howarth KL, Hampton S, Ramsden RT. Cochlear implantation following temporal bone fracture. J Laryngol Otol 1999;113(5):454–457

[34] Lyos AT, Marsh MA, Jenkins HA, Coker NJ. Progressive hearing loss after transverse temporal bone fracture. Arch Otolaryngol Head Neck Surg 1995;121(7):795–799

[35] ten Cate W-JF, Bachor E. Autoimmune-mediated sympathetic hearing loss: a case report. Otol Neurotol 2005;26(2):161–165

[36] Bajin MD, Yılmaz T, Günaydın RÖ, Kuşçu O, Sözen T, Jafarov S. Management of acquired atresia of the external auditory canal. J Int Adv Otol 2015;11(2):147–150

[37] Sudhoff H, Linthicum FH Jr. Temporal bone fracture and latent meningitis: temporal bone histopathology study of the month. Otol Neurotol 2003;24(3):521–522

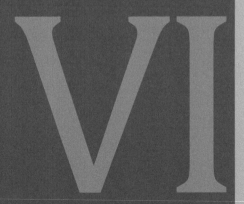

Section VI

Reconstruction

VI

56 Regional and Local Flaps in Children

Justin Loloi, Meghan Wilson, Jessyka G. Lighthall

Summary

When primary closure of facial defects is not an option, local and regional flaps are instrumental to re-establishing function and providing a highly cosmetic result. Local flaps have also been used in the treatment of secondary cleft lip and palate deformities, congenital orbitofacial deformities, velopharyngeal insufficiency, and in the posttraumatic or postablative treatment of children. A careful analysis of the defect characteristics and flap planning will optimize the reconstructive result and help restore psychosocial well-being in this population. Although an exhaustive review of all flaps is beyond the scope of this chapter, the authors will review the most commonly used local and regional flaps currently used in children.

Keywords: Pediatric, reconstruction, local flaps, regional flaps, facial reconstruction, Abbé flap, FAMM flap, tongue flap

56.1 Introduction

The face plays a significant role in the recognition of the individual, social interaction, and critical functions such as communication, smell, sight, taste, respiration, and nutrition intake. Special consideration to social and emotional development must be given in pediatrics. At around 5 years of age, children begin to develop self-esteem and a sense of self-image.[1] Consequently, defects of the face may result in devastating emotional and psychological disturbances in this sensitive population.[2] Although children may exhibit a more vigorous healing response and fewer complications of chronic disease such as those in smoking and diabetes mellitus, treatment of maxillofacial defects in this population presents challenges not otherwise encountered in the adult population. This is partly credited to the unique anatomic and physiological variations in the growing facial skeleton.[3] Common etiologies of head-and-neck defects in the pediatric population include maxillofacial trauma, neoplasm (benign or malignant), infection, inflammation, and congenital malformations.

There are important differences between the adult and pediatric head-and-neck region that need to be accounted for in reconstruction. Generally, the skin of a child's face has increased elasticity and is growing with growth centers located throughout the facial skeleton. The lack of sun damage and rhytids along with indistinct borders between aesthetic subunits makes it more difficult to adequately hide a surgical scar in the pediatric population.

The goal of any reconstruction is to restore functionality and provide an aesthetic result with minimal donor site morbidity.[4] The reconstructive ladder is a useful concept utilized in the pediatric population to characterize and assess the degree of treatment required.[5] When possible, reconstruction with primary closure should be performed. Secondary intention healing is slow and may lead to contractures, scarring, and restriction of movements. In children, adjuncts to facilitate reconstruction of large defects may include temporary closure with skin grafting and placement of tissue expanders to recruit additional tissue to allow local flap transfer. Tissue expansion is a powerful surgical modality that can be especially useful in growing skin and soft tissue in the pediatric population.[6] Rather than replacing tissue, tissue expanders are placed under adjacent tissue with slow expansion to allow for secondary local flap procedures to provide improved aesthetic results. Given that pediatric patients, when compared to adults, have a scarcity of usable tissue, the implementation of pretransfer expansion of donor sites to increase the amount of available tissue is a helpful tool in the reconstruction of large defects (▶ Fig. 56.1). Although children have thinner and less available soft tissue for expansion, their skin inherently has a better blood supply and is more easily expandable than that of adults. Nevertheless, a recent study suggested there is no difference in complication rates between adult and pediatric populations who underwent tissue expansion.[7]

Local flaps are the workhorse for reconstruction of pediatric craniofacial defects and will be discussed in detail in this chapter. If adequate local tissue is not available, the use of a regional flap may allow for closure of larger

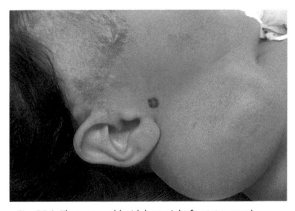

Fig. 56.1 Three-year-old with large right frontotemporal defect secondary to dog bite injury. Tissue expander in place in preparation for local flap closure with cervicofacial flap. Patient also has a left scalp expander in place for combined scalp rotation flap.

defects and will also be reviewed below. However, large regional flaps (e.g., pectoralis myocutaneous flaps) are used less often due to significant donor and recipient site morbidity and poor aesthetic outcomes. With the advent of free tissue transfer, microvascular reconstruction has surpassed regional flaps as the preferred reconstruction for large or composite defects in the pediatric population. This chapter will focus on more commonly used local and regional flap reconstruction in the pediatric population.

56.2 Local and Regional Flaps

A local flap is defined as transfer of skin and subcutaneous tissue with its blood supply to an immediately adjacent defect. It is important when designing a local flap to try to minimize wound closure tension by utilizing skin extensibility when recruiting skin and to align resultant scars along the borders of subunits or parallel to the relaxed skin tension lines.[8] The definition of a regional flap is less concise and debated. Although many authors consider a flap that is not adjacent to the defect to be a regional flap, the true definition of a regional flap is a pedicled flap from outside the head-and-neck region. Regional flaps are typically reserved for defects which cannot be adequately reconstructed with the sole use of a local flap and are used far less often than local flaps, particularly in the pediatric population, as they are associated with a higher donor site morbidity and tend to have worse aesthetic outcomes with poor tissue match.[9] Additionally, for large or composite pediatric facial defects, free tissue transfer has largely replaced regional flap reconstruction.

Regardless of the definition utilized, local and regional flaps may be classified in many different ways (▶Table 56.1). Flaps may have a random pattern design in which the vascular supply is from the dermal and subdermal plexus or an axial design based off a named arterial supply in the subcutaneous fat. They may

Table 56.1 Classification of local and regional flaps.

Method of transfer
- **Advancement** Unipedicle
- Bipedicle
- V-Y and Y-V
- Island
- **Pivotal** Rotation
- Transposition
- Interpolated
- Island
- **Hinge** "Turn-over"

Vascular supply
Random pattern Based off of dermal and subdermal plexus from perforators
Axial pattern Based off of a named vessel typically in the subcutaneous tissue

Interpolated
- Must cross under (tunneled) or over intact skin
- Flap is not adjacent to the defect

rotate, advance linearly, or use a combination of these movements to fill a defect. The secondary defect caused by the flap is then closed primarily. Flaps may also be transposed over or under an intact bridge of skin, typically requiring a secondary procedure to divide the vascular supply. Local and regional flaps have large clinical value in head-and-neck reconstructions as the vascular conditions in the region allow for excellent viability along with superior color and facial skin quality match.[10]

There are many factors that play a role in the selection of a reasonable flap, including the size and location of the defect and the intrinsic viability of the flap.[8,11] Although both categories of flaps are relatively safe and reliable, they do have a risk of postoperative complications such as wound infection, hemorrhage, hematoma, flap loss with necrosis, and poor cosmetic outcomes with need for revision surgery. Although a detailed discussion of every possible flap is beyond the scope of this chapter, the more common local and regional flaps used in pediatric head-and-neck reconstruction will be reviewed.

56.3 Cervicofacial Flap

The cervicofacial flap is a random pattern local flap that recruits soft tissue from surrounding facial and cervical skin to reconstruct moderate (1.5 cm) to large defects (>3.0 cm) of the cheek, periorbital region, temple, and posterior neck.[12,13] It typically incorporates a combination of rotation and advancement movements. Incisions are placed in borders of subunits or existing rhytids to minimize visibility of scars. This flap is classically elevated in a subcutaneous plane but may be modified by dissecting the flap in a deeper, sub-superficial musculoaponeurotic system (SMAS) and subplatysmal plane to enhance flap thickness, increase the vascular supply, and improve viability of the flap (▶Fig. 56.2a–d).[14,15] The surgeon may elevate the entire flap deep to the SMAS in the face and platysma in the neck or may choose to elevate in a subcutaneous plane in the face and deep to the platysma in the neck. Regardless of the preferred level of elevation, the surgeon should stay superficial to the parotidomasseteric fascia and care should be taken when elevating anterior to the anterior border of the parotid gland to protect distal branches of the facial nerve.

The cervicofacial flap provides several advantages in facial reconstruction aside from those related to an enhanced blood supply. It offers an excellent cosmetic profile including good skin texture, color, and flexibility match to the recipient skin. This is particularly useful in the pediatric population because of the relative importance of appearance in the psychosocial development of a child. Second, the mobile nature of the flap makes it a more reliable and adaptable option in reconstructive efforts. Finally, the cervicofacial flap can be employed in

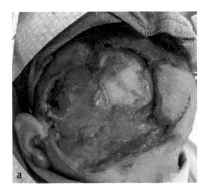
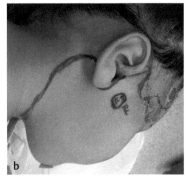

Fig. 56.2 Three-year-old with delayed reconstruction of right frontotemporal defect. **(a)** Initial defect. **(b)** Skin markings for planned cervicofacial flap after tissue expansion. **(c)** Cervicofacial flap rotated and advanced into defect. **(d)** Postoperative result 20 months after flap closure with intervening scar revision.

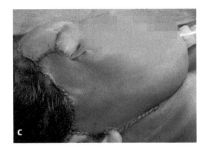
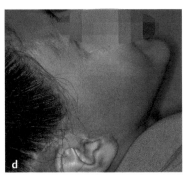

conjunction with procedures that require simultaneous parotidectomy or facial reanimation. This flap typically results in a standing cutaneous deformity. Although this can often be safely removed at the time of initial surgery, care should be taken not to narrow the flap base as this will exacerbate vascular insufficiency.

A major drawback of the extensively mobilized cervicofacial flap is the risk of distal flap necrosis secondary to compromised blood supply.[12,15] This risk is minimized in children as there are fewer comorbidities such as smoking or diabetes. Flap necrosis in children may occur due to hematoma, thin flap elevation, infection, or excessive tension. Minimizing wound closure tension is also key to decreasing the risk of widened, unattractive, or hypertrophic scars.

56.4 Scalp Rotation Flap

The scalp is a richly perfused multilayered region of the head that can be strategically rotated to reconstruct hair-bearing defects of the head and neck. The major contributing vessels are the supratrochlear, occipital, supraorbital, superficial temporal, occipital, and posterior auricular arteries.[16] The scalp is relatively inelastic and stiff relative to other facial tissues and therefore requires a larger flap to be harvested than from other areas of the face. If necessary, the entirety of the scalp may be elevated and rotated, or multiple rotation flaps may be employed depending on the size and location of the defect. The scalp flap may be elevated in either a subgaleal or subperiosteal

plane depending on the defect characteristics. The indispensable nature of the scalp, mostly due to the fibrous galea aponeurosis, serves a beneficial means of attenuating the distension of the pertinent vasculature which may otherwise compromise the viability of the tissue.[16] If necessary, galeotomies or incisions in the pericranium may be created to aid in the rotation of this flap.

Scalp rotation flaps are most commonly used to treat defects secondary to tumor resection, congenital abnormalities, osteomyelitis, and traumas/burn injuries.[17] The scalp rotational flap is a relatively simple and quick technique in repairing small and moderate defects of the head. It is especially valuable because of the excellent color, skin, and texture characteristics of the scalp tissue. This flap is useful to reconstruct a defect at the hairline and may be combined with facial flaps to optimize results (▶ Fig. 56.3a,b).

Careful attention must be given when working with scalp rotational flaps on the pediatric population. Although the scalp has a vigorous blood supply, long axial flaps are at a higher risk of necrosis in children because the galea aponeurosis is not fully developed, which puts the relevant vasculature in jeopardy of distension and stretching.[16] In addition, the lack of distensibility in the scalp may necessitate supplementary skin grafting for donor site closure.[18] Scalp expansion is a useful adjunct to increase the amount of available tissue for rotation prior to reconstruction and allow primary closure of donor site. Excessive stretch on the scalp may lead to temporary hair loss due to telogen shock, which may take months to show regrowth. This flap also redistributes hair and may

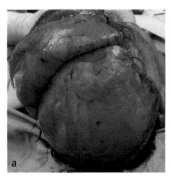
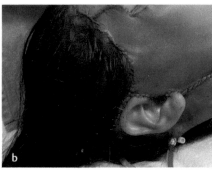

Fig. 56.3 Same patient as in ▶ Fig. 56.1 and ▶ Fig. 56.2 with planned scalp rotation flap. **(a)** Scalp rotation flap elevated (note depression of left parietal cranium from tissue expander). **(b)** Scalp flap inset to recreate frontotemporal hair line.

cause alterations in the direction of hair growth. Other risks of surgery include hematoma, adverse scarring with alopecia, and numbness of the scalp.

56.5 Geometric Flaps

Geometric flaps tend to be rotational and transposition random pattern flaps based off of the subdermal vascular plexus. They incorporate distinct geometric shapes in the planning and execution of the flap. Although useful for reconstructions of the temple, cheek, and nose in adults, they are used less frequently in children due to the inability to hide the geometric scars and local tissue distortion.[14] Although relatively simple to execute, the geometric flaps require careful assessment and planning as incisions cannot be placed within relaxed tension lines or along subunit borders which may elicit high degrees of tension at the closure point and lead to adverse scarring. These flaps also require excision of standing cutaneous deformities, which may be addressed at the time of flap transposition.

A major advantage in the use of these flaps is preservation of the skin characteristics of the recipient site. In addition, they offer greater flexibility in the use of available tissue when compared to many other local flaps. With respect to the pediatric population, the bilobed and rhombic flaps are rarely used due to irregularity and prominence of scars in conjunction with the inability to place scars along aesthetic subunits.

56.5.1 Bilobe Flap

The bilobed flap consists of two lobes that recruit tissue from areas of increased skin mobility. The first lobe is adjacent to the defect, is generally the same size of the defect, and may incorporate a 45° to 90° arc of rotation depending on the design. The second lobe may be half of the width of the defect and also incorporates a 45° to 90° arc of rotation.[8,19,20] The flap is elevated in a supraperichondrial plane in the nose and a subcutaneous plane in the cheek and neck and transposed into the defect. It should be noted that a standing cutaneous deformity will have to be excised at the base of the defect adjacent to the first lobe.

56.5.2 Rhombic Flap

The rhombic flap is a transposition flap that also pivots over intact skin to reconstruct defect in the head and neck. This flap requires the defect to be converted into a rhombic shape and utilizes straight-lined limbs based on the short- and long-axis of the defect to create a rhombic-shaped donor flap.[14,20] The design may be modified to alter the angles between the defect limbs or to incorporate a W-plasty based on the characteristics of the defect. The flap is elevated in a subcutaneous plane and transposed into the defect. Note the irregularity of the resulting scar, making this a largely unfavorable flap in the pediatric population.

56.6 Interpolated Flaps for Cutaneous Defects

56.6.1 Paramedian Forehead Flap

The pediatric nose is unique and will change drastically throughout puberty and into adulthood. Although smaller defects may be treated with adjacent tissue, larger defects necessitate repair with a forehead flap as the first-line method.[21,22] The forehead is richly perfused by the supraorbital, supratrochlear, superficial temporal, occipital, and posterior auricular arteries.[23] The paramedian forehead flap is composed of skin, subcutaneous fat, frontalis muscle, and a thin layer of areolar tissue overlying the periosteum. It offers an excellent color and texture match with which to resurface the nose when adjacent tissue may not be used. Following the subunit approach to nasal reconstruction, often the defect is enlarged with resection of uninvolved tissue such that the entire subunit is reconstructed.[11] This will ultimately result in a more aesthetic reconstruction.

Although when initially described the median forehead was used as a donor site, this has largely been replaced by the paramedian forehead flap supplied by the supratrochlear artery. It is generally used as an interpolated flap transposed over an intact bridge of skin, requiring at least one additional stage for division and inset of the flap.[21] During the first phase of reconstruction, the flap is elevated, the frontalis muscle and subcutaneous fat are typically excised distally to thin the flap, and the flap is secured to the recipient site. Although some authors will incorporate an intervening stage for flap contouring, at a minimum the reconstruction will require a second stage to divide the pedicle, further contour the flap, and complete the inset at the nose.[24]

In order to maximize the viability of the flap and to prevent fibrosis, contraction, and fat necrosis, additional steps may be taken between the time of inset and division.[22] During this intermediate stage, the flap and recipient site is further polished. This is accomplished via soft tissue excision and cartilage grafting. Primary cartilage grafts serve as the ideal method in not only minimizing the risk of contraction and collapse but also creating an ideal, rigid subsurface architecture prior to division.

The forehead flap has been extensively used in the adult population with extensive research available in the literature. In children, publications on the use of the forehead flap is sparse, likely secondary to the fact that large nasal defects in children are not common.[1,23,25,26] The procedure for forehead flap reconstruction is similar to that of adults (▶Fig. 56.4).[27] The authors refer readers to the text "Aesthetic Reconstruction of the Child's Nose" by Dr. Gary Burget for a comprehensive review of pediatric forehead flap reconstruction.[22]

With a low pivot point, the flap is more able to reach the recipient site without transferring hair-bearing scalp, which may compromise the aesthetic result and require delayed

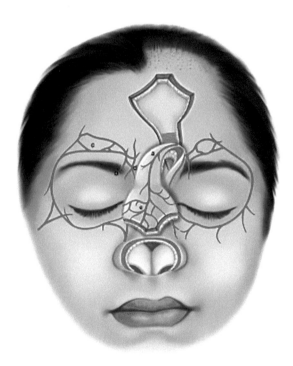

Fig. 56.4 Elevation of a left paramedian forehead flap for nasal tip defect based on the supratrochlear vascular pedicle. (Reproduced with permission from Reckley LK, Peck JJ, Roofe SB. Flap Basics III: Interpolated Flaps. *Facial plastic surgery clinics of North America.* 2017;25(3):337–346.)

techniques of hair removal. Disadvantages to the forehead flap are the multiple stages required, vertical scarring on the forehead, possible eyebrow malposition, flap loss, poor color or contour match, and potential need for resurfacing.

56.7 Oral and Perioral Flaps

56.7.1 Tongue Flap

Tongue flaps were introduced for intraoral reconstruction in the early 1900s and serve as a useful technique in repairing defects of the lips and palate in both children and adults.[28,29] In children, the tongue flap is frequently indicated for the closure of large or recurrent oronasal fistulae in the cleft population[29-31] however other conditions that may benefit from a tongue flap include loss of lip tissue in dog bites, oral thermal trauma, or repair of oral mucosa following resection of intraoral tumors.[32] Tongue flaps have a rich blood supply and may be based anteriorly, posteriorly, or laterally. The anteriorly based dorsal tongue flap is commonly employed due to its rich blood supply (dorsal lingual arteries of the ranine arch) and low morbidity associated with its use.[33] However, the location of the defect and flap mechanics will dictate the type of dorsal tongue flap to be used as either anterograde or retrograde flow is adequate to perfuse the flap.[28] Posteriorly based flaps incorporate the dorsal lingual artery, and laterally based flaps utilize the lingual artery. The flap is generally designed slightly longer and wider than the defect to account for contraction. Additionally, 2 to 3 mm of tongue musculature is included to include vasculature inflow and venous outflow. The flap is left pedicled, requiring a second stage to divide the pedicle and inset 2 to 3 weeks later (▶Fig. 56.5).[31]

Tongue flap closure has been associated with high success rate in both children and adults. Potential complications include articulation disturbances, mastication of the pedicle leading to flap loss, dehiscence due to excess tension, and an abnormal appearance of the reconstructed site due to differences in appearance of the tongue and oral mucosa.

56.7.2 Facial Artery Myomucosal Flap

The facial artery myomucosal (FAMM) flap, first described by Pribaz et al in 1992, combines the principles of nasolabial and buccal mucosal flaps to treat a variety of oronasal defects such as those of the palate, nasal septum, and upper and lower lips.[34] With a distinct regard to the pediatric population, the FAMM flap has been used extensively in cleft palate surgery, particularly for closure of persistent or large oronasal fistulae, but has also been described for nasal cavity, skull base, and oropharyngeal defect reconstruction.[35-38] The flap is composed of mucosa, submucosa, buccinator muscle, orbicularis muscle, and the facial artery along with its venous drainage.[34]

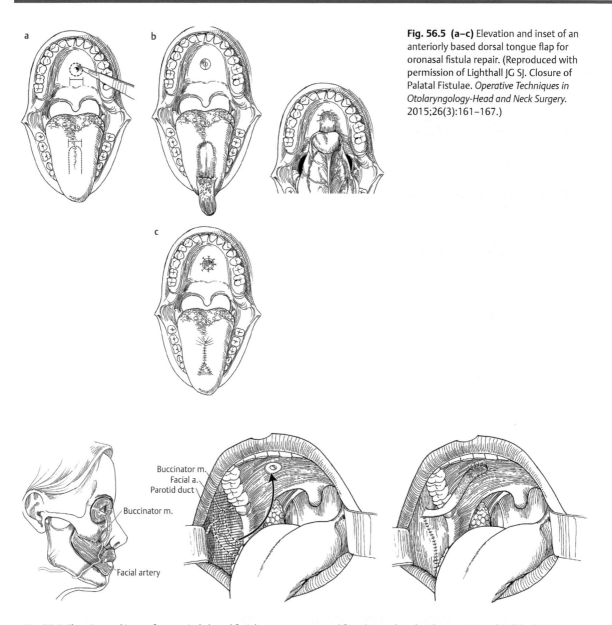

Fig. 56.5 (a–c) Elevation and inset of an anteriorly based dorsal tongue flap for oronasal fistula repair. (Reproduced with permission of Lighthall JG SJ. Closure of Palatal Fistulae. *Operative Techniques in Otolaryngology-Head and Neck Surgery.* 2015;26(3):161–167.)

Buccinator m.
Facial a.
Parotid duct

Buccinator m.

Facial artery

Fig. 56.6 Elevation and inset of a superiorly based facial artery myomucosal flap. (Reproduced with permission of Lighthall JG SJ. Closure of Palatal Fistulae. *Operative Techniques in Otolaryngology-Head and Neck Surgery* 2015;26(3):161–167.)

Typically, the course of the facial artery is confirmed using a hand-held Doppler. Dissection begins with an incision through the mucosa, submucosa, and buccinator muscle with subsequent identification of the facial artery distally. After the facial artery is identified, ligated, and cut, the flap is elevated to precisely include the facial vessels (▶Fig. 56.6).[31] The FAMM flap is versatile and may measure 9 cm × 2 cm or more and may be based either inferiorly (anterograde flow) or superiorly (retrograde flow).[31,34] It may also be raised as an interpolated or island flap to meet the specific needs of the defect. Interpolated flaps typically require division and inset 2 to 3 weeks later. For children undergoing reconstruction

with a FAMM flap, it is important to keep in mind that if they have teeth, biting into or through the flap is a real possibility and so proper precautions should be taken.

The FAMM flap is highly vascularized soft tissue which remains soft postoperatively with minimal risk of contracture. Therefore, it serves as a useful technique with low donor site morbidity in those requiring large amounts of vascularized tissue. A major disadvantage of the FAMM flap is loss of tissue due to pedicle thrombosis, venous congestion, and traumatic division of the pedicle from biting or infection.[34] In addition, the flap width is limited by the presence of Stensen duct so additional flaps may be needed to reconstruct a wider area of defect.

Finally, because the flap revolves around the presence of the facial artery, patients in whom the facial artery is transected (e.g., malignancy) may not be eligible for this type of reconstruction.

56.7.3 Abbé–Sabattini Cross-Lip Flap

The Abbé–Sabattini flap (often referred to as the Abbé flap) is a full-thickness composite flap classically involving the transfer of tissue of the central lower lip to the upper lip during secondary cleft repair.[39] First described by Sabattini in 1838 and then later popularized by Robert Abbé in 1898, it is effective in replacing functional and structural components in a plethora of defects in the upper and lower lips. In children, defects are typically due to a congenital deformity (e.g., bilateral cleft deformity) or secondary to trauma, though in adults this is generally due to tumor resection. Traditionally, the flap is full-thickness, composed of skin, muscle, and mucosa with a pedicle containing the superior or inferior labial artery. A Doppler ultrasound may be employed to ensure proper identification of the pedicle artery, though it is rarely necessary.

For cleft, the length of the Abbé flap is designed to approximate the length of the defect and to replace the philthral aesthetic unit with healthy soft tissue.[39] For other defects, the flap height should equal the defect height, while the flap width is typically one-half the defect width. When necessary, a lower lip Abbé flap may be extended to incorporate additional length from the chin to also provide columellar reconstruction. The pedicle is generally found at the level of the vermillion border posterior to the orbicularis oris muscle. Typically, after the flap is outlined centrally in the lower lip, all the layers on one side are divided while on the other, a pedicle with the superior or inferior labial artery is maintained. Flap design is versatile and may be used for either upper or lower lip reconstruction (▶ Fig. 56.7). The flap is rotated with respect to the pedicle and sutured into place with division and inset following a 2- to 3-week period of adequate healing.[39]

In cleft surgery, the Abbé flap is useful in reconstruction of secondary cleft lip deformities such as whistle deformity, lack of a Cupid's bow, columellar shortening, and lack of upper lip bulk and vermillion tubercle.[40,][41] Possible complications of the Abbé flap are limited amount of flap available, scarring, microstomia, poorly aligned vermillion border or dry-wet border, flap loss, wound dehiscence, and oral incompetence.

56.7.4 Pharyngeal Flap

Another frequently used flap in the pediatric population is the pharyngeal flap for the treatment of velopharyngeal dysfunction after prior palatoplasty, in submucous cleft, or after tumor removal. This flap is most often used as a superiorly based flap and incorporates posterior pharyngeal wall mucosa and muscle. The flap width and length will vary based on patient needs. Typically the posterior palate is split and the flap is elevated from distal to proximal off of the prevertebral fascia toward the velum and inset (▶ Fig. 56.8).[42]

Nasopharyngeal stents are placed bilaterally to maintain ports and decrease the risk of total nasopharyngeal stenosis or obstructive sleep apnea. Complications are generally uncommon but may include flap dehiscence, flap contracture resulting in recurrent velopharyngeal dysfunction, snoring, or hemorrhage.

56.8 Temporoparietal Fascia Flap

In the temporal region, the temporoparietal fascia (TPF) is the most superficial fascial layer underneath the subcutaneous fat. The temporoparietal fascial flap (TPFF) is a pliable, well-vascularized regional flap often used in orbitomaxillary and auricular reconstruction.[43–45] The TPF is a lateral extension of the galea of the scalp and is continuous with the SMAS of the face. The predominant vasculature supplying the region is the superficial temporal artery.[46] Especially in the pediatric population, the TPFF has become a workhorse flap for external ear reconstruction, notably, in the treatment of hemifacial microsoma and auricular defects (e.g., microtia). However, it may also be used for posttraumatic defects, scalp

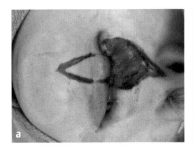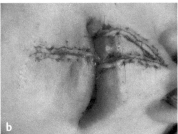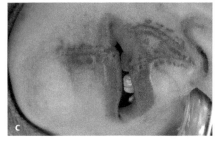

Fig. 56.7 The Abbé–Sabattini flap in an 11-year-old who sustained a dog bite injury to the right upper lip. **(a)** Flap markings for flap from lower lip to upper lip. **(b)** Flap inset. **(c)** At time of division and inset of flap.

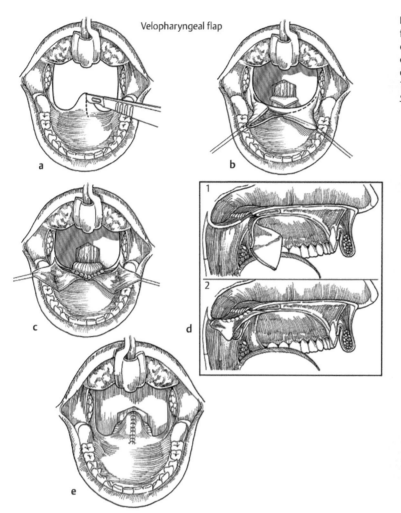

Velopharyngeal flap

Fig. 56.8 (a–e) Superiorly based pharyngeal flap for treatment of velopharyngeal dysfunction. (Reproduced with permission of Setabutr D. Sc. Surgical management of Velopharyngeal Dysfunction; *Operative Techniques in Otolaryngology-Head and Neck Surgery.* 2015;26[1]:33–38.)

reconstruction, and maxillofacial volume augmentation and may be used as an isolated TPFF or a composite flap as needed.

Generally, the superficial temporal vessels are easily identified by palpation and a Doppler is not necessary. The incision design and location will vary based on indication of use and harvesting type (e.g., open vs. endoscopic). An open incision may be made starting in the preauricular sulcus and extending to the superficial temporal line. Sharp dissection in the subcutaneous plane will allow for preservation of the thin TPFF while minimizing injury to the hair follicles. The flap can be extended approximately 3 to 4 cm superior to the superior temporal line if additional length is necessary. Care should be taken with anterior flap elevation not to injure the frontal branch of the facial nerve. Once the TPF is exposed, the flap may be incised anteriorly, posteriorly, and superiorly to leave an inferiorly based flap with a pedicle width of at least 2 cm (▶ Fig. 56.9). The flap is typically tunneled to the recipient site and therefore does not require a second stage for division and inset.

The TPFF is a versatile flap primarily due to its thinness, rich vascularity, and extensive reach. It is ideal for smaller orbitomaxillary and auricular defects and leaves inconspicuous donor scars. It not only has the advantage of proximity and minimal donor site morbidity but also has a wide arc of rotation, making it a versatile flap in the repair of a multitude of defects. A primary limitation is that it often does not provide the bulk that is required in larger volume defects. Some of the encountered complications more commonly seen with the TPFF are hematoma formation, alopecia, flap failure, and bulk along the pedicle tunnel.

56.9 Pericranial Flap

The pericranium corresponds to the periosteum of the cranium in the forehead and scalp. The pericranial flap serves as a thin, reliable, versatile flap in reconstruction of the head and neck and is associated with minimal donor site morbidity. In children, pericranial flaps may be used for reconstruction in hemicraniofacial microsma, facial fractures, hemifacial atrophy, auricular reconstruction,

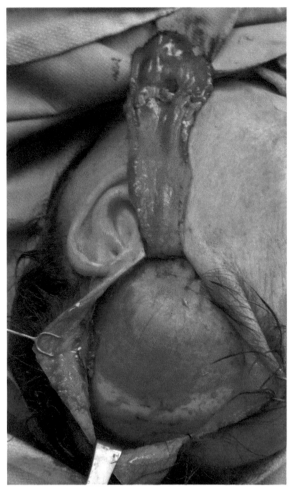

Fig. 56.9 Demonstration of reach and arc of rotation of a temporoparietal flap.

anterior skull base defects, frontal sinus cranialization, nasal defects, and orbital reconstruction.[47–50]

The pericranial flap may be unilateral or bilateral and has a rich vascular supply from the supraorbital and supratrochlear vessels. It may be harvested in an open approach through a coronal incision or a minimally invasive endoscopic approach and tunneled to its recipient site. For the open approach, a coronal incision is made and deepened to a subgaleal plane to expose the pericranium. The frontal flap is elevated from superior temporal line on one side to superior temporal line on the other side and may be elevated inferiorly over the supraorbital rims. If additional length is needed on the flap, the superior skin flap may also be elevated. The lateral and superior incisions are then made and a periosteal elevator is used to elevate the pericranium inferiorly, preserving the supraorbital and supratrochlear vascular supply. The flap may then be rotated into the recipient site.

The success of the pericranial flap is high, although flap failure may occur if injury to the vascular pedicle is encountered during flap elevation or during forehead trauma. Compression of the pedicle may occur as can excess tension. Damage to the frontal branch of the facial nerve indicates an incorrect plane of dissection as does alopecia due to hair follicle injury.

56.10 Submental Island Flap

The submental island flap is a fasciocutaneous entity that is useful in the reconstruction of soft tissue defects of the lower face and intraoral region. It is not commonly used in the pediatric population due to lack of excess submental tissue limiting the size of the skin paddle and visible external scars and contour deformities. It may, however, be useful for smaller anterior intraoral defects. The characteristic perforating artery is the submental artery, a branch of the facial artery along the superior aspect of the submandibular gland, accompanied by drainage via the facial vein.[51]

Following identification of the submental artery (often with the aid of ultrasound), the flap is elevated by making the superior skin incision on the distal part of the flap. During the dissection, muscular attachments of the anterior digastric and mylohyoid muscles are often harvested. When approaching the submandibular gland, it may be ideal to raise a subplatysmal flap to allow for visual inspection and dissection of the facial artery and marginal mandibular branch of the facial nerve. Following the dissection, the submandibular gland may be removed to aid in complete dissection of the submental artery. The unique design of the submental island flap allows for it to achieve good mobility and predictability along with ideal skin color characteristics. Overall, the submental island flap is rarely used in children due to lack of submental tissue excess and the availability of other local and distant flap options that offer improved cosmesis.

56.11 Pectoralis Major Muscle or Myocutaneous Flap

The pectoralis major muscle has bundles that run both horizontally and obliquely across the chest. The primary blood supply to the muscle is through the thoracoacromial artery, a branch of the subclavian artery. In adult head-and-neck reconstruction, the pectoralis major myocutaneous flap (PMMF) is useful in the repair of postoncological defects of the oral cavity, cheek, and neck.[52] It is rarely employed in the pediatric population due to significant donor site morbidity.[53] This flap has largely been replaced by free tissue transfer in children. In fact, it is now considered a salvage mechanism after failure of a free flap and is mostly indicated in those who are considered poor candidates for free flaps or for complex low neck and chest defects.

This flap may be elevated as a muscle only or a myocutaneous flap. The pectoralis major muscle may be approached through an anterior incision in the chest.

After the muscle is visualized, its fascia is incised and its horizontal and oblique fibers are split. Careful consideration must be taken when elevating the flap off the pectoralis minor muscle chest wall to ensure preservation of the neurovascular bundle on the undersurface of the flap. A skin paddle may be included overlying the pectoralis major muscle. Once the flap is elevated, it can be advanced to the head-and-neck region through a subcutaneous tunnel.[52]

The major benefit in implementing the PMMF is its ability to provide a large volume of vascularized tissue with a flap that is quick and simple to raise. It has enough bulk to fill large cavities, augment contour, and provide reasonable support. Due to its axial vessels, it has a robust vascular network and nerve bundle, lessening the risk of flap atrophy and contraction. Risks of the PMMF are adverse scarring and contour, altered nipple position, hematoma, wound infection, altered shoulder function, and wound dehiscence.

56.12 Conclusion

Treatment of pediatric facial defects and deformities is largely accomplished with local tissue rearrangement and flaps when primary closure is not a viable option. These procedures are generally well-tolerated in children and have few adverse effects. Large regional flaps are rarely used due to advances in microvascular free tissue transfer. As in adults, a careful analysis of the defect and planning of flap closure is essential to optimize aesthetic and functional results.

56.13 Highlights

a. Indications
   - Repair of defects when primary closure is not an option.
   - Restore functionality and provide an aesthetic result.
b. Contraindications
   - Not medically cleared for a surgical procedure.
   - Contraindication to local flaps: lack of sufficient local tissue.
c. Complications
   - Skin infection or wound breakdown.
   - Flap loss.
   - Poor cosmesis, hypertrophic scaring, keloid.
   - Additional site specific complications (i.e., microstomia for an oral commissure defect reconstruction or alopecia in scalp reconstruction).
d. Special preoperative considerations
   - General endotracheal anesthesia.
e. Special intraoperative considerations
   - Pre-incision planning and careful measurements.
   - Elevation of flap in the correct plane.
   - Avoidance of tension at closure.

f. Special postoperative considerations
   - Larger flaps may require overnight monitoring.
   - Education on wound care for caretakers.
   - In some children dressings or restraints to avoid would manipulation.

References

[1] Giugliano C, Andrades PR, Benitez S. Nasal reconstruction with a forehead flap in children younger than 10 years of age. Plast Reconstr Surg 2004;114(2):316–325, discussion 326–328

[2] Kung TA, Gosain AK. Pediatric facial burns. J Craniofac Surg 2008;19(4):951–959

[3] Meier JD, Tollefson TT. Pediatric facial trauma. Curr Opin Otolaryngol Head Neck Surg 2008;16(6):555–561

[4] Squaquara R, Kim Evans KF, Spanio di Spilimbergo S, Mardini S. Intraoral reconstruction using local and regional flaps. Semin Plast Surg 2010;24(2):198–211

[5] Boyce DE, Shokrollahi K. Reconstructive surgery. BMJ 2006;332 (7543):710–712

[6] Braun TL, Hamilton KL, Monson LA, Buchanan EP, Hollier LH Jr. Tissue expansion in children. Semin Plast Surg 2016;30(4):155–161

[7] Adler N, Elia J, Billig A, Margulis A. Complications of nonbreast tissue expansion: 9 years experience with 44 adult patients and 119 pediatric patients. J Pediatr Surg 2015;50(9):1513–1516

[8] Baker SR, ed. Local Flaps in Facial Reconstruction. 3rd ed. Philadelphia, PA: Elsevier/Saunders; 2014:71–107

[9] Blackwell KE, Buchbinder D, Biller HF, Urken ML. Reconstruction of massive defects in the head and neck: the role of simultaneous distant and regional flaps. Head Neck 1997;19(7):620–628

[10] Heymans O, Verhelle N. Local and regional flaps. In: Téot L, Banwell PE, Ziegler UE, eds. Surgery in Wounds. Berlin, Heidelberg: Springer; 2004:187–193

[11] Menick FJ. Principles and planning in nasal and facial reconstruction: making a normal face. Plast Reconstr Surg 2016;137 (6):1033e–1047e

[12] Menick FJ. Reconstruction of the cheek. Plast Reconstr Surg 2001;108(2):496–505

[13] Moore BA, Wine T, Netterville JL. Cervicofacial and cervicothoracic rotation flaps in head and neck reconstruction. Head Neck 2005;27(12):1092–1101

[14] Chu EA, Byrne PJ. Local flaps I: bilobed, rhombic, and cervicofacial. Facial Plast Surg Clin North Am 2009;17(3):349–360

[15] Tan ST, MacKinnon CA. Deep plane cervicofacial flap: a useful and versatile technique in head and neck surgery. Head Neck 2006;28(1):46–55

[16] Hoffman JF. Management of scalp defects. Otolaryngol Clin North Am 2001;34(3):571–582

[17] Earnest LM, Byrne PJ. Scalp reconstruction. Facial Plast Surg Clin North Am 2005;13(2):345–353, vii

[18] Kroll SS, Margolis R. Scalp flap rotation with primary donor site closure. Ann Plast Surg 1993;30(5):452–455

[19] Pepper JP, Baker SR. Local flaps: cheek and lip reconstruction. JAMA Facial Plast Surg 2013;15(5):374–382

[20] Starkman SJ, Williams CT, Sherris DA. Flap basics I: rotation and transposition flaps. Facial Plast Surg Clin North Am 2017;25 (3):313–321

[21] Menick FJ. Nasal reconstruction. Plast Reconstr Surg 2010;125 (4):138e–150e

[22] Burget GC. Aesthetic Reconstruction of the Child's Nose. Chicago, IL: Gary Burget; 2012

[23] Burget GC. Preliminary review of pediatric nasal reconstruction with detailed report of one case. Plast Reconstr Surg 2009; 124(3):907–918

[24] Menick FJ. Forehead flap: master techniques in otolaryngology-head and neck surgery. Facial Plast Surg 2014;30(2):131–144

[25] Caspara Uth C, Boljanovic S. Nasal reconstruction in a child after a dog bite: 9 years later. Plast Reconstr Surg Glob Open 2015;3(5):e398

[26] Pittet B, Montandon D. Nasal reconstruction in children: a review of 29 patients. J Craniofac Surg 1998;9(6):522–528

[27] Reckley LK, Peck JJ, Roofe SB. Flap basics III: interpolated flaps. Facial Plast Surg Clin North Am 2017;25(3):337–346

[28] Buchbinder D, St-Hilaire H. Tongue flaps in maxillofacial surgery. Oral Maxillofac Surg Clin North Am 2003;15(4):475–486, v

[29] Jackson IT. Use of tongue flaps to resurface lip defects and close palatal fistulae in children. Plast Reconstr Surg 1972;49(5):537–541

[30] Sohail M, Bashir MM, Khan FA, Ashraf N. Comparison of clinical outcome of facial artery myomucosal flap and tongue flap for closure of large anterior palatal fistulas. J Craniofac Surg 2016;27(6):1465–1468

[31] Lighthall JGSJ. Closure of palatal fistulae. Oper Tech Otolaryngol: Head Neck Surg 2015;26(3):161–167

[32] Deshmukh A, Kannan S, Thakkar P, Chaukar D, Yadav P, D'Cruz A. Tongue flap revisited. J Cancer Res Ther 2013;9(2):215–218

[33] Al-Qattan MM. A modified technique of using the tongue tip for closure of large anterior palatal fistula. Ann Plast Surg 2001;47(4):458–460

[34] Pribaz J, Stephens W, Crespo L, Gifford G. A new intraoral flap: facial artery musculomucosal (FAMM) flap. Plast Reconstr Surg 1992;90(3):421–429

[35] Ferrari S, Ferri A, Bianchi B, Varazzani A, Giovacchini F, Sesenna E. Oncologic safety of facial artery myomucosal flaps in oral cavity reconstruction. Head Neck 2016;38(Suppl 1):E1200–E1202

[36] Rahpeyma A, Khajehahmadi S. Facial artery musculomucosal (FAMM) flap for nasal lining in reconstruction of large full thickness lateral nasal defects. Ann Med Surg (Lond) 2015;4(4):351–354

[37] Shetty R, Lamba S, Gupta AK. Role of facial artery musculomucosal flap in large and recurrent palatal fistulae. Cleft Palate Craniofac J 2013;50(6):730–733

[38] Xie L, Lavigne P, Lavigne F, Ayad T. Modified facial artery musculomucosal flap for reconstruction of posterior skull base defects. J Neurol Surg Rep 2016;77(2):e98–e101

[39] Bagatin M, Most SP. The Abbe flap in secondary cleft lip repair. Arch Facial Plast Surg 2002;4(3):194–197

[40] Koshy JC, Ellsworth WA, Sharabi SE, Hatef DA, Hollier LH Jr, Stal S. Bilateral cleft lip revisions: the Abbe flap. Plast Reconstr Surg 2010;126(1):221–227

[41] Lo LJ, Kane AA, Chen YR. Simultaneous reconstruction of the secondary bilateral cleft lip and nasal deformity: Abbé flap revisited. Plast Reconstr Surg 2003;112(5):1219–1227

[42] Setabutr D. Sc. Surgical management of velopharyngeal dysfunction Oper Tech Otolaryngol: Head Neck Surg 2015;26(1):33–38

[43] Kim JY, Buck DW II, Johnson SA, Butler CE. The temporoparietal fascial flap is an alternative to free flaps for orbitomaxillary reconstruction. Plast Reconstr Surg 2010;126(3):880–888

[44] Reinisch J, Tahiri Y. Polyethylene ear reconstruction: a state-of-the-art surgical journey. Plast Reconstr Surg 2018;141(2):461–470

[45] Brent B, Byrd HS. Secondary ear reconstruction with cartilage grafts covered by axial, random, and free flaps of temporoparietal fascia. Plast Reconstr Surg 1983;72(2):141–152

[46] David SK, Cheney ML. An anatomic study of the temporoparietal fascial flap. Arch Otolaryngol Head Neck Surg 1995;121(10):1153–1156

[47] Bastaninejad S, Karimi E, Saeedi N, Amirizad E. Endoscopic pericranial flap design for the restoration of nasal mid-vault lining defects. Int J Oral Maxillofac Surg 2018;47(7):865–868

[48] Fadle KN, Hassanein AG, Kasim AK. Orbitocranial fibrous dysplasia: outcome of radical resection and immediate reconstruction with titanium mesh and pericranial flap. J Craniofac Surg 2016;27(8):e719–e723

[49] Majer J, Herman P, Verillaud B. "Mailbox Slot" pericranial flap for endoscopic skull base reconstruction. Laryngoscope 2016;126(8):1736–1738

[50] Ravindra VM, Neil JA, Shah LM, Schmidt RH, Bisson EF. Surgical management of traumatic frontal sinus fractures: case series from a single institution and literature review. Surg Neurol Int 2015;6:141

[51] Cheng A, Bui T. Submental island flap. Oral Maxillofac Surg Clin North Am 2014;26(3):371–379

[52] Patel K, Lyu DJ, Kademani D. Pectoralis major myocutaneous flap. Oral Maxillofac Surg Clin North Am 2014;26(3):421–426

[53] Adekeye EO, Lavery KM, Nasser NA. The versatility of pectoralis major and latissimus dorsi myocutaneous flaps in the reconstruction of cancrum oris defects of children and adolescents. J Maxillofac Surg 1986;14(2):99–102

57 Facial Paralysis in the Pediatric Patient

Eyal Gur, Daniel J. Kedar

Summary

The face through facial expressions is the center of our entire emotional life. Facial nerve paralysis is a devastating condition with profound functional, aesthetic and psychological consequences. It's ethnology in the pediatric population derive from both congenital and acquired conditions. Reconstruction of the paralyzed face focuses on restoring both form and function. The surgical plan may vary depending on the severity of the facial paralysis and the timing from which the facial nerve damage was diagnosed to the time of intervention.

In this chapter we describe the common facial reanimation procedures, considerations in choosing the appropriate reconstruction procedure, and the general approach for treatment of facial paralysis.

Keywords: Facial palsy, facial paralysis, facial reanimation, cross face nerve graft, gracillis free flap

57.1 Introduction

Paralysis of the facial mimetic muscles causes loss of voluntary facial movements, loss of involuntary facial expression, and dysfunction in facial tone. It is a devastating condition with a profound functional, aesthetic, and psychological consequences.

Symptoms may include ocular dryness and tearing, speech difficulties, oral incontinence, impairment in mastication, and obstruction of nasal air way. Significant emotional distress is the result of facial disfigurement, impaired communication, and social dysfunction.

Facial paralysis manifests as a spectrum of conditions, presenting as either unilateral or bilateral, and range from partial to complete weakness.

57.2 Etiology and Epidemiology

Etiology is either congenital or acquired. The latter include idiopathic causes, infection, trauma, iatrogenic, and neoplasms.

57.2.1 Congenital Facial Nerve Palsy

This is present at birth. This is the most common form of facial paralysis seen in pediatric setting. It may be isolated with the involvement of the facial nerve and its musculature only, or it may be part of a syndrome. It may be the result of developmental defects or of traumatic etiology.

It is estimated that facial paralysis occurs in 2.0% of live births[1]

Birth weight greater than 3500 grams, forceps-assisted delivery, and prematurity are all risk factors associated with traumatic facial palsy. The presence of multisystem dysmorphia and multiple cranial nerve abnormalities tend to favor developmental abnormalities, although isolated facial palsy can be of developmental origin.[2]

A well-recognized form of congenital facial palsy is Möbius syndrome, which is typically accompanied by impairment of ocular abduction. In addition, two loci for isolated facial palsy of developmental origin have been identified, designated hereditary congenital facial paresis 1 and 2 on chromosomes 3q21–22 and 10q21.3–22.1, respectively.[3-5] Other syndromes are also associated with facial palsies, including hemifacial microsomia (the most common unilateral syndromatic facial palsy), Poland syndrome, osteopetrosis, trisomy 13 and 18.[6]

The difference between developmental and traumatic facial palsies in the perinatal period is that some or complete recovery of function favors traumatic lesions. Early motor nerve conduction study also helps distinguish these etiologies.

57.2.2 Möbius Syndrome

This syndrome, sometimes called Möbius sequence, is a congenital facial palsy (unilateral or bilateral) with abnormalities of abducens nerve (cranial nerve VI) function, though other cranial nerves (III, IV, V, VIII) may be involved.[7,8] Postmortem analysis has shown hypoplasia of the motor nucleus of the facial nerve with small or absent facial nerve rootlets exiting the brainstem.[9] Möbius syndrome is also associated with trunk and limb anomalies in about one-third of patients. The incidence of Möbius syndrome is estimated to be about 1 in 200,000 live births. A genetic cause has not yet been identified,[10] but linkage points to a distinct locus at 13q12.2–13.[11] There is some overlap with the hereditary congenital facial paresis syndromes.

57.2.3 Acquired Facial Nerve Palsy

Approximately one-half of all acquired cases qualify for the label "Bell's palsy," previously defined as an acute facial nerve palsy of unknown cause.

The diagnosis of idiopathic (Bell's) facial nerve palsy is based upon the following criteria:

- A diffuse involvement of all of the distal branches of the facial nerve is present.
- Onset is acute, over a day or two; the course is progressive, reaching maximal clinical weakness/paralysis within 3 weeks or less from the first day of visible

weakness; recovery of some degree of function usually occurs within 6 months.

- Associated prodrome, ear pain, or dysacusis may be reported.

The most common identified cause of acute onset facial nerve palsy in children has in the past been acute otitis media. However, Lyme disease may be a more common cause in endemic areas than otitis media.[12]

Patients with Lyme disease and facial nerve palsy may have other clinical features of Lyme disease, but many have no other symptoms, nor a history of tick bite or erythema migrans.[13] Painless, nontender swelling and erythema of the face preceding the facial palsy are distinctive features that may be present and help confirm the clinical diagnosis.[14] The likelihood that Lyme disease is the cause of a seventh nerve palsy diminishes in either nonendemic areas or at a time of year when Lyme disease is not prevalent. In pediatric patients with low immunization rates and acute facial paralysis, varicella-zoster virus reactivation has been identified in up to 37 percent of cases.[15] Most such cases are characterized by the absence of rash (i.e., zoster sine herpete) while a few are notable for the presence of typical zoster lesions in the auditory canal and auricle, termed the Ramsay Hunt syndrome. HIV infection rarely causes facial palsy. If it does, onset is at the time of seroconversion, when a CSF lymphocytosis usually is present.[16]

Several other disorders should be considered in the differential diagnosis of facial nerve palsy. Cholesteatoma should be suspected if the onset of facial palsy is gradual.[17] The Melkersson–Rosenthal syndrome is characterized by facial paralysis, episodic facial swelling, and a fissured tongue, typically beginning in adolescence but with recurrent episodes of facial palsy.[18] Sarcoidosis should be considered, especially in patients with bilateral facial palsy. Severe systemic hypertension has been linked to unilateral primary facial nerve palsy in children and adolescents and rarely in adults.[19] Hypertension should be suspected in a pediatric patient, if facial palsy is associated with headache, altered level of consciousness, vomiting, convulsions, or focal central nervous system deficit.

Other acquired causes for facial paralysis are temporal bone trauma and cranial neoplasm (whether from the primary tumor or due to iatrogenic cause following treatment).

57.3 Prognosis

Congenital facial palsies, including Möbius syndrome, have a poor prognosis for recovery of function because of insufficient development of the facial nerve, or canal.

Traumatic facial paralysis in the perinatal period has an excellent prognosis, with 100 percent of patients showing some degree of improvement of function on the affected side.

Most children with Bell's palsy recover with minimal, if any, dysfunction.[20] The prognosis of Bell's palsy is favorable if some recovery is seen within the first 21 days of onset.[21] A diagnosis of Bell's palsy is doubtful if some facial function, however small, has not returned within 3 to 4 months, and additional evaluation to determine the etiology is warranted.[22]

57.4 Treatment

The treatment of facial nerve palsy in children is guided by the etiology and the severity of the condition. In the case of idiopathic acquired facial palsy, treatment options include glucocorticoids with or without antivirals (e.g., Acyclovir or Valacyclovir). The treatment of facial nerve palsy due to a specific cause involves treatment of the underlying disorder.

Treatment options for congenital or permanently acquired lesions include surgical interventions for facial reanimation.

57.5 Surgery

Reanimation of the paralyzed face focuses on restoration of form and function. Goals are to achieve protection of the eye, facial symmetry at rest, voluntary symmetric facial movement and to restore involuntary mimetic facial expression.[23]

The most significant unit for reconstruction, from a functional and aesthetic perspective, is the buccal-zygomatic muscle complex (BZMC), which is responsible for smiling and for the tone of the cheeks. This complex includes the risorius, the zygomaticus major and minor, and the levator anguli oris muscles, and is normally innervated by tributaries of the zygomatic and buccal branches of the facial nerve. Significant functional problems are associated with paralysis of the oral musculature, including drooling and speech difficulties. Flaccid lip and cheek can lead to difficulties with chewing food, cheek biting, and pocketing food in the buccal sulcus. However, the main emphasis of surgery is usually centered on reconstruction of a smile.

Three elements are required for the formation of a smile: neural input, a functioning muscle innervated by the nerve, and a proper muscle orientation. All three factors contribute to the decision as to which reconstruction will be performed.

The timing from which the facial nerve damage is diagnosed to the time of intervention is a key factor for the choice of reconstruction.

In an acute facial nerve damage, primary repair or cable nerve grafting must be considered. In recent paralysis (in which the mimetic musculature may be reactivated by provision of neural input), a nerve graft is used to relay facial input. A long standing paralysis necessitates both new nerve input and muscle transfer.

57.6 Primary Repair

57.6.1 Indications

Acute traumatic/iatrogenic facial paralysis should be reconstructed within 72 hours from injury onset, if proximal and distal facial nerve stumps are present on the paralyzed side.

In an acute facial nerve damage such as in trauma or operation, immediate primary repair must be considered within 72 hours. For acute traumatic injuries primary repair of the nerve, direct or using nerve grafts, renders the best outcome.[24]

The advantages of acute repair include the ability to perform intraoperative nerve stimulation (which aids in locating the nerve stumps), to optimize motor nerve recovery, and to adequately gain exposure and mobilize nerve ends without the interference of scar tissue.

Nerve ends have been reported to still contain neurotransmitters within 72 hours of injury, and from a histopathologic standpoint, nerve ends have symmetrically apposed fascicles immediately after transection but then become increasingly difficult to match, as Schwann cell proliferation, fibrosis, and angiogenesis occur at each end.[25]

In cases of immediate injury due to penetrating trauma, surgical exploration should be undertaken. The wound should be copiously irrigated and appropriate antibiotics should be administered.

57.6.2 Technique

An operative microscope is usually used for all nerve repair cases as it aids in accurate placement of epineural sutures and minimize damage to nerve tissue.

The proximal and distal portions of the nerve must be identified. The use of an electric nerve stimulator can be useful in identification of distal branches. The nerve ends must be neurolyzed from the surrounding scar tissue bed. During this step, it is critical to avoid physical damage (i.e., crushing or tearing) to the nerve ends.

Adequate exposure also entails injured nerve end resection in order to find healthy nerve tissue and facilitate fascicle apposition. Given the healing process initiated at the nerve ends after traumatic injury, more end resection is required as the time from injury increases. In cases whereby there is uncertainty of the viability of the nerve, an intraoperative histology is used.

Repair must be achieved with minimal tension. Even in the setting of a fresh nerve laceration, some tension exists because of the elastic nature of nerves. A failure to hold an end-to-end repair with a single 9–0 suture is a sign of undue tension.[26] As tension on the neurorrhaphy seems to diminish perfusion and neural regeneration, if there is insufficient length of nerve for primary repair, an interpositional graft from the great auricular nerve,

sural nerve, or other suitable donor nerve should be performed.

A few epineural sutures are placed, the preferred suture material being nylon with caliber typically 9–0 or 10–0. The repair should be on the looser rather than the tighter side. The most destructive error is a repair that is too tight, whereby opposing fascicles are forced to pass each other. Repairing the back wall first in a slightly loose fashion is helpful to initially align the nerve ends and to keep the back wall fascicles contained. Repairing the remainder of the nerve so that the fascicles *barely* touch is the goal. At the end of the repair, there should be no deformity to the nerve. At the repair site, the edges of the nerve should be flushed without any kinks. No fascicles should be escaping the repair site. If minimal, this situation can be salvaged by a minimal trimming of escaping fascicles. Otherwise, the repair should be repeated but in a looser fashion.

Coaptation of the nerve at a site more proximal than the stylomastoid foramen should be avoided, when possible, as the arrangement of nerve fibers in this region is less organized in terms of geographical distribution to the face; thus, wrong re-routing can lead to greater synkinesia.

57.7 Nerve Grafting: Ipsilateral and Cross-Facial

See ▶ Fig. 57.1.

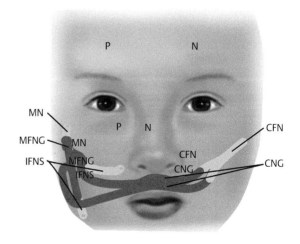

Fig. 57.1 The "babysitter" procedure: two cross-face cable grafts together with cable graft from motor master nerve to facial nerve. CFN, contralateral facial nerve; CNG, cross-face nerve graft; IFNS, ipsilateral facial nerve stumps; MFNG, masseter-to-facial nerve grafts; N, normal; NM, nerve to masseter; P, paralyzed.

57.7.1 Indications

Recent facial paralysis reconstruction should be managed not later than a year after injury onset.

Recent Paralysis is defined for a paralysis in which the mimetic musculature may be reactivated by provision of neural input, and the time limit is generally 18 to 24 months.

Preoperative EMG may help to rule out early irreversible atrophy, which seldom develops earlier than 12 months after the onset of palsy, particularly in cases of recurrent facial palsy, palsy caused by radiotherapy, and Ramsay–Hunt syndrome. Patients with recent paralyses have fibrillations of the mimetic musculature, and if these fibrillations cannot be recorded, the paralysis must be considered long-standing.

By reactivation of the mimetic musculature of the face, the muscle tone can be preserved. The patient will gain better facial symmetry by preventing the dogmatic facial sagging of the affected side, better eye closure (with innervation of the orbicularis occuli) and better oral continence (with innervation of the orbicularis oris).

In the past, if a functional facial nerve branch was available only on the contralateral face, a cross-face nerve graft was used to relay facial nerve input across the face to the BZMC.

Axons from the contralateral facial nerve regenerate through the sheath of the graft and innervate the muscle over 4 to 6 months.[27–29]

Because muscle atrophy could develop while the facial nerve regenerates, an ipsilateral motor nerve (nerve to the masseter muscle) was transposed and connected to the facial nerve to serve as a temporary innervator ("babysitter") to the muscle. In that way muscle tone was preserved while waiting for the cross-face grafts to grow across, and eventually spontaneous smiling would be restored.[23,30] Yet from the author's experience, this type of reanimation by itself will usually result in a strong, unsightly, mass action created by the masseter-to-facial nerve anastomosis but a weak muscle contraction coming from the cross-face grafting, so even with the preservation of muscle tone and the added compliance of the orbicularis oris and occuli, a poor, nonspontaneous, and unsightly smile will result.

Since we have noticed that a cross-face nerve graft did not deliver a strong smile in the last-described situation, it is now the author's choice, even in recent paralysis, to use masseter-to-facial anastomosis, which will be responsible for the eye and mouth tone, together with a cross-face nerve graft followed by a second-stage free gracilis muscle transfer that will be responsible for the spontaneity of the smile.

In this approach, in the first stage the distal stump of the facial nerve at the affected side is re-innervated. This innervation can be either based on an ipsilateral facial nerve if present (in cases where the nerve was cut or partially dissected) or by a cross-cranial nerve re-innervation (mostly facial-to-masseter nerve) as a permanent innervation.

At the same surgery, a cross-face nerve graft is coapted to the lower trunks of the normal contralateral facial nerve, and then tunneled across the face through the upper lip and banked for the second stage.

Within 2 to 3 months, the paralyzed facial muscles will regain tone and then will begin to function in a mass pattern motion.

At a second stage (9 months later), a free muscle is transferred and the cross-face nerve graft is used to innervate the free muscle. Within 3 to 6 months, spontaneous facial motion is initiated by the contralateral facial nerve that should take control of the transferred muscle.

In cases where the masseter nerve was used to innervate the mimetic muscles, if the masseter nerve action is still noticeable at the BZMC and unsightly, the facial nerve branches to the BZMC can be transected at a later procedure so that the smile will be solely produced by the transferred muscle.

57.7.2 Technique

Sural nerve harvest (▶ Fig. 57.2): The sural nerve comes out from the tibial nerve at the popliteal region, from there it moves deep in between the two heads of the gastrocnemius muscle, emerges superficially along their course to the heal, and is directed subcutaneously to the posterior aspect of the lateral malleolus. Around the malleolus, it splits into several small branches that give sensation to the lateral aspect of the foot up to two-thirds the distance to the toes.

Dissection starts with a 1.5 horizontal or longitudinal incision about 3 cm from the popliteal fossa. The nerve is detected usually with the lesser saphenous vein escorting it along its course. The nerve is transected proximally and a dull edge vein stripper is introduced, which bluntly dissects the nerve to a branching point where another skin opening is taken. The process is repeated until adequate nerve length is achieved (usually 11–14 cm). The other

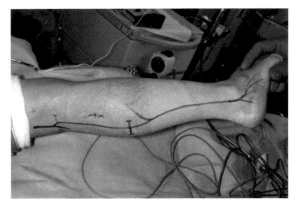

Fig. 57.2 Surface landmarks for sural nerve harvest.

option, the nerve can be dissected from distal to proximal by identifying it 1.5 cm lateral and proximal to the lateral malleolus. From there, dissection moves cephalically using the same vein stripper. The drawback of the last-described option is that there is a higher chance for loss of the lateral foot sensation.

Cross-face nerve graft: On the nonaffected side, through a modified face lift incision extending slightly to the neck, superficial dissection of the superficial muscular aponeurotic system (SMAS) is taken until the anterior border of the parotid gland is reached. At that point, the dissection goes deeper to the thin fascia that covers the masseter muscle. Facial nerve branches run just under that transparent fascia. Dissection of facial nerve branches at that level is limited to the space between the lower border of the zygoma and the Stenson duct because all nerve branches that reach the zygomatic muscle complex and are responsible for the smile will be located at that tiny zone.

Using a nerve stimulator, usually two relatively large facial nerve branches responsible for the motion of the BZMC are identified (▶ Fig. 57.3). The one with less intense stimulus on the BZMC and, even more important, less effect on the orbicularis oculi is sacrificed and serves as the donor motor nerve branch for the cross-face graft. In some cases, if there is an aim to reanimate the orbicularis occuli muscle as well, with an independent action from the BZMC, a second nerve graft is transferred from an ocular branch on the nonaffected side to the affected side.

The sural nerve graft is then tunneled in a subcutaneous level across the cheek and the upper lip to the

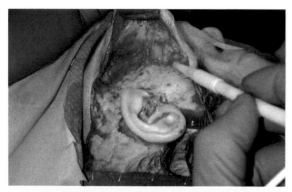

Fig. 57.3 Mapping and identification of the normal contralateral facial nerve branch to be sacrificed.

contralateral upper buccal sulcus right above the first molar tooth (▶ Fig. 57.4a, b). Through a buccal sulcus incision, it is verified that the nerve graft reached its place. If banked, the nerve is marked with a 3–0 blue nylon suture and sometimes using a small piece of colored vessel loop, to help with identifying that nerve end during the second-stage procedure. If a babysitter procedure is intended, the sural nerve is anastomosed to the facial nerve branch in an interfascicular fashion and the facial incisions are closed over a Penrose drain.

Masseter (branch of trigeminal-fifth cranial nerve) innervation procedure: The following description applies for both masseter-to-facial nerve anastomosis and masseter-to-gracilis muscle nerve anastomosis.

The masseter nerve dissection area is outlined by the anterior border of the parotid gland, posterior border of the masseter muscle, zygomatic arch cranially, and parotid duct inferiorly. Dissection starts using an L-shaped incision at the SMAS in an imaginary junction between the lower border of the zygoma and the ramus of the mandible; the masseteric branch of the trigeminal nerve is exposed with blunt dissection, usually close to the deep surface of the muscle. The nerve is then sectioned as distally as possible to facilitate approximation of its stump to the facial nerve or gracilis nerve branches (depending on the procedure) located more superficially. If a masseter nerve to facial nerve is performed, the facial nerve branches are sectioned as close as possible to the stump of the masseter nerve. In a case where there is a gap, a short nerve cable graft is used (either from the sural nerve or the great auricular nerve).[23,28,31] Masseter nerve is coapted to the distal facial nerve stump or stumps using the microscope and interrupted epineural sutures of 10–0 nylon.

In case of a cross-face facial reanimation without the intention to use a free muscle transfer, when the cable graft is coapted at the same procedure (as a true babysitter one-stage procedure), the coaptation of the cross-facial nerve is done distally to the masseter-facial nerve repair, to a nerve branch responsible for the motion of the BZMC.

57.8 Innervated Free Flaps

See ▶ Fig. 57.5.

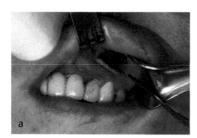
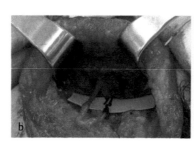

Fig. 57.4 (a, b) Anastomosing and tunneling of the sural nerve graft to the paralyzed side upper buccal sulcus.

57.8.1 Indications

- Long-standing facial paralysis can be reconstructed at any time using the staged cross-face nerve graft and free gracilis muscle transfer for patients younger than 60 years.
- Long-standing facial paralysis can be reconstructed at any time using free gracilis transfer connected to the masseter motor nerve for patients older than 60 years or for bilateral facial paralysis (including Möbius syndrome) patients.
- Long-standing incomplete facial paralysis can be reconstructed at any time using the free gracilis transfer connected to a viable ipsilateral facial nerve stump (if present) at any age.
- In cases where a distal segment of the facial nerve was sacrificed for oncologic purposes, a free gracilis transfer is needed for the reconstruction.
- For the most optimal results concerning a smile, even in recent facial paralysis, a muscle transfer procedure is indicated.
- Patients with partial facial weakness, where there is a good neural input yet weak muscle contraction and a week smile due to muscle atrophy, can benefit from a free muscle transfer to an ipsilateral facial branch.

Facial nerve–based reanimation for long-lasting paralysis (in which sufficient time has passed since onset of the facial nerve injury that the facial muscle motor end plates have undergone fibrosis) necessitates both re-innervation and a free muscle transfer.

In the author's point of view, so do recent facial paralysis patients that seek the most optimal result surgically possible.

Various muscles are available for muscle transfer. However, the gracilis muscle is the preferred of all. The neuromuscular pedicle is reliable and relatively easy to dissect and prepare. A segment of the muscle can be tailored to any desired size (width and length) and also split into several segments, based on the neurovascular pedicle anatomy. These characteristics make the flap customizable to the patient's facial proportions and needs. There is no functional loss in the thigh adduction and the scar is reasonably well hidden.[32]

When an ipsilateral nerve is available, a one-stage free gracilis muscle flap transfer is performed (▶Fig. 57.6). The flap is inset subcutaneously in the paralyzed cheek from the modiolus to the temporal fascia above the auricle. The blood vessels of the flap are anastomosed to facial or superficial temporal vessels and its motor nerve is sutured to the residual ipsilateral facial nerve zygomatic branch that creates a smile.

When an ipsilateral nerve is unavailable, a two-stage procedure is used, with the first being a cross-face sural nerve graft and the second a free gracilis muscle transfer connected to the previously transferred cross-face sural nerve graft.

In the first stage, the nerve graft is harvested, coapted to a contralateral facial branch responsible for a smiling stimulus (with as little blink action as possible), tunneled across the face, through the upper lip to the paralyzed side, and banked in the upper buccal sulcus, above the first upper molar tooth on the paralyzed side. In the second stage (which is scheduled around 9 months later), the free gracilis muscle flap is harvested and transferred to the paralyzed cheek and its motor nerve is sutured to the cable graft that was previously banked. Reanimation

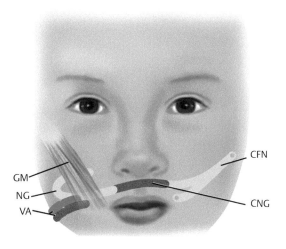

Fig. 57.5 Two-stage cross-face nerve graft and free gracilis muscle transfer shown at the end of the process. CFN, contralateral facial nerve; CNG, cross-face nerve graft; GM, gracilis muscle; N, normal; NG, nerve of gracilis (part of obturator nerve); P, paralyzed; VA, venous and arterial anastomoses.

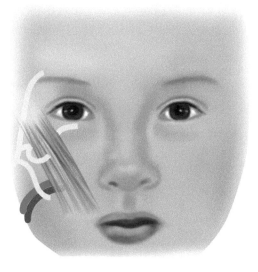

Fig. 57.6 One-stage free gracilis muscle transfer to ipsilateral facial nerve stump.

of the muscle commences after 4 to 8 months and reaches full capacity within a year.[27,28]

When facial nerves are absent on both sides or the patient is over 60 years of age and nerve growth is slow and weak, a nonfacial nerve–based reanimation procedure is performed and is usually based on the ipsilateral motor nerve to the masseter that is connected to a free muscle transfer. Thus, the stimulus to create a smile movement will depend on a voluntary action such as teeth clenching or chewing. These unsightly synkinetic actions of chewing and smiling simultaneously may become more natural over time. In this procedure there is hardly any donor nerve morbidity, unless the temporalis muscle is not functioning on the operated side, thus leaving the mandible with no functioning muscles. It is important to mention that a hypoglossal or accessory nerve can be used as well but have greater morbidity and give inferior aesthetic and functional results.

Patients who are unsuitable or do not wish to undergo a microsurgical procedure to achieve facial dynamic reconstruction may be reconstructed by the transfer of a local muscle flap, namely the temporalis or masseter muscle.[33] The temporalis muscle procedure usually achieves fare static and dynamic results. However, it does not provide a spontaneous smile.

57.8.2 Technique

The sural nerve harvest and the cross-face nerve grafting techniques are described earlier in this chapter.

57.8.3 Second-Stage Free Gracilis Transfer

Surface landmarks for gracilis muscle harvest (▶Fig. 57.7): A line is drawn in the medial side of the thigh, from the pubic tubercle to the medial condyle of the femur. The gracilis muscle lies 2 cm posteriorly to that line. The neurovascular pedicle should be found about 8 cm from the tubercle.

An 8- to 10-cm incision is performed on the assumed location of the muscle. After the superficial and deep fascias of the thigh are incised longitudinally, the muscle should be present right under, with several perforating vessels coming from its surface to the skin (▶Fig. 57.8). The muscle is dissected lengthwise and the fascia between the gracilis and the adductor longus is incised.

Right behind that fascia, the neurovascular pedicle is identified and serves to identify and verify the gracilis muscle. At that stage, the nerve is dissected to its origin from the obturator foramen and then transected to give the longest nerve pedicle as possible. The gracilis vascular pedicle is then dissected between the adductor longus and the adductor magnus up to its origin to the profunda femoris vessels (▶Fig. 57.9). The gracilis muscle is further dissected and freed 360°. The muscle is then tailored by splitting it longitudinally to fit the narrow space of the cheek (▶Fig. 57.10). The muscle strip that is harvested may occasionally weigh no more than 10 g. The length of the needed muscle unit is measured in the cheek from the oral modiolus to the superficial temporal fascia superior to the auricular helix takeoff and marked in the thigh when the knee is stretched. The knee is then flexed. And the muscle is transected caudally and cephalically.

Along the transected muscle edge to be sutured to the modiolus, five 4–0 vicryl sutures are aligned to create a

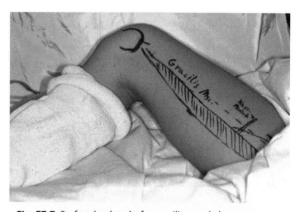

Fig. 57.7 Surface landmarks for gracilis muscle harvest.

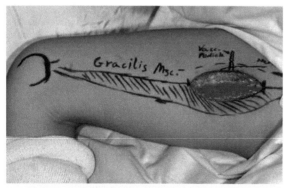

Fig. 57.8 Identification of the gracilis muscle in the thigh.

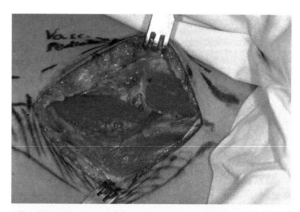

Fig. 57.9 Dissection of the neurovascular pedicle.

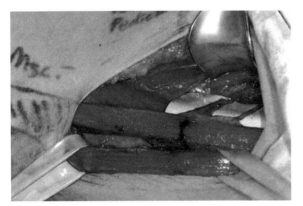

Fig. 57.10 Tailoring of the gracilis muscle.

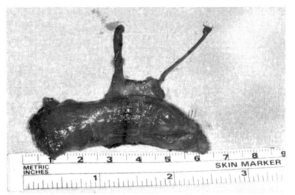

Fig. 57.11 Flap vessels are transected following placement of blocking stitches along muscle edge.

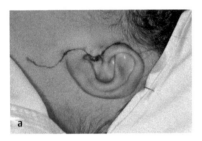

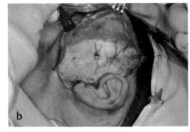

Fig. 57.12 Dissection of recipient paralyzed cheek. **(a)** Incision landmarks; **(b)** subcutaneous flap dissection; **(c)** resection of fat pad; **(d)** facial vessels dissected.

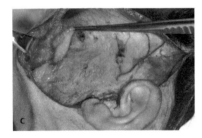

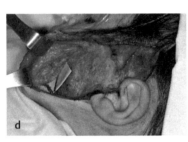

blocking point to the main stitches that will later connect the muscle to the modiolus.

Only when the cheek recipient vessels are fully dissected and flow verified, the gracilis vessels are transected (▶ Fig. 57.11).

On the affected side of the face, a modified face lift incision is marked with an upward extension of 5 cm superior to the helix takeoff and a short 2-cm curved neck extension about 1 cm caudal to the mandible angle (▶ Fig. 57.12a). The incision line is infiltrated with lidocaine 2%–adrenalin 1:100,000 solution.

Subcutaneous dissection is carried out, leaving thin fatty layer under the skin flap (▶ Fig. 57.12b). The dissection area covers a fan-shaped space from the full length of the skin incision to the modiolus and 1.5 cm along the upper and lower lips. It is important to notice the facial/angular artery near the oral commissure as a landmark for the appropriateness of the level of dissection.

At that stage, the facial artery and vein are dissected at their cross-over point with the mandible, where the artery will usually go anteriorly toward the commissure

and the vein cephalically toward the anterior border of the masseter muscle. By compressing the cheek bulk from the inside, the buccal fat pad is identified, dissected, and resected to free space for the gracilis (▶ Fig. 57.12c, d).

Four 0 white vicryl sutures are looped through the remnants and fibrotic layer of the orbicularis oris: one at the modiolus, two (0.5 cm apart) at the upper lip, and one at the lower lip. Careful placement of those stitches will determine the right natural pull of the mouth at motion and the accurate creation of the nasolabial fold (▶ Fig. 57.13).

The intraoral upper buccal sulcus old scar from the cross-face procedure is reincised carefully, revealing the marking stitch and the nerve ending of the cross-face nerve graft (▶ Fig. 57.14a, b). The very end of the cross-face graft is transected and sent for frozen section identification of viable peripheral nerve axons. A tunnel is created between the facial and the intraoral dissections and a vessel loop is transferred from one space to the other.

The gracilis muscle after being detached from the thigh is transferred to the face. The 0 vicryl sutures are looped twice through it and through the old orbicularis to serve as a pulley that will help in mobilizing the

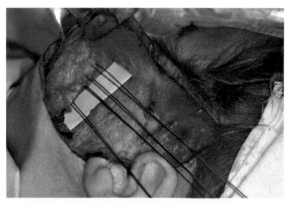

Fig. 57.13 Placement of anchoring vicryl sutures at the modiolus.

flap to the modiolus and for securing it properly into place.

Only after arterial and venous anastomosis in the face and neural anastomosis in the buccal sulcus, the muscle is stretched to reach its origin in the temporal region above the auricle (▶Fig. 57.15 and ▶Fig. 57.16). It is secured by four to five, 0 vicryl sutures that are placed by pulling the muscle and fixating the muscle at the point where the lip or modiolus move just slightly with the muscle pull. At the end of that part the oral commissure should be slightly pulled obliquely and upwards, exposing the lateral upper teeth (▶Fig. 57.17a, b).

At the end of the procedure, a Penrose drain is left in the operated cheek and a vacuum drain in the donor site in the thigh (▶Fig. 57.18).

The skin is closed meticulously and a protecting sticker and a hook-splint are sutured to the patient's scalp and its hook

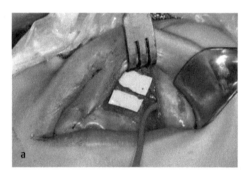
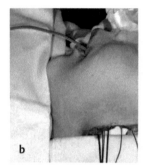

Fig. 57.14 (a, b) Dissection of the cross-face nerve graft.

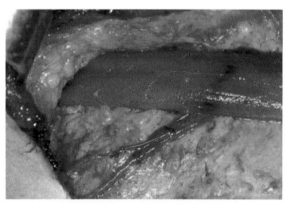

Fig. 57.15 Vessels and nerve anastomosis.

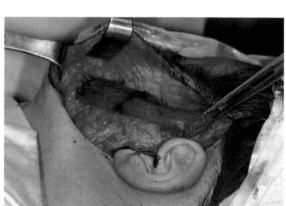

Fig. 57.16 Positioning and tension measurement of the gracilis muscle.

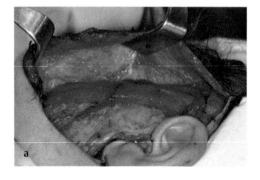
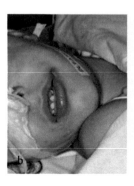

Fig. 57.17 (a, b) Muscle flap secured with correct tension.

is inserted to the oral commissure to protect the cheek from extra external pressure. See (▶Fig. 57.19 and ▶Fig. 57.20) for pre- and postoperative photos of the patients.

57.8.4 One-Stage Free Gracilis to Masseter Facial Reanimation

In cases such as Möbius syndrome, since most of the patients have a bilateral weakness, the contralateral facial nerve is not a viable option. In these cases, a one-stage procedure is performed.

The ipsilateral masseter nerve is exposed as mentioned above in cross cranial nerve innervation procedure, while

the gracilis flap is harvested from the contralateral side. Later the gracilis free flap transfer is performed as mentioned above with coaptation of the obturator nerve to the masseter nerve.

57.9 Conclusion

Even though it remains impossible to correct long-standing facial paralysis completely, facial nerve paralysis surgery presents with a very high success rate.

Most operated patients even with a near-normal or even weak smiles results are relatively satisfied only from the subtle presence of slight motion in their paralyzed faces.[34]

Immediate facial nerve neurorrhaphy yields the best reanimation results. Re-innervation of the mimetic muscles at the affected side either with an ipsilateral facial nerve stump or a cross cranial nerve innervation with a simultaneous cross-face nerve graft followed by a free muscle transfer is the gold standard for treatment of recent paralysis. Re-innervation of the BZMC should not be attempted beyond 12 months of paralysis without muscle transfer. Re-innervation based on facial nerve should be aspired for, even at the cost of conducting a cross-face procedure and the two-stage cross-face nerve graft and gracilis muscle transfer. This procedure is a validated reliable procedure and plays pivotal role in dynamic reanimation for facial paralysis.

57.10 Highlights

a. Contraindications
   - Current oncologic disease.
   - Medical status not permitting long anesthesia.
   - Major depression.
   - Unrealistic expectations.

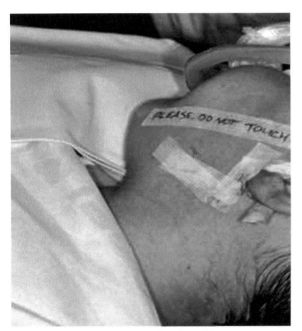

Fig. 57.18 A Penrose drain is left in the operated cheek.

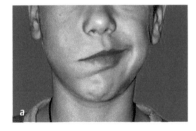
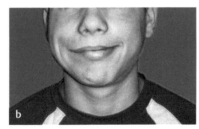

Fig. 57.19 (a, b) Patient 1—congenital right complete facial paralysis treated with a two stage procedure: first a cross face nerve graft, then gracilis muscle transfer.

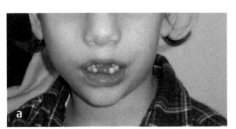
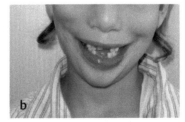
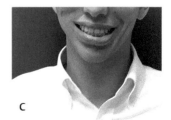

Fig. 57.20 (a) Bilateral mobius syndrome, treated first for the left side with gracillis transfer to masseter nerve, then to the right side three months later. **(b)** One year following the two procedures. **(c)** 10 years follow-up.

b. Complications
   - Injury to functioning facial nerve.
   - Recipient or donor site wound infection.
   - Recipient or donor site hematoma.
   - Failure to achieve facial motion or symmetry.
   - Facial bulge over gracilis muscle.
   - Inadequate motion or spastic transplanted muscle.
c. Special preoperative considerations
   - Assess whether there is a viable facial nerve stump on the paralyzed side.
   - If there is no viable ipsilateral facial nerve, assess whether there is a functioning facial nerve on the contralateral side.
   - Assess whether there are viable facial muscles on the paralyzed side.
   - Choose the appropriate surgical approach for patients over 60 years.
   - Assure that the patient understands the nature of those long procedures and the long time lag until the final result shows. Assure reasonable expectations of the final results.
d. Special intraoperative considerations
   - At first stage cross-face nerve graft, pick a reasonably large nerve branch, but assure it does have a stronger nerve that does the same action.
   - Assure that the selected normal branch to be sacrificed does not play a major role in orbicularis oculi action.
   - Bank the cross-face nerve stump in a constant location and mark it with a thick (3–0) nylon suture for the ease of retrieving it at the second stage.
   - At the second stage, treat the muscle gently and preserve its epimysium. Tailor the muscle to be transferred, to make it as thin, gentle, and long as possible and needed, while not compromising the neurovascular pedicle that penetrates it.
   - Place the muscle obliquely from the modiolus to the fascia superior to the auricle.
e. Special postoperative considerations
   - Immediate extubation.
   - Admit the patient to a step-down unit for 24 hours after surgery.
   - Protect the operated cheek by proper signaling and the designated splint.
   - When motion starts, several months after the procedure, the patient should practice daily, in front of a mirror, to strengthen the muscle action and create more symmetry with the healthy side smile.

References

[1] Falco NA, Eriksson E. Facial nerve palsy in the newborn: incidence and outcome. Plast Reconstr Surg 1990;85(1):1–4

[2] Thomas JG. Facial nerve palsy in children. In: Post TW, ed. UpToDate. Waltham, MA: Up-ToDate Inc. http://www.uptodate.com. Accessed October 7, 2017

[3] Kremer H, Kuyt LP, van den Helm B, et al. Localization of a gene for Möbius syndrome to chromosome 3q by linkage analysis in a Dutch family. Hum Mol Genet 1996;5(9):1367–1371

[4] Verzijl HT, van der Zwaag B, Lammens M, ten Donkelaar HJ, Padberg GW. The neuropathology of hereditary congenital facial palsy vs Möbius syndrome. Neurology 2005;64(4):649–653

[5] Verzijl HT, van den Helm B, Veldman B, et al. A second gene for autosomal dominant Möbius syndrome is localized to chromosome 10q, in a Dutch family. Am J Hum Genet 1999;65(3):752–756

[6] Jankauskienė A, Azukaitis K. Congenital unilateral facial nerve palsy as an unusual presentation of BOR syndrome. Eur J Pediatr 2013;172(2):273–275

[7] Verzijl HT, van der Zwaag B, Cruysberg JR, Padberg GW. Möbius syndrome redefined: a syndrome of rhombencephalic maldevelopment. Neurology 2003;61(3):327–333

[8] Cattaneo L, Chierici E, Bianchi B, Sesenna E, Pavesi G. The localization of facial motor impairment in sporadic Möbius syndrome. Neurology 2006;66(12):1907–1912

[9] Hanissian AS, Fuste F, Hayes WT, Duncan JM. Möbius syndrome in twins. Am J Dis Child 1970;120(5):472–475

[10] MacKinnon S, Oystreck DT, Andrews C, Chan WM, Hunter DG, Engle EC. Diagnostic distinctions and genetic analysis of patients diagnosed with moebius syndrome. Ophthalmology 2014;121(7):1461–1468

[11] Slee JJ, Smart RD, Viljoen DL. Deletion of chromosome 13 in Moebius syndrome. J Med Genet 1991;28(6):413–414

[12] Cook SP, Macartney KK, Rose CD, Hunt PG, Eppes SC, Reilly JS. Lyme disease and seventh nerve paralysis in children. Am J Otolaryngol 1997;18(5):320–323

[13] Smouha EE, Coyle PK, Shukri S. Facial nerve palsy in Lyme disease: evaluation of clinical diagnostic criteria. Am J Otol 1997;18(2):257–261

[14] Markby DP. Lyme disease facial palsy: differentiation from Bell's palsy. BMJ 1989;299(6699):605–606

[15] Furuta Y, Ohtani F, Aizawa H, Fukuda S, Kawabata H, Bergström T. Varicella-zoster virus reactivation is an important cause of acute peripheral facial paralysis in children. Pediatr Infect Dis J 2005;24(2):97–101

[16] Murr AH, Benecke JE Jr. Association of facial paralysis with HIV positivity. Am J Otol 1991;12(6):450–451

[17] Jackson CG, von Doersten PG. The facial nerve: current trends in diagnosis, treatment, and rehabilitation. Med Clin North Am 1999;83(1):179–195, x

[18] Levenson MJ, Ingerman M, Grimes C, Anand KV. Melkersson-Rosenthal syndrome. Arch Otolaryngol 1984;110(8):540–542

[19] Jörg R, Milani GP, Simonetti GD, Bianchetti MG, Simonetti BG. Peripheral facial nerve palsy in severe systemic hypertension: a systematic review. Am J Hypertens 2013;26(3):351–356

[20] Peitersen E. Bell's palsy: the spontaneous course of 2,500 peripheral facial nerve palsies of different etiologies. Acta Otolaryngol Suppl 2002;549:4–30

[21] Jabor MA, Gianoli G. Management of Bell's palsy. J La State Med Soc 1996;148(7):279–283

[22] Hashisaki GT. Medical management of Bell's palsy. Compr Ther 1997;23(11):715–718

[23] Aviv JE, Urken ML. Management of the paralyzed face with microneurovascular free muscle transfer. Arch Otolaryngol Head Neck Surg 1992;118(9):909–912

[24] Terzis JK, Konofaos P. Nerve transfers in facial palsy. Facial Plast Surg 2008;24(2):177–193

[25] Trehan SK, Model Z, Lee SK. Nerve repair and nerve grafting. Hand Clin 2016;32(2):119–125

[26] de Medinaceli L, Prayon M, Merle M. Percentage of nerve injuries in which primary repair can be achieved by end-to-end approximation: review of 2,181 nerve lesions. Microsurgery 1993;14(4):244–246

[27] Terzis JK, Noah ME. Analysis of 100 cases of free-muscle transplantation for facial paralysis. Plast Reconstr Surg 1997;99(7):1905–1921

[28] Tate JR, Tollefson TT. Advances in facial reanimation. Curr Opin Otolaryngol Head Neck Surg 2006;14(4):242–248

[29] Braam MJ, Nicolai JP. Axonal regeneration rate through cross-face nerve grafts. Microsurgery 1993;14(9):589–591

[30] Yoleri L, Songür E, Mavioğlu H, Yoleri O. Cross-facial nerve grafting as an adjunct to hypoglossal-facial nerve crossover in reanimation of early facial paralysis: clinical and electrophysiological evaluation. Ann Plast Surg 2001;46(3):301–307

[31] Manktelow RT, Tomat LR, Zuker RM, Chang M. Smile reconstruction in adults with free muscle transfer innervated by the masseter motor nerve: effectiveness and cerebral adaptation. Plast Reconstr Surg 2006;118(4):885–899

[32] Manktelow RT. Microvascular reconstruction: anatomy, applications, and surgical technique. New York, NY: Springer-Verlag; 1986

[33] Gillies H. Experiences with fascia lata grafts in the operative treatment of facial paralysis. Proceedings of the Royal Society of Medicine, London, England, August 1934. London, England, John Bale, Sons, and Danielsson; 1935

[34] Terzis JK, Olivares FS. Long-term outcomes of free-muscle transfer for smile restoration in adults. Plast Reconstr Surg 2009;123(3):877–888

58 Free Flap Transfers in Head-and-Neck Reconstructions of Pediatric Patients

David Ben-Nun, Ravit Yanko, Arik Zaretski, Dan M. Fliss, Nidal Muhanna

Summary

Free flap transfer in reconstructive head-and-neck microsurgeries in the pediatric patient is overall a rare and underreported phenomenon in the literature. Moreover, the research that can be found usually references studies that include a limited number of subjects, making their conclusions less strong than one would like. However, abundant information about free flap procedures among adult patients does exist and while there are obviously several issues with attempting to interchange adult and pediatric parameters, there are many key pieces of information that can be gleaned from that research and be applied to children. Microsurgeons can gain considerable information about the effectiveness of various flaps in restoring functionality to specific regional structures of the head and neck, including the maxilla, hemimandible, TMJ, tongue, oral cavity, orbit of the eye, skull base, and more. Moreover, the information provided on donor-site morbidity can help surgeons rule out or rule in specific flaps for application in the pediatric patient when considering long-term morbidities that may be caused as a result of the reconstructive surgery. Doctors can also better understand the likelihood of flap loss, thrombotic complications, wound dehiscence, osseointegration, nerve sensation, and bone resorption at the recipient site. Also, key information about surgical techniques, such as feasibility of a two-team approach, locating perforating vessels and nerves, and patient recovery, can be useful in the pediatric patient as well.

Pediatric patients are not the same as adult patients in the case of free flap transfers. They possess fewer comorbidities, a smaller anatomy, they are expected to continue to grow, and the ailments that afflict them are different than those that afflict adult patients. However, using the vast information that has been generated and documented in adult patients as well as the limited research on pediatric patients can be extremely useful in guiding new procedures that will hopefully add to the current volume of literature on free flap reconstruction of the head and neck in the pediatric patient.

Keywords: Head and neck reconstructions, free flaps, pediatric head and neck surgery, free tissue transfer, pediatric microsurgery

58.1 Introduction

Free flap tissue transfers are an important part of head-and-neck reconstructions, and they are often carried out following resections of tumors, trauma, and burn injuries. The first vascularized free-tissue transfer in a head-and-neck reconstruction was performed in an adult in 1959 when a vascularized flap of jejunum was transplanted into the cervical esophagus.[1] In the early 1970s, the first free-tissue transfers were initiated in pediatric patients.[2-4] Since then, a significant body of research that has documented the use of free flap reconstruction of the head and neck has emerged. However, the available research on free flap reconstruction of the head and neck in children is limited compared to the amount of information on similar procedures carried out in adults.[5] This is understandable for several reasons. In general, there is less time for a child to undergo such a complicated procedure in terms of lifespan compared to an adult. Additionally, children are typically in better health than adults and are less likely to become afflicted by some of the diseases that damage the body in a manner that necessitates free flap reconstruction.[6] Children also have fewer comorbidities that result in defects which require repair via free flap reconstruction. Historically, some surgeons have been less likely to undertake the complex free flap reconstructive surgeries in children due to concerns regarding inadequate size of recipient vessels for microvascular anastomoses, among other factors.[7]

Although free flap reconstruction is generally described as an effective method for surgical reconstruction in the pediatric population, it represents a particularly challenging practice for a number of reasons. Since the anatomy of the pediatric patient is smaller and less developed, reconstructive surgery requires the manipulation of small, narrow vessels which can make performing venous anastomoses particularly challenging. It also means that the size of potential tissue and bone donor sites for the free-tissue flap may also be limited, although, by extension, this also means that the recipient sites would also be smaller. Additionally, the patient's future growth patterns may be severely impacted either at the site of reconstruction or the donor site, which may lead to lasting functional impairment or aesthetic harm.[7] Another factor that must be weighed in any pediatric reconstruction is that any impairment or physical damage also has the potential to have a lasting psychosocial impact.[8] Lastly, there are psychosocial factors of free flap reconstructions in children, whereby the pressures of complex microvascular reconstruction surgery are invariably compounded by concerned parents and family members who are anxious for a favorable outcome for the child.[6] There are some "advantages" that microsurgeons may encounter when performing reconstructive procedures in the pediatric population: these patients often have fewer comorbidities than adults, they may undergo more uniform and predictable wound healing, and their anatomy may be more clearly defined and unaltered.[9]

Another element that differentiates free flap reconstruction in adults and children is the pathology that typically precipitates the ablative defect that creates the need for a reconstructive procedure. In adults, the predominant cause of surgical resections of the head and neck that require free flaps is squamous cell carcinoma. In children, the most frequent cause of malignant tumors that require reconstruction is a sarcoma, particularly rhabdomyosarcoma, osteosarcoma, and Ewing's sarcoma.[5] This difference also has implications on the reconstruction that is performed following the tumor resection since sarcomas are present in the bone, cartilage, blood vessels, and other connective tissues and thus may require more aggressive and invasive surgical procedures for a complete cure. In turn, these more aggressive procedures require more robust reconstructions. Moreover, pediatric patients with these malignancies often receive preoperative neoadjuvant therapy, which is intended to facilitate a complete surgical resection of the tumor by shrinking it and targeting micrometastases that may already have occurred.[10] However, this form of therapy often complicates the microreconstructive procedure and makes manipulation of the vessels more challenging. Finally, while the adult head-and-neck tumors may develop from comorbidities, such as smoking, alcohol consumption, or HPV, tumor development in children is more likely to be sporadic or genetic.[6,11]

There are many options to choose from when it comes to donor sites for free flap reconstruction in both adults and children. Selection should primarily be based on the functional requirement of the area that is being reconstructed. The main emphasis should be placed on designing a surgical plan that will ensure the integrity of the anatomical structures in question at both the donor and recipient sites. For example, in the case of a skull base reconstruction, maintaining a separation between intracranial contents and the paranasal sinuses is a primary functional concern.[8,12] Once the integrity of anatomical regions has been addressed, attention should be paid to maintaining functions, such as facial expression, swallowing, and speech. Lastly, if integrity and function of the relevant structures can be maintained, the form or aesthetics of the region being reconstructed should be addressed to ensure optimal cosmetic appearance. For instance, it is possible to use various flaps for reconstruction of the mandible or the maxilla. However, the use of a segmented free fibular flap might be preferred over a scapula free flap (SFF) since the fibula may provide more structural support and allow for the use of dental implants.[13] It is also important to address the potential morbidity at the site of tissue elevation, since each free flap carries with it its own set of potential long-term morbidities. For example, if a free flap procedure does not explicitly require muscle at the recipient site, it may be best to use a fasciocutaneous flap in order to lessen the likelihood of future muscular dysfunction at the donor site in children. Selection of the proper free flap for each procedure is crucial. Great care should be taken to ensure

that total reconstruction can be accomplished using a single free flap. Procedures involving multiple free flaps are rare and should be avoided whenever possible.

Free flaps can be classified in a number of different ways, including their donor or recipient site, primary blood supply, type of tissue, and proximity to the site of reconstruction. In pediatric patients, free flaps can be divided into two main categories, soft tissue free flaps and osseous free flaps. Specifically, the former contains soft tissue, such as skin, fat, muscle, cartilage, and other connective tissue, and the latter includes all of these along with a section of bone from the donor site. Soft tissue free flaps that are used in the pediatric population include the radial forearm flap, the abdominis rectus flap, the anterolateral thigh flap, the parascapular flap, and the latissimus dorsi. free flaps that include bone include the fibula flap, the SFF, and the iliac flap.

58.2 Soft Tissue Free Flaps

58.2.1 Anterolateral Thigh Flap

The anterolateral thigh (ALT) flap has emerged as a workhorse flap for reconstructions that require ample soft tissue without a component of bone. The ALT was first described by Song et al in 1984 and originates from the descending branch of the lateral circumflex femoral artery.[14] It is considered as being a versatile flap, and one that is easy to raise with low donor-site morbidity.[15] The ALT offers many advantages. First, it is very reliable and has low reported levels of total and partial failure.[16] Second, it appears to be favored by many patients due to the fact that the scar left behind by its elevation can be easily concealed due to its location compared to other free flaps, such as those from the radial forearm and fibula.[17] Additionally, the ALT offers surgeons the option of creating a "chimeric" flap that can incorporate surrounding tissue.[12]

In order to raise an ALT flap, an incision is made above the rectus femoris along a line that runs from the anterior superior iliac spine to the lateral angle of the patella. The rectus femoris and tensor fascia lata are separated from one another in the proximal third by retracting the rectus femoris medially, which should expose the vascular pedicle to the tensor fascia lata. The space between the rectus femoris and vastus lateralis is then identified and opened at the middle third to reveal the vascular pedicle to the vastus lateralis. Once the perforators are located, the skin flap is circumcised and the rectus femoris can be released from its insertion at the quadriceps tendon to the patella[18,19] (▶ Fig. 58.1).

In the pediatric population, one particularly relevant area of head-and-neck reconstruction in which the ALT is effective is among burn patients. Yu et al reported a 100% success rate in 11 procedures involving fasciocutaneous ALT flaps that were transplanted onto the scalps of pediatric burn patients. Those authors advocated the ALT for these cases because it can be used to reconstruct large-scale

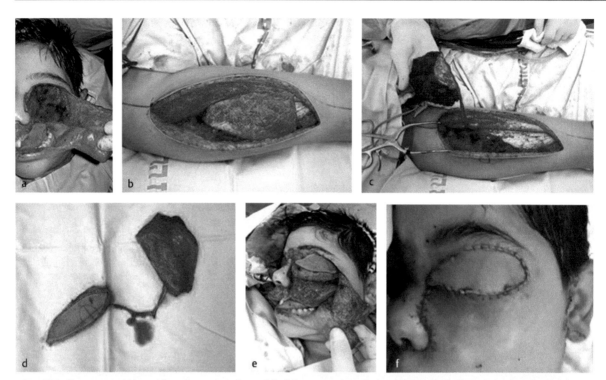

Fig. 58.1 Eleven-year-old boy with malignant neoplasm of the left paranasal sinuses involving the left orbit. An eleven-year-old boy with malignant neoplasm of the left paranasal sinuses involving the left orbit who underwent left orbital exenteration, maxillectomy, infratemporal, and pterygopalatine fossa resection with anterolateral thigh (ALT) free flap reconstruction. **(a)** Defect after resection. **(b–d)** Chimeric ALT flap harvesting using the right thigh. **(e–f)** Flap inset—flap skin was used to cover the outer orbital defect and the muscle to fill in the maxillary cavity and pterygopalatine area.

defects with a single-stage procedure that can be conducted using a "two team" approach.[20] According to Yu et al one difference between adult and pediatric patients is that the vessels used in anastomoses in the ALT flap in children must be selected carefully since only selected ones, such as the temporal artery, possess the necessary caliber for anastomosis with the flap's vascular pedicle.

The ALT is currently used to repair many defects that were formally repaired using a radial forearm free flap (RFFF).[15] The thigh flap is preferred over the radial forearm flap since harvesting of the RF flap requires destruction of a major blood vessel in the arm and the closure of the donor site necessitates a skin graft, both of which may compromise the function of the arm.[21] However, it should be noted that RFFF flaps are considered easier to raise since the ALT has a more complex anatomy owing mostly to a thin perforator that originates from the descending branch of the lateral circumflex femoral artery.[21] As mentioned above, for pediatric patients, the ALT appears to be a much more suitable option than the RFFF flap for head-and-neck reconstructions that require soft tissue, given the risk of donor-site morbidity with which the radial flap is associated.

The ALT flap can be used in a number of head-and-neck reconstruction procedures. Bianchi et al reported that the ALT is particularly well suited to partial or total glossectomies.[22] The flap is able to provide the muscular "bulk" that is necessary to allow for the lingual-palatal contact that is an important part of the oral phase of deglutition, as well as necessary obliteration of any submandibular dead spaces, ensuring a complete separation between the oral cavity and the neck. Moreover, the option to harvest chimeric ALT flaps makes the ALT flap especially flexible in terms of where it can be used in head-and-neck reconstructions. The ALT flap has been described as being effective in the reconstruction of radical parotidectomy defects due to its ample skin and neural tissue and ability to avoid the need for a second donor site.[23–25] Haynes et al reported that the ALT flap is useful for severe deformities of the pediatric anophthalmic orbit, adding that it also aids in the retention of an ocular prosthesis.[26] Lastly, Garfein et al indicated that the ALT flap is recommended for use in midface reconstruction of the pediatric patient, noting that the procedure should be conducted in children the same way it is in adults since the goals of the procedure are the same in both populations: to maintain facial dimensions, provide a framework for soft tissues of the cheek, and isolate the oral cavity from the neck.[27]

Donor-site morbidity of the ALT flap has been consistently reported as low, although this may depend on several factors, including the surgical technique used, the specific outline of the ALT that is selected and the flap size.[28,29] In a systematic review that analyzed 42 articles which included 2324 patients, Collins et al determined that the most common donor-site morbidity reported by patients who underwent ALT free flap surgery was lateral thigh paresthesia, most likely due to damage to lateral femoral cutaneous nerve of the thigh.[30] Additionally, some damage has been reported to occur to the vastus lateralis muscle as a result of the dissection of perforator vessels of the ALT flap, which can lead to problems with knee extension.[31] Flap losses were reported at a rate of 7% in a study by Horn et al that examined 41 ALT transfers conducted over a 9-year period.[32] Overall, however, the ALT is associated with limited donor-site morbidity, thus making it a good candidate for pediatric head-and-neck reconstruction procedures.

58.2.2 Radial Forearm Free Flap

The RFFF was traditionally one of the most commonly used fasciocutaneous free flaps. First described in 1981 by Yang et al, the RFFF has many advantages for use in head-and-neck reconstructions, including long pedicle length, sparsity of hair, high vessel caliber and appropriate thickness.[33–35] The RFFF is often preferred for small- to medium-sized defects in buccal, floor of mouth, lower lip and soft palate reconstructions.[36] The radial flap also provides two venous drainage systems: one is a superficial system of veins that drain to the cephalic and basilic veins and the other is a deep system that drains via venae comitantes that travel alongside the radial artery. This duality confers an advantage during flap harvest since it offers surgeons a choice of vessels from which to select for micro anastomoses.[37] However, the RFFF is associated with many significant donor-site morbidities, which have made it less preferable in many reconstruction cases in children, with some sources indicating a specific preference of the ALT flap over the RFFF.[36,38–40]

The RFFF is raised with an incision along the ulnar border to expose the flexor carpi ulnaris tendon. The subfascia is dissected until the flexor carpi radialis tendon is reached and identification of the radial vessels is possible. The vascular pedicle is then dissected superiorly along the brachioradialis muscle and the appropriate length of flap is elevated.[18]

One of the main considerations for donor-site morbidity associated with the RFFF is the aesthetic appearance of the residual scar. In a review of 56 patients who had undergone RFFF procedures with a mean post-procedure follow-up of 7.9 years, Li et al found that patients felt that the donor-site scar significantly impacted their appearance and most of them did not feel comfortable wearing short-sleeved shirts.[33] Smith et al reported that 90% of patients who underwent an RFFF procedure viewed their arm as "disfigured."[41] This factor should be considered when weighing free flap reconstruction options, especially in younger patients.

Another concern highly relevant to the pediatric patient is that RFFF volumes have been reported to become significantly reduced in the long term. Joo et al observed that RFFF volumes were reduced by 42.7% on average during post-procedure follow-ups from 3 months to 5 years, leading those researchers to conclude that RFFF procedures should be undertaken with flaps that are 40% larger than the recipient site for which they are intended.[42] Finally, harvesting the RFFF results in complete interruption of the radial artery, an important vessel of the arm, causing perfusion of the limb to occur via the ulnar artery, which does not always allow for equal perfusion of all parts of the hand.[18] Additional donor-site complications, such as edema formation, reduced strength and extension of the hand, and cold intolerance have also been reported.[43]

58.2.3 Rectus Abdominis Flap

Originating from the deep inferior epigastric vessels, the rectus abdominis flap (RAF) can be harvested with the rectus abdominis muscle as an RMFF or without muscle (or limited muscle) as a musculo-adipose rectus free flap (MARF). The muscle is often included in the flap in order to provide increased volume and pliability for decreasing the likelihood of infection when used in the oral cavity or the orbit, or for decreasing the likelihood of cerebrospinal fluid leakage when used in the skull base. RMFFs are useful for repairing a defect within a contained space that requires ample subcutaneous fat tissue. Some examples of a possible defect that would be suitable for a rectus free flap transplant include the orbit of the eye, glossectomy defects, maxillary reconstruction, and other soft tissue defects of the oral cavity.[44,45]

The RAF is elevated with a vertical incision from the distal ribs to the pubic ramus. The muscle is then progressively liberated from the rectus sheath that surrounds it anteriorly. The muscle is then posteriorly separated to reveal the inferior epigastric vessels distally, which serve as the vascular pedicle, and excised. Finally, the muscle is released from its origin at the pubic crest and symphysis pubis.[19]

The MARF has many advantages, including an ample supply of subcutaneous fat, which can be helpful in a reconstructive procedure of an obese patient that requires ample subcutaneous fat at the recipient site. Conversely, some surgeons avoid the rectus flap in obese patients for the same reason, since it may require thinning of the flap once it is removed.[46] This may be less applicable in the case of pediatric patients who tend to have lower body mass indices than adult patients. The RMFF offers an ample pedicle length, which has been described as being as long as 18 cm, and it is useful for patients with defects distant from recipient vessels or damaged vessels at the recipient site.[45] This is typically less of an issue in the pediatric patient due to the smaller anatomy and fewer comorbidities, such as atherosclerosis or previous tissue transplants. Use of the MARF may be preferred over the RMFF in the pediatric patient undergoing maxillary defect repair given that many sources have shown that vascularized fat has a much lower rate of atrophy than muscle.[47–49] Thus, for a pediatric patient, it may be more prudent to opt for the MARF, which contains less muscle than the RMFF, with the hope of preventing future atrophy and preserving function and aesthetics in the long-term.

The RMFF has been described as a suitable flap for use in complex midfacial defects, including maxillectomy defects that require medium-to-large surface area volume flaps with muscle to provide bulk. One of the advantages of the rectus flap in those cases is the ease with which surgeons can create multiple skin islands that can be used to repair defects in the nasal and palatal tissues concurrently as, for example, in the case of a maxilla defect repair.[13] The RMFF has also been described as useful in the repair of a skull base defect in the pediatric patient. Iida et al described a case in which an RMFF was used to repair an anterior skull base defect in a one-year-old child. The surgeons opted to include 3 cm of the rectus abdominis muscle in the flap while leaving 1 cm of the muscle in place in that case.[50] By doing so, they used a thicker, more substantive barrier while attempting to limit the potential for long-term complications at the donor site. In contrast, Duek et al described the MARF as being particularly suitable for reconstruction of pediatric anterior skull base defects, specifically because the vascularized adipose tissue in the flap is less likely to atrophy over time, as mentioned above.[8]

Donor-site morbidity for the rectus free flap has been reported as being low by many sources in the literature, but patients who have undergone abdominal surgery in the past need special consideration since the blood supply to their rectus flap may be compromised.[51–54] The risk of an abdominal hernia may also be increased if donor-site repair is not adequately accomplished, which is something that should be borne in mind in the pediatric patient whose body is still developing.[44]

58.2.4 Latissimus Dorsi Free Flap

The latissimus dorsi free flap (LDFF) was first described by Tansini in 1896 for use in reconstruction of the chest wall after mastectomy.[55] It is often used as a pedicled flap as well as a free transfer flap. The vascular supply of the LDFF is provided by the thoracodorsal artery, which is a branch of the subscapular artery. It also receives blood supply from the intercostal arteries that extend laterally from the midline. The LDFF offers a large selection of skin, muscle, the ability to create a sensate flap via use of the intercostal nerves, and a long pedicle that can reach up to 18 cm.[56] It also offers multiple small

perforator arteries that can be useful for procedures that require anastomoses with multiple blood vessels. Additionally, the LDFF allows for a concealed scar, which is often preferred, especially by women undergoing autologous breast reconstruction, and we can assume that it would be desirable for most patients, including children.[55]

The LDFF is raised via a longitudinal incision from the axilla to the posterior iliac crest. The lateral border of the muscle is exposed by reflection of the posterior skin flap. Then, the anterior border of the latissimus dorsi muscle is retracted to expose the vasculature. The thoracodorsal vessels are then dissected superiorly to provide the vascular pedicle. The muscle is then released from its origins at the vertebrae and from the iliac crest in a distal-to-proximal manner.[19]

The LDFF has been reported to be effective in various head-and-neck reconstructive surgeries, including repair of large defects greater than 7 cm that require voluminous tissue transfer.[57] It has also been reported to be effective in facial reanimation surgery to treat facial palsy, which requires a long neurovascular pedicle as well as a significant muscular component to allow for facial movement.[58] Biglioli et al advocated the use of the LDFF for the purposes of correcting unilateral facial palsy in order to recover the emotional smiling function in the pediatric population. In their retrospective study, they showed that out of 40 patients who received an LDFF innervated by the contralateral facial nerve over a 9-year period, 92.5% were able to recover voluntary and spontaneous smiling abilities following the procedure.[59] Lastly, Girod et al reported success with LDFF transfers in anterior and middle skull base defect repair in the pediatric population, specifically in the case of reconstructive procedures following resection of rhabdosarcomas and osteosarcomas.[60]

The LDFF involves the extraction of a large, central back muscle that assists in performing numerous movements of the arms. For this reason, its use in pediatric patients should be carefully considered, although donor-site morbidity has been reported to be minimal by some investigators. A study by Osinga et al that followed pediatric patients 8 years after they underwent LDFF harvesting indicated that the patients suffered no specific or significant impairment of the shoulder joint.[61] However, some recent research has shown that most patients report significant difficulty with vigorous activity after the latissimus dorsi muscle has been removed.[62–64] One potential solution to decreasing the likelihood of significant donor-site morbidity would be to use the fasciocutaneous flap instead of the myocutaneous flap, since the former is associated with less donor-site morbidity if no muscle is required in the free flap transfer.[56] Complications have been described in relation to free-tissue transfer of the LDFF, in particular, dorsal seroma, capsular contracture, skin necrosis and hematoma. Pinsolle et al reported a complication rate of 49% and a 3.8% flap failure rate in a study that examined 249 patients who underwent latissimus dorsi transfer procedures over 12 years.[65]

58.2.5 Parascapular Fasciocutaneous Free Flap

The parascapular fasciocutaneous free flap (PFFF) originates from the descending branch of the circumflex scapular artery along the lateral border of the upper back. This flap was first described by Nassif et al in 1982, and has been shown to provide a skin paddle length of up to 25 cm in length.[66,67] The flap is often categorized as part of the scapular/parascapular system of the back that can be used to craft chimeric flaps with or without an osteocutaneous component.[68] Similar to its scapular flap counterpart, the PFFF is often selected for use in head-and-neck reconstructions due to the abundance of skin surface area, the length and caliber of the pedicle, low donor-site morbidity, and the thickness and complexion of skin.[19,66]

The PFFF is raised in the same manner as the SFF with an incision along the infraspinatus muscle. It is dissected from the infraspinatus and teres minor muscles until the circumflex scapular artery is seen to emerge from the posterior triangle. This position should be identified ahead of time via Doppler so that it is clearly marked. From this point, the descending branch of the circumflex scapular artery should be identified and dissected inferiorly as it travels underneath the teres major muscle.[19]

The PFFF should be considered for pediatric patients since it has been shown to possess low donor-site morbidity, high patient satisfaction, and a concealed scar. In a study of parascapular transfer patients, In a study of parascapular transfer patients, Roll et al showed no shoulder girdle deformity post-procedure, with a limited range of motion experienced by only 2 of the 20 patients in their survey.[69] Moreover, Klinkenberg et al reported high patient satisfaction in a survey that reviewed patients who underwent ALT, lateral arm, and parascapular free flap transfers. Few complications have been reported in parascapular free flap transfer and chief among them is seroma, which should be viewed as a minor complication.[70,71] One disadvantage to using the PFFF in head-and-neck reconstructions is that the flap cannot be harvested using a "two team" approach. In most cases, tumor resection must be completed first, and then the patient must be re-positioned in a lateral decubitus position for harvesting of the flap.[19] Additionally, the flap cannot be harvested as an innervated flap.[70]

58.2.6 Osteocutaneous Free Flaps

Fibula Free Flap

The fibula free flap (FFF) is often selected for use in pediatric surgical reconstruction procedures due to its anatomic reliability, ease of elevation, and robust blood supply.[72] It also provides access to a long length of vascularized bone, and has been shown to result in acceptable donor-site morbidity figures.[73] It has become the most popular flap for reconstruction in head-and-neck patients. An article released on behalf of the American Academy of Otolaryngology showed that the FFF was the most common flap used in pediatric surgeries.[74] Similarly, in a study period of approximately 14 years that included 109 free flap cases, Starnes-Roubaud et al found that the FFF, followed by the ALT flap, was the most common flap used in pediatric patients.[6] The FFF flap procedure was first developed by Taylor et al in 1975, and it was first used in a pediatric setting by Posnick et al in 1993.[75,76] The elevation procedure involves making a lateral incision into the calf and raising a skin paddle from the peroneus brevis and longus muscles in the lateral leg compartment. Once the skin paddle is separated, muscles attached to the fibula are dissected away and the desired bone segment is removed along with the peroneal vessels (▸ Fig. 58.2). The FFF, along with costochondral grafts, are the most common options used in reconstruction of the temporomandibular joint (TMJ) and mandible in children, and they have been used for decades. In the general population, TMJ reconstruction is usually indicated in cases of chronic destruction secondary to osteoarthritis.[77] In the pediatric population, the most common precipitating factor for TMJ reconstruction is usually congenital deformities, ankyloses, and progressive condylar resorption. The most common congenital deformity is hemifacial microsomnia, a relatively common occurrence with an incidence of approximately 1 in every 4000 births.[78]

Another reason that makes the FFF popular in free flap reconstructions is that it provides a vascularized tissue bed that is less likely to be resorbed when compared with a graft, which should be an especially major concern in reconstructive procedures in the pediatric patient.[79] Costochondral grafts have been reported to undergo partial or complete resorption over time and to display unpredictable growth patterns, and reports of overgrowth on the reconstructed side are common.[80] The FFF is widely accepted as one of the best options for reconstruction of the mandible in a pediatric patient and has been for some time. The key to a successful procedure in a growing patient is ensuring that the fibula endochondral growth centers are preserved and transplanted at the recipient site to allow for the potential of continued growth. Additionally, the height of the fibula bone will not be sufficient to mimic the height of the original mandible in some cases for which it may be recommended to use a "double-barrel" technique by folding the fibula onto itself to create the appropriate height.[81]

Potential donor morbidities in the setting of FFFs can include the "standard" complications of graft transplantation surgery, such as skin graft loss, paresthesias, wound dehiscence, and cellulitis, as well as more anatomically

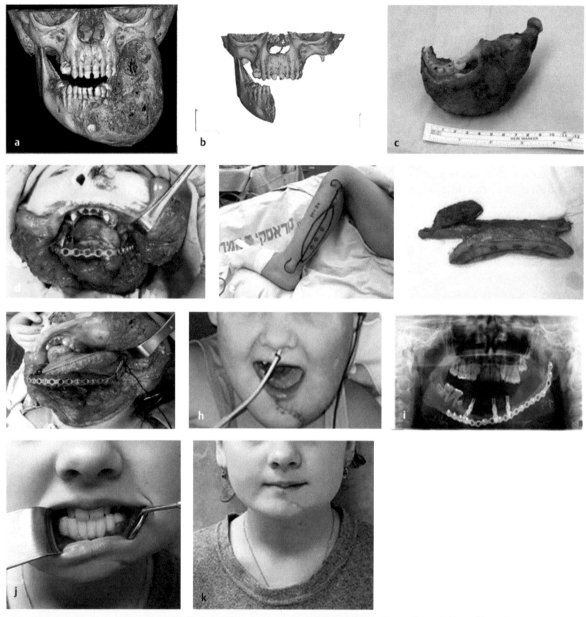

Fig. 58.2 Mandibular reconstruction with fibula free flap reconstruction in a 6-year-old patient with ameloblastic fibroodontosarcoma. **(a)** 3D rendering of CT image showing the tumor site in the left mandible. **(b)** Left mandibular defect after right mandibulectomy. **(c)** The left mandibular resected specimen. **(d)** The titanium plate was adjusted to reconstruct the mandibular defect. **(e–f)** The left leg was used to harvest the left fibula with the overlying skin and muscle. **(g)** The flap was inserted with the skin overlying the inner side of the flap to reconstruct the oral cavity. **(h)** Mouth opening few weeks after reconstruction. **(i)** Panorex—post-dental implantation showing the fibula with the dental implants. **(j, k)** A few years post-surgery showing the dental implants with very good functional and cosmetic results.

specific complications, such as valgus ankle deformity and flexion contracture of the great toe.[82] It should be noted that the FFF procedure has been shown convincingly to have no effect on fibular growth or load-bearing ability—both of which are important considerations, especially in children and active adults—as long as proximal bone segments of 4 cm and distal bone segments of 6 cm are preserved.[83] In adults, the most common donor-site morbidity has been reported as flexion contracture of the great toe. This occurs when the fibula flap elevation includes removal of a portion of the flexor hallucis longus muscle, which is situated directly posterior to the fibula bone and the peroneal vessels and thus is often excised or nicked during the procedure. This complication was shown to occur in 4.3% of adult patients who underwent an FFF procedure in a study that examined 946 patients over 16 years.[84] In comparison, in a study that examined 31 pediatric patients who underwent FFF procedures over 10 years, the reported rate of flexion contracture of the great toe was significantly higher (12.9% of the patients).[82] Clearly, surgical skill and precision must be considered as an important factor in the morbidity of this donor site, given that it is a result of damage to a muscle that needs not be excised in the procedure but often is damaged due to its close proximity to the desired bone and vascular segments. Moreover, one might hypothesize that one reason for this increased rate of donor-site morbidity in FFF procedures in children is due to the fact that the more compact anatomy in a pediatric patient makes it even more difficult to avoid impinging on the flexor hallucis longus muscle during graft removal. Neurological impairments were also reported frequently; however, they very rarely resulted in permanent neurological damage.[82]

Perhaps the most overwhelming consideration in FFF reconstruction, especially in the case of the pediatric patient undergoing mandibular reconstruction, is flap growth at the recipient site. The whole free flap transplantation procedure would seem somewhat futile if the transplanted flap could not grow with the patient since this would necessitate future interventions as the patient ages. A recent study published by Temiz et al addressed this matter and convincingly showed that 10 pediatric patients who underwent mandibular reconstruction via an FFF demonstrated clear signs of flap growth in the transplanted sections at a mean follow-up of 57.7 months post-procedure.[72] Additionally, a systematic review compiled by Zhang et al reported that 81.5% of the 51 patients that were discussed in the reviewed articles demonstrated postoperative growth potential of the reconstructed fibula segment. It is worth noting that this number was reduced to 50% in patients whose condyle of the jaw was not preserved during the reconstructive procedure, thereby apparently implicating the condyle in the potential for the regenerative bone growth process.[35]

Scapula Free Flap (SFF)

The scapula region provides another useful option for free flap reconstructions of the head and neck in pediatric patients. The scapula offers a plentiful selection of soft tissue, muscle, and bone that can be included in a graft that is designed exactly according to the recipient site's needs, given its large surface area. There are two principal donor sites associated with osseous free flaps of the scapula: lateral scapular border flaps and scapular tip free flaps. The SFF provides an excellent option for use in patients requiring short-segment linear defects or an abundance of soft tissue. However, it may be less

amenable to procedures that are required to fix a defect of greater than 12 cm.[73] The SFF also carries the advantage of providing a long pedicle of up to 17 cm, which can be useful in certain procedures.[73] The scapula has been found to provide from 6 cm up to 14 cm of bone stock, depending upon which parts of the bone are included.[85,86] The SFF allows for generous sculpting of tissue segments, given the large amount of surface area and tissue that can be harvested from one donor site, thus making it especially useful for procedures that require a large skin paddle. Finally, use of the scapula in reconstructive procedures provides the benefit of allowing earlier ambulation of the patient during recovery from surgery when compared to the FFF flap, and thus may be preferred for this reason.

The SFF is elevated with horizontal incisions above the infraspinatus muscle. The fasciocutaneous flap is then separated from the infraspinatus and teres minor muscles until the posterior muscle triangle and the circumflex scapular artery are visible. After the circumflex scapular artery and its branches are dissected, the infraspinatus and teres minor muscles are incised, and the teres major and subscapularis muscles are transected to allow access to the scapula bone. Osteotomy is performed and the flap is raised.[19]

The SFFs can be designed to include the circumflex scapular artery and the thoracodorsal artery, both branches of the subscapular branch of the axillary artery, its main vascular pedicle, resulting in a type of "chimeric" flap with two pedicles leading to a single pedicle. This makes it very versatile.

Some research indicates that SFFs are not used as frequently as the FFFs or the iliac crest flap (discussed below) in reconstructive procedures that require bone free flaps.[87] One reason for this could be that the scapula bone does not become fully ossified until approximately the age of 10 years in most pediatric patients, before which the inferior 7 to 8 cm of the bone are composed primarily of hyaline cartilage.[88] A review of the literature indicates that the use of the SFF is rare in pediatric patients. Another reason for this could be a result of the fact that the scapula is often used in adults only when comorbidities, such as atherosclerosis, prevent the fibula flap from being harvested, and these comorbidities are rarely present in children. The SFF does provide numerous advantages for reconstructive procedures and may be preferred over the FFF in cases of complex soft tissue requirements.

One important note that is particularly relevant to the pediatric patient who will continue to grow is that bone resorption has been reported to be more significant in cases that used SFFs compared to the resorption seen with FFFs and iliac crest flaps. In a study conducted by Wilkman et al that analyzed 186 head-and-neck cancer patients who had undergone reconstructive surgery with microvascular free flaps, the SFFs retained only 69% of their original volume at 48 months post-procedure. In comparison, FFFs maintained 95% of their original volume, and iliac crest flaps maintained 88% of their original volume.[89] This finding seems particularly pertinent to pediatric patients who are likely to live with transplanted flaps far longer than the average adult patient and thus would benefit from a flap that has a high likelihood of retaining its original volume.

With regard to the SFF's ability to provide adequate functionality in the pediatric patient, there is some disagreement as to whether or not the SFF will support dental implants. While the FFF is well known as being able to accept dental implants, there is less support for dental implants in an SFF, although the lateral scapular border has been reported to have this capacity.[73,90]

Donor-site morbidity has been reported to be particularly low in the case of the SFF transfer for head-and-neck reconstructions.[91] However, some have reported limited shoulder function as well as potential damage to the brachial plexus as morbidities to be aware of.[87] In a meta-analysis of 47 studies in which 646 children received 694 free flaps, Markiewicz et al reported there was no difference in survival among free flaps used in head-and-neck reconstruction in children, specifically vis-à-vis SFFs and fibula free flaps. The survival rate for both types of flaps was reported to be 96.4%.[7]

Iliac Crest Free Flap

The iliac crest free flap (ICFF) is another osteocutaneous flap that is used in microsurgical reconstruction of the head and neck in children. Based on the deep circumflex iliac artery, the ICFF provides ample bone from the pelvis as well as a large skin paddle. The ICFF can be harvested without a skin paddle, and this is often done since the skin paddle can be especially thick and may not be suitable for the recipient site. The ICFF is a complicated flap to raise and has been gradually replaced by the FFF in most cases.[19] However, the ICFF is considered particularly useful for reconstruction of the hemi-mandible, especially in young patients, as well as curved bones, such as the pelvis and short, straight bone defects between 6 and 8 cm in length.[92] The iliac crest is effective for mandible reconstruction, since it allows the surgeon to design the appropriate piece of bone required from the pelvis in order to match the shape of the mandible that is missing, and it is reported to provide up to 15 cm of bone.[93] Finally, the ICFF can be harvested using a "two team" approach, which decreases operating time, expenses and morbidity and is thus generally favored over alternative sources.[94]

In order to elevate the ICFF, an incision is made that follows the course of the femoral artery, exposing the iliac crest and the inguinal ligament. The inguinal ligament is then released from the anterior superior iliac spine. The three muscles that comprise the abdominal wall, the external oblique, internal oblique, and transversus abdominis, are released from the iliac crest, which should expose the deep circumflex iliac artery. The iliacus muscle is also transected. Osteotomy is performed and the ICFF is raised.[29]

Some disadvantages of using the iliac crest are that the surgical procedure is more complicated than elevating the fibula, for example. Additionally, as mentioned above, the skin paddle that is harvested along with the iliac crest may be too thick or otherwise inappropriate for the recipient site. For example, the iliac skin flap is reported to be too thick for intraoral reconstructive surgery.[95] In general, the ICFF procedure is reported to result in more complications when compared to the FFF, for example. From a sample size of 156 osteocutaneous free flap procedures, Mücke et al reported that the iliac crest had a higher percentage of flap losses and delayed wound healing when compared with the FFF.[94]

In spite of this increased risk of complications, Politi et al have reported that quality of life was reported to be higher in patients that underwent mandibular reconstruction with an ICFF compared to patients who received an FFF. Patients reported higher scores when asked about aesthetics, speech, eating, and donor-site morbidity.[96] This could be an especially important outcome to consider in the pediatric patient that is expected to live for several decades following the procedure. The iliac crest has been reported to maintain its shape several years post-procedure, which is an important consideration in a reconstructive procedure for young patients. Moreover, Taylor et al provided evidence that the growth of transplanted ICFFs occurred in children who underwent iliac crest hemimandible reconstructions.[92] The iliac crest is widely reported to allow anchorage for dental implants, which is an important consideration in a pediatric patient.[94] Wang et al described a novel procedure in which the ilioinguinal nerve is grafted along with the ICFF, which leads to a decrease in resorption of bone at the recipient site in the setting of mandibular reconstructive surgery, leading to a higher chance of a successful graft with successful dental implants.[97]

The ICFF procedure entails significant donor-site morbidity. Notably, the lateral cutaneous nerve of the thigh has been reported to have been damaged in some procedures for raising an ICFF. Hernia may result at the donor site in some cases if too much of the muscle is removed with the free flap.[92] Iliac donor-site morbidity is also known to include gait disturbances, given that the bone is harvested from the pelvis, which is crucial in ambulation.[98] This cause for donor-site morbidity alone may alert for caution in choosing this free flap in the pediatric patient.

58.3 Highlights

a. Overview
   - Free flap transfer in reconstructive head-and-neck microsurgeries in the pediatric patient is overall a rare and underreported phenomenon.
   - Free flap surgery differs in pediatric patients due to smaller anatomy, desire to accommodate for future growth, complicating psychosocial factors, distinctive pathologies responsible for defect that requires repair.
   - Soft tissue free flaps used in pediatric head and neck reconstruction include: radial forearm flap, abdominis rectus flap, anterolateral thigh flap, parascapular flap, and latissimus dorsi flap.
   - Osseous free flaps include: fibula free flap, SFF, and iliac free flap.

b. Soft tissue free flaps
   - Anterolateral thigh flap (ALT):
     ○ Second most commonly used free flap in pediatric surgeries.
     ○ Often used in pediatric burn patients.
     ○ Low reported donor site morbidity in pediatric patients.
   - Radial forearm free flap (RFFF):
     ○ Preferred for small-to medium-sized defects in buccal, floor of mouth, lower lip and soft palate reconstructions.
     ○ Largely replaced by ALT free flap for many indications because of significant donor-site morbidity, particularly as it relates to aesthetic appearance and hand perfusion complications.
   - Rectus abdominis flap (RAF):
     ○ Useful for repairing orbit of the eye, glossectomy, maxillary reconstruction, and other soft tissue defects of the oral cavity.
     ○ Low reported donor site morbidity, however abdominal hernia may be a concern especially in pediatric patients.
   - Latissimus dorsi free flap (LDFF):
     ○ May be used for facial reanimation surgery, anterior and middle skull base defect repair.
     ○ Pediatric donor site morbidity has been reported to be minimal.
   - Parascapular fasciocutaneous free flap (PFFF):
     ○ May be used for ability to craft chimeric flap, large, thick skin surface, and low donor site morbidity.

c. Osteocutaneous free flaps
   - Fibula free flap (FFF):
     ○ Most commonly used flap in pediatric free flap transfer.
     ○ Often used for TMJ and mandible reconstruction in pediatric patients.
     ○ Procedure does not commonly affect fibular growth or load-bearing.
   - Scapula free flap (SFF):
     ○ Not commonly used in pediatric patients.
     ○ Large flap volume loss at follow up has been reported.
     ○ Low failure rate in pediatric patients.
   - Iliac crest free flap (ICFF):
     ○ May be used for reconstruction of hemi-mandible.
     ○ Higher percentage of flap failure compared to FFF.
     ○ Significant donor site morbidity including hernia, gait disturbances, nerve damage.

References

[1] Seidenberg B, Rosenak SS, Hurwitt ES, Som ML. Immediate reconstruction of the cervical esophagus by a revascularized isolated jejunal segment. Ann Surg 1959;149(2):162–171

[2] Ohmori K, Harii K, Sekiguchi J, Torii S. The youngest free groin flap yet? Br J Plast Surg 1977;30(4):273–276

[3] Ducic Y, Young L. Improving aesthetic outcomes in pediatric free tissue oromandibular reconstruction. Arch Facial Plast Surg 2011;13(3):180–184

[4] Harii K, Ohmori K. Free groin flaps in children. Plast Reconstr Surg 1975;55(5):588–592

[5] Weizman N, Gil Z, Wasserzug O, et al. Surgical ablation and free flap reconstruction in children with malignant head and neck tumors. Skull Base 2011;21(3):165–170

[6] Starnes-Roubaud MJ, Hanasono MM, Kupferman ME, Liu J, Chang EI. Microsurgical reconstruction following oncologic resection in pediatric patients: a 15-year experience. Ann Surg Oncol 2017;24(13):4009–4016

[7] Markiewicz MR, Ruiz RL, Pirgousis P, et al. Microvascular free tissue transfer for head and neck reconstruction in children: part I. J Craniofac Surg 2016;27(4):846–856

[8] Duek I, Pener-Tessler A, Yanko-Arzi R, et al. Skull base reconstruction in the pediatric patient. J Neurol Surg B Skull Base 2018;79(1):81–90

[9] Upton J, Guo L. Pediatric free tissue transfer: a 29-year experience with 433 transfers. Plast Reconstr Surg 2008;121(5):1725–1737

[10] Davidoff AM, Fernandez-Pineda I, Santana VM, Shochat SJ. The role of neoadjuvant chemotherapy in children with malignant solid tumors. Semin Pediatr Surg 2012;21(1):88–99

[11] Gradoni P, Giordano D, Oretti G, Fantoni M, Ferri T. The role of surgery in children with head and neck rhabdomyosarcoma and Ewing's sarcoma. Surg Oncol 2010;19(4):e103–e109

[12] Chim H, Salgado CJ, Seselgyte R, Wei FC, Mardini S. Principles of head and neck reconstruction: an algorithm to guide flap selection. Semin Plast Surg 2010;24(2):148–154

[13] Cordeiro PG, Chen CMA. A 15-year review of midface reconstruction after total and subtotal maxillectomy: part I. Algorithm and outcomes. Plast Reconstr Surg 2012;129(1):124–136

[14] Song YG, Chen GZ, Song YL. The free thigh flap: a new free flap concept based on the septocutaneous artery. Br J Plast Surg 1984;37(2):149–159

[15] Husso A, Mäkitie AA, Vuola J, Suominen S, Bäck L, Lassus P. Evolution of head and neck microvascular reconstructive strategy at an academic centre: an 18-year review. J Reconstr Microsurg 2016;32(4):294–300

[16] Wei FC, Jain V, Celik N, Chen HC, Chuang DC, Lin CH. Have we found an ideal soft-tissue flap? An experience with 672 anterolateral

thigh flaps. Plast Reconstr Surg 2002;109(7):2219–2226, discussion 2227–2230

[17] Brown JS, Thomas S, Chakrabati A, Lowe D, Rogers SN. Patient preference in placement of the donor-site scar in head and neck cancer reconstruction. Plast Reconstr Surg 2008;122(1):20e–22e

[18] Wolffe KD, Holzle F. Raising of microvascular flaps: a systematic approach. Berlin, Germany: Springer; 2005

[19] Masquelet A, Gilbert A. An atlas of flaps in limb reconstruction. London, England: Martin Dunitz Ltd; 1995

[20] Yu JA, Lin HJ, Jin ZH, Shi K, Niu ZH, Zhao JC. Free anterolateral thigh flap for coverage of scalp large defects in pediatric burn population. J Burn Care Res 2012;33(4):e180–e185

[21] Liu WW, Li H, Guo ZM, et al. Reconstruction of soft-tissue defects of the head and neck: radial forearm flap or anterolateral thigh flap? Eur Arch Otorhinolaryngol 2011;268(12):1809–1812

[22] Bianchi B, Ferri A, Ferrari S, et al. The free anterolateral thigh musculocutaneous flap for head and neck reconstruction: one surgeon's experience in 92 cases. Microsurgery 2012;32(2):87–95

[23] Iida T, Nakagawa M, Asano T, Fukushima C, Tachi K. Free vascularized lateral femoral cutaneous nerve graft with anterolateral thigh flap for reconstruction of facial nerve defects. J Reconstr Microsurg 2006;22(5):343–348

[24] Elliott RM, Weinstein GS, Low DW, Wu LC. Reconstruction of complex total parotidectomy defects using the free anterolateral thigh flap: a classification system and algorithm. Ann Plast Surg 2011;66(5):429–437

[25] Cannady SB, Seth R, Fritz MA, Alam DS, Wax MK. Total parotidectomy defect reconstruction using the buried free flap. Otolaryngol Head Neck Surg 2010;143(5):637–643

[26] Hynes SL, Forrest CR, Borschel GH. Use of the anterolateral thigh flap for reconstruction of the pediatric anophthalmic orbit. J Plast Reconstr Aesthet Surg 2016;69(1):84–90

[27] Garfein E, Doscher M, Tepper O, Gill J, Gorlick R, Smith RV. Reconstruction of the pediatric midface following oncologic resection. J Reconstr Microsurg 2015;31(5):336–342

[28] Mureau MA, Posch NA, Meeuwis CA, Hofer SO. Anterolateral thigh flap reconstruction of large external facial skin defects: a follow-up study on functional and aesthetic recipient- and donor-site outcome. Plast Reconstr Surg 2005;115(4):1077–1086

[29] Wolff KD, Kesting M, Thurmüller P, Böckmann R, Hölzle F. The anterolateral thigh as a universal donor site for soft tissue reconstruction in maxillofacial surgery. J Craniomaxillofac Surg 2006;34(6):323–331

[30] Collins J, Ayeni O, Thoma A. A systematic review of anterolateral thigh flap donor site morbidity. Can J Plast Surg 2012;20(1):17–23

[31] Weise H, Naros A, Blumenstock G, et al. Donor site morbidity of the anterolateral thigh flap. J Craniomaxillofac Surg 2017;45(12):2105–2108

[32] Horn D, Jonas R, Engel M, Freier K, Hoffmann J, Freudlsperger C. A comparison of free anterolateral thigh and latissimus dorsi flaps in soft tissue reconstruction of extensive defects in the head and neck region. J Craniomaxillofac Surg 2014;42(8):1551–1556

[33] Li P, Zhang X, Luo RH, et al. Long-term quality of life in survivors of head and neck cancer who have had defects reconstructed with radial forearm free flaps. J Craniofac Surg 2015;26(2):e75–e78

[34] Yang G, Chen B, Gao W, et al. Forearm free skin flap transplantation. Zhonghua Yi Xue Za Zhi 1981;61:139–141

[35] Zhang WB, Liang T, Peng X. Mandibular growth after paediatric mandibular reconstruction with the vascularized free fibula flap: a systematic review. Int J Oral Maxillofac Surg 2016;45(4):440–447

[36] Knott PD, Seth R, Waters HH, et al. Short-term donor site morbidity: a comparison of the anterolateral thigh and radial forearm fasciocutaneous free flaps. Head Neck 2016;38(Suppl 1):E945–E948

[37] Zhai QK, Dai W, Tan XX, Sun J, Zhang CP, Qin XJ. Proper choice of donor site veins for patients undergoing free radial forearm flap reconstruction for the defects of head and neck. J Oral Maxillofac Surg 2018;76(3):664–669

[38] de Bree R, Hartley C, Smeele LE, Kuik DJ, Quak JJ, Leemans CR. Evaluation of donor site function and morbidity of the fasciocutaneous radial forearm flap. Laryngoscope 2004;114(11):1973–1976

[39] Kerawala CJ, Martin IC. Sensory deficit in the donor hand after harvest of radial forearm free flaps. Br J Oral Maxillofac Surg 2006;44(2):100–102

[40] Skoner JM, Bascom DA, Cohen JI, Andersen PE, Wax MK. Short-term functional donor site morbidity after radial forearm fasciocutaneous free flap harvest. Laryngoscope 2003;113(12):2091–2094

[41] Smith GI, Yeo D, Clark J, et al. Measures of health-related quality of life and functional status in survivors of oral cavity cancer who have had defects reconstructed with radial forearm free flaps. Br J Oral Maxillofac Surg 2006;44(3):187–192

[42] Joo YH, Hwang SH, Sun DI, Park JO, Cho KJ, Kim MS. Assessment of volume changes of radial forearm free flaps in head and neck cancer: long-term results. Oral Oncol 2011;47(1):72–75

[43] Timmons MJ, Missotten FE, Poole MD, Davies DM. Complications of radial forearm flap donor sites. Br J Plast Surg 1986;39(2):176–178

[44] Uusitalo M, Ibarra M, Fulton L, et al. Reconstruction with rectus abdominis myocutaneous free flap after orbital exenteration in children. Arch Ophthalmol 2001;119(11):1705–1709

[45] Kang SY, Spector ME, Chepeha DB. Perforator based rectus free tissue transfer for head and neck reconstruction: new reconstructive advantages from an old friend. Oral Oncol 2017;74:163–170

[46] Low TH, Lindsay A, Clark J, Chai F, Lewis R. Reconstruction of maxillary defect with musculo-adipose rectus free flap. Microsurgery 2017;37(2):137–141

[47] Tran NV, Chang DW, Gupta A, Kroll SS, Robb GL. Comparison of immediate and delayed free TRAM flap breast reconstruction in patients receiving postmastectomy radiation therapy. Plast Reconstr Surg 2001;108(1):78–82

[48] Sakamoto Y, Takahara T, Ota Y, et al. MRI analysis of chronological changes in free flap volume in head and neck reconstruction by volumetry. Tokai J Exp Clin Med 2014;39(1):44–50

[49] Yamaguchi K, Kimata Y, Onoda S, Mizukawa N, Onoda T. Quantitative analysis of free flap volume changes in head and neck reconstruction. Head Neck 2012;34(10):1403–1407

[50] Iida T, Mihara M, Yoshimatsu H, et al. Reconstruction of an extensive anterior skull base defect using a muscle-sparing rectus abdominis myocutaneous flap in a 1-year-old infant. Microsurgery 2012;32(8):622–626

[51] Kroll SS, Baldwin BJ. Head and neck reconstruction with the rectus abdominis free flap. Clin Plast Surg 1994;21(1):97–105

[52] Cordeiro PG, Disa JJ. Challenges in midface reconstruction. Semin Surg Oncol 2000;19(3):218–225

[53] Agochukwu N, Bonaroti A, Beck S, Liau J. Laparoscopic harvest of the rectus abdominis for perineal reconstruction. Plast Reconstr Surg Glob Open 2017;5(11):e1581

[54] Kim EK, Evangelista M, Evans GRD. Use of free tissue transfers in head and neck reconstruction. J Craniofac Surg 2008;19(6):1577–1582

[55] Schaverien M, Wong C, Bailey S, Saint-Cyr M. Thoracodorsal artery perforator flap and Latissimus dorsi myocutaneous flap: anatomical study of the constant skin paddle perforator locations. J Plast Reconstr Aesthet Surg 2010;63(12):2123–2127

[56] Yang LC, Wang XC, Bentz ML, et al. Clinical application of the thoracodorsal artery perforator flaps. J Plast Reconstr Aesthet Surg 2013;66(2):193–200

[57] Zhu G, Li C, Chen J, Cai Y, Li L, Wang Z. Modified free latissimus dorsi musculocutaneous flap in the reconstruction of extensive postoncologic defects in the head and neck region. J Craniofac Surg 2015;26(2):572–576

[58] Leckenby J, Butler D, Grobbelaar A. The axillary approach to raising the latissimus dorsi free flap for facial re-animation: a descriptive surgical technique. Arch Plast Surg 2015;42(1):73–77

[59] Bigliolo F, Colombo V, Tarabbia F, et al. Recovery of emotional smiling function in free flap facial reanimation. J Oral Maxillofac Surg 2012;70(10):2413–2418

[60] Girod A, Boissonnet H, Jouffroy T, Rodriguez J. Latissimus dorsi free flap reconstruction of anterior skull base defects. J Craniomaxillofac Surg 2012;40(2):177–179

[61] Osinga R, Mazzone L, Meuli M, Meuli-Simmen C, von Campe A. Assessment of long-term donor-site morbidity after harvesting the latissimus dorsi flap for neonatal myelomeningocele repair. J Plast Reconstr Aesthet Surg 2014;67(8):1070–1075

[62] Adams WP Jr, Lipschitz AH, Ansari M, Kenkel JM, Rohrich RJ. Functional donor site morbidity following latissimus dorsi muscle flap transfer. Ann Plast Surg 2004;53(1):6–11

[63] Koh CE, Morrison WA. Functional impairment after latissimus dorsi flap. ANZ J Surg 2009;79(1–2):42–47

[64] Clough KB, Louis-Sylvestre C, Fitoussi A, Couturaud B, Nos C. Donor site sequelae after autologous breast reconstruction with an extended latissimus dorsi flap. Plast Reconstr Surg 2002;109(6):1904–1911

[65] Pinsolle V, Grinfeder C, Mathoulin-Pelissier S, Faucher A. Complications analysis of 266 immediate breast reconstructions. J Plast Reconstr Aesthet Surg 2006;59(10):1017–1024

[66] Nassif TM, Vidal L, Bovet JL, Baudet J. The parascapular flap: a new cutaneous microsurgical free flap. Plast Reconstr Surg 1982;69(4):591–600

[67] Chiu DT, Sherman JE, Edgerton BW. Coverage of the calvarium with a free parascapular flap. Ann Plast Surg 1984;12(1):60–66

[68] Urken M. Scapular and parascapular fasciocutaneous and osteofasciocutaneous and subscapular mega flap. In: Urken M, ed. Atlas of Regional Free Flaps for Head and Neck Reconstruction. Baltimore, MD: Lippincott Williams & Wilkins; 2012:292–325

[69] Roll C, Prantl L, Feser D, Nerlich M, Kinner B. Functional donor-site morbidity following (osteo-) fasciocutaneous parascapular flap transfer. Ann Plast Surg 2007;59(4):410–414

[70] Klinkenberg M, Fischer S, Kremer T, Hernekamp F, Lehnhardt M, Daigeler A. Comparison of anterolateral thigh, lateral arm, and parascapular free flaps with regard to donor-site morbidity and aesthetic and functional outcomes. Plast Reconstr Surg 2013;131(2):293–302

[71] Kucera Marcum K, Browne JD. Parascapular free flaps in skin malignancies. Laryngoscope 2011;121(3):538–540

[72] Temiz G, Bilkay U, Tiftikçioğlu YO, Mezili CT, Songür E. The evaluation of flap growth and long-term results of pediatric mandible reconstructions using free fibular flaps. Microsurgery 2015;35(4):253–261

[73] Dowthwaite SA, Theurer J, Belzile M, et al. Comparison of fibular and scapular osseous free flaps for oromandibular reconstruction: a patient-centered approach to flap selection. JAMA Otolaryngol Head Neck Surg 2013;139(3):285–292

[74] Arnold DJ, Wax MK; Microvascular Committee of the American Academy of Otolaryngology—Head and Neck Surgery. Pediatric microvascular reconstruction: a report from the Microvascular Committee. Otolaryngol Head Neck Surg 2007;136(5):848–851

[75] Taylor GI, Miller GD, Ham FJ. The free vascularized bone graft: a clinical extension of microvascular techniques. Plast Reconstr Surg 1975;55(5):533–544

[76] Posnick JC, Wells MD, Zuker RM. Use of the free fibular flap in the immediate reconstruction of pediatric mandibular tumors: report of cases. J Oral Maxillofac Surg 1993;51(2):189–196

[77] Resnick CM. Temporomandibular joint reconstruction in the growing child. Oral Maxillofac Surg Clin North Am 2018; 30(1):109–121

[78] Figueroa AA, Pruzansky S. The external ear, mandible and other components of hemifacial microsomia. J Maxillofac Surg 1982;10(4):200–211

[79] Davis BR, Powell JE, Morrison AD. Free-grafting of mandibular condyle fractures: clinical outcomes in 10 consecutive patients. Int J Oral Maxillofac Surg 2005;34(8):871–876

[80] Yang YT, Li YF, Jiang N, et al. DirectGrafts of autogenous coronoid process to reconstruct the mandibular condyle in children with unilateral ankylosis of the temporomandibular joint: long-term effects on mandibular growth. Br J Oral Maxillofac Surg 2017;1–6

[81] Fowler NM, Futran ND. Utilization of free tissue transfer for pediatric oromandibular reconstruction. Facial Plast Surg Clin North Am 2014;22(4):549–557

[82] Barla M, Polirsztok E, Peltié E, et al. Free vascularised fibular flap harvesting in children: an analysis of donor-site morbidity. Orthop Traumatol Surg Res 2017;103(7):1109–1113

[83] Shpitzer T, Neligan P, Boyd B, Gullane P, Gur E, Freeman J. Leg morbidity and function following fibular free flap harvest. Ann Plast Surg 1997;38(5):460–464

[84] Gaskill TR, Urbaniak JR, Aldridge JM III. Free vascularized fibular transfer for femoral head osteonecrosis: donor and graft site morbidity. J Bone Joint Surg Am 2009;91(8):1861–1867

[85] Seneviratne S, Duong C, Taylor GI. The angular branch of the thoracodorsal artery and its blood supply to the inferior angle of the scapula: an anatomical study. Plast Reconstr Surg 1999;104(1):85–88

[86] Clark JR, Vesely M, Gilbert R. Scapular angle osteomyogenous flap in postmaxillectomy reconstruction: defect, reconstruction, shoulder function, and harvest technique. Head Neck 2008;30(1):10–20

[87] Gibber MJ, Clain JB, Jacobson AS, et al. Subscapular system of flaps: an 8-year experience with 105 patients. Head Neck 2015;37(8):1200–1206

[88] Genden EM, Buchbinder D, Chaplin JM, Lueg E, Funk GF, Urken ML. Reconstruction of the pediatric maxilla and mandible. Arch Otolaryngol Head Neck Surg 2000;126(3):293–300

[89] Wilkman T, Apajalahti S, Wilkman E, Törnwall J, Lassus P. A comparison of bone resorption over time: an analysis of the free scapular, iliac crest, and fibular microvascular flaps in mandibular reconstruction. J Oral Maxillofac Surg 2017;75(3):616–621

[90] Schultes G, Gaggl A, Kärcher H. Stability of dental implants in microvascular osseous transplants. Plast Reconstr Surg 2002;109(3):916–921, discussion 922–924

[91] Ferrari S, Ferri A, Bianchi B, Varazzani A, Perlangeli G, Sesenna E. Donor site morbidity after scapular tip free flaps in head-and-neck reconstruction. Microsurgery 2015;35(6):447–450

[92] Taylor GI, Corlett RJ, Ashton MW. The evolution of free vascularized bone transfer: a 40-year experience. Plast Reconstr Surg 2016;137(4):1292–1305

[93] Goh BT, Lee S, Tideman H, Stoelinga PJ. Mandibular reconstruction in adults: a review. Int J Oral Maxillofac Surg 2008;37(7): 597–605

[94] Mücke T, Loeffelbein DJ, Kolk A, et al. Comparison of outcome of microvascular bony head and neck reconstructions using the fibular free flap and the iliac crest flap. Br J Oral Maxillofac Surg 2013;51(6):514–519

[95] Moubayed SP, L'Heureux-Lebeau B, Christopoulos A, et al. Osteocutaneous free flaps for mandibular reconstruction: systematic review of their frequency of use and a preliminary quality of life comparison. J Laryngol Otol 2014;128(12): 1034–1043

[96] Politi M, Toro C. Iliac flap versus fibula flap in mandibular reconstruction. J Craniofac Surg 2012;23(3):774–779

[97] Wang L, Wei JH, Yang X, et al. Preventing early-stage graft bone resorption by simultaneous innervation: innervated iliac bone flap for mandibular reconstruction. Plast Reconstr Surg 2017;139(5):1152e–1161e

[98] Genden EM. Reconstruction of the mandible and the maxilla: the evolution of surgical technique. Arch Facial Plast Surg 2010;12(2):87–90

59 Otoplasty

David Leshem, Sivan Zissman

Summary

Prominent ear is a relatively common disorder, which can be caused by different anatomical variations. Preoperative evaluation should include the child's capability of understanding and accepting the surgical procedure and postoperative care. Prominent ears may be addressed by molding, mostly initiated within the first 72 hours of life, or later by surgical technique starting at the age of 6 to 7 years. We prefer performing the Chongchet technique to avoid relapse due to suture failure, suture extrusion, and the surgical result is more predictable. Complications are quite rare. The most common complication is hematoma.

Keywords: Prominent ear, ear molding, otoplasty

59.1 Introduction

Prominent ear is a relatively common disorder suggested to be approximately in 5% of the population.[1]

It may be caused by several reasons including underdeveloped or absent antihelix, overdevelopment of the conceal wall, increased concho-scaphal angle more than 90 degrees, and increased cephalo-auricular distances; these causes may be isolated or combined.[2,3]

Prominent ear may be associated with other secondary deformities such as macrotia, constricted ear, Stahl ear (extra crus/fold), Darwin tubercle (thickening at the junction of upper and middle third of the helix), and mastoid prominence which may have impact on surgical planning.

The transmission pattern of protruding ears is suggested to be autosomal dominant inheritance. The pathogenesis is not so clear; however, point genetic mutations and some environmental factors such as hypoxia, radiation exposure, and certain drugs like thalidomide[4] may play a role in this process.

Although most of the operations are secondary to aesthetical problems, children who suffer from this condition may develop social and psychological difficulties, lack of self-confidence, emotional stress, and social isolations during young childhood.[5,6]

59.2 Anatomy of the Ear

The main anatomical structures of the ear are illustrated in ▶ Fig. 59.1.

In normal anatomy, the helix should project beyond the antihelix. The superior part of the ear typically correlates with the brow, and the inferior part usually descends to the level of the columellar base. Ear length reaches 5.5 to 6.5 cm and width increases to approximately 50% to 60% of length by adulthood. On the vertical axis, the ear normally projects postero-laterally by 15 to 30 degrees.

The helix-to-mastoid distance should be at the range of 10 to 12 mm in the upper third, 16 to 18 mm in the middle third, 20 to 22 mm in the lower third.[7] In anatomically normal shaped ears, the angle between the mastoid and the helix should not exceed 30 degrees.[8,9] In prominent ears, deviations may be seen at the antihelix, conchea, lobule, and helix-mastoid angle.

59.3 Preoperative Assessment

Preoperative evaluation should include the child capability of understanding and accepting the surgical procedure and postoperative care.

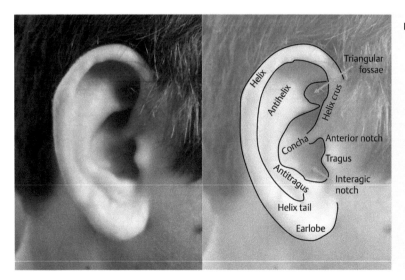

Fig. 59.1 Anatomy of external ear.

The following measurements should be always assessed prior to the day of surgery: the degree of antihelical fold, helical rim projection, conchal depth, mastoid helix degree, lobule deformity, maturity and quality of auricular cartilage, and the presence of other associated anomalies.

59.4 Timing of Surgery

By the age of 6 to 7 years auricle length will reach to about 90% of its mature size.

It has been shown that otoplasty in the pediatric population has no significant influence on later auricular growth.[10]

The surgical timing may depend on several factors such as auricular growth, cartilage size and stability, child developmental status and psychological willingness, and before school age.

We prefer performing otoplasty surgery starting at the age of 6 to 7, always keeping in mind that noncooperative patient or unrealistic expectations should not be operated.

59.5 Nonsurgical Treatment

59.5.1 Ear Molding

Ear molding has been known to be an optional treatment in the newborn, mostly initiated within the first 72 hours of life. The effect of circulating maternal hormones in the baby's blood enables cartilage molding and design.

Mechanical force is used to hold the pinna in a position, by using different soft, elastic, and moldable materials in combination with surgical tape continuously for the first 6 to 8 weeks of life.[11,12]

When the initiation of the treatment is delayed by more than two months, less favorable results are achieved and the duration of the treatment needed is longer.

59.6 Otoplasty Surgical Technique

In 1845 Dieffenbach[13] was the first who performed otoplasty for correction of posttraumatic prominent ears. He described an excision of retroauricular skin and creating a concho-mastoidal suture for fixation. In 1910 Luckett[14] combined the skin and cartilage excision along the length of the antihelical fold with a horizontal mattress suture in order to achieve a better contouring of the scapha.

In 1963 Converse and Wood-Smith described a combination technique of incomplete cartilage incisions from the posterior aspect with additional fixation sutures for contour improving.[15]

In 1963 and 1967 Mustardé introduced a new approach to create an antihelical fold.[16,17] It is the most common technique designated to correct upper-third deformity, primarily inadequate antihelical fold definition, using concho-scaphal mattress permanent sutures. It is especially suitable for children up to 10 years old due to their soft and pliable cartilage. During this procedure, the new antihelical fold and concha is marked with methylene blue dipped needles through the full-thickness cartilage, and ellipse skin excision is made and the antihelix is formed with a mattress suture anchored in the cartilage.

For conchal reduction, in 1968 Furnas described a concha-mastoid fixation mattress suture technique that may be used in combination with the Mustardé technique.[18]

In 1963 Stenström and Chongchet presented the incision scoring techniques.

Stenström[19] described anterior scaphal scoring using a rasp blindly to produce an antihelical fold. He later modified his technique with the addition of a posterior approach for simultaneous concha reduction with spindle-shaped anterior excision.

In contrast, Chongchet technique[20] uses sharp scalpel for anterior scoring of the ear cartilage along the line of the future antihelix through a posterior approach. Both techniques involve retroauricular spindle-shaped skin excisions.

Earfold is a new technique for minimally invasive otoplasty repair introduced by Norbert Kang[21] using a clip made up of super elastic nickel titanium implant that is usually inserted under local anesthesia in subperichondral plane.

We prefer the Chongchet technique because it stops relapse due to suture failure or suture extrusion, and the surgical result is more predictable in the long run.

We choose to present our preferred Chongchet technique of an 8-year-old boy in the following steps (▶ Fig. 59.2):
- Ear symmetry is measured followed by marking the desired antihelical fold before and after pushing the helical fold to its normal position (▶ Fig. 59.2a, b).
- The ear is infiltrated with lidocaine 2% and epinephrine 1:100,000 ampules at the anterior and posterior aspects in order to reduce bleeding and ease the dissection between the skin and the cartilage.
- Retroauricular ellipse skin is marked and excised almost along the whole length of the helix (▶ Fig. 59.2c).
- Exposure and undermining between the skin edges to the helical border is done followed by opening incision of the cartilage (▶ Fig. 59.2d, e).
- The new site of the antihelix is marked by stabbing inked 23 gauged needles in three to four different locations through the full-thickness cartilage, and the incision is made accordingly (▶ Fig. 59.2f, h).
- Parallel incisions are made on the outer layer of the cartilage to form the new antihelix; concha excess cartilage is evaluated and excised if needed.

As part of the conceal definition Furnas mattress suture is placed in order to attach the conchal cartilage to the mastoid fascia followed by subcuticular suture for skin closure (▶ Fig. 59.2i–k).

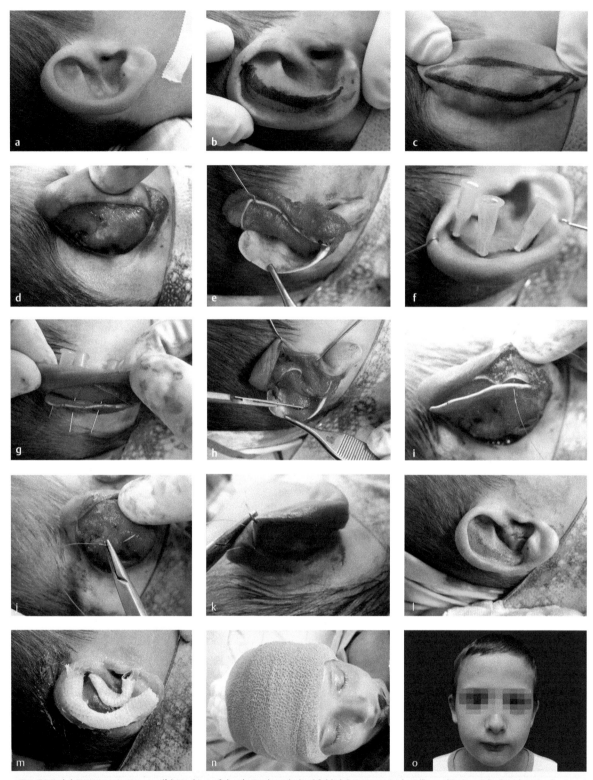

Fig. 59.2 **(a)** Preoperative image. **(b)** Marking of the desired antihelical fold. **(c)** Retroauricular ellipse skin is marked and excised. **(d)** Exposure and undermining between the skin edges to the helical border. **(e)** Opening incision of the cartilage. **(f)** Marking of the new antihelix with inked needles. **(g)** The inked needles go through the full-thickness cartilage up to the postauricular skin. **(h)** Excision of cartilage according to the marking. **(i)** Closure of the new cartilage edges. **(j)** Furnas mattress sutures, between the conchal cartilage to the mastoid fascia. **(k)** Subcuticular suture for skin closure. **(l)** Postoperative image. **(m)** Fixation of the new antihelix by placement of rapped vaseline gaze. **(n)** Postoperative head bandage. **(o)** 6-week postoperative image.

- Fixation of the new antihelix is done by placement of rapped vaseline gaze, covered with head bandage (▶ Fig. 59.2l–o).

Postoperative head dressing change is usually done after 4 to 5 days; possible hematoma or infection signs are evaluated followed by head band for additional 10 days. After the dressing is removed, maintaining good hygiene and avoiding contact sports till the healing process is completed are recommended.

Ear shape is observed in long-term follow-up starting 2 weeks postop followed by regular visits after 1, 3, 6, 12, 18, 24 months.

59.7 Complications

Otoplasty complication can be divided into early and late.

Early complications: Hematomas (most common), infections that may lead to perichondritis, pain, itching, and skin and cartilage necrosis.

Late complications: Hypertrophic scars, keloids, dysesthesias, suture material rejection with fistula formation, asymmetry, and recurrence.[3,22]

59.8 Highlights

a. Indications
   - Prominent ear.
b. Contraindications
   - Child incapability of understanding and accepting the surgical procedure and postoperative care.
   - Non-cooperative patient.
   - Unrealistic expectations.
c. Complications
   - Early:
     ◦ Hematomas.
     ◦ Infections.
     ◦ Perichondritis.
     ◦ Pain.
     ◦ Itching.
     ◦ Skin and cartilage necrosis.
   - Late:
     ◦ Hypertrophic scars.
     ◦ Keloids.
     ◦ Dysesthesias.
     ◦ Suture material rejection with fistula formation.
     ◦ Asymmetry.
     ◦ Recurrence.
d. Special preoperative considerations
   - Child's age.
   - Developed and stable cartilage.
   - Prophylaxis preoperative antibiotics.
e. Special intraoperative considerations
   - Ear anatomy and surgical marking.
   - Atraumatic cartilage handling.
f. Special postoperative considerations
   - Local antibiotic ointment.
   - Bulky head dressing.
   - Head band support for 2 weeks.

References

[1] Kelley P, Hollier L, Stal S. Otoplasty: evaluation, technique, and review. J Craniofac Surg 2003;14(5):643–653

[2] Salgarello M, Gasperoni C, Montagnese A, Farallo E. Otoplasty for prominent ears: a versatile combined technique to master the shape of the ear. Otolaryngol Head Neck Surg 2007;137(2):224–227

[3] Janis JE, Rohrich RJ, Gutowski KA. Otoplasty. Plast Reconstr Surg 2005;115(4):60e–72e

[4] Takemori S, Tanaka Y, Suzuki JI. Thalidomide anomalies of the ear. Arch Otolaryngol 1976;102(7):425–427

[5] Olivier B, Mohammad H, Christian A, Akram R. Retrospective study of the long-term results of otoplasty using a modified Mustardé (cartilage-sparing) technique. J Otolaryngol Head Neck Surg 2009;38(3):340–347

[6] Coltro PS, Alves HR, Gallafrio ST, Busnardo FF, Ferreira MC. Sensibility of the ear after otoplasty. Ann Plast Surg 2012;68(2):120–124

[7] Janz BA, Cole P, Hollier LH Jr, Stal S. Treatment of prominent and constricted ear anomalies. Plast Reconstr Surg 2009;124 (1, Suppl):27e–37e

[8] Farkas LG. Anthropometry of normal and anomalous ears. Clin Plast Surg 1978;5(3):401–412

[9] Farkas LG. Anthropometry of the normal and defective ear. Clin Plast Surg 1990;17(2):213–221

[10] Balogh B, Millesi H. Are growth alterations a consequence of surgery for prominent ears? Plast Reconstr Surg 1992;90(2):192–199

[11] Sorribes MM, Tos M. Nonsurgical treatment of prominent ears with the Auri method. Arch Otolaryngol Head Neck Surg 2002;128(12):1369–1376

[12] Woo JE, Park YH, Park EJ, Park KY, Kim SH, Yim SY. Effectiveness of ear splint therapy for ear deformities. Ann Rehabil Med 2017;41(1):138–147

[13] Dieffenbach JE. Die operative Chirurgie. Leipzig: F. A. Brockhaus; 1845

[14] Luckett WH. A new operation for prominent ears based on the anatomy of the deformity. Surg Gynecol Obstet 1910;10:635

[15] Converse JM, Wood-Smith D. Technical details in the surgical correction of the lop ear deformity. Plast Reconstr Surg 1963;31:118–128

[16] Mustardé JC. The correction of prominent ears using simple mattress sutures. Br J Plast Surg 1963;16:170–178

[17] Mustardé JC. The treatment of prominent ears by buried mattress sutures: a ten-year survey. Plast Reconstr Surg 1967;39(4):382–386

[18] Furnas DW. Correction of prominent ears by conchamastoid sutures. Plast Reconstr Surg 1968;42(3):189–193

[19] Stenstroem SJA. "natural" technique for correction of congenitally prominent ears. Plast Reconstr Surg 1963;32:509–518

[20] Chongchet V. A method of antiheliz reconstruction. Br J Plast Surg 1963;16:268–272

[21] Kang NV, Sojitra N, Glumicic S, et al. Earfold implantable clip system for correction of prominent ears: analysis of safety in 403 patients. Plast Reconstr Surg Glob Open 2018;6(1):e1623

[22] Sadhra SS, Motahariasl S, Hardwicke JT. Complications after prominent ear correction: a systematic review of the literature. J Plast Reconstr Aesthet Surg 2017;70(8):1083–1090

Index

Note: Page numbers set in **bold** or *italic* indicate headings or figures, respectively.